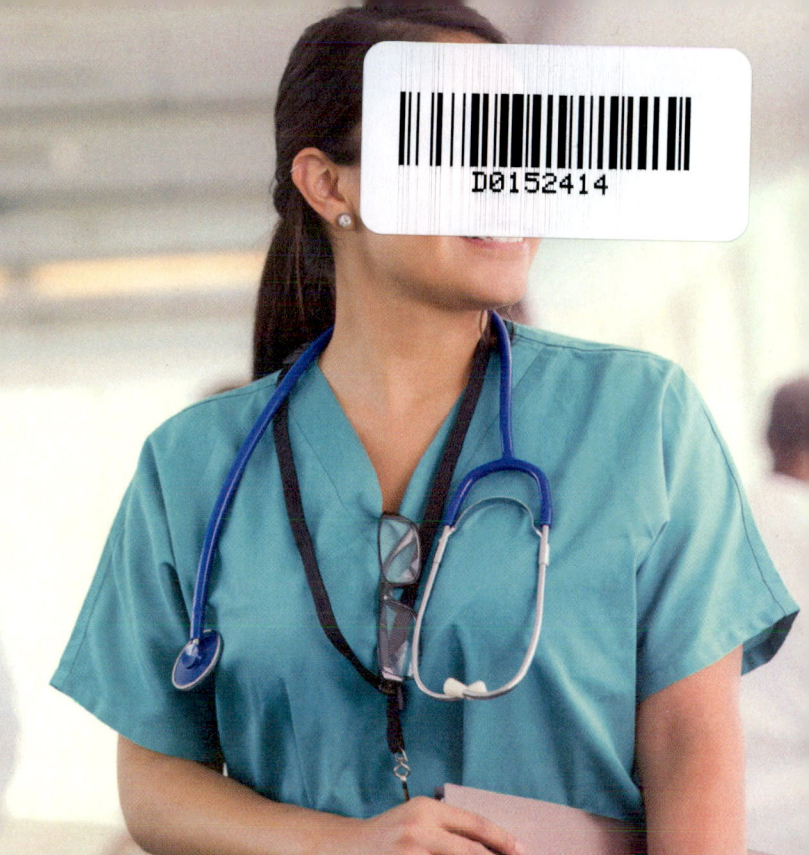

Help your students learn to **Think Like a Nurse** with **new digital learning resources** in Maternal and Pediatric Nursing!

MyNursingLab®

MyNursingLab's personalized learning path helps students master and retain course information more quickly so they can focus on higher-level decision-making skills.

NEW! Clinical Decision-Making Cases in MyNursingLab provide opportunities for students to practice analyzing information and making important decisions at key moments in patient care scenarios.

Learn more at mynursinglab.com

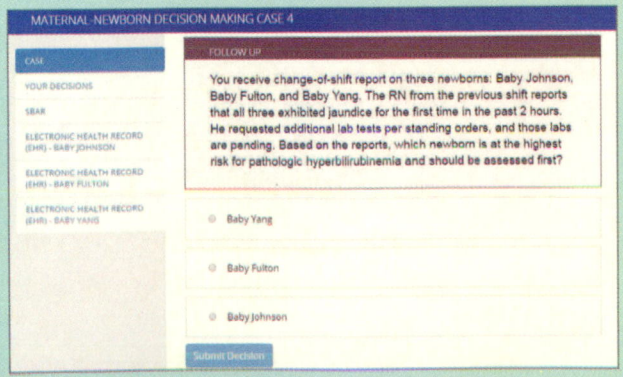

NEW! Maternity & Pediatric Nursing Reference App

The Maternity & Pediatric Nursing Reference App provides a collection of handy tools and additional content, previously only available in text format, for quick reference in the clinical setting. Students can now easily access this vital content in a useful mobile format wherever and whenever they need it! Now available for free on both the Apple App Store and Google Play.

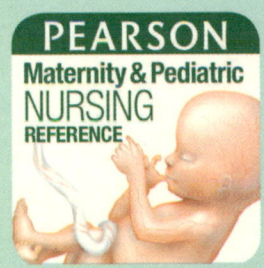

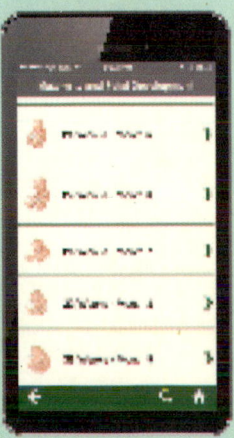

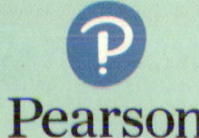

Pearson

CONTEMPORARY
MATERNAL-NEWBORN NURSING CARE

9e

Patricia A. Wieland Ladewig, RN, PhD
Provost Emerita
Regis University
Denver, Colorado

Marcia L. London, RN, MSN, APRN, CNS, NNP-BC
Guest Lecturer and Director of Neonatal Nurse Practitioner Program (Ret.)
Helen and Arthur E. Johnson Beth-El College of Nursing and Health Sciences
University of Colorado
Colorado Springs, Colorado

Michele R. Davidson, RN, PhD, CNM, CFN
Associate Professor of Nursing and Women's Studies
Postpartum Psychosis Coordinator, Postpartum Support International
George Mason University
Fairfax, Virginia

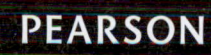

Boston   Columbus   Indianapolis   New York   San Francisco
Amsterdam   Cape Town   Dubai   London   Madrid   Milan   Munich   Paris   Montréal   Toronto

Publisher: Julie Levin Alexander
Editorial Coordinator: Sarah Henrich
Portfolio Manager: Katrin Beacom
Editorial Assistant: Erin Sullivan
Content Producer: Erin Rafferty
Development Editor: Lynda Hatch
Vice President of Sales & Marketing: David Gesell
Vice President, Director of Marketing: Margaret Waples
Senior Product Marketing Manager: Christopher Barry
Field Marketing Manager: Brittany Hammond
Director, Publishing Operations: Paul DeLuca

Team Lead, Project Management: Cynthia Zonneveld
Team Lead, Program Management: Melissa Bashe
Full-Service Vendor: SPi Global
Full-Service Senior Production Editor: Patty Donovan
Manufacturing Manager: Maura Zaldivar-Garcia
Senior Producer: Amy Peltier
Media Producer and Project Manager: Lisa Rinaldi
Art Director: Mary Siener
Cover Credit: Shutterstock, vlavetal
Printer/Binder: RR Donnelley, Willard
Cover Printer: RR Donnelley, Willard

Notice: Care has been taken to confirm the accuracy of information presented in this book. The authors, editors, and the publisher, however, cannot accept any responsibility for errors or omissions or for consequences from application of the information in this book and make no warranty, express or implied, with respect to its contents.

The authors and publisher have exerted every effort to ensure that drug selections and dosages set forth in this text are in accord with current recommendations and practice at time of publication. However, in view of ongoing research, changes in government regulations, and the constant flow of information relating to drug therapy and reactions, the reader is urged to check the package inserts, pharmacy information, or current online information of all drugs for any change in indications or dosage and for added warning and precautions. This is particularly important when the recommended agent is a new and/or infrequently administered drug.

A note about nursing diagnoses: Nursing diagnoses in this text are taken from *Nursing Diagnoses—Definitions and Classification 2015–2017*. Herdman, T.H. & Kamitsuru, S. (Eds.) Nursing Diagnosis—Definitions and Classification 2015–2017. Copyright © 2014, 1994–2014 NANDA International. Used by arrangement with John Wiley & Sons Limited. Companion website: www.wiley.com/go/nursingdiagnoses. In order to make safe and effective judgments using NANDA-I nursing diagnoses it is essential that nurses refer to the definitions and defining characteristics of the diagnoses listed in this work.

Library of Congress Cataloging-in-Publication Data

Names: Ladewig, Patricia W., author. | London, Marcia L., author. | Davidson, Michele R., author.
Title: Contemporary maternal-newborn nursing care / Patricia A. Wieland Ladewig, Marcia L. London, Michele R. Davidson.
Description: Ninth edition. | Hoboken, NJ : Pearson Education, [2017] | Includes bibliographical references and index.
Identifiers: LCCN 2016035090| ISBN 9780134257020 | ISBN 0134257022
Subjects: | MESH: Maternal-Child Nursing
Classification: LCC RG951 | NLM WY 157.3 | DDC 618.2/0231—dc23 LC record available at https://lccn.loc.gov/2016035090

1 16

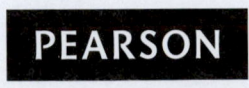

ISBN-13: 978-0-13-425702-0
ISBN-10:   0-13-425702-2

Dedication

We dedicate this book to parents—

Who love, cherish, and protect their children
Who guide, nurture, and shape them

So that they grow to be compassionate, loving, responsible adults.
Such parents know that the reward comes when
The children you love become adults you also like and enjoy as people!
And, as always, we dedicate our work to our beloved families

To Tim Ladewig; Ryan, Amanda, Reed, and Addison; Erik, Kedri, Emma, and Camden

To David London, Craig, Jennifer, Hannah, and Matthew

To Nathan Davidson, Hayden, Chloe, Caroline, and Grant

About the Authors

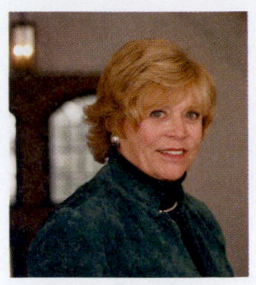

PATRICIA A. WIELAND LADEWIG received her BS from the College of Saint Teresa in Winona, Minnesota; her MSN from Catholic University of America in Washington, DC; and her PhD in higher education administration from the University of Denver in Colorado. She served as an Air Force nurse and discovered her passion for teaching as a faculty member at Florida State University. Over the years, she has taught at several schools of nursing. In addition, she became a women's health nurse practitioner and maintained a part-time clinical practice for many years. In 1988, Dr. Ladewig became the first director of the nursing program at Regis College in Denver. In 1991, when the college became Regis University, she became academic dean of the Rueckert-Hartman College for Health Professions. Under her guidance, the School of Nursing added a graduate program. In addition, the college added a School of Physical Therapy and a School of Pharmacy. In 2009 Dr. Ladewig became the Chief Academic Officer at Regis University. She retired from the position in 2016. She and her husband, Tim, enjoy skiing, baseball games, and traveling. However, their greatest pleasure comes from their family: son Ryan, his wife Amanda, and grandchildren Reed and Addison; and son Erik, his wife Kedri, and grandchildren Emma and Camden.

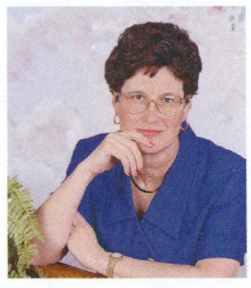

MARCIA L. LONDON received her BSN and School Nurse Certificate from Plattsburgh State University in Plattsburgh, New York, and her MSN in pediatrics as a clinical nurse specialist from the University of Pittsburgh in Pennsylvania. She worked as a pediatric nurse and began her teaching career at Pittsburgh Children's Hospital Affiliate Program. Mrs. London began teaching at Beth-El School of Nursing and Health Science in 1974 (now part of the University of Colorado, Colorado Springs) after opening the first intensive care nursery at Memorial Hospital of Colorado Springs. She has served in many faculty positions at Beth-El, including assistant director of the School of Nursing. Mrs. London obtained her postmaster's Neonatal Nurse Practitioner certificate in 1983 and subsequently developed the Neonatal Nurse Practitioner (NNP) certificate and the master's NNP program at Beth-El. She is active nationally in neonatal nursing and was involved in the development of National Neonatal Nurse Practitioner educational program guidelines. Mrs. London pursued her interest in college student learning by taking doctoral classes in higher education administration and adult learning at the University of Denver in Colorado.

She feels fortunate to be involved in the education of her future colleagues and teaches undergraduate education. Mrs. London and her husband, David, enjoy reading, travel, and hockey games. They have two sons. Craig, who lives in Florida with his wife, Jennifer, and daughter Hannah, works with Internet companies. Matthew works in computer teleresearch. Both are more than willing to give Mom helpful hints about computers.

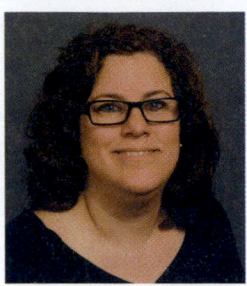

MICHELE R. DAVIDSON completed undergraduate nursing degrees at Marymount University (ADN) and George Mason University (BSN) and worked in multiple women's health specialty areas including postpartum, newborn nursery, high-risk nursery, labor and delivery, reproductive endocrinology, gynecology medical–surgical, and oncology units. Dr. Davidson earned her MSN and a nurse-midwifery certificate from Case Western Reserve University and worked as a nurse-midwife for 16 years, during which time she delivered more than 1,000 babies. She completed her PhD in nursing administration and healthcare policy at George Mason University (GMU) and began teaching at GMU in 1999 while continuing practice as a nurse-midwife. Dr. Davidson serves as the coordinator for postpartum psychosis for Postpartum Support International (PSI), the largest organization providing resources for women with postpartum mood and anxiety disorders. She has an interest in women's mental health and focuses her research on perinatal and postpartum mood and anxiety disorders along with an interest in the care of individuals with disabilities. She was a member of the American College of Nurse-Midwives Certification Council, the body that writes the national certification examination for certified nurse-midwives. She serves on several national committees where she provides expertise in maternal mortality and postpartum mood disorders. She is a member of numerous editorial and advisory boards. Dr. Davidson has certifications in lactation consulting, forensic nursing, and surgical first assistant. In 2012, her book, *A Nurse's Guide to Women's Mental Health*, won an American Journal of Nursing Book Award. Dr. Davidson and her husband, Nathan, a family nurse practitioner, have provided commuity health care services on Smith Island, Maryland, a small island in the Chesapeake Bay, for the past two decades. In her free time, she enjoys gardening, pinteresting, baking, decorating, entertaining, and spending time on Smith Island with her husband, and their four children: Hayden, Chloe, Caroline, and Grant. Dr. Davidson and her family love the Eastern Shore of Maryland and Virginia and continue to be part-time residents of Smith Island, Maryland.

Thank You!

Contributors

We extend a sincere thank you to our contributors, who gave their time, effort, and expertise so tirelessly to develop and write resources that help provide students with the latest information by extending our content beyond the book.

Janet Houser, PhD, RN
Evidence-Based Practice features
Regis University
Denver, Colorado

Nathan S. Davidson, II, CFNP, MSN, RN
Concept Maps
George Mason University
Fairfax, VA

Reviewers

With each revision, our goal remains constant—to ensure that our text reflects the most current research and the latest information about nursing. This would not be possible without the support of our colleagues in clinical practice and nursing education. Their suggestions, contributions, and words of encouragement help us achieve this goal. In publishing, as in health care, quality assurance is an essential part of this process—and this is the dimension that reviewers add. We extend a sincere thanks to all those who reviewed the manuscript for this text.

Barbara L. Cannella, PhD, RNC-OB, APN
Clinical Associate Professor
Rutgers University
Newark, New Jersey

Tonya Chapin, RN, MSN
Associate Professor
of Nursing
Colorado Mesa University
Grand Junction, Colorado

Laura Clemens, BSN, RN, C-EFM
Clinical Nurse I
New York-Presbyterian
Hospital
New York, New York

Kelley Connor, RN, MS, CNE, CHSE
Associate Professor
Boise State University
Boise, Idaho

Elizabeth Cordero, RN, BSN, MBA
Nursing Instructor
Western Nevada College
Carson City, Nevada

Margot R. De Sevo, PhD, LCCE, IBCLC, RNC
Professor
Adelphi University
Garden City, New York

Holly J. Diesel, PhD, RN
Associate Professor
Academic Chair:
Accelerated and
RN-to-BSN Programs
Goldfarb School of
Nursing Barnes Jewish
College
St. Louis, Missouri

Karan Dublin, MEd, BSN, RN
Professor of Nursing
Tyler Junior College
Tyler, Texas

Julie Fitzgerald, PhD, RN
Assistant Professor of Nursing
Ramapo College
of New Jersey
Mahwah, New Jersey

Julie C. Garcia, MSN, APRN, CNS, CCRP
Clinical Research Project
Manager
University of Texas Health
Science Center
San Antonio, Texas

Jolynn Greenhalgh, DNP, ARNP
Teaching Faculty II
Florida State University
Tallahassee, Florida

Brenda K. Hoolapa, RNC-OB, MS, BSN
Clinical Instructor
University of Texas
Arlington, Texas

Kathleen N. Krov, PhD, CNM, RN, CNE
Associate Professor
Raritan Valley Community
College
Somerville, New Jersey

Meredith Krutar, MSN, FNP-BC
Assistant Professor
of Nursing
Carroll College
Helena, Montana

Robyn Leo, MS, RN
Associate Professor and
Chairperson for
Nursing
Worcester State University
Worcester, Massachusetts

Carolyn Levi, MSN, RN
Nursing Faculty
Grand Rapids Community
College
Grand Rapids, Michigan

Diane E. Mosqueda, DNP, APRN, FNP-C, CNE
Assistant Professor
University of Texas
Medical Branch
Galveston, Texas

Patricia Novak, RN, BSN, MSN
Instructor
Gateway Community
College
Phoenix, Arizona

Valerie O'Dell, DNP,RN, CNE
Associate Professor
of Nursing
MSN Program Director
Youngstown State
University
Youngstown, Ohio

Wendi Strauss Pulse, DNP, MSN, RNC-OB, C-EFM
Affiliate Faculty
Regis University
Denver, Colorado

Amy Roberts, MSN, RN
Assistant Professor
Minot State University
Minot, North Dakota

Joanne Silbert-Flagg, DNP, CPNP, IBCLC
Assistant Professor, Director, Baccalaureate Nursing Program
Johns Hopkins University School of Nursing
Baltimore, Maryland

Eleanor Lowndes Stevenson, PhD, RN
Assistant Professor
Duke University School of Nursing
Durham, North Carolina

Linda Stone, MS, RN
Adjunct Clinical Instructor
Labouré College
Milton, Masssachusetts

Patricia Suplee, PhD, RNC-OB
Associate Professor
Rutgers University
Camden, New Jersey

Brenda Tanner, MSN, RNC-OB
Associate Professor
Greenville Technical College
Greenville, South Carolina

Wanda Williams, PhD, RN, WHNP-BC
Assistant Professor
Rutgers University
Camden, New Jersey

Donna Wilsker, MSN, RN
Assistant Professor
Lamar University
Beaumont, Texas

Preface

Maternal–newborn nursing is multifaceted, challenging, rewarding, and endlessly varied. Opportunities abound to touch lives and to make a difference. Many nurses opt for a career in mother–baby care and clinic or office nursing so that they can work closely with childbearing families. As these nurses continue their education, they may embrace the role of nurse practitioner, nurse-midwife, genetic counselor, lactation consultant, or childbirth educator. Those nurses who find the most reward by working in intense, highly technical situations are often drawn to the neonatal intensive care unit, to high-risk pregnancy units, or to work with laboring families. As these nurses advance their education, they often choose the clinical specialist role. Some nurses become enthralled by the possibility of shaping the profession for years to come, and so they become nurse managers or administrators, nursing faculty, advocates, influential leaders in national associations such as AWHONN, or even authors. We applaud them, too!

Because of the varied and rich opportunities for nurses, the theme we emphasize in this edition is the many facets of maternal–newborn nursing. This thread is subtly woven throughout the book. You will find it in the chapter opening quotes from nurses in a variety of roles and settings, in the photographs on the cover and part openers, and in the text itself. As authors and educators, it is our hope that we can encourage and inspire students to consider a rewarding career in maternal–newborn nursing.

As always, the underlying philosophy of *Contemporary Maternal–Newborn Nursing Care* remains unchanged. We see pregnancy and childbirth as normal life processes with the family members as co-participants in care. We remain committed to providing a text that is accurate and readable, a text that helps students develop the skills and abilities they need now and in the future in an ever-changing healthcare environment.

Organization—A Nursing Care Management Framework

Nurses today must be able to think critically and to solve problems effectively. For these reasons, we begin with an introductory unit to set the stage by providing information about maternal–newborn nursing and important related concepts. Subsequent units progress in a way that closely reflects the steps of the nursing process. We clearly delineate the nurse's role within this framework. Thus, the units related to pregnancy, labor and birth, the newborn period, and postpartum care begin with a discussion of basic theory followed by chapters on nursing assessment and nursing care for essentially healthy women or infants. Within the nursing care chapters and content areas, we use the heading **Nursing Management** and the subheadings **Nursing Assessment and Diagnosis, Planning and Implementation**, and **Evaluation**.

Complications of a specific period appear in the last chapter or chapters of each unit. The chapters also use the nursing process as an organizational framework. We believe that students can more clearly grasp the complicated content of the high-risk conditions once they have a good understanding of the normal processes of pregnancy, birth, and postpartum and newborn care. However, to avoid overemphasizing the prevalence of complications in such a wonderfully normal process as pregnancy and birth, we avoid including an entire unit that focuses only on complications. To aid student study, Chapter 21, Childbirth at Risk: Labor-Related Complications, focuses on issues that impact both pregnancy and labor and birth. We think you will find this very helpful.

More specialized or distinctive material is sometimes focused in a single chapter, such as the chapters on maternal nutrition, pregnancy in selected populations, and special diagnostic procedures. For faculty, we provide detailed syllabus suggestions and reading assignments for your course, whether you teach high-risk conditions at the end of the course or integrate them throughout the course.

Themes for the Ninth Edition
Evidence-Based Practice

The use of reliable information as the basis for planning and providing effective care—evidence-based practice (EBP)—is becoming a hallmark of skillful, proficient care. EBP draws on information from a variety of sources including nursing research. To help nurses become more comfortable in using evidence-based practice, we include a brief discussion of it in Chapter 1, Contemporary Maternal–Newborn Care, and then provide examples of evidence-based practice as it relates to maternal–newborn nursing throughout the textbook.

Critical Thinking and Clinical Decision Making

It is a challenge and a responsibility to help students use evidence, analyze information, and make sound decisions that result in safe, effective patient care. In this edition, we provide new tools to support this learning process. The use of **concept maps** is an exciting trend in nursing care management. Concept maps are visual depictions of the relationships that exist among a variety of concepts and ideas related to a patient's specific health problem. The relationship "picture" created by the map allows the nurse to plan interventions that can address multiple problems more effectively. To help students understand how the concept maps can influence care planning, we have included four concept maps in this edition.

Scenarios provide a realistic way of enabling students to apply concepts. Throughout this edition a feature titled **Clinical Reasoning** presents a brief **Case Study** and asks critical thinking questions to help students formulate how they would handle the issues raised. To further reinforce the importance of critical thinking, each chapter ends with a section entitled **Clinical Reasoning in Action**, which presents a patient scenario with questions to help students apply concepts they have learned in the chapter.

Community-Based Nursing Care

Although pregnancy, birth, and the postpartum period cover a period of many months, in reality most women spend only 2 to 3 days, if any, in the hospital. Thus, by its very nature, maternal-newborn nursing is primarily community-based nursing care. This emphasis on nursing care provided in community-based settings is a driving force in healthcare today and, consequently, forms a dominant theme throughout this edition. We address this topic in focused, user-friendly ways. For example, **Community-Based Nursing Care** is a special heading used throughout this text. Because we consider home care to be one form of community-based care, it often has a separate heading under Community-Based Nursing Care. Even more important, Chapter 29, The Postpartum Family: Early Care Needs and Home Care, provides a thorough explanation of home care, both from a theoretical perspective and as a significant tool in caring for childbearing families.

Emphasis on Health Promotion and Family Teaching

As nurses and educators, we are supportive of the goals and objectives of *Healthy People 2020*. This science-based effort provides a 10-year agenda for improving the health and well-being of the nation. Throughout the text, we have incorporated content reflecting the objectives of the project as they relate to women, newborns and infants, and childbearing families.

Patient and family teaching remains a critical element of effective nursing care, one that we continue to emphasize. Our focus is on the teaching that nurses do at all stages of pregnancy and the childbearing process—including the important postpartum teaching that is done before and after families are discharged from the hospital. With this in mind, in this edition we have incorporated a new feature, **Health Promotion**, that assists students to focus on important areas of health teaching with women and families. Also, more detailed discussions of client and family teaching are summarized in **Teaching Highlights** guides, such as the one on sexual activity during pregnancy. These teaching guides help students plan and organize their thoughts for preparing to teach women and their families.

Women With Special Needs

In this edition we have refocused the content on selected populations by including it in a single chapter. Chapter 12, Pregnancy in Selected Populations, addresses the distinct needs of pregnant adolescents and women over age 35. In addition, it contains a discussion of the special needs of women with physical and/or intellectual disabilities. A new feature, **Women With Special Needs**, is incorporated throughtout the text to expand on this content as it relates to specific conditions.

Safety is Essential

Patient safety is an essential element of effective patient care. It is the focus of The Joint Commission and one of the key elements of the Quality and Safety Education for Nurses (QSEN) project, which is discussed in Chapter 1. To help keep safety in the forefront, a special feature called *SAFETY ALERT!* is found throughout the text. This feature calls attention to issues that could place a client at risk. Another feature, **Clinical Tip**, relates to many nursing concepts, including safety, by providing readers with concrete suggestions for safe, effective practice.

Professionalism

Professionalism in Practice, another new feature, focuses on topics such as legal considerations, contemporary nursing practice issues, professional accountability, patient advocacy, and home and community care considerations. This reflects our belief that professionalism requires that the astute nurse demonstrate professional standards of moral, ethical, and legal conduct and model the values of the nursing profession as he or she cares for childbearing and childrearing families.

Commitment to Cultural Competence

As nurses and educators, we feel a strong commitment to the importance of acknowledging and respecting diversity and multiculturalism. Thus, we strive continually to make our textbook ever more inclusive, integrating diversity in our photographs, illustrations, case scenarios, and content. Chapter 2, Family, Culture, and Complementary Health Approaches, lays the foundational concepts for students to develop cultural competence, whereas the **Developing Cultural Competence** feature carries the concept forward by providing insights into specific issues related to culture. In addition, integrated into our narrative are a variety of issues and scenarios affecting maternal–newborn nursing care.

Women's Health Care

Women's health care is specifically addressed in Chapter 5, Health Promotion for Women, and Chapter 6, Common Gynecologic Problems. Because of the nature of this textbook, we do not address gynecologic cancers.

Resources for Student Success

- **Online Resources** are available at www.pearson highered.com/nursingresources and aim to further enhance the student's learning experience, build on knowledge gained from this textbook, prepare students for the NCLEX-RN® examination, and foster clinical reasoning.

- The *Clinical Skills Manual for Maternity and Pediatric Nursing*, ISBN 0134257006, is a useful resource to assist students in successful planning and performance of essential nursing skills. This manual helps to translate theoretic concepts into performance while caring for clients in a variety of settings.

- NEW! Pearson's *Maternity and Pediatric Nursing Reference App*, now available for both iPhone and Android devices, provides a collection of handy tools and additional content for students and professionals looking for a quick reference in maternity or pediatrics nursing. The maternity content includes a section on **Patient/Family Teaching**, which supplies useful information, tips, and strategies for educating parents and families in a variety of situations and settings. The colorful **Maternal–Fetal Growth and Development Timeline** depicts maternal/fetal development month by month and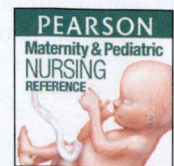

provides specific teaching guidelines for each stage of pregnancy.

- **MyNursingLab for Maternal–Newborn Nursing** is designed to engage students with maternal–newborn content while offering data-driven guidance that helps them better absorb course material and understand difficult concepts. The Pearson eText version of this text is available with MyNursingLab for Maternal–Newborn Nursing.

Resources for Faculty Success

Pearson is pleased to offer a complete suite of resources to support teaching and learning, including:

- **TestGen Test Bank**
- **Lecture Note PowerPoints**
- **Classroom Response System PowerPoints**
- **Instructor's Resource Manual**

Features to Help You Use This Textbook Successfully

Instructors and students alike value the in-text learning aids that we include in our textbooks. The following guide will help you use the features and resources from *Contemporary Maternal-Newborn Nursing*, Ninth Edition, to be successful in the classroom, in the clinical setting, on the NCLEX-RN® examination, and in nursing practice.

Each chapter begins with **Learning Outcomes** and a chapter opening **Quote**. These personal stories from nurses illustrate the challenging scope of the work, the satisfaction derived from helping women and their families, and the sheer joy of assisting new babies into the world.

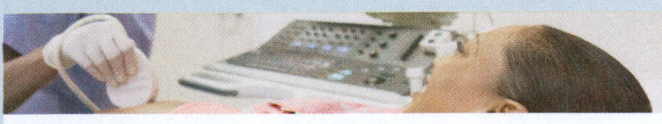

Chapter 8
Physical and Psychologic Changes of Pregnancy

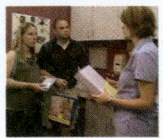

In my experience, few women are ever really prepared for all the changes they experience during pregnancy, especially a first pregnancy. That is why early prenatal care is important. Yes, starting care early gives us a better chance to identify risk factors, but it also enables us to do a better job of prenatal education. I am constantly amazed by what a difference it makes for a woman when she has a good idea of what to expect and why.
—A Nurse Working with an Obstetrician in Private Practice

Learning Outcomes

8.1 Identify the anatomic and physiologic changes that occur during pregnancy.

8.2 Relate the physiologic and anatomic changes that occur in the body systems during pregnancy to the signs and symptoms that develop in the woman.

8.3 Compare subjective (presumptive), objective (probable), and diagnostic (positive) changes of pregnancy.

8.4 Contrast the various types of pregnancy tests.

8.5 Examine the emotional and psychologic changes that commonly occur in a woman, her partner, and her family during pregnancy.

8.6 Summarize cultural factors that may influence a family's response to pregnancy.

Assessment Guides assist you with diagnoses by incorporating physical assessment and normal findings, alterations and possible causes, and guidelines for nursing interventions.

ASSESSMENT GUIDE	Initial Prenatal Assessment		
Physical Assessment/Normal Findings	**Alterations and Possible Causes***	**Nursing Responses to Data†**	
Vital Signs			
Blood Pressure (BP): Less than or equal to 120/80 mmHg	High BP (essential hypertension; renal disease; pregestational hypertension, apprehension; preeclampsia if initial assessment not done until after 20 weeks' gestation)	BP of 120–139/80–89 is considered prehypertensive. BP greater than 140/90 requires immediate consideration; establish woman's BP; refer to healthcare provider if necessary. Assess woman's knowledge about high BP; counsel on self-care and medical management.	
Pulse: 60–100 beats/min; rate may increase 10 beats/min during pregnancy	Increased pulse rate (excitement or anxiety, dehydration, infection, cardiac disorders)	Count for 1 full minute; note irregularities. Evaluate temperature, increase fluids.	
Respirations: 12–20 breaths/min (or pulse rate divided by four); pregnancy may induce a degree of hyperventilation; thoracic breathing predominant	Marked tachypnea or abnormal patterns	Assess for respiratory disease.	
Temperature: 36.2°–37.6°C (97°–99.6°F)	Elevated temperature (infection)	Assess for infection process or disease state if temperature is elevated; refer to healthcare provider.	
Weight			
Gain depends on body build Underweight: 12.5–18.0 kg (28–40 lb) Normal weight: 11.5–16.0 kg (25–35 lb) Overweight: 7.0–11.5 kg (15–25 lb) Obese: 5.0–9.1 kg (11–20 lb)	Weight less than 45.4 kg (100 lb) or greater than 91.1 kg (200 lb); rapid, sudden weight gain (preeclampsia)	Evaluate need for nutritional counseling; obtain information on eating habits, cooking practices, food regularly eaten, food allergies, income limitations, need for food supplements, pica and other abnormal food habits. Note initial weight to establish baseline for weight gain throughout pregnancy. Determine body mass index (BMI) and recommend weight gain for pregnancy.	

Clinical Reasoning   Hot Tub Use in Pregnancy

Karen Blade, a 23-year-old woman, G1P0, is 10 weeks pregnant when she sees you for her first prenatal examination. She has been experiencing some mild nausea and fatigue but otherwise is feeling well. She asks you about continuing with her routine exercises (walking 3 miles a day and lifting light weights). She also asks about using the heated pool and a hot tub.

What should you tell her?

Clinical Reasoning boxes provide brief case scenarios that ask you to determine the appropriate response.

Clinical Skill boxes offer step-by-step techniques of some tasks expected of nurses in clinical situations, preparing you for your clinical experience. Included are the preparation steps, with rationales; equipment and supplies needed; and steps for the skill itself.

Clinical Skill 5-1
Assisting with a Pelvic Examination

NURSING ACTION

Preparation

- Ensure that the room is sufficiently warm by checking room temperature and adjusting the thermostat if necessary. If overhead heat lamps are available, turn them on.
- Explain the procedure to the woman. If she has never had a pelvic examination, show her the equipment to be used as part of the explanation.

Rationale: Explaining the procedure helps reduce anxiety and increase cooperation.

- Ask the woman to empty her bladder and to remove clothing below the waist.

Rationale An empty bladder promotes comfort during the internal examination.

- Have padding on the stirrups. If stirrups are not padded, the woman may prefer to leave her shoes on during the procedure.

Rationale: Stirrups are padded to ease the pressure of the feet against the metal and to decrease the discomfort associated with cold stirrups. If they are not padded, wearing shoes accomplishes the same purpose.

- Give the woman a disposable drape or sheet to use during the exam. Ask her to sit at the end of the examining table with the drape opened across her lap.
- Position the woman in the lithotomy position with her thighs flexed and abducted. Place her feet in the stirrups. Her buttocks should extend slightly beyond the edge of the examining table.

Rationale: This position provides the exposure necessary to conduct the examination effectively.

- Drape the woman with the sheet, leaving a flap so that the perineum can be exposed.

Rationale: The drape helps preserve the woman's sense of dignity and privacy.

Equipment and Supplies

- Vaginal specula of various sizes, warmed with water or on a heating pad prior to insertion
- Sterile gloves
- Water-soluble lubricant
- Materials for Pap smear or ThinPrep® Pap test and cultures
- Good light source

Note: Lubricant may alter the results of tests and cultures and is not used during the speculum examination. Its use is reserved for the bimanual examination.

Procedure: Sterile Gloves

1. The examiner dons gloves for the procedure. Explain each part of the procedure as the examiner performs it. Let the woman know that the examiner begins with an inspection of the external genitalia. The speculum is then inserted to allow visualization of the cervix and vaginal walls and to obtain specimens for testing (e.g., Pap smear). After the speculum is withdrawn, the examiner performs a bimanual examination of the internal organs using the fingers of one hand inserted in the woman's vagina while the other hand presses over the woman's uterus and ovaries. The final step of the procedure is generally a rectal examination.
2. Ask the woman to breathe slowly and regularly and to use any method she finds effective in helping her to remain relaxed.

Rationale: Relaxation helps decrease muscle tension.

3. Let her know when the examiner is ready to insert the speculum and ask her to bear down.

Rationale: Bearing down helps open the vaginal orifice and relaxes the perineal muscles.

4. After the speculum is withdrawn, lubricate the examiner's fingers prior to the bimanual examination.

Rationale: Lubrication decreases friction and eases insertion of the examiner's fingers.

5. After the examiner has completed the examination and moved away from the woman, move to the end of the examination table and face the woman. Cover her with the drape. Apply gentle pressure to her knees and encourage her to move toward the head of the table. Assist her to remove her feet from the stirrups, then offer your hand to her and assist her to sit up.

Rationale: Assistance is important because the lithotomy position is an awkward one and many women, especially those who are pregnant, obese, or older, may find it difficult to get out of the stirrups.

6. Provide her with tissues to wipe the lubricant from her perineum.

Rationale: Vaginal secretions and lubricant may be discharged from the vagina when the woman sits upright.

7. Provide the woman with privacy while she dresses. Be sure that she is not dizzy and that she is standing or sitting safely before leaving the room.

Rationale: Lying supine may cause postural hypotension.

Clinical Tip features offer hands-on suggestions for specific procedures and interventions. The authors' wealth of clinical knowledge is reflected in these "real world" insights.

Clinical Tip

When advising clients that a screening test, such as the NTT, is abnormal, be sure to explain that this does *not* mean their baby definitely has the disorder, but rather indicates that the baby *may* be at risk. It is imperative for parents to understand that an abnormal NTT, or any type of screening test, is only an indication that more testing is needed to make the actual diagnosis. Advise parents that some women with abnormal test results have normal fetuses and that because the test only screens and does not actually diagnosis the fetus, a fetus that screens within the normal criteria could have an unrecognized anomaly.

Concept Maps provide a visual description of data you can analyze as you plan and provide care.

Concept Map

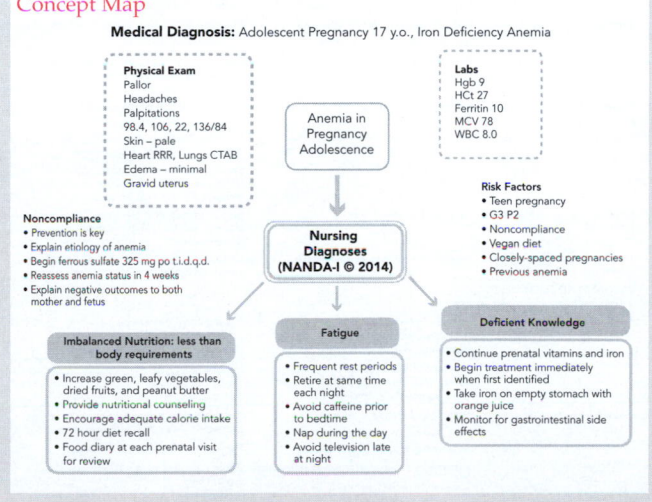

Developing Cultural Competence boxes highlight specific cultural issues and their application to nursing care.

Developing Cultural Competence Female Relatives as Caregivers

In most Middle Eastern countries, childbirth is exclusively attended to by women. A woman in labor is most commonly surrounded by female relatives and friends. Most Arab Muslim women prefer to have a female healthcare provider attend the labor and birth (Abushaikha & Massah, 2013).

Evidence-Based Practice boxes present recent nursing research, discuss implications, and challenge you to incorporate this information into your nursing practice through nursing actions.

| EVIDENCE-BASED PRACTICE | Validity of the Noninvasive Prenatal Test for the Detection of Chromosomal Abnormalities |

Clinical Question

Does the Noninvasive Prenatal Test (NIPT) detect chromosomal abnormalities with a strong degree of accuracy? Which abnormalities are best detected with the NIPT?

The Evidence

Noninvasive methods for testing for fetal abnormalities reduce the risk of procedural complications for the mother and baby, and lower costs. Since becoming clinically available in 2011, the tests have been rapidly adopted. Evidence is widely available for the specificity and accuracy of these tests. One group of researchers retrieved data from more than 31,000 clients that received the NIPT, and studied the rate of true positives, false positives, and false negatives for the conditions of trisomies 21, 18, 13, and X. Another study of a statewide prenatal screening program determined how many would be accurately diagnosed in a comparison of noninvasive and invasive diagnostic tests (amniocentesis). A third group of researchers studied more than 3400 clients to determine the relative sensitivity of the test. The samples included women who were both high- and low-risk for fetal aneuploidy. Taken together, these large-data studies support the strongest level of evidence.

The NIPT was as sensitive in the detection of chromosomal abnormalities as the invasive amniocentesis (Porreco,

Garite, Maurel, et al., 2014). Norton, Currier, & Jeliffe-Pawlowski (2014) determined that 80% of chromosomal abnormalities were detected by NIPT; 17% were missed and were false negatives. In the large-scale report, the predictive value was 83%, with only 2 of 500 false negatives (Dar, Curnow, Gross, et al., 2014). Both specificity and sensitivity of the test were validated at very high rates for trisomy 21 in 2 of the 3 studies, but had less sensitivity for trisomies 18 and 13 and low sensitivity for trisomy X.

Best Practice

Mothers at high risk for chromosomal aneuploidy can be counseled that noninvasive testing is as accurate as the more invasive amniocentesis. In any case, the test will detect the abnormality at least 80% of the time, and false negatives are low. The test will be most accurate, though, for trisomy 21, and will have little accuracy for trisomy X. Mothers at risk of trisomy 21 will be find the test most useful.

Clinical Reasoning

How would you construct an educational program for counseling women about their options for noninvasive prenatal testing for chromosomal abnormalities? What are the characteristics of a mother for whom the test would be most informative?

Healthy People 2020

(MICH-1.9) Reduce the rate of infant deaths from sudden unexpected infant deaths (includes SIDS, unknown cause, accidental suffocation, and strangulation in bed).

Healthy People 2020 goals are cited throughout the text to acquaint you with national public health efforts that have direct relevance to maternal, newborn, and women's health care.

A feature entitled **Health Promotion** provides client teaching information that will help you empower your clients in ways to enhance their own health care.

Health Promotion Self-Care Measures for Common Discomforts of Pregnancy

Discomfort	Influencing Factors	Self-Care Measures
FIRST TRIMESTER		
Nausea and vomiting	Increased levels of human chorionic gonadotropin	Avoid odors or causative factors.
	Changes in carbohydrate metabolism	Eat dry crackers or toast before arising in morning.
	Emotional factors	Have small but frequent meals.
	Fatigue	Avoid greasy or highly seasoned foods.
		Take dry meals with fluids between meals.
		Drink carbonated beverages.
		Avoid lying supine for 2 hours after eating.
Urinary frequency	Pressure of uterus on bladder in both first and third trimesters	Void when urge is felt.
		Increase fluid intake during the day.
		Decrease fluid intake only in the evening to decrease nocturia.
Fatigue	Specific causative factors unknown	Plan time for a nap or rest period daily.
	May be aggravated by nocturia due to urinary frequency	Go to bed earlier.
		Seek family support and assistance with responsibilities so that more time is available to rest.
Breast tenderness	Increased levels of estrogen and progesterone	Wear well-fitting, supportive bra.
Increased vaginal discharge	Hyperplasia of vaginal mucosa and increased production of mucus by the endocervical glands due to the increase in estrogen levels	Promote cleanliness by daily bathing. Avoid douching, nylon underpants, and pantyhose; use cotton underpants, which are more absorbent; can use powder to maintain dryness, if not allowed to cake.
Nasal stuffiness and nosebleed (epistaxis)	Elevated estrogen levels	May be unresponsive, but cool air vaporizer may help; avoid use of nasal sprays and decongestants.
Ptyalism (excessive, often bitter salivation)	Specific causative factors unknown	Use astringent mouthwashes, chew gum, or suck hard candy.
SECOND AND THIRD TRIMESTERS		
Heartburn (pyrosis)	Increased production of progesterone, decreasing gastrointestinal motility and increasing relaxation of cardiac sphincter	Eat small and more frequent meals. Use low-sodium antacids.
	Displacement of stomach by enlarging uterus, thus regurgitation of acidic gastric contents into the esophagus	Avoid overeating, fatty and fried foods, lying down after eating, and sodium bicarbonate.
Ankle edema	Prolonged standing or sitting	Practice frequent dorsiflexion of feet when prolonged sitting or standing is necessary.
	Increased levels of sodium due to hormonal influences	Elevate legs when sitting or resting.
	Circulatory congestion of lower extremities	Avoid tight garters or restrictive bands around legs.
	Increased capillary permeability	
	Varicose veins	
Varicose veins	Venous congestion in the lower veins that increases with pregnancy	Elevate legs frequently. Wear supportive hose.
	Hereditary factors (weakening of walls of veins, faulty valves)	Avoid crossing legs at the knees, standing for long periods, garters, and hosiery with constrictive bands.
	Increased age and weight gain	

Key Facts to Remember boxes summarize the elements of particular importance related to a specific topic.

KEY FACTS TO REMEMBER
Nursing Responsibilities in Genetic Counseling

- Identify families at risk for genetic problems.
- Determine how the genetic problem is perceived and what information is desired before proceeding.
- Assist families in acquiring accurate information about the specific problem.
- Act as a liaison between the family and genetic counselor.
- Assist the family in understanding and dealing with information received.
- Provide information on support groups.
- Aid families in coping with this crisis.
- Provide information about known genetic factors.
- Ensure continuity of nursing care to the family.

Medications Used To Treat: Endometriosis

- **Combined oral contraceptives (COCs)**, which suppress menstruation, can be used in women who do not desire fertility.
- **Progestins** such as medroxyprogesterone acetate (MPA) and Dienogest exert an antiendometriotic effect and ultimate atrophy. The medication is administered intramuscularly every 3 months; the effectiveness of the treatment is evaluated every 3 to 6 months. Side effects may include nausea, weight gain, fluid retention, and breakthrough bleeding.
- **Danazol** is a testosterone derivative that suppresses ovulation and causes amenorrhea. It is intended for short-term therapy. Because of adverse effects on lipid metabolism and significant side effects such as weight gain, hirsutism, acne, oily skin, vaginal dryness, hot flushes, reduced libido, voice changes, clitoral enlargement, and decreased breast size, many clinicians have moved away from danazol to other treatment options.
- **Gonadotropin-releasing hormone (GnRH) analogs** such as *nafarelin acetate* (given as a metered nasal spray twice daily) and *leuprolide acetate* (Lupron, given once a month as an intramuscular injection), are gaining popularity because many women tolerate them better than danazol and their results in treating endometriosis are comparable. GnRH analogs suppress the menstrual cycle through estrogen antagonism. This may result in the hypoestrogen side effects of hot flushes, vaginal dryness, headache, breast reduction, and loss of bone density. Consequently, the use of GnRH agonists should be limited to 6 months (Hogg & Vyas, 2015).

Medications Used to Treat is a feature in tabular format that provides an overview of medications used for specific conditions.

Also provided are **Nursing Care Plans** that address nursing care for women who have complications such as preeclampsia or diabetes mellitus, as well as for high-risk newborns. We designed this information to enhance your preparation for the clinical setting.

Nursing Care Plan: Language Barriers at First Prenatal Visit

Nursing Diagnosis: *Health Maintenance, Ineffective,* related to alteration in verbal and written communication skills (NANDA-I ©2014)

GOAL: Client will demonstrate understanding of health information received during prenatal visits.

INTERVENTION	RATIONALE
If no interpreter is available, refer to posters with pictures to explain routine care and procedures during the prenatal examination.	Posters put words into verbal images and are helpful in communicating information.
Provide handouts and brochures about prenatal care in the woman's native language.	Translated handouts provide information that the client can refer to at home. This reinforces information discussed during the visit and helps the family understand what the woman will experience during the pregnancy and at each visit.
Use teaching models to demonstrate procedures. Teaching models may include plastic pelvis, knitted uterus, fetal model, breast model, birth control devices, ultrasound equipment, and so forth.	Visual aids help to communicate information during the examination.
Schedule an interpreter for subsequent prenatal visits.	If a family member cannot translate the health information to the client, an independent translator is essential to ensure that information is accurately provided. When an interpreter is used (especially a family member), the nurse should be sure that the interpreter is translating information received from the woman and not simply answering the questions for her.
Refer the woman to prenatal classes taught in her own language, if available.	Prenatal classes taught in the woman's language enable her to receive health information that is easily understood, which will provide a better understanding of what she should expect during pregnancy, birth, and postpartum. Prenatal classes may also provide a social outlet for clients.
Involve other members of the healthcare team in planning and providing care.	Cultures vary in language, nonverbal expression, dietary habits, use of time, spatial expectations, and so forth. Use of medication and blood products may also be influenced by cultural beliefs. Social workers who are familiar with the client's cultural beliefs, for example, may help the client adjust to different healthcare practices while providing suggestions to ensure prenatal care that is more in line with the woman's cultural beliefs. Dietitians may help the woman plan meals that are aligned with her cultural practices while meeting the nutritional needs of pregnancy.

EXPECTED OUTCOME: Effective communication occurs. The client will gain an understanding of basic prenatal information as evidenced by using hand gestures, by pointing to pictures on posters and translated phrases on handouts, and through an interpreter, if one is available.

Professionalism in Practice **Emancipated Minors**

It is important to remember that if a pregnant minor is considered emancipated, she has the right and responsibility to consent to health care for herself and later for her child. She is entitled to respect and confidentiality in her dealings with healthcare providers. Only with her consent can other adults, including her parents, be included in communication.

Professionalism in Practice focuses on important topics related to contemporary nursing practice issues, including legal and ethical considerations. This feature reflects a commitment to quality improvement in all aspects of care.

The *SAFETY ALERT!* features present essential information that calls attention to issues that could place a client or a nurse at risk and provide guidance on maintaining a safe environment for all clients and healthcare providers.

SAFETY ALERT!

CST testing should be conducted only in a setting where tocolytic medications are available in case a hypersystole pattern occurs or if labor is stimulated from the test. Prompt administration of a tocolytic agent may be needed to ensure that the fetus and mother maintain a safe and healthy status.

TEACHING HIGHLIGHTS | What to Tell the Pregnant Woman About Assessing Fetal Activity

CONTENT	TEACHING METHOD
• Explain that fetal movements are first felt around 18 weeks' gestation. From that time the fetal movements get stronger and easier to detect. A slowing or stopping of fetal movement may be an indication that the fetus needs some attention and evaluation.	Describe procedures and demonstrate how to assess fetal movement. Sit beside the woman and show her how to place her hand on the fundus to feel fetal movement.
• Explain the procedure for the Cardiff Count-to-Ten method or for the fetal movement record (FMR). For both methods, advise the woman as follows:	Provide a written teaching sheet for the woman's use at home. Demonstrate how to record fetal movements on a Cardiff Count-to-Ten scoring card or on an FMR.
• Beginning at about 28 weeks' gestation, keep a daily record of fetal movement. • Try to begin counting at about the same time each day, about 1 hour after a meal if possible. • Lie quietly in a side-lying position.	Watch the woman fill out the record as examples are provided. Encourage her to complete the record each day and bring it with her to each prenatal visit. Assure her that the record will be discussed at each prenatal visit, and questions may be addressed at that time if desired.
• Using the Cardiff card, have the woman place an X for each fetal movement until she has recorded 10. Movement varies considerably, but most women feel fetal movement at least 10 times in 3 hours.	Provide the woman with a name and phone number in case she has further questions.
• Using the FMR, have the woman count three times a day for 20 to 30 minutes each session. If there are fewer than three movements in a session, have the woman count for 1 hour or more.	
• Explain when to contact the care provider: • If there are fewer than 10 movements in 3 hours. • If overall the fetus's movements are slowing, and it takes much longer each day to note 10 movements. • If there are no movements in the morning.	

Teaching Highlights present special healthcare issues or problems and the related key teaching points to address with women and their families.

Women With Special Needs boxes serve as reminders that women with individualized needs may require modified plans of care.

Women With Special Needs Intimate Partner Violence

Women with disabilities are at greater risk of being victimized and of sustaining intimate partner violence. Women who rely on their partner for assistance with activities of daily living are at risk for having care withheld and being neglected, in addition to physical and mental abuse. They are also at risk for financial abuse. The nurse should provide an extensive intimate partner assessment with the woman without the partner present to determine if abuse is occurring.

Clinical Reasoning In Action

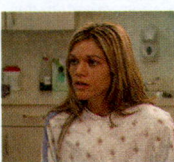

Marie Neives, age 19, presents while you are working at a Planned Parenthood clinic. She is there for a GYN exam and tells you that she is sexually active with her boyfriend but doesn't want to become pregnant. Since she lives at home with her parents, she does not want to use "the pill" because her mother might find out. Marie tells you she has a family history of cystic fibrosis (CF) and is concerned that she will pass the disease on. Marie asks you for information concerning fertility awareness. You obtain a menstrual history as follows: menarche age 12, cycle every 28 days for 5 days, dysmenorrhea the first 2 days with moderate flow. She has had one sexual partner. She states her boyfriend, also 19 years of age and of Northern European ancestry, doesn't like to use condoms and that she has been lucky so far in not getting pregnant. You assist the nurse practitioner with a physical and pelvic examination. The results show that Marie is essentially healthy. The nurse practitioner asks you to review with Marie fertility awareness and discuss her risk of having a child with CF.

1. Explore with Marie "natural family planning." How would you explain this to her?
2. What is the chance that Marie is a carrier for CF? Given that her boyfriend does not have a family history of CF, could the couple still have an affected child if Marie were a carrier and were to become pregnant?
3. After figuring out her menstruation cycle, to avoid conception when would you tell Marie to abstain from unprotected intercourse?
4. Explain carrier screening for CF to Marie. In what circumstances would you refer Marie and her boyfriend to genetic counseling?

Clinical Reasoning in Action features at the end of each chapter propose a real-life scenario and a series of clinical reasoning questions so that you can apply to the clinical setting what you learned in class.

Each chapter ends with **Focus Your Study**, which outlines the main points of the chapter and a list of **References**.

Focus Your Study

• Virtually all systems of a woman's body are altered in some way during pregnancy.

• Blood pressure decreases slightly during pregnancy. It reaches its lowest point in the second trimester and gradually increases to near normal levels in the third trimester.

• The enlarging uterus may cause pressure on the vena cava when the woman lies supine, causing supine hypotensive syndrome.

• A physiologic anemia may occur during pregnancy because the total plasma volume increases more than the total number of erythrocytes. This difference produces a drop in the hematocrit.

• The glomerular filtration rate increases somewhat during pregnancy. Glycosuria may be caused by the body's inability to reabsorb all the glucose filtered by the glomeruli.

• Changes in the skin include the development of chloasma; linea nigra; darkened nipples, areola, and vulva; striae; and spider nevi.

• Insulin needs increase during pregnancy. A woman with a latent deficiency state may respond to the increased stress on the islets of Langerhans by developing gestational diabetes.

• The subjective (presumptive) signs of pregnancy are symptoms experienced and reported by the woman, such as amenorrhea, nausea and vomiting, fatigue, urinary frequency, breast changes, and quickening.

• The objective (probable) signs of pregnancy can be perceived by the examiner but may be caused by conditions other than pregnancy.

• The diagnostic (positive) signs of pregnancy can be perceived by the examiner and can be caused only by pregnancy.

Acknowledgments

We are especially grateful to Janet Houser, PhD, RN, for contributing the **Evidence-Based Practice** features to this edition. She has a wide and varied background in nursing and is a born teacher. A special thank you to Nathan S. Davidson, II, CFNP, MSN, RN, for creating the **Concept Maps** for this edition.

A project of this scope is not possible without the skill and expertise of many. And so we extend special thanks to the following people.

First and foremost, we thank Portfolio Manager, Katrin Beacom, for her support and encouragement. We are very grateful to Content Producer, Erin Rafferty, for her unfailing efficiency and leadership in helping guide this project. Julie Alexander, our publisher, has delineated a vision for the future and a commitment to excellence for Pearson Health Science. Her energy, responsiveness, and forward thinking are awe-inspiring and challenge us to give our best. We have valued our long, rewarding relationship with this very special woman.

We cannot adequately express our deep gratitude to our developmental editor, Lynda Hatch. She brings a fresh, discerning perspective that helped us update content and streamline narrative. More importantly, she remains calm when things are rushed and is unfailingly supportive. She is a crucial part of our team and we are truly blessed to have her!

We also extend our deep appreciation to Patty Donovan of SPi Global. She steered the book through all phases of production and was always effective in her role, patient and gracious in her interactions, and responsive to our needs.

This is a time of possibilities for nursing. The need for skilled nurses has never been higher, nor have the opportunities to make a real difference in the lives of childbearing families ever been greater. Time and again we have seen the difference a skilled nurse can make in the lives of people in need. We, like you, are committed to helping all nurses recognize and take pride in that fact. Thank you for your letters, your comments, and your suggestions. We feel embraced by your support.

PWL
MLL
MRD

Contents

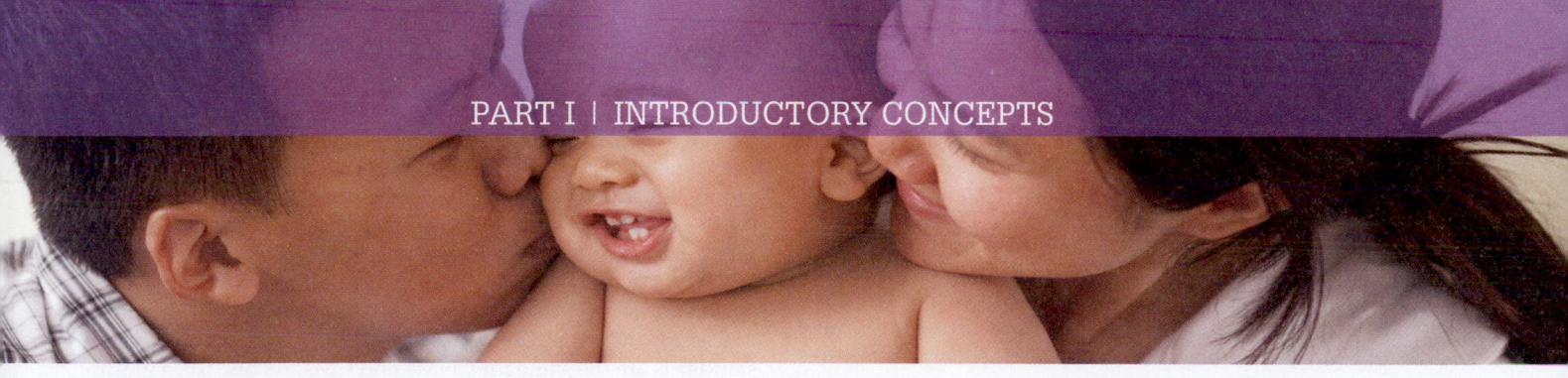

Chapter 1
Contemporary Maternal-Newborn Care

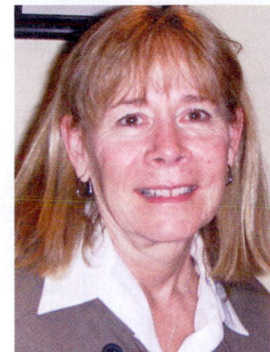

The opportunities I've had as a nurse are amazing. I've been an Air Force nurse and a hospital staff nurse. I thought I could never love any type of nursing more than I loved the mother-baby unit, but then I became a nurse practitioner and found wonderful new challenges. At the same time, I became a faculty member at a local university and learned the joy of helping to shape future nurses' lives. Do you know how lucky I am? I am 57, I've been a nurse for 36 years, and I am still passionate about what I do!

—A Nurse Educator

⌄ Learning Outcomes

1.1 Summarize the current status of factors related to health insurance and access to health care.

1.2 Describe the use of community-based nursing care in meeting the needs of childbearing families.

1.3 Identify the nursing roles available to the maternal-newborn and women's healthcare nurses.

1.4 Delineate significant legal and ethical issues that influence the practice of maternal-newborn nursing.

1.5 Discuss the role of evidence-based practice in improving the quality of nursing care for childbearing families.

1.6 Explain how nurses can use descriptive and inferential statistics in clinical practice in maternal-child health nursing.

The practice of most nurses is filled with special moments, shared experiences, times in which they know they have practiced the essence of nursing and, in so doing, touched a life. What is the essence of nursing? Simply stated, nurses care *for* people, care *about* people, and use their expertise to help people help themselves. Skilled nurses view clients and families holistically, with a clear realization that a myriad of factors have shaped each individual's perceptions.

The following situation demonstrates the impact a skilled nurse can have by practicing from a framework that considers a client holistically:

My first pregnancy had ended in a miscarriage at 8 weeks' gestation, so when I became pregnant again we decided to wait until I was a full 3 months along to tell our families. We had just told

both families the preceding day when it happened again. We rushed to the hospital and, a short time later, I passed a small fetus in the Johnny cap the nurse had placed in the commode. My poor baby was so tiny, only about 3 inches long. We called the nurse, who came and took my baby away.

I sat on the side of the bed and sobbed as my husband sought to console me. The nurse returned a few minutes later and said, "I saw on your record that you are Catholic. Would you like me to baptize your baby?" I was amazed and humbled by her suggestion. She had thought of something that I had not yet even considered. I said, "Oh, yes, please." And she left. Even in my grief, I recognized the meaningfulness of her act. I realized that I had been incredibly fortunate to have a nurse who showed me so very clearly that I was a person, an individual in need of personalized care. I vowed that I would practice nursing in the same holistic way. I also began sharing my story with the students I taught so that they could recognize the difference an expert, caring nurse can make.

We believe that many nurses who work with childbearing families are experts: They are sensitive, intuitive, and technically skilled. They view clients holistically and can support the efforts of childbearing families to make decisions about their needs and desires. Such nurses do make a difference in the quality of care that childbearing families receive.

Contemporary Childbirth

Contemporary childbirth is characterized by an emphasis on the family. Today the concept of family-centered childbirth is accepted and encouraged. Fathers and partners are active participants, not simply bystanders (Figure 1–1); siblings are encouraged to visit and meet the newest family member, and they may even attend the birth. New definitions of family are evolving. The family of a single mother may include her mother, her sister, another relative, a close friend, the father of the child, or a same-sex partner. Many cultures also recognize the importance of extended families, in which the expectant woman's mother, sister, or other family member may provide care and support (see Chapter 2).

Contemporary childbirth is also characterized by an increasing number of choices about the birth experience. The family can make choices about the primary healthcare provider (physician, certified nurse-midwife, or certified midwife), the use of a *doula* to provide labor support, the place of birth (hospital, birthing center, or home), and birth-related experiences (e.g., method of childbirth preparation, position for birth, and use of analgesia and anesthesia), as well as breastfeeding and child care choices.

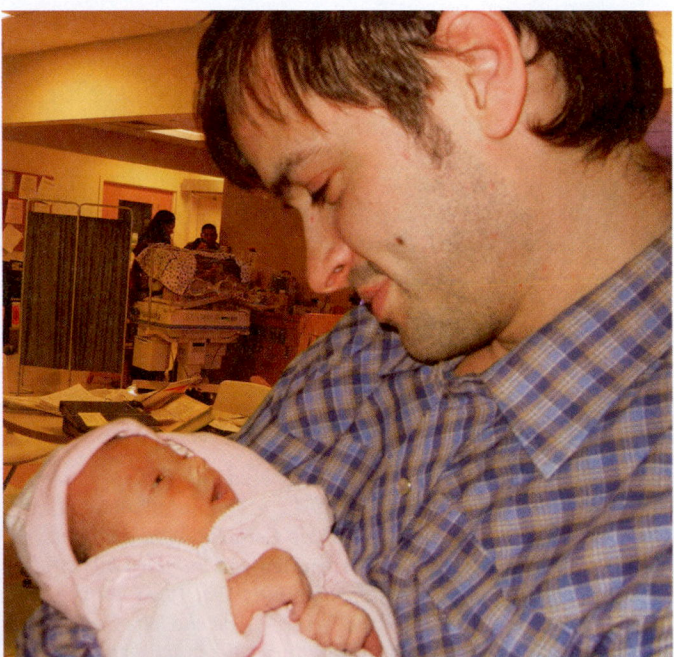

Figure 1–1 This new father enjoys some private time with his daughter just minutes after her birth.

SOURCE: Val M. Emmich.

Many women elect to have their pregnancy and birth managed by a certified nurse-midwife (CNM). Midwives who are not registered nurses but who complete a direct-entry midwifery education program that meets the standards established by the American College of Nurse-Midwives (ACNM) may take a certification exam to become a *certified midwife (CM)*. In 2012 CNMs and CMs attended 7.9% of all births in the United States and 11.8% of all vaginal births (American College of Nurse-Midwives [ACNM], 2014). Education and certification standards are the same for CNMs and CMs. As of 2010, a graduate degree is required (ACNM, 2014).

The North American Registry of Midwives (NARM) is also a certification agency. Midwives certified through NARM may have been prepared through a formal educational program at a college, university, or midwifery school, or through apprenticeship or self-study. They are eligible to use the credential *certified professional midwife (CPM)* (North American Registry of Midwives [NARM], 2014).

The place of birth is an important decision. Birthing centers and special homelike labor–delivery–recovery–postpartum (LDRP) rooms in hospitals have become increasingly popular. Some women choose to give birth at home, although healthcare professionals do not generally recommend this approach. Most professionals are concerned that, in the event of an unanticipated complication, delay in receiving emergency care might jeopardize the well-being of the mother or her baby. Some CNMs do attend home births; however, the majority of home births are attended by CMs, CPMs, or lay midwives. In 2013, 1.4% of births occurred outside of a hospital. Of these, 64% were home births, while the remainder occurred in a freestanding birthing center; this is the highest number of home births reported since this information began to be collected in 1989 (Martin, Hamilton, Osterman, et al., 2015).

Health Teaching and Contemporary Care

The physical and psychologic changes of pregnancy are dramatic and occasionally disconcerting, even for women who have planned their pregnancies. Effective, thoughtful, and carefully timed teaching can help prepare women for the changes they will encounter throughout the trimesters of pregnancy. In addition, anticipatory guidance can help women and their loved ones plan for the birth of the baby and beyond.

In the early 1990s, women who gave birth vaginally remained in the hospital for about 3 days. This provided time for nurses to assess the family's knowledge and skill and to complete essential teaching. In an effort to control costs, discharge within 12 to 24 hours after birth became the norm. This practice did not necessarily cause problems for women with supportive families, thorough prenatal preparation, and adequate resources for necessary follow-up care. However, because early discharge severely limits the time available for patient teaching, women with little knowledge, experience, or support were often inadequately prepared to care for themselves and their newborns. Fortunately, the negative impact of this practice gained recognition nationwide and resulted in legislation that provides for a postpartum stay of up to 48 hours following a vaginal birth and up to 96 hours following a cesarean birth at the discretion of the mother and her healthcare provider. Nevertheless, nurses are challenged to prepare parents adequately—especially first-time parents—for postpartum and newborn care. For this reason, the ability to provide concise and effective teaching is especially

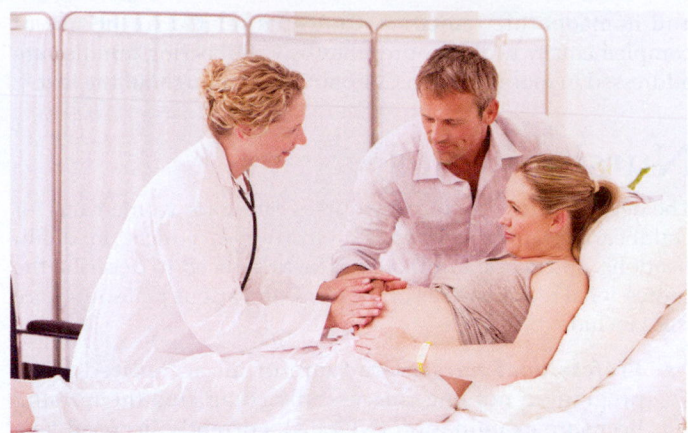

Figure 1–2 Individualized education for childbearing couples is one of the prime responsibilities of the maternal-newborn nurse.

SOURCE: © WavebreakMediaMicro/Fotolia.

important (Figure 1–2). Nurses can also supplement the teaching they complete with informational handouts and referral to community agencies when indicated.

The Healthcare Environment

In 2011, healthcare expenditures in the United States were $2.3 trillion, a 4.1% increase over the previous year (National Center for Health Statistics [NCHS], 2014). Cost, access, and quality of health care have become the "bywords" of the times. Almost all adults over age 65 are covered by Medicare, so the vast majority of the uninsured are under age 65.

The Affordable Care Act bridges a portion of the gap. It ends pre-existing condition exclusions for children and adults, eliminates annual limits on insurance coverage, and keeps young adults covered for a longer period. It also provides more affordable health insurance options, including tax credits for middle- and low-income families. These credits cover a major portion of the cost (U.S. Department of Health and Human Services, 2015).

For women who become pregnant, early prenatal care is one of the most important approaches available to reduce adverse pregnancy outcomes. In 2012, 74.1% of pregnant women in the United States began prenatal care in the first trimester; almost 20% began care in the second trimester; and 6% began prenatal care in the third trimester or received no prenatal care (U.S. Dept. of Health and Human Services, 2014).

Community-Based Nursing Care

Primary care is the focus of much attention as caregivers search for a new, more effective direction for health care. Primary care includes a focus on health promotion, illness prevention, and individual responsibility for one's own health. These services are best provided in community-based settings. Community-based healthcare systems providing primary care and some secondary care are becoming available in schools, workplaces, homes, churches, clinics, transitional care programs, and other ambulatory settings.

The growth and diversity of health payer plans offer both opportunities and challenges for women's and children's health care. Opportunities for improved delivery of screening and preventive services exist in community-based models of coordinated and comprehensive well-woman and well-child

care. A challenge that health payer plans face is how to relate to essential community providers of care, such as family-planning clinics, women's health centers, and child health centers, that offer a unique service or serve groups of women and children with special needs (adolescents, women and children with disabilities, and ethnic or racial minorities).

Community-based care is also part of a trend initiated by consumers, who are asking for a "seamless" system of family-centered, comprehensive, coordinated health care, health education, and social services. This type of system requires coordination as clients move from primary care services to acute care facilities and then back into the community. Nurses can assume this care-management role and perform an important service for individuals and families.

Community-based care is especially important in maternal-child nursing because the vast majority of health care provided to childbearing women and their families takes place outside of hospitals in clinics, offices, community-based organizations, and private homes. In addition, maternal-child nurses offer specialized services such as childbirth preparation classes and postpartum exercise classes that typically take place outside of hospitals. In essence, we are expert at providing community-based nursing care.

HOME CARE

Providing health care in the home is an especially important dimension of community-based nursing care. Shorter hospital stays end in the discharge of individuals who still require support, assistance, and teaching. Home care helps fill this gap. Conversely, home care enables some individuals to remain at home with conditions such as pregnancy-related complications that formerly would have required hospitalization.

Nurses are the major providers of home care services. Home care nurses perform direct nursing care and also supervise unlicensed assistive personnel who provide less-skilled levels of service. In a home setting, nurses use their skills in assessment, therapeutics, communication, teaching, problem solving, and organization to meet the needs of childbearing women and their families. They also play a major role in coordinating services from other providers, such as physical therapists and lactation consultants.

Postpartum and newborn home visits help ensure a satisfactory transition from the birthing center to the home. Chapter 29 discusses home care and provides guidance about making a home visit. Throughout the text we have also provided information on the use of home care to meet the needs of pregnant women with health problems, such as diabetes or preterm labor. We believe that home care offers nurses the opportunity to function in an autonomous role and make a significant difference for individuals and families.

Healthy People 2020 Goals

For 30 years the federal government's *Healthy People* initiative has been providing science-based, national agendas for improving the health of all Americans. This effort is based on the recognition that it is possible to motivate action by setting national objectives and monitoring progress. Analysis indicates that this approach has led to significant progress in many areas.

Healthy People 2020 is grouped by topic area and objectives. Maternal-newborn and women's health nurses focus directly on many of the topics, including maternal, infant, and child health; adolescent health (new to the list); family planning; injury and violence prevention; lesbian, gay, bisexual, and transgender health (new); and sexually transmitted infections. Because of the role women play in maintaining their family's health, many other topics may also be of importance to women, such as immunization and infectious diseases; diabetes; and nutrition and weight status, to name but a few. Nurses of all disciplines will find it helpful to become familiar with the 2020 topics and objectives, which may be found at the *Healthy People* website. To increase your familiarity with the objectives, look for the *Healthy People 2020* feature that identifies relevant objectives for topics presented throughout the text.

Culturally Competent Care

The U.S. population becomes more diverse every day. Approximately 47% of all children less than 18 years of age are from families of minority populations (Federal Interagency Forum on Child and Family Statistics, 2013). Thus, it is vitally important that nurses who care for women and for childbearing families recognize the importance of a family's cultural values and beliefs, which may be quite different from those of the nurse.

Specific elements that contribute to a family's value system include the following:

- Religious and social beliefs
- Presence and influence of the extended family, as well as socialization within the ethnic group
- Communication patterns
- Beliefs and understanding about the concepts of health and illness
- Beliefs about propriety of physical contact with strangers
- Education

Developing Cultural Competence   Values Conflicts

Conflicts can occur with a childbearing woman and her family when the traditional rituals and practices of the family's elders do not conform to current healthcare practices (Spector, 2013). Nurses need to be sensitive to the potential implications for the woman's health and that of her newborn, especially after they are discharged home. When cultural values are not part of the nursing care plan, a woman and her family may be forced to decide whether the family's beliefs should take priority over the healthcare professional's guidance.

When the family's cultural and social values are incorporated into the plan of care, the family is more likely to embrace the plan, especially in the home setting. By learning about the values, religious beliefs, traditions, and practices of local ethnic groups, nurses can develop an individualized nursing care plan for each childbearing woman and her family.

Because of the importance of culturally competent care, this topic is discussed in more depth in Chapter 2 and throughout the text.

Complementary Health Approaches

Interest in complementary health approaches, sometimes called complementary and alternative medicine (CAM), continues to grow nationwide and affects the care of childbearing families. CAM includes a wide array of therapies such as acupuncture, acupressure, aromatherapy, therapeutic touch, biofeedback, massage therapy, meditation, yoga, herbal therapies,

and homeopathic remedies. Concepts related to the use of complementary health approaches by childbearing families are addressed in more detail in Chapter 2 and throughout the text.

Nursing Roles

The depth of care provided by nurses caring for women and for childbearing families depends on the nurses' education, qualifications, and scope of practice. The titles used to describe the professional requirements of the nurse in various maternity care roles include:

- *Professional nurse:* Graduate of an accredited basic program in nursing; successfully completed the nursing licensure examination (NCLEX); currently licensed as a registered nurse (RN); may work as labor nurse, mother-baby nurse, lactation consultant, clinic nurse, newborn nursery nurse, home health nurse, adult or newborn intensive care nurse, gynecology unit nurse. See Figure 1–3.
- *Certified registered nurse (RNC):* Passed a national certification exam showing expertise in a field.
- *Nurse practitioner (NP):* Received specialized education in a Doctor of Nursing Practice (DNP) program or a master's degree program; can function in an advanced practice role. Provides ambulatory care services to expectant families; if a neonatal nurse practitioner (NNP), cares for newborns; may function in acute care, high-risk settings. NPs focus on physical and psychosocial assessments, including history, physical examination, and certain diagnostic tests and procedures; make clinical judgments and begin appropriate treatments, seeking physician consultation when necessary.
- *Clinical nurse specialist (CNS):* Has a master's degree and specialized knowledge and competence in a specific clinical area; often found on mother-baby units, on pediatric units, and in intensive care units assisting staff to provide excellent, evidence-based care.
- *Certified nurse-midwife (CNM):* Educated in the two disciplines of nursing and midwifery; certified by the American College of Nurse-Midwives (ACNM); prepared to manage

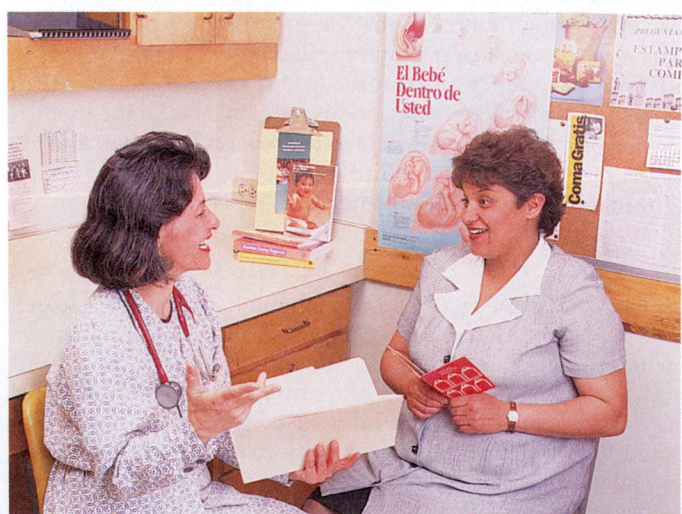

Figure 1–3 At each prenatal visit, the professional nurse reviews important areas of health teaching and provides opportunities for the pregnant woman to ask questions and raise concerns.

SOURCE: George Dodson/Pearson Education, Inc.

independently the care of women at low risk for complications during pregnancy and birth and the care of healthy newborns.

- *Nurse researcher:* Has an advanced doctoral degree, typically a Ph.D, and assumes a leadership role in generating new research; generally found in university settings, although more and more hospitals are employing them to conduct research relevant to health care, administrative issues, and other concerns.

Legal Considerations

Scope of Practice

The *scope of practice* is defined as the limits of nursing practice set forth in state statutes. Although some state practice acts continue to limit nursing practice to the traditional responsibilities of providing client care related to health maintenance and disease prevention, most state practice acts cover expanded practice roles that include collaboration with other health professionals in planning and providing care, physician-delegated diagnosis and prescriptive privilege, and the delegation of client care tasks to other specified licensed and unlicensed personnel. A nurse must function within the scope of practice or risk being accused of practicing medicine without a license.

Standards of Nursing Care

Standards of care establish minimum criteria for competent, proficient delivery of nursing care. Such standards are designed to protect the public and are used to judge the quality of care provided. Legal interpretation of actions within standards of care is based on what a reasonably prudent nurse with similar education and experience would do in similar circumstances.

The American Nurses Association (ANA) has published standards of professional practice for maternal-child health. Organizations such as the Association of Women's Health, Obstetric and Neonatal Nurses (AWHONN), the National Association of Neonatal Nurses (NANN), and the Association of periOperative Registered Nurses (AORN) have developed standards for specialty practice. Agency policies, procedures, and protocols also provide appropriate guidelines for care standards. For example, **clinical practice guidelines** are comprehensive interdisciplinary care plans for a specific condition that describe the sequence and timing of interventions that should result in expected client outcomes. Clinical practice guidelines are adopted within a healthcare setting to reduce variation in care management, to limit costs of care, and to evaluate the effectiveness of care.

While standards of care do not carry the force of law, they have important legal significance. Any nurse who fails to meet appropriate standards of care invites allegations of negligence or malpractice. Practicing within the guidelines established by an agency or following local or national standards decreases the potential for litigation.

Patients' Rights

Patients' rights encompass such topics as safety, informed consent, and the right to privacy.

PATIENT SAFETY

The Joint Commission, a nongovernmental agency that audits the operation of hospitals and healthcare facilities, has identified patient safety as an important responsibility of healthcare professionals, and provides an annual list of specific patient safety goals. These goals and requirements, which are updated regularly, can be found on The Joint Commission website.

Safety is a major focus of nursing education programs. The Quality and Safety Education for Nurses (QSEN) project, established in 2005, is designed "to meet the challenge of preparing future nurses who will have the knowledge, skills and attitudes (KSAs) necessary to continuously improve the quality and safety of the healthcare systems within which they work" (Quality and Safety Education for Nurses [QSEN], 2011, p. 1). The project focuses on competencies in six areas:

1. Patient-centered care
2. Teamwork and collaboration
3. Evidence-based practice
4. Quality improvement
5. Safety
6. Informatics

To support the efforts of The Joint Commission and to draw special attention to the importance of the QSEN project's emphasis on safety, key issues related to safety are noted throughout this text in the feature **SAFETY ALERT!**

INFORMED CONSENT

Informed consent is a legal concept that protects a client's right to autonomy and self-determination by specifying that no action may be taken without that person's prior understanding and freely given consent. Although this policy is usually enforced for such major procedures as surgery or regional anesthesia, it pertains to any nursing, medical, or surgical intervention. To touch a person without consent (except in an emergency) constitutes battery. Consent is not informed unless the woman understands the recommended procedures or treatments, their rationales, the benefits of each, and any associated risks. When possible, it is important to have translators available for non–English-speaking women.

The person, usually the physician, who is ultimately responsible for the treatment or procedure should provide the information necessary to obtain informed consent. In such cases, the nurse's role is to witness the client's signature giving consent. If the nurse determines that the client does not understand the procedure or risks, the nurse must notify the physician, who must then provide additional information to ensure that the consent is informed. Anxiety, fear, pain, and medications that alter consciousness may influence an individual's ability to give informed consent. An oral consent is legal, but written consent is easier to defend in a court of law.

Society grants parents the responsibility and authority to give consent for their minor children (generally under age 18). Special problems can occur in maternal-newborn nursing when a minor gives birth. It is possible that, depending on state law, the very young mother may consent to treatment for her newborn but not for herself. In most states, however, a pregnant teenager is considered an emancipated minor and may therefore give consent for herself as well.

Refusal of a treatment, medication, or procedure after appropriate information is provided also requires that a client sign a form releasing the doctor and clinical facility from liability resulting from the effects of such a refusal. The refusal of blood transfusions or Rh immune globulin by Jehovah's Witnesses is an example of such refusal.

Nurses are responsible for educating clients about any nursing care provided. Before each nursing intervention, the maternal-newborn nurse lets the woman know what to expect, thus ensuring her cooperation and obtaining her consent. Afterward, the nurse documents the teaching and the learning outcomes in the woman's healthcare record. The importance of clear, concise, and complete nursing records cannot be overemphasized. These records are evidence that the nurse obtained consent, performed prescribed treatments, reported important observations to the appropriate staff, and adhered to acceptable standards of care.

RIGHT TO PRIVACY

The *right to privacy* is the right of a person to keep her or his person and property free from public scrutiny. To protect a client, only those responsible for her care should examine her or discuss her case.

Most states have recognized the right to privacy through statutory or common law, and some states have written that right into their constitutions. The ANA, the National League for Nursing (NLN), and The Joint Commission have adopted professional standards protecting clients' privacy. Healthcare agencies should also have written policies dealing with client privacy. The Health Insurance Portability and Accountability Act (HIPAA) of 1996, which was fully implemented in 2002, has a provision that guarantees the security and privacy of health information.

Laws, standards, and policies about privacy specify that information about an individual's treatment, condition, and prognosis can be shared only by health professionals responsible for that person's care. Information considered as vital statistics (name, age, occupation, and so on) may be revealed legally but is often withheld because of ethical considerations. The client should be consulted regarding what information may be released and to whom.

Special Ethical Issues in Maternity Care

Although ethical dilemmas confront nurses in all areas of practice, those related to pregnancy, birth, and the newborn seem especially difficult to resolve.

Maternal-Fetal Conflict

Until fairly recently, the fetus was viewed legally as a nonperson. Mother and fetus were viewed as one complex client—the pregnant woman—of which the fetus was an essential part. However, advances in technology have permitted the physician to treat the fetus and monitor fetal development. The fetus is increasingly viewed as a client separate from the mother. This focus on the fetus intensified in 2002 when President George W. Bush announced that "unborn children" would qualify for government healthcare benefits. This move was designed to promote prenatal care but it represented the first time that any U.S. federal policy had defined childhood as starting at conception.

Most women are strongly motivated to protect the health and well-being of their fetus. In some instances, however, women have refused interventions on behalf of the fetus, and forced interventions have occurred. These include forced cesarean birth; coercion of mothers who practice high-risk behaviors such as substance abuse to enter treatment; and, perhaps most controversial, mandating experimental in utero therapy or surgery in an attempt to correct a specific birth defect. These interventions infringe on the mother's autonomy. They may also be detrimental to the baby if, as a result, maternal bonding is hindered, the mother is afraid to seek prenatal care, or the mother is herself harmed by the actions taken.

Attempts have also been made to criminalize the behavior of women who fail to follow a physician's advice or who engage in behaviors (such as substance abuse) that are considered harmful to the fetus. This raises two thorny questions:

1. What practices should be monitored?
2. Who will determine when the behaviors pose such a risk to the fetus that the courts should intervene?

The American College of Obstetricians and Gynecologists (ACOG) (2005) has affirmed the fundamental right of pregnant women to make informed, uncoerced decisions about medical interventions and has taken a direct stand against coercive and punitive approaches to the maternal-fetal relationship.

Both ACOG and the American Academy of Pediatrics (AAP) recognize that cases of maternal-fetal conflict involve two clients, both of whom deserve respect and treatment. Such cases are best resolved using internal hospital mechanisms including counseling, the intervention of specialists, and consultation with an institutional ethics committee. Court intervention should be considered a last resort, appropriate only in extraordinary circumstances.

Abortion

Since the 1973 *Roe v. Wade* Supreme Court decision, abortion has been legal in the United States. Abortion can be performed until the *period of viability*, that is, the point at which the fetus can survive independently of the mother. After that time, abortion is permissible only when the life or health of the mother is threatened. Before viability, the rights of the mother are paramount; after viability, the rights of the fetus take precedence.

Personal beliefs, cultural norms, life experiences, and religious convictions shape people's attitudes about abortion. Ethicists have thoughtfully and thoroughly argued positions supporting both sides of the question. However, few issues spark the intensity of response seen when the issue of abortion is raised.

At present the decision about abortion is to be made by the woman and her physician. Nurses (and other caregivers) have the right to refuse to assist with the procedure if abortion is contrary to their moral and ethical beliefs. However, if a nurse works in an institution where abortions may be performed, the nurse can be dismissed for refusing to assist. To avoid being placed in a situation contrary to their ethical values and beliefs, nurses should determine the philosophy and practices of an institution before going to work there. A nurse who refuses to participate in an abortion because of moral or ethical beliefs has a responsibility to ensure that someone with similar qualifications is available to provide appropriate care for the woman. Clients must never be abandoned, regardless of a nurse's beliefs.

Intrauterine Fetal Surgery

Intrauterine fetal surgery, generally considered experimental, is a therapy for certain anatomic lesions that can be corrected surgically and are incompatible with life if not treated. The procedure involves opening the uterus during the second trimester (before viability), performing the planned surgery, and replacing the fetus in the uterus. The risks to the fetus are substantial, and the mother is committed to cesarean births for this and subsequent pregnancies (because the upper, active segment of the uterus is entered). The parents must be informed of the experimental nature of the treatment, the risks of the surgery, the commitment to cesarean birth, and alternatives to the treatment.

As in other aspects of maternity care, caregivers must respect the pregnant woman's autonomy. The procedure involves health risks to the woman, and she retains the right to refuse any surgical procedure. Healthcare providers must be careful that their zeal for new technology does not lead them to focus unilaterally on the fetus at the expense of the mother.

Reproductive Assistance

Assisted reproductive technology (ART) is the term used to describe highly technologic approaches used to produce pregnancy. *In vitro fertilization and embryo transfer (IVF-ET)*, a therapy offered to selected infertile couples, is perhaps the best-known ART technique.

Multifetal pregnancy may occur with ART because the use of ovulation-inducing medications typically triggers the release of multiple eggs. When fertilized, they produce multiple embryos, which are then implanted. Multifetal pregnancy increases the risk of miscarriage, preterm birth, and neonatal morbidity and mortality. It also increases the mother's risk of complications, including cesarean birth. To help prevent a high-order multifetal pregnancy (presence of three or more fetuses), the American Society for Reproductive Medicine (ASRM) and the Society for Assisted Reproductive Technology have issued guidelines to limit the number of embryos transferred. These guidelines are designed to decrease risk while also allowing for individualized care (ASRM & Society for Assisted Reproductive Technology, 2013).

This practice raises ethical considerations about the handling of the unused embryos. When a multifetal pregnancy does occur, the physician may suggest that the woman consider fetal reduction, in which some fetuses are aborted to give the remaining ones a better chance for survival. This procedure raises ethical concerns about the sacrifice of some so that the remainder can survive.

Prevention should be the first approach to the problem of multifetal pregnancy. Prevention begins with careful counseling about the risks of multiple gestation and the ethical issues that relate to fetal reduction. No physician who is morally opposed to fetal reduction should be expected to perform the procedure; however, physicians should be aware of the ethical and medical issues involved and be prepared to respond to families in a professional and ethical manner (ACOG, 2013).

Surrogate childbearing is another approach to infertility. Surrogate childbearing occurs when a woman agrees to become pregnant for a childless couple. She may be artificially inseminated with the male partner's sperm or a donor's sperm or may receive a gamete transfer, depending on the infertile couple's needs. If fertilization occurs, the woman carries the fetus to term and releases the baby to the couple after birth.

These methods of resolving infertility raise ethical issues about candidate selection, responsibility for a child born with a congenital defect, and religious objections to artificial conception. Other ethical questions include the following:

- What should be done with surplus fertilized oocytes?
- To whom do frozen embryos belong?
- Who is liable if a woman or her offspring contracts HIV from donated sperm?
- Should children be told about their conception?

Embryonic Stem Cell Research

Human stem cells can be found in embryonic tissue and in the primordial germ cells of a fetus. Research has demonstrated that in tissue cultures these cells can be made to differentiate into other types of cells such as blood, nerve, or heart cells, which might then be used to treat problems such as diabetes, Parkinson and Alzheimer diseases, spinal cord injury, or metabolic disorders. The availability of specialized tissue or even organs grown from stem cells might also decrease society's dependence on donated organs for organ transplants.

Positions about embryonic stem cell research vary dramatically, from the view that any use of human embryos for research is wrong to the view that any form of embryonic stem cell research is acceptable, with a variety of other positions that fall somewhere in between these extremes. Other questions also arise: What sources of embryonic tissue are acceptable for research? Is it ever ethical to clone embryos solely for stem cell research? Is there justification for using embryos remaining after fertility treatments?

The question of how an embryo should be viewed—with the status in some way of a person or in some sense of property (and, if property, whose?)—is a key question in the debate. Ethicists recognize that it is not necessary to advocate full moral status or personhood for an embryo to have significant moral qualms about the instrumental use of a human embryo in the "interests" of society. The issue of consent, which links directly to an embryo's status, also merits consideration. In truth, the ethical questions and dilemmas associated with embryonic stem cell research are staggeringly complex and require careful analysis and thoughtful dialogue.

Evidence-Based Practice in Maternal-Newborn Nursing

Evidence-based practice—that is, nursing care in which all interventions are supported by current, valid research evidence—is emerging as a force in health care. It provides a useful approach to problem solving and decision making and to self-directed, client-centered, lifelong learning. Evidence-based practice builds on the actions necessary to transform research findings into clinical practice by also considering other forms of evidence that can be useful in making clinical practice decisions. These other forms of evidence may include statistical data, quality measurements, risk management measures, and information from support services such as infection control.

As clinicians, nurses need to meet three basic competencies related to evidence-based practice:

1. To recognize which clinical practices are supported by sound evidence, which practices have conflicting findings as to their effect on client outcomes, and which practices have no evidence to support their use

2. To use data in their clinical work to evaluate outcomes of care

3. To appraise and integrate scientific bases into practice.

Nurses need to know what data are being tracked in their workplaces and how care practices and outcomes are improved as a result of quality improvement initiatives. However, there is more to evidence-based practice than simply knowing what is being tracked and how the results are being used. Competent, effective nurses learn to question the very basis of their clinical work.

We have provided *snapshots* of evidence-based practice related to childbearing women and families in the *Evidence-Based Practice* feature throughout this text. We believe that these snapshots will help you understand the concept more clearly. We also expect that these examples may challenge you to question the usefulness of some of the routine care you observe in clinical practice. That is the impact of evidence-based practice—it moves clinicians beyond practices of habit and opinion to practices based on high-quality, current science.

Nursing Research

Research is vital to expanding the science of nursing, fostering evidence-based practice, and improving client care. Research also plays an important role in advancing the profession of nursing. For example, nursing research can help determine the psychosocial and physical risks and benefits of both nursing and medical interventions.

The gap between research and practice is being narrowed by the publication of research findings in popular nursing journals, the establishment of departments of nursing research in hospitals, and collaborative research efforts by nurse researchers and clinical practitioners. Interdisciplinary research between nurses and other healthcare professionals is also becoming more common. This ever-increasing recognition of the value of nursing research is important because well-done research supports the goals of evidence-based practice.

Nursing Care Plans

Nursing care plans, which use the nursing process as an organizing framework, are invaluable in planning and organizing care. Care plans are especially useful for nursing students and novice nurses. To help organize care, this text provides several examples of nursing care plans.

Clinical Reasoning

It can be challenging to use evidence, analyze information, and make sound decisions that result in safe, effective patient care.

Scenarios provide a realistic way of enabling students to apply concepts. The *Clinical Reasoning* feature found throughout the chapters and the *Clinical Reasoning in Action* feature at the end of every chapter in this text presents a patient scenario and asks clinical reasoning questions to help students formulate how they would handle the issues raised and how they would apply concepts they have learned in the chapter.

Statistical Data and Maternal-Infant Care

Increasingly nurses are recognizing the value and usefulness of statistics. Health-related statistics provide an objective basis for projecting client needs, planning the use of resources, and determining the effectiveness of specific treatments.

The two major types of statistics are descriptive and inferential. *Descriptive statistics* describe or summarize a set of data. They report the facts—what is—in a concise and easily retrievable way. An example of a descriptive statistic is the birth rate in the United States. Although these statistics support no conclusions about why some phenomenon has occurred, they identify certain trends and high-risk target groups and generate possible research questions. *Inferential statistics* allow the investigator to draw conclusions or inferences about what is happening between two or more variables in a population and to suggest or refute causal relationships between them.

Descriptive statistics are the starting point for the formation of research questions. Inferential statistics answer specific questions and generate theories to explain relationships between variables. Theory applied in nursing practice can help to change the specific variables that may be causing or at least contributing to certain health problems.

The following sections discuss descriptive statistics that are particularly important to maternal-newborn health care. Inferential considerations are addressed as possible research questions that may assist in identifying relevant variables.

Birth Rate

Birth rate refers to the number of live births per 1000 people. In the United States, the birth rate in 2013 was 12.4. Birth rates decreased for women in their twenties, increased slightly for women in their thirties and women in their fifties, and remained unchanged for women in their forties. The birth rate for teens 15 to 19 years of age was 26.5 births per 1000 teenagers, a record low for the country. Overall rates declined slightly for White, Hispanic, and Asian/Pacific Islander women and remained unchanged for non-Hispanic Black women and American Indian/Alaskan Native women. The birth rate for unmarried women declined for the fifth consecutive year to 44.3 per 1000 as compared to the peak rate of 51.8 in 2007 and 2008 (Martin et al., 2015).

In 2013 the cesarean birth rate decreased slightly to 32.7% of all U.S. births, down from 32.8% in 2010–2012 (Martin et al., 2015).

Table 1–1 identifies infant mortality rates for selected countries based on 2014 estimates. As the data indicate, the range is dramatic among the countries listed. Information about birth

TABLE 1–1 Live Birth Rates and Infant Mortality Rates for Selected Countries

COUNTRY	BIRTH RATE	INFANT MORTALITY RATER
Afghanistan	38.8	117.2
Argentina	16.9	10.0
Australia	12.2	4.4
Cambodia	24.4	51.4
Canada	10.3	4.7
China	12.2	14.8
Egypt	23.4	22.4
France	12.5	3.3
Germany	8.4	3.5
Ghana	31.4	38.5
India	19.9	43.2
Iraq	26.9	37.5
Japan	8.1	2.1
Mexico	19.0	12.6
Russia	11.9	7.1
Sweden	11.9	2.6
United Kingdom	12.2	4.4
United States	12.6*	6.0**

*Source: Martin et al. (2015).
**Source: Kochanek, Murphy, Xu, et al. (2014).
Source: Data from The World Fact Book 2014. Washington, DC: The Central Intelligence Agency. Retrieved from https://www.cia.gov/library/publications/the-world-factbook/geos/uk.html.

rates and mortality rates is limited for some countries because of a lack of organized reporting mechanisms.

Research questions that can be posed about birth rates include the following:

- Is there an association between birth rates and changing social values?
- Do the differences in birth rates among various countries reflect cultural differences, availability of contraceptive information, or other factors?

Infant Mortality

The **infant mortality rate** is the number of deaths of infants under 1 year of age per 1000 live births in a given population. *Neonatal mortality* is the number of deaths of newborns less than 28 days of age per 1000 live births, *perinatal mortality* includes both neonatal deaths and fetal deaths per 1000 live births, and *fetal death* is death in utero at 20 weeks or more gestation.

In 2013, the infant mortality rate in the United States was 6.0 per 1000 live births. The three leading causes of infant deaths were congenital malformations, low birth weight, and maternal complications (Kochanek, Murphy, Xu, et al., 2014).

The U.S. infant mortality rate continues to be of concern because the United States' rate is higher than that of most European countries as well as Australia, New Zealand, Japan, Korea, and Israel. Much of the infant mortality rate can be attributed to the high percentage of preterm births in the United States (MacDorman, Mathews, Mohangoo, et al., 2014). Healthcare professionals, policy makers, and the public continue to stress the need for better prenatal care, coordination of health services, and provision of comprehensive maternal-child services in the United States.

The data in Table 1–1 raise questions about access to health care during pregnancy and after birth and about standards of living, nutrition, and sociocultural factors. Additional factors affecting the infant mortality rate may be identified by considering the following research questions:

- What are the leading causes of infant mortality in each country?
- Why do mortality rates differ among racial groups?

Maternal Mortality

Maternal mortality rate is the number of deaths from any cause related to or aggravated by pregnancy or pregnancy management during the pregnancy cycle (including the 42-day postpartum period) per 100,000 live births. It does not include deaths of pregnant women because of external causes such as accidents, homicides, and suicides. Since 1986, the Centers for Disease Control and Prevention (CDC) has tracked pregnancy-related deaths. A **pregnancy-related death** is defined as the death of a woman while pregnant or within 1 year of the termination of pregnancy (regardless of the length of the pregnancy or the site of implantation) from any cause aggravated by pregnancy or related to it (Centers for Disease Control and Prevention [CDC], 2014).

Healthy People 2020

(MICH-5) Reduce the rate of maternal mortality

The pregnancy-related mortality rate in the United States in 2009 and 2011 was 17.8 deaths per 100,000 live births. This number has increased steadily from 7.2 per 100,000 live births in 1987. Black women have a significantly higher risk of maternal death than white women: 42.8 deaths per 100,000 live births as compared to 12.5 deaths for white women, and 17.3 deaths for women of other races (CDC, 2014). This apparent increase in maternal deaths may be due to improved identification of pregnancy-related causes or to changes in the way maternal deaths are coded. Some research suggests that an increasing number of women in the United States with chronic health conditions such as hypertension, diabetes, and chronic heart disease are becoming pregnant (CDC, 2014).

Additional factors may be identified by asking the following research questions:

- Is there a correlation between maternal mortality and age?
- Is there a correlation between maternal mortality and availability of health care?
- Is there a correlation between maternal mortality and economic status?

Implications for Nursing Practice

Nurses can use statistics in a number of ways. For example, they can use statistical data to:

- Determine populations at risk
- Assess the relationship between specific factors
- Help establish databases for specific client populations
- Determine the levels of care needed by particular client populations
- Evaluate the success of specific nursing interventions
- Determine priorities in caseloads
- Estimate staffing and equipment needs of hospital units and clinics

Statistical information is available through many sources, including professional literature; state and city health departments; vital statistics sections of private, county, state, and federal agencies; special programs or agencies (such as family planning); demographic profiles of specific geographic areas; and the internet.

Nurses who use this information are better prepared to promote the health needs of maternal-newborn clients and their families.

Focus Your Study

- Contemporary childbirth is family centered, recognizing the needs and roles of the woman and her partner, siblings, grandparents, and other family members.

- Community-based care is especially important in maternal-child nursing because the vast majority of care provided to childbearing women and their families takes place outside of hospitals in clinics, offices, community-based organizations, and private homes.

- The Affordable Care Act ends pre-existing condition exclusions for children and adults, eliminates annual limits on insurance coverage, and keeps young adults covered for a longer period.

- The nurse who provides culturally competent care recognizes the importance of the childbearing family's value system, acknowledges that differences occur among people, and seeks to respect and respond to ethnic diversity in a way that leads to mutually desirable outcomes.

- Interest in complementary health approaches continues to grow nationwide and affects the care of childbearing families.

- A nurse must perform within the scope of practice or be subject to the accusation of practicing medicine without a license. The standard of care of individual nursing practice is based on a comparison with the care provided by a reasonably prudent nurse.

- Nursing standards provide information and guidelines for nurses in their own practice, in developing policies and protocols in healthcare settings, and in directing the development of quality nursing care.

- Informed consent—based on knowledge of a procedure and its benefits, risks, and alternatives—must be secured before providing treatment.

- Maternal-fetal conflict may arise when the fetus is viewed as a person with equal rights to those of the mother's and external agents attempt to restrict a mother's actions to support the well-being of the fetus.

- Abortion can legally be performed until the fetus reaches the age of viability. The decision to have an abortion is made by a woman in consultation with her physician.

- A variety of procedures are available to help infertile couples achieve a pregnancy. However, some of these procedures provoke serious ethical dilemmas.

- Evidence-based practice refers to clinical practice based on research findings and other available data. It increases nurses' accountability and results in better client outcomes.

- Nursing research plays a vital role in adding to the nursing knowledge base, expanding clinical practice, and further developing nursing theory.

- Descriptive statistics describe a set of data. Inferential statistics allow the investigator to draw conclusions about what is happening between two or more variables in a population.

Clinical Reasoning in Action

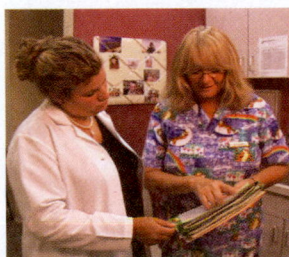

You are working as a prenatal nurse in a local clinic. Before entering a client's room, you review her medical record for pertinent information such as cultural background, significant family members, weeks of gestation, test results, birth plan, and her education for health promotion. You greet the client and her family members by name and ask how they are coping with the pregnancy. Depending on the trimester of the pregnancy, you review the discomforts or concerns of the mother/family and what they may expect. You examine the mother, including fundal height, fetal heart rate and fetal position if appropriate, maternal blood pressure, weight gain, and urine analysis. With each client, you discuss the community resources available such as prenatal classes, lactation consultants, and prenatal exercise/yoga classes. Based upon the information you obtain, you might refer the mother to social services or the WIC program as appropriate. At the end of the clinic session, you review the clients with the collaborating physician.

1. How would you define the terms *family* and *family-centered care*?

2. Describe how the nursing process provides the framework for the delivery of direct nursing care.

3. How would you describe the concept of community-based care?

4. How would you describe culturally competent care?

References

American College of Nurse-Midwives (ACNM). (2014). *Essential facts about midwives.* Retrieved from http://www.midwife.org/Essential-Facts-about-Midwives

American College of Obstetricians and Gynecologists (ACOG). (2005). *Maternal decision making, ethics, and the law* (Committee Opinion No. 321). Washington, DC: Author.

American College of Obstetricians and Gynecologists (ACOG). (2013). *Multifetal pregnancy reduction* (Committee Opinion No. 553). Washington, DC: Author.

American Society for Reproductive Medicine and the Society for Assisted Reproductive Technology. (2013). Criteria for number of embryos to transfer: a committee opinion. *Fertility and Sterility, 99,* 44–46.

Centers for Disease Control and Prevention (CDC). (2014). *Pregnancy mortality surveillance system.* Retrieved from http://www.cdc.gov/reproductivehealth/maternalinfanthealth/pmss.html

Federal Interagency Forum on Child and Family Statistics. (2013). *America's children: Key national indicators of well-being, 2013.* Retrieved from http://childstats.gov/americaschildren/index.asp

Kochanek, K. D., Murphy, S. L., Xu, J., & Arias, E. (2014). Mortality in the United States, 2013. *NCHS Data Brief,* No. 178. Retrieved from http://www.cdc.gov/nchs/data/databriefs/db178.pdf.

MacDorman, M. F., Mathews, T. J., Mohangoo, A. D., & Zeitlin, J. (2014). International comparisons of infant mortality and related factors: United States and Europe, 2010. *National Vital Statistics Reports, 63*(5), 1–7.

Martin, J. A., Hamilton, B. E., Osterman, M. J. K., Curtin, S. C., & Mathews, T. J. (2015). Births: Final data for 2013. *National Vital Statistics Reports, 64*(1), 1–68.

National Center for Health Statistics (NCHS). (2014). *Health, United States, 2013: With special feature on prescription drugs.* Hyattsville, MD: Author.

North American Registry of Midwives (NARM). (2014). *Equivalency applicants: Important: Updates to CPM eligibility requirements.* Retrieved from http://narm.org/equivalency-applicants/

Quality and Safety Education for Nurses (QSEN). (2011). *About QSEN.* Retrieved from http://www.qsen.org/about_qsen.php

Spector, R. E. (2013). *Cultural diversity in health and illness* (8th ed.). Upper Saddle River, NJ: Prentice Hall Health.

U.S. Department of Health and Human Services. (2014). *Child Health USA 2014.* Rockville, MD: Author.

U.S. Department of Health and Human Services. (2015). Key features of the Affordable Care Act by year. Retrieved from http://www.hhs.gov/healthcare/facts/timeline/timeline-text.html

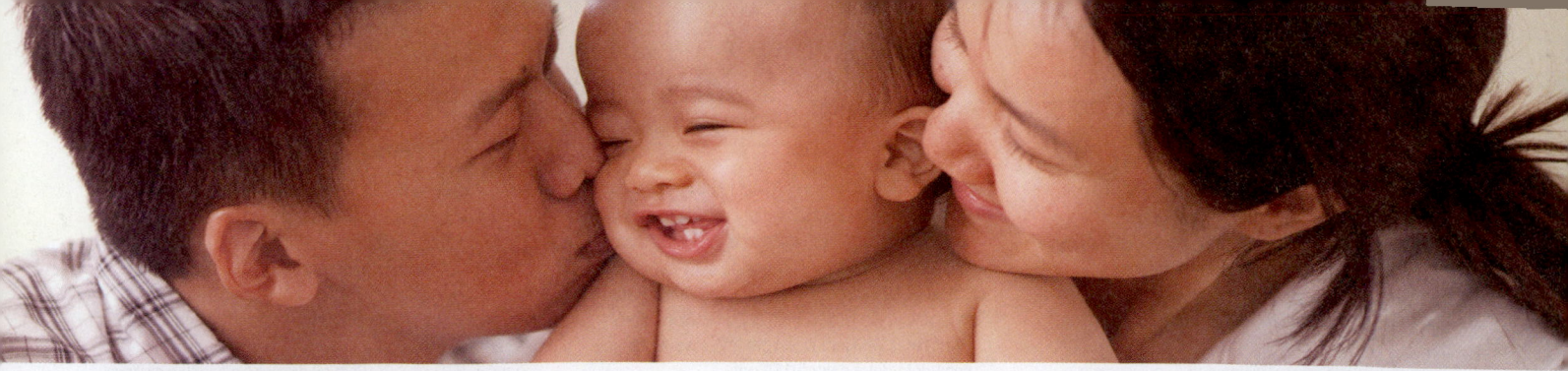

Chapter 2
Family, Culture, and Complementary Health Approaches

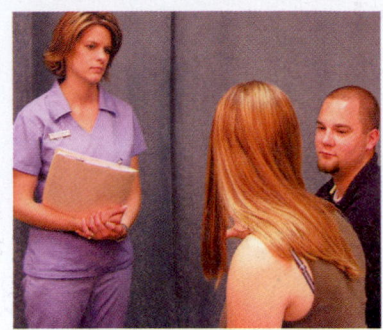

When I first began working at this prenatal clinic I was not very tuned in to the nuances of families. Now I am much better at picking up cues about a family's functioning—who makes decisions, who controls the finances, how power is distributed. I have also come to realize that, unless the family trusts me, they tell me only what they think I need to know. It's not that they mean to be devious, but they may not tell me about the complementary therapies they use or the cultural practices that are important to them if they think I will be judgmental. As I have become more open and accepting, I have become a far better nurse.

—A Nurse Working in a Prenatal Clinic

⌄ Learning Outcomes

2.1 Describe how family type may influence nursing care of the childbearing family.

2.2 Explain the changes that a childbearing family will undergo based on the developmental tasks to be completed.

2.3 Identify information that would be useful to collect when performing a family assessment.

2.4 Integrate the prevalent cultural norms that affect childbearing and childrearing when providing care to that family.

2.5 Explain the importance of cultural competency in providing nursing care to the childbearing family.

2.6 Interpret the information collected from a cultural assessment to provide culturally sensitive care.

2.7 Identify ways a nurse might accommodate the religious rituals and practices of the childbearing family.

2.8 Distinguish among complementary and alternative therapies.

2.9 Describe the benefits and risks of the various complementary and alternative therapies to the childbearing family.

2.10 Formulate nursing care within the nurse practice act and with the informed consent of the client when using appropriate complementary health approaches with childbearing families.

Individuals do not live in isolation. Their values, beliefs, behaviors, decisions, attitudes, and biases are shaped by many factors including their families, their culture, and their religious beliefs. Nurses who provide effective, holistic care recognize this reality and seek to learn about and care for the entire childbearing family.

This chapter begins with a discussion of family types, functioning, and assessment. It then addresses the impact of culture on the childbearing family, and concludes with a brief examination of the complementary health approaches a family might use.

The Family

The U.S. Census Bureau (2013) defines a **family** as individuals who are joined together by marriage, blood, adoption, or residence in the same household. More broadly, however, families are generally characterized by bonds of emotional closeness, sharing, and support. Many practitioners and professionals are moving away from traditional definitions and instead identify as family members those individuals whom the client wants to be included in the family unit. Family is now commonly defined as members of an individual's identified group, both related and unrelated, who comprise the individual's social network, often assisting with family duties, such as childrearing.

Within families, members are guided by a common set of values that bind them together. These family values are greatly influenced by external factors including cultural background, social norms, education, environmental influences, socioeconomic status, and beliefs held by peers, coworkers, political and community leaders, and other individuals outside the family unit. Because of the influence of these external factors, a family's values may change considerably over the years.

Types of Families

Various types of families exist in contemporary American society. The following list identifies common types of family structures:

- The *nuclear family* consists of a husband-provider, a wife who stays home, and children. Although the nuclear family was once the norm in the United States, it is no longer the most common type of family.

- In the *dual-career/dual-earner family*, both parents work, either by choice or by necessity. Today, two thirds of all two-parent families are this type. Dual-career families have to address issues related to child care, household chores, and spending time together.

- The *child-free family* is a growing trend. In some cases a family is child free by choice; in other cases, a family is child free because of issues related to infertility.

- In an *extended family*, a couple shares household and childrearing responsibilities with parents, siblings, or other relatives. Multigenerational arrangements of this sort are more common in non–U.S. cultures and in working-class families.

- An *extended kin network family* is a specific form of extended family in which two nuclear families of primary or unmarried kin live near each other. The family shares a social support network, chores, goods, and services. This type of family model is common in the Latino community.

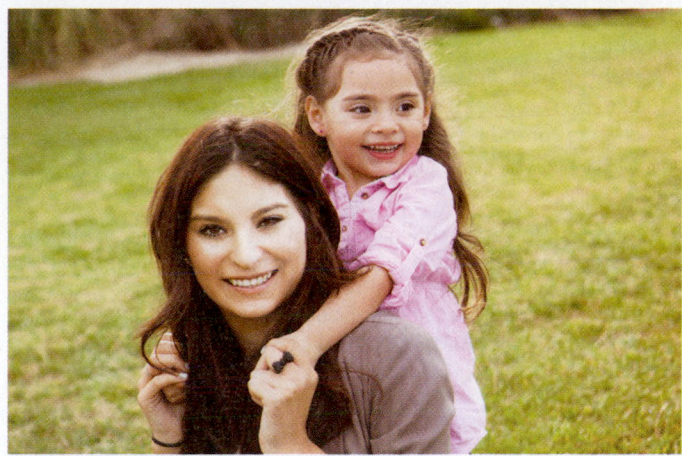

Figure 2–1 **Single-parent families account for nearly one third of all U.S. families.**

SOURCE: © Phase4Photography/Fotolia.

- The *single-parent family* is becoming increasingly common. In some cases, the head of the household is widowed, divorced, abandoned, or separated. In other cases, the head of the household, most often the mother, was never married. Single-parent families often face difficulties because the sole parent may lack social and emotional support, need assistance with childrearing issues, and face financial strain (Figure 2–1).

- A *stepfamily* consists of a biologic parent with children and a new spouse who may or may not have children. This family structure has become increasingly common because of high rates of divorce and remarriage. These families are also known as *remarried*, *reconstituted*, or *blended families*. Stepfamily models have both strengths and challenges. Stepfamilies may have fewer financial issues and may offer a child a new support person and role model. Remarriage also provides a new opportunity for a successful relationship for the parents; however, the relationship between stepparents and stepchildren can be strained. Stresses can include discipline issues, adjustment problems, role ambiguity, strain with the other biologic parent, and communication issues.

- A *binuclear family* is a post-divorce family in which the biologic children are members of two nuclear households, both that of the father and that of the mother. The children alternate between the two homes. This is also called coparenting and involves joint custody. In joint custody, both parents have equal responsibility and legal rights, regardless of where the children live. The binuclear family model enables both parents to be involved in a child's upbringing and provides additional support and role models from extended family members. However, it often requires negotiation and compromise between the parents about childrearing decisions.

- A *nonmarital heterosexual cohabitating family* describes a heterosexual couple who may or may not have children and who live together outside of marriage. This may include never-married individuals as well as divorced or widowed persons. Although some individuals choose this model for personal reasons, others do so for financial reasons. *Gay and lesbian families* include those in which two or more people who share a same-sex orientation live together (with or without children), those who are legally married, and those in which a gay or lesbian single parent rears a child. In 2015, the Supreme Court of the United States ruled that marriage was a constitutional right, which allowed same sex couples to marry. The ruling is expected to expand the number of reported families and change common perceptions on marriage (Petrow, 2015).

Clinical Tip

It is important to establish which parent has legal custody, current visitation policies, and other variables (restraining orders, supervised visitation, etc.) when communicating information to parents about their children. Certain legal issues may prohibit the nurse from sharing some information with the noncustodial parent.

Family Development Frameworks

Family development refers to the dynamics or changes that a family experiences over time, including changes in relationships, communication patterns, roles, and interactions. Although each family is unique, the members go through a set of fairly predictable changes. For example, Duvall (1977) developed an eight-stage family life cycle that describes the developmental process that each family encounters. This model is based on the nuclear family (Table 2–1). The oldest child serves as a marker for the family's developmental stages except in the last two stages, when children are no longer present. Couples with more than one child may find themselves in overlapping stages with developmental advances occurring simultaneously.

Other family development models have been developed to address the stages and developmental tasks facing the unattached young adult, the gay and lesbian family, those who divorce, and those who remarry. For further information on this topic, readers are referred to textbooks on families and on developmental psychology.

Family Assessment

The nurse's understanding of a family's structure helps provide insight into the family's support system and needs. A *family assessment* is a collection of data about the family's type and structure, current level of functioning, support system, sociocultural background, environment, and needs.

To obtain an accurate and concise family assessment, the nurse needs to establish a trusting relationship with the woman and her family. Data are best collected in a comfortable, private environment, free from interruptions.

Basic information should include the following:

- Name, age, sex, and family relationship of all people residing in the household
- Family type, structure, roles, and values
- Cultural associations, including cultural norms and customs related to childbearing, childrearing, and newborn/infant feeding (This might include expected activities, forbidden activities, the role of the father, the role of the maternal grandmother, and the like.)
- Religious affiliations, including specific religious beliefs and practices related to childbearing
- Support network, including extended family, friends, and religious and community associations
- Communication patterns, including verbal and written language barriers.

In addition, the nurse gathers information about the health of individual family members and the home environment. In many cases this information is gathered during client interviews. However, a home visit provides far more data about family relationships, roles, needs, and preparation for a new baby.

Cultural Influences Affecting the Family

When caring for families it is critical to consider the influence of culture, which may affect how a family responds to health-related issues. **Culture** can be defined as the beliefs, values, attitudes, and practices that are accepted by a population, a community, or an individual. Culture is learned and not ingrained in our genetic material, yet it can be passed on from

TABLE 2–1 The Eight-Stage Family Life Cycle

Stage I	Beginning families	Marriage between partners, identification as partners, establishing goals for future, interaction and building relationships with kin.
Stage II	Childbearing families	Birth of first child, new role as parents, integrating new family member into existing family.
Stage III	Families with preschool children	Establishing family network, socialization of children, reinforcing independence in children when separating from parents.
Stage IV	Families with school-age children	Facilitating peer relationships while maintaining family dynamics, adjusting to outside influences.
Stage V	Families with teenagers	Increase in children's independence and autonomy; parents' concerns shift to aging parents, careers, and marital relationship.
Stage VI	Families launching young adults	Readjustment of marital relationship; parents and children establish separate identities outside the family unit.
Stage VII	Middle-aged parents	Renewed marital relationship; new outside interests; fewer family responsibilities; new roles as grandparents and as in-laws; increased concern for aging parents, death, and disability of older generation.
Stage VIII	Retirement and old age	End of career; shift to retirement; maintain functioning during the aging process; maintain marital relationship; adjust to potential loss of spouse, friends, and siblings; prepare for eventual death.

Source: Adapted from Duvall, E. M. (1977). Marriage and family development (5th ed.). Philadelphia, PA: Lippincott; Duvall, E. M., & Miller, B. C. (1985). Marriage and family development (6th ed.). New York, NY: Harper Row; Coehlo, D. P. (2015). Family child health nursing. In J. R. Kaakinen, D. P. Coehlo, R. Steele, A. Tabacco, & S. M. H. Hanson, Family health care nursing: Theory, practice, and research (5th ed., pp. 387–432). Philadelphia, PA: F. A. Davis.

generation to generation by means of *enculturation*. When a group is isolated, either geographically or economically, culture is often reinforced.

Ethnicity is a social identity that is associated with shared behaviors and patterns. These include family structure, religious affiliation, language, dress, eating habits, and health behaviors. Many Americans define ethnicity by physical characteristics such as skin color. However, many people consider themselves to be biracial or identify themselves with a specific group not because of skin color but because of a shared ideology or attitudes. More and more, individuals are blends of ethnic and racial backgrounds and it is often difficult to assign a specific ethnic or racial identity to someone. Although some beliefs and practices are common among certain ethnic or racial groups, one must be careful to avoid stereotyping individuals. It is important not to assume that because individuals identify themselves as a specific ethnicity or race they must practice certain customs.

Acculturation is the process by which people adapt to a new cultural norm. When a group completely changes its cultural identity to become part of the majority culture, *assimilation* occurs.

Acculturation frequently occurs when people leave their country of origin and immigrate to a new country. It is often associated with improved health status and health behaviors, especially if the immigration is associated with improved socioeconomic status, which leads to better nutrition and access to health care. This is frequently true, for example, for people who emigrate from a developing country. Some negative health behaviors may occur such as obesity. Problems may also occur if a person emigrates from a country with universal health care to a country in which he or she is not eligible for health care or cannot afford it.

Developing Cultural Competence   Culture Shock

The experience that people have in attempting to understand or adapt to a culture that is fundamentally different from their own culture is known as *culture shock*, which can be associated with feelings of discomfort, powerlessness, anxiety, and disorientation. Immigrants may experience culture shock when differences or conflicts arise between their own values, beliefs, and customs and the ways of their new surroundings (Spector, 2013). The nurse should assess childbearing women and their families who have recently immigrated for indications of culture shock. Referring the family to counseling or support from representatives of the family's culture, such as a translator or community group, may be helpful.

Cultural Influences on Childbearing and Childrearing

A family's culture may influence its beliefs about and practices surrounding many aspects of childbearing and childrearing.

BELIEFS AND ATTITUDES ABOUT PREGNANCY

Children are generally valued all over the world, not only for the joy they bring but also because they ensure continuation of the family and cultural values. This valuing of children may manifest itself in different ways, however. Families in the United States and many Western countries commonly have only one or two children out of a desire to provide the children with the best home and education they can afford and to spend as much free time with them as possible. In contrast, in many cultures throughout the world, it is common to have as many children as possible.

In some cultures, a woman who gives birth achieves a higher status, especially if the child is male. This is especially true in the traditional Chinese culture and in some Middle Eastern cultures. Similarly, in the United States individuals of the Mormon faith view motherhood as the most important aspect of a woman's life, comparable with the male role of priest (Chen, 2014). In Latino groups, having children is evidence of the male's virility and is a sign of manliness or *machismo*, a desired trait.

Culture may also influence attitudes and beliefs about contraception. For example, many Muslims from the Middle East may use birth control but do not believe in sterilization because it is a permanent method (Javed, 2015). Other Muslims might not practice contraception because children are highly valued and it is believed that the traditional role of women is to bear children. In Chinese society, in contrast, where state policy limits the number of children a couple can have, contraception is common.

Health values and beliefs are also important in understanding reactions and behavior. Certain behaviors can be expected if a culture views pregnancy as a sickness, whereas other behaviors can be expected if the culture views pregnancy as a natural occurrence. For example, because Native Americans, African Americans, and Mexican Americans generally view pregnancy as a natural and desirable condition, prenatal care may not be a priority. In other cultures, pregnancy may be seen as a time of increased vulnerability. In Orthodox Judaism, for example, it is a man's responsibility to procreate, but it is a woman's right, not her obligation, to do so. This is because, according to Orthodox Jewish law, the health of the mother, both physically and mentally, is of primary concern, and she should never be obliged to do something that threatens her life.

Individuals of many cultures take certain protective precautions based on their beliefs. For example, many Southeast Asian women fear that they will have a complicated labor and birth if they sit in a doorway or on a step. Thus they tend to avoid areas near doors in waiting rooms and examining rooms. In the Mexican American culture, the belief is common that *mal aire*, or bad air, may enter the body and cause harm. Preventive measures such as keeping the windows closed or covering the head are used. Some Latinos place a raisin on the cord stump of newborns to prevent drafts from entering their bodies. A **taboo** is a behavior or thing that is to be avoided. Many cultures, including those found in the United States, have taboos centered on the unborn baby and/or newborn that are meant to ensure that the baby will survive. For example, it is common among Muslims to avoid naming the baby until after birth; similarly, many Orthodox Jewish women wait to set up the nursery until after the baby is born.

In developing countries, mortality rates among newborns, infants, and young children are extremely high; thus, certain traditions focus on protecting the baby from evil spirits. For example, many Muslim parents will pin an amulet to the newborn's clothes as protection. The amulet may represent a palm, an eye, a blue stone, or a verse from the Quran. Following birth, it is common for a male family member to whisper prayers in the newborn baby's ear to declare faith and protect the baby (Walton, Akram, & Hossain, 2014).

The *equilibrium model of health* is based on the concept of balance between light and dark, heat and cold. Some Eastern philosophies focus on the notion of *yin* and *yang*. Yin represents the female, passive principle—darkness, cold, wetness; yang is the masculine, active principle—light, heat, and dryness. When the two are combined, they are all that can be. The hot–cold classification is seen in cultures in Latin America, the Near East, and Asia.

Some Mexican Americans may consider illness to be an excess of either hot or cold. To restore health, imbalances are often corrected by the proper use of foods, medications, or herbs. These substances are also classified as hot or cold. For example, an illness attributed to an excess of cold will be treated with only hot foods or medications (Purnell, 2014). The classification of foods is not always consistent, but it conforms to a general structure of traditional knowledge. Certain foods, spices, herbs, and medications are perceived to cool or heat the body. These perceptions do not necessarily correspond to the actual temperature; some hot dishes are said to have a cooling quality.

Southeast Asians believe it is important to keep the woman "warm" after birth, because blood, which is considered "hot," has been lost, and the woman is at risk of becoming "cold." Therefore, they avoid cold drinks and foods following birth. In contrast, many women in India consider pregnancy a "hot" period and eat "cool" foods to balance the hot state (Purnell, 2014).

The concepts of hot and cold are not as important in Native American or African American beliefs. Similarities exist in all of these groups, however, because of their emphasis on a balance in nature.

Clinical Tip

When offering your clients fluids, ask if they would prefer them hot, warm, or iced. This can help ensure both proper hydration and support of cultural beliefs.

HEALTH PRACTICES DURING PREGNANCY AND POSTPARTUM

Healthcare practices during pregnancy are influenced by numerous factors, such as the prevalence of traditional home remedies and folk beliefs, the importance of indigenous healers, and the influence of professional healthcare workers. In an urban setting, the age, length of time in the city, marital status, and strength of the family may affect these patterns. Socioeconomic status is also important, because modern medical services are more accessible to those who can afford them.

An awareness of alternative health sources is crucial for health professionals, because these practices affect health outcomes. For example, in the traditional Mexican American culture, mothers are often influenced by *familism*, a close-knit, interdependent network of nuclear and extended family members who are connected for the good of the family. Close intergenerational networks exist and young mothers often seek the advice of their mothers or older women about childbirth. In many cases, decisions about health care are made by the family.

Indigenous healers are also important to specific cultures. In the Mexican American culture, the healer is called a *curandero* or *curandera*, whereas the *partera* is a lay midwife who gives advice and treats illnesses during pregnancy and also attends labor and birth (Spector, 2013). In some Native American tribes, the medicine man or woman may fulfill the healing role. Herbalists are often found in Asian cultures, and faith healers, root doctors, and spiritualists are sometimes consulted by members of some African cultures.

Among many people there is a period of isolation postpartum. Chinese women, for example, observe *zuoyuezzi*, often referred to as "doing the month," after childbirth. During this time the mother is typically supported by the baby's grandmother or a close family member. She is encouraged to rest and avoid domestic chores and outside activities. She also avoids bathing, brushing her teeth, and washing her hair. She strives to maintain a balance of hot and cold foods (Cutler & Callister, 2013). Similarly, many Muslim women stay in the house for 40 days following a birth, cared for by female relatives (Walton et al., 2014).

CULTURAL FACTORS AND NURSING CARE

Healthcare providers are often unaware of the cultural characteristics they themselves demonstrate. Without cultural awareness, caregivers tend to project their own cultural responses onto foreign-born clients; clients from different socioeconomic, religious, or educational groups; or clients from different regions of the country. This projection leads caregivers to assume that the clients are demonstrating a specific behavior for the same reason that they themselves would. Moreover, healthcare providers often fail to realize that medicine has its own culture, which has been dominated historically by traditional middle-class values and beliefs. Madeleine Leininger (1973) developed the cultural care diversity and universality nursing theory that specifically addresses caring and the impact that culture plays on nursing care (Leininger & MacFarland, 2006).

Ethnocentrism is the conviction that the values and beliefs of one's own cultural group are the best or only acceptable ones. It is characterized by an inability to understand the beliefs and worldview of another culture. To a certain extent, all of us are guilty of ethnocentrism, at least some of the time. Thus, the nurse who values stoicism during labor may be uncomfortable with the more vocal response of some Latin American women. Another nurse may be disconcerted by a Southeast Asian woman who believes that pain is something to be endured rather than alleviated and who is intent on maintaining self-control during labor.

Healthcare providers sometimes believe that if members of other cultures do not share Western values and beliefs, they should adopt them. For example, a nurse who believes strongly in equality of the sexes may find it difficult to remain silent if a woman from a Middle Eastern culture defers to her husband in decision making. It is important to remember that pressure to defy cultural values and beliefs can be stressful and anxiety provoking for many women.

To address issues of cultural diversity in the provision of health care, emphasis is being placed on developing *cultural competence*, that is, the skills and knowledge necessary to appreciate, respect, and work with individuals from different cultures. It requires self-awareness, awareness and understanding of cultural differences, and the ability to adapt clinical skills and practices as needed (Spector, 2013).

The nurse can begin developing cultural competence by becoming knowledgeable about the cultural practices of local groups. For example, is it considered courteous to avoid eye contact? Should last names be used in conversations as a sign of respect? Is a female healthcare provider necessary? Do communication and language barriers exist? If so, how can they be addressed?

Generalization about cultural characteristics or values is difficult because not every individual in a culture may display these characteristics. Just as variations are seen among cultures, variations are also seen within cultures. For example, because of their exposure to the American culture, a third-generation Chinese American family might have very different values and beliefs from those of a Chinese family that has recently immigrated to America. For this reason, the nurse needs to supplement a general knowledge of cultural values and practices with a complete assessment of each individual's values and practices.

Cultural Assessment   Cultural assessment is an important aspect of prenatal care. Healthcare professionals are becoming increasingly aware that they must address cultural needs in the prenatal assessment to provide culturally sensitive health care during pregnancy. Healthcare providers should conduct a cultural assessment to obtain information about health practices based on the client's beliefs, values, customs, and behaviors related to pregnancy and childbearing. This includes information about ethnic background, amount of affiliation with the ethnic group, patterns of decision making, religious preference, language, communication style, and common etiquette practices (National Institutes of Health, 2013). The nurse can also explore the woman's (or family's) expectations of the healthcare system. Once this information is gathered, the nurse can then plan and provide care that is appropriate and responsive to family needs.

A cultural assessment might include questions such as the following:

- Who in the family must be consulted before decisions are made about a person's care?
- Does the client see primarily in the present or does she have a futuristic time orientation?
- What type of healthcare provider is most appropriate for the client?
- Does the client have beliefs or traditions that may affect the plan of care?

Clinical Tip

When you care for a family in which the grandparents play a key role in decision making, be sure that they are present if you are teaching something that is important for the family to understand.

Several cultural assessment tools are available to assist the nurse in gathering this information to ensure the provision of culturally competent care. The nurse who respects cultural diversity while building trust is an asset to childbearing families as they adjust to new roles.

Impact of Religion and Spirituality

The terms *religion* and *spirituality* mean different things to different people. Many people consider *religion* to be an institutionalized system that shares a common set of beliefs and practices; others define it more simply as a belief in a transcendent power. The latter definition, however, approaches most people's understanding of *spirituality* as a concern with the spirit or soul.

A childbearing family's religious beliefs, affiliation, and practices can influence deeply their experiences and attitudes toward health care, childbearing, and childrearing. Members of certain religious groups such as Christian Scientists may attempt to avoid all medical interventions whereas others such as Jehovah's Witnesses may refuse specific interventions such as blood transfusions. Roman Catholics may refuse contraception. In most cases, the woman and her family gain comfort from acknowledgment of and respect for their religious beliefs and practices in the healthcare setting. However, the agnostic (one who has doubts about the existence of a transcendent being) or the atheist (one who believes that there is no higher power) may be offended if care providers assume references to God or to a higher power will be comforting.

A religious or spiritual history is often completed when a woman is admitted to a clinic or labor setting. The assessment can include questions about current spiritual beliefs and practices that will affect the mother and baby during the hospital stay or preferences for religious rituals during labor and birth. When possible, the nurse should attempt to accommodate religious rituals and practices requested by the childbearing family.

Considering the diversity of religious beliefs, it is not unusual for nurses to encounter childbearing families whose beliefs conflict with their own. This is not problematic as long as the nurse avoids attempts to influence the client's decision making. For example, a nurse who does not believe in baptism should avoid revealing this to a Catholic mother seeking baptism for her stillborn baby. Nurses should also examine their religious beliefs related to genetic screening procedures, use of assisted reproductive technology to achieve pregnancy, use of technology to support life in a severely compromised newborn, abortion, and even less dramatic issues such as methods of contraception, circumcision, and infant feeding. In many institutions nurses can ask to be reassigned to a different client if their religious beliefs are in conflict; however, if other personnel are not available, it is the nurse's responsibility to provide sensitive, appropriate, and nonjudgmental care to that client.

Complementary Health Approaches and the Childbearing Family

Throughout most of the 20th century in the United States, it was rare for European American childbearing families to consult anyone except their obstetrician for advice about their pregnancy, birth, and the postpartum period. Though such clients are still encountered today, perinatal nurses are more likely to care for childbearing families who integrate other types of practitioners and therapies with traditional Western medicine.

A **complementary therapy** may be defined as any procedure or product that is used as an adjunct to conventional medical treatment. The term *integrative health* describes the use of complementary therapies within mainstream health care (National Center for Complementary and Integrated Health [NCCIH], 2015). Although complementary therapies were entirely absent from clinics and hospitals until the past few decades, therapies such as acupuncture, acupressure, and massage therapy are now often used together with conventional medical care, and many health insurance plans cover at least a portion of the cost of such therapies.

In contrast, an **alternative therapy** is usually considered a substance or procedure that is used in place of conventional medicine (Micozzi, 2014; NCCIH, 2015). Thus, alternative therapies are not usually available in conventional clinics and hospitals, and their costs are not typically covered under most health insurance policies. Consequently, a client may be reluctant to discuss them with a mainstream physician or nurse.

The dramatic increase in complementary and alternative therapies that began in the 1990s has probably resulted from a combination of several factors:

- Increased consumer awareness of the limitations of conventional Western medicine
- Increased international travel
- Increased media attention
- Advent of the internet

It seems clear that the future of American health care will reveal an ever-increasing integration between mainstream medicine and complementary health approaches. Some obvious examples of this new integration in perinatal settings include the acceptance of certain herbal teas for antepartum discomforts; the use of massage, Reiki, or therapeutic touch during the first stage of labor; music during childbirth; and the increased emphasis on skin-to-skin mother-to-baby bonding in the immediate postpartum period.

Further evidence of this increased integration is the establishment in 1992 of the Office of Alternative Medicine (OAM) at the National Institutes of Health. The OAM was mandated by Congress to promote research into complementary and alternative therapies and dissemination of information to consumers. In 1998, the OAM was incorporated into a new National Center for Complementary and Alternative Medicine (NCCAM) with an expanded mission and increased funding. Over time NCCAM recognized a new domain of *integrative medicine*, an approach that combines mainstream medical therapies with complementary therapies for which there is some high-quality scientific evidence of safety and effectiveness (NCCIH, 2015). In 2014, NCCAM changed its name to the National Center for Complementary and Integrated Health (NCCIH). Many studies of complementary and alternative therapies are currently under way and can be accessed via the NCCIH website.

Benefits and Risks

Complementary health approaches have many benefits for the childbearing family and other healthcare consumers. Many complementary and alternative therapies emphasize prevention and wellness, and place a higher value on holistic healing than on physical cure. In addition, many are noninvasive, have few side effects, and are more affordable and available than conventional therapies.

However, many of these remedies have associated risks that must be considered thoughtfully before a decision is made to use them. These risks include lack of standardization, lack of regulation and research substantiating safety and effectiveness, inadequate training and certification of some healers, and financial and health risks of unproven methods.

SAFETY ALERT!

Complementary and alternative therapies must be assessed for safety, including positive and negative benefits, cost, efficacy, and clinical usefulness. The use of herbs and natural products raises many issues, of which these are just a few: standards of products, misleading claims, and safety related to megadoses of some products.

Types of Complementary Health Approaches

Numerous forms of complementary and alternative therapies are available. Only a few of the most commonly used approaches are presented here.

HOMEOPATHY

Homeopathy is best understood in contrast to conventional Western medicine, which is also called *allopathic medicine*. The term *allopathy* is derived from the Greek words *allos* meaning "different" and *pathos* meaning "suffering." Thus, allopathic medicine uses remedies that produce effects differing from—or in opposition to—those of the disease being treated. For example, conventional healthcare practitioners may prescribe an anti-inflammatory to reduce swelling or a sedative to relieve insomnia.

In contrast, the term *homeopathy* is derived from the Greek word *homos* meaning "the same." It is based on the "law of similars," which says that a substance that can cause symptoms when taken by healthy people can help treat those who are experiencing similar symptoms (Micozzi, 2014). Thus, it is often described as a healing system that uses like to cure like; specifically, homeopathic remedies are minute dilutions of substances that, if ingested in larger amounts, would produce effects *similar* to the symptoms of the disorder being treated. For example, *Cantharis vesicatoria* is a species of beetle (commonly called Spanish fly) whose poison causes, among other symptoms, burning pains and a frantic urge to urinate. Homeopathic *Cantharis* is a minute dilution of this toxin, and is thus a remedy of choice for women suffering from cystitis. Homeopathy is widely used in pregnancy, labor, birth, and postpartum, and in newborns (Micozzi, 2014).

NATUROPATHY

Naturopathy is commonly referred to as *natural medicine*. It is more precisely defined as a healing system that combines safe and effective traditional means of preventing and treating human disease with the most current advances in modern medicine (American Association of Naturopathic Physicians [AANP], 2015). Many naturopathic physicians are eclectic, employing a variety of therapies in their practice. These might include clinical nutrition, botanical medicine, homeopathy, natural childbirth, traditional Chinese medicine, hydrotherapy, naturopathic manipulative therapy, pharmacology, minor surgery, and counseling for lifestyle modification (AANP, 2015).

TRADITIONAL CHINESE MEDICINE

Traditional Chinese medicine (TCM) developed more than 3000 years ago in the Chinese culture and then gradually spread with modifications to other Asian countries. The underlying focus of TCM is prevention, although diagnosis and treatment of disease also play important roles.

TCM seeks to ensure the balance of energy, which is called *chi* or *qi* (pronounced "chee"). Chi is the invisible flow of energy in the body that maintains health and vitality and enables the body to carry out its physiologic functions. Chi flows along certain pathways or meridians.

Another important concept in TCM (mentioned earlier) is that of *yin* and *yang*, opposing internal and external forces that, together, represent the whole.

TCM includes the following therapeutic techniques:

- *Acupuncture* uses very fine (hairlike) stainless steel needles to stimulate specific acupuncture points depending on the person's medical assessment and condition.

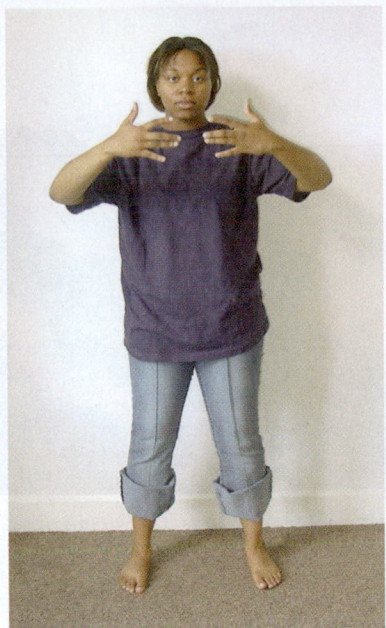

Figure 2–2 Pregnant woman practices the movements of Qigong.

SOURCE: Michele Davidson.

- *Acupressure* (Chinese massage) uses pressure from the fingers and thumbs to stimulate pressure points.
- *Herbal therapy* is an important part of TCM but it is sometimes difficult to locate a skilled herbalist because there are relatively few in the United States.
- *Qigong* (pronounced "chee-goong") is a self-discipline that involves the use of breathing, meditation, self-massage, and movement. Typically practiced daily, the movements are non-tiring and are designed to stimulate the flow of chi (Figure 2–2).
- *T'ai chi* (pronounced "ty chee") is a form of martial art. It originally focused on physical fitness and self-defense, but is currently used to improve overall health as well.
- *Moxibustion* involves the application of heat from a small piece of burning herb called *moxa (Artemesia vulgaris)*. The moxa stick is typically burned at the lateral side of the little toe. In TCM moxibustion has many uses. For example, studies from China demonstrate good success when moxibustion is used to help turn a fetus that is breech to a vertex presentation (Vas, Aranda-Regules, Modesto, et al., 2013).

MIND-BASED THERAPIES

Biofeedback is a method used to help individuals learn to control their physiologic responses based on the concept that the mind controls the body. An individual is hooked up to a system of highly sensitive instruments that relay information about the body back to that person. Currently biofeedback has more than 150 applications for disease prevention and the restoration of health. The effectiveness of biofeedback has been proven in countless studies and it is now considered a conventional therapy more than a complementary one.

Hypnosis, whether guided by a trained hypnotherapist or induced through self-hypnosis, is a state of great mental and physical relaxation during which a person is very open to suggestions. In this state, the individual is able to modify body responses. Pregnant women who receive hypnosis before childbirth have reported shorter, less painful labors and births.

Visualization is a complementary therapy in which a person goes into a relaxed state and focuses on or "visualizes" soothing or positive scenes such as a beach or a mountain glade. Visualization helps reduce stress and encourage relaxation. For example, a therapist may work with a woman before childbirth to help the woman create positive images of labor.

Guided imagery is a state of intense, focused concentration used to create compelling mental images. It is sometimes considered a form of hypnosis. Guided imagery is useful in imagining a desired effect such as weight loss or in mentally rehearsing a new procedure or activity.

CHIROPRACTIC THERAPY

Chiropractic, the third largest independent health profession in the United States (behind medicine and dentistry), is based on concepts of manipulation to address health problems that are thought to be the result of abnormal nerve transmissions caused by misalignment of the spine (subluxation). In the United States doctors of chiropractic perform more than 90% of all spinal manipulations (American Chiropractic Association, 2015). Chiropractors also stress the importance of proper nutrition and regular exercise to good health. Chiropractic is widely available and popular demand has earned it a higher level of insurance coverage than most other alternative therapies have.

MASSAGE THERAPY

Massage has been used for centuries as a form of therapy. *Massage therapy* involves the manipulation of the soft tissues of the body to reduce stress and tension, increase circulation, diminish pain, and promote a sense of well-being. Different techniques have been developed, including Swedish massage, shiatsu massage, Rolfing, and trigger point massage. Most forms use techniques such as pressing, kneading, gliding, circular motion, tapping, and vibrational strokes.

Certain massage therapists specialize in massage for women during pregnancy. Massage is often helpful as women adapt to the discomforts of their changing bodies. In addition, certified nurse-midwives often use perineal massage before labor to stretch the muscles of the perineum around the vaginal opening and thereby prevent tearing of the tissues during childbirth. During labor, massage of the back and buttocks by the nurse, labor coach, or *doula* can help the woman relax and may help decrease her discomfort. Infant massage is also growing in popularity in the United States (Figure 2–3).

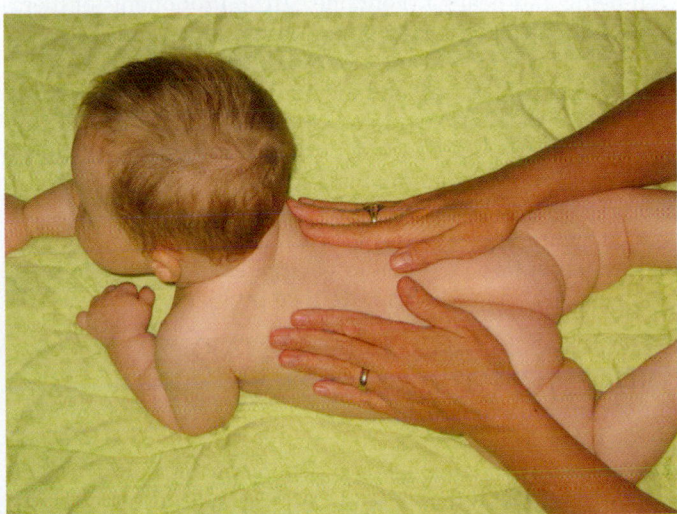

Figure 2–3 The calm, soothing strokes of infant massage can help comfort a baby and minimize crying.

SOURCE: Michele Davidson.

HERBAL THERAPIES

Herbal therapy or herbal medicine has been used since ancient times to treat illnesses and ailments. Like vitamins and minerals, herbs are a form of dietary supplement, but they are often used to treat the symptoms of specific ailments rather than simply to enhance overall health. Well-known herbal remedies include ginger, rosemary, ginseng, ginkgo, chamomile, oil of evening primrose, *echinacea*, garlic, lemon balm, and black cohosh.

Currently about 1500 botanical substances are sold in the United States as dietary supplements or as part of traditional ethnic medications. Herbal formulations, however, are not subject to Food and Drug Administration (FDA) premarket testing for safety and effectiveness. Thus, these products can be sold over the counter with little control. Herbs are categorized as dietary supplements and are controlled by the Dietary Supplement Health and Education Act of 1994. They do not require approval by the Food and Drug Administration (FDA) as do prescription and over-the-counter medications; however, the FDA does have the authority to pull a product from the market if it is proven to be dangerous (Food and Drug Administration [FDA], 2014). Consequently most of what is known about herbs comes from Europe, where they have been studied for some time. Herbal products from Germany, France, England, and Australia are reasonably safe because in these countries herbs are regulated as if they were drugs.

The use of herbs during pregnancy is an especially important consideration for nurses working with childbearing families. Pregnant and lactating women interested in using herbs are best advised to consult with their healthcare providers before taking any herbs, even as teas. Lists identifying common herbs that women are advised to avoid or use with caution during pregnancy and lactation are available.

THERAPEUTIC TOUCH

Therapeutic touch is a complementary therapy meant to be used with conventional medical care. It was developed in the early 1970s by Dr. Delores Krieger, a nursing professor at New York University, and Dora Kunz, a clairvoyant healer. Therapeutic touch is grounded in the belief that people are a system of energy with a self-healing potential. The therapeutic touch practitioner, often a nurse, can unite his or her energy field with that of the recipient's, directing it in a specific way to promote well-being and healing (Fontaine, 2015). Proponents of therapeutic touch believe that a strong desire to help the recipient is essential, as is a conscious use of self to act as a link between the universal life energy and the other person (Micozzi, 2014). Impressive anecdotal evidence and many small studies suggest that therapeutic touch is effective in a variety of conditions; however, large randomized trials are needed to establish effectiveness.

Like many other conventional and complementary therapies, therapeutic touch should be applied cautiously to pregnant women and newborns by trained providers (Figure 2–4).

OTHER TYPES OF COMPLEMENTARY AND ALTERNATIVE THERAPIES

This discussion only touched on some of the most common forms of complementary and alternative therapies. Other examples include Ayurveda (the traditional medicine of India), meditation, craniosacral therapy, reflexology, hydrotherapy, Hatha yoga, regular physical exercise, aromatherapy, color and light therapy, music and sound therapies, magnetic therapy, and Reiki, to name a few. Readers interested in these therapies are referred to specialty texts.

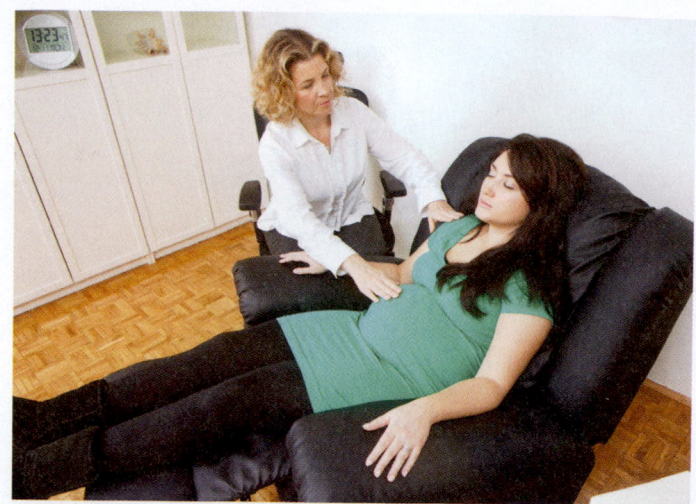

Figure 2–4 During pregnancy, therapeutic touch is often helpful in easing pain and reducing anxiety.

SOURCE: Dean bertoncelj/Shutterstock.

Developing Cultural Competence Herbalism

The World Health Organization estimates that 80% of Earth's population depends on plants to treat common ailments. Herbalism is an essential part of traditional Indian, Asian, Native American, and naturopathic medicines. Many homeopathic remedies are also developed from herbs.

Nursing Care of the Childbearing Family Using Complementary Health Approaches

Some form of complementary health approach is currently being used by more than 33% of adults in the United States. Women use complementary methods more often than men do, as do people with higher educational levels and people who have been hospitalized within the past year. By race, when megavitamin therapy and prayer are included in the definition, African Americans are the greatest users of complementary methods. When those elements are excluded, Asians are the greatest users, followed by Whites (NCCIH, 2015).

The reality that women may use complementary methods and not reveal it raises some concern. Certain modalities such as biofeedback, acupuncture, aromatherapy, and massage are not likely to cause adverse effects during pregnancy. The possibility exists, however, that interactions may occur between herbal therapies and medications prescribed by the caregiver. Complications may also develop from the use of vitamin supplements.

Nurses who create a climate of respect and openness tend to be more effective in gathering information about a woman's use of complementary methods. The following recommendations may be useful to nurses when taking a history:

• Ask questions that are direct and nonjudgmental in seeking information about the client's use of complementary methods.

- Include questions related to complementary methods in a listing with other treatment modalities, such as, "What prescription, over-the-counter, herbal, or homeopathic remedies or nutritional supplements are you currently taking?"
- Avoid making negative or disparaging comments about complementary methods. Such comments send the message that complementary health approaches are not desirable and may discourage people from disclosing their use of complementary therapies.
- Ask questions related to nontraditional care using straightforward questions, such as, "Do you regularly engage in any alternative therapies such as yoga, massage, chiropractic care, or biofeedback?"

In working with childbearing families, or indeed with any clients, nurses who use complementary therapies should choose those methods that are within the scope of nursing practice in their state and not limited by the licensure of other providers (such as massage therapists). Nurses are also best advised to use complementary therapies that are considered somewhat mainstream and that are supported by evidence about their safety and effectiveness. For example, a nurse working with a pregnant woman might suggest acupressure wristbands for the treatment of nausea. Other therapies that nurses often employ include progressive relaxation, exercise and movement, therapeutic touch, visualization and guided imagery, prayer, meditation, music therapy, massage, storytelling, aromatherapy, and journaling.

Nurses who use complementary modalities should document their use within the context of nursing practice. This is most effective when the modality is identified as an intervention to address a specific nursing diagnosis or identified client need. Thus, music therapy might be used for a laboring woman to address the identified nursing diagnosis of acute pain.

Nurses have a role in conducting and supporting research on complementary therapies. Because of the variety of therapies in use, research is needed in a host of areas. The results of research on complementary health approaches can be found in professional journals and at the National Center for Complementary and Integrated Health website. As the evidence supporting the use of certain interventions grows, nurses and other healthcare providers are incorporating the results as part of their evidence-based practice.

Focus Your Study

- Family values, roles, and power are important to consider when attempting to provide holistic health care to childbearing families.
- Nuclear families consist of a mother, father, and children.
- Dual-career/dual-earner families comprise the majority of contemporary families in the United States.
- Child-free families are a growing trend in American culture.
- Extended family members can play an active role in family life, decision making, and family roles.
- Single-parent families account for almost one third of all U.S. families, and stepparent and binuclear families are increasingly common.
- The developmental framework looks at a family over time as it progresses through predictable stages within the life cycle.
- A family assessment provides an in-depth tool to collect pertinent family life information that can assist the nurse in planning care.
- Culture plays a significant part in a family's development, assignment of roles, and observance of traditions, customs, and taboos.
- Cultural norms influence a family's beliefs about the importance of children, pregnancy, health practices, and infant feeding.
- A cultural assessment can assist the nurse in identifying cultural norms and in providing culturally appropriate nursing care. It should focus on factors that will influence the practices of the childbearing family with regard to health needs.
- A religious history is included when assessing contemporary families. When possible, the nurse accommodates the family's religious-based preferences for care.
- A complementary therapy is an adjunct to mainstream medical treatment, whereas an alternative therapy is used in place of prescribed medical therapy.
- The National Center for Complementary and Integrated Health promotes research into complementary health approaches and integrative health and disseminates the information to consumers.
- Complementary therapies have several benefits. Many of them emphasize prevention and wellness, place a higher value on holistic healing than on physical cure, are noninvasive, and have few side effects. In addition, many are more affordable and available than conventional therapies.
- Risks of using complementary or alternative therapies include lack of standardization, lack of regulation and research substantiating safety and effectiveness, inadequate training and certification of some healers, and financial and health risks of unproven methods.
- The term *homeopathy* is derived from the Greek word *homos,* meaning "the same." It is a healing system that uses like to cure like; that is, homeopathic remedies are minute dilutions of substances that, if ingested in larger amounts, would produce effects similar to the symptoms of the disorder being treated.
- Traditional Chinese medicine (TCM) seeks to ensure the balance of energy, called *chi* or *qi.* TCM techniques include acupuncture, acupressure, herbal therapy, Qigong, t'ai chi, and moxibustion.
- Biofeedback is a method used to help individuals learn to control their physiologic responses based on the concept that the mind controls the body.

- Hypnosis, whether guided by a trained hypnotherapist or induced through self-hypnosis, is a state of great mental and physical relaxation during which a person is very open to suggestions.

- Guided imagery is a state of intense, focused concentration used to create compelling mental images.

- Chiropractic, a profession practiced by licensed chiropractors, is based on concepts of manipulation, especially spinal manipulation.

- Therapeutic touch is based on the belief that people are a system of energy with a self-healing potential. The therapeutic touch practitioner, often a nurse, can unite his or her energy field with that of the client's, directing it in a specific way to promote well-being and healing.

- Many nurses are open to and supportive of complementary and alternative therapies. Nurses who incorporate such therapies into their practice must be certain that they are practicing within the framework of their nurse practice act and with the informed consent of their clients.

Clinical Reasoning in Action

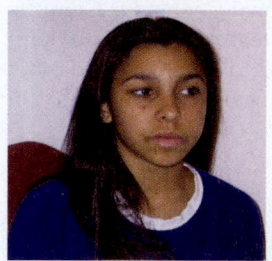

While working in an inner-city clinic for adolescents, you meet a new client, a 14-year-old Latina girl named Juanita. She is accompanied by her parents. None of them speak English. Through an interpreter, Juanita tells you that she recently moved here with her parents. They have brought her here today because she has a sore throat. The *curandera* they took her to see prescribed the herbal remedy *echinacea*, but her throat is still sore. The rapid test you perform for strep throat is positive and the nurse practitioner prescribes an antibiotic.

SOURCE: Pearson Education, Inc.

1. According to the national standards for culturally and linguistically appropriate services in health care set by the government, what are examples of important standards of care that you, as the nurse, can provide in the care of this adolescent?

2. How can you, as the nurse, take steps to achieve cultural competence?

3. How would you, as the nurse, be able to address some of the disparities that can exist when this client comes to the clinic?

4. What are some examples of common food preferences in the Latino American culture?

References

American Association of Naturopathic Physicians (AANP). (2015). *What is naturopathic medicine?* Retrieved from http://naturopathic.org/content.asp?contentid=59

American Chiropractic Association. (2015). *Spinal manipulation.* Retrieved from http://www.acatoday.org

Chen, C. H. (2014). Diverse yet hegemonic: Expressions of motherhood in "I'm a Mormon" ads. *Journal of Media and Religion, 13*(1), 1–47. doi:10.1080/15348423.2014.871973

Cutler, M., & Callister, L. C. (2013). Perceptions of giving birth and adherence to cultural practices in Chinese women. *Brigham Young University Journal of Undergraduate Research,* August 27, 2013. Retrieved from http://jur.byu.edu/?p=3636

Duvall, E. M. (1977). *Marriage and family development* (5th ed.). New York, NY: Harper Row.

Fontaine, K. L. (2015). *Complementary and alternative therapies for nursing practice* (4th ed.). Upper Saddle River, NJ: Pearson.

Food & Drug Administration (FDA). (2014). *Dietary supplements: What you need to know.* Retrieved from http://www.fda.gov/Food/ResourcesForYou/Consumers/ucm109760.htm

Javed, F. (2015). The sterilized and subjugated: Population control and the plight of Indian women. *Harvard International Review,* April 15, 2014. Retrieved from http://hir.harvard.edu/the-sterilized-and-subjugated-population-control-and-the-plight-of-indian-women

Leininger, M. (1973). *Cultural care theory: An evaluation process.* Paper presented at the group meeting of the Minnesota National League of Nursing, Northfield, MN.

Leininger, M., & MacFarland, M. R. (2006). *Cultural care diversity and universality: A worldwide nursing theory* (2nd ed.). Sudbury, MA: Jones & Bartlett.

Micozzi, M. S. (2014). *Fundamentals of complementary & alternative medicine* (5th ed.). St. Louis, MO: Elsevier Saunders.

National Center for Complementary and Integrated Health (NCCIH). (2015). *What is CAM?* Retrieved from http://nccam.nih.gov/health/whatiscam

National Institutes of Health. (2013). *Cultural competency.* Retrieved from http://www.nih.gov/clearcommunication/culturalcompetency.htm

Petrow, S. (2015). Life after Supreme Court's decision to legalize same-sex marriage. *Washington Post.* Retrieved from http://www.washingtonpost.com/lifestyle/style/civilities-life-after-supreme-courts-decision-to-legalize-same-sex-marriage/2015/07/13/f0625bc4-2733-11e5-b77f-eb13a215f593_story.html

Purnell, L. D. (2014). *Guide to culturally competent health care* (3rd ed.). Philadelphia, PA: F. A. Davis.

Spector, R. E. (2013). *Cultural diversity in health and illness* (8th ed.). Upper Saddle River, NJ: Pearson.

U.S. Census Bureau. (2013). *Definition: Household and family.* Retrieved from https://www.census.gov/prod/2013pubs/p20-570.pdf

Vas, J., Aranda-Regules, J. M., Modesto, M., Ramos-Monserrat, M., Barón, M., Aguilar, I., . . . Rivas-Ruiz, F. (2013). Using moxibustion in primary health care to correct non-vertex presentation: A multicentre randomised controlled trial. *Accupuncture Medicine, 31*(1), 31–38. doi:10.1136/acupmed-2012-010261

Walton, L. M., Akram, F., & Hossain, F. (2014). Health beliefs of Muslim women and implications for health care providers: Exploratory study on the health beliefs of Muslim women. *Online Journal of Health Ethics, 10*(2), 5. Retrieved from http://aquila.usm.edu/ojhe/vol10/iss2/5/

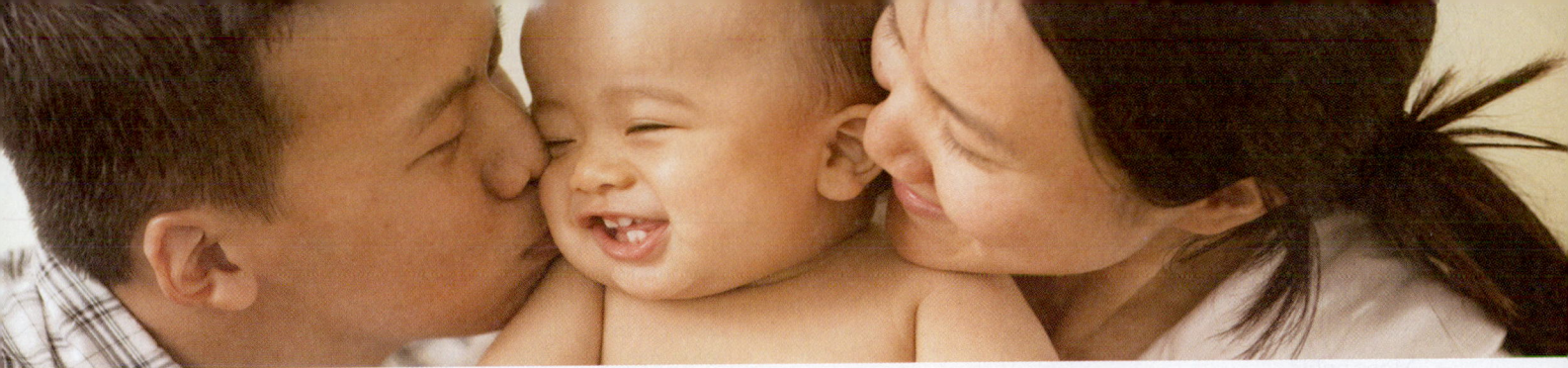

Chapter 3
Reproductive Anatomy and Physiology

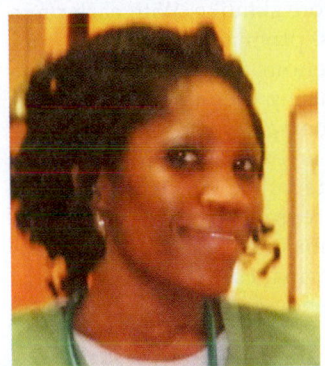

I am amazed by how little many of our students know about anatomy, physiology, and reproduction. As nurses, we must use every opportunity we have to teach young people about their bodies and those of their partners. Information is the key to helping keep them safe and well!

—University Health Clinic Nurse

∨ Learning Outcomes

3.1 Identify the structures and functions of the female reproductive system.

3.2 Explain the significance of specific female reproductive structures during pregnancy and childbirth.

3.3 Summarize the actions of the hormones estrogen and progesterone, and the prostaglandins that affect reproductive functioning.

3.4 Identify the two phases of the ovarian cycle and the changes that occur in each phase.

3.5 Describe the phases of the menstrual cycle, their dominant hormones, and the changes that occur in each phase.

3.6 Identify the structures and functions of the male reproductive system.

Understanding childbearing requires more than understanding sexual intercourse or the process by which the female and male sex cells unite. The nurse must also become familiar with the structures and functions that make childbearing possible and the phenomena that initiate it. This chapter presents the anatomic, physiologic, and sexual aspects of the female and male reproductive systems.

The female and male reproductive organs are *homologous*; that is, they are fundamentally similar in structure and function. The primary functions of both female and male reproductive systems are to produce sex cells and to transport them to locations where their union can occur. The sex cells, called *gametes*, are produced by specialized organs called *gonads*. A series of ducts and glands within both male and female reproductive systems contributes to the production and transport of the gametes.

Female Reproductive System

The female reproductive system consists of the external and internal genitals and the accessory organs of the breasts. Because of its importance to childbearing, the bony pelvis is also discussed in this chapter.

23

External Genitals

All the external reproductive organs except the glandular structures can be directly inspected. The appearance of the external genitalia varies greatly among women. Heredity, age, race, and the number of children a woman has borne influence the size, color, and shape of her external organs. The female external genitals, also referred to as the **vulva**, include the following structures (Figure 3–1):

- Mons pubis
- Labia majora
- Labia minora
- Clitoris
- Urethral meatus and opening of the paraurethral (Skene) glands
- Vaginal vestibule (vaginal orifice, vulvovaginal [Bartholin] glands, hymen, and fossa navicularis)
- Perineal body.

Although they are not true parts of the female reproductive system, the urethral meatus and perineal body are considered here because of their proximity and relationship to the vulva. The vulva has a generous supply of blood and nerves. As a woman ages estrogen secretions decrease, causing the vulvar organs to atrophy.

MONS PUBIS

The *mons pubis* is a softly rounded mound of subcutaneous fatty tissue beginning at the lowest portion of the anterior abdominal wall (see Figure 3–1). Also known as the *mons veneris*, this structure covers the front portion of the symphysis pubis. The mons pubis is covered with pubic hair, typically with the hairline forming a transverse line across the lower abdomen. The mons pubis protects the pelvic bones, especially during coitus.

LABIA MAJORA

The *labia majora* are longitudinal, raised folds of pigmented skin, one on either side of the vulvar cleft. Their chief function is to protect the structures lying between them. The labia majora are covered by hair follicles and sebaceous glands, with underlying adipose and muscle tissue.

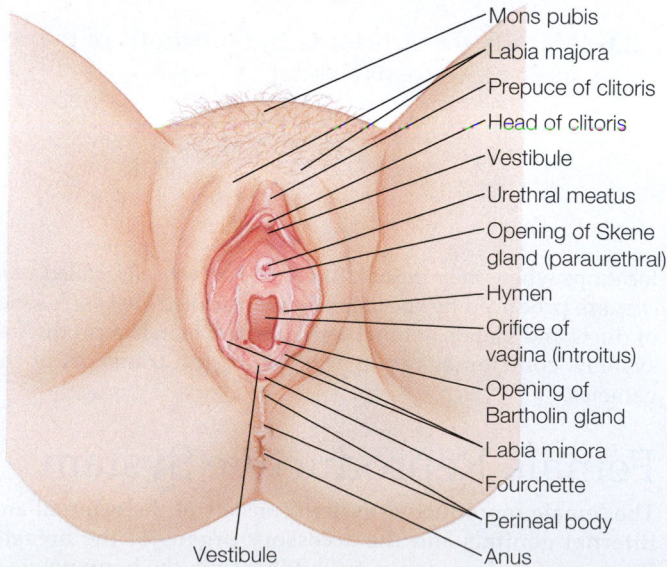

Mons pubis
Labia majora
Prepuce of clitoris
Head of clitoris
Vestibule
Urethral meatus
Opening of Skene gland (paraurethral)
Hymen
Orifice of vagina (introitus)
Opening of Bartholin gland
Labia minora
Fourchette
Perineal body
Anus
Vestibule

Figure 3–1 Female external genitals, longitudinal view.

The inner surface of the labia majora in women who have not had children is moist and looks like mucous membrane, whereas after many births it is more skinlike. With each pregnancy, the labia majora become less prominent.

Because of the extensive venous network in the labia majora, varicosities may occur during pregnancy, and obstetric or sexual trauma may cause hematomas (Cunningham et al., 2014). The labia majora share an extensive lymphatic supply with the other structures of the vulva, which can facilitate the spread of cancer in the female reproductive organs. Because of the nerves supplying the labia majora (from the first lumbar and third sacral segment of the spinal cord), certain regional anesthesia blocks will affect them and cause numbness.

LABIA MINORA

The *labia minora* are soft folds of skin within the labia majora that converge near the anus, forming the *fourchette*. Each labium minus has the appearance of shiny mucous membrane, moist and devoid of hair follicles. The labia minora are rich in sebaceous glands, which lubricate and waterproof the vulvar skin and provide bactericidal secretions. Because the sebaceous glands do not open into hair follicles but open directly onto the surface of the skin, sebaceous cysts commonly occur in this area. The labia minora are composed of erectile tissue and involuntary muscle tissue. Vulvovaginitis in this area is irritating because the labia minora have many tactile nerve endings. The labia minora increase in size at puberty and decrease after menopause because of changes in estrogen levels.

CLITORIS

The *clitoris,* located between the labia minora, is about 5 to 6 mm long and 6 to 8 mm across. Its tissue is essentially erectile. The glans of the clitoris is partly covered by a fold of skin called the *prepuce,* or clitoral hood. This area resembles an opening to an orifice and may be confused with the urethral meatus. Accidental attempts to insert a catheter in this area produce extreme discomfort. The clitoris has rich blood and nerve supplies and is the primary erogenous organ of women. In addition, it secretes *smegma,* which along with other vulval secretions has a unique odor that may be sexually stimulating to the male.

URETHRAL MEATUS AND PARAURETHRAL GLANDS

The *urethral meatus* is located 1 to 2.5 cm beneath the clitoris in the midline of the vestibule; it often appears as a puckered, slitlike opening. At times the meatus is difficult to visualize because of the presence of blind dimples, small mucosal folds, or wide variations in location.

The paraurethral glands, or *Skene glands,* open into the posterior wall of the urethra close to its opening (see Figure 3–1). Their secretions lubricate the vaginal opening, facilitating sexual intercourse.

VAGINAL VESTIBULE

The vaginal vestibule is a boat-shaped depression enclosed by the labia majora that is visible when they are separated (see Figure 3–1). The vestibule contains the vaginal opening, or *introitus,* which is the border between the external and internal genitals.

The *hymen* is a thin, elastic collar or semicollar of tissue that surrounds the vaginal opening. The appearance changes during the woman's lifetime. At birth, the hymen is essentially avascular. For thousands of years, some societies have perpetuated the belief that the hymen covers the vaginal opening and thus an intact hymen is a sign of virginity. However, modern studies of female genital anatomy have revealed that the hymen surrounds rather than entirely covers the vaginal opening, and can be torn not only through sexual intercourse but also through strenuous physical activity, masturbation, menstruation, or the use of tampons, thus dispelling old beliefs. For more information on the nurse's role in discussing these topics, see Chapter 5.

External to the hymen at the base of the vestibule are two small papular elevations containing the openings of the ducts of the *vulvovaginal (Bartholin) glands.* They lie under the constrictor muscle of the vagina. These glands secrete a clear, thick, alkaline mucus that enhances the viability and motility of the sperm deposited in the vaginal vestibule. These gland ducts can harbor *Neisseria gonorrhea* and other bacteria, which can cause pus formation and abscesses in the Bartholin glands.

The vestibular area is innervated mainly by the perineal nerve from the sacral plexus. The area is not sensitive to touch generally; however, the hymen contains numerous free nerve endings as receptors to pain.

PERINEAL BODY

The **perineal body** is a wedge-shaped mass of fibromuscular tissue found between the lower part of the vagina and the anus (see Figure 3–1). The superficial area between the anus and the vagina is referred to as the *perineum.*

The muscles that meet at the perineal body are the external sphincter ani, both levator ani (the superficial and deep transverse perineal), and the bulbocavernosus. These muscles mingle with elastic fibers and connective tissue in an arrangement that allows a remarkable amount of stretching. During the last part of labor, the perineal body thins out until it is just a few centimeters thick. This tissue is often the site of an episiotomy or lacerations during childbirth (see Chapter 21).

Female Internal Reproductive Organs

The female internal reproductive organs—the vagina, uterus, fallopian tubes, and ovaries—are target organs for estrogenic hormones and they play a unique part in the reproductive cycle (Figure 3–2). Certain internal reproductive organs can

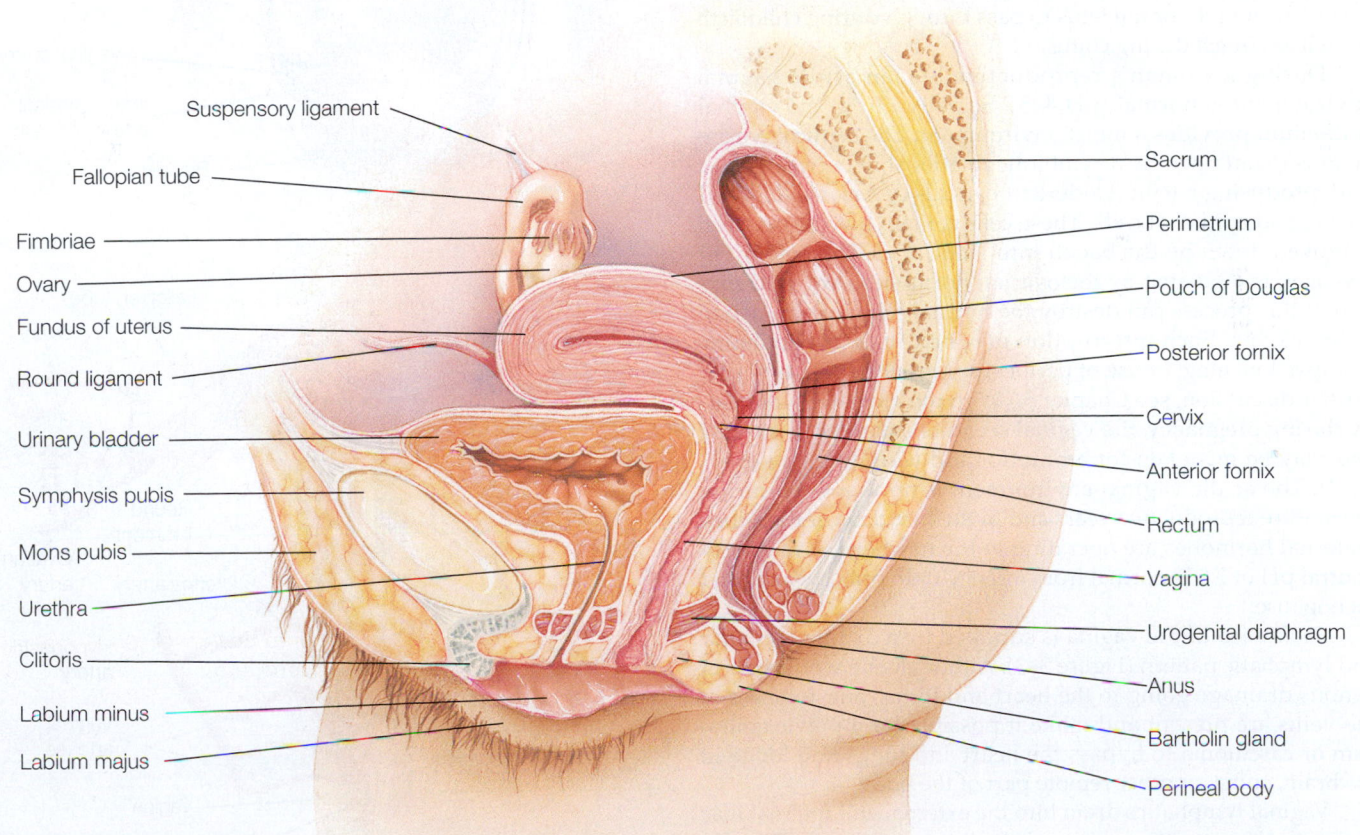

Figure 3–2 **Female internal reproductive organs.**

be palpated during vaginal examination and assessed with various instruments.

VAGINA

The **vagina** is a muscular and membranous tube that connects the external genitals with the uterus. It extends from the vulva to the uterus in a position nearly parallel to the plane of the pelvic brim. The vagina is often called the *birth canal* because it forms the lower part of the pelvic axis through which the fetus must pass during birth.

Because the cervix of the uterus projects into the upper part of the anterior wall of the vagina, the anterior wall is approximately 2.5 cm shorter than the posterior wall. Measurements range from 6 to 8 cm for the anterior wall and from 7 to 10 cm for the posterior wall (Cunningham et al., 2014).

In the upper part of the vagina, which is called the vaginal vault, there is a recess or hollow around the cervix. This area is called the *vaginal fornix.* Since the walls of the vaginal vault are very thin, various structures can be palpated through them, including the uterus, a distended bladder, the ovaries, the appendix, the cecum, the colon, and the ureters. The upper fourth of the vagina is separated from the rectum by the pouch of Douglas (sometimes referred to as the *cul-de-sac of Douglas*). This deep pouch or recess is posterior to the cervix.

When a woman lies on her back after intercourse, the space in the fornix permits the pooling of semen. The collection of a large number of sperm near the cervix at or near the time of ovulation increases the chances of pregnancy.

The walls of the vagina are covered with ridges, or *rugae,* crisscrossing each other. These rugae allow the vaginal tissues to stretch enough for the fetus to pass through during childbirth as well as stretch during coitus.

During a woman's reproductive life, an acidic vaginal environment is normal (pH 4–5). Secretion from the vaginal epithelium provides a moist environment. The acidic environment is maintained by a symbiotic relationship between lactic acid–producing bacilli (Döderlein bacillus or *lactobacillus*) and the vaginal epithelial cells. These cells contain glycogen, which is broken down by the bacilli into lactic acid. The amount of glycogen is regulated by the ovarian hormones. Any interruption of this process can destroy the normal self-cleaning action of the vagina. Such interruption may be caused by antibiotic therapy, douching, or use of perineal sprays or deodorants. (For further discussion, see Chapter 5.) With the increased vascularity during pregnancy, the vaginal secretions markedly increase and may be mistaken for amniotic fluid (Cunningham et al., 2014). The acidic vaginal environment is normal only during the mature reproductive years and in the first days of life, when maternal hormones are operating in the newborn. A relatively neutral pH of 7.5 is normal from infancy until puberty and after menopause.

Each third of the vagina is supplied by a distinct vascular and lymphatic pattern (Figure 3–3). Although one would expect venous drainage going to the heart and lungs, anastomoses of the veins are present and make it possible for a pelvic embolism or carcinoma to bypass the heart and lungs and lodge in the brain, spine, or other remote part of the body.

Vaginal lymphatics drain into the external and internal iliac nodes, the hypogastric nodes, and the inguinal glands. The posterior wall drains into nodes lying in the rectovaginal septum. Any vaginal infection follows these routes.

The pudendal nerve supplies what relatively little somatic innervation there is to the lower third of the vagina.

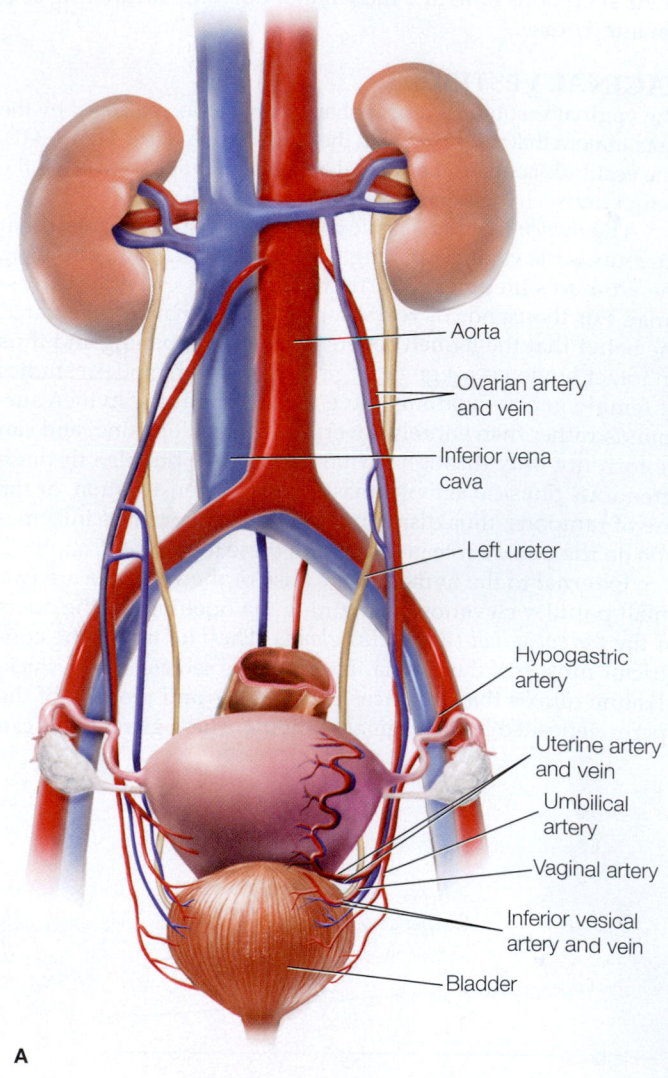

A

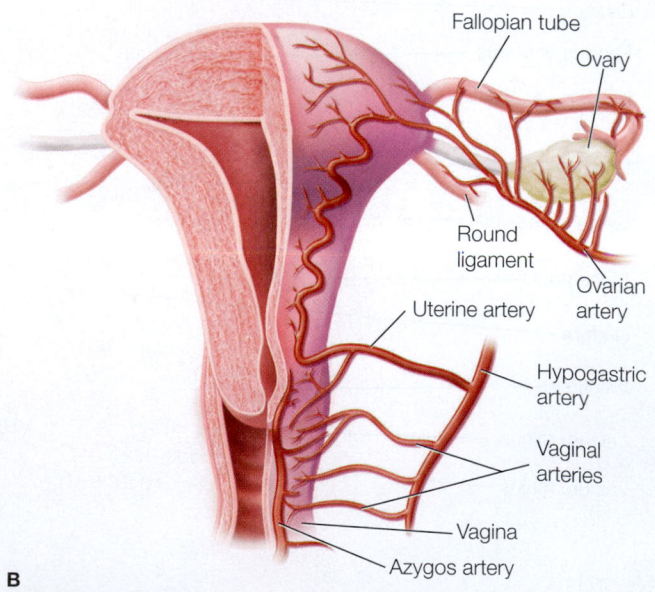

B

Figure 3–3 Blood supply to internal reproductive organs. A. Pelvic blood supply. B. Blood supply to vagina, ovaries, uterus, and fallopian tube.

Thus sensation during sexual excitement and coitus is reduced in this area, as is vaginal pain during the second stage of labor.

The vagina has three functions:

- To serve as the passage for sperm during coitus and for the fetus during birth
- To provide passage for the menstrual products from the uterine endometrium to the outside of the body
- To protect against trauma from sexual intercourse and infection from pathogenic organisms.

UTERUS

The **uterus** is a hollow, muscular, thick-walled organ shaped like an upside-down pear (Figure 3–4). It lies in the center of the pelvic cavity between the base of the bladder and the rectum and above the vagina. It is level with or slightly below the brim of the pelvis, with the external opening of the cervix (external os) about level with the ischial spines. In the never pregnant (nulligravid) mature woman, the uterus weighs about 60 g; it weighs more in a woman who has been pregnant. The uterus measures 6 to 8 cm in length in the nulligravid woman and 9 to 10 cm in multiparous women (Cunningham et al., 2014).

The body of the uterus can move freely forward or backward. Only the cervix is anchored laterally. Thus the position of the uterus can vary, depending on a woman's posture and musculature, number of children borne, bladder and rectal fullness, and even normal respiratory patterns. Generally, the uterus bends forward, forming a sharp angle with the vagina. Four pairs of ligaments (i.e., the cardinal, uterosacral, round, and broad) support the uterus. Single anterior and posterior ligaments also support the uterus.

The uterus is divided into two major parts: the upper triangular portion called the **corpus** or uterine body; and the lower cylindrical portion called the cervix. The corpus comprises the upper two thirds of the uterus and is composed mainly of a smooth muscle layer (myometrium). The lower third is the cervix or neck. The rounded uppermost portion of the corpus that extends above the points of attachment of the fallopian tubes is called the **fundus**. The elongated portion of the uterus where the fallopian tubes enter is called the **cornua**.

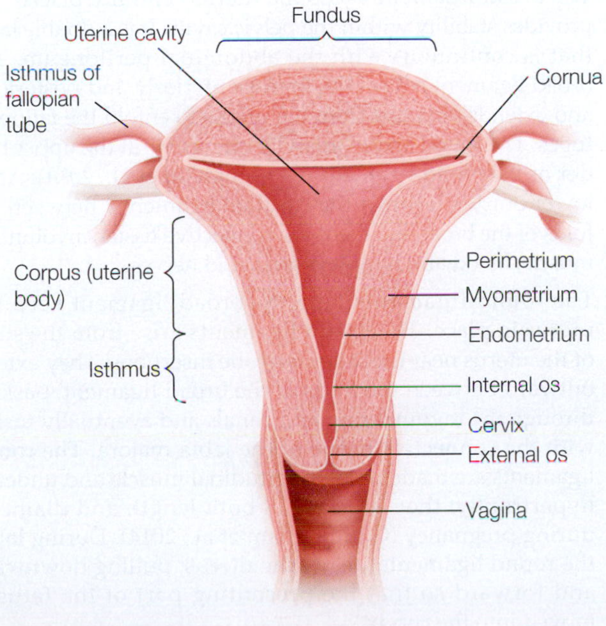

The *isthmus* is that portion of the uterus between the internal cervical os and the endometrial cavity. The isthmus is about 6 mm above the uterine opening of the cervix (the internal os), and it is in this area that the uterine lining changes into the mucous membrane of the cervix; it joins the corpus to the cervix. The isthmus takes on importance in pregnancy because it becomes the lower uterine segment. At birth, this thin lower segment, situated behind the bladder, is the site for lower segment cesarean births (see Chapter 22).

The blood and lymphatic supplies to the uterus are extensive. Innervation of the uterus is entirely by the autonomic nervous system. Even without an intact nerve supply, the uterus can contract adequately for birth; for example, hemiplegic women have adequate uterine contractions.

Pain of uterine contractions is carried to the central nervous system by the 11th and 12th thoracic nerve roots. Pain from the cervix and upper vagina passes through the ilioinguinal and pudendal nerves. The motor fibers to the uterus arise from the 7th and 8th thoracic vertebrae. Because the sensory and motor levels are separate, epidural anesthesia can be used during labor and birth.

The function of the uterus is to provide a safe environment for fetal development. The uterine lining is cyclically prepared by steroid hormones for implantation of the embryo, a process known as **nidation**. Once the embryo is implanted, the developing fetus is protected until it is expelled.

Both the body of the uterus and the cervix are changed permanently by pregnancy. The body never returns to its prepregnant size, and the external os changes from a circular opening of about 3 mm to a transverse slit with irregular edges.

UTERINE CORPUS

The uterine corpus is made up of three layers. The outermost layer is the *serosal layer*, or **perimetrium**, which is composed of peritoneum. The middle layer is the *muscular uterine layer,* or **myometrium**. This muscular uterine layer is continuous with the muscle layers of the fallopian tubes and the vagina. This characteristic helps these organs present a unified reaction to various stimuli—ovulation, orgasm, or the deposition of sperm in the vagina. These muscle fibers also extend into the ovarian, round, and cardinal ligaments and minimally into the uterosacral ligaments, which helps explain the vague but disturbing pelvic "aches and pains" reported by many pregnant women.

The myometrium has three distinct layers of uterine (smooth) involuntary muscles (Figure 3–5). The outer layer, found mainly over the fundus, is made up of longitudinal muscles that cause the descent of the fetus, which places pressure on the cervical fibers leading to cervical effacement and delivery of the fetus. The thick middle layer is made up of interlacing muscle fibers in figure-eight patterns that assist the longitudinal fibers in expelling the fetus. These muscle fibers surround large blood vessels, and their contraction produces a hemostatic action (a tourniquet-like action on blood vessels to stop bleeding after birth). The inner muscle layer consists of circular fibers that form sphincters at the fallopian tube attachment sites and at the internal os. The internal os sphincter inhibits the expulsion of the uterine contents during pregnancy but stretches in labor as cervical dilatation occurs. An incompetent cervical os can be caused by a torn, weak, or absent sphincter at the internal os. The sphincters at the fallopian tubes prevent menstrual blood from flowing backward into the fallopian tubes from the uterus.

Uterine cavity

Fundus

Isthmus of fallopian tube

Cornua

Corpus (uterine body)

Isthmus

Perimetrium

Myometrium

Endometrium

Internal os

Cervix

External os

Vagina

Figure 3–4 **Structures of the uterus.**

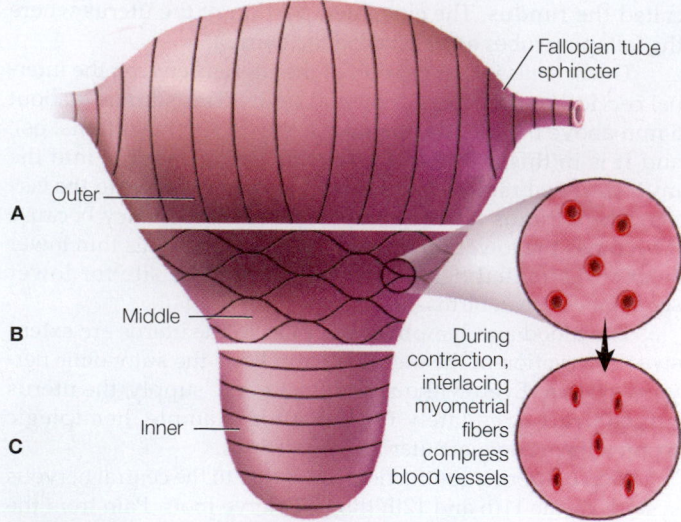

Fallopian tube sphincter

A Outer

B Middle

C Inner

During contraction, interlacing myometrial fibers compress blood vessels

Figure 3–5 Myometrium uterine muscle layers placement and function. A. Outer layer (longitudinal muscles) suited to expel fetus. B. Middle layer (interlacing muscle fibers in figure-eight pattern) surrounds and constricts blood vessels to stop bleeding. C. Inner layer (circular muscle fibers form sphincters at fallopian tubes and internal os) prevents backflow of menstrual blood into fallopian tubes and cervical dilatation during labor/delivery.

Although each layer of muscle has been discussed as having a unique function, it must be remembered that the uterine musculature works as a whole. The uterine contractions of labor are responsible for the dilatation of the cervix and provide the major force for the passage of the fetus through the pelvis and vaginal canal at birth.

The *mucosal layer,* or **endometrium**, of the uterine corpus is the innermost layer. This single layer consists of columnar epithelium, glands, and stroma. From menarche to menopause, the endometrium undergoes monthly degeneration and renewal in the absence of pregnancy. As it responds to the governing hormonal cycle and prostaglandin influence as well, the endometrium varies in thickness from 0.5 to 5 mm.

The glands of the endometrium produce a thin, watery, alkaline secretion that keeps the uterine cavity moist. This endometrial milk not only helps sperm travel to the fallopian tubes but also nourishes the developing embryo before it implants in the endometrium(for a discussion of implantation see Chapter 4).

The blood supply to the endometrium is unique. In the myometrium, the radial arteries branch off from the arcuate arteries at right angles. Once inside the endometrium, they become the basal arteries supplying the zona basalis (a layer of the endometrium) and ultimately become the coiled arteries supplying the zona functionalis (also part of the endometrium). The basal arteries are not sensitive to cyclic hormonal control; hence, the zona basalis portion remains intact and is the site of new endometrial tissue generation. The coiled arteries are extremely sensitive to hormonal control. Their response is alternate relaxation and constriction during the ischemic, or terminal, phase of the menstrual cycle. These differing responses allow part of the endometrium to remain intact while other endometrial tissue is shed during menstruation.

When pregnancy occurs and the endometrium is not shed, the reticular stromal cells surrounding the endometrial glands become the decidual cells of pregnancy. The stromal cells are highly vascular, channeling a rich blood supply to the endometrial surface.

CERVIX

The narrow neck of the uterus is the **cervix**. It meets the body of the uterus at the internal os and descends about 2.5 cm to 4.0 cm in a nonpregnant woman to connect with the vagina at the external os (Heitmann, 2013) (see Figure 3–4). Thus it provides a protective entrance for the body of the uterus. The cervix is divided by its line of attachment into the vaginal and supravaginal areas. The *vaginal cervix* projects into the vagina at an angle of from 45 to 90 degrees. The *supravaginal cervix* is surrounded by the attachments that give the uterus its main support: the uterosacral ligaments, the transverse ligaments of the cervix (Mackenrodt ligaments), and the pubocervical ligaments.

The vaginal cervix appears pink and ends at the external os. The cervical canal appears rosy red and is lined with columnar ciliated epithelium, which contains mucus-secreting glands. Most cervical cancer begins at this *squamocolumnar* junction. The specific location of the junction varies with age and number of pregnancies.

Elasticity is the chief characteristic of the cervix. It is able to stretch because of the high fibrous and collagenous content of the supportive tissues and also because of the vast number of folds in the cervical lining.

The cervical mucus has three functions:

- To lubricate the vaginal canal
- To act as a bacteriostatic agent
- To provide an alkaline environment to shelter deposited sperm from the acidic vaginal secretions.

At ovulation, cervical mucus is clearer, thinner, more profuse, and more alkaline than at other times.

UTERINE LIGAMENTS

The uterine ligaments support and stabilize the various reproductive organs. The ligaments shown in Figure 3–6 are described as follows:

1. The **broad ligament** keeps the uterus centrally placed and provides stability within the pelvic cavity. It is a double layer that is continuous with the abdominal peritoneum. The broad ligament covers the uterus anteriorly and posteriorly and extends outward from the uterus to enfold the fallopian tubes. The round and ovarian ligaments are at the upper border of the broad ligament (Cunningham et al., 2014). At its lower border, it forms the cardinal ligaments. Between the folds of the broad ligament are connective tissue, involuntary muscle, blood and lymph vessels, and nerves.

2. The **round ligaments** help the broad ligament keep the uterus in place. The round ligaments arise from the sides of the uterus near the fallopian tube insertions. They extend outward between the folds of the broad ligament, passing through the inguinal ring and canals and eventually fusing with the connective tissue of the labia majora. The round ligaments are made up of longitudinal muscle and undergo hypertrophy; they increase in both length and diameter during pregnancy (Cunningham et al., 2014). During labor the round ligaments steady the uterus, pulling downward and forward so that the presenting part of the fetus is moved into the cervix.

3. The **ovarian ligaments** anchor the lower pole of the ovary to the cornua of the uterus. They are composed of muscle

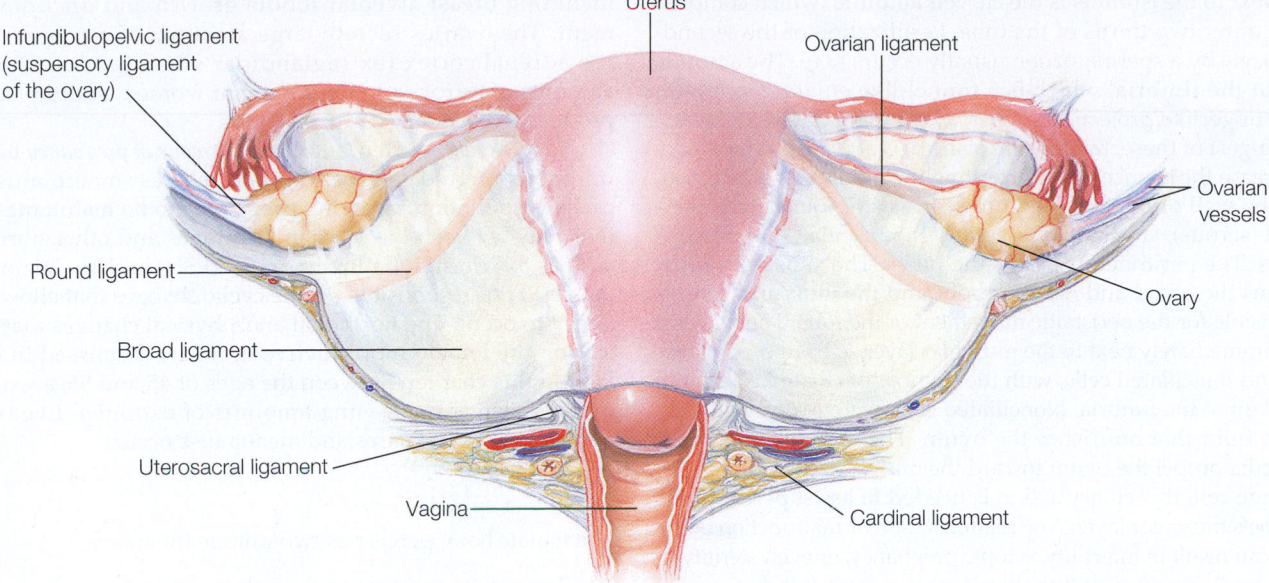

Figure 3–6   Uterine ligaments.

fibers that allow the ligaments to contract. This contractile ability influences the position of the ovary to some extent, thus helping the fimbriae of the fallopian tubes to "catch" the ovum as it is released each month.

4. The **cardinal ligaments** are the chief uterine supports and suspend the uterus from the side walls of the true pelvis. These ligaments, also known as Mackenrodt or transverse cervical ligaments, arise from the sides of the pelvic walls and attach to the cervix in the upper vagina. These ligaments prevent uterine prolapse and also support the upper vagina.

5. The **infundibulopelvic ligament** suspends and supports the ovaries. Arising from the outer third of the broad ligament, the infundibulopelvic ligament contains the ovarian vessels and nerves.

6. The **uterosacral ligaments** provide support for the uterus and cervix at the level of the ischial spines. Arising on each side of the pelvis from the posterior wall of the uterus, the uterosacral ligaments sweep back around the rectum and insert on the sides of the first and second sacral vertebrae.

The uterosacral ligaments contain smooth muscle fibers, connective tissue, blood and lymph vessels, and nerves. They also contain sensory nerve fibers that contribute to dysmenorrhea (painful menstruation) (see Chapter 5).

FALLOPIAN TUBES

The two **fallopian tubes**, also known as the *oviducts* or *uterine tubes*, arise from each side of the uterus and reach almost to the sides of the pelvis, where they turn toward the ovaries (Figure 3–7). Each tube is approximately 8 to 13.5 cm long. A short section of each fallopian tube is inside the uterus; its opening into the uterus is only 1 mm in diameter. The fallopian tubes link the peritoneal cavity with the uterus and vagina. This linkage increases a woman's biologic vulnerability to disease processes.

Each fallopian tube may be divided into three parts: the *isthmus*, the *ampulla*, and the infundibulum or *fimbria*. The fallopian tube **isthmus** is straight and narrow, with a thick muscular wall and an opening (lumen) 2 to 3 mm in diameter. It is the site of tubal ligation, a surgical procedure to prevent pregnancy (see Chapter 5).

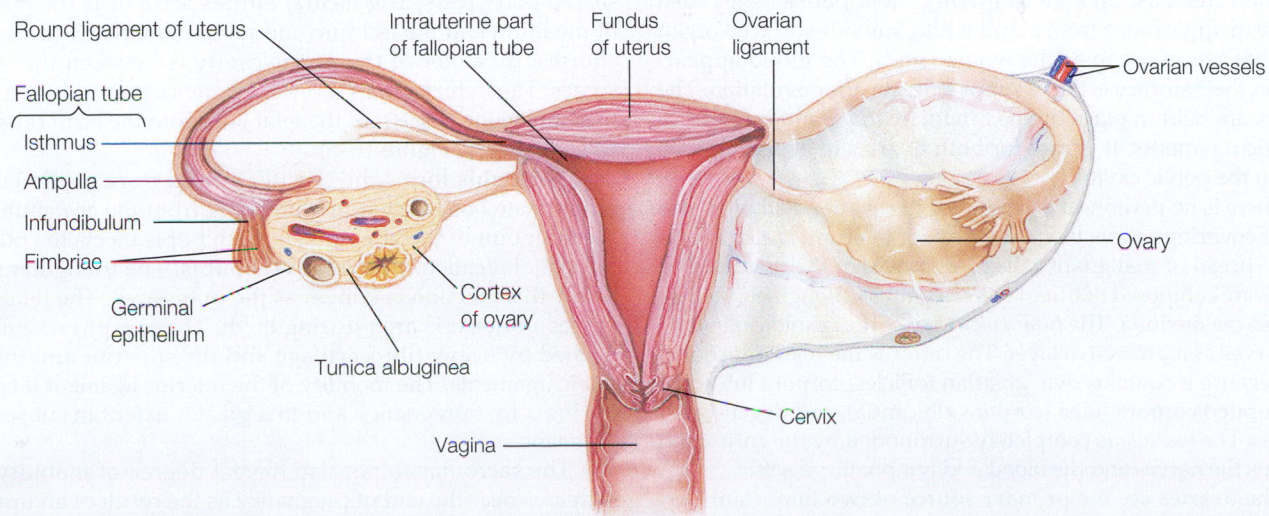

Figure 3–7   Fallopian tubes and ovaries.

Next to the isthmus is the curved **ampulla**, which comprises the outer two thirds of the tube. Fertilization of the secondary oocyte by a spermatozoon usually occurs here. The ampulla ends at the **fimbria**, which is a funnel-like enlargement with many fingerlike projections (*fimbriae*) reaching out to the ovary. The longest of these, the fimbria ovarica, is attached to the ovary to increase the chances of intercepting the ovum as it is released.

The wall of the fallopian tube consists of four layers: peritoneal (serous), subserous (adventitial), muscular, and mucous tissues. The peritoneum covers the tubes. The subserous layer contains the blood and nerve supply, and the muscular layer is responsible for the peristaltic movement of the tube. The mucosal layer, immediately next to the muscular layer, is composed of ciliated and nonciliated cells, with the number of ciliated cells more abundant at the fimbria. Nonciliated cells secrete a protein-rich, serous fluid that nourishes the ovum. The constantly moving tubal cilia propel the ovum toward the uterus. Because the ovum is a large cell, this ciliary action is needed to assist peristalsis in the tube's muscular layer. Any malformation or malfunction of the tubes can result in infertility, ectopic pregnancy, or even sterility.

A well-functioning tubal transport system involves active fimbriae close to the ovary, peristalsis of the tube created by the muscular layer, ciliated currents beating toward the uterus, and the proximal contraction and distal relaxation of the tube caused by different types of prostaglandins.

A rich blood and lymphatic supply serves each fallopian tube. Thus the tubes have an unusual ability to recover from an inflammatory process (see Figure 3–3). The fallopian tubes have three functions:

- To provide transport for the ovum from the ovary to the uterus (transport time through the fallopian tubes varies from 3 to 4 days)
- To provide a site for fertilization
- To serve as a warm, moist, nourishing environment for the ovum or zygote (fertilized egg) (See Chapter 4 for further discussion.)

OVARIES

The **ovaries** are two almond-shaped structures just below the pelvic brim. One ovary is located on each side of the pelvic cavity. Their size varies among women and with the stage of the menstrual cycle. Each ovary weighs approximately 6 to 10 g and is 1.5 to 3.0 cm wide, 2 to 5 cm long, and 1.0 to 1.5 cm thick. The ovaries of girls are small, but they become larger after puberty and then decrease in size following menopause. They also change in appearance from a dull white, smooth-surfaced organ to a pitted gray organ as the woman ages. The pitted appearance on their surface is the result of scarring after ovulation. The ovaries are held in place by the broad, ovarian, and infundibulopelvic ligaments. It is rare for both ovaries to be at the same level in the pelvic cavity.

There is no peritoneal covering for the ovaries. Although this lack of covering assists the mature ovum to erupt, it also allows easier spread of malignant cells from cancer of the ovaries. The ovaries are composed of three layers: the tunica albuginea, the cortex, and the medulla. The *tunica albuginea* is dense and dull white and serves as a protective layer. The *cortex* is the main functional part because it contains ova, graafian follicles, corpora lutea, the degenerated corpora lutea (corpora albicantia), and degenerated follicles. The *medulla* is completely surrounded by the cortex and contains the nerves and the blood and lymphatic vessels.

The ovaries are the primary source of two important hormones: the estrogens and progesterone. *Estrogens* are associated with those characteristics contributing to femaleness, including breast alveolar lobule growth and duct development. The ovaries secrete large amounts of estrogen, while the adrenal cortex (extraglandular sites) produces minute amounts of estrogen in nonpregnant women, and the fat cells produce a secondary estrogen.

Progesterone is often called the *hormone of pregnancy* because it inhibits uterine contractions and relaxes smooth muscle to cause vasodilation, allowing pregnancy to be maintained. The interplay between the ovarian hormones and other hormones such as follicle-stimulating hormone (FSH) and luteinizing hormone (LH) is responsible for the cyclic changes that allow pregnancy to occur. The hormonal and physical changes that occur during the female reproductive cycle are discussed in depth later in this chapter. Between the ages of 45 and 55, a woman's ovaries secrete decreasing amounts of estrogen. Eventually, ovulatory activity ceases and menopause occurs.

Bony Pelvis

The female bony pelvis has two unique functions:

- To support and protect the pelvic contents
- To form the relatively fixed axis of the birth passage.

Because the pelvis is so important to childbearing, its structure must be understood clearly.

BONY STRUCTURE

The pelvis is made up of four bones: two innominate bones, the sacrum, and the coccyx (or tailbone). The pelvis resembles a bowl or basin; its sides are the innominate bones, and its back is the sacrum and coccyx. Lined with fibrocartilage and held tightly together by ligaments (Figure 3–8), the four bones join at the symphysis pubis, the two sacroiliac joints, and the sacrococcygeal joints.

The *innominate bones,* also known as the hip bones, are made up of three separate bones: the ilium, ischium, and pubis. These bones fuse to form a circular cavity, the *acetabulum,* which articulates with the femur.

The *ilium* is the broad, upper prominence of the hip. The iliac crest is the margin of the ilium. The ischial spines, the foremost projections nearest the groin, are the site of attachment for ligaments and muscles.

The *ischium,* the strongest bone, is under the ilium and below the acetabulum. The L-shaped ischium ends in a marked protuberance, the ischial tuberosity, on which the weight of a seated body rests. The **ischial spines** arise near the junction of the ilium and the ischium and jut into the pelvic cavity. The shortest diameter of the pelvic cavity is between the ischial spines. The ischial spines serve as reference points during labor to evaluate the descent of the fetal head into the birth canal (see Chapter 16 and Figure 16–7).

The **pubis** forms the slightly bowed front portion of the innominate bone. Extending medially from the acetabulum to the midpoint of the bony pelvis, each pubis meets the other to form a joint called the **symphysis pubis**. The triangular space below this junction is known as the pubic arch. The fetal head passes under this arch during birth. The symphysis pubis is formed by heavy fibrocartilage and the superior and inferior pubic ligaments. The mobility of the inferior ligament increases during a first pregnancy and to a greater extent in subsequent pregnancies.

The sacroiliac joints also have a degree of mobility that increases near the end of pregnancy as the result of an upward, gliding movement. The pelvic outlet may be increased by 1.5 to 2 cm in the squatting, sitting, and dorsal lithotomy positions.

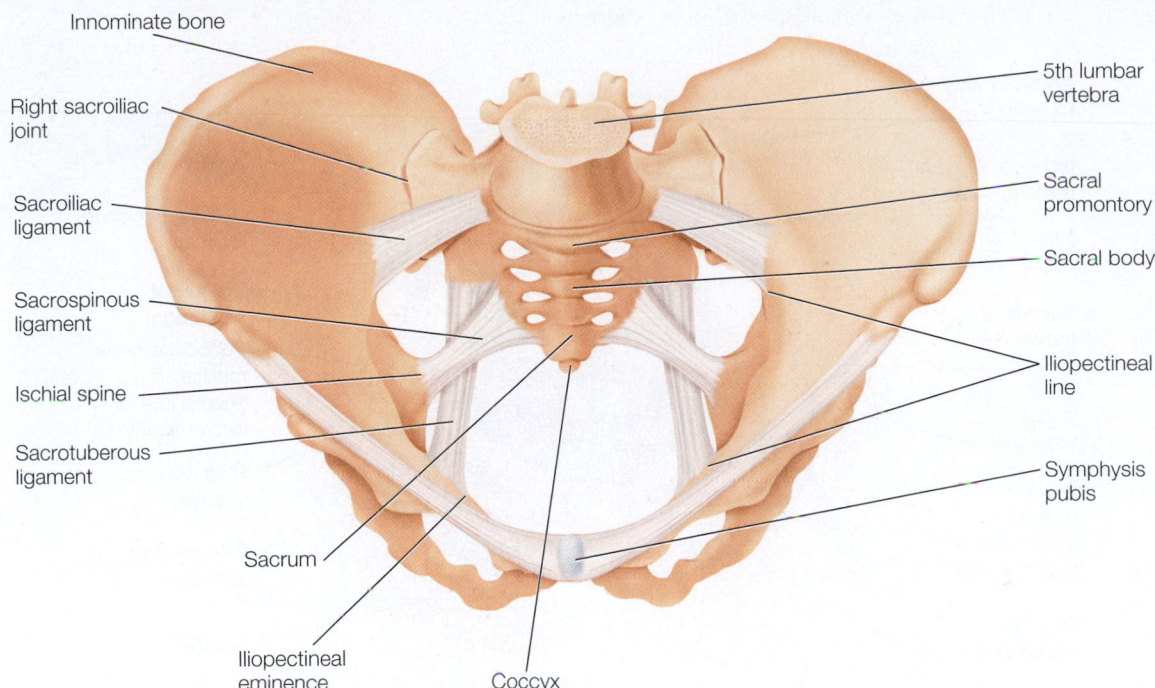

Innominate bone

Right sacroiliac
joint

Sacroiliac
ligament

Sacrospinous
ligament

Ischial spine

Sacrotuberous
ligament

Sacrum

Iliopectineal
eminence

Coccyx

5th lumbar
vertebra

Sacral
promontory

Sacral body

Iliopectineal
line

Symphysis
pubis

Figure 3–8 Pelvic bones with supporting ligaments.

These relaxations of the joints are induced by the hormones of pregnancy.

The *sacrum* is a wedge-shaped bone formed by the fusion of five vertebrae. The anterior upper portion of the sacrum has a projection into the pelvic cavity known as the **sacral promontory**. This projection is another obstetric guide in determining pelvic measurements. (For a discussion of pelvic measurements, see Chapter 9.)

The small triangular bone last on the vertebral column is the coccyx. It articulates with the sacrum at the sacrococcygeal joint. The coccyx usually moves backward during labor to provide more room for the fetus.

PELVIC FLOOR

The muscular floor of the bony pelvis is designed to overcome the force of gravity exerted on the pelvic organs. It acts as a supporting structure to the irregularly shaped pelvic outlet, thereby providing stability and support for surrounding structures.

Deep fascia, the levator ani, and coccygeal muscles form the part of the pelvic floor known as the **pelvic diaphragm**. The components of the pelvic diaphragm function as a whole, yet they are able to move over one another. This feature provides an exceptional capacity for dilatation during birth and return to prepregnancy condition following birth. Above the pelvic diaphragm is the pelvic cavity; below and behind it is the perineum. The sacrum is located posteriorly.

The levator ani muscle makes up the major portion of the pelvic diaphragm. It consists of four muscles: the iliococcygeus, pubococcygeus, puborectalis, and pubovaginalis. The iliococcygeal muscle, a thin muscular sheet underlying the sacrospinous ligament, helps the levator ani support the pelvic organs. Muscles of the pelvic floor are shown in Figure 3–9 and discussed in Table 3–1.

PELVIC DIVISION

The **pelvic cavity** is divided into the false pelvis and the true pelvis (Figure 3–10A). The **false pelvis**, the portion above the pelvic brim, or linea terminalis, serves to support the weight of the enlarged pregnant uterus and direct the presenting fetal part into the true pelvis below.

The **true pelvis** is the portion that lies below the pelvic brim. The bony circumference of the true pelvis is made up of the sacrum, coccyx, and innominate bones and represents the bony limits of the birth canal. The relationship between the true pelvis and the fetal head is of paramount importance: The size and shape of the true pelvis must be adequate for normal fetal passage during labor and at birth. The true pelvis consists of three parts: the inlet, the pelvic cavity, and the outlet (Figure 3–10B). Each part has distinct measurements that aid in evaluating the adequacy of the pelvis for childbirth. The effects of inadequate or abnormal pelvic diameters on labor and birth are discussed in Chapter 16.

The **pelvic inlet** is the upper border of the true pelvis and is typically rounded in the female. The size and shape of the pelvic inlet are determined by assessing three anteroposterior diameters: the diagonal conjugate, obstetric conjugate, and conjugate vera. The **diagonal conjugate** extends from the subpubic angle to the middle of the sacral promontory and is typically 12.5 cm. The diagonal conjugate can be measured manually during a pelvic examination. The **obstetric conjugate** extends from the middle of the sacral promontory to an area approximately 1 cm below the pubic crest. Its length is estimated by subtracting 1.5 cm from the length of the diagonal conjugate (Figure 3–11). The fetus passes through the obstetric conjugate, and the size of this diameter determines whether the fetus can move down into the birth canal in order for engagement to occur. The true (anatomic) conjugate, or **conjugate vera**, extends from the middle of the sacral promontory to the middle of the pubic crest (superior surface of the symphysis). One additional measurement, the transverse diameter, helps determine the shape of the inlet. The **transverse diameter** is the largest diameter of the inlet and is measured by using the linea terminalis as the point of reference.

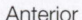

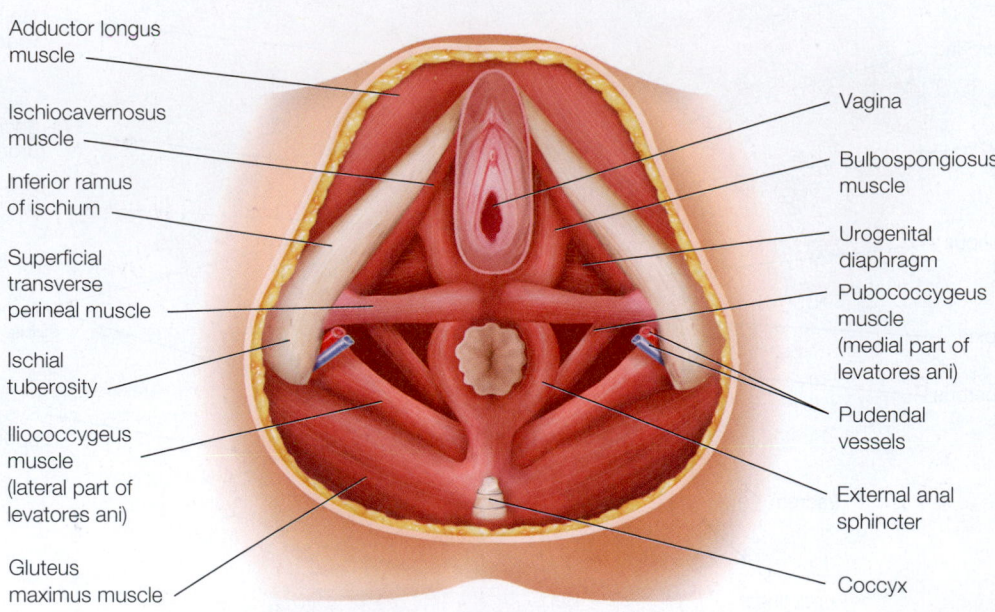

Anterior

Adductor longus muscle

Ischiocavernosus muscle

Inferior ramus of ischium

Superficial transverse perineal muscle

Ischial tuberosity

Iliococcygeus muscle (lateral part of levatores ani)

Gluteus maximus muscle

Vagina

Bulbospongiosus muscle

Urogenital diaphragm

Pubococcygeus muscle (medial part of levatores ani)

Pudendal vessels

External anal sphincter

Coccyx

Posterior

Figure 3–9 **Muscles of the pelvic floor. (The puborectalis, pubovaginalis, and coccygeal muscles cannot be seen from this view.)**

The mid-pelvis or *pelvic cavity* (canal) is a curved canal with a longer posterior than anterior wall. During labor, the descent of the fetal head into the true pelvis can be described by station and the midpelvis and ischial spines serve to mark zero station (Cunningham et al., 2014). A change in the lumbar curve can increase or decrease the tilt of the pelvis and can influence the progress of labor because the fetus has to adjust itself to this curved path as well as to the different diameters of the true pelvis.

The **pelvic outlet** is at the lower border of the true pelvis. The size of the pelvic outlet can be determined by assessing the outlet *transverse diameter*. The anteroposterior diameter of the pelvic outlet increases during birth as the presenting part pushes the coccyx posteriorly at the mobile sacrococcygeal joint.

Decreased mobility, a large head, and/or a forceful birth can cause the coccyx to break. As the baby's head emerges, the long diameter of the head (occipital frontal) parallels the long diameter of the outlet (anteroposterior).

The transverse diameter (*bi-ischial* or *intertuberous*) extends from the inner surface of one ischial tuberosity to the other. In the pelvic outlet, the transverse diameter is the shortest diameter and becomes even shorter if the woman has a narrowed pubic arch. The pubic arch is of great importance because the fetus must pass under it during birth. If it is narrow, the baby's head may be pushed backward toward the coccyx, making extension of the head difficult. This situation, known as *outlet dystocia*, may require the use of forceps or a cesarean birth. The shoulders of a large baby may also become wedged under the

TABLE 3–1 Muscles of the Pelvic Floor

MUSCLE	ORIGIN	INSERTION	INNERVATION	ACTION
Levator ani	Pubis, lateral pelvic wall, and ischial spine	Blends with organs in pelvic cavity	Inferior rectal, second, and third sacral nerves, plus anterior rami of third and fourth sacral nerves	Supports pelvic viscera; helps form pelvic diaphragm
Iliococcygeus	Pelvic surface of ischial spine and pelvic fascia	Central point of perineum, coccygeal raphe, and coccyx		Assists in supporting abdominal and pelvic viscera
Pubococcygeus	Pubis and pelvic fascia	Coccyx		
Puborectalis	Pubis	Blends with rectum; meets similar fibers from opposite side		Forms sling for rectum, just posterior to it; raises anus
Pubovaginalis	Pubis	Blends into vagina		Supports vagina
Coccygeus	Ischial spine and sacrospinous ligament	Lateral border of lower sacrum and upper coccyx	Third and fourth sacral nerves	Supports pelvic viscera; helps form pelvic diaphragm; flexes and abducts coccyx

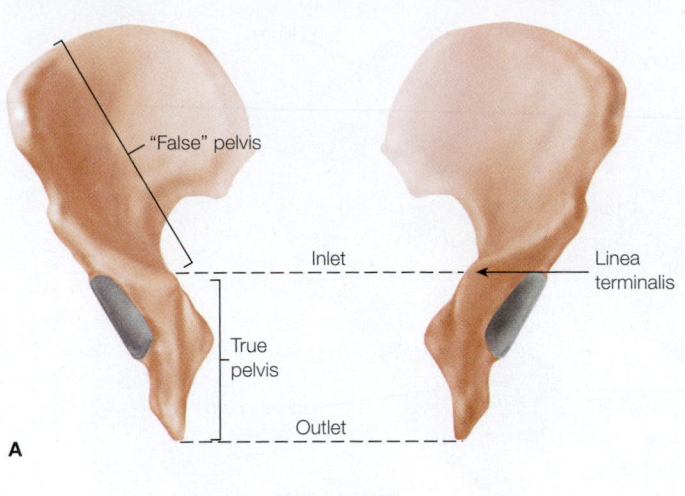

A

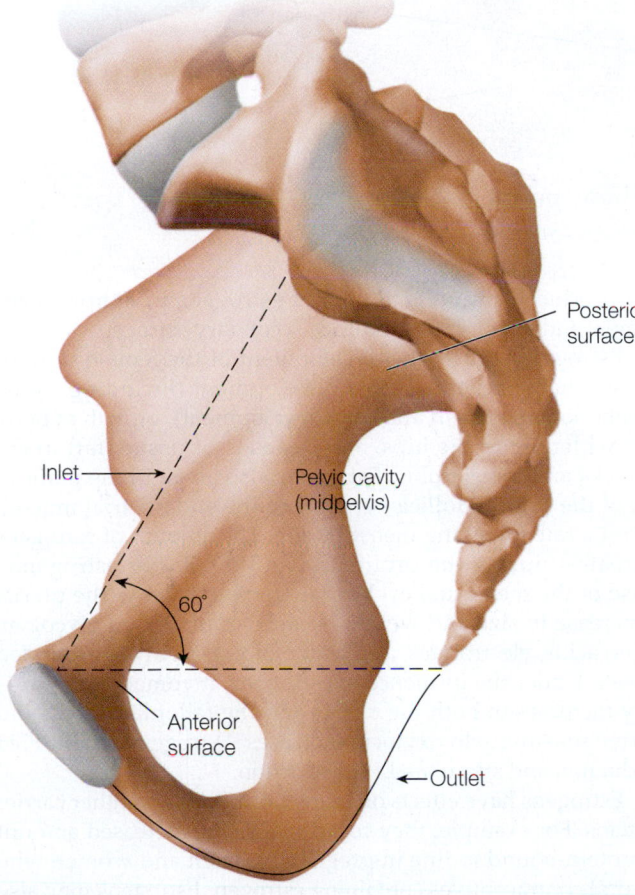

B

Figure 3–10   Female pelvis. A. False pelvis is a shallow cavity above the inlet; true pelvis is the deeper portion of the cavity below the inlet. B. True pelvis consists of inlet, cavity (midpelvis), and outlet.

pubic arch, making birth more difficult (see Chapter 22). The clinical assessment of each of these obstetrical diameters is discussed further in Chapter 9.

PELVIC TYPES

The Caldwell–Moloy classification of pelvises is widely used to differentiate bony pelvic types (Caldwell & Moloy, 1933). The four basic types are *gynecoid, android, anthropoid,* and *platypelloid* (see Figure 16–1). However, variations in the female pelvis are so great that classic types are not usual. Each type has a

characteristic shape, and each shape has implications for labor and birth, as discussed in detail in Chapter 21.

Breasts

The **breasts**, or *mammary glands,* considered accessories of the reproductive system, are specialized sebaceous glands (Figure 3–12). They are conical and symmetrically placed on the sides of the chest. The greater pectoral and anterior serratus muscles underlie each breast. Suspending the breasts are fibrous tissues, called *Cooper ligaments*, which extend from the deep fascia in the chest outward to just under the skin covering the breast. The left breast is frequently larger than the right. In different racial groups breasts develop at slightly different levels in the pectoral region of the chest.

In the center of each mature breast is the **nipple**, a protrusion about 0.5 to 1.3 cm in diameter. The nipple is composed mainly of erectile tissue, which becomes more rigid and prominent during the menstrual cycle, sexual excitement, pregnancy, and lactation. The nipple is surrounded by the heavily pigmented **areola**, which is 2.5 to 10 cm in diameter. Both the nipple and the areola are roughened by small papillae called *tubercles of Montgomery*. As a baby suckles, these tubercles secrete a fatty substance that helps lubricate and protect the nipple (Karam, 2013).

The breasts are composed of glandular, fibrous, and adipose tissue. The glandular tissue consists of acini, or alveoli, which are arranged in a series of 15 to 24 lobes separated from each other by adipose and fibrous tissue. Each lobe is made up of several lobules that are made up of many grapelike clusters of alveoli clustered around tiny ducts. The lining of these ducts secretes the various components of milk. The ducts from several lobules share common openings, commonly called nipple pores, and open on the surface of the nipple. The smooth muscle of the nipple causes erection of the nipple on contraction (Karam, 2013).

The biologic function of the breasts is to:

- Provide nourishment
- Provide protective maternal antibodies to babies through the lactation process
- Be a source of pleasurable sexual sensation.

Female Reproductive Cycle

The **female reproductive cycle (FRC)** is composed of the ovarian cycle, during which ovulation occurs, and the menstrual cycle, during which menstruation occurs. These two cycles take place simultaneously (Figure 3–13).

Effects of Female Hormones

After menarche, a woman undergoes a cyclic pattern of ovulation and menstruation, which is disrupted only by pregnancy for a period of 30 to 40 years. This cycle is an orderly process under neurohormonal control. Each month, multiple oocytes mature, with one rupturing from the ovary and entering the fallopian tube. The ovary, vagina, uterus, and fallopian tubes are major target organs for female hormones.

The ovaries produce mature gametes and secrete hormones (see discussion in Chapter 4). Ovarian hormones include estrogen, progesterone, and testosterone. The ovary is sensitive to follicle-stimulating hormone (FSH) and luteinizing hormone (LH). The uterus is sensitive to estrogen and

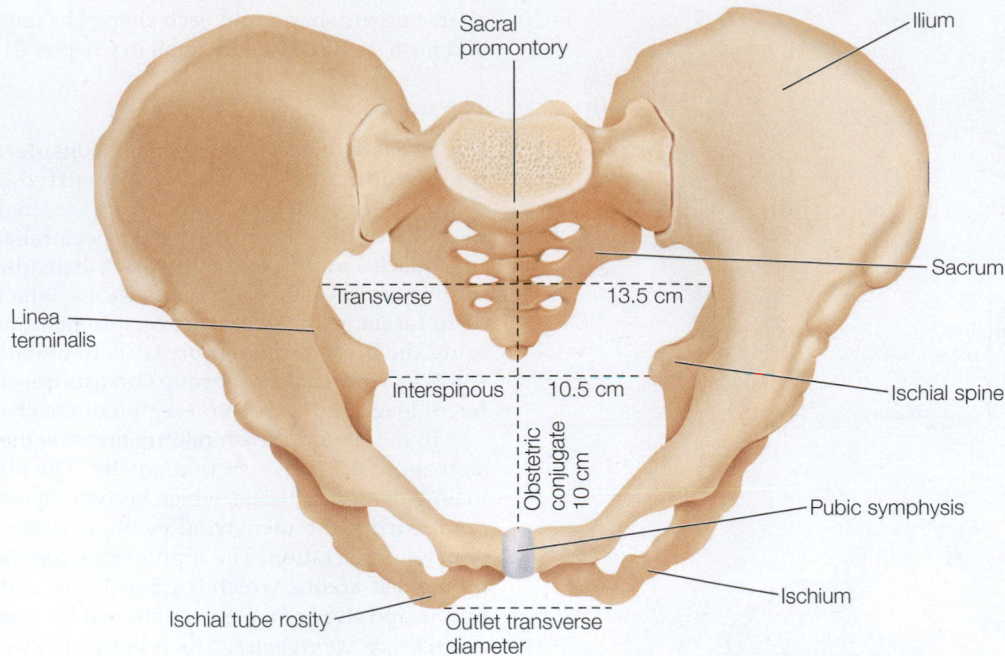

Figure 3–11 Pelvic planes: coronal section and diameters of the bony pelvis.

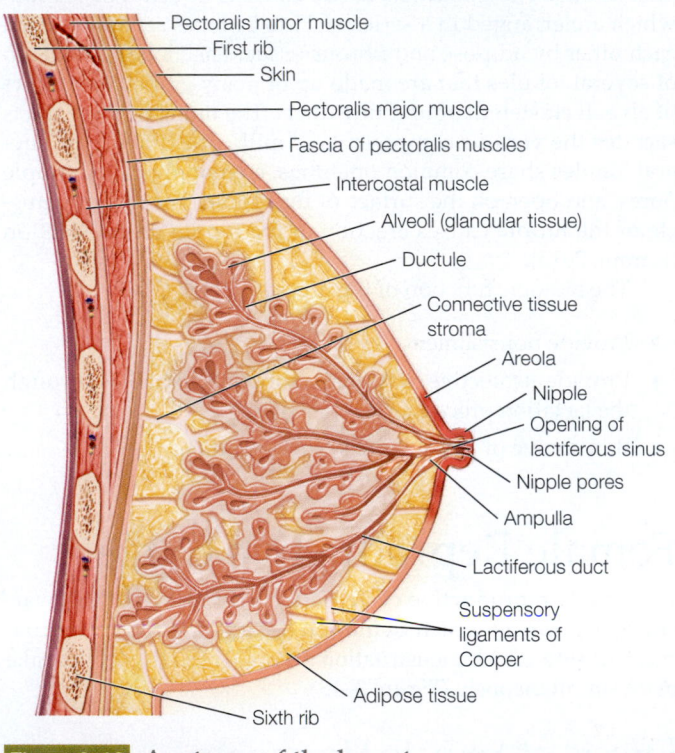

Figure 3–12 Anatomy of the breast.

progesterone. The relative proportion of these hormones to each other controls the events of both ovarian and menstrual cycles.

ESTROGENS

Estrogens are hormones associated with characteristics contributing to "femaleness." The major estrogenic effects are due primarily to three classical estrogens: estrone, β-estradiol, and estriol. The major estrogen is β-estradiol. The ovaries secrete large amounts of estrogen, while the adrenal cortex (extraglandular

site) produces minute amounts of estrogens in nonpregnant women, and the fat cells produce a secondary estrogen.

Estrogens control the development of the female secondary sex characteristics: breast development (including breast alveolar lobule growth and duct development), growth of body hair, widening of the hips, and deposits of tissue (fat) in the buttocks and mons pubis. Estrogens also assist in the maturation of the ovarian follicles and cause the endometrial mucosa to proliferate following menstruation. The amount of estrogens is greatest during the proliferative (follicular or estrogenic) phase of the menstrual cycle. Estrogens also cause the uterus to increase in size and weight because of increased glycogen, amino acids, electrolytes, and water. Blood supply is expanded as well. Under the influence of estrogens, myometrial contractility increases in both the uterus and the fallopian tubes, and uterine sensitivity to oxytocin increases. Estrogens inhibit FSH production and stimulate LH production.

Estrogens have effects on many hormones and other carrier proteins. For example, they contribute to the increased amount of protein-bound iodine in pregnant women and women who use oral contraceptives containing estrogen. Estrogens may also increase libidinal feelings in humans. They decrease the excitability of the hypothalamus, which may cause an increase in sexual desire.

PROGESTERONE

Progesterone is secreted by the corpus luteum and is found in greatest amounts during the secretory (luteal or progestational) phase of the menstrual cycle. Under the influence of progesterone the following occur:

- Vaginal epithelium proliferates
- Cervix secretes thick, viscous mucus
- Breast glandular tissue increases in size and complexity
- Breasts prepare for lactation
- Temperature rise of about 0.5 to 1.0°F (0.3 to 0.6°C) accompanies ovulation and persists throughout the secretory phase of the menstrual cycle.

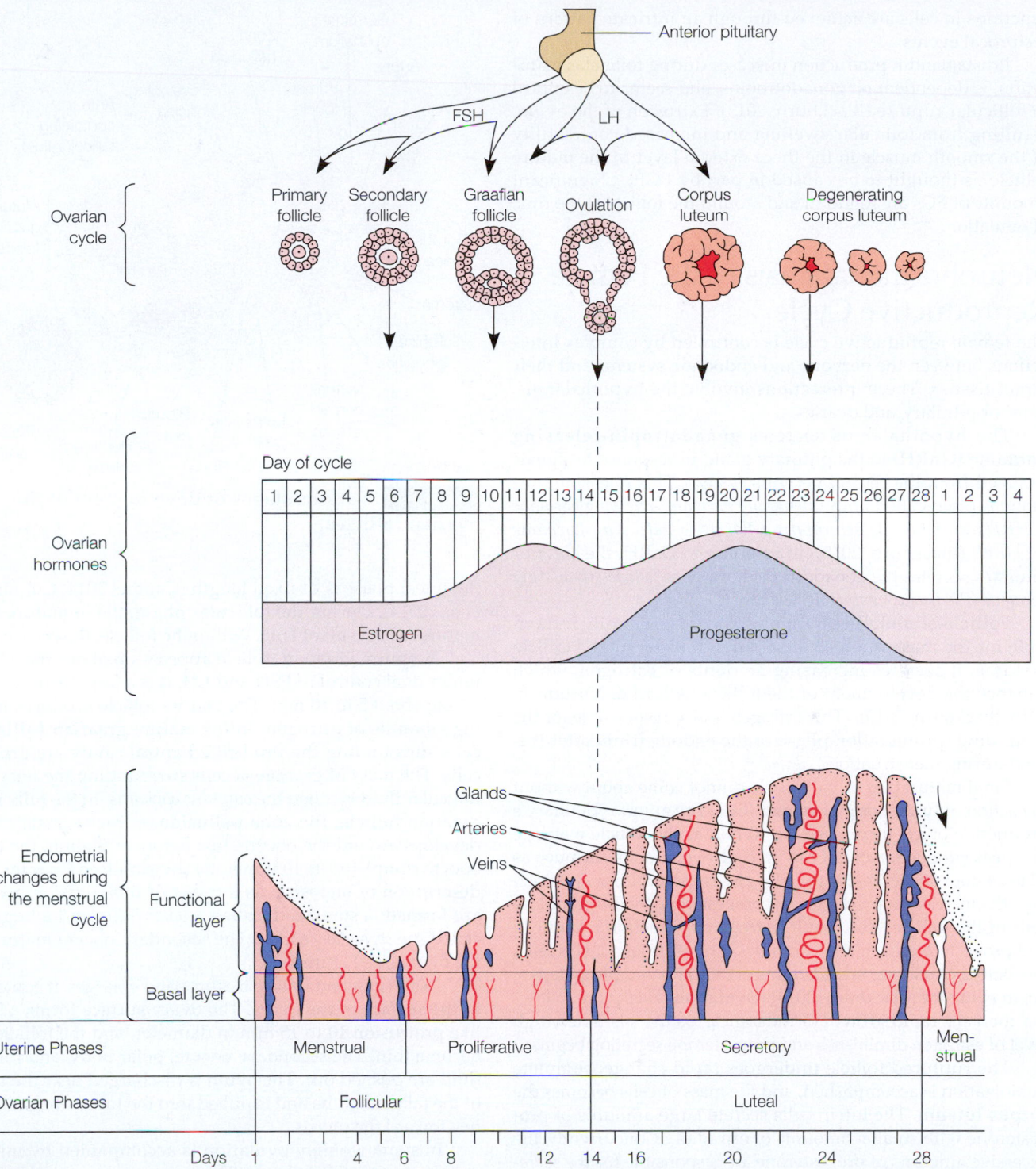

Figure 3–13 Female reproductive cycle: interrelationships of hormones with the three phases of the uterine cycle and the two phases of the ovarian cycle in an ideal 28-day cycle.

Progesterone is often called the hormone of pregnancy because it decreases the uterine motility and contractility caused by estrogens, and it relaxes smooth muscle to cause vasodilation, thereby preparing the uterus for implantation after the ovum is fertilized and maintaining pregnancy. The placenta is the primary source of progesterone during pregnancy. Progesterone also inhibits the action of prolactin in α-lactalbumin synthesis, thereby preventing lactation during pregnancy.

PROSTAGLANDINS

Prostaglandins (PGs) are oxygenated fatty acids that are produced by the cells of the endometrium and are also classified as hormones. Prostaglandins have varied action in the body. The two primary types of prostaglandins are groups E and F. Generally PGE relaxes smooth muscles and is a potent vasodilator; PGF is a potent vasoconstrictor and increases the contractility of muscles and arteries. Although the primary actions of PGE and PGF seem antagonistic, their basic regulatory functions in cells are achieved through an intricate pattern of reciprocal events.

Prostaglandin production increases during follicular maturation, is dependent on gonadotropins, and seems to be critical to follicular rupture (Blackburn, 2013). Extrusion of the ovum, resulting from follicular swelling and increased contractility of the smooth muscle in the theca externa layer of the mature follicle, is thought to be caused in part by $PGF_{2\alpha}$. Significant amounts of PGs are found in and around the follicle at the time of ovulation.

Neurohormonal Basis of the Female Reproductive Cycle

The female reproductive cycle is controlled by complex interactions between the nervous and endocrine systems and their target tissues. These interactions involve the hypothalamus, anterior pituitary, and ovaries.

The hypothalamus secretes **gonadotropin-releasing hormone (GnRH)** to the pituitary gland in response to signals received from the central nervous system. This releasing hormone is often called both *luteinizing hormone–releasing hormone (LHRH)* and *follicle-stimulating hormone–releasing hormone (FSHRH)* (Blackburn, 2013). In response to GnRH, the anterior pituitary secretes the gonadotropic hormones *follicle-stimulating hormone (FSH)* and *luteinizing hormone (LH)*.

Follicle-stimulating hormone (FSH) is primarily responsible for the maturation of the ovarian follicle. As the follicle matures, it secretes increasing amounts of estrogen, which enhance the development of the follicle (Alford & Nurudeen, 2013; Blackburn, 2013). (This estrogen is also responsible for the rebuilding/proliferation phase of the endometrium after it is shed during menstruation.)

Final maturation of the follicle cannot come about without the action of **luteinizing hormone (LH)**. The anterior pituitary's production of LH increases 6- to 10-fold as the follicle matures. The peak production of LH can precede ovulation by as much as 12 to 24 hours (Caudle, 2014). LH is also responsible for "luteinizing" the increase in production of progesterone by the granulose cells of the follicle. As a result, estrogen production is reduced and progesterone secretion continues. Thus estrogen levels fall a day before ovulation; tiny amounts of inhibitin and progesterone are in evidence (Blackburn, 2013). **Ovulation** takes place following the very rapid growth of the follicle, as the sustained high level of estrogen diminishes and progesterone secretion begins.

The ruptured follicle undergoes rapid change, complete luteinization is accomplished, and the mass of cells becomes the **corpus luteum**. The lutein cells secrete large amounts of progesterone with smaller amounts of estradiol. (Concurrently, the excessive amounts of progesterone are responsible for the secretory phase of the uterine cycle.) On day 7 or 8 following ovulation, the corpus luteum begins to involute, losing its secretory function. The production of both progesterone and estrogen is severely diminished. The anterior pituitary responds with increasingly large amounts of FSH; a few days later LH production begins. As a result, new follicles become responsive to another ovarian cycle and begin maturing.

Ovarian Cycle

The ovarian cycle has two phases: the *follicular phase* (days 1–14) and the *luteal phase* (days 15–28 in a 28-day cycle). Figure 3–14 depicts the changes that the follicle undergoes during the ovarian cycle. In women whose menstrual cycles vary, usually only the length of the follicular phase varies, because

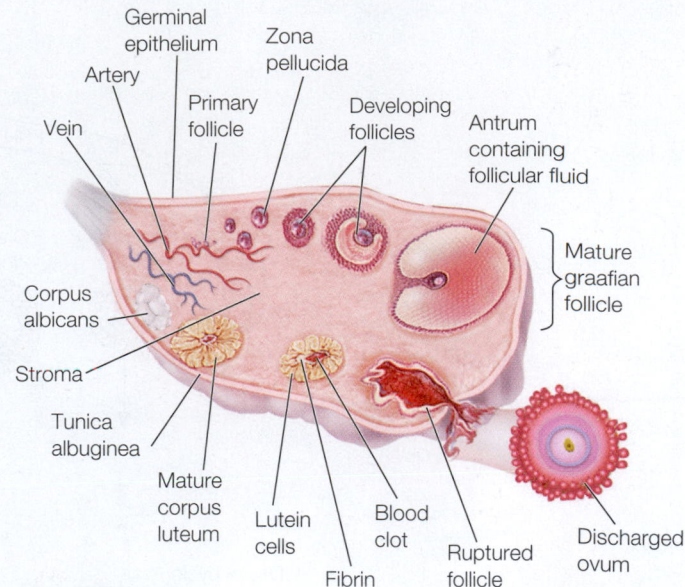

Figure 3–14 **Various stages of development of the ovarian follicles.**

the luteal phase is of fixed length (Caudle, 2014; Cunningham et al., 2014). During the follicular phase, the immature follicle matures as a result of FSH. Within the follicle, the oocyte grows.

A mature graafian follicle appears on about the 14th day under dual control of FSH and LH. It is a large structure, measuring about 5 to 10 mm. The mature follicle produces increasing amounts of estrogen. In the mature **graafian follicle**, the cells surrounding the fluid-filled antral cavity are granulosa cells. The mass of granulosa cells surrounding the oocyte and follicular fluid is called the *cumulus oophorus*. In the fully mature graafian follicle, the zona pellucida, a thick elastic capsule, develops around the oocyte. Just before ovulation, the mature oocyte completes its first meiotic division (see Chapter 4 for a description of meiosis). As a result of this division, two cells are formed: a small cell, called a *polar body*, and a larger cell, called the *secondary oocyte*. The secondary oocyte matures into the ovum (see Figure 4–1).

As the graafian follicle matures and enlarges, it comes close to the surface of the ovary. The ovary surface forms a blister-like protrusion 10 to 15 mm in diameter, and the follicle walls become thin. The secondary oocyte, polar body, and follicular fluid are pushed out. The ovum is discharged near the fimbria of the fallopian tube and is pulled into the tube to begin its journey toward the uterus.

In some women, ovulation is accompanied by midcycle pain known as *mittelschmerz*. This pain may be caused by a thick tunica albuginea or by a local peritoneal reaction to the expelling of the follicular contents. Vaginal discharge may increase during ovulation, and a small amount of blood (midcycle spotting) may be discharged as well.

The body temperature increases about 0.3° to 0.6°C (0.5° to 1.0°F) 24 to 48 hours after the time of ovulation. It remains elevated until the day before menstruation begins. There may be an accompanying sharp basal body temperature drop before the increase. These temperature changes are useful clinically to determine the approximate time ovulation occurs (Blackburn, 2013).

Generally the ovum takes several minutes to travel through the ruptured follicle to the fallopian tube opening. The contractions of the tube's smooth muscle and its ciliary action propel the ovum through the tube. The ovum remains in the ampulla, where, if it is fertilized, cleavage can begin. The ovum is thought to be fertile for only 6 to 24 hours. It reaches the uterus 72 to 96 hours after its release from the ovary.

The luteal phase begins when the ovum leaves its follicle. Under the influence of LH, the corpus luteum develops from the ruptured follicle. Within 2 or 3 days, the corpus luteum becomes yellowish and spherical and increases in vascularity. If the ovum is fertilized and implants in the endometrium, the fertilized egg begins to secrete **human chorionic gonadotropin (hCG)**, which is needed to maintain the corpus luteum. If fertilization does not occur, within about a week after ovulation the corpus luteum begins to degenerate, eventually becoming a connective tissue scar called the *corpus albicans*. With degeneration comes a decrease in estrogen and progesterone. This allows for an increase in LH and FSH, which triggers the hypothalamus.

Uterine (Menstrual) Cycle

Menstruation is cyclic uterine bleeding in response to cyclic hormonal changes. Menstruation occurs when the ovum is not fertilized and begins about 14 days after ovulation (in an ideal 28-day cycle), in the absence of pregnancy. The menstrual discharge, also referred to as the *menses*, or *menstrual flow*, is composed of blood mixed with fluid, cervical and vaginal secretions, bacteria, mucus, leukocytes, and other cellular debris. The menstrual discharge is dark red and has a distinctive odor.

Menstrual parameters vary greatly among individuals. Generally, menstruation occurs every 29 days, but it varies from 21 to 35 days. Some women normally have longer cycles, which can skew standard calculations of the estimated date of birth (EDB) when they become pregnant. Emotional and physical factors such as illness, excessive fatigue, stress or anxiety, and vigorous exercise programs can alter the cycle interval. Certain environmental factors such as temperature and altitude may also affect the cycle. The duration of menses is from 2 to 7 days, with the blood loss averaging 25 to 60 mL, and the loss of iron averaging 0.5 to 1 mg daily.

The uterine (menstrual) cycle has three phases: menstrual, proliferative, and secretory (see Figure 3–13). Menstruation occurs during the *menstrual phase*. Some endometrial areas are shed, although others remain. Some of the remaining tips of the endometrial glands begin to regenerate. The endometrium is in a resting state following menstruation. Estrogen levels are low, and the endometrium is 1 to 2 mm deep. During this part of the cycle, the cervical mucosa is scanty, viscous, and opaque.

The *proliferative phase* begins when the endometrial glands enlarge, becoming twisted and longer in response to increasing amounts of estrogen. The blood vessels become prominent and dilated, and the endometrium increases in thickness six- to eightfold. This gradual process reaches its peak just before ovulation. The cervical mucosa becomes thin, clear, watery, and more alkaline, making the mucosa more receptive to spermatozoa. As ovulation nears, the cervical mucosa shows increased elasticity (see Figure 5–4A). The cervical mucosa pH increases from below 7.0 to 7.5 at the time of ovulation. On microscopic examination, the mucosa shows a characteristic ferning pattern (Caudle, 2014) (see Figure 5–4B). See Teaching Highlights: Methods of Determining Ovulation in Chapter 7.

The *secretory phase* follows ovulation. The endometrium, under estrogenic influence, undergoes slight cellular growth. Progesterone, however, causes such marked swelling and growth that the epithelium is warped into folds. The amount of tissue glycogen increases. The glandular epithelial cells begin to fill with cellular debris, become twisted, and dilate. The glands

secrete small quantities of endometrial fluid in preparation for a fertilized ovum. The vascularity of the entire uterus increases greatly, providing a nourishing bed for implantation. If implantation occurs, the endometrium, under the influence of progesterone, continues to develop and become even thicker (see Chapter 4 for a discussion of implantation).

If fertilization does not occur, the *menstrual phase* (days 27–28) begins. The corpus luteum begins to degenerate, and as a result both estrogen and progesterone levels fall. Areas of necrosis appear under the epithelial lining. Extensive vascular changes also occur. Small blood vessels rupture, and the spiral arteries constrict and retract, causing a deficiency of blood in the endometrium, which becomes pale. Blood then escapes into the stromal cells of the uterus. The menstrual flow (days 1–6) begins, thus beginning the menstrual cycle again. After menstruation the basal layer remains, so that the tips of the glands can regenerate the new functional endometrial layer. See *Key Facts to Remember: Summary of the Female Reproductive Cycle*.

KEY FACTS TO REMEMBER
Summary of Female Reproductive Cycle

Ovarian Cycle

- *Follicular phase* (days 1–14): Primordial follicle matures under influence of FSH and LH up to the time of ovulation.
- *Luteal phase* (days 15–28): Ovum leaves follicle; corpus luteum develops under LH influence and produces high levels of progesterone and low levels of estrogen.

Menstrual Cycle

- *Menstrual phase* (days 1–6): Estrogen levels are low.
  Cervical mucus is scant, viscous, and opaque.
  Endometrium is shed.
- *Proliferative phase* (days 7–14): Endometrium and myometrium thickness increases.
  Estrogen peaks just before ovulation.
- Cervical mucus at ovulation:
  Is clear, thin, watery, alkaline.
  Is more favorable to sperm, shows ferning pattern, and has increased elasticity on microscopic exam.
  Just before ovulation, body temperature may drop slightly; then at ovulation basal body temperature increases 0.3° to 0.6°C (0.5° to 1.0°F).
  Mittelschmerz and/or midcycle spotting may occur.
- *Secretory phase* (days 15–26): Estrogen drops sharply, and progesterone dominates.
  Vascularity of entire uterus increases.
  Tissue glycogen increases, and the uterus is made ready for implantation.
- *Menstrual phase begins* (days 27–28): Both estrogen and progesterone levels drop.
  Spiral arteries undergo vasoconstriction.
  Endometrium becomes pale, blood vessels rupture.
  Blood escapes into uterine stromal cells, gets ready to be shed.

Male Reproductive System

The primary reproductive functions of the male genitals are to produce and transport sex cells (sperm) through and eventually out of the male genital tract and into the female genital tract. The external and internal genitals of the male reproductive system are shown in Figure 3–15.

External Genitals

The two external reproductive organs are the penis and scrotum.

PENIS

The *penis* is an elongated, cylindrical structure consisting of a body, called the *shaft*, and a cone-shaped end, called the *glans*. The penis lies in front of the scrotum. The shaft of the penis is made up of three longitudinal columns of erectile tissue: the paired *corpora cavernosa* and the *corpus spongiosum*. These columns are covered by dense fibrous connective tissue and then enclosed by elastic tissue. The penis is covered by a thin outer layer of skin.

The corpus spongiosum contains the urethra and becomes the glans at the distal end of the penis. The urethra widens within the glans and ends in a slitlike opening, located in the tip of the glans, called the *urethral meatus*. A circular fold of skin arises just behind the glans and covers it. Known as the *prepuce*, or *foreskin*, it may be removed by the surgical procedure of circumcision (see Chapter 25). If the corpus spongiosum does not surround the urethra completely, the urethral meatus may occur on the ventral aspect of the penile shaft (hypospadias) or on the dorsal aspect (epispadias).

The penis is innervated by the pudendal nerve. Sexual stimulation causes the penis to elongate, thicken, and stiffen, a process called *erection*. The penis becomes erect when its blood vessels become engorged, a consequence of parasympathetic nerve stimulation. If sexual stimulation is intense enough, the forceful and sudden expulsion of semen occurs through the rhythmic contractions of the penile muscles. This phenomenon is called *ejaculation*.

The penis serves both the urinary and the reproductive systems. Urine is expelled through the urethral meatus. The reproductive function of the penis is to deposit sperm in the vagina so that fertilization of the ovum can occur.

SCROTUM

The *scrotum* is a pouchlike structure that hangs in front of the anus and behind the penis. Composed of skin and the *dartos* muscle, the scrotum shows increased pigmentation and scattered hairs. The sebaceous glands open directly onto the scrotal surface; their secretion has a distinctive odor. Contraction of the dartos and cremasteric muscles shortens the scrotum and draws it closer to the body, thus wrinkling its outer surface. The degree of wrinkling is greatest in young men and at cold temperatures and is least in older men and at warm temperatures.

Inside the scrotum are two lateral compartments. Each compartment contains a testis with its related structures. Because the left spermatic cord grows longer, the left testis and its scrotal sac hang lower than the right. A ridge (raphe) on the external scrotal surface marks the position of the medial septum and continues anteriorly on the urethral surface of the penis, disappearing in the perineal area.

The function of the scrotum is to protect the testes and the sperm by maintaining a temperature lower than that of the body. Spermatogenesis cannot occur if the testes fail to descend and thus remain at body temperature. Because it is sensitive to touch, pressure, temperature, and pain, the scrotum defends against potential harm to the testes.

Male Internal Reproductive Organs

The male internal reproductive organs include the gonads (testes or testicles), a system of ducts (epididymides, vas deferens, ejaculatory duct, and urethra), and accessory glands (seminal vesicles, prostate gland, bulbourethral glands, and urethral glands).

TESTES

The *testes* are a pair of oval, compound glandular organs contained in the scrotum. In the sexually mature male, they are the site of spermatozoa production and the secretion of several male sex hormones.

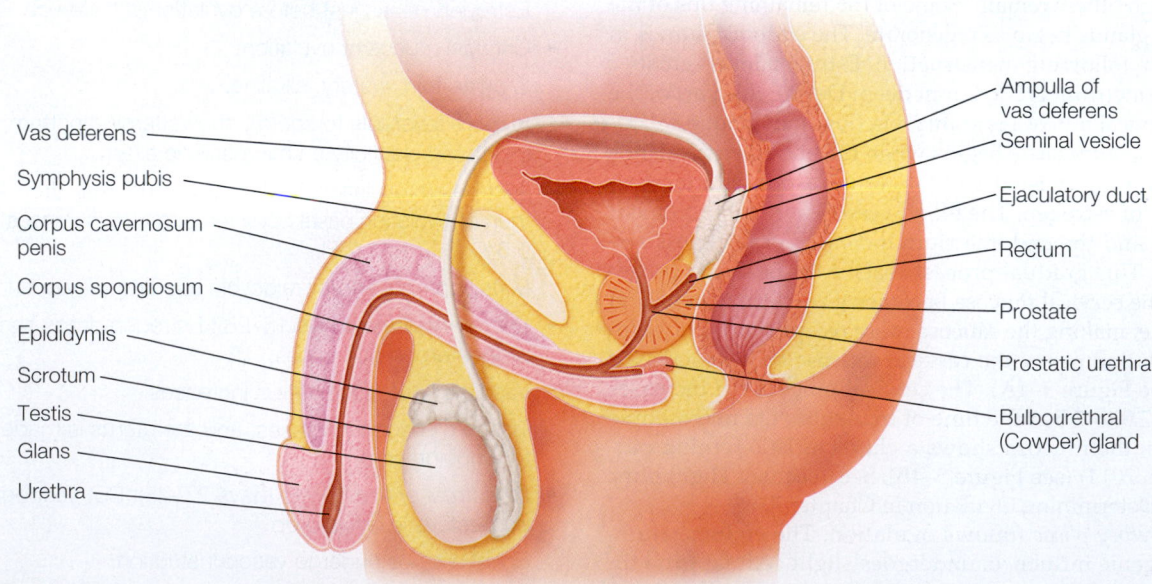

Vas deferens
Symphysis pubis
Corpus cavernosum penis
Corpus spongiosum
Epididymis
Scrotum
Testis
Glans
Urethra

Ampulla of vas deferens
Seminal vesicle
Ejaculatory duct
Rectum
Prostate
Prostatic urethra
Bulbourethral (Cowper) gland

Figure 3–15 Male reproductive system, sagittal view.

Each testis is 4 to 6 cm long, 2 to 3 cm wide, and 3 to 4 cm thick and weighs about 10 to 15 g. Each is covered by an outer serous membrane and an inner capsule that is tough, white, and fibrous. The connective tissue sends projections inward to form septa, dividing the testis into 250 to 400 lobules. Each lobule contains one to three tightly packed, convoluted *seminiferous tubules* containing sperm cells in all stages of development.

The seminiferous tubules are surrounded by loose connective tissue that houses abundant blood and lymph vessels and *interstitial (Leydig) cells*. The interstitial cells produce testosterone, the primary male sex hormone. The tubules also contain Sertoli cells, which nourish and protect the spermatocytes (for the phase between spermatids and spermatozoa—see Chapter 4).

The seminiferous tubules come together to form 20 to 30 straight tubules, which in turn form an anastomotic network of thin-walled spaces, the *rete testis*. The rete testis forms 10 to 15 efferent ducts that empty into the duct of the epididymis.

Most of the cells lining the seminiferous tubules undergo **spermatogenesis**, a process of maturation in which spermatocytes become spermatozoa. (Chapter 4 further discusses the process of spermatogenesis.) Sperm production varies among and within the tubules, with cells in different areas of the same tubule undergoing different stages of spermatogenesis. The sperm are eventually released from the tubules into the epididymis, where they mature further.

Like the female reproductive cycle, the process of spermatogenesis and other functions of the testes are the result of complex neural and hormonal controls. The hypothalamus secretes releasing factors that stimulate the anterior pituitary to release the gonadotropins—FSH and LH. These hormones cause the testes to produce **testosterone**, which maintains spermatogenesis, increases sperm production by the seminiferous tubules, and stimulates production of seminal fluid.

Testosterone is the most prevalent and potent of the testicular hormones. It is also responsible for the development of secondary male characteristics and certain behavioral patterns. The effects of testosterone include structural and functional development of the male genital tract, emission and ejaculation of seminal fluid, distribution of body hair, promotion of growth and strength of long bones, increased muscle mass, and enlargement of the vocal cords. The action of testosterone on the central nervous system is thought to produce aggressiveness and sexual drive. The action of testosterone is constant, not cyclic like that of the female hormones. Its production is not limited to a certain number of years, but it is thought to decrease with age.

The testes have two primary functions:

- Serve as the site of spermatogenesis
- Produce testosterone.

EPIDIDYMIS

The *epididymis* (plural, *epididymides*) is a duct about 5.6 m long, although it is convoluted into a compact structure about 3.75 cm long. An epididymis lies behind each testis. It arises from the top of the testis, courses downward, and then passes upward, where it becomes the vas deferens.

The epididymis provides a reservoir for maturing spermatozoa. When discharged from the seminiferous tubules into the epididymis, the sperm are immotile and incapable of fertilizing an ovum. The spermatozoa usually remain in the epididymis for 2 to 10 days but can be stored in the body for up to 42 days. As the sperm move along the tortuous course of the epididymis they become both motile and fertile.

VAS DEFERENS AND EJACULATORY DUCTS

The *vas deferens*, also known as the *ductus deferens*, is about 40 cm long and connects the epididymis with the prostate. One vas deferens arises from the posterior border of each testis. It joins the spermatic cord and weaves over and between several pelvic structures until it meets the vas deferens from the opposite side. Each vas deferens terminus expands to form the *terminal ampulla*. It then unites with the seminal vesicle duct (a gland) to form the ejaculatory duct, which enters the prostate gland and ends in the prostatic urethra. The ejaculatory ducts serve as passageways for semen and fluid secreted by the seminal vesicles. The main function of the vas deferens is to rapidly squeeze the sperm from their storage sites (the epididymis and distal part of the vas deferens) into the urethra.

Men who choose to take total responsibility for birth control may elect to have a vasectomy. In this procedure, the scrotal portion of the vas deferens is surgically incised or cauterized. Although sperm continue to be produced for the next several years, they can no longer reach the outside of the body. Eventually, the sperm deteriorate and are reabsorbed.

URETHRA

The *male urethra* is the passageway for both urine and semen. The urethra begins in the bladder and passes through the prostate gland, where it is called the *prostatic urethra*. The urethra emerges from the prostate gland to become the *membranous urethra*. It terminates in the penis, where it is called the *penile urethra*. In the penile urethra, goblet secretory cells are present, and smooth muscle is replaced by erectile tissue.

ACCESSORY GLANDS

The male accessory glands secrete a unique and essential component of the total seminal fluid in an ordered sequence.

The *seminal vesicles* are two glands composed of many lobes. Each vesicle is about 7.5 cm long. They are situated between the bladder and the rectum, immediately above the base of the prostate. The epithelium lining the seminal vesicles secretes an alkaline, viscous, clear fluid rich in high-energy fructose, prostaglandins, fibrinogen, and amino acids. During ejaculation, this fluid mixes with the sperm in the ejaculatory ducts. This fluid helps provide an environment favorable to sperm motility and metabolism.

The *prostate gland* encircles the upper part of the urethra and lies below the neck of the bladder. Made up of several lobes, it measures about 4 cm in diameter and weighs 20 to 30 g. The prostate is made up of both glandular and muscular tissue. It secretes a thin, milky, alkaline fluid containing high levels of zinc, calcium, citric acid, and acid phosphatase. This fluid protects the sperm from the acidic environment of the vagina and the male urethra, which would otherwise be spermicidal.

The *bulbourethral (Cowper) glands* are a pair of small, round structures on either side of the membranous urethra. The glands secrete a clear, thick, alkaline fluid rich in mucoproteins that becomes part of the semen. This secretion also lubricates the penile urethra during sexual excitement and neutralizes the acid in the male urethra and the vagina, thereby enhancing sperm motility.

The *urethral (Littré) glands* are tiny mucus-secreting glands found throughout the membranous lining of the penile urethra. Their secretions add to those of the bulbourethral glands. See *Key Facts to Remember: Summary of Male Reproductive Organ Functions.*

KEY FACTS TO REMEMBER
Summary of Male Reproductive Organ Functions

- The testes house seminiferous tubules and gonads.
- Seminiferous tubules contain sperm cells in various stages of development and undergoing meiosis.
- Sertoli cells nourish and protect spermatocytes (phase between spermatids and spermatozoa).
- Leydig cells are the main source of testosterone.
- Epididymides provide an area for maturation of sperm and a reservoir for mature spermatozoa.
- The vas deferens connects the epididymis with the prostate gland, then connects with ducts from the seminal vesicle to become an ejaculatory duct.
- Ejaculatory ducts provide a passageway for semen and seminal fluid into the urethra.
- Seminal vesicles secrete yellowish fluid rich in fructose, prostaglandins, and fibrinogen. This provides nutrition that increases motility and the fertilizing ability of sperm. Prostaglandins also aid fertilization by making the cervical mucus more receptive to sperm.
- The prostate gland secretes thin, alkaline fluid containing calcium, citric acid, and other substances. This alkalinity counteracts the acidity of ductus and seminal vesicle secretions.
- Bulbourethral (Cowper) glands secrete alkaline, viscous fluid into semen, aiding in neutralization of acidic vaginal secretions.

SEMEN

The male ejaculate, *semen* or *seminal fluid*, is made up of spermatozoa and the secretions of all the accessory glands. The seminal fluid transports viable and motile sperm to the female reproductive tract. Effective transportation of sperm requires adequate nutrients, an adequate pH (about 7.5), a specific concentration of sperm to fluid, and an optimal osmolarity.

A spermatozoon is made up of a head and a tail (Figure 3–16). The head's main components are the acrosome and the nucleus.

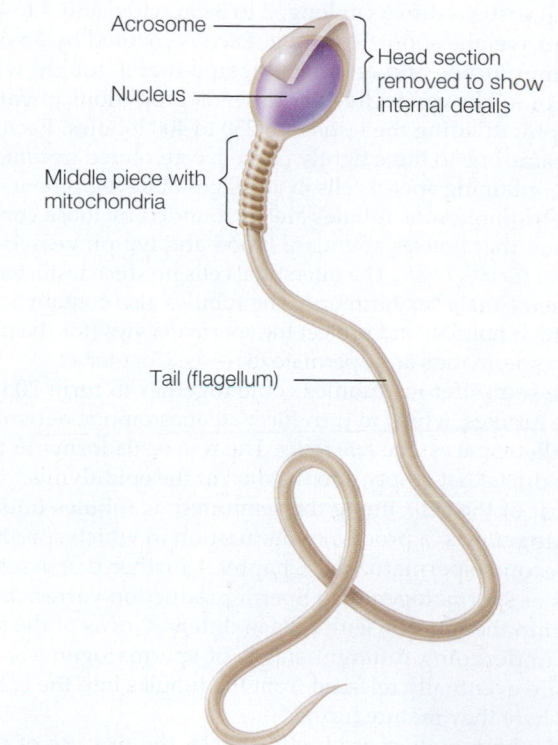

Figure 3–16 Schematic representation of a mature spermatozoon.

The head carries the male's haploid number of chromosomes (23), and it is the part that enters the ovum at fertilization (see Chapter 4). The tail, or *flagellum*, is specialized for motility. The tail is divided into the middle and the end piece.

Sperm may be stored in the epididymis and distal vas deferens for up to 42 days, depending primarily on the frequency of ejaculations. The average volume of ejaculate following abstinence for several days is 2 to 5 mL but may vary from 1 to 10 mL. Repeated ejaculation results in decreased volume. Once ejaculated, sperm can live for 2 or 3 days in the female genital tract.

Focus Your Study

- Reproductive activities require complex interactions between the reproductive structures, the central nervous system, and such endocrine glands as the pituitary, hypothalamus, testes, and ovaries.

- The female reproductive system consists of the ovaries, where female germ cells and female sex hormones are formed; the fallopian tubes, which capture the ovum and allow transport to the uterus; the uterus, which is the implantation site for the fertilized ovum; the cervix, which is a protective portal for the body of the uterus and the connection between the vagina and the uterus; and the vagina, which is the passageway from the external genitals to the uterus and provides for discharge of menstrual products out of the body.

- The pelvic structure of the true pelvis consists of an inlet, cavity (midpelvis), and outlet and must be adequate for normal fetal passage during labor and birth. The midpelvis (cavity) structure includes the ischial spines, which are used to mark the descent of the fetal head into the true pelvis.

- Estrogen causes endometrial mucosa to proliferate following menstruation and increases the size and weight of the uterus. It increases uterine sensitivity to oxytocin and therefore increases myometrial contractility in both the uterus and the fallopian tubes. Estrogen inhibits FSH production while stimulating LH production. Progesterone decreases uterine motility and contractility. It causes uterine endometrium to increase its nutrient store and arterial blood supply.

The vaginal epithelium proliferates and the cervix secretes thick, viscous mucus. Progesterone increases breast glandular tissue and prepares the breasts for lactation. Prostaglandins are necessary for follicular rupture.

- The female reproductive cycle may be described in terms of the ovarian cycle, during which ovulation occurs, and the menstrual cycle, during which menstruation occurs. These two cycles take place simultaneously and are under neurohormonal control.

- The ovarian cycle has two phases: the follicular phase and the luteal phase. During the follicular phase, the primordial follicle matures under the influence of FSH and LH until ovulation occurs. The luteal phase begins when the ovum leaves the follicle and the corpus luteum develops under the influence of LH. The corpus luteum produces high levels of progesterone and low levels of estrogen.

- The menstrual cycle has three phases: menstrual, proliferative, and secretory. Menstruation is characterized by degeneration of the corpus luteum, decreases in both estrogen and progesterone levels, constriction of the spiral arteries, and escape of blood into the stromal cells of the endometrium. Then begins the actual shedding of the endometrial lining, when estrogen levels are low. The proliferative phase begins when the endometrial glands begin to enlarge under the influence of estrogen and cervical mucosal changes occur; the changes peak at ovulation. The secretory phase follows ovulation, and, influenced primarily by progesterone, the uterus increases its vascularity to make ready for possible implantation.

- The male reproductive system consists of the testes, where male germ cells and male sex hormones are formed; a series of continuous ducts through which spermatozoa are transported outside the body; accessory glands that produce secretions important to sperm nutrition, survival, and transport; and the penis, which serves as the reproductive organ of intercourse.

Clinical Reasoning in Action

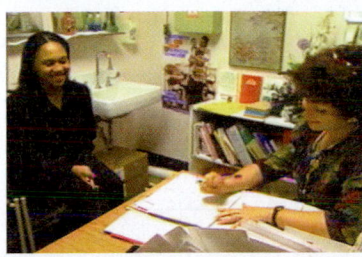

You are working in the OB/GYN clinic when Sally Smith, a 17-year-old teenager, comes in complaining of irregular menses. She believes her periods are really "messed up" and interfering with her active schedule. She wants them to be more regular and asks you for birth control. She tells you that she is a member of the swimming team and is a senior in high school. She says she is planning to start community college next year to obtain an associate degree in computer technology. You assess Sally's history as follows: menarche began at age 12; periods occur every 28 to 32 days. She usually experiences cramping in the first 2 days and the flow lasts 4 to 5 days. She uses an average of 4 to 5 tampons a day during her period. She has never been hospitalized, has no prior medical problems, and is up to date on her immunizations except for meningitis.

1. Based on your knowledge of menstruation, how would you describe Sally's menstrual cycle?

2. What is your primary goal in discussing Sally's menstrual cycle with her?

3. What information would you give Sally relating to her menstrual cycle?

4. What important request does Sally have?

5. Sally expresses problems dealing with the cramping she experiences with the first 2 days of her menses. What would you suggest to Sally to cope with the discomfort?

References

Alford, C., & Nurudeen, S. (2013). Physiology of reproduction in women. In A. H. DeCherney, L. Nathan, N. Lauffer, & A. S. Roman (Eds.), *Current diagnosis and treatment: Obstetrics & gynecology* (10th ed.). Boston, MA: McGraw-Hill.

Blackburn, S. T. (2013). *Maternal, fetal, & neonatal physiology: A clinical perspective* (4th ed.). St. Louis, MO: Saunders.

Caldwell, W. E., & Moloy, H. C. (1933). Anatomical variations in the female pelvis and their effect on labor with a suggested classification [Historical article]. *American Journal of Obstetrics and Gynecology, 26*, 479–505.

Caudle, P. W. (2014). Reproductive tract structure and function. In R. G. Jordan, J. L. Engstrom, J. A. Marfell, & C. L. Farley (Eds.), *Prenatal and postnatal care: A women-centered approach*. Ames, IA: Wiley Blackwell.

Cunningham, F. G., Leveno, K. J., Bloom, S. L., Spong, C. Y., Dashe, J. S., Hoffman, B. L., . . . Sheffield, J. S. (2014). *Williams obstetrics* (24th ed.). New York, NY: McGraw-Hill.

Heitmann, R. J. (2013). Anatomy of the female reproductive system. In A. H. DeCherney, L. Nathan, N. Lauffer, & A. S. Roman (Eds.), *Current diagnosis and treatment: Obstetrics & gynecology* (10th ed.). Boston, MA: McGraw-Hill.

Karam, A. (2013). The breast. In A. H. DeCherney, L. Nathan, N. Lauffer, & A. S. Roman (Eds.), *Current diagnosis and treatment: Obstetrics & gynecology* (10th ed.). Boston, MA: McGraw-Hill.

Morris, D. (2007). The pubic hair. In D. Morris, *The naked woman: A study of the female body*. New York, NY: Thomas Dunne Books.

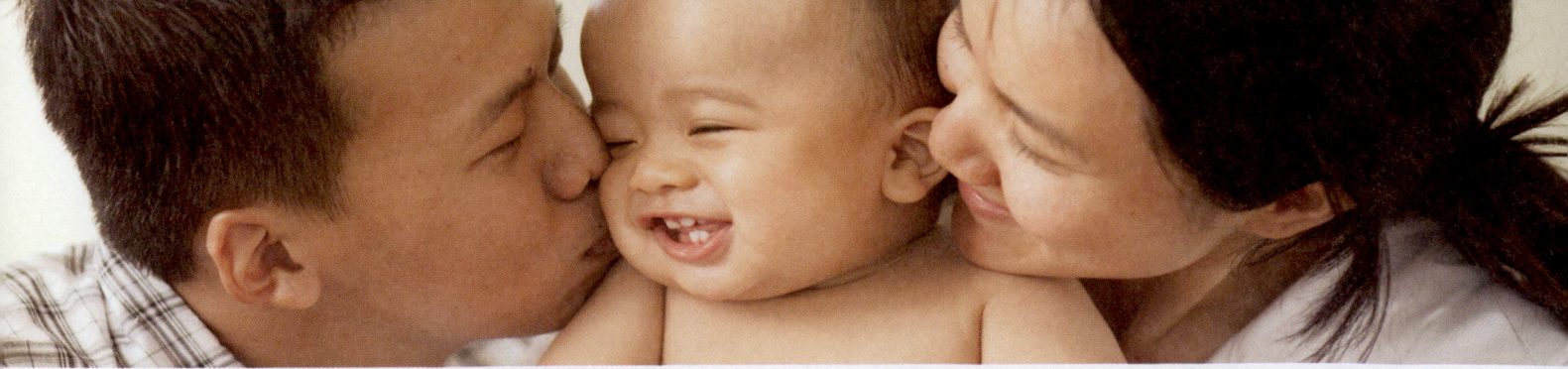

Chapter 4
Conception and Fetal Development

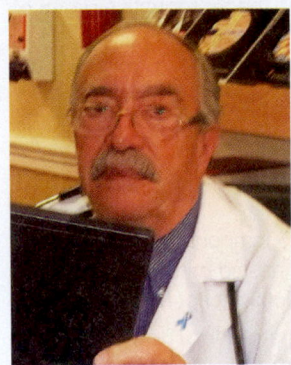

I love teaching the course content on conception and fetal development. Each time, I am struck anew by the absolute magic of human reproduction.

—Department of Nursing Faculty Member

⌄ Learning Outcomes

4.1 Differentiate between meiotic cellular division and mitotic cellular division.

4.2 Compare the processes by which ova and sperm are produced.

4.3 Analyze the components of the fertilization process and how each may impact fertilization.

4.4 Summarize the processes that occur during the cellular multiplication and differentiation stages of intrauterine development and their effect on the structures that form.

4.5 Compare the factors and processes by which fraternal (dizygotic) and identical (monozygotic) twins are formed.

4.6 Describe the development, structure, and functions of the placenta and umbilical cord during intrauterine life (embryonic and fetal development).

4.7 Contrast the significant changes in growth and development of the fetus at 4, 6, 12, 16, 20, 24, 28, 36, and 40 weeks' gestation.

4.8 Identify the factors that influence congenital malformations of the various organ systems.

The human genome contains *genes*, which are units of genetic information. Genes are encoded in the DNA that makes up the chromosomes in the nucleus of each cell. These chromosomes, which determine the structure and function of organ systems and traits, are of the same biochemical substances. How then does each person become unique? The answer lies in the physiologic mechanisms of heredity, the processes of cellular division, and the environmental factors that influence our development from the moment we are conceived. This chapter explores the processes involved in conception and fetal development—the basis of human uniqueness.

Cellular Division

Each human begins life as a single cell called a *fertilized ovum* or **zygote**. This single cell reproduces itself, and in turn each resulting cell also reproduces itself in a continuing process. The new cells are similar to the cells from which they came. Cells are reproduced by either mitosis or meiosis, two different but related processes.

Mitosis

Mitosis results in the production of diploid body (somatic) cells, which are exact copies of the original cell. During mitosis, the cell undergoes several changes ending in cell division. As the last phase of cell division nears completion, a furrow develops in the cell cytoplasm, which divides it into two daughter cells, each with its own nucleus. Daughter cells have the same **diploid number of chromosomes** (46) and same genetic makeup as the cell from which they came. After a cell with 46 chromosomes goes through mitosis, the result is two identical cells, each with 46 chromosomes. Mitosis makes growth and development possible, and in mature individuals it is the process by which our body cells continue to divide and replace themselves.

Meiosis

Meiosis is a special type of cell division by which diploid cells in the testes and ovaries give rise to **gametes** (sperm and ova). These cells are different from somatic (body) cells because they contain half the genetic material of the parent cell—only 23 chromosomes—the **haploid number of chromosomes**.

Meiosis consists of two successive cell divisions. In the first division, the chromosomes replicate. Next, a pairing takes place between homologous chromosomes (Sadler, 2015). Instead of separating immediately, as in mitosis, the chromosomes become closely intertwined. At each point of contact, there is a physical exchange of genetic material between the chromatids (the arms of the chromosomes). New combinations are provided by the newly formed chromosomes; these combinations account for the wide variation of traits in people (e.g., hair or eye color). The chromosome pairs then separate, and the members of the pair move to opposite sides of the cell. (In contrast, during mitosis the chromatids of each chromosome separate and move to opposite poles.) The cell divides, forming two daughter cells, each with 23 double-structured chromosomes—the same amount of deoxyribonucleic acid (DNA) as a normal somatic cell. In the second division, the chromatids of each chromosome separate and move to opposite poles of each of the daughter cells. Cell division occurs, resulting in the formation of four cells, each containing 23 single chromosomes (the haploid number of chromosomes). These daughter cells contain only half the DNA of a normal somatic cell (Sadler, 2015).

Chromosomal mutations may occur during the second meiotic division, for example, if two of the chromatids do not move apart rapidly enough when the cell divides. The still-paired chromatids are carried into one of the daughter cells and eventually form an extra chromosome. Another type of chromosomal mutation can occur if chromosomes break during meiosis. The effects of the chromosomal mutations of *nondisjunction* and *translocation* are described in Chapter 7. See *Key Points to Remember: Comparison of Mitosis and Meiosis.*

Gametogenesis

Meiosis occurs during **gametogenesis**, the process by which germ cells, or gametes (ovum and sperm), are produced. Each gamete must have only the haploid number (23) of chromosomes so that when the female gamete (egg or ovum) and the male gamete (sperm or spermatozoon) unite to form the zygote (fertilized ovum), the normal human diploid number of chromosomes (46) is reestablished.

Oogenesis

Oogenesis is the process that produces the female gamete, called an ovum (egg). As discussed in Chapter 3, the ovaries begin to develop early in the fetal life of the female. All the ova that the female will produce in her lifetime are present at birth. The ovary gives rise to oogonial cells, which develop into oocytes. Meiosis (cell replication by division) begins in all oocytes before the

female fetus is born but stops before the first division is complete and remains in this arrested phase until puberty. During puberty, the mature primary oocyte proceeds (by oogenesis) through the first meiotic division in the graafian follicle of the ovary.

The first meiotic division produces two cells of unequal size with different amounts of cytoplasm but with the same number of chromosomes. These two cells are the *secondary oocyte* and a minute *polar body*. Both the secondary oocyte and the polar body contain 22 double-structured autosomal chromosomes and one double-structured sex chromosome (X).

At the time of ovulation, a second meiotic division begins immediately and proceeds as the secondary oocyte moves down the fallopian tube. Division is again not equal, and the secondary oocyte moves into the metaphase stage of cell division, where its meiotic division is arrested until and unless the oocyte is fertilized.

When the secondary oocyte completes the second meiotic division after fertilization, the result is a mature ovum with the haploid number of chromosomes and virtually all the cytoplasm. In addition, the second polar body (also haploid) forms at this time. The first polar body has now also divided, producing two additional polar bodies. Thus, at the completion of meiosis, four haploid cells have been produced: the three polar bodies, which eventually disintegrate, and one ovum (Sadler, 2015) (Figure 4–1A).

Spermatogenesis

During puberty, the germinal epithelium in the seminiferous tubules of the testes begins the process of spermatogenesis, which produces the male gamete (sperm). The diploid spermatogonium replicates before it enters the first meiotic division, during which it is called the *primary spermatocyte*. During this first meiotic division, the spermatogonium replicates and forms two cells called *secondary spermatocytes*, each of which contains

KEY FACTS TO REMEMBER
Comparison of Mitosis and Meiosis

Mitosis

Purpose

Produce cells for growth and tissue repair. Cell division characteristic of all somatic cells.

Cell Division

One-stage cell division.

Number of Daughter Cells

Two daughter cells identical to the mother cell, each with the diploid number of chromosomes (46).

Meiosis

Purpose

Produce reproductive cells (gametes). Reduction of chromosome number by half (from diploid [46] to haploid [23]), so that when fertilization occurs the normal diploid number is restored. Introduces genetic variability.

Cell Division

Two-stage reduction.

Number of Daughter Cells

Four daughter cells, each containing one-half the number of chromosomes as the mother cell, or 23 chromosomes. Non-identical to original cell.

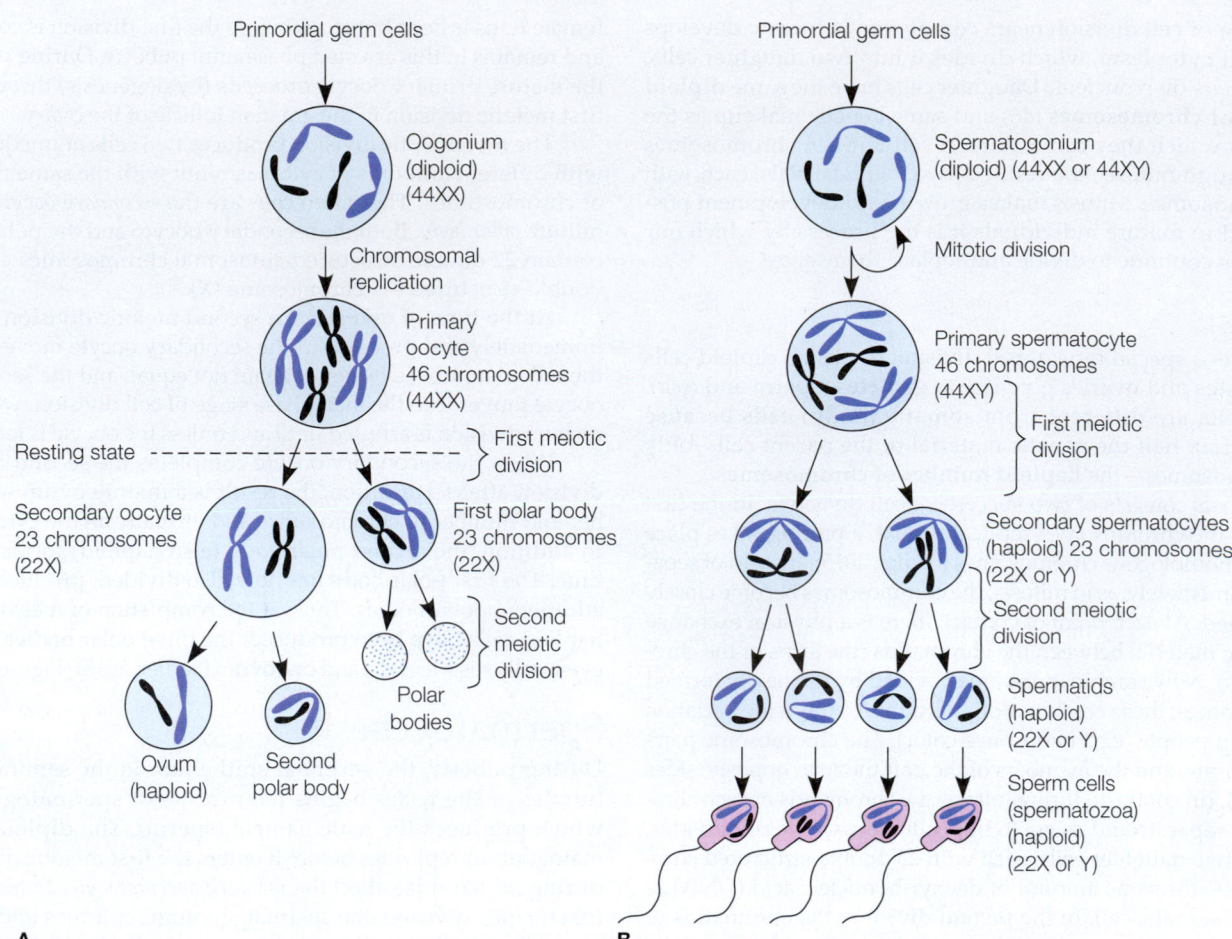

Figure 4–1 Gametogenesis involves meiosis within the ovary and the testis. A. During meiosis each oogonium produces a single haploid ovum once some cytoplasm moves into the polar bodies. B. Each spermatogonium, in contrast, produces four haploid spermatozoa.

22 double-structured autosomal chromosomes and either a double-structured X sex chromosome or a double-structured Y sex chromosome. During the second meiotic division, they divide to form four spermatids, each with the haploid number of chromosomes. The spermatids undergo a series of changes during which they lose most of their cytoplasm and become sperm (spermatozoa) (see Figure 4–1B). The nucleus becomes compacted into the head of the sperm, which is covered by a cap called an *acrosome* that is, in turn, covered by a plasma membrane. A long tail is produced from one of the centrioles.

The Process of Fertilization

Fertilization is the process by which a sperm fuses with an ovum to form a new diploid cell, or zygote. The zygote begins life as a single cell with a complete set of genetic material, 23 chromosomes from the mother's ovum and 23 chromosomes from the father's sperm for a total of 46 chromosomes. The following events lead to fertilization.

Preparation for Fertilization

The mature ovum and spermatozoa have only a brief time to unite. Ova are considered fertile for about 12 to 24 hours after ovulation. Sperm can survive in the female reproductive tract for 48 to 72 hours, but are believed to be healthy and highly fertile for only about 24 hours.

The ovum's cell membrane is surrounded by two layers of tissue. The layer closest to the cell membrane is called the *zona pellucida*.

It is a clear, noncellular layer whose thickness influences the fertilization rate. Surrounding the zona pellucida is a ring of elongated cells, called the *corona radiata* because the cells radiate from the ovum like the gaseous corona around the sun. These cells are held together by hyaluronic acid. The ovum has no inherent power of movement. During ovulation, high estrogen levels increase peristalsis within the fallopian tubes, which helps move the ovum through the tube toward the uterus. The high estrogen levels also cause a thinning of the cervical mucus, facilitating movement of the sperm through the cervix, into the uterus, and up the fallopian tube.

The process of fertilization takes place in the ampulla (outer third) of the fallopian tube. In a single ejaculation, the male deposits approximately 200 to 500 million spermatozoa into the vagina, of which only hundreds of sperm actually reach the ampulla (Sadler, 2015; Caudle, 2014). Fructose in the semen, secreted by the seminal vesicles, is the energy source for the sperm. The spermatozoa propel themselves up the female tract by the flagellar movement of their tails. Transit time from the cervix into the fallopian tube can be from as short as 30 minutes to as long as 6 days (Sadler, 2015). Prostaglandins in the semen may increase uterine smooth muscle contractions, which help transport the sperm. The fallopian tubes have a dual ciliary action that facilitates movement of the ovum toward the uterus and movement of the sperm from the uterus toward the ovary.

The sperm must undergo two processes before fertilization can occur: capacitation and the acrosomal reaction. **Capacitation** is the removal of the plasma membrane overlying the spermatozoa's acrosomal area and the loss of seminal plasma proteins. If the glycoprotein coat is not removed, the sperm will not be able to fertilize the ovum (Sadler, 2015). Capacitation occurs in the female reproductive tract (aided by uterine enzymes) and is thought to take about 7 hours. Sperm that undergo capacitation now take on three characteristics: (1) the ability to undergo the acrosomal reaction, (2) the ability to bind to the zona pellucida, and (3) the acquisition of hypermotility.

The **acrosomal reaction** follows capacitation, whereby the acrosomes of the sperm surrounding the ovum release their enzymes (hyaluronidase, a protease called acrosin, and trypsin-like substances) and thus break down the hyaluronic acid in the ovum's corona radiata (Sadler, 2015). Hundreds of acrosomes must rupture before enough hyaluronic acid is cleared for a single sperm to penetrate the ovum's zona pellucida successfully.

At the moment of penetration by a fertilizing sperm, the zona pellucida undergoes cortical and zona reactions that release lysosomal enzymes. These enzymes prevent additional sperm from entering a single ovum (Caudle, 2014). This is known as the *block to polyspermy*. This cellular change is mediated by release of materials from the cortical granules, organelles found just below the ovum's surface, and is called the *cortical reaction* (Figure 4–2).

The Moment of Fertilization

After the sperm enters the ovum, a chemical signal prompts the secondary oocyte to complete the second meiotic division, forming the nucleus of the ovum and ejecting the second polar body. Then the nuclei of the ovum and sperm swell and approach each other. The true moment of fertilization occurs as the nuclei unite. Their individual nuclear membranes disappear, and their chromosomes pair up to produce the diploid zygote. Because each nucleus contains a haploid number of chromosomes (23), this union restores the diploid number (46). The zygote contains a new combination of genetic material that results in an individual different from either parent and from anyone else.

At the moment of fertilization, the sex of the zygote is determined. The two chromosomes (the sex chromosomes) of the 23rd pair—either XX or XY—determine the sex of an individual. The X chromosome is larger and bears more genes than the Y chromosome. Females have two X chromosomes, and males have an X and a Y chromosome. The mature ovum produced by oogenesis can have only one type of sex chromosome—an X. Spermatogenesis produces two sperm with an X chromosome and two

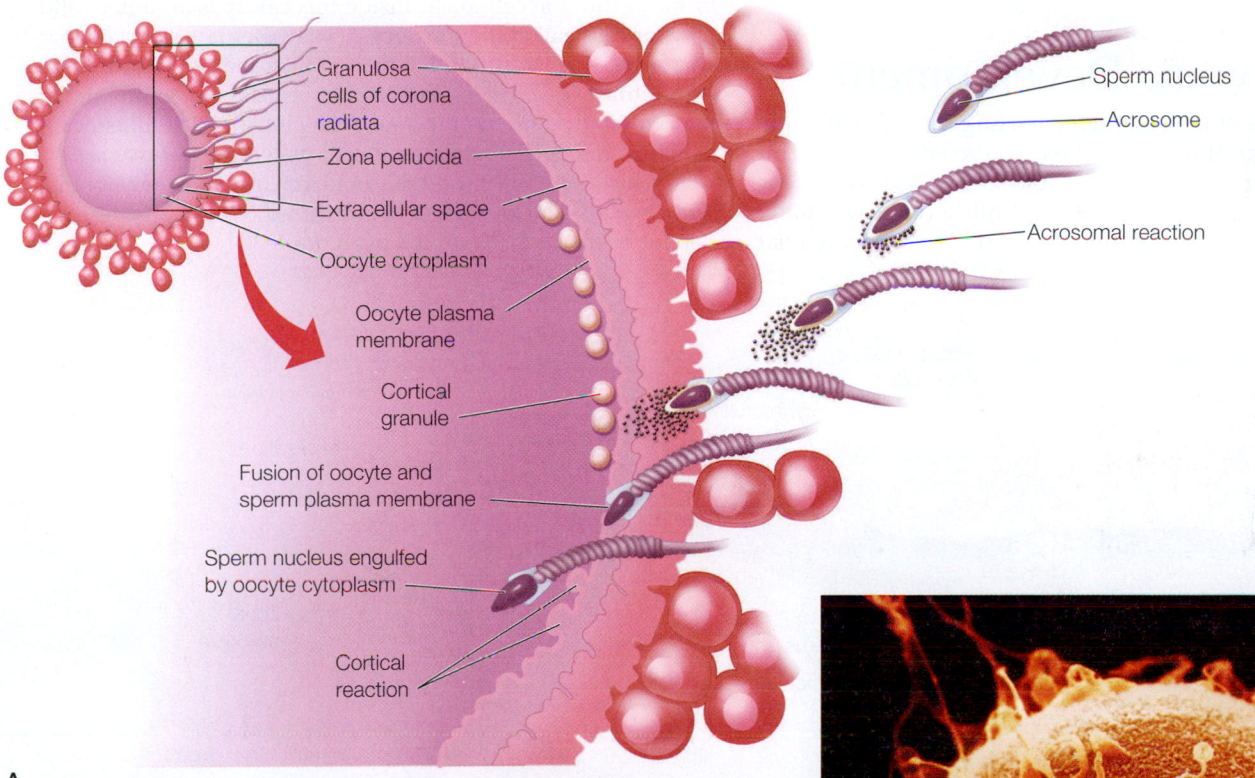

Granulosa cells of corona radiata

Zona pellucida

Extracellular space

Oocyte cytoplasm

Oocyte plasma membrane

Cortical granule

Fusion of oocyte and sperm plasma membrane

Sperm nucleus engulfed by oocyte cytoplasm

Cortical reaction

Sperm nucleus

Acrosome

Acrosomal reaction

A

B

Figure 4–2 Sperm penetration of an ovum. A. The sequential steps of oocyte penetration by a sperm are depicted moving from top to bottom. B. Scanning electron micrograph of human sperm surrounding a human ovum (750X). The smaller spherical cells are granulosa cells of the corona radiata.

sperm with a Y chromosome. When each gamete contributes an X chromosome, the resulting zygote is female. When the ovum contributes an X and the sperm contributes a Y chromosome, the resulting zygote is male. As discussed in more detail in Chapter 7, certain traits are termed *sex linked* because they are controlled by the genes on the X sex chromosome. Two examples of sex-linked traits are color blindness and hemophilia.

Developing Cultural Competence Iraqi Childbirth Customs

"My sister, she did not have baby for very, very long time, you see. This is very sad where I am from [Iraq]. Her husband's family wanted him to leave her and we so feared he would. Then my sister became pregnant and it was very nice, we all so happy to see. Then I learned my sister birthed a baby girl and I cried and cried for a week. My mother cried too, so sad at this time no baby come and then finally to have a girl. I still feel sad for her."

(Excerpt from author's interview with Iraqi on customs in Iraq)

Preembryonic Development

The first 14 days of development, starting the day the ovum is fertilized (conception), are called the *preembryonic stage*, or the *stage of the ovum*. Development after fertilization can be divided into two phases: cellular multiplication and cellular differentiation. These phases are characterized by rapid cellular multiplication, and differentiation and establishment of the primary germ layers and embryonic membranes. Synchronized development of both the endometrium and the embryo is a prerequisite for implantation to succeed (Moore, Persaud, & Torchia, 2016). These phases and the process of implantation (nidation), which occurs between them, are discussed next.

Cellular Multiplication

Cellular multiplication begins as the zygote moves through the fallopian tube toward the cavity of the uterus. This transport takes 3 days or more and is accomplished mainly by a very weak fluid current in the fallopian tube resulting from the beating action of the ciliated epithelium that lines the tube.

The zygote now enters a period of rapid mitotic divisions called **cleavage**, during which it divides into two cells, four cells, eight cells, and so on. These cells, called *blastomeres*, are so small that the developing cell mass is only slightly larger than the original zygote. The blastomeres are held together by the zona pellucida, which is under the corona radiata. The blastomeres eventually form a solid ball of 12 to 32 cells called the **morula** (Moore et al., 2016).

As the morula enters the uterus, two things happen: The intracellular fluid in the morula increases, and a central cavity forms within the cell mass. Inside this cavity is an inner solid mass of cells called the **blastocyst**. The outer layer of cells that surrounds the cavity and replaces the zona pellucida is the **trophoblast**. Eventually, the trophoblast develops into one of the two embryonic membranes, the chorion. The blastocyst develops into a double layer of cells called the *embryonic disk*, from which the embryo and the amnion (embryonic membrane) will develop. The journey of the fertilized ovum to its destination in the uterus is illustrated in Figure 4–3.

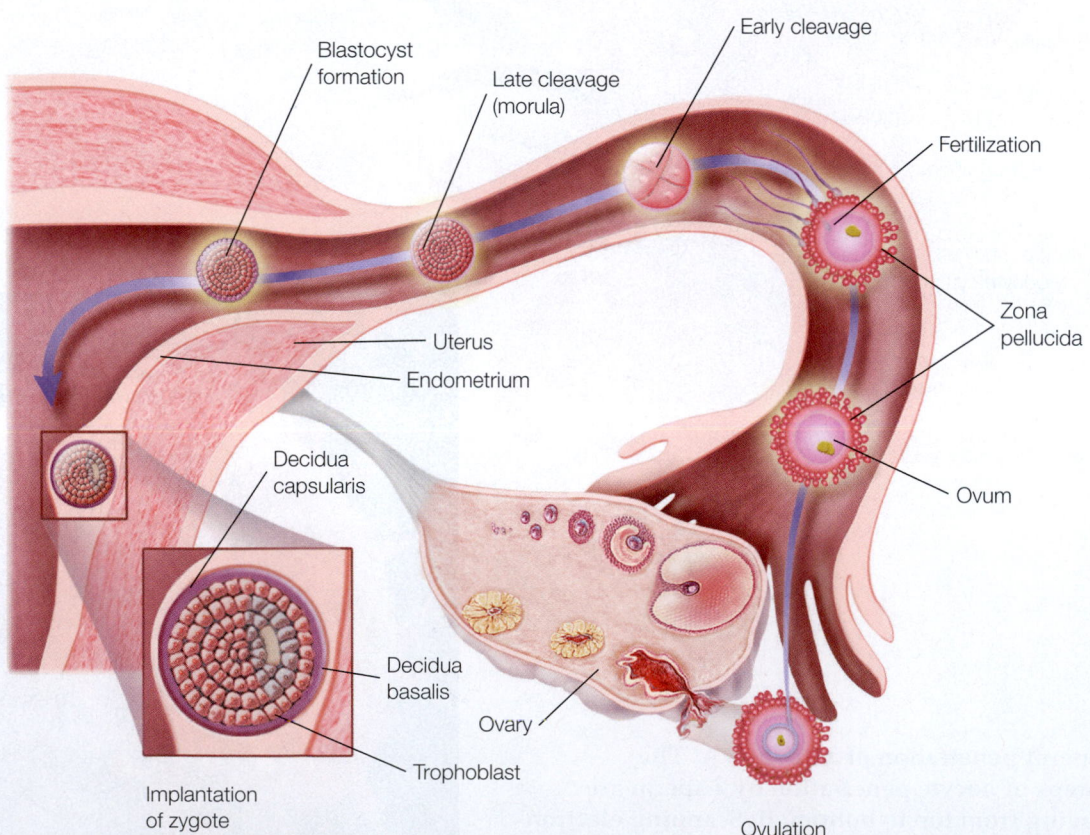

Figure 4–3 During ovulation, the ovum leaves the ovary and enters the fallopian tube. Fertilization generally occurs in the outer third of the fallopian tube. Subsequent changes in the fertilized ovum from conception to implantation are depicted.

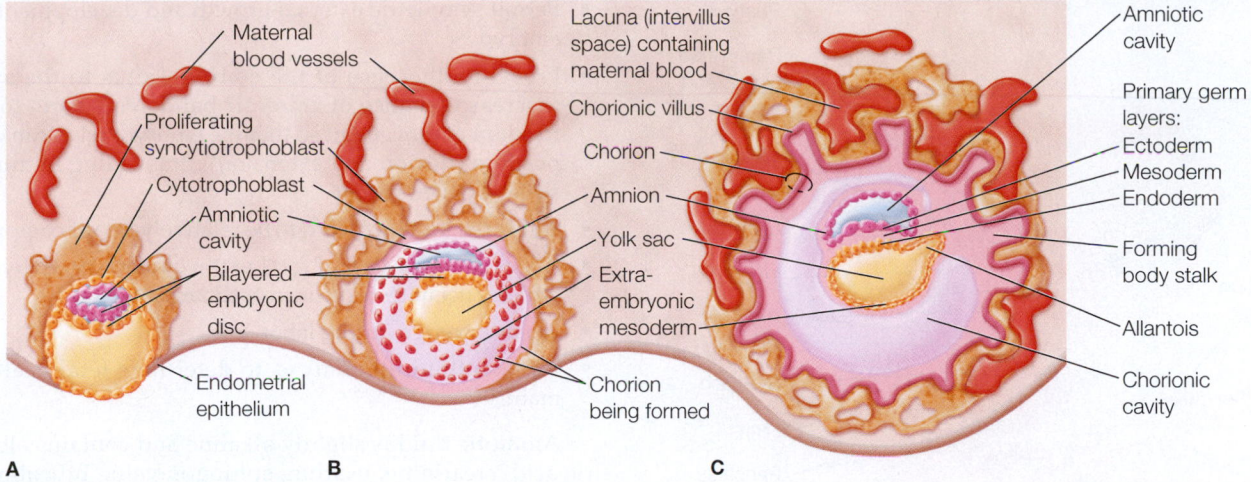

Figure 4–4 Formation of primary germ layers. A. Implantation of a 7 1/2-day blastocyst in which the cells of the embryonic disk are separated from the amnion by a fluid-filled space. The erosion of the endometrium by the syncytiotrophoblast is ongoing. B. Implantation is completed by day 9, and extraembryonic mesoderm is beginning to form a discrete layer beneath the cytotrophoblast. C. By day 16, the embryo shows all three germ layers, a yolk sac, and an allantois (an outpouching of the yolk sac that forms the structural basis of the body stalk, or umbilical cord). The cytotrophoblast and associated mesoderm have become the chorion, and chorionic villi are developing.

Early pregnancy factor (EPF), an immunosuppressant protein, is secreted by the trophoblastic cells. This factor appears in the maternal serum within 24 to 48 hours after fertilization and forms the basis of a pregnancy test during the first 10 days of development (Caudle, 2014; Moore et al., 2016).

Implantation (Nidation)

While floating in the uterine cavity, the blastocyst is nourished by the uterine glands, which secrete a mixture of lipids, mucopolysaccharides, and glycogen. The trophoblast attaches itself to the surface of the endometrium for further nourishment. The most frequent site of attachment is the upper part of the posterior uterine wall. Between days 7 and 10 after fertilization, the zona pellucida disappears and the blastocyst implants itself by burrowing into the uterine lining and penetrating down toward the maternal capillaries until it is completely covered (Moore et al., 2016). The blastocyst will orient itself so that the embryonic pole is closest to the endometrial lining (Blackburn, 2013; Caudle, 2014). The lining of the uterus thickens below the implanted blastocyst, and the cells of the trophoblast grow down into the thickened lining, forming processes that will be called chorionic villi.

Under the influence of progesterone, the endometrium increases in thickness and vascularity in preparation for implantation and nutrition of the ovum. After implantation, the endometrium is called the decidua. The portion of the decidua that covers the blastocyst is called the **decidua capsularis**, the portion directly under the implanted blastocyst is the **decidua basalis**, and the portion that lines the rest of the uterine cavity is the **decidua vera (parietalis)** (see magnified inset in Figure 4–3) (Blackburn, 2013). The maternal part of the placenta develops from the decidua basalis, which contains large numbers of blood vessels. The chorionic villi (discussed shortly) in contact with the decidua basalis will form the fetal portion of the placenta.

Cellular Differentiation

PRIMARY GERM LAYERS

About the 10th to 14th day after conception, the homogeneous mass of blastocyst cells differentiates into the primary germ layers (Figure 4–4). These three layers, the **ectoderm**, **mesoderm**, and **endoderm**, are formed at the same time as the embryonic membranes. All tissues, organs, and organ systems will develop from these primary germ cell layers (Table 4–1). For example,

TABLE 4–1 Derivation of Body Structures from Primary Cell Layers

ECTODERM	MESODERM	ENDODERM
Epidermis	Dermis	Respiratory tract epithelium
Sweat glands	Wall of digestive tract	Epithelium (except nasal), including pharynx, tongue, tonsils, thyroid, parathyroid, thymus, tympanic cavity
Sebaceous glands	Kidneys and ureter (suprarenal cortex)	
Nails	Reproductive organs (gonads, genital ducts)	
Hair follicles	Connective tissue (cartilage, bone, joint cavities)	Lining of digestive tract
Lens of eye		Primary tissue of liver and pancreas
Sensory epithelium of internal and external ear, nasal cavity, sinuses, mouth, anal canal	Skeleton	Urethra and associated glands
Central and peripheral nervous systems	Muscles (all types)	Urinary bladder (except trigone)
Nasal cavity	Cardiovascular system (heart, arteries, veins, blood, bone marrow)	Vagina (parts)
Oral glands and tooth enamel	Pleura	
Pituitary gland	Lymphatic tissue and cells	
Mammary glands	Spleen	

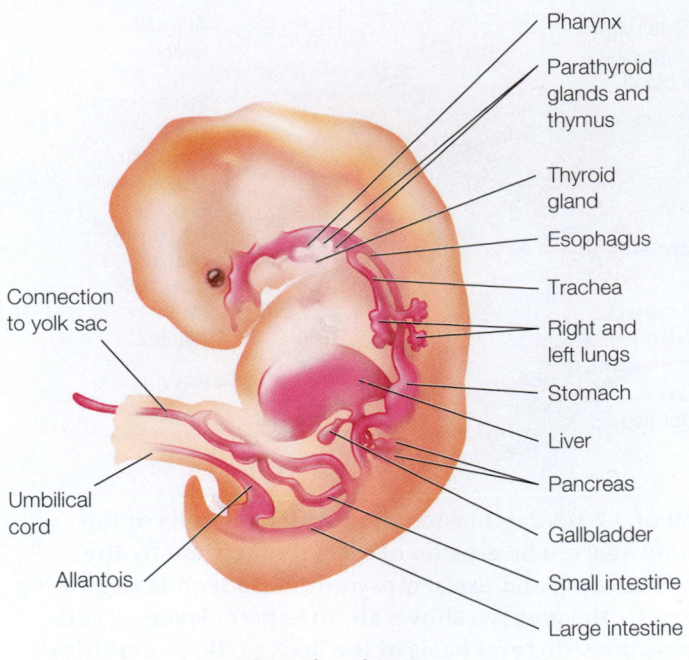

Connection to yolk sac

Umbilical cord

Allantois

Pharynx
Parathyroid glands and thymus
Thyroid gland
Esophagus
Trachea
Right and left lungs
Stomach
Liver
Pancreas
Gallbladder
Small intestine
Large intestine

5-week embryo

Figure 4–5 Endoderm differentiates to form the epithelial lining of the digestive and respiratory tracts and associated glands.

differentiation of the endoderm results in the formation of epithelium lining the respiratory and digestive tracts (Figure 4–5).

EMBRYONIC MEMBRANES

The **embryonic membranes** begin to form at the time of implantation (Figure 4–6). These membranes protect and support the embryo as it grows and develops inside the uterus. The first and outermost membrane to form is the **chorion**. This thick membrane develops from the trophoblast, and has many fingerlike projections called *chorionic villi* on its surface. These chorionic villi can be used for early genetic testing of the embryo at 8 to 11 weeks' gestation by chorionic villi sampling (CVS) (see Chapter 13 for a detailed discussion of CVS). As the pregnancy progresses, the chorionic villi begin to degenerate, except for those just under the embryo, which grow and branch into depressions in the uterine wall, forming the fetal portion of the placenta. By the fourth month of pregnancy, the surface of the chorion is smooth except at the place of attachment to the uterine wall.

The second membrane to form, the amnion, originates from the ectoderm, a primary germ layer, during the early stages of embryonic development. The **amnion** is a thin protective membrane that contains amniotic fluid. The space between the membrane and the embryo is the *amniotic cavity*. This cavity surrounds the embryo and yolk sac, except where the developing embryo (germ-layer disk) attaches to the trophoblast via the umbilical cord. As the embryo grows, the amnion expands until it comes into contact with the chorion. These two slightly adherent membranes form the fluid-filled amniotic sac, also called the **bag of waters (BOW)**, which protects the floating embryo.

AMNIOTIC FLUID

The primary functions of **amniotic fluid** are to:

- Act as a cushion to protect the embryo against mechanical injury
- Help control the embryo's temperature (relies on the mother to release heat)

- Permit symmetric external growth and development of the embryo
- Prevent adherence of the embryo/fetus to the amnion (decreases chance of amniotic band syndrome) to allow freedom of movement so that the embryo/fetus can change position (flexion and extension), thus aiding in musculoskeletal development
- Allow the umbilical cord to be relatively free of compression
- Act as an extension of fetal extracellular space (hydropic fetuses/neonates have increased amniotic fluid)
- Act as a wedge during labor
- Provide fluid for analysis to determine fetal health and maturity

Amniotic fluid is slightly alkaline and contains albumin, uric acid, creatinine, lecithin, sphingomyelin, bilirubin, vernix, leukocytes, epithelial cells, enzymes, and fine hair called **lanugo**. The amount of amniotic fluid at 10 weeks is about 30 mL, and it increases to 210 mL at 16 weeks (Cunningham et al., 2014). After 28 weeks, the amniotic fluid volume changes little until 39 weeks, after which it decreases dramatically (Blackburn, 2013). The average volume ranges from 700 to 1000 mL in the third trimester. As the pregnancy continues, the fetus influences the volume of amniotic fluid by swallowing the fluid, excreting lung fluid, and excreting urine into the amniotic fluid.

Abnormal variations in amniotic fluid volume are referred to as *oligohydramnios* (less than 400 mL of amniotic fluid) or *hydramnios* (more than 2000 mL or amniotic fluid index greater than 97.5 percentile for the corresponding gestational age). Hydramnios is also called *polyhydramnios*. See Chapter 21 for an in-depth discussion of alterations in amniotic fluid volume during childbirth.

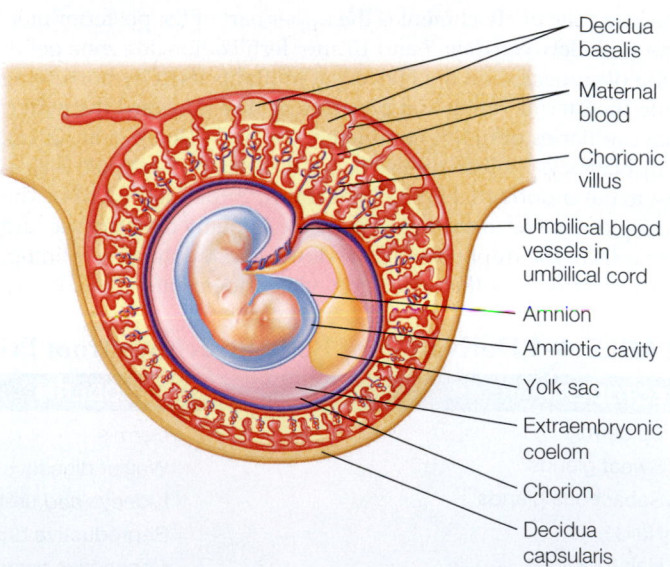

Decidua basalis
Maternal blood
Chorionic villus
Umbilical blood vessels in umbilical cord
Amnion
Amniotic cavity
Yolk sac
Extraembryonic coelom
Chorion
Decidua capsularis

Figure 4–6 Early development of primary embryonic membranes. At 4 1/2 weeks, the decidua capsularis (placental portion enclosing the embryo on the uterine surface) and decidua basalis (placental portion encompassing the elaborate chorionic villi and maternal endometrium) are well formed. The chorionic villi lie in blood-filled intervillous spaces within the endometrium. The amnion and yolk sac are well developed.

YOLK SAC

In humans, the yolk sac is small and functions early in embryonic life. It develops as a second cavity in the blastocyst on about day 8 or 9 after conception. It forms primitive red blood cells during the first 6 weeks of development, until the embryo's liver takes over the process. As the embryo develops, the yolk sac is incorporated into the umbilical cord, where it can be seen as a degenerated structure after birth.

UMBILICAL CORD

As the placenta is developing, the **umbilical cord** is also being formed from the amnion (Caudle, 2014). The *body stalk*, which attaches the embryo to the yolk sac, contains blood vessels that extend into the chorionic villi. The body stalk fuses with the embryonic portion of the placenta to provide a circulatory pathway from the chorionic villi to the embryo. As the body stalk elongates to become the umbilical cord, the vessels in the cord decrease to one large vein and two smaller arteries. About 1 in 200 umbilical cords have only two vessels, an artery and a vein; this condition may be associated with congenital malformations primarily of the renal, gastrointestinal, and cardiovascular systems (Sadler, 2015). A specialized connective tissue known as **Wharton jelly** surrounds the blood vessels in the umbilical cord (Caudle, 2014; Moore et al., 2016). This tissue, plus the high blood volume pulsating through the vessels, prevents compression of the umbilical cord in utero. The umbilical cord has no sensory or motor innervation, so cutting the cord after birth is not painful. At term (37 to 42 weeks' gestation), the average cord is 2 cm (0.8 in.) across and about 55 cm (22 in.) long. The cord can attach itself to the placenta in various sites. Central insertion into the placenta is considered normal. (See Chapter 21 for a discussion of the various attachment sites.)

Umbilical cords appear twisted or spiraled, which is most likely caused by fetal movement. A true knot in the umbilical cord rarely occurs; if it does, the cord is longer than usual. More common are so-called false knots, caused by the folding of cord vessels. A *nuchal cord* is said to exist when the umbilical cord encircles the fetal neck.

Twins

Twins normally occur in approximately 33 per 1000 live births in the United States (Blackburn, 2013). The current rate of twinning is attributed to delayed childbearing and use of artificial reproductive treatments.

Twins may be either fraternal or identical (Figure 4–7). If twins are fraternal, they are dizygotic, which means they arise from two separate ova fertilized by two separate spermatozoa. There are two placentas, two chorions, and two amnions (see Figure 4–7A); however, the placentas sometimes fuse and look as if they are one. Despite their birth relationship, fraternal twins are no more similar to each other than they would be to siblings born singly. They may be of the same or different sex.

Dizygotic twinning increases with maternal age up to about age 35 and then decreases abruptly. The chance of dizygotic twins increases with parity, and with coital frequency. The chance of dizygotic twinning decreases during periods of malnutrition and during winter and spring for women living in the Northern Hemisphere.

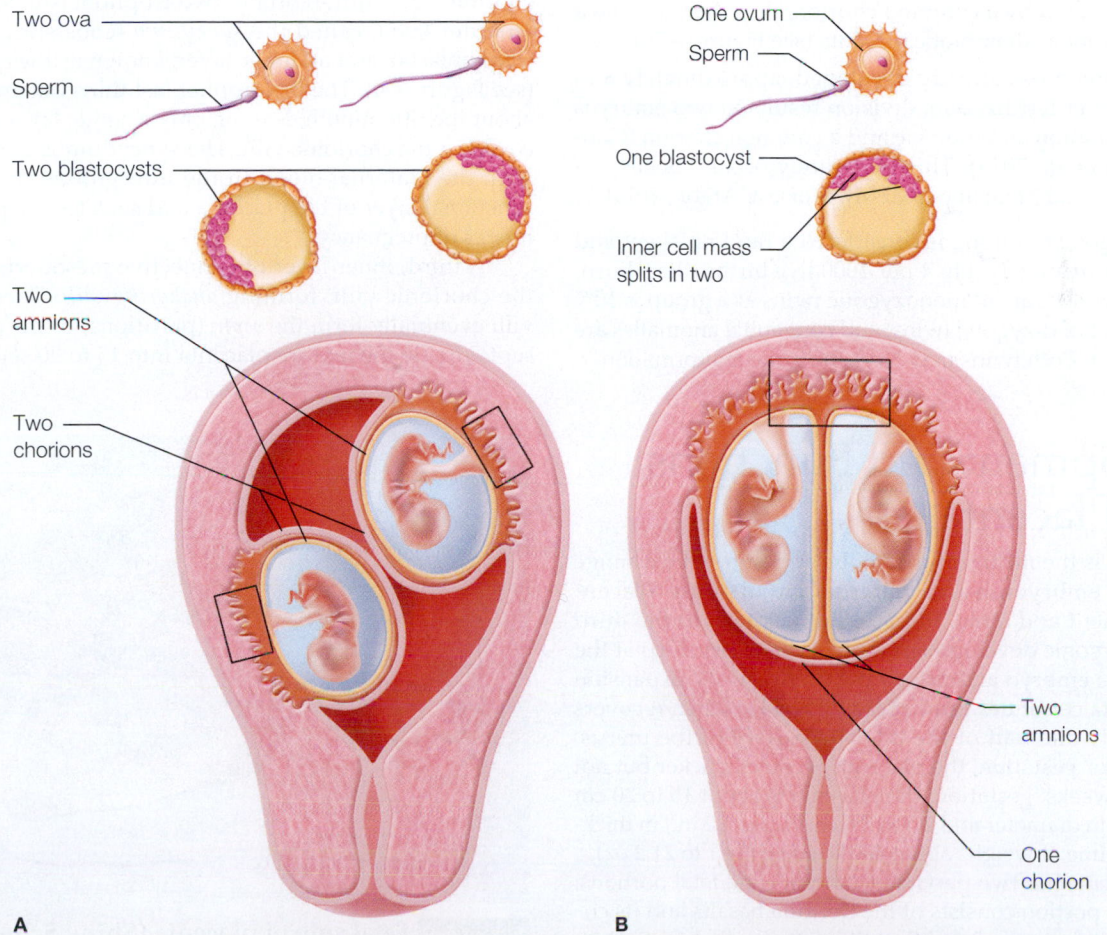

Figure 4–7 **A. Formation of fraternal twins. (Note separate placentas.) B. Formation of identical twins.**

Studies indicate that dizygotic twins occur in certain families, perhaps because of genotype (genetic constitution) of the mother that results in elevated serum gonadotropin levels leading to double ovulation (Moore et al., 2016). Fraternal (nonidentical or dizygotic) twins have been reported to occur more often among women of African ancestry than among White women and more often among White women than among women of Asian origin (Moore et al., 2016). Among all groups, as parity (having given birth to a viable baby) increases, so does the chance for multiple births.

Identical, or monozygotic, twins develop from a single fertilized ovum. They are of the same sex and have the same phenotype (appearance). Identical twins usually have a common placenta. Monozygosity is not affected by environment, race, physical characteristics, or fertility.

Monozygotic twins originate from division of the fertilized ovum at different stages of early development, after the zygote consists of thousands of cells. Complete separation of the cellular mass into two parts is necessary for twin formation. The number of amnions and chorions present depends on the timing of the division:

1. If division occurs within 3 days of fertilization (before the inner cell mass and chorion are formed), two embryos, two amnions, and two chorions will develop. This dichorionic–diamniotic situation occurs about 20% to 30% of the time, and there may be two distinct placentas or a single fused placenta.

2. If division occurs about 5 days after fertilization (when the inner cell mass is formed and the chorion cells have differentiated but those of the amnion have not), two embryos develop with separate amnion sacs. These sacs will eventually be covered by a common chorion; thus there will be a monochorionic–diamniotic placenta (see Figure 4–7B).

3. If the amnion has already developed, approximately 8 to 12 days after fertilization, division results in two embryos with a common amniotic sac and a common chorion (Cunningham et al., 2014). This type rarely occurs (Society of Maternal-Fetal Medicine [SMFM]; Moise & Argon, 2013).

Monozygotic twinning is considered a random event and occurs in approximately 3 to 4 per 1000 live births (Blackburn, 2013). The survival rate of monozygotic twins as a group is 10% lower than that of dizygotic twins, and congenital anomalies are more prevalent. Both twins may have the same malformation.

Development and Functions of the Placenta

The **placenta** is the means of metabolic and nutrient exchange between the embryonic and maternal circulations. Placental development and circulation do not begin until the third week of embryonic development. The placenta develops at the site where the embryo attaches to the uterine wall. Expansion of the placenta continues until about 20 weeks, when it covers approximately one-half of the internal surface of the uterus. After 20 weeks' gestation, the placenta becomes thicker but not wider. At 40 weeks' gestation, the placenta is about 15 to 20 cm (5.9 to 7.9 in.) in diameter and 2.5 to 3.0 cm (1.0 to 1.2 in.) in thickness. At that time, it weighs about 400 to 600 g (14.1 to 21.2 oz).

The placenta has two parts: the maternal and fetal portions. The maternal portion consists of the decidua basalis and its circulation. Its surface is red and fleshlike (often called *Dirty Duncan*) (Figure 4–8). The fetal portion consists of the chorionic villi

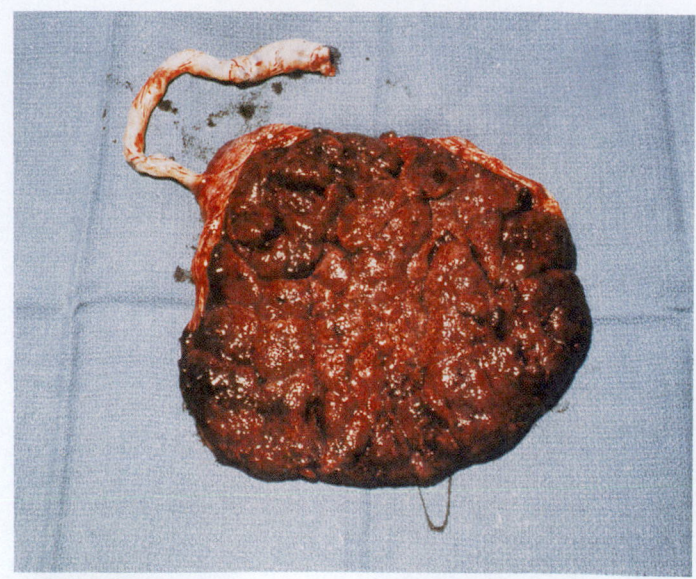

Figure 4–8 Maternal side of placenta (Dirty Duncan).
SOURCE: M. London.

and their circulation. The fetal surface of the placenta is covered by the amnion, which gives it a shiny, gray appearance (often called *Shiny Schultze*) (Figure 4–9).

Development of the placenta begins with the chorionic villi. The trophoblastic cells of the chorionic villi form spaces in the tissue of the decidua basalis. These spaces fill with maternal blood, and the chorionic villi grow into them. As the chorionic villi differentiate, two trophoblastic layers appear: an outer layer, called the *syncytium* (consisting of syncytiotrophoblasts), and an inner layer, known as the *cytotrophoblast* (see Figure 4–4). The cytotrophoblast thins out and disappears about the fifth month, leaving only a single layer of syncytium covering the chorionic villi. The syncytium is in direct contact with the maternal blood in the intervillous spaces. It is the functional layer of the placenta and secretes the placental hormones of pregnancy.

A third, inner layer of connective mesoderm develops in the chorionic villi, forming *anchoring villi*. These anchoring villi eventually form the *septa* (partitions) of the placenta. The septa divide the mature placenta into 15 to 20 segments called

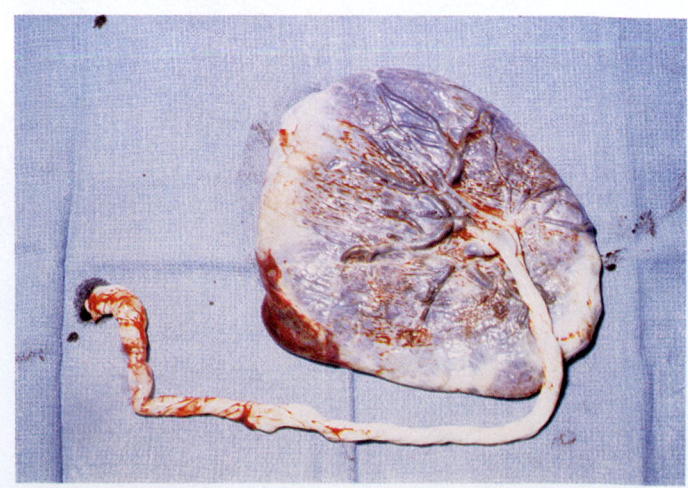

Figure 4–9 Fetal side of placenta (Shiny Schultze).
SOURCE: M. London.

cotyledons (subdivisions of the placenta made up of anchoring villi and decidual tissue). In each cotyledon, the *branching villi* form a highly complex vascular system that allows compartmentalization of the uteroplacental circulation. The exchange of gases and nutrients takes place across these vascular systems.

Exchange of substances across the placenta is minimal during the first 3 to 5 months of development because the villous membrane is initially too thick, which limits its permeability. As the villous membrane thins, placental permeability increases until about the last month of pregnancy, when permeability begins to decrease as the placenta ages. In the fully developed placenta, fetal blood in the villi and maternal blood in the intervillous spaces are separated by three to four thin layers of tissue.

Placental Circulation

The completion of the maternal–placental–fetal circulation occurs about 17 days after conception, when the embryonic heart begins functioning (Moore et al., 2016). By the end of the fourth week, embryonic blood is circulating between the embryo and the chorionic villi. In the intervillous spaces, maternal blood supplies oxygen and nutrients to the embryonic capillaries in the villi. The placenta has begun to function as a means of metabolic exchange between embryo and mother. By 14 weeks, the placenta is a discrete organ. It has grown in thickness as a result of growth in the length and size of the chorionic villi and accompanying expansion of the intervillous space.

In the fully developed placenta's umbilical cord, fetal blood flows through the two umbilical arteries to the capillaries of the villi, and oxygen-enriched blood flows back through the umbilical vein into the fetus (Figure 4–10). Late in pregnancy, a soft blowing sound (*funic souffle*) can be heard over the area of the umbilical cord. The sound is synchronous with the fetal heartbeat and fetal blood flow through the umbilical arteries.

Maternal blood, rich in oxygen and nutrients, spurts from the arcuate artery to the radial artery to the uterine spiral arteries and then spurts into the intervillous spaces. These spurts are produced by the maternal blood pressure. The spurt of blood is directed toward the chorionic plate, and as the blood loses pressure, it becomes lateral (spreads out). Fresh blood enters continuously and exerts pressure on the contents of the intervillous spaces, pushing blood toward the exits in the basal plate. The blood then drains through the uterine and other pelvic veins. A *uterine souffle*, timed precisely with the mother's pulse, is also heard just above the mother's symphysis pubis during the last months of pregnancy. This souffle is caused by the augmented blood flow entering the dilated uterine arteries.

Braxton Hicks contractions are intermittent painless uterine contractions that may occur every 10 to 20 minutes and occur more frequently near the end of pregnancy (see Chapter 16). These contractions are believed to facilitate placental circulation by enhancing the movement of blood from the center of the cotyledon through the intervillous space. Placental blood flow is enhanced when the woman is lying on her side because venous return from the lower extremities is not compromised (Blackburn, 2013).

Placental Functions

Placental exchange functions occur only in those fetal vessels that are in intimate contact with the covering syncytial membrane. The syncytium villi have brush borders containing many microvilli, which greatly increase the exchange rate between maternal and fetal circulation (Sadler, 2015).

The placental functions, many of which begin soon after implantation, include fetal respiration, nutrition, and excretion. To carry out these functions, the placenta is involved in metabolic and transfer activities. In addition, it has endocrine

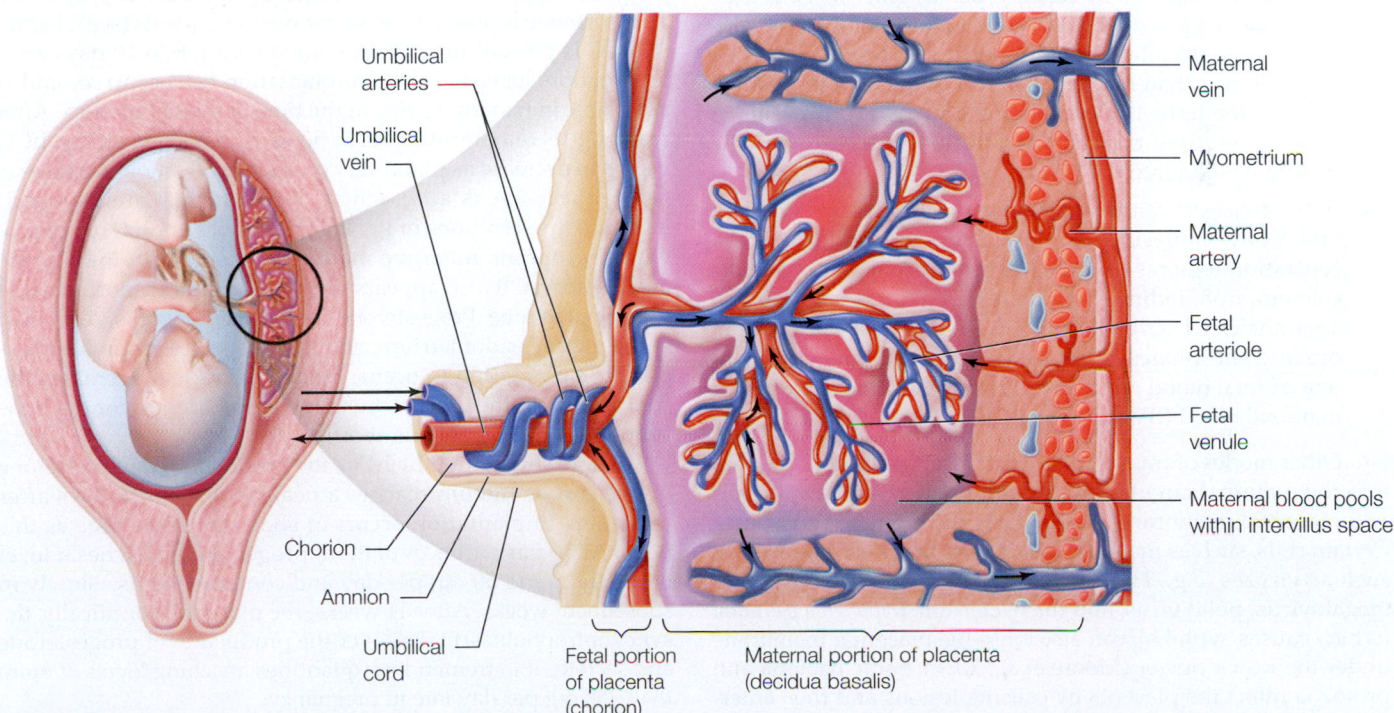

Umbilical arteries
Umbilical vein
Chorion
Amnion
Umbilical cord
Fetal portion of placenta (chorion)
Maternal portion of placenta (decidua basalis)
Maternal vein
Myometrium
Maternal artery
Fetal arteriole
Fetal venule
Maternal blood pools within intervillus space

Figure 4–10 Vascular arrangement of the placenta. Arrows indicate the direction of blood flow. Maternal blood flows through the uterine arteries to the intervillous spaces of the placenta and returns through the uterine veins to maternal circulation. Fetal blood flows through the umbilical arteries into the villous capillaries of the placenta and returns through the umbilical vein to the fetal circulation.

functions and special immunologic properties; see discussion later in this section.

METABOLIC ACTIVITIES

The placenta performs several essential metabolic activities:

- Continuously produces glycogen, cholesterol, and fatty acids for fetal use and hormone production
- Produces numerous enzymes required for fetoplacental transfer, including sulfatase, which enhances excretion of fetal estrogen precursors, and insulinase, which increases the barrier to insulin
- Breaks down certain substances such as epinephrine and histamine (Blackburn, 2013)
- Stores glycogen and iron

TRANSPORT FUNCTION

The placental membranes actively control the transfer of a wide range of substances by a variety of transport mechanisms:

1. *Simple diffusion* moves substances from an area of higher concentration to an area of lower concentration. Substances that move across the placenta by simple diffusion include water, oxygen, carbon dioxide, electrolytes (sodium and chloride), anesthetic gases, and drugs. Insulin, steroid hormones originating from the adrenals, and thyroid hormones cross the placenta at a very slow rate. Unfortunately, many substances of abuse, such as cocaine and heroin, cross the placenta via simple diffusion. The rate of oxygen transfer across the placental membrane is greater than that allowed by simple diffusion, indicating that oxygen is also transferred by some type of facilitated diffusion transport.

2. *Facilitated transport* involves a carrier system to move molecules from an area of greater concentration to an area of lower concentration. Molecules such as glucose, galactose, and some oxygen are transported by this method. The glucose level in the fetal blood ordinarily is approximately 20% to 30% lower than the glucose level in the maternal blood, because the fetus is metabolizing glucose rapidly. This in turn causes rapid transport of additional glucose from the maternal blood into the fetal blood.

3. *Active transport* can work against a concentration gradient and allows molecules to move from areas of lower concentration to areas of higher concentration. Amino acids, calcium, iron, iodine, water-soluble vitamins, and glucose are transferred across the placenta in this way. The calcium, organic phosphates levels, and measured amino acid content of fetal blood are in greater concentration than that of maternal blood (Blackburn, 2013).

Other modes of transfer also exist. Fetal red blood cells pass into the maternal circulation through breaks in the capillaries and placental membrane, particularly during labor and birth. Certain cells, such as maternal leukocytes, and microorganisms, such as viruses (e.g., HIV, which causes AIDS), rubella, cytomegalovirus, polio virus, and the bacterium *Treponema pallidum* (which causes syphilis), can also cross the placental membrane under their own power (Moore et al., 2016). Some bacteria and protozoa infect the placenta by causing lesions and then entering the fetal blood system.

Reduction of the placental surface area, as with abruptio placentae (partial or complete premature separation of an abnormally implanted placenta), lessens the area that is functional for exchange. Placental diffusion distance also affects exchange. In conditions such as diabetes and placental infection, edema of the villi increases the diffusion distance, thus increasing the distance the substance has to be transferred. Blood flow alteration changes the transfer rate of substances. Decreased blood flow in the intervillous space is seen in labor and with certain maternal diseases such as hypertension. Mild fetal hypoxia increases the umbilical blood flow, but severe hypoxia results in decreased blood flow.

As the maternal blood picks up fetal waste products and carbon dioxide, it drains back into the maternal circulation through the veins in the basal plate. Fetal blood is hypoxic by comparison; it therefore attracts oxygen from the mother's blood. Affinity for oxygen increases as the fetal blood gives up its carbon dioxide, which also decreases its acidity.

ENDOCRINE FUNCTIONS

The placenta produces hormones that are vital to the survival of the fetus. These include human chorionic gonadotropin (hCG), human placental lactogen (hPL) [also referred to as human chorionic somatomammotropin (hCS)], relaxin, inhibitin, and two steroid hormones, estrogen and progesterone.

The hormone hCG is similar to luteinizing hormone (LH) and prevents the normal involution of the corpus luteum at the end of the menstrual cycle. If the corpus luteum stops functioning before the 11th week of pregnancy, spontaneous abortion occurs. hCG also causes the corpus luteum to secrete increased amounts of estrogen and progesterone.

After the 11th week, the placenta produces enough progesterone and estrogen to maintain pregnancy. In the male fetus, hCG also exerts an interstitial cell–stimulating effect on the testes, resulting in the production of testosterone. This small secretion of testosterone during embryonic development is the factor that causes male sex organs to grow. hCG may play a role in the trophoblast's immunologic capabilities (ability to exempt the placenta and embryo from rejection by the mother's system). This hormone is used as a basis for pregnancy tests (see Chapter 8). hCG is present in maternal blood serum 8 to 10 days after fertilization, just as soon as implantation has occurred, and is detectable in maternal urine at the time of missed menses. After reaching its maximum level at 50 to 70 days' gestation, hCG begins to decrease as placental hormone production increases.

Progesterone is an essential hormone for pregnancy. It increases the secretions of the fallopian tubes and uterus to provide appropriate nutritive matter for the developing morula and blastocyst. It also appears to aid in ovum transport through the fallopian tube. Progesterone causes decidual cells to develop in the uterine endometrium, and it must be present in high levels for implantation to occur. Progesterone also decreases the contractility of the uterus, thus preventing uterine contractions from causing spontaneous abortion.

Before stimulation by hCG, the production of progesterone by the corpus luteum reaches a peak about 7 to 10 days after ovulation. Implantation occurs at about the same time as this peak. At 16 days after ovulation, progesterone reaches a level between 25 and 50 mg per day and continues to rise slowly in subsequent weeks. After 11 weeks, the placenta (specifically, the syncytiotrophoblast) takes over the production of progesterone and secretes it in tremendous quantities, reaching levels of more than 250 mg per day late in pregnancy.

By 7 weeks, the placenta produces more than 50% of the estrogens in the maternal circulation. *Estrogens* serve mainly a proliferative function, causing enlargement of the uterus, breasts, and breast glandular tissue. Estrogens also have a significant role in increasing vascularity and vasodilation, particularly in the villous capillaries toward the end of pregnancy. Placental estrogens increase markedly toward the end of pregnancy, to as much as 30 times the daily production in the middle of a normal monthly menstrual cycle. The primary estrogen secreted by the placenta (*estriol*) is different from the estrogen secreted by the ovaries (*estradiol*). The placenta cannot synthesize estriol by itself. Essential precursors such as dehydroepiandrosterone sulfate (DHEA-S) are provided by the fetal adrenal glands, are processed by the fetal liver, and are transported to the placenta for the final conversion to estrone, estradiol, and estriol (Blackburn, 2013).

The hormone *human placental lactogen (hPL)*, is similar to human pituitary growth hormone; hPL stimulates certain changes in the mother's metabolic processes. These changes ensure that more protein, glucose, and minerals are available for the fetus. Secretion of hPL can be detected about 4 weeks after conception.

IMMUNOLOGIC PROPERTIES

The placenta and the embryo are transplants of living tissue within the same species and are therefore considered *homografts*. Unlike other homografts, the placenta and the embryo appear exempt from immunologic reaction by the host. Most recent data suggest that there is a suppression of cellular immunity by the placental hormones (progesterone and hCG) during pregnancy. One theory suggests that chorionic villi syncytiotrophoblastic tissue is immunologically inert. The chorionic villi may lack major histocompatibility (MHC) antigens and thus do not evoke rejection responses. They do, however, protect against antibody formation. Extravillous trophoblast (EVT) cells, which invade the uterine deciduas, have human leukocyte antigen (HLA-G), which is not readily recognized by sensitized T lymphocytes and natural killer cells (Blackburn, 2013; Cunningham et al., 2014).

Development of the Fetal Circulatory System

The circulatory system of the fetus has several unique features that, by maintaining the blood flow to the placenta, provide the fetus with oxygen and nutrients while removing carbon dioxide and other waste products.

Most of the blood supply bypasses the fetal lungs because they do not carry out respiratory gas exchange. The placenta assumes the function of the fetal lungs by supplying oxygen and allowing the fetus to excrete carbon dioxide into the maternal bloodstream. Figure 4–11 shows the fetal circulatory system. The blood from the placenta flows through the umbilical vein, which enters the abdominal wall of the fetus at the site that, after birth, is the umbilicus (belly button). As umbilical venous blood approaches the liver, a small portion of the blood enters the liver sinusoids, mixes with blood from the portal circulation, and then enters the inferior vena cava via hepatic veins. Most of the umbilical vein's blood flows through the **ductus venosus** directly into the fetal inferior vena cava, bypassing the liver. This blood then enters the right atrium, passes through the **foramen ovale** into the left atrium, and pours into the left ventricle, which pumps blood into the aorta. Some blood returning from the head and upper extremities by way of the superior vena cava is emptied into the right atrium and passes through the tricuspid valve into the right ventricle. This blood is pumped into the pulmonary artery, and a small amount passes to the lungs for nourishment only. The larger portion of blood passes from the pulmonary artery through the **ductus arteriosus** into the descending aorta, bypassing the lungs. Finally, blood returns to the placenta through the two umbilical arteries, and the process is repeated.

The fetus obtains oxygen via diffusion from the maternal circulation because of the gradient difference of PO_2 of 50 mm Hg in maternal blood in the placenta to 30 mm Hg PO_2 in the fetus. At term the fetus receives oxygen from the mother's circulation at a rate of 20 to 30 mL per minute (Sadler, 2015). Fetal hemoglobin facilitates obtaining oxygen from the maternal circulation, because it carries as much as 20% to 30% more oxygen than adult hemoglobin.

Fetal circulation delivers the highest available oxygen concentration to the head, neck, brain, and heart (coronary circulation) and a lesser amount of oxygenated blood to the abdominal organs and the lower body. This circulatory pattern leads to cephalocaudal (head-to-tail) development in the fetus.

Embryonic and Fetal Development

Pregnancy is calculated to last an *average* of 10 lunar months: 40 weeks, or 280 days. This period of 280 days is calculated from the onset of the last normal menstrual period to the time of birth. Many obstetric units in the United States and Australia use a combination of menstrual dates and ultrasonographic dates to perform this calculation. Estimated date of birth (EDB), sometimes referred to as the *estimated date of delivery (EDD)*, is usually calculated by this method. Most fetuses are born within 10 to 14 days of the calculated date of birth. The postconception age (fertilization age) of the fetus is calculated to be *about* 2 weeks less, or 266 days (38 weeks), or 9.5 calendar months. The latter measurement is more accurate because it measures time from the fertilization of the ovum, or conception. See Chapter 9 for a detailed discussion of due date determination, including the Nägele rule.

The basic events of organ development in the embryo and fetus are outlined in Table 4–2. The time periods in the table are **postconception age periods**. During the period from fertilization to the end of the embryonic period (8 weeks), age is often expressed in days but can be given in weeks. During the fetal period (9th week until birth), age is given in weeks (Moore et al., 2016). The National Institute for Health and Clinical Excellence (NICE) (National Institute for Health and Clinical Excellence, 2011) guidelines state that the *crown–rump length (CRL)* should be used to determine gestational age, and if the CRL is greater than 84 mm, the *head circumference (HC)* should be used instead.

In review, human development follows three stages. The preembryonic stage, as discussed earlier in the chapter, consists of the first 14 days of development after the ovum is fertilized; then the embryonic stage covers the period from day 15 until approximately the end of the eighth week, and the fetal stage extends from the end of the eighth week until birth.

Embryonic Stage

The stage of the **embryo** starts on day 15 (the beginning of the third week after conception) and continues until approximately the eighth week, or until the embryo reaches a CRL of 3 cm (1.2 in.). This length is usually reached about 56 days after fertilization (the end of the eighth gestational week).

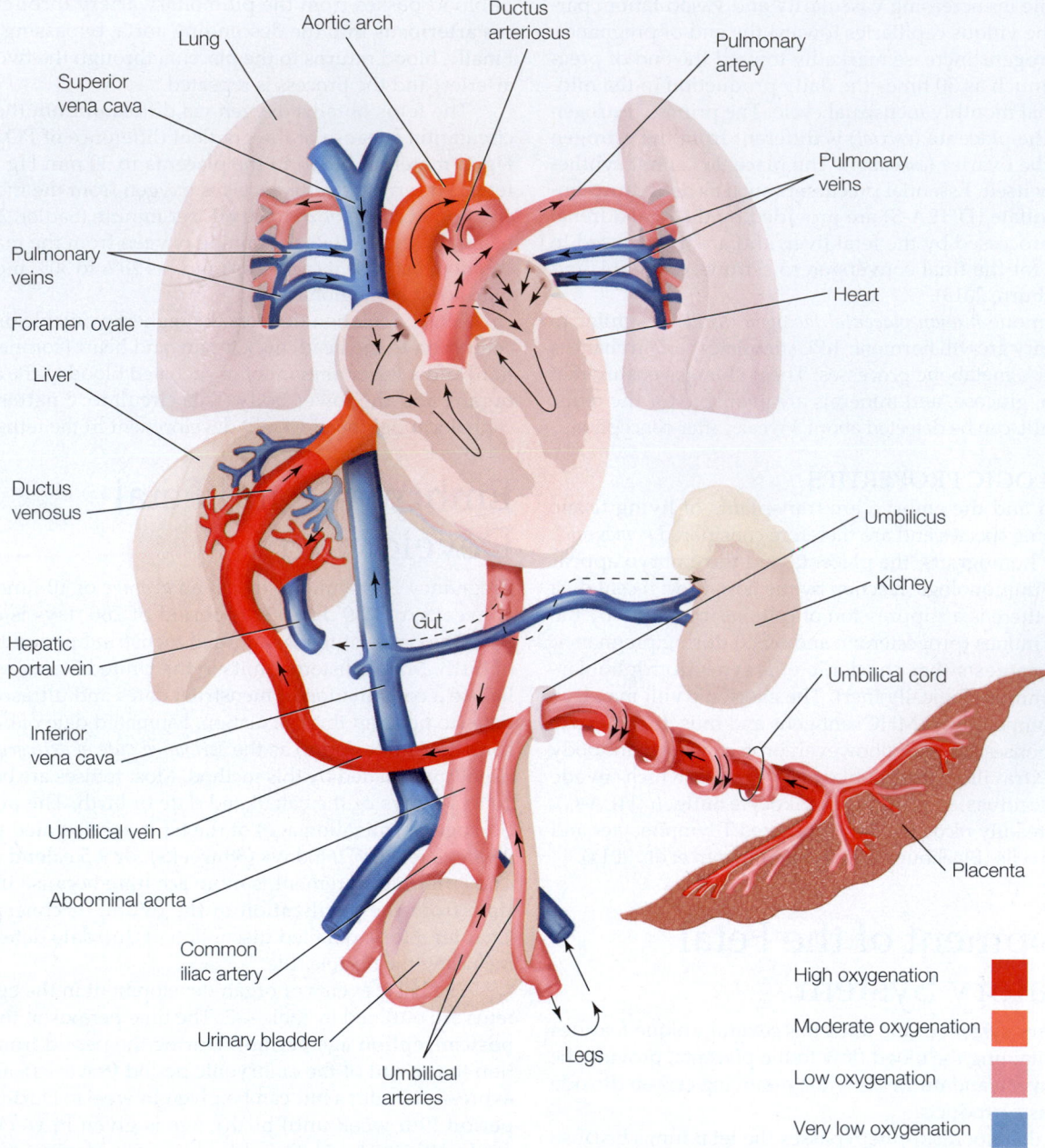

Lung
Aortic arch
Ductus arteriosus
Pulmonary artery
Superior vena cava
Pulmonary veins
Pulmonary veins
Foramen ovale
Heart
Liver
Ductus venosus
Umbilicus
Kidney
Hepatic portal vein
Gut
Umbilical cord
Inferior vena cava
Umbilical vein
Placenta
Abdominal aorta
Common iliac artery
Urinary bladder
Umbilical arteries
Legs

High oxygenation
Moderate oxygenation
Low oxygenation
Very low oxygenation

Figure 4–11 Fetal circulation. Blood leaves the placenta and enters the fetus through the umbilical vein. After circulating through the fetus, the blood returns to the placenta through the umbilical arteries. The ductus venosus, the foramen ovale, and the ductus arteriosus allow the blood to bypass the fetal liver and lungs.

During the embryonic stage, tissues differentiate into essential organs and the main external features develop (Figure 4–12). The embryo is the most vulnerable to *teratogens* during this period. These are discussed in more depth later in the chapter.

3 WEEKS

In the third week, the embryonic disk becomes elongated and pear shaped, with a broad cephalic end and a narrow caudal end. The ectoderm has formed a long cylindrical tube for brain and spinal cord development. The gastrointestinal tract, created from the endoderm, appears as another tubelike structure communicating with the yolk sac. The most advanced organ is the heart. At 3 weeks, a single tubular heart forms just outside the body cavity of the embryo.

4 TO 5 WEEKS

During days 21 to 32, *somites* (a series of mesodermal blocks) form on either side of the embryo's midline. The vertebrae that form the spinal column will develop from these somites. Before 28 days, arm and leg buds are not visible, but the tail bud is present. The pharyngeal arches—which will form the lower jaw, hyoid bone, and larynx—develop at this time. The pharyngeal pouches also appear; these pouches will form the eustachian tube and cavity of the middle ear, the tonsils, and the parathyroid and thymus glands. The primordia of the ear and eye are also present. By the end of 28 days, the tubular heart is beating at a regular rhythm and pushing its own primitive blood cells through the main blood vessels.

During the fifth week, the optic cups and lens vessels of the eye form and the nasal pits develop. Partitioning in the

TABLE 4–2 Timeline of Organ System Development in the Embryo and Fetus

Age: 2–3 Weeks

Length: 2 mm (0.08 in.) CRL

Nervous system: Groove forms along middle back as cells thicken; neural tube forms from closure of neural groove.

Cardiovascular system: Beginning of blood circulation; tubular heart begins to form during third week.

Gastrointestinal system: Liver begins to function.

Genitourinary system: Formation of kidneys beginning.

Respiratory system: Nasal pits forming.

Endocrine system: Thyroid tissue appears.

Eyes: Optic cup and lens pit have formed; pigment in eyes.

Ears: Auditory pit is now enclosed structure.

Age: 4 Weeks

Length: 4–6 mm (0.16–0.24 in.) CRL

Weight: 0.4 g (0.014 oz)

Nervous system: Anterior portion of neural tube closes to form brain; closure of posterior end forms spinal cord.

Musculoskeletal system: Noticeable limb buds.

Cardiovascular system: Tubular heartbeats at 28 days, and primitive red blood cells circulate through fetus and chorionic villi.

Gastrointestinal system: Mouth: formation of oral cavity; primitive jaws present; esophagotracheal septum begins division of esophagus and trachea.

Digestive tract: Stomach forms; esophagus and intestine become tubular; ducts of pancreas and liver forming.

Age: 5 Weeks

Length: 8 mm (0.32 in.) CRL

Weight: Only 0.5% of total body weight is fat (to 20 weeks).

Nervous system: Brain has differentiated and cranial nerves are present.

Musculoskeletal system: Developing muscles have innervation.

Cardiovascular system: Atrial division has occurred.

Age: 6 Weeks

Length: 12 mm (0.47 in.) CRL

Musculoskeletal system: Bone rudiments present; primitive skeletal shape forming; muscle mass begins to develop; ossification of skull and jaws begins.

Cardiovascular system: Chambers present in heart; groups of blood cells can be identified.

Gastrointestinal system: Oral and nasal cavities and upper lip formed; liver begins to form red blood cells.

Respiratory system: Trachea, bronchi, and lung buds present.

Ears: Formation of external, middle, and inner ear continues.

Sexual development: Embryonic sex glands appear.

Age: 7 Weeks

Length: 18 mm (0.71 in.) CRL

Cardiovascular system: Fetal heartbeats can be detected.

Gastrointestinal system: Mouth: tongue separates; palate folds. Digestive tract: stomach attains final form.

Genitourinary system: Separation of bladder and urethra from rectum.

Respiratory system: Diaphragm separates abdominal and thoracic cavities.

Eyes: Optic nerve formed; eyelids appear, thickening of lens.

Sexual development: Differentiation of sex glands into ovaries and testes begins.

Age: 8 Weeks

Length: 2.5–3.0 cm (0.98–1.2 in.) CRL

Weight: 2 g (0.07 oz.)

Musculoskeletal system: Digits formed; further differentiation of cells in primitive skeleton; cartilaginous bones show first signs of ossification; development of muscles in trunk, limbs, and head; some movement of fetus now possible.

Cardiovascular system: Development of heart essentially complete; fetal circulation follows two circuits—four extraembryonic and two intraembryonic. Heartbeat can be heard with Doppler at 8–12 weeks.

Gastrointestinal system: Mouth: completion of lip fusion. Digestive tract: rotation in midgut; anal membrane has perforated.

Ears: External, middle, and inner ear assuming final forms.

Sexual development: Male and female external genitals appear similar until end of ninth week.

Age: 10 Weeks

Length: 5–6 cm (1.97–2.36 in.) CRL

Weight: 14 g (0.49 oz.)

Nervous system: Neurons appear at caudal end of spinal cord; basic divisions of brain present.

Musculoskeletal system: Fingers and toes begin nail growth.

Gastrointestinal system: Mouth: separation of lips from jaw; fusion of palate folds.

Digestive tract: Developing intestines enclosed in abdomen.

Genitourinary system: Bladder sac formed.

Endocrine system: Islets of Langerhans differentiated.

Eyes: Eyelids fused closed; development of lacrimal duct.

Sexual development: Males: production of testosterone and physical characteristics between 8 and 12 weeks.

(continued)

TABLE 4–2 Timeline of Organ System Development in the Embryo and Fetus (*continued*)

Age: 12 Weeks

Length: 8 cm (3.15 in.) CRL; 11.5 cm (4.53 in.) CHL (crown–heel length [CHL])

Weight: 45 g (1.59 oz)

Musculoskeletal system: Clear outlining of miniature bones (12–20 weeks); process of ossification is established throughout fetal body; appearance of involuntary muscles in viscera.

Gastrointestinal system: Mouth: completion of palate.

Digestive tract: Appearance of muscles in gut; bile secretion begins; liver is major producer of red blood cells.

Respiratory system: Lungs acquire definitive shape.

Skin: Pink and delicate.

Endocrine system: Hormonal secretion from thyroid; insulin present in pancreas.

Immunologic system: Appearance of lymphoid tissue in fetal thymus gland.

Age: 16 Weeks

Length: 13.5 cm (5.3 in.) CRL; 15 cm (5.9 in.) CHL

Weight: 200 g (7 oz)

Musculoskeletal system: Teeth beginning to form hard tissue that will become central incisors.

Gastrointestinal system: Mouth: differentiation of hard and soft palate.

Digestive tract: Development of gastric and intestinal glands; intestines begin to collect meconium.

Genitourinary system: Kidneys assume typical shape and organization.

Skin: Appearance of scalp hair; lanugo present on body; transparent skin with visible blood vessels; sweat glands developing.

Eyes, ears, and nose: Formed.

Sexual development: Sex determination possible.

Age: 18 Weeks

Musculoskeletal system: Teeth beginning to form hard tissue (enamel and dentine) that will become lateral incisors.

Cardiovascular system: Fetal heart tones audible with fetoscope at 16–20 weeks.

Age: 20 Weeks

Length: 19 cm (7.5 in.) CRL; 25 cm (9.84 in.) CHL

Weight: 435 g (15.34 oz) (6% of total body weight is fat).

Nervous system: Myelination of spinal cord begins.

Musculoskeletal system: Teeth beginning to form hard tissue that will become canines and first molars. Lower limbs are of final relative proportions.

Gastrointestinal system: Fetus actively sucks and swallows amniotic fluid; peristaltic movements begin.

Skin: Lanugo covers entire body; brown fat begins to form; vernix caseosa begins to form.

Immunologic system: Detectable levels of fetal antibodies (IgG type).

Blood formation: Iron is stored and bone marrow is increasingly important.

Age: 24 Weeks

Length: 23 cm (9.06 in.) CRL; 28 cm (11.02 in.) CHL

Weight: 780 g (1.72 lb)

Nervous system: Brain looks like mature brain.

Musculoskeletal system: Teeth are beginning to form hard tissue that will become the second molars.

Respiratory system: Respiratory movements may occur (24–40 weeks). Nostrils reopen. Alveoli appear in lungs and begin production of surfactant; gas exchange possible.

Skin: Reddish and wrinkled; vernix caseosa present.

Immunologic system: IgG levels reach maternal levels.

Age: 28 Weeks

Length: 27 cm (10.63 in.) CRL; 35 cm (13.8 in.) CHL

Weight: 1200–1250 g (2.65–2.76 lb)

Nervous system: Begins regulation of some body functions.

Skin: Adipose tissue accumulates rapidly; nails appear; eyebrows and eyelashes present.

Eyes: Eyelids open (26–29 weeks).

Sexual development: Males: testes descend into inguinal canal and upper scrotum.

Age: 32 Weeks

Length: 31 cm (12.2 in.) CRL; 38–43 cm (15.0–17.0 in.) CHL

Weight: 2000 g (4.4 lb)

Nervous system: More reflexes present.

Age: 36 Weeks

Length: 35 cm (13.78 in.) CRL; 42–48 cm (16.5–18.9 in.) CHL

Weight: 2500–2750 g (5.5–6.1 lb)

Musculoskeletal system: Distal femoral ossification centers present.

Skin: Pale; body rounded, lanugo disappearing, hair fuzzy or woolly; few sole creases; sebaceous glands active and helping to produce vernix caseosa (36–40 weeks).

Ears: Earlobes soft with little cartilage.

Sexual development: Males: scrotum small and few rugae present; descent of testes into upper scrotum to stay (36–40 weeks). Females: labia majora and minora equally prominent.

Age: 38–40 Weeks

Length: 40 cm (15.75) CRL; 48–52 cm (18.9–20.5 in.) CHL

Weight: 3000–3600 g+ (6.6–7.9 lb+) (16% of total body weight is fat).

Respiratory system: At 38 weeks, lecithin–sphingomyelin (L/S) ratio approaches 2:1 (indicates decreased risk of respiratory distress from inadequate surfactant production if born now).

Skin: Smooth and pink; vernix present in skin folds; moderate to profuse silky hair; lanugo on shoulders and upper back; nails extend over tips or digits; creases cover sole.

Ears: Earlobes firmer because of increased cartilage.

Sexual development: Males: rugous scrotum. Females: labia majora well developed and minora small or completely covered.

Note: *Age refers to postfertilization or postconception age. Measurements are an average.*

Sources: Data from Moore, K. L., Persaud, T. V. N., & Torchia, M. G. (2016). *The developing human: Clinical oriented embryology* (10th ed.). Philadelphia, PA: Saunders/Elsevier; Sadler, T. W. (2015). *Langman's medical embryology* (13th ed.). Philadelphia, PA: Lippincott Williams & Wilkins.

heart occurs with the dividing of the atrium. The embryo has a marked C-shaped body, accentuated by the rudimentary tail and the large head folded over a protuberant trunk (Figure 4–13). By day 35, the arm and leg buds are well developed, with paddle-shaped hand and foot plates. The heart, circulatory system, and brain show the most advanced development. The brain has differentiated into five areas, and 10 pairs of cranial nerves are recognizable.

6 WEEKS

At 6 weeks the head structures are more highly developed and the trunk is straighter than in earlier stages. The upper and lower jaws are recognizable, and the external nares are well formed. The trachea has developed, and its caudal end

is bifurcated for beginning lung formation. The upper lip has formed, and the palate is developing. The ears are developing rapidly. The arms have begun to extend ventrally across the chest, and both arms and legs have digits, although they may still be webbed. There is a slight elbow bend in the arms, which are more advanced in development than the legs. Beginning at this stage, the prominent tail will recede. The heart now has most of its definitive characteristics, and fetal circulation begins to be established. The liver starts to produce blood cells.

7 WEEKS

At 7 weeks the head of the embryo is rounded and nearly erect (Figure 4–14). The eyes have shifted and are closer together, and the eyelids are beginning to form. The palate is near completion,

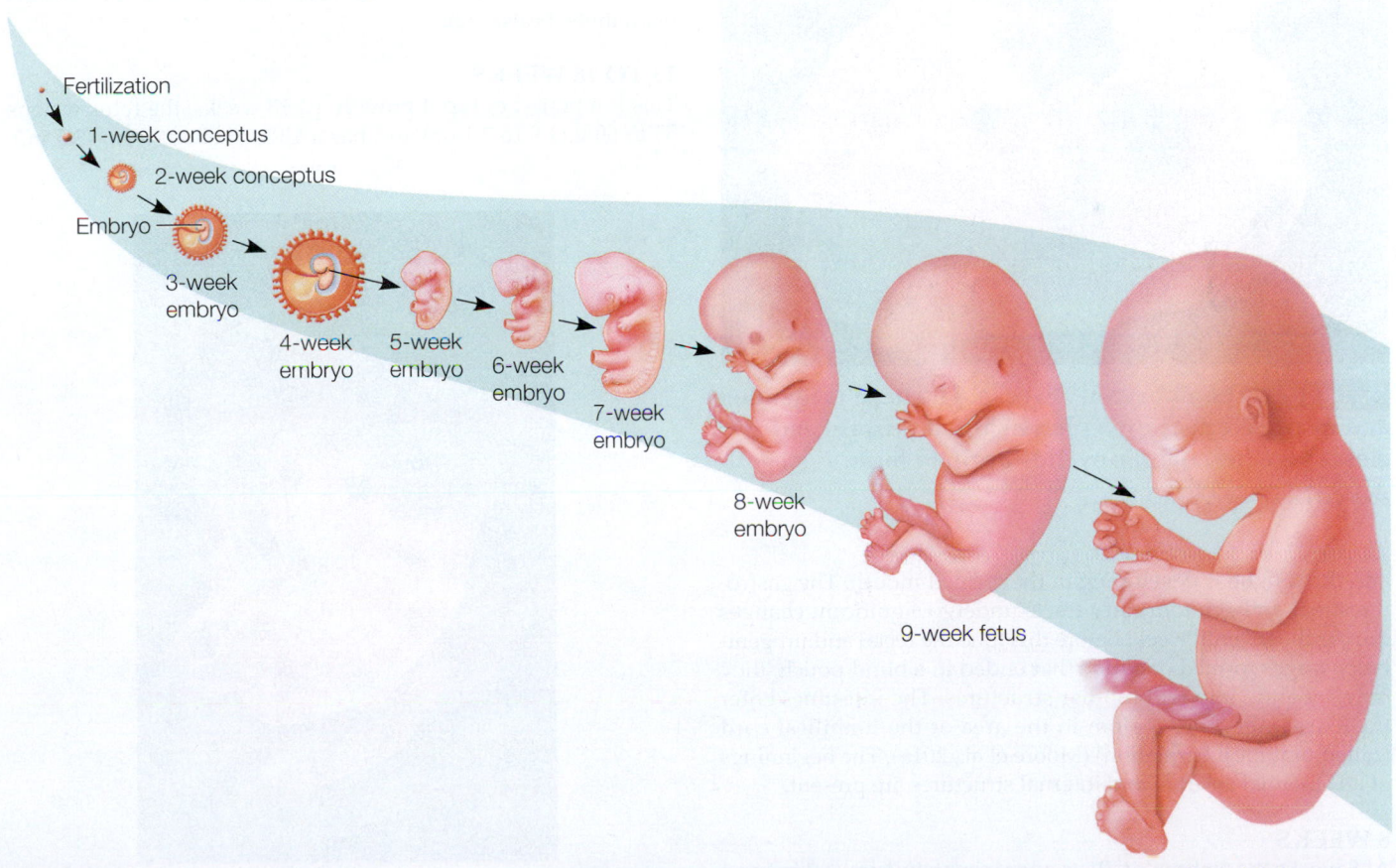

Fertilization

1-week conceptus

2-week conceptus

Embryo

3-week embryo

4-week embryo

5-week embryo

6-week embryo

7-week embryo

8-week embryo

9-week fetus

12-week fetus

Figure 4–12 **The actual size of a human conceptus from fertilization to the early fetal stage. The embryonic stage begins in the third week after fertilization; the fetal stage begins in the ninth week.**

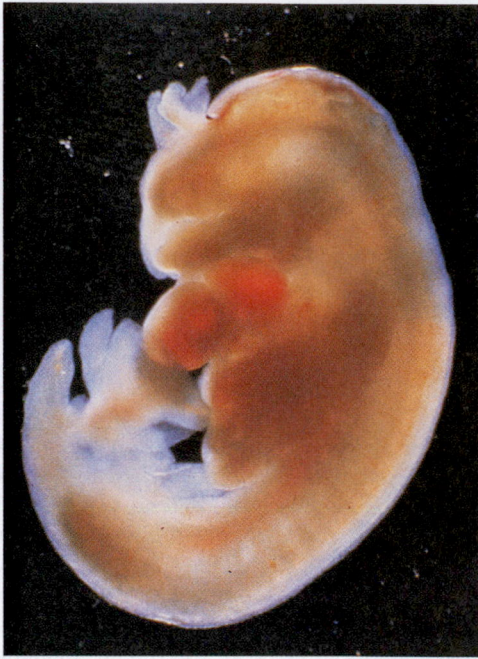

Figure 4–13 The embryo at 5 weeks. The embryo has a marked C-shaped body and a rudimentary tail.

SOURCE: Omikron/Getty Images.

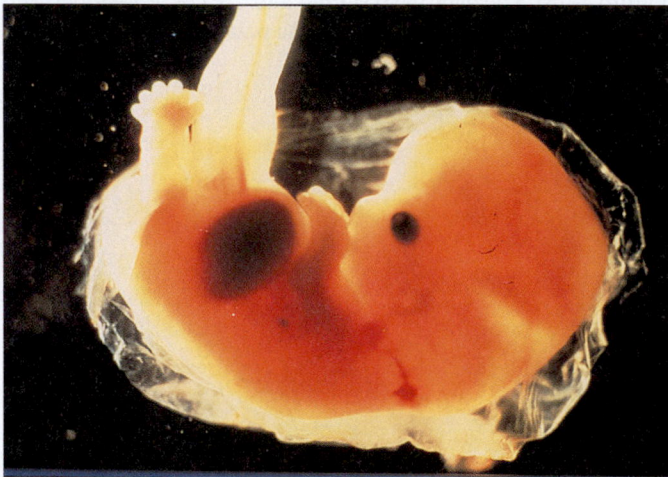

Figure 4–14 The embryo at 7 weeks. The head is rounded and nearly erect. The eyes have shifted forward and closer together, and the eyelids begin to form.

SOURCE: Petit Format/Science Source.

and the tongue is developing in the formed mouth. The gastrointestinal and genitourinary tracts undergo significant changes during the seventh week. Before this time the rectal and urogenital passages formed one tube that ended in a blind pouch; they now separate into two tubular structures. The intestines enter the extraembryonic coelom in the area of the umbilical cord (called umbilical herniation) (Moore et al., 2016). The beginnings of all essential external and internal structures are present.

8 WEEKS

At 8 weeks the embryo's CRL is approximately 3 cm (1.2 in.) and it clearly resembles a human being. Facial features continue to develop. The eyelids begin to fuse. Auricles of the external ears begin to assume their final shape, but they are still set low (Moore

et al., 2016). External genitals appear, but the embryo's sex is not clearly identifiable. The rectal passage opens with the perforation of the anal membrane. The circulatory system through the umbilical cord is well established. Long bones are beginning to form, and the large muscles are now capable of contracting.

Fetal Stage

By the end of the eighth week, the embryo is sufficiently developed to be called a **fetus**. Every organ system and external structure that will be found in the full-term newborn is present. The remainder of gestation is devoted to refining structures and perfecting function.

9 TO 12 WEEKS

By the end of the ninth or tenth week the fetus reaches a CRL of 5 cm (2 in.) and weighs about 14 g (0.5 oz). The head is large and comprises almost half of the fetus's entire size (Figure 4–15). At 12 weeks, the fetus reaches 8 cm (3.2 in.) CRL and weighs about 45 g (1.6 oz). The face is well formed, with the nose protruding, the chin small and receding, and the ears acquiring a more adult shape. The eyelids close at about the 10th week and will not reopen until about the 26- to 29-week period. Some movement of the lips suggestive of the sucking reflex has been observed at 3 months. Tooth buds now appear for all 20 of the child's first teeth (baby teeth). The limbs are long and slender, with well-formed digits. The fetus can curl its fingers toward the palm and begins to make a tiny fist. The legs are still shorter and less developed than the arms. The urogenital tract completes its development, well-differentiated genitals appear, and the kidneys begin to produce urine. Red blood cells are produced primarily by the liver. Spontaneous movements of the fetus now occur. Fetal heart rates can be ascertained by electronic devices between 8 and 12 weeks. The rate is 120 to 160 beats per minute (beats/min).

13 TO 16 WEEKS

This is a period of rapid growth. At 13 weeks, the fetus weighs 55 to 60 g (1.9 to 2.1 oz) and has a CRL of about 9 cm (3.5 in.).

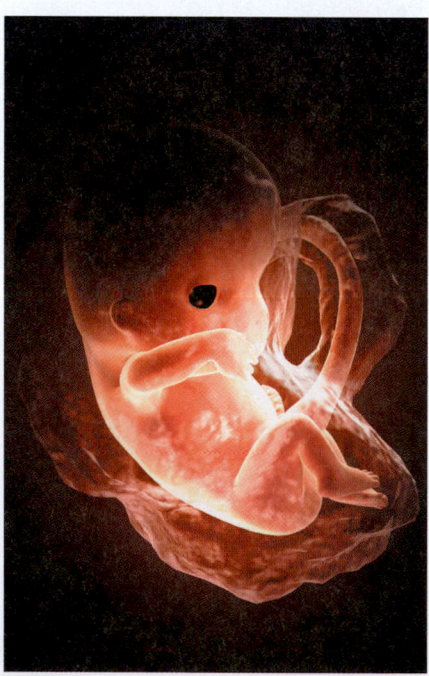

Figure 4–15 The fetus at 9 weeks. Every organ system and external structure is present.

SOURCE: MedicalRF.com/Corbis.

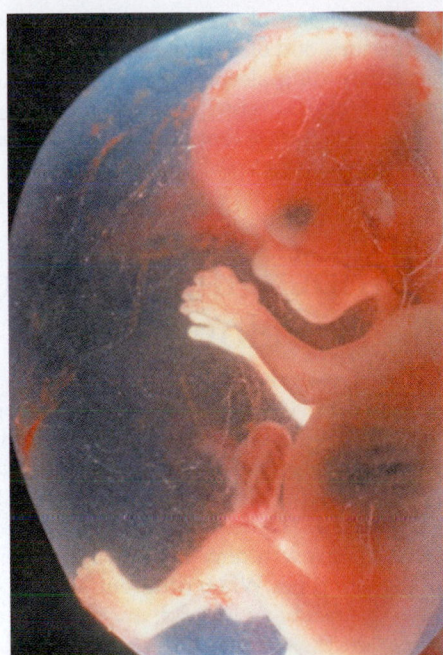

Figure 4–16 The fetus at 14 weeks. During this period of rapid growth the skin is so transparent that blood vessels are visible beneath it. More muscle tissue and body skeleton have developed, and they hold the fetus more erect.

SOURCE: Claude Edelmann/Science Source.

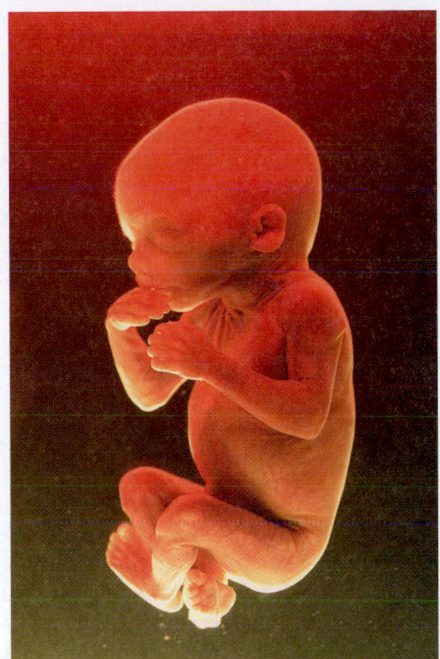

Figure 4–17 The fetus at 20 weeks. The fetus now weighs about 435 g (15.34 oz) and measures about 19 cm (7.5 in.). Subcutaneous deposits of brown fat make the skin a little less transparent. "Woolly" hair may cover the head, and nails have developed on the fingers and toes.

SOURCE: James Stevenson/Science Source.

Lanugo, or fine hair, begins to develop, especially on the head. The skin is so transparent that blood vessels are clearly visible beneath it. More muscle tissue and body skeleton have developed and hold the fetus more erect (Figure 4–16). Active movements are present; the fetus stretches and exercises its arms and legs. It makes sucking motions, swallows amniotic fluid, and produces meconium in the intestinal tract. Bronchial tubes are branching out in the primitive lungs, and sweat glands are developing. The liver and pancreas now begin production of their appropriate secretions. By the beginning of week 16, skeletal ossification is clearly identifiable.

20 WEEKS
The fetus doubles its CRL and now measures 19 cm (7.5 in.) long. Fetal weight is between 435 and 465 g (15.3 and 16.4 oz). Lanugo covers the entire body and is especially prominent on the shoulders. Subcutaneous deposits of brown fat, which has a rich blood supply, make the skin less transparent. Brown fat is found chiefly at the root of the neck, posterior to the sternum and in the perirenal area. Nipples now appear over the mammary glands. The head is covered with fine, "woolly" hair, and the eyebrows and eyelashes are beginning to form. Nails are present on both fingers and toes. Muscles are well developed, and the fetus is active (Figure 4–17). The mother feels fetal movement, known as *quickening*. The fetal heartbeat is audible through a fetoscope. Quickening and fetal heartbeat can help in validating the EDB.

24 WEEKS
The fetus at 24 weeks reaches a CRL of 23 cm (9.06 in.) or CHL of 28 cm (11.02 in.). It weighs about 780 g (1.72 lb). The hair on the head is growing long, and eyebrows and eyelashes have formed. The eye is structurally complete and will soon open. The fetus has a reflex hand grip (grasp reflex) and, by the end of

6 months, a startle reflex. Skin covering the body is reddish and wrinkled, with little subcutaneous fat. Skin on the hands and feet has thickened, with skin ridges on palms and soles forming distinct footprints and fingerprints. The skin over the entire body is covered with **vernix caseosa**, a protective cheeselike, fatty substance secreted by the sebaceous glands. The alveoli in the lungs are just beginning to form.

25 TO 28 WEEKS
At about 25 weeks, the fetal skin is still red, wrinkled, and covered with vernix caseosa. The brain is developing rapidly, and the nervous system is complete enough to provide some degree of regulation of body functions. The eyelids, under neural control, open and close. The fetus has nails on both fingers and toes. In the male fetus, the testes begin to descend into the scrotal sac. Even though the lungs are still physiologically immature, they are sufficiently developed to provide gas exchange. A fetus born at this time will require immediate and prolonged intensive care to survive and then to decrease the risk of major handicap. The fetus at 28 weeks is about 27 cm (10.6 in.) CRL or 35 to 38 cm (13.8 to 15.0 in.) CHL and weighs 1200 to 1250 g (2.65 lb, to 2.75 lb).

29 TO 32 WEEKS
At 30 weeks the pupillary light reflex is present (Moore et al., 2016). The fetus is gaining weight from an increase in body muscle and fat and weighs about 2000 g (4.4 lb), with a CRL of 31 cm (12.2 in.) or with a CHL of about 38 to 43 cm (15 to 17 in.), by 32 weeks of age. The central nervous system (CNS) has matured enough to direct rhythmic breathing movements and partially control body temperature. However, the lungs are not yet fully mature. Bones are fully developed but soft and flexible. The fetus begins storing iron, calcium, and phosphorus. In

males the testicles may be located in the scrotal sac but are often still high in the inguinal canals.

35 TO 36 WEEKS

The fetus begins to become plump, and less wrinkled skin covers the deposits of subcutaneous fat. Lanugo begins to disappear, and the nails reach the edge of the fingertips. By 35 weeks of age the fetus has a firm grasp and exhibits spontaneous orientation to light. By 36 weeks of age its weight is usually 2500 to 2750 g (5.5 to 6 lb), and the CHL of the fetus is about 42 to 48 cm (16.5 to 18.9 in.) or CRL is about 35 cm (13.78 in.). A baby born at this time has a good chance of surviving but may require special care, especially if intrauterine growth restriction is occurring.

38 TO 40 WEEKS

The fetus is considered full term at 38 weeks and up to 40 weeks after conception. The CHL varies from 48 to 52 cm (18.9 to 20.5 in.), or CRL of about 40 cm (15.75 in.), with males usually longer than females. Males also usually weigh more than females. The weight at term is about 3000 to 3600 g (6.6 to 7.9 lb) and varies in different ethnic groups. The skin is pink and has a smooth, polished look. The only lanugo left is on the upper arms and shoulders. The hair on the head is no longer woolly but is coarse and about 1 in. long. Vernix caseosa is present, with heavier deposits remaining in the creases and folds of the skin. The body and extremities are plump, with good skin turgor, and the fingernails extend beyond the fingertips. The chest is prominent but still a little smaller than the head, and mammary glands protrude in both sexes. In males, the testes are in the scrotum or palpable in the inguinal canals.

As the fetus enlarges, amniotic fluid diminishes to about 400 mL or less, and the fetal body mass fills the uterine cavity (Blackburn, 2013). The fetus assumes what is called its *position of comfort*, or lie. The head is generally pointed downward, following the shape of the uterus (and possibly because the head is heavier than the feet). The extremities, and often the head, are well flexed. After 5 months, patterns in feeding, sleeping, and activity become established, so at term the fetus has its own body rhythms and individual style of response. See *Key Facts to Remember: Fetal Development: What Parents Want to Know*. For a detailed discussion of each body system's transition to full functioning in the newborn, see Chapter 23.

Factors Influencing Embryonic and Fetal Development

Factors that may affect embryonic development include the quality of the sperm or ovum from which the zygote was formed, the genetic code established at fertilization, and the adequacy of the intrauterine environment. If the environment is unsuitable before cellular differentiation occurs, all the cells of the zygote are affected. The cells may die, which causes spontaneous abortion, or growth may be slowed, depending on the severity of the situation. When differentiation is complete and the fetal membranes have formed, an injurious agent has the greatest effect on those cells undergoing the most rapid growth. Thus the time of injury is critical in the development of anomalies.

Because organs are formed primarily during embryonic development, the growing organism is considered most vulnerable to hazardous agents during the first months of pregnancy. Any agent (e.g., drug, virus, or radiation) that can cause development of abnormal structures in an embryo is called a **teratogen**. It is important to remember that the effects of teratogens depend on the (1) maternal and fetal genotype, (2) stage of development when exposure occurs, and (3) dose and duration of exposure of the agent. Potential teratogens can cause malformations of the heart, limbs, eyes, and other organ systems as early as 3 weeks postconception (Moore et al., 2016). Chapter 8 discusses the effects of specific teratogenic agents on the developing fetus.

Adequacy of the maternal environment is also important during the periods of rapid embryonic and fetal development. Maternal nutrition can affect brain and neural tube development. The period of maximum brain growth and myelination begins with the fifth lunar month before birth and continues into adulthood (Blackburn, 2013). Amino acids, glucose, and fatty acids are considered to be the primary dietary factors in brain growth. A subtle type of damage that affects the associative capacity of the brain, possibly leading to learning disabilities, may be caused by nutritional deficiency at this stage.

KEY FACTS TO REMEMBER
Fetal Development: What Parents Want to Know

4 weeks:	The fetal heart begins to beat.
8 weeks:	All body organs are formed.
8 to 12 weeks:	Fetal heart rate can be heard by ultrasound Doppler device.
16 weeks:	Baby's sex can be seen. Although thin, the fetus looks like a baby.
20 weeks:	Heartbeat can be heard with fetoscope. Mother feels movement (quickening). Baby develops a regular schedule of sleeping, sucking, and kicking. Hands can grasp. Baby assumes a favorite position in utero. Vernix caseosa (lanolin-like covering) protects the body, and lanugo (fine hair) keeps oil on skin. Head hair, eyebrows, and eyelashes present.
24 weeks:	Weighs 780 g (1 lb, 10 oz). Activity is increasing. Fetal respiratory movements begin.
28 weeks:	Eyes open and close. Baby can breathe at this time. Surfactant needed for breathing at birth is formed. Baby is two thirds its final length.
32 weeks:	Baby has fingernails and toenails. Subcutaneous fat is being laid down. Baby appears less red and wrinkled.
38+ weeks:	Baby fills total uterus. Baby gets antibodies from mother.

SAFETY ALERT!

Vitamins and folic acid supplements taken before conception can reduce the incidence of neural tube defects.

Healthy People 2020

MICH-14 Increase the proportion of women of childbearing potential with daily intake of at least 400 mcg of folic acid from fortified foods or dietary supplementation to 26.2% from the current level of 23.8%

Poor maternal nutrition may also predispose babies who were small or disproportionate at birth to the development of adult coronary heart disease, hypertension, and diabetes (Moore et al., 2016). Maternal nutrition is discussed in depth in Chapter 11.

Another prenatal influence on the intrauterine environment is maternal hyperthermia associated with sauna or hot tub use. Studies of the effects of maternal hyperthermia during the first trimester have raised concern about possible CNS defects and failure of neural tube closure. Maternal substance abuse also affects the intrauterine environment and is discussed in Chapter 14 and Chapter 26. Cigarette smoking during pregnancy is a well-established cause of intrauterine growth restriction (IUGR) (Moore et al., 2016).

> **Clinical Reasoning** **Illness During Pregnancy**
> Melodie Chong, in her third week of pregnancy, develops a fever of 40°C (104°F) and flulike symptoms but refuses to take any medication because she is afraid that drugs will harm her baby. Most factors—maternal, fetal, and environmental—may affect prenatal growth.
>
> *Melodie asks when her baby is most vulnerable for abnormal growth or structure. How would you answer?*

Focus Your Study

- Humans have 46 chromosomes, which are divided into 23 pairs: 22 pairs of autosomes and 1 pair of sex chromosomes.

- Mitosis is the process by which somatic (body) cells are formed. It provides growth and development of the organisms and replacement of body cells.

- Meiosis is the process by which gametes (ova and sperm) are formed. It occurs during gametogenesis (oogenesis and spermatogenesis) and consists of two successive cell divisions (reduction division), which produce a gamete with 23 chromosomes (22 autosomal chromosomes and 1 sex chromosome), the haploid number of chromosomes.

- Gametes must have a haploid number of chromosomes (23) so that when the female gamete (ovum) and the male gamete (spermatozoon) unite (fertilization) to form the zygote, the normal human diploid number of chromosomes (46) is reestablished.

- An ovum is to be considered fertile for about 12 to 24 hours after ovulation, and the sperm is capable of fertilizing the ovum for only about 24 hours after it is deposited in the female reproductive tract.

- Fertilization usually takes place in the ampulla (outer third) of the fallopian tube. Both capacitation and acrosomal reaction must occur for the sperm to fertilize the ovum. Capacitation is the removal of the plasma membrane, which exposes the acrosomal covering of the sperm head. Acrosomal reaction is the deposit of hyaluronidase in the corona radiata, which allows the sperm head to penetrate the ovum.

- Sex chromosomes are referred to as X and Y. Females have two X chromosomes, and males have an X and a Y chromosome. Y chromosomes are carried only by the sperm. To produce a female child, both the mother and the father contribute an X chromosome. To produce a male child, the mother contributes an X chromosome and the father contributes a Y chromosome.

- Intrauterine development first proceeds via cellular multiplication in which the zygote undergoes rapid mitotic division called cleavage. As a result of cleavage, the zygote divides and multiplies into cell groupings called blastomeres, which are held together by the zona pellucida. The blastomeres eventually become a solid ball of cells called the morula. When a cavity forms in the morula cell mass, the inner solid cell mass is called the blastocyst.

- Implantation usually occurs in the upper part of the posterior uterine wall when the blastocyst burrows into the uterine lining.

- After implantation, the endometrium is called the decidua. Decidua capsularis is the portion that covers the blastocyst. Decidua basalis is the portion that is directly under the blastocyst. Decidua vera is the portion that lines the rest of the uterine cavity.

- Embryonic membranes are called the amnion and the chorion. The amnion is formed from the ectoderm and is a thin protective membrane that contains the amniotic fluid and the embryo. The chorion is a thick membrane that develops from the trophoblast and encloses the amnion, embryo, and yolk sac.

- Amniotic fluid cushions the fetus against mechanical injury, maintains the embryo's temperature, allows symmetric external growth, prevents adherence to the amnion, and permits freedom of movement.

- Primary germ layers will give rise to all tissues, organs, and organ systems. The three primary germ cell layers are ectoderm, endoderm, and mesoderm.

- The umbilical cord contains two umbilical arteries, which carry deoxygenated blood from the fetus to the placenta, and one umbilical vein, which carries oxygenated blood from the placenta to the fetus. The umbilical cord normally has a central insertion into the placenta. Wharton jelly, a specialized connective tissue, helps prevent compression of the umbilical cord in utero.

- Twins are either monozygotic (identical) or dizygotic (fraternal). Dizygotic twins arise from two separate ova fertilized by two separate spermatozoa. Monozygotic twins develop from a single ovum fertilized by a single spermatozoon.

- The placenta develops from the chorionic villi and decidua basalis and has two parts:
  - The maternal portion, consisting of the decidua basalis, is red and fresh looking.
  - The fetal portion, consisting of chorionic villi, is covered by the amnion and appears shiny and gray.

- The placenta is made up of 15 to 20 segments called cotyledons.

- The placenta serves endocrine (hPL, hCG, estrogen, and progesterone), metabolic, and immunologic functions. It acts as the fetus's respiratory organ, is an organ of excretion, and aids in the exchange of nutrients.

- Stages of fetal development include the preembryonic stage (the first 14 days of human development starting at the time of fertilization), the embryonic stage (from day 15 after fertilization, or the beginning of the third week, until approximately 8 weeks), and the fetal stage (from 8 weeks until birth, at approximately 38+ weeks post–conception).

- Significant events that occur during the embryonic stage include the fetal heart beginning to beat at 4 weeks and the establishment of fetal circulation at 6 weeks. Fetal circulation is a specially designed circulatory system that provides for oxygenation of the fetus while bypassing the fetal lungs.

- The fetal stage is devoted to refining structures and perfecting function. The following are some significant developments during the fetal stage:
  - At 8 to 12 weeks: all organ systems are formed and now require maturation.
  - At 16 weeks: the sex of the fetus can be determined visually.
  - At 20 weeks: the fetus measures 19 cm (7.5 in.) CRL, myelination of spinal cord begins. Suck and swallow begins, lanugo covers body, vernix caseosa begins to form; fetal heartbeat can be auscultated by a fetoscope, and the mother can feel movement (quickening).

- At 24 weeks: 23 cm (9.06 in.) CRL, respiratory movement and surfactant production begins, brain appears mature. Vernix caseosa covers the entire body.
- At 26 to 29 weeks: the eyes reopen after closing at around 10 weeks.
- At 28 weeks: 27 cm (10.63 in.) CRL, nervous system begins regulation of some functions, adipose tissue accumulates rapidly. Nails, eyebrows, and eyelids are present. Eyes open and close.
- At 32 weeks: skin appears less wrinkled and red because subcutaneous fat has been laid down.
- At 35 to 36 weeks: 35 cm (13.78 in.) CRL, earlobes soft with little cartilage, fingernails reach the ends of fingers, few sole creases.
- At 38 weeks: vernix caseosa is apparent only in the creases and folds of skin, and lanugo remains on upper arms and shoulders only.
- At 38 to 40 weeks: 40 cm (15.75 in.) CRL, adequate surfactant, vernix caseosa in skin folds and lanugo on shoulders, earlobes firm, sex apparent.

- The embryo is particularly vulnerable to teratogenesis during the first 8 weeks of cell differentiation and organ system development. Effects of teratogens depend on the (1) maternal and fetal genotype, (2) stage of development when exposure occurs, and (3) dose and duration of exposure of the agent.

Clinical Reasoning in Action

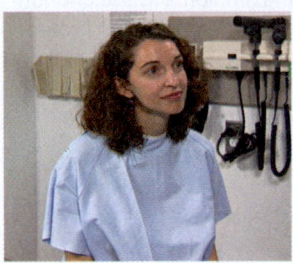

You are working at the local clinic when Frances, a 28-year-old G2 P1001 at 11 weeks' gestation, comes into the office. Frances tells you that early in the first trimester, her husband experienced a flulike syndrome and that he was later diagnosed with cytomegalovirus (CMV) pneumonia. She tells you that his physician found an enlarged supraclavicular lymph node and an ulcer on one tonsil. Laboratory testing revealed elevated liver enzymes. Further testing led to the discovery of positive IgM levels. She has come today with symptoms including night sweats, persistent sore throat, joint pain, headache, vomiting, and fatigue.

You obtain vital signs of temperature 99°F (37.2°C), pulse 90, respirations 14, BP 110/70. Her physical exam is normal; no lymphadenopathy are present. Her weight gain is 2 lb even though she has experienced nausea and some vomiting. She is worried that her husband's illness could be related to her current symptoms.

1. How would you respond to Frances's concern?

2. Frances asks you if her baby is formed. How would you discuss the three stages of development?

3. Frances asks when her baby is most vulnerable for abnormal growth or structure. How would you answer?

4. Frances asks what stage her baby is in. What would you tell her?

References

Blackburn, S. T. (2013). *Maternal, fetal, & neonatal physiology: A clinical perspective* (4th ed.). St. Louis, MO: Saunders/Elsevier.

Caudle, P. W. (2014). Physiological foundations of prenatal and postnatal care. In R. G. Jordan, J. L. Engstrom, J. A. Marfell, & C. L. Farley (Eds.) *Prenatal and postnatal care: A women-centered approach.* Ames, IA: Wiley Blackwell.

Cunningham, F. G., Leveno, K. J., Bloom, S. L., Spong, C. Y., Dashe, J. S., Hoffman, B. L., . . . & Sheffield, J. S. (2014). *Williams obstetrics* (24th ed.). New York, NY: McGraw-Hill.

Moore, K. L., Persaud, T. V. N., & Torchia, M. G. (2016). *The developing human: Clinical oriented embryology* (10th ed.). Philadelphia, PA: Saunders/Elsevier.

National Institute for Health and Clinical Excellence (NICE) (2011). *Antenatal care: Routine care for the healthy pregnant woman.* Retrieved from http://www.nice.org.uk/CG62

Sadler, T. W. (2015). *Langman's medical embryology* (13th ed.). Philadelphia, PA: Lippincott Williams & Wilkins.

Society of Maternal-Fetal Medicine (SMFM); Moise, K. J., & Argon, P. S. (2013). The importance of determining chorionicity in twin gestations. *Contemporary OB/GYN,* February 3, 2013, 35–43.

Chapter 5
Health Promotion for Women

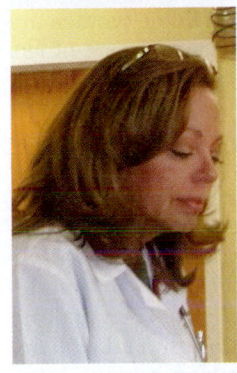

I have started caring for the teenage daughters of many of my longtime clients. Making each teen's first pelvic exam a positive experience has become something of a mission for me. Yesterday I completed a young woman's first GYN exam and as I finished she said, "That was easy. Why do women make such a fuss about a pelvic?" I wanted to jump up and shout, "Yes!" Attitudes are changed one person at a time.

—A Women's Health Nurse Practitioner

⌄ Learning Outcomes

5.1 Describe accurate information to be provided to girls and women so that they can implement effective self-care measures for dealing with menstruation.

5.2 Contrast the signs, symptoms, and nursing management of women with dysmenorrhea and those with premenstrual syndrome.

5.3 Compare the advantages, disadvantages, and effectiveness of the various methods of contraception available today.

5.4 Summarize major health measures to address in providing preconception counseling.

5.5 Identify basic gynecologic screening procedures indicated for well women.

5.6 Explain the physical and psychologic aspects and clinical treatment options of menopause when caring for menopausal women.

5.7 Describe the phases of the cycle of violence.

5.8 Identify the phases of the rape trauma syndrome.

5.9 Discuss the nurse's role in screening and caring for women who have experienced domestic violence or rape.

A woman's healthcare needs change throughout her lifetime. As a young girl she needs health teaching about menstruation, sexuality, and personal responsibility. As a teen she needs information about reproductive choices and safe sexual activity. During this time she should also be introduced to the importance of healthcare practices such as regular Pap smears. The mature woman may need to be reminded of these self-care issues and prepared for physical changes that accompany childbirth and aging. By educating women about their bodies, their healthcare choices, and their right to be knowledgeable consumers, nurses can help women assume responsibility for the health care they receive.

This chapter provides information about selected aspects of women's health care with an emphasis on conditions typically addressed in a community-based setting.

Community-Based Nursing Care

Women's health refers to a holistic view of women and their health-related needs within the context of their everyday lives. It is based on the awareness that a woman's physical, mental, and spiritual status are interdependent and affect her state of health or illness. The woman's view of her situation, her assessment of her needs, her values, and her beliefs are valid and important factors to be incorporated into any healthcare intervention.

Nurses can work with women to provide health teaching and information about self-care practices in schools, during routine examinations in a clinic or office, at senior centers, at meetings of volunteer organizations, through classes offered by local agencies or schools, or in the home. This community-based focus is the key to providing effective nursing care to women of all ages. Nurses oriented to community-based care are especially effective in recognizing the autonomy of each individual and in dealing with clients holistically. A holistic approach is important in addressing not only physical problems but also major health issues such as violence against women, which may go undetected unless healthcare providers are alert for signs of it.

The Nurse's Role in Addressing Issues of Sexuality

Because sexuality and its reproductive implications are such an intrinsic and emotion-laden part of life, people have many concerns, problems, and questions about sex roles, behaviors, education, inhibitions, morality, and related areas such as family planning. Health factors are another consideration. The increase in the incidence of sexually transmitted infections, especially HIV/AIDS and genital herpes, has caused many people to modify their sexual practices and activities. Women frequently ask questions or voice concerns about these issues to the nurse in a clinic or ambulatory setting. Thus the nurse may need to assume the role of counselor on sexual and reproductive matters.

Nurses who assume this role must recognize their own feelings, values, and attitudes about sexuality so they can be more sensitive when they encounter the values and beliefs of others. Nurses need to have accurate, up-to-date information about anatomy and physiology and about topics related to sexuality, sexual practices, and common gynecologic problems. In addition, when a woman is accompanied by her partner, it is important that the nurse be sensitive to the dynamics of the relationship and communication patterns between the two.

Taking a Sexual History

Nurses are often responsible for taking a woman's initial history, including her gynecologic and sexual history. To be effective in this role, the nurse must have effective communication skills and ideally should conduct the interview in a quiet, private place free of distractions.

Clinical Tip

When taking a history, start your interview with less intimate areas, such as medical and surgical history, and then proceed to the sexual history toward the end of the history-taking session. This approach helps the woman develop a comfort level with you before disclosing personal information.

Opening the discussion with a brief explanation of the purpose of such questions is often helpful. For example, the nurse might say, "As your nurse I'm interested in all aspects of your well-being. Often women have concerns or questions about sexual matters, especially as their life situations change. I will be asking you some questions about your sexual history as part of your general health history." This explanation will help women understand the nature of this part of the history and allow for more open, honest answers.

It may be helpful to use direct eye contact as much as possible unless the nurse knows it is culturally unacceptable to the woman. The nurse should do little, if any, writing or typing into a computer during the interview, especially if the woman seems ill at ease or is discussing very personal issues. Open-ended questions are often useful in eliciting information. For example, "What, if anything, would you change about your sex life?" will elicit more information than "Are you happy with your sex life now?" The nurse needs to clarify terminology and proceed from easier topics to those that are more difficult to discuss.

Throughout the interview the nurse should be alert to body language and nonverbal cues. It is important that the nurse not assume that the woman is heterosexual. Some women are open about lesbian relationships or transgender surgery; others are more reserved until they develop a sense of trust in their caregivers.

After completing the sexual history, the nurse assesses the information obtained. If there is a problem that requires further medical tests and assessments, the nurse refers the woman to a nurse practitioner, certified nurse-midwife, physician, or counselor as necessary. In many instances the nurse alone will be able to develop a nursing diagnosis and then plan and implement therapy. The nurse needs to be realistic when making assessments and planning interventions. Insight and skill are necessary to recognize when a woman's problem requires interventions that are beyond a nurse's preparation and ability. In such situations, the nurse must make appropriate referrals.

Menstruation

Girls today begin to learn about puberty and menstruation at a young age. Unfortunately, the source of their "education" is sometimes their peers or the media; thus the information is often incomplete, inaccurate, and sensationalized. Nurses who work with young girls and adolescents recognize this and work hard to provide accurate health teaching and to correct misinformation that has been given about menarche (the onset of menses) and the menstrual cycle.

Cultural, religious, and personal attitudes about menstruation are part of the menstrual experience. Currently in the Western world there are few restrictions associated with menstruation. Sexual intercourse during menses is a common practice and is not generally contraindicated. For most couples, the decision is one of personal preference. (The physiology of menstruation is discussed in Chapter 3.)

Counseling the Premenstrual Girl About Menarche

Many young women find it embarrassing or stressful to discuss the menstrual experience, both because of the many taboos associated with the subject and because of their immaturity. However, the most critical factor in successful adaptation to menarche is the adolescent's level of preparedness. Information should be given to premenstrual girls over time rather than all at once. This allows them to absorb information and develop questions.

The following basic information is helpful for girls and young women:

- **Cycle length.** Cycle length is determined from the first day of one menses to the first day of the next menses. Initially, cycle length may be irregular. Once established, a female's cycle length is about 29 days, but the normal length may vary from 24 to 38 days. Cycle length often varies by a day or two from one cycle to the next, although greater normal variations may also occur.

- **Amount of flow.** The average flow is approximately 25 to 60 mL per period. Usually women characterize the amount of flow in terms of the number of pads or tampons used. Flow is often heavier at first and lighter toward the end of the period.

- **Length of menses.** Menses normally lasts from 3 to 5 days, although it may vary and may last up to 7 days.

The nurse should make it clear that variations in age at menarche, length of cycle, and duration of menses are normal because adolescents may worry if their experiences vary from those of their peers. It also is helpful to acknowledge the negative aspects of menstruation (messiness and embarrassment) while stressing its positive role as a symbol of maturity and womanhood.

Cultural factors may play an important role in menstruation for girls and women of some cultures. See *Developing Cultural Competence: Islamic Women and Menstruation.*

Developing Cultural Competence Islamic Women and Menstruation

Islamic women who are menstruating are not required to fast during the month of Ramadan but if they elect not to fast, they are expected to make up the missed fasting days before the next Ramadan. Because it may be harder to fast alone, many Muslim women use oral contraceptives to delay their menses until Ramadan ends (Kridli, 2011). Others choose to fast even when menstruating.

Educational Topics

PADS AND TAMPONS

Since early times women have made pads and tampons from cloth or rags, which required washing but were reusable. Commercial tampons were introduced in the 1930s.

Today adhesive-stripped, disposable minipads and maxipads and flushable tampons are available. However, the deodorants and increased absorbency that manufacturers have added to both sanitary napkins and tampons may prove harmful. The chemical used to deodorize can create irritation of the vulva and inner aspects of the vagina. This irritation may cause an external rash or internal sores from trauma to the tender mucosal lining of the vagina.

Interest is growing in the use of eco-friendly menstrual products including reusable menstrual pads made of washable cotton, menstrual cups, and menstrual sponges. These products are becoming more readily available at pharmacies and major discount stores. (See Figure 5–1.)

The use of superabsorbent tampons has been linked to the development of toxic shock syndrome (TSS)(see Chapter 6). Women may prevent problems by using tampons with the minimum absorbency necessary to control menstrual flow, changing them every 3 to 6 hours, and avoiding using them for vaginal discharge or very light bleeding. Because *Staphylococcus aureus*, the causative organism of TSS, is frequently found on the hands,

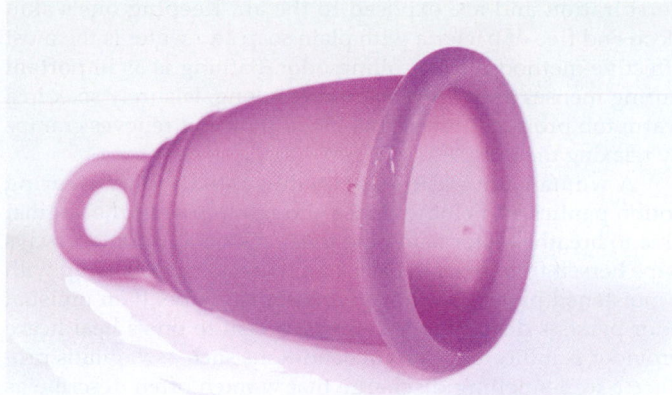

Figure 5–1 **A menstrual cup is an eco-friendly way to manage menstrual flow.**

SOURCE: Aguadeluna/Fotolia.

a woman should wash her hands before inserting a fresh tampon and should avoid touching the tip of the tampon when unwrapping it or before insertion.

In the absence of a heavy menstrual flow, tampons absorb moisture, leaving the vaginal walls dry and subject to injury. The absorbency of regular tampons varies. If the tampon is hard to pull out or shreds when removed, or if the vagina becomes dry, the tampon is probably too absorbent.

A woman may want to use tampons only during the day and switch to napkins at night to avoid vaginal irritation. If a woman experiences vaginal irritation, itching, or soreness or notices an unusual odor while using tampons, she should stop using them and be evaluated for infection. The choice of sanitary protection—whether napkins or tampons—must meet the individual's needs and feel comfortable. Cultural factors may play a role in this decision.

Clinical Tip

If you work with teens and preteens, keep a variety of pads and tampons on hand so that you can help these young girls become familiar with the options available for dealing with menstruation. You can also put colored water in a small glass and insert a tampon to show a girl how much fluid a tampon absorbs. Girls often think that they lose far more blood with a period than they actually do.

VAGINAL SPRAYS, DOUCHING, AND CLEANSING

Vaginal sprays are unnecessary and can cause infections, itching, burning, rashes, and other problems. Generally healthcare providers do not recommend them. If a woman chooses to use a spray, she needs to know that these sprays are for external use only, should be used infrequently, and should never be applied to irritated or itching skin.

Douching as a hygiene practice is unnecessary because the vagina cleanses itself. Douching washes away the natural mucus and upsets the vaginal flora, which can make the vagina more susceptible to infection. Douching with perfumed douches can cause allergic reactions. Propelling water up the vagina may force bacteria and germs from the vagina into the uterus. Women should avoid douching during menstruation because the cervix is dilated to permit the downward flow of menstrual fluids from the uterine lining. Douching is also contraindicated during pregnancy.

The secretions that bathe the vagina are odorless while they are in the vagina; odor develops when they mingle with perspiration and are exposed to the air. Keeping one's skin clean and free of bacteria with plain soap and water is the most effective method of controlling odor. Bathing is as important during menses as at any other time. A long, leisurely soak in a warm tub promotes menstrual blood flow and relieves cramps by relaxing the muscles.

A woman can ensure adequate ventilation by wearing cotton panties and clothes loose enough to permit the vaginal area to breathe. After using the toilet, a woman should always wipe herself from front to back and, if necessary, follow up with a moistened paper towel or premoistened wipe. If an unusual odor persists despite these efforts, a visit to one's healthcare provider is indicated. Certain conditions such as vaginitis produce a foul-smelling discharge that women often describe as having a "fishy" odor.

Associated Menstrual Conditions

New self-explanatory terminology has been developed to define a variety of menstrual irregularities. These include the following:

- Abnormal uterine bleeding (AUB)
- Heavy menstrual bleeding (HMB)
- Heavy and prolonged menstrual bleeding (HPMB)
- Intermenstrual bleeding (IMB)
- Postmenopausal bleeding (PMB)

The following terms may still be used among some caregivers to define various menstrual irregularities; however, an International Review Panel has recommended that they be phased out (Garza-Cavazos & Loret de Mola, 2012):

- Hypomenorrhea: *abnormally* short duration of menses
- Hypermenorrhea: abnormally long duration of menses
- Oligomenorrhea: infrequent menses
- Polymenorrhea: too frequent menses
- Menorrhagia: excessive menstrual flow
- Metrorrhagia: bleeding between periods
- Menometrorrhagia: bleeding that is excessive in amount and duration, which occurs at either regular or irregular intervals

AMENORRHEA

Amenorrhea, the absence of menses, is classified as primary or secondary. Primary amenorrhea (menstruation has not been established by 16 years of age or within 4 years of breast development) necessitates a thorough assessment to determine its cause. Possible causes include congenital obstructions; Turner syndrome; congenital absence of the uterus, ovaries, or vagina; testicular feminization (external genitals appear female but uterus and ovaries are absent and testes are present); chronic anovulation related to polycystic ovarian syndrome, thyroid, or adrenal disorders; or absence or imbalance of hormones. Treatment depends on the causative factors. Some causes are not correctable.

Secondary amenorrhea is caused most frequently by pregnancy. Additional causes include lactation, hormonal imbalances, poor nutrition (anorexia nervosa, obesity, and fad dieting), ovarian lesions, strenuous exercise (associated with long-distance runners, dancers, and other athletes with low body fat ratios), debilitating systemic diseases, stress of high intensity and/or long duration or stressful life events, changes in season or climate, use

---

EVIDENCE-BASED PRACTICE | Amenorrhea in Female Athletes

Clinical Question
What is the incidence of amenorrhea in female athletes? What is the attitude of athletes toward amenorrhea, particularly elite athletes?

The Evidence
Hormonal changes brought about by extreme exercise and related low energy may result in menstrual dysfunction in female athletes, even those with normal eating patterns. Two studies focused on amenorrhea in female athletes. One study included 245 female athletes in National Collegiate Athletics Association (NCAA) Division 1 sports and focused on both the prevalence of menstrual irregularities and the attitudes of athletes toward amenorrhea. A second, year-long study conducted in Sweden focused on 149 elite athletes—those ranked in the top 10 nationally for their sport. These are descriptive studies, but taken together form a strong level of evidence.

In the general population, the prevalence of amenorrhea is approximately 1%. In contrast, 18% of the NCAA Division I athletes reported amenorrhea and 36% reported fewer than 10 cycles in a year (oligomenorrhea.) Twenty-five percent of the elite athletes reported a history of amenorrhea (Rost, Jacobsson, Dahlstrom, et al., 2014). Runners with lower body mass index (BMI) had a higher prevalence of amenorrhea, as did women who participated in sports with high demands on aerobic performance such as long distance running.

Missed or irregular menses are often the first sign of a health disturbance, yet some athletes interpret missed menses as a sign of fitness. Fifty-seven percent of the NCAA athletes believed missing menses was normal, 58% believed it was not harmful, and 67% believed it is common among all women (Myrisk, Reinn, & Harkins, 2014). This normalization of amenorrhea is problematic from a clinical standpoint in that amenorrhea is one element of the "female athlete triad" that includes menstrual dysfunction, eating disorders, and osteoporosis. The long-term consequences of menstrual irregularities can include loss of bone mineral density and a three-fold greater risk of musculoskeletal injury.

Best Practice
Coaches, athletic trainers, and athletes need education regarding the serious consequences of menstrual dysfunction and the "female athlete triad" in general. The most common reported cause of amenorrhea among athletes is energy deficiency brought on by consuming too few calories relative to energy expenditure. Adequate nutrition for female athletes is essential to avoid the long-term consequences of menstrual dysfunction.

Clinical Reasoning
How can the nurse affect the attitudes of athletes about normal menstrual function and the importance of adequate nutrition? How can coaches and athletic trainers be motivated to attend to menstrual dysfunction as a signal of a health disturbance?

of oral contraceptives or the phenothiazine and chlorpromazine group of tranquilizers, exposure to radiation or chemotherapy, viral infection, and syndromes such as Cushing and Sheehan.

Treatment is dictated by the causative factors. The nurse can explain that once the underlying condition has been corrected—for example, when sufficient body weight has been gained—menses will resume. Female athletes and women who participate in strenuous exercise routines may be advised to increase their caloric intake or reduce their exercise levels for a month or two to see whether a normal cycle ensues. If it does not, medical referral is indicated.

DYSMENORRHEA

Dysmenorrhea, or painful menstruation, occurs at, or a day before, the onset of menstruation and disappears by the end of menses. Dysmenorrhea is classified as primary or secondary. Primary dysmenorrhea is defined as cramps without underlying disease. Prostaglandins E_2 and F_{2a}, which are produced by the uterus in higher concentrations during menses, are the primary cause. They increase uterine contractility and decrease uterine artery blood flow, causing ischemia. The end result is the painful sensation of cramps. Dysmenorrhea typically disappears after a first pregnancy and may not occur if cycles are anovulatory.

Treatment of primary dysmenorrhea includes combined oral contraceptives, which inhibit ovulation, and nonsteroidal anti-inflammatory drugs (NSAIDs) such as ibuprofen, aspirin, and naproxen, which act as prostaglandin inhibitors. See *Health Promotion: Self-Care Measures for Dysmenorrhea.*

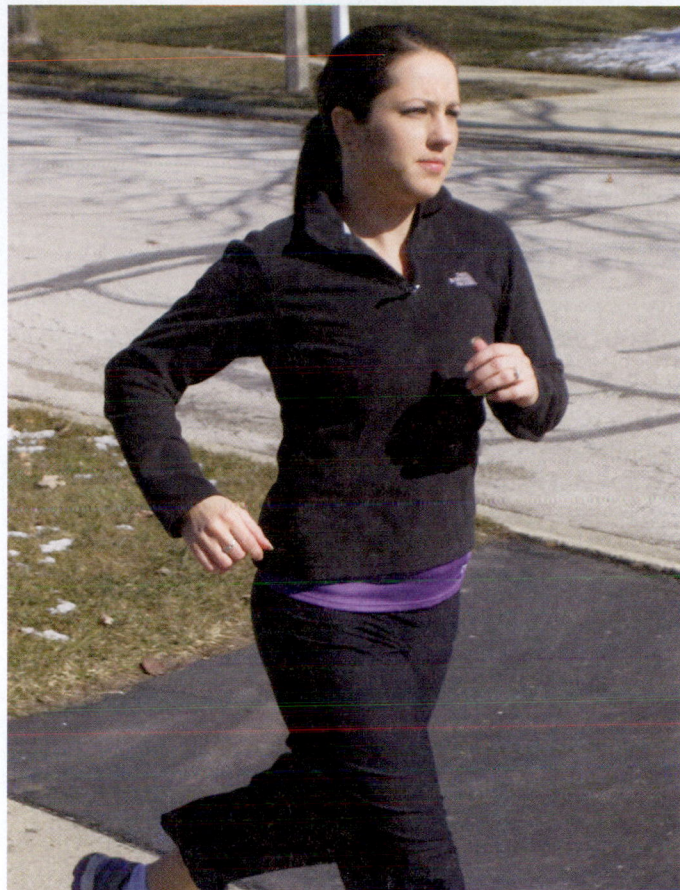

Figure 5–2 Regular exercise is an important part of therapy for dysmenorrhea.

SOURCE: Erik Ladewig.

Health Promotion **Self-Care Measures for Dysmenorrhea**

- Regular exercise, rest, application of heat, and good nutrition (Figure 5–2).

- Avoidance of salt to decrease discomfort from fluid retention.

- Vitamin B_6 may help relieve the premenstrual bloating and irritability some women experience.

- Vitamin E, a mild prostaglandin inhibitor, may ease cramping.

Secondary dysmenorrhea is associated with pathology of the reproductive tract and usually appears after menstruation has been established. Conditions that most often cause secondary dysmenorrhea include endometriosis, residual pelvic inflammatory disease (PID), cervical stenosis, uterine fibroids, ovarian cysts, benign or malignant tumors of the pelvis or abdomen, and the presence of an intrauterine device. Because primary and secondary dysmenorrhea may coexist, accurate diagnosis is essential for appropriate treatment.

For women with severe dysmenorrhea, use of continuous oral contraceptive therapy, which does not allow ovulation or menstruation to occur, may help. Hysterectomy may be the treatment of choice if there are anatomic disorders and child-bearing is not desired.

PREMENSTRUAL SYNDROME

Premenstrual syndrome (PMS) refers to a symptom complex associated with the luteal phase of the menstrual cycle (2 weeks before the onset of menses). The symptoms must, by definition, occur between ovulation and the onset of menses. They repeat at the same stage of each menstrual cycle and include some or all of the following:

- *Psychologic:* irritability, lethargy, depression, low morale, anxiety, sleep disorders, crying spells, and hostility
- *Neurologic:* classic migraine, vertigo, and syncope
- *Respiratory:* rhinitis, hoarseness, and occasionally asthma
- *Gastrointestinal:* nausea, vomiting, constipation, abdominal bloating, and craving for sweets
- *Urinary:* retention and oliguria
- *Dermatologic:* acne
- *Mammary:* swelling and tenderness
- *Musculoskeletal:* joint or muscle pain

Most women experience only some symptoms. They usually are most pronounced 2 or 3 days before the onset of menstruation and subside as menstrual flow begins, with or without treatment.

The exact cause of PMS is unknown although evidence suggests that progesterone and estradiol levels are involved in some way. Central nervous system–mediated interactions between neurohormones and sex steroids may also account for the occurrence of PMS. Certain risk factors such as stress, traumatic life events, genetics, obesity, or a history of depression or other psychiatric disorders may predispose women to these disorders (Matsumoto, Asakura, & Hayashi, 2013).

Premenstrual dysphoric disorder (PMDD), a more serious form of PMS, is a diagnosis that may be applied to a small subgroup of women with PMS whose symptoms are primarily mood related and severe. Women with PMDD may benefit from combined oral contraceptives that contain drospirenone such as Yaz, which has received FDA approval for use as a treatment. Selective serotonin reuptake inhibitors (SSRIs) such as fluoxetine hydrochloride (Prozac), sertraline hydrochloride (Zoloft), and paroxetine CR (Paxil CR) may also be effective (Kelderhouse & Taylor, 2013).

Nursing Management

The focus of management for the woman with PMS, at least initially, involves lifestyle changes and natural approaches. After assessment, counseling for PMS may include advising the woman to restrict her intake of foods containing methylxanthines such as chocolate, cola, and coffee; restrict her intake of alcohol, nicotine, red meat, and foods containing salt and sugar; increase her intake of complex carbohydrates and protein; and increase the frequency of meals. For women whose primary symptoms are psychologic, supplementation with B-complex vitamins, especially B_6, may decrease anxiety and depression. Vitamin E supplements may help reduce cramping and breast tenderness. A calcium supplement of 1200 mg per day may help relieve certain physical and psychologic symptoms. Magnesium supplements may help reduce fluid retention and bloating. These women may also gain relief from complementary therapies such as *vitex agnus castus* (fruit of the chaste tree) and acupuncture (Kelderhouse & Taylor, 2013).

A program of aerobic exercise such as fast walking, jogging, and aerobic dancing is generally beneficial. In addition to vitamin supplements, pharmacologic treatments for PMS include diuretics and prostaglandin inhibitors.

An empathic relationship with a healthcare professional to whom the woman feels free to voice concerns is highly beneficial. Encourage the woman to keep a diary to help track activities, diet, exercise, stressful events, and symptoms associated with PMS. Self-care groups and self-help literature can help women feel they have control over their bodies.

Contraception

The decision to use a method of contraception may be made individually by a woman (or, in the case of vasectomy, by a man) or jointly by a couple. The decision may be motivated by a desire to avoid pregnancy, to gain control over the number of children conceived, or to determine the spacing of future children. In choosing a specific method, consistency of use outweighs the absolute reliability of the given method.

Decisions about contraception should be made voluntarily, with full knowledge of advantages, disadvantages, effectiveness, side effects, contraindications, and long-term effects. Many outside factors influence this choice, including cultural practices, religious beliefs, attitudes and personal preferences,

---

Professionalism in Practice **Family Planning**

The United Nations Population Fund (UNFPA) has determined that in developing regions of the world, satisfying the unmet need for modern contraception would result in a 70% decrease in unintended pregnancies, from 74 million to 22 million. Moreover, for every additional dollar used to fund contraception, the cost of pregnancy-related care is decreased by $1.47.

Source: Guttmacher Institute, 2014.

---

cost, effectiveness, misinformation, practicality of method, and self-esteem. Different methods of contraception may be appropriate at different times for couples.

Healthy People 2020

(FP-1) Increase the proportion of pregnancies that are intended

(FP-2) Reduce the proportion of females experiencing pregnancy despite use of a reversible contraceptive method.

Fertility Awareness Methods

Fertility awareness–based (FAB) methods, also known as *natural family planning (NFP)*, include methods that require a woman to monitor her *fertile window* (generally between days 8–19 of 26- to 32-day cycles) and abstain from intercourse or use a barrier method during that time. A woman is most fertile from 3 to 6 days before ovulation until 1 day post-ovulation (Zieman, Hatcher, & Allen, 2015). In conjunction with FAB, women may choose to improve identification of their fertile days by use of an over-the-counter ovulation prediction kit (e.g., OvuKit). They may also use a temperature computer (e.g., Bioself 2000) or a hormone computer (e.g., Persona) to help predict fertile days.

Fertility awareness methods are free, safe, and acceptable to many whose religious beliefs prohibit other methods. They provide an increased awareness of the body, involve no artificial substances or devices, encourage a couple to communicate about sexual activity and family planning, and are useful in helping a couple plan a pregnancy.

To be used effectively, all FAB methods require extensive initial counseling and are best suited for women with regular menstrual cycles. FAB/NFP methods may interfere with sexual spontaneity, require the couple to maintain records for several menstrual cycles (months) before beginning use, may be difficult or impossible for women with irregular menstrual cycles or who are breastfeeding to use, and may not be as reliable in preventing pregnancy as other methods.

The *basal body temperature (BBT) method* to detect ovulation requires that a woman take her BBT every morning upon awakening (before any activity) and record the readings on a temperature graph. To do this, she uses a basal body temperature thermometer. After 3 to 4 months of recording temperatures, a woman with regular cycles should be able to predict when ovulation will occur. The method is based on the fact that the temperature sometimes drops just before ovulation and almost always rises and remains elevated for several days after. The temperature rise occurs in response to the increased progesterone levels that occur in the second half of the cycle. Figure 5–3 shows a sample BBT chart. To avoid conception, the couple abstains from intercourse on the day of the temperature rise and for 3 days after. Because the temperature rise does not occur until after ovulation, a woman who had intercourse just before the rise is at risk of pregnancy.

The *Billings ovulation method*, sometimes called the *cervical mucus method*, involves the assessment of cervical mucus changes that occur during the menstrual cycle. The amount and character of cervical mucus change because of the influence of estrogen and progesterone. At the time of ovulation the mucus (estrogen-dominant mucus) is clearer, more stretchable (a quality called *spinnbarkeit*), and more permeable to sperm. It also shows a characteristic fern pattern when placed on a glass slide and allowed to dry (see Figure 5–4). During the luteal phase, the cervical mucus is thick and sticky (progesterone-dominant mucus) and forms a network that traps sperm, making their passage more difficult.

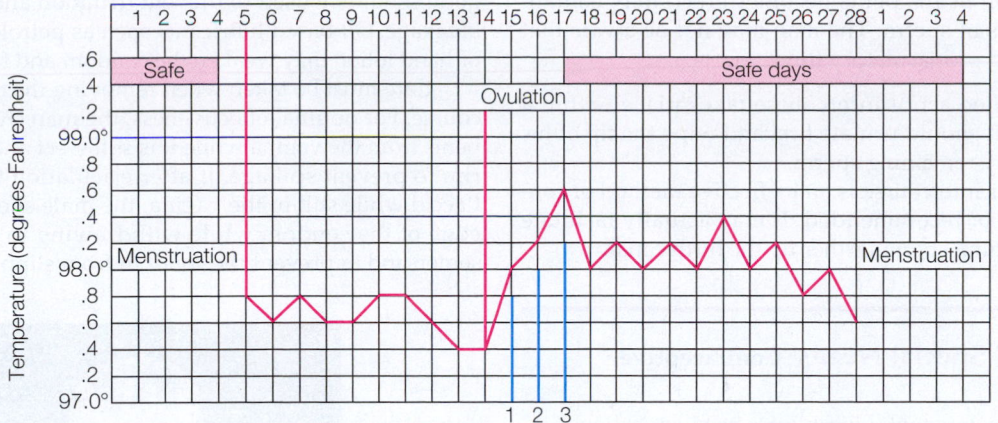

Days of menstrual cycle

Figure 5–3 Sample basal body temperature chart.

SOURCE: DAVIDSON, MICHELE C.; LONDON, MARCIA L.; LADEWIG, PATRICIA W., OLDS' MATERNAL-NEWBORN NURSING & WOMEN'S HEALTH ACROSS THE LIFESPAN, 10th Ed., ©2016. Reprinted and Electronically reproduced by permission of Pearson Education, Inc., New York, NY.

To use the cervical mucus method, the woman abstains from intercourse for the first menstrual cycle. Each day she assesses her cervical mucus for amount, feeling of slipperiness or wetness, color, clearness, and spinnbarkeit, as she becomes familiar with varying characteristics. The peak day of wetness and clear, stretchable mucus is assumed to be the time of ovulation. To use this method correctly, the woman should abstain from intercourse from the time she *first* notices that the mucus is becoming clear, more elastic, and slippery until 4 days *after* the last wet mucus (ovulation) day. Because this method evaluates the effects of hormonal changes, it can be used by women with irregular cycles.

The *symptothermal method* consists of various assessments made and recorded by the couple. These include information regarding cycle days, coitus, cervical mucus changes, and secondary signs such as increased libido, abdominal bloating, *mittelschmerz* (midcycle abdominal pain), and basal body temperature. Through the various assessments, the couple learns to recognize signs that indicate ovulation.

The *TwoDay Method* is based on a woman's ability to distinguish the difference between progesterone-mediated and estrogen-mediated cervical mucus that is present at her introitus before she urinates, preferably in the afternoon and evening. If she notices cervical secretions of any type either yesterday or today, she is fertile *today*. If no secretions were noted for two consecutive days, she is not fertile *today*—hence the name (Zieman et al., 2015).

The *calendar rhythm method* is based on the assumptions that ovulation tends to occur about 14 days before the start of the next menstrual period. To use this method, the woman must record her menstrual cycles for 6 months to identify the shortest and longest cycles. The first day of menstruation is the first day of the cycle. The fertile phase is calculated from 18 days before the end of the shortest recorded cycle through 11 days from the end of the longest recorded cycle. For example, if a woman's cycle lasts from 24 to 28 days, the fertile phase would be calculated as day 6 through day 17. For effective use of this method, she must abstain from intercourse during the fertile phase.

Situational Contraceptives

Abstinence can be considered a method of contraception, and, partly because of changing values and the increased risk of infection with intercourse, it is gaining increased acceptance.

Coitus interruptus, or withdrawal, is one of the oldest and least reliable methods of contraception. This method requires that the male withdraw from the female's vagina when he feels that ejaculation is impending. He then ejaculates away from the external genitalia of the woman. Failure tends to occur for two reasons:

- This method demands great self-control on the part of the man, who must withdraw just as he feels the urge for deeper penetration with impending orgasm.

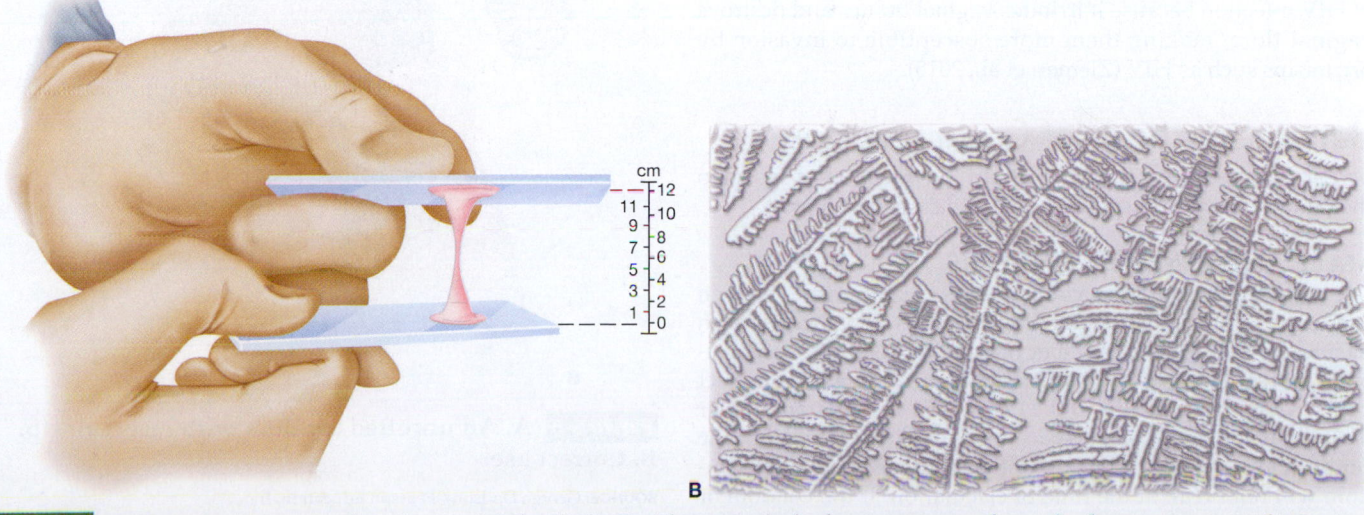

Figure 5–4 A. Cervical mucus showing spinnbarkeit. B. Characteristic fern pattern of cervical mucus at ovulation.

- In some men, the preejaculatory fluid, which a man may release as soon as his penis becomes erect, may contain small numbers of sperm. The man may not be aware that he has released preejaculatory fluid.

If more than one act of intercourse takes place within a short time, the man should urinate first and wipe the tip of his penis to remove any remaining sperm.

Douching after intercourse is an ineffective method of contraception and is *not* recommended. It may actually facilitate conception by pushing sperm farther up the birth canal.

> ### Women With Special Needs Contraceptive Counseling
>
> Women with developmental disabilities need education on sexual issues including conception and pregnancy prevention. A level of functioning assessment should be performed to determine if the woman is capable of using different types of contraceptives effectively. Contraceptive choices should be discussed and provided as needed.

Spermicides

The **spermicide** approved for use in the United States, non-oxynol-9 (N-9), is available as a cream, jelly, foam, vaginal film, and suppository. Spermicide is inserted into the vagina before intercourse. It destroys sperm by disrupting the cell membrane. A spermicide that effervesces in a moist environment offers more rapid protection, and coitus may take place immediately after it is inserted. Suppositories may require up to 30 minutes to dissolve and will not offer protection until they do so. The nurse instructs the woman to insert these spermicide preparations high in the vagina and to maintain a supine position.

N-9 is minimally effective when used alone, but its effectiveness increases in conjunction with a barrier method of contraception such as a diaphragm, cervical cap, or male or female condom. The cervical sponge is both a spermicide and a barrier method, as it contains N-9 and its matrix traps sperm.

The major advantages of spermicides are their wide availability and low toxicity. Skin irritation and allergic reactions to spermicides are the primary disadvantages. N-9 does not offer protection against infection from the human immunodeficiency virus (HIV) or against any other sexually transmitted infection. Moreover, N-9 may actually increase a woman's risk of HIV infection because it irritates vaginal tissues and destroys vaginal flora, making them more susceptible to invasion by organisms such as HIV (Zieman et al., 2015).

Barrier Methods of Contraception

Barrier methods of contraception prevent the transport of sperm to the ovum, immobilize sperm, or are lethal against sperm.

MALE AND FEMALE CONDOMS

The male **condom** offers a viable means of contraception when used consistently and properly (Figure 5–5). Acceptance has been increasing as a growing number of men are assuming responsibility for regulation of fertility. The condom is applied to the erect penis, rolled from the tip to the end of the shaft, before vulvar or vaginal contact. A small space must be left at the end of the condom to allow for collection of the ejaculate, so that the condom will not break at the time of ejaculation. If the condom or

vagina is dry, water-soluble lubricants such as K-Y jelly or Astroglide should be used to prevent irritation and possible condom breakage. Oil-based lubricants such as petroleum jelly, baby oil, or hand lotion may weaken the condom and facilitate breakage.

Care must be taken when removing the condom after intercourse. For optimal effectiveness, the man should withdraw his penis from the vagina while it is still erect and hold the condom rim to prevent spillage. If after ejaculation the penis becomes flaccid while still in the vagina, the male should hold on to the edge of the condom while withdrawing to avoid spilling the semen and to prevent the condom from slipping off.

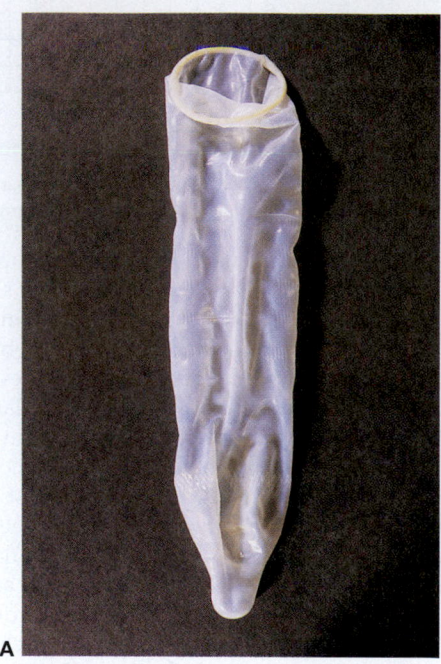

A

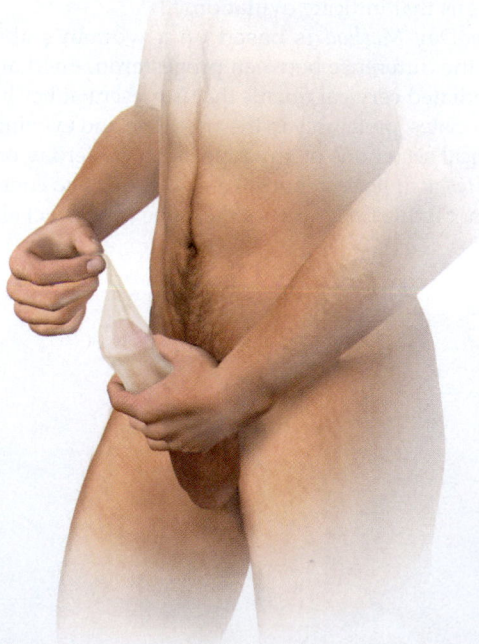

B

Figure 5–5 A. An unrolled condom with reservoir tip. B. Correct use.

SOURCE: George Dodson/ Pearson Education, Inc.

The effectiveness of male condoms is largely determined by their use. The condom is small, disposable, and inexpensive; it has no side effects (if not allergic to latex), requires no medical examination, and offers visual evidence of effectiveness. Most condoms are made of latex, although polyurethane and silicone rubber condoms are available for individuals allergic to latex. All condoms except natural "skin" condoms, made from lamb's intestines, offer protection against both pregnancy and sexually transmitted infections (STIs). Breakage, displacement, perineal or vaginal irritation, and dulled sensation are possible disadvantages. Condoms deteriorate in hot conditions, making them susceptible to breaking. Thus, men should avoid placing them in their car glove boxes or in their wallets in a rear pants pocket.

The male condom is becoming increasingly popular because of the protection it offers from infections. For women, sexually transmitted infection increases the risk of pelvic inflammatory disease (PID) and resultant infertility. Many women are beginning to insist that their sexual partners use condoms, and many women carry condoms with them.

The *Reality female condom* is a thin sheath with a flexible ring at each end (Figure 5–6). The inner ring, at the closed end of the condom, serves as the means of insertion and fits over

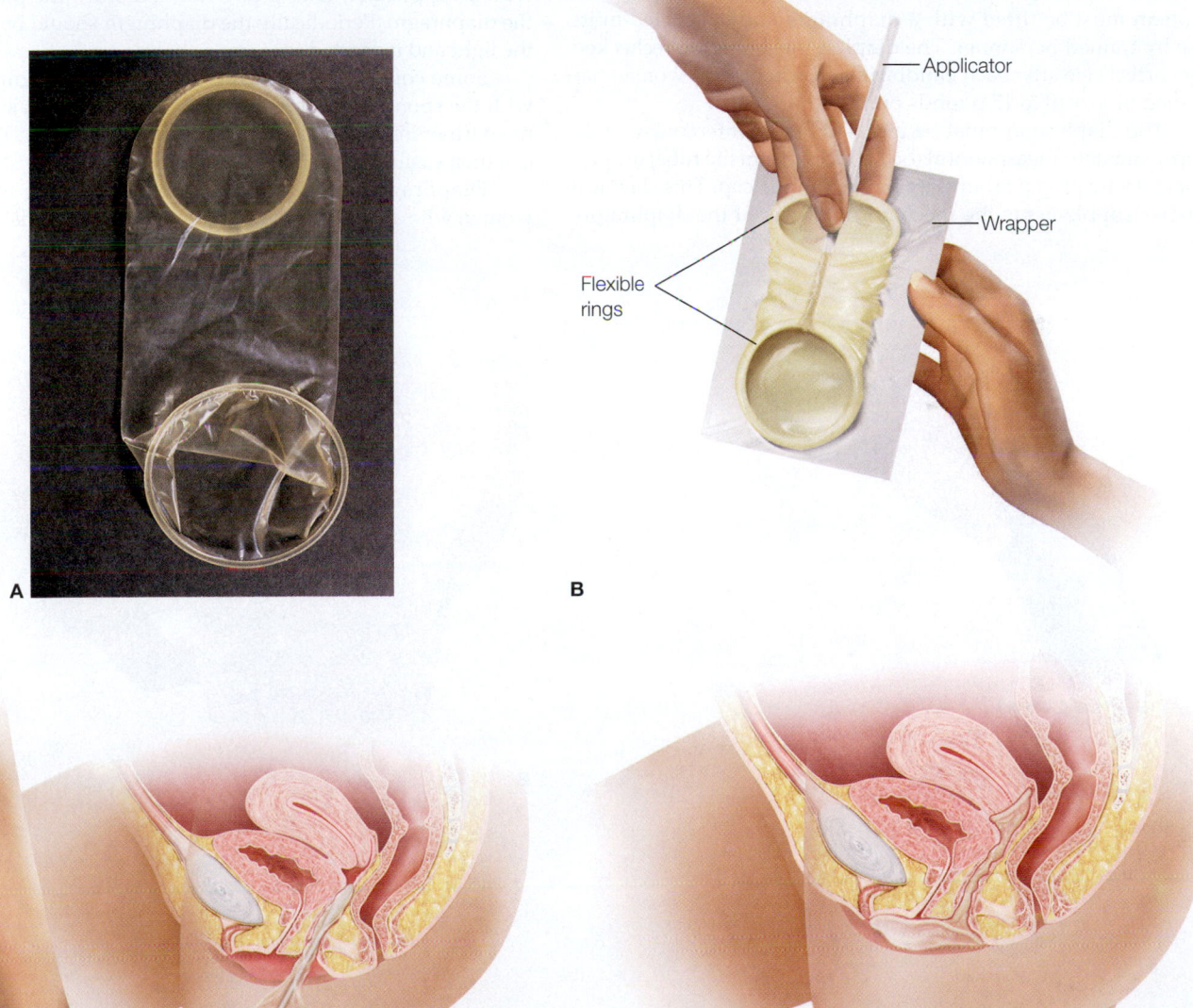

Figure 5–6 A. The female condom. To insert the condom: B. Remove condom and applicator from wrapper by pulling up on the ring. C. Insert condom slowly by gently pushing the applicator toward the small of the back. D. When properly inserted, the outer ring should rest on the folds of skin around the vaginal opening, and the inner ring (closed end) should fit loosely against the cervix.

SOURCE: George Dodson/Pearson Education, Inc.

the cervix like a diaphragm. The second ring remains outside the vagina and covers a portion of the woman's perineum. It also covers the base of the man's penis during intercourse. Available over the counter and designed for one-time use, the condom may be inserted up to 8 hours before intercourse. The inner sheath is prelubricated but does not contain spermicide and is not designed to be used with a male condom. Because it also covers a portion of the vulva, it probably provides better protection than other contraceptive methods against some pathogens. High cost, noisiness during intercourse, and the cumbersome feel of the device make acceptability a problem for some couples.

DIAPHRAGM AND CERVICAL CAP

The **diaphragm** (Figure 5–7) is used with spermicidal cream or jelly and offers a good level of protection from conception. The woman must be fitted with a diaphragm and instructed in its use by trained personnel. The diaphragm should be rechecked for correct size after each childbirth and whenever a woman has gained or lost 10 to 15 pounds or more.

The diaphragm must be inserted before intercourse, with approximately 1 teaspoonful (or 1.5 inches from the tube) of spermicidal jelly placed around its rim and in the cup. This chemical barrier supplements the mechanical barrier of the diaphragm.

The diaphragm is inserted through the vagina and covers the cervix. The last step in insertion is to push the edge of the diaphragm under the symphysis pubis, which may result in a "popping" sensation. When fitted properly and correctly in place, the diaphragm should not cause discomfort to the woman or her partner. Correct placement of the diaphragm can be checked by touching the cervix with a fingertip through the cup. The cervix feels like a small, firm, rounded structure and has a consistency similar to that of the tip of the nose. The center of the diaphragm should be over the cervix. If more than 6 hours elapse between insertion of the diaphragm and intercourse, additional spermicidal cream or jelly should be used. It is necessary to leave the diaphragm in place for at least 6 hours after coitus. If intercourse is desired again within the 6 hours, another type of contraception must be used or additional spermicidal jelly placed in the vagina with an applicator, taking care not to disturb the placement of the diaphragm. Periodically the diaphragm should be held up to the light and inspected for tears or holes.

Some couples feel that the use of a diaphragm interferes with the spontaneity of intercourse. The nurse can suggest that the partner insert the diaphragm as part of foreplay. The woman can then easily verify the placement herself.

Diaphragms are an excellent contraceptive method for women who are lactating, who cannot or do not wish to use the

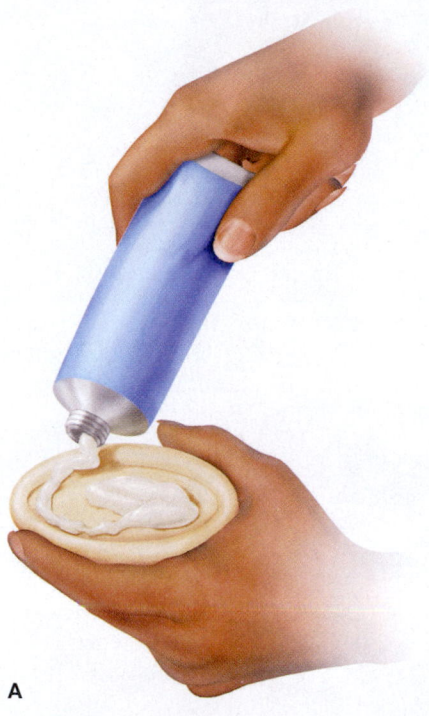

A

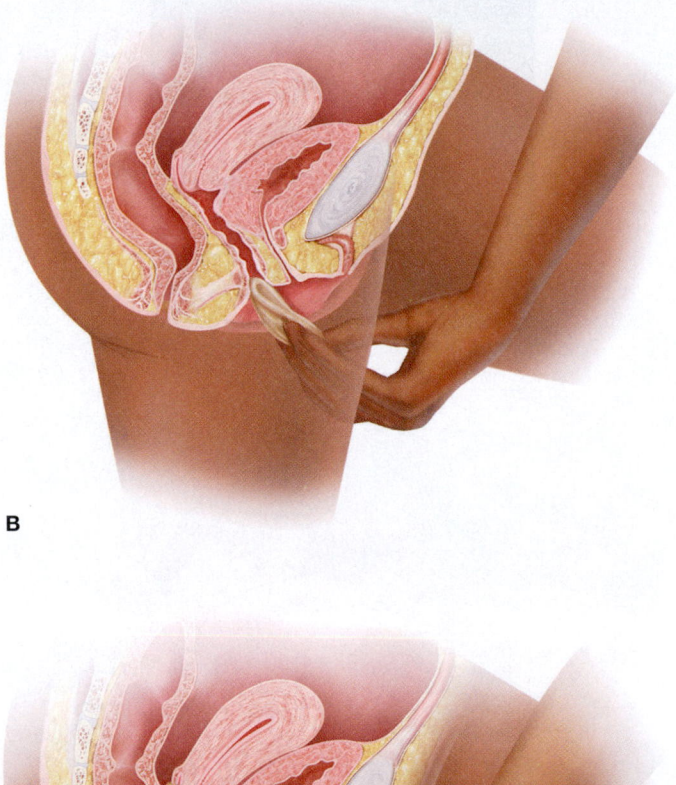

B

C

Figure 5–7 Inserting the diaphragm. A. Apply jelly to the rim and center of the diaphragm. B. Insert the diaphragm. C. Push the rim of the diaphragm under the pubic symphysis. Then check placement of the diaphragm. The cervix should be felt through the diaphragm.

NOTE: the diaphragm shown here is no longer manufactured, but many women who use a diaphragm will still have this model.

pill (oral contraceptives), who are smokers over age 35, or who wish to avoid the increased risk of PID associated with intrauterine devices. A silicone diaphragm is available for women with a latex allergy.

Women who object to touching their genitals to insert the diaphragm, check its placement, and remove it may find this method unsatisfactory. It is not recommended for women with a history of urinary tract infection (UTI), because pressure from the diaphragm on the urethra may interfere with complete bladder emptying and lead to recurrent UTIs.

SAFETY ALERT!

Women with a history of toxic shock syndrome should not use diaphragms or any of the barrier methods because they are left in place for prolonged periods. For the same reason, the diaphragm should not be used during a menstrual period or if a woman has abnormal vaginal discharge.

The *FemCap* is a latex cup-shaped device, used with spermicidal cream or jelly, that fits snugly over the cervix and is held in place by suction. Advantages, disadvantages, and contraindications are similar to those associated with the diaphragm.

VAGINAL SPONGE

The *Today vaginal sponge*, available without a prescription, is a pillow-shaped, soft, absorbent synthetic sponge containing spermicide. It is made with a concave or cupped area on one side that fits over the cervix, and has a loop for easy removal. The sponge is moistened thoroughly with water before insertion to activate the spermicide, and then inserted into the vagina with the cupped side against the cervix (Figure 5–8). It should be left in place for 6 hours following intercourse and may be worn for up to 24 hours, then removed and discarded.

The sponge has the following advantages: professional fitting is not required, it may be used for multiple acts of coitus for up to 24 hours, one size fits all, and it acts as both a barrier and a spermicide. Problems associated with the sponge include difficulty removing it and irritation or allergic reactions. Some women report a problem because the sponge absorbs vaginal secretions, contributing to vaginal dryness. The sponge is more effective for women who have never given birth. Overall, it is slightly less effective than a diaphragm.

Long-Acting Reversible Contraception (LARC)

Long-acting reversible contraceptive methods include those that are used for an extended period of time, do not require user compliance, and are reversible upon discontinuation. These cost-effective methods, which include intrauterine contraception and the subdermal implant, are especially well suited for adolescents and are more effective than other contraceptive methods in preventing unplanned pregnancy over time (Deal, Moore, & Sutton, 2014). However, they are significantly underutilized.

INTRAUTERINE CONTRACEPTION

Intrauterine contraception (IUC) refers to the use of an *intrauterine device (IUD)* that is designed to be inserted into the uterus by a qualified healthcare provider and left in place for an extended period, providing continuous contraceptive protection for 3 to 10 years (Figure 5–9). The following devices are available in the United States:

- The *Copper IUC (ParaGard T 380A)* is a small, T-shaped device that has copper covering parts of its stem and arms. It provides effective contraception for 10 years.

- The *Mirena levonorgestrel intrauterine system (LNg-IUC)* is a small, T-shaped frame with a reservoir that releases levonorgestrel gradually. The Mirena provides 5 years of protection.

- The *Skyla LNg-IUC* gradually releases levonorgestrel and has a 3-year indication. Sklya is smaller than the Mirena and may fit into the uterus of nulliparous women more easily. Skyla also has a radiopaque silver ring at the top of the "T" (if the woman needs an MRI, she must notify the technician).

Both Mirena and Sklya are progestin-only; thus the primary cause of discontinuation is unscheduled bleeding. The

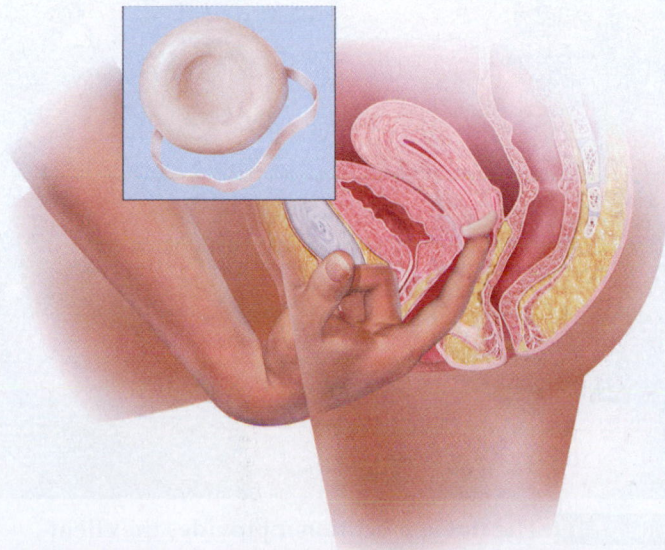

Figure 5–8 The vaginal sponge is moistened well with water and inserted into the vagina with the concave portion positioned over the cervix.

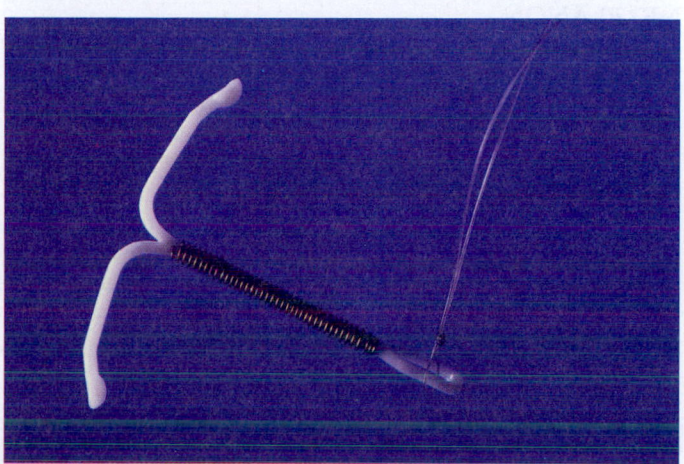

Figure 5–9 An example of an IUD.

SOURCE: Boucharlat/AGE Fotostock America Inc.

LNg-IUCs are an excellent choice for women who are allergic to copper or who have heavy menses and desire decreased bleeding or amenorrhea.

Traditionally, IUC was believed to be an abortifacient (abortion-causing) method. This belief is not accurate. All IUC is truly contraceptive. It creates a foreign body response in the uterus that prevents fertilization. The Copper T IUD repels sperm and impairs sperm from functioning properly. The Mirena and Skyla LNg-IUCs cause the lining of the uterus (endometrium) to become atrophic and cause changes in the cervical mucus that form a barrier preventing sperm penetration (Cheng & Van Leuven, 2015).

Advantages of IUC include a high rate of effectiveness, continuous contraceptive protection, no coitus-related activity, and relative inexpensiveness over time. Possible adverse reactions to the IUD include discomfort to the wearer, increased bleeding during menses, increased risk of pelvic inflammatory disease (PID), uterine perforation, intermenstrual bleeding, dysmenorrhea, and expulsion of the device.

IUC is an excellent method of contraception for most women including adolescents. IUCs are contraindicated in women who are pregnant and in women who have an active pelvic infection (PID, endometritis, cervicitis, or pelvic tuberculosis). IUCs should not be inserted in women with cervical or endometrial cancer, or gestational choriocarcinoma. The risk for IUC expulsion is greater in women with anatomic abnormalities of the uterus.

An IUC device is inserted into the uterus with its strings or tail protruding through the cervix into the vagina. It may be inserted at any time during a woman's cycle providing she is not pregnant or during the 4- to 6-week postpartum check. After insertion, the clinician instructs the woman to check for the presence of the strings once a week for the first month and then after each menses. She is told that she may have some cramping or bleeding intermittently for 2 to 6 weeks and that her first few menses may be irregular. Follow-up examination is suggested 4 to 8 weeks after insertion.

Women with IUCs should contact their healthcare providers if they are exposed to an STI or if they develop the following warning signs: late period, abnormal spotting or bleeding, pain with intercourse, abdominal pain, abnormal discharge, signs of infection (fever, chills, and malaise), or missing string. If the woman becomes pregnant with an IUD in place, the device should be removed as soon as possible to prevent infection and miscarriage (Cunningham et al., 2014).

NEXPLANON

Nexplanon is a single-capsule implant inserted subdermally in the woman's nondominant upper underarm. It is impregnated with etonogestrel, a progestin, and is effective for 3 years. It acts by preventing ovulation. Nexplanon also stimulates the production of thick cervical mucus, which inhibits sperm penetration past the cervix.

Nexplanon provides effective continuous contraception removed from the act of coitus. Possible side effects include spotting, irregular bleeding or amenorrhea, an increased incidence of ovarian cysts, weight gain, headaches, fluid retention, acne, hair loss, mood changes, and depression.

Hormonal Contraceptives

Hormonal contraceptives are available in a variety of forms. They may be progestin-only hormones, most often using a synthetic form of progesterone called progestin, or a combination of estrogen and a progestin.

COMBINED ESTROGEN–PROGESTIN APPROACHES

Combined hormonal approaches work by inhibiting the release of an ovum, by creating an atrophic endometrium, and by maintaining a thick cervical mucus that slows sperm transport and inhibits the process that allows sperm to penetrate the ovum.

COMBINED ORAL CONTRACEPTIVES

Combined oral contraceptives (COCs), also called *birth control pills*, are a combination of estrogen and progestin. COCs are safe, highly effective, and rapidly reversible (Figure 5–10). COCs are generally taken daily for 21 days, typically beginning on the Sunday after the first day of the menstrual cycle although the woman can also start on day 1 of her menstrual cycle. In most cases menses occurs 1 to 4 days after the last pill is taken. Seven days after taking her last pill, the woman restarts the pill. Thus the woman always begins the pill on the same day. Some companies offer a 28-day pack with seven "blank" pills so that the woman never stops taking a pill. The pill should be taken at approximately the same time each day—usually upon arising or before retiring in the evening.

Three COC formulations for extended use are available in the United States. Women taking extended use COCs have four withdrawal bleeds per year (rather than 12), or no withdrawal bleeding at all. Extended use COCs reduce the side effects of COCs such as bloating, headache, breast tenderness, cramping, and swelling (Lentz, Lobo, Gershenson, et al., 2012). Many of these formulations are now generic, but were previously marketed as Seasonale, Seasonique, and Lybrel. Irregular pill taking is one of the major causes of unscheduled bleeding, a side effect that leads many women to discontinue COCs.

Although they are highly effective when taken correctly, COCs may produce a variety of side effects, which may be either

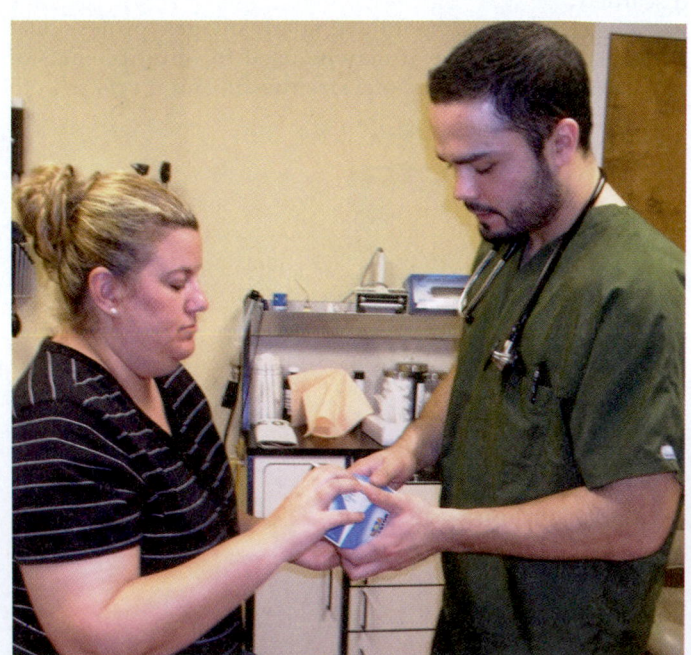

Figure 5–10 The nurse practitioner provides the client with combined oral contraceptives (COCs). He discusses their use with her and addresses any questions or concerns she has about using birth control pills.

SOURCE: Nathan Davidson.

TABLE 5–1 Side Effects Associated With Oral Contraceptives

ESTROGEN EFFECTS	PROGESTIN EFFECTS
Alterations in lipid metabolism	Acne, oily skin
Breast tenderness; engorgement; increased breast size	Breast tenderness; increased breast size
Cerebrovascular accident	Decreased high-density lipoprotein (HDL) cholesterol levels
Changes in carbohydrate metabolism	
Chloasma	Decreased libido
Fluid retention; cyclic weight gain	Depression
Headache	Fatigue
Hepatic adenomas	Hirsutism
Hypertension	Increased appetite; weight gain
Leukorrhea, cervical erosion, ectopia	Increased low-density lipoprotein (LDL) cholesterol levels
Nausea	
Nervousness, irritability	Oligomenorrhea, amenorrhea
Telangiectasia	
Thromboembolic complications: thrombophlebitis, pulmonary embolism	Pruritus
	Sebaceous cysts

progesterone or estrogen related (Table 5–1). The use of low-dose (35 mcg or less estrogen) preparations has reduced many of the side effects. The newer 20-mcg pills have even fewer side effects but they may result in less contraceptive effectiveness.

Absolute contraindications to the use of oral contraceptives include:

- Pregnancy
- Previous history of thrombophlebitis or thromboembolic disease
- Acute or chronic liver disease of cholestatic type with abnormal function
- Presence of estrogen-dependent carcinomas
- Undiagnosed uterine bleeding
- Heavy smoking
- Gallbladder disease
- Hypertension
- Diabetes
- Hyperlipidemia

In addition to the absolute contraindications, women with the following relative contraindications who use COCs need to be monitored frequently: migraine headaches, epilepsy, depression, oligomenorrhea, and amenorrhea. Women who choose this method of contraception should be fully advised of its potential side effects.

COCs also have some important noncontraceptive benefits. Many women experience relief of uncomfortable menstrual symptoms. Cramps are lessened, flow is decreased, and cycle regularity is increased. Mittelschmerz is eliminated. More important, there is a reduction in the incidence of ovarian cancer, endometrial cancer, colorectal cancer, menstrual migraines, and iron deficiency anemia. In addition, hormonal contraceptives can be effective in improving bone mineral density and in treating acne or hirsutism, pelvic pain due to endometriosis, and bleeding due

to leiomyomas (American College of Obstetricians and Gynecologists [ACOG], 2012a). In addition, COCs are considered a good solution to the physiologic problems some women experience during the perimenopause, such as hot flashes. Because of the increased risk of myocardial infarction (heart attack), women over age 35 who smoke should not take COCs. The woman using oral contraceptives should contact her healthcare provider if she becomes depressed, becomes jaundiced, develops a breast lump, or experiences any of the following warning signs: severe abdominal pain, severe chest pain or shortness of breath, severe headaches, dizziness, changes in vision (vision loss or blurring), speech problems, or severe leg pain.

OTHER COMBINED HORMONAL METHODS

Hormones can now be administered transdermally using a *contraceptive skin patch* called Ortho Evra. Roughly the size of a silver dollar, but square, the patch is applied weekly for 3 weeks to one of four sites: abdomen, buttocks, upper outer arm, or trunk (excluding the breasts). During the fourth week, no patch is worn and menses occurs. The patch is highly effective in women who weigh less than 198 pounds. It is as safe and reliable as COCs and has a better rate of compliance. Product labeling specifies that there is a greater risk of venous thromboembolism (VTE) for women using the patch versus those taking COCs. The U.S. Food and Drug Administration considers the patch a safe method of contraception for women not at risk of a VTE (U.S. Food and Drug Administration (FDA), 2015).

The *NuvaRing vaginal contraceptive ring*, another form of low-dose, sustained-release hormonal contraceptive, is a flexible soft ring that the woman inserts into her vagina (Figure 5–11). The ring is left in place for 3 weeks and then removed for 1 week to allow for withdrawal bleeding. One size fits virtually all women. The ring is highly effective and has minimal side effects. The ring can be worn during intercourse and is comfortable for both the woman and her partner. Replacement rings should be kept in the refrigerator to maintain integrity.

PROGESTIN CONTRACEPTIVES

The progestin-only pill, also called the *minipill,* is another oral contraceptive. It is used primarily by nursing mothers, because it does not interfere with breast milk production. It is also used by women who have a contraindication to the estrogen component of the combination preparation, such as history of thrombophlebitis

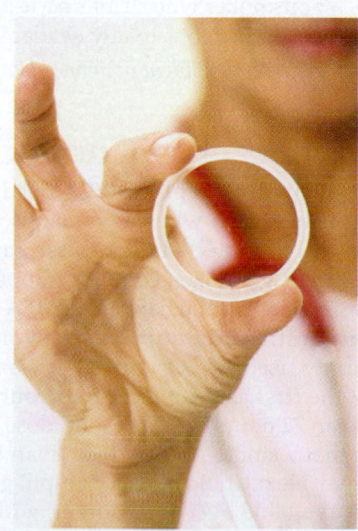

Figure 5–11   The NuvaRing vaginal contraceptive ring.
SOURCE: © N. Aubrier/Getty Images.

or hypertension, but who are strongly motivated to use this form of contraception. The major problems with progesterone-only pills are amenorrhea or irregular bleeding patterns.

Long-acting progestin-only contraceptives include Nexplanon and Depo-Provera. Nexplanon is also considered a LARC method and was discussed previously.

Depot-medroxyprogesterone acetate (DMPA) (**Depo-Provera**) is administered by injection, and provides highly effective contraception for 3 months after administration, with subsequent injections every 10 to 14 weeks. It is available in two dosings: DMPA-IM 150 mg for intramuscular use or DMPA-SC 104 mg for subcutaneous use.

DMPA, which acts primarily by suppressing ovulation, is safe, convenient, private, and relatively inexpensive. It also separates birth control from the act of coitus. It can be given to nursing mothers because it contains no estrogen. Side effects include menstrual irregularities, headache, weight gain, breast tenderness, and depression. Return of fertility may be delayed for an average of 10 months.

DMPA is associated with bone demineralization, especially during the first 2 years of use. The rate of calcium loss slows after this time, and bone loss is reversible after discontinuation of DMPA. All women on DMPA should exercise daily and take 1200 mg of calcium with vitamin D.

Clinical Reasoning Choosing a Method of Contraception

Monique Hermann, age 37, was divorced 3 years ago. Her only son, now 19, is away at college. Recently, with some trepidation, Monique began dating, and she is now enjoying an active social life. She is being seen today for advice about contraception, which had not been an issue during her marriage because her husband had had a vasectomy. She reports that she is a little nervous about becoming sexually active because until this point her husband had been her only sexual partner. She is very attracted to two different men but does not prefer one over the other at this point. She states that she wants a reliable method that would permit her to have intercourse at any time without having to take action beforehand because she thinks that would be embarrassing for her. Similarly she is not interested in the patch, which is visible. She is not willing to consider a tubal ligation. She is a nonsmoker who drinks occasionally. She has no known contraindications to any available methods. *Which methods of contraception might be appropriate for Monique?*

Postcoital Emergency Contraception

Postcoital **emergency contraception (EC),** once known as the *morning after pill,* is indicated when a woman is worried about pregnancy because of unprotected intercourse, rape, or possible contraceptive failure (e.g., broken condom, slipped diaphragm, missed COCs, or too long a time between DMPA injections).

Plan B, a progestin-only approach (levonorgestrel), is the most commonly used EC. Originally it was given in two 0.75-mg doses—the first as soon after intercourse as possible (but not longer than 72 hours) and a second dose 12 hours later. Studies suggest that a single 1.5-mg dose (Plan B One-Step™) may be as effective. Next Choice™ is a two-pill generic form of Plan B. Both are available over the counter, without prescription, to any woman 15 years or older. A new FDA-approved EC, ulipristal acetate (ella™), available by prescription only, is highly effective, especially after unprotected intercourse.

A selective progesterone receptor modulator, ella™ can be taken up to 5 days after unprotected intercourse, thus providing two additional days for use (Levy, Jager, Kapp, et al., 2014).

Placement of the Copper T IUD within 5 days after unprotected intercourse is the most effective postcoital contraceptive available (Zieman et al., 2015). However, the cost is high if the IUD is used only for EC.

Operative Sterilization

Operative **sterilization** is an inclusive term that refers to surgical procedures that permanently prevent pregnancy. Before sterilization is performed on either partner, the physician provides a thorough explanation of the procedure to both. Each needs to understand that sterilization is not a decision to be taken lightly or entered into when psychologic stresses, such as separation or divorce, exist. Even though both male and female procedures are theoretically reversible, the permanency of the procedure should be stressed and understood.

Male sterilization is achieved through a relatively minor procedure called a **vasectomy**. This procedure involves surgically severing the vas deferens in both sides of the scrotum. It takes about 4 to 6 weeks and 6 to 36 ejaculations to clear the remaining sperm from the vas deferens. During that period, the couple is advised to use another method of birth control and to bring in two or three semen samples for a sperm count. The man is rechecked at 6 and 12 months to ensure that fertility has not been restored by recanalization. Side effects of a vasectomy include pain, infection, hematoma, sperm granulomas, and spontaneous reanastomosis (reconnecting).

Female sterilization is most frequently accomplished by **tubal ligation**. The tubes are located through a small subumbilical incision or by mini-laparotomy techniques and are clipped, ligated, electrocoagulated, banded, or plugged. Tubal ligation may be done at any time; however, the postpartum period is an ideal time to perform the procedure because the tubes are somewhat enlarged and easily located.

Complications of female sterilization procedures include coagulation burns on the bowel, perforation of the bowel, pain, infection, hemorrhage, and adverse anesthesia effects. Reversal of a tubal ligation depends on the type of procedure performed.

The *Essure* method of permanent sterilization requires no surgical incision and yields no scar. Under hysteroscopy, a stainless steel microinsert is placed into the proximal section of each fallopian tube. Within 3 months, these microinserts create a benign tissue response that occludes the fallopian tubes. Three months after placement, tubal occlusion is confirmed by hysterosalpingogram.

Male Contraception

The vasectomy and the condom, discussed previously, are currently the only forms of male contraception available in the United States. Hormonal contraception for men has yet to be developed, although studies are under way. Developing safe, effective, and reversible male contraceptives is challenging: It is easier to interrupt a woman's cyclic process than to interrupt a man's continuous fertility.

Nursing Management

In most cases, you will work with the female partner providing information and guidance about contraceptive methods because most contraceptive methods are for women. A man can purchase condoms without seeing a healthcare provider; thus, only with vasectomy does a man require counseling and interaction with a nurse. You can play an important role in helping a woman choose a method of contraception that is acceptable to her and her partner.

In addition to completing a history and assessing for any contraindications to specific methods, spend time with a woman learning about her lifestyle, personal attitudes about particular contraceptive methods, religious beliefs, personal biases, and plans for future childbearing, before helping her select a particular contraceptive method. Once the method is chosen, help the woman learn to use it effectively. Table 5–2 summarizes factors to consider when choosing an appropriate method of contraception.

Also review any possible side effects and warning signs related to the method chosen and counsel the woman about what action to take if she suspects she is pregnant. In many cases you will be involved in telephone counseling of women who call with questions and concerns about contraception. Thus it is vital to be knowledgeable about this topic and to have resources available to find answers to less common questions. *Teaching Highlights: Using a Method of Contraception* provides guidelines for helping women use a method of contraception effectively.

Clinical Interruption of Pregnancy

Although abortion was legalized in the United States in 1973, the associated controversy over moral and legal issues continues. Many people are opposed to abortion for religious, ethical, or personal reasons. Others feel that access to a safe, legal abortion is every woman's right. A number of physical and psychosocial factors influence a woman's decision to seek an abortion. Some situations may involve lack of knowledge about contraceptive options, contraceptive failure, rape, or incest.

Medical abortion provides an effective alternative to surgical abortion for many women with unintended pregnancies. The combination of *mifepristone* (Mifeprex or RU 486), an anti-progesterone, and *misoprostol*, a prostaglandin analogue that causes smooth muscle to contract, leads to complete abortion in approximately 92% of women (ACOG, 2011). The regimen of mifepristone 200 mg orally followed in 24 to 48 hours by misoprostol 800 mcg buccally (in the cheek pouch) is the FDA approved regimen for use up to 70 days after the last menstrual period. About 7 to 14 days after taking the misoprostol, the woman is seen by her healthcare provider to confirm that the abortion was successful (FDA, 2016). Other regimens are used in an attempt to decrease cost, decrease time to expulsion of the products of conception, and decrease side effects but ACOG (2011) affirms that mifepristone-misoprostol

TABLE 5–2 Factors to Consider When Choosing a Method of Contraception

- Effectiveness of method in preventing pregnancy
- Safety of the method:
  Are there inherent risks?
  Does it offer protection against STIs or other conditions?
- Client's age and future childbearing plans
- Any contraindications in client's health history
- Religious or moral factors influencing choice
- Personal preferences, biases
- Lifestyle:
  How frequently does client have intercourse?
  Does she have multiple partners?
  Does she have ready access to medical care in the event of complications?
- Is cost a factor?
- Partner's support and willingness to cooperate
- Personal motivation to use method

regimens are preferable to those using methotrexate-misoprostol or misoprostol alone for medical abortion.

In the first trimester, surgical abortion may be performed by dilation and curettage (D&C), minisuction, or vacuum curettage. The major risks include perforation of the uterus, laceration of the cervix, systemic reaction to the anesthetic agent, hemorrhage, and infection. Second-trimester abortion may be done using dilation and extraction (D&E), hypertonic saline, systemic prostaglandins, and intrauterine prostaglandins. Surgical abortion in the first trimester is technically easier and safer than abortion in the second trimester.

Nursing Management

Recognize that the decision to have an abortion is a major one with psychologic implications for the woman and her partner, if he is involved. In caring for a woman who decides to have an abortion, it is important to do the following:

- Provide information about the methods of abortion and associated risks
- Counsel the woman about available alternatives to abortion and their implications

---

TEACHING HIGHLIGHTS | Using a Method of Contraception

- Discuss factors a woman should consider when choosing a method of contraception (see Table 5–2). Note that different methods may be appropriate at different times in a woman's life.
- Review the woman's reasons for choosing a particular method and confirm the absence of any contraindications to specific methods.
- Give a step-by-step description of the correct procedure for using the method chosen. Provide opportunities for questions.
- If a technique is to be learned, such as charting BBT or inserting a diaphragm, demonstrate and then have the woman do a return demonstration as appropriate. (*Note:* If certain aspects are beyond your level of expertise, such as fitting a cervical cap, review the content about its use and confirm that the woman understands what she is to do.)
- Provide information on what the woman should do if unusual circumstances arise (for example, she misses a pill or forgets to take a morning temperature). These can be presented in a written handout as well.
- Stress warning signs that may require immediate action by the woman and explain why these signs indicate a risk. (These should also be covered in the handout.)
- Arrange to talk with the woman again soon, either by phone or at a return visit, to see if she has any questions or has encountered any problems.

- Encourage the woman to talk about her feelings related to her decision
- Provide support before, during, and after the procedure
- Monitor vital signs, intake, and output
- Provide for physical comfort and privacy throughout the procedure
- Teach about self-care, the importance of the postabortion checkup, and contraception review

Preconception Counseling

One of the first questions a couple should ask before conception is whether they wish to have children. At times one individual wishes to have a child, whereas the other does not. In such situations, an open discussion is essential to reach a mutually acceptable decision. In some cases, professional counseling for the couple may be necessary.

Couples who wish to have children face a decision about the timing of pregnancy. At what point in their lives do they believe it would be best to become parents? For couples who have religious beliefs that do not support contraception or who feel that family planning is unnatural and wrong, planning the timing of pregnancy is unacceptable and irrelevant. These couples can still take steps to ensure that they are in the best possible physical and mental health when pregnancy occurs.

Preconception Health Measures

Preconception planning typically begins with a careful health assessment, including a consideration of known or suspected risks.

MODIFIABLE RISK FACTORS

The nurse encourages the woman to address modifiable health risks including the following:

- *Smoking.* Pregnancy often provides a strong incentive for women to quit smoking.
- *Alcohol.* Alcohol consumed during pregnancy can result in fetal alcohol syndrome, birth defects, and low birth weight.
- *Social drugs and street drugs.* These substances pose a real threat to the fetus and are associated with a variety of complications.
- *Caffeine.* The effects of caffeine are less clearly understood; however, as a precaution the woman is advised to limit her daily intake.
- *Medications.* A woman who uses any prescription or over-the-counter medications needs to discuss the implications of their use with her healthcare provider. It is best to avoid using any medication if possible.
- *Environmental hazards.* Because of the possible teratogenic effects of environmental hazards in the workplace, the couple contemplating pregnancy needs to determine whether they are exposed to any environmental hazards at work or in their community.

PHYSICAL EXAMINATION

It is advisable for both partners to have a physical examination to identify any health problems that might affect pregnancy so that they can be corrected if possible. These might include medical conditions, such as high blood pressure or obesity; problems that pose a threat to fertility, such as certain sexually transmitted infections; or conditions that keep the individual from achieving optimal health, such as anemia or colitis. If the family history indicates previous genetic disorders, or if the couple is planning pregnancy when the woman is over age 35, the healthcare provider may suggest that the couple consider genetic counseling. Some ethnic groups have higher incidences of certain genetic conditions; therefore, testing should be offered when risks are identified.

In addition to the history and physical exam, the woman may have the following laboratory tests: urinalysis, complete blood count, blood type and Rh factor, venereal disease research laboratory (VDRL) test, Pap smear, gonorrhea culture, chlamydia screen, and rubella and hepatitis screens. Women who are not immune to rubella should be counseled about the possible effects on the fetus should infection occur during the first trimester of pregnancy. If a woman decides to receive the rubella vaccine, the nurse needs to advise her to wait 3 months before conceiving to eliminate the risk of prenatal infection. These women should be counseled to use contraception during the 3-month period to prevent pregnancy. Before conception, the woman is also advised to have a dental examination and any necessary dental work completed to avoid exposure to X-rays and the risk of infection.

Women should also be asked questions regarding their psychologic history and assessed for mental illness. Certain classes of medications may be contraindicated during pregnancy, and drug changes may be needed prior to conception to prevent adverse maternal or fetal effects.

NUTRITION

Before conception, it is advisable for the woman to be at an average weight for her body build and height. The nurse can discuss nutrition and recommend that the woman follow a nutritious diet that contains ample quantities of all the essential nutrients. Some nutritionists advocate emphasizing the following nutrients: calcium, protein, iron, B complex vitamins, vitamin C, magnesium, and folic acid. Folic acid supplementation should be initiated before conception because it decreases the incidence of neural tube defects in newborns. The CDC estimates that most of these birth defects could be prevented if all women of childbearing age consumed 400 mcg of folic acid daily (Centers for Disease Control and Prevention [CDC], 2012).

Consumption of a balanced diet with the appropriate distribution of the basic food groups is especially important during pregnancy. Excessive intake of certain vitamins can cause severe fetal problems and should be avoided. Nutritional counseling is warranted for women with a history of eating disorders.

EXERCISE

A woman is advised to establish a regular exercise plan beginning at least 3 months before she plans to attempt to become pregnant. The exercise should be one she enjoys and will continue. It needs to provide some aerobic conditioning and some general toning. Exercise improves the woman's circulation and general health and tones her muscles. Once an exercise program is well established, the woman is generally encouraged to continue it during pregnancy. Prepregnancy obesity, defined as a body mass index (BMI) of 30 or above, puts the woman at risk for a variety of complications; therefore, it is advisable to advocate weight reduction for obese women who want to become pregnant.

Contraception

A woman who takes birth control pills is advised to stop the pill and have two or three normal menses before attempting to conceive. This allows the natural hormonal cycle to return and facilitates dating the subsequent pregnancy. A woman using an intrauterine device is advised to have it removed and wait 1 month before attempting to conceive. This allows the endometrium to be resterilized. Other methods of contraception that women can use during the waiting period include a variety of barrier methods of contraception (condoms, diaphragm, or cervical cap with a spermicide).

Conception

Most preconception recommendations focus on helping the couple attain their best possible health states so that they do not enter pregnancy with unnecessary risks. Conception is a personal and emotional experience, and, even if a couple is prepared, the individuals may feel some ambivalence. This is a normal response, but they may require reassurance that the ambivalence will pass. The prospective parents may get so caught up in preparation and in their efforts to "do things right" that they lose sight of the pleasure they derive from each other and their life together and cease to value the joy of spontaneity in their relationship. It is often helpful for the healthcare provider to remind an overly zealous couple that moderation is always appropriate and that there is value in "taking time to smell the roses."

Health Promotion Activities

Healthcare providers and consumers alike are becoming increasingly aware of the importance of activities that promote health and prevent illness, and the value of regular screenings to detect any health problems early. Health screening recommendations vary by age. General screening and immunization guidelines for women can be found on the website of the CDC's Office of Women's Health. This section focuses on some of the most commonly used screening procedures: breast self-examination and breast examination by a trained healthcare provider, mammography, Pap smear, and pelvic examination.

Breast Examination

Like the uterus, the breast undergoes regular cyclic changes in response to hormonal stimulation. Each month, in rhythm with the cycle of ovulation, the breasts become engorged with fluid in anticipation of pregnancy, and the woman may experience sensations of tenderness, lumpiness, or pain. If conception does not occur, the accumulated fluid drains away via the lymphatic network. *Mastodynia* or *mastalgia* (premenstrual swelling and tenderness of the breasts) is common. It usually lasts for 3 to 4 days before the onset of menses, but the symptoms may persist throughout the month.

After menopause, adipose breast tissue atrophies and is replaced by connective tissue. Elasticity is lost, and the breasts may droop and become pendulous. The recurring breast engorgement associated with ovulation ceases. If estrogen replacement therapy is used to counteract other symptoms of menopause, breast engorgement may resume.

Clinical breast examination (CBE) by a trained healthcare provider, such as a physician, nurse practitioner, or nurse-midwife, has typically been an essential element of a routine gynecologic examination. ACOG (2014) recommends a CBE every 1 to 3 years for women ages 20 to 39 years and annually for women age 40 and older. However, the American Cancer Society (ACS) no longer recommends CBE among average risk women at any age (Oeffinger, Fontham, Etzioni, et al., 2015).

BREAST SELF-EXAMINATION

Breast self-examination (BSE) plays a small role in breast cancer detection because a woman who is familiar with the look and feel of her breasts is more likely to detect a change early. The American Cancer Society (ACS) recommends BSE be presented to the client as an option, which a woman can do occasionally or on a regular basis, typically monthly. Women who choose to do BSE should have their technique reviewed during the annual examination (American Cancer Society [ACS], 2014). The American College of Obstetricians and Gynecologists stresses *breast self-awareness,* the need for a woman to be aware of how her breasts normally look and feel. ACOG (2012c) identifies breast self-examination as one way for a woman to develop self-awareness. The BSE procedure is typically taught in the course of a routine physical examination or during an initial visit to a caregiver.

Therefore, in light of the conflicting recommendations, in the course of a routine physical examination, or during an initial visit to the caregiver, women are generally taught BSE technique. If done, breast self-examination can be performed periodically or on a regular monthly basis about 1 week after each menstrual period, when the breasts are typically not tender or swollen. After menopause, BSE should be performed on the same day each month (chosen by the woman for ease of remembrance). See *Teaching Highlights: Breast Self-Examination.*

MAMMOGRAPHY

A **mammogram** is a soft tissue X-ray of the breast without the injection of a contrast medium (Figure 5–12). It can detect lesions before they can be felt and has gained wide acceptance as an effective screening tool for breast cancer. ACOG (2014) recommends that all women ages 40 and older be offered annual screening mammograms while the American Cancer Society recommends that women of average risk for breast cancer begin having regular mammograms at age 45. Women between ages 40 and 44 should be given the opportunity to begin annual

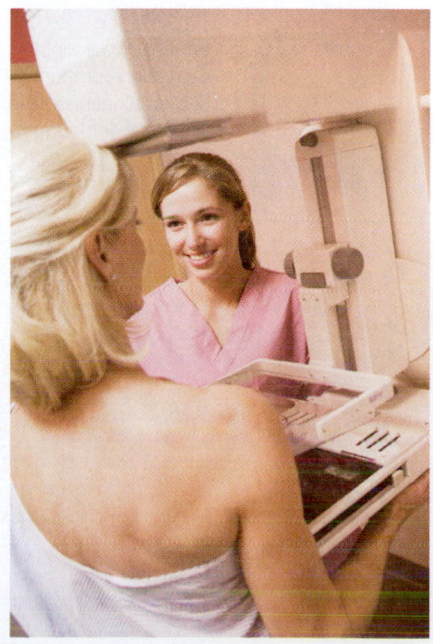

TEACHING HIGHLIGHTS | Breast Self-Examination

Describe and demonstrate the correct procedure for BSE

Inspection

The woman should inspect her breasts by standing or sitting in front of a mirror. She should inspect them in three positions: both arms relaxed at her sides, both arms raised straight over her head, and both hands placed on her hips while she leans forward. Instruct her to note the following:

- Size and symmetry of the breasts, and their shape, contours, and direction. Have her check for redness or inflammation, rashes, ulceration, or nipple discharge. A blue hue with a marked venous pattern that is focal or unilateral may indicate an area of increased blood supply due to tumor. Symmetric venous patterns are normal.

- Thickening or edema. Skin edema is seen as thickened skin with enlarged pores ("orange peel"). It may indicate blocked lymph drainage due to tumor.

- Surface of the skin. Skin dimpling, puckering, or retraction when the hands are pressed together in front of the chest or against the hips suggests malignancy.

- The nipples. Note any deviation, flattening, broadening, or recent inversion.

Palpation

The woman should be instructed to palpate her breasts as follows:

- Lie down. Put one hand behind your head. With the other hand, fingers flattened, gently feel your breast. Press lightly (Figure 5–13A).

- Still lying down, check each breast as shown in Figure 5–13B. Follow the arrows shown in the image, moving in an up and down pattern, feeling gently for a lump or thickening. Remember to feel all parts of each breast, including the "tail" of tissue near the armpit. Repeat the process on the second breast.

- Now repeat the same process on each breast while sitting up, with your hand still behind your head.

- Squeeze the nipple between your thumb and forefinger. Look for any discharge—clear, bloody, or milky (Figure 5–13C).

Determine whether the client has any questions about her findings during this examination. If she has questions, palpate the area and attempt to identify whether it is normal.

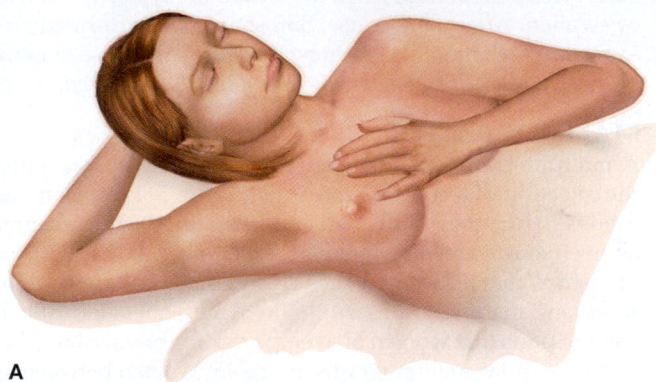

A

With one hand behind your head, flatten your fingers and press lightly on your breast, feeling gently for a lump or thickening.

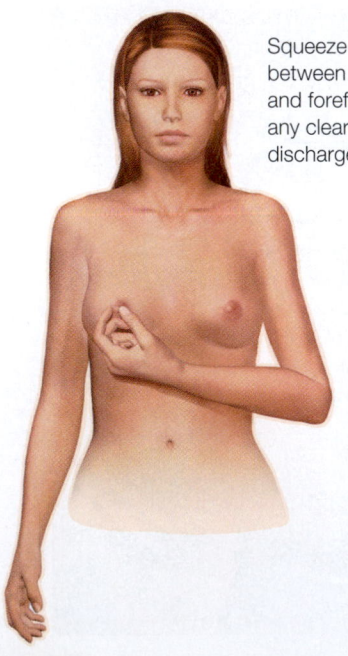

Squeeze your nipple between your thumb and forefinger; look for any clear or bloody discharge.

C

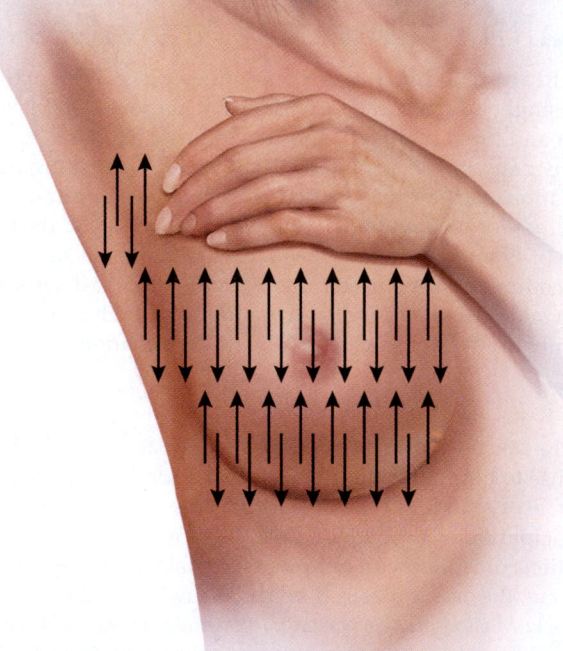

B

Check each breast in an up-and-down pattern, feeling all parts of the breast.

Figure 5–13 Procedure for breast self-examination.

screening. For women between 45 and 54 years of age, the ACS recommends annual mammograms; women age 55 and older may transition to biennial mammograms or continue receiving annual mammograms if they choose (Oeffinger et al., 2015). In addition, the ACS (2014) now recommends both mammogram and magnetic resonance imaging (MRI) beginning at age 30 in women who are at a high risk for breast cancer due to gene mutations and/or a strong family history of breast cancer and in women who had radiation to the chest between the ages of 10 and 30 years, because they often develop breast cancer at a younger age. On the other hand, the U.S. Preventive Services Task Force on Breast Cancer Screening (USPSTF, 2015) recommends biennial screening for women ages 50 to 74 years. The Task Force also states that prior to age 50 the decision to start mammography should be an individual one.

Pap Smear and Pelvic Examination

The *Papanicolaou smear* (**Pap smear**) is a form of cervical cytology testing used to screen for cellular abnormalities by obtaining a sample containing cells from the cervix and the endocervical canal. Traditionally the test has been done by preparing a Pap smear slide. Currently, a liquid-based medium Pap smear is used more often. In this test, no slide is prepared; instead, the Pap smear is obtained using a plastic spatula on the surface of the cervix and a cytobrush, which is inserted into the cervical os or opening to obtain cells in the cervical canal. The brush and spatula are swished in the solution to release cells. The specimen is sent to a laboratory where a special processor prepares a slide. This test has become the method of choice for cervical cancer screening. Liquid-based Pap smear preparations allow for removal of debris from the sample, such as blood and mucus, thereby increasing accuracy. Additionally, these preparations allow for human papillomavirus (HPV) screening and for some STI infection screening. Pap smear findings are reported using the Bethesda system (see Table 6–1).

In 2012 new guidelines for cervical cancer screening (Table 5–3) were issued by the U.S. Preventive Services Task Force, the American Cancer Society, and other groups. These are population-based guidelines and, as such, they are not appropriate for all women. The final decision on the frequency of screening is best made by the caregiver in light of the woman's history and physical findings.

Women should be advised to avoid douching, intercourse, female hygiene products, and spermicidal agents immediately before a specimen is obtained for screening. Specimens should not be obtained during menstruation or when visible cervicitis exists.

The *pelvic examination* enables the caregiver to assess a variety of factors about the woman's vagina, uterus, ovaries, and lower abdominal area. It is often performed after cervical cytology testing but may be performed without it for diagnostic purposes. Women sometimes perceive the pelvic exam as uncomfortable and embarrassing and may delay having yearly gynecologic examinations. This avoidance may pose a threat to life and health.

TABLE 5–3 Screening for Cervical Cancer

POPULATION	TEST AND FREQUENCY
Women under age 21	No screening
Women ages 21 to 29	Screening with cytology alone every 3 years (Note: co-testing for HPV is not recommended for this group because of the high prevalence of HPV).
Women ages 30 to 65	Preferred approach: screen with cytology and HPV testing every 5 years Acceptable approach: test with cytology alone every 3 years
Women over 65 who have had adequate prior screening and are not at high risk	Do not screen
Women who have undergone hysterectomy and have no history of high-grade pre-cancer or cervical cancer	Do not screen

Source: U.S. Preventive Services Task Force (USPSTF). (2012). Cervical Cancer Screening Guidelines for Average-Risk Women. http://www.cdc.gov/cancer/cervical/pdf/guidelines.pdf

Clinical Tip

When you teach about pelvic examination and cervical cytology testing, be certain that the woman understands that she should not douche for at least 24 hours beforehand. Douching is the use of a medicated solution or water to clean the vagina. Douching can interfere with the accuracy of the test. Occasionally a caregiver will specifically request that a woman use a douche before cervical cytology testing; douching should be done only in this circumstance.

To make the pelvic examination less threatening and thus improve the woman's health-seeking behavior, caregivers can offer the woman a mirror to watch the procedure, point out anatomic parts to her, and position and drape her to allow eye-to-eye contact with the practitioner. Caregivers can encourage the woman to participate by asking questions and giving feedback.

Nurse practitioners, certified nurse-midwives, and physicians all perform pelvic examinations. Nurses assist the practitioner and the woman during the examination. See *Clinical Skill: Assisting with a Pelvic Examination.*

Menopause

Menopause, defined as the absence of menstruation for 1 full year, is a time of transition for a woman, marking the end of her reproductive abilities. *Climacteric*, or *change of life* (often used synonymously with menopause), refers to the host of psychologic and physical alterations that occur around the time of menopause.

Although menopause usually occurs between 45 and 52 years of age, the current median age at menopause is 50 to 51 years. The average life span of a woman in the United States is over 80 years; thus, the average woman will live approximately one third of her life after menopause.

A woman's psychologic adaptation to menopause and the climacteric is multifactorial. She is influenced by her own

Clinical Skill 5-1
Assisting with a Pelvic Examination

NURSING ACTION

Preparation

- Ensure that the room is sufficiently warm by checking room temperature and adjusting the thermostat if necessary. If overhead heat lamps are available, turn them on.

- Explain the procedure to the woman. If she has never had a pelvic examination, show her the equipment to be used as part of the explanation.

Rationale: Explaining the procedure helps reduce anxiety and increase cooperation.

- Ask the woman to empty her bladder and to remove clothing below the waist.

Rationale An empty bladder promotes comfort during the internal examination.

- Have padding on the stirrups. If stirrups are not padded, the woman may prefer to leave her shoes on during the procedure.

Rationale: Stirrups are padded to ease the pressure of the feet against the metal and to decrease the discomfort associated with cold stirrups. If they are not padded, wearing shoes accomplishes the same purpose.

- Give the woman a disposable drape or sheet to use during the exam. Ask her to sit at the end of the examining table with the drape opened across her lap.

- Position the woman in the lithotomy position with her thighs flexed and abducted. Place her feet in the stirrups. Her buttocks should extend slightly beyond the edge of the examining table.

Rationale: This position provides the exposure necessary to conduct the examination effectively.

- Drape the woman with the sheet, leaving a flap so that the perineum can be exposed.

Rationale: The drape helps preserve the woman's sense of dignity and privacy.

Equipment and Supplies

- Vaginal specula of various sizes, warmed with water or on a heating pad prior to insertion

- Sterile gloves

- Water-soluble lubricant

- Materials for Pap smear or ThinPrep® Pap test and cultures

- Good light source

Note: Lubricant may alter the results of tests and cultures and is not used during the speculum examination. Its use is reserved for the bimanual examination.

Procedure: Sterile Gloves

1. The examiner dons gloves for the procedure. Explain each part of the procedure as the examiner performs it. Let the woman know that the examiner begins with an inspection of the external genitalia. The speculum is then inserted to allow visualization of the cervix and vaginal walls and to obtain specimens for testing (e.g., Pap smear). After the speculum is withdrawn, the examiner performs a bimanual examination of the internal organs using the fingers of one hand inserted in the woman's vagina while the other hand presses over the woman's uterus and ovaries. The final step of the procedure is generally a rectal examination.

2. Ask the woman to breathe slowly and regularly and to use any method she finds effective in helping her to remain relaxed.

Rationale: Relaxation helps decrease muscle tension.

3. Let her know when the examiner is ready to insert the speculum and ask her to bear down.

Rationale: Bearing down helps open the vaginal orifice and relaxes the perineal muscles.

4. After the speculum is withdrawn, lubricate the examiner's fingers prior to the bimanual examination.

Rationale: Lubrication decreases friction and eases insertion of the examiner's fingers.

5. After the examiner has completed the examination and moved away from the woman, move to the end of the examination table and face the woman. Cover her with the drape. Apply gentle pressure to her knees and encourage her to move toward the head of the table. Assist her to remove her feet from the stirrups, then offer your hand to her and assist her to sit up.

Rationale: Assistance is important because the lithotomy position is an awkward one and many women, especially those who are pregnant, obese, or older, may find it difficult to get out of the stirrups.

6. Provide her with tissues to wipe the lubricant from her perineum.

Rationale: Vaginal secretions and lubricant may be discharged from the vagina when the woman sits upright.

7. Provide the woman with privacy while she dresses. Be sure that she is not dizzy and that she is standing or sitting safely before leaving the room.

Rationale: Lying supine may cause postural hypotension.

---

expectations and knowledge, physical well-being, family views, marital stability, and sociocultural expectations. As the number of women reaching menopause increases, the negative emotional connotations society once attached to menopause are diminishing, enabling menopausal women to cope more effectively and even encouraging them to view menopause as a time of personal growth.

Perimenopause refers to the period of time before menopause when ovarian function wanes and hormonal deficiencies begin to produce symptoms. Perimenopause is characterized by decreasing ovarian function, unstable endocrine physiology, and highly variable hormone profiles. Symptoms of perimenopause may be nonexistent or bothersome. They may include PMS, hot flashes, irregular periods, insomnia, decreased libido, vaginal dryness, and mood changes.

Contraception remains a concern during perimenopause. Combined hormonal methods (the pill, patches, and vaginal rings) are popular among healthy nonsmokers because many women also benefit from the noncontraceptive effects, including regulation of menses, treatment of anovulatory bleeding, relief of symptoms of estrogen deficiency, and a decreased risk of endometrial and ovarian cancers. Other contraceptive options for perimenopausal women include sterilization, IUCs, progestin-only methods, and barrier methods such as male and female condoms, diaphragm, cervical cap, and spermicides.

Physical Aspects

The physical characteristics of menopause are linked to the shift from a cyclic to a noncyclic hormonal pattern. The age at onset may be influenced by nutritional, cultural, or genetic factors. The onset of menopause occurs when estrogen levels become so low that menstruation stops.

Generally ovulation ceases 1 to 2 years before menopause, but individual variations exist. Atrophy of the ovaries occurs gradually. Follicle-stimulating hormone (FSH) levels rise, and less estrogen is produced. Menopausal symptoms include atrophic changes in the vagina, vulva, and urethra and in the trigonal area of the bladder.

Many menopausal women experience a vasomotor disturbance commonly known as a *hot flash*, a feeling of heat arising from the chest and spreading to the neck and face. Hot flashes are often accompanied by profuse sweating, night sweats, and sleep disturbances. These episodes may occur as often as 20 to 30 times a day and generally last 3 to 5 minutes. Some women also experience dizzy spells, palpitations, and weakness. Many women find their own most effective ways to deal with the hot flashes. Some report that using a fan or drinking a cool liquid helps relieve distress; others seek relief through hormone therapy or complementary therapies.

The uterine lining (endometrium) and the uterine muscle layer (myometrium) atrophy, as do the cervical glands. The uterine cavity constricts. The fallopian tubes and ovaries atrophy extensively. The vaginal mucosa becomes smooth and thin, and the rugae disappear, leading to loss of elasticity. As a result, intercourse can be painful, but this problem may be overcome by using lubricating gel. Dryness of the mucous membrane can lead to burning and itching. The vaginal pH level increases as the number of Döderlein bacilli decreases.

Vulvar atrophy occurs late, and the pubic hair thins, turns gray or white, and may ultimately disappear. The labia shrivel and lose their heightened pigmentation. Pelvic fascia and muscles atrophy, resulting in decreased pelvic support. The breasts become pendulous and decrease in size and firmness.

Sexual functioning generally declines with age although more than 75% of the middle-aged women in the Study of Women's Health Across the Nation (SWAN) cited sex as being moderately to extremely important (Santoro & Sutton-Tyrrell, 2011). Factors contributing to the decline in both interest and occurrence of sexual activity are widespread. Pain during intercourse due to lack of lubrication and thinning vaginal walls is a common cause. Other factors may include a lack of partners, stress in current relationships, psychosocial factors, and a decline in general health. Completing a good sexual history will help the nurse to assess the woman's sexual health and allow the woman to ask questions and express concerns or frustrations. Long-range physical changes may include **osteoporosis**,

a decrease in the bony skeletal mass. This change is associated with lowered estrogen levels, lack of physical exercise, inadequate vitamin D, and a chronic low intake of calcium. The greatest influencing factor, however, is a family history of osteoporosis. Moreover, the estrogen deprivation that occurs in menopausal women may significantly increase their risk of coronary heart disease, which is the number one killer of women in the United States. Loss of protein from the skin and supportive tissues causes wrinkling. Postmenopausal women frequently gain weight, which may be because of excessive caloric intake or due to lower caloric need with the same level of intake.

Women With Special Needs Assisting the Older Woman with a Physical Disability

More than 50% of women over the age of 65 have a physical disability. The most common disabilities in this age group are related to arthritis or rheumatism. Older women with physical disabilities may need assistance getting onto the examination table for a gynecologic examination. The nurse should assist the woman into a semi-Fowler position and move both legs simultaneously to stirrups to prevent muscle strain or injury.

Psychologic Aspects

A woman's psychologic adaptation to menopause and the climacteric is multifactorial. It is often complicated because women of this age may be dealing with other life circumstances such as adjustment to an "empty nest" or caring for aging parents. Numerous personal factors influence a woman's ability to deal with these changes, such as self-concept, physical health, marital stability, relationships with others, and cultural values. Some women express disappointment in approaching this time of their lives, whereas many others may see it as a positive transition that offers freedom from menses or concern about contraception.

Memory and cognitive function change with advancing age. It may be that declining estrogen levels contribute to loss of this function as well as to the development of dementia. In the United States, Alzheimer disease (AD) is the most common form of dementia, estimated to affect 5.2 million Americans. Projections indicate that by the year 2025, 7.1 million Americans over the age of 65 will have AD (Alzheimer's Association, 2013). This projected increase represents a major health concern for the country.

Clinical Therapy

MENOPAUSAL HORMONE THERAPY

Menopausal hormone therapy (MHT), formerly called *hormone replacement therapy (HRT)*, refers to the administration of specific hormones, usually estrogen therapy (ET) alone or combined estrogen–progestogen therapy (EPT), to alleviate menopausal symptoms. ET is used for women who have had a hysterectomy, whereas EPT is used for women with an intact uterus. When estrogen is given alone, it can produce endometrial hyperplasia and increase the risk of endometrial cancer. Thus, in women who still have a uterus, estrogen is opposed by giving a progestin.

For over a decade, the use of MHT had decreased significantly because of a large study that suggested that the risks of MHT outweighed the benefits, particularly the increased risk of breast cancer, thromboembolic disease, and stroke. In light of findings from more recent clinical trials, that study has been called into question. In late 2012, the International Menopause Society convened a global panel to develop recommendations about the clinical management of menopausal hormone therapy. Among their recommendations were the following (deVilliers, Gass, Haines, et al., 2013):

- MHT remains the most effective therapy for moderate to severe menopausal vasomotor symptoms (hot flashes and night sweats). For symptomatic women younger than age 60 or within 10 years after menopause, the benefits are likely to outweigh the risks.

- The decision to use MHT is an individual one based on quality of life, health priorities, and personal risk factors (age, time since onset of menopause, risk of venous ischemic heart disease, thromboembolism, and breast cancer).

MHT is effective for the prevention of fractures related to osteoporosis in women who are at risk before age 60 or within 10 years of menopause. MHT can be prescribed in a number of ways, including orally; transdermally (patch); intramuscularly; topically as a gel, lotion, or vaginal cream; or through a vaginal ring. It is given in a continuous manner as a daily administration of both estrogen and progestogen, or as a cyclic or sequential therapy, with estrogen use daily and a progestogen added on a set sequence. Combination estrogen-progestogen preparations are also available.

Postmenopausal women experiencing decreased libido may experience improved sexual desire, responsiveness, and frequency when testosterone is added to their MHT. Options for providing testosterone in doses low enough for women are still limited. Estratest, a combined estrogen–androgen pill, is used by some women. Custom-compounded testosterone preparations are available by prescription.

Before starting MHT a woman should undergo a thorough health history; physical examination, including Pap smear; measurement of cholesterol, lipids, and liver enzyme levels; and baseline mammogram. An initial endometrial biopsy is indicated for women with an increased risk of endometrial cancer; biopsy is also indicated if excessive, unexpected, or prolonged vaginal bleeding occurs. Women taking estrogen should be advised to stop immediately if they develop headaches, visual changes, signs of thrombophlebitis, or chest pain.

COMPLEMENTARY HEALTH APPROACHES

For women who do not wish to take MHT or who have medical contraindications to it, a variety of approaches have been proposed as complementary or alternative treatment or preventive measures for the discomforts of the perimenopausal and postmenopausal years. Research suggests that mind-body practices such as yoga, t'ai chi, and meditation are helpful in reducing many of the common symptoms of menopause for some women; acupuncture may also help reduce the severity of symptoms. Ginseng may help relieve mood symptoms and sleep disturbances but has not been effective in treating hot flashes (National Center for Complementary and Alternative Medicine [NCCAM], 2012). Women may also seek relief through diet and nutrition, specifically a high-fiber, low-fat diet with supplements of calcium and vitamins D, E, and B complex.

Phytoestrogens, plant substances with estrogen-like properties, have been studied extensively to determine their effectiveness in relieving menopausal symptoms. The two main classes of phytoestrogens are isoflavones such as soy, and lignans, found in flaxseed, legumes, whole grains, fruits, and vegetables. The use of phytoestrogens is associated with a decrease in hot flash frequency but not in other symptoms of menopause when compared to a placebo (Chen, Lin, & Liu, 2014). Research into the use of phytoestrogens continues.

A bioidentical hormone refers to a hormone that is structurally identical to those found in the body, more specifically, those produced by the ovaries. They have received attention because of current views, which are not supported by medical literature, that these "more natural" hormones are safer and more effective. These hormones are compounded by a specialty pharmacy and are not approved by the FDA; their use is not recommended (deVilliers et al., 2013).

DHEA is a dietary supplement that is changed in the body to the hormones estrogen and testosterone. It has been suggested that DHEA might have anti-aging effects and might help in improving decreased sexual arousal, mood, cognition, and bone density, although the results of randomized controlled trials are mixed and further study is needed (Rutkowski, Sowa, Rutkowski-Talipska, et al., 2014).

Weight-bearing exercises such as walking, jogging, tennis, and low-impact aerobics help increase bone mass and decrease the risk of osteoporosis. Exercise also improves cholesterol profiles and contributes to overall health. Pelvic floor, or Kegel, exercises can help maintain vaginal muscle tone and increase blood circulation to the perineal area. Vaginal lubricants and adequate foreplay can be helpful in maintaining a satisfactory sexual experience. Stress management and relaxation techniques such as biofeedback, meditation, yoga, visualization, and massage may provide a sense of well-being.

PREVENTION AND TREATMENT OF OSTEOPOROSIS

One out of every two White women over age 50 and one in five men in the United States will have an osteoporosis-related fracture. Osteoporosis is less common in African American women but those with the diagnosis have the same fracture risk (National Osteoporosis Foundation [NOF], 2013). Table 5–4 identifies risk factors associated with osteoporosis.

Healthy People 2020

(AOCBC-10) Reduce the proportion of adults with osteoporosis

(AOCBC-11) Reduce hip fractures among older adults

TABLE 5–4 Risk Factors for Osteoporosis

- Advanced age
- Being female
- European or Asian ethnic origin
- Small-boned and thin body type (weight less than 127 lb)
- Family history of osteoporosis
- Lack of regular weight-bearing exercise
- Nulliparity
- Early onset of menopause
- Consistently low intake of calcium
- Cigarette smoking
- Moderate to heavy alcohol intake
- Use of certain medications such as anticonvulsants, corticosteroids, chemotherapy, barbiturates

Bone mineral density (BMD) testing is useful in identifying individuals who are at risk for osteoporosis. The NOF (2013) recommends BMD testing for all women ages 65 and older and all men ages 70 and older. BMD testing may also be indicated for premenopausal or postmenopausal women with risk factors, certain medical conditions such as eating disorders, thyroid disorders, leukemia, rheumatoid arthritis, and multiple sclerosis, and for those women on certain medications such as corticosteroids or anticonvulsants.

Prevention of osteoporosis is a primary goal of care. Peri- and postmenopausal women are advised to have a calcium intake of at least 1200 mg per day. Most women require supplements to achieve this level. Vitamin D supplements (800 to 1000 international units per day) may also be indicated for those at risk of deficiency. In addition, women are advised to participate regularly in weight-bearing exercise, to consume only modest quantities of alcohol and caffeine, and to stop smoking. Alcohol and smoking have a negative effect on the rate of bone resorption. In caring for women at menopause and beyond, it is important to ensure that the woman's height is measured at each visit, because a loss of height is often an early sign that vertebrae are being compressed because of reduced bone mass.

The effectiveness of estrogen in preventing osteoporosis is well documented. Women with no contraindications to estrogen who are showing evidence of bone loss are good candidates for HT. For women who are unable or unwilling to take estrogen, other medications available to treat or help prevent osteoporosis include the following:

- *Bisphosphonates* are calcium regulators that act by inhibiting bone resorption and increasing bone mass. Alendronate (Fosamax) and risedronate (Actonel) are commonly prescribed. Zoledronic acid (Zometa) is administered intravenously once a year and seems to achieve the same results in treating osteoporosis as other bisphosphonates taken daily or weekly without the troublesome gastrointestinal side effects.

- *Selective estrogen receptor modulators (SERMs)* such as raloxifene (Evista) preserve the beneficial effects of estrogen, including its protection against osteoporosis, but do not stimulate uterine or breast tissue.

- *Salmon calcitonin* is a calcium regulator that may inhibit bone loss. Administered as a nasal spray, its value is less clear than that of the other medications listed.

- *Parathyroid hormone*, taken daily as a subcutaneous injection, activates bone formation, which results in substantial increases in bone density.

- *Receptor activator of nuclear factor kappa-B ligand (RANKL) inhibitor* (denosumab, brand name Prolia®) decreases bone resorption and increases bone mass and strength. It is administered subcutaneously every 6 months.

Nursing Management

Most menopausal women deal well with this developmental phase of life, although some women may need counseling to adjust successfully. Reaction to menopause is determined to a large extent by the life the woman has lived, by the security she has in her feminine identity, and by her feelings of self-worth and self-esteem.

Nurses and other healthcare professionals can help the menopausal woman achieve high-level functioning at this time in her life. Of paramount importance is your ability to understand and provide support for the woman's views and feelings.

Whether the woman expresses relief and delight or tearfulness and fear, use an empathic approach in counseling, health teaching, and providing physical care.

Explore the question of the woman's comfort during sexual intercourse. In counseling, you may say, "After menopause many women notice that their vagina seems dryer and intercourse can be uncomfortable. Have you noticed any changes?" This gives the woman information and may open discussion. Then go on to explain that dryness and shrinking of the vagina can be addressed by use of a water-soluble jelly. Use of estrogen, orally or in vaginal creams, may also be indicated. Increased frequency of intercourse will maintain some elasticity in the vagina. When assessing the menopausal woman, address the question of sexual activity openly but tactfully, because the woman may have been socialized to be reticent about discussing sex.

The crucial need of women in the perimenopausal period of life is for adequate information about the changes taking place in their bodies and their lives. Supplying that information provides both a challenge and an opportunity for nurses.

Violence Against Women

Violence against women has become endemic in society today. Violence affects women of all ages, races, ethnic backgrounds, socioeconomic levels, educational levels, and walks of life. Two of the most common forms of violence are domestic violence, also called *intimate partner violence* or *relationship violence*, and sexual assault. Worldwide, 35% of women have experienced intimate partner violence or non-partner sexual violence at some time in their lives; estimates suggest that 38% of all female murders are committed by an intimate partner (World Health Organization [WHO], 2013).

Violence against women is a major health concern: In addition to causing injuries, associated physical and mental health outcomes, and fatalities, violence costs the healthcare system millions of dollars annually. In response to this epidemic, healthcare providers are becoming more knowledgeable about actions they should take to identify women at risk, implement preventive measures, and provide effective care.

Healthy People 2020

IVP-39 (Developmental) Reduce violence by current or former partners

IVP-40 (Developmental) Reduce sexual violence

Domestic Violence

Domestic violence or **intimate partner violence (IPV)** is defined as a pattern of coercive behaviors and methods used to exert power and control by one individual over another in an adult domestic or intimate relationship. This section focuses on domestic violence experienced by women in heterosexual relationships, although gay and lesbian individuals experience domestic violence in their relationships as well.

Although the incidence has decreased significantly in the past decade, domestic violence is still staggeringly common in the United States, where almost one in four women (22.3%) will experience at least one act of severe physical violence during her lifetime. Psychologic aggression by an intimate partner is even more common—47.1% of women will experience at least one act of psychologic aggression during their lifetimes (Breiding, Smith, Basile, et al., 2014).

The woman may be married to her abuser, or she may be living with, dating, or divorced from him. Domestic violence takes many forms, including verbal attacks, insults, intimidation, threats, sexual violence, emotional abuse, social isolation, economic deprivation, intellectual derision, ridicule, stalking, and physical attacks and injury. Physical battering includes slapping, kicking, shoving, punching, forms of torture, attacks with objects or weapons, and sexual assault. Women who are physically abused can also suffer psychologic and emotional abuse.

CYCLE OF VIOLENCE

In an effort to explain the experience of battered women, Walker (1984) developed the theory of the cycle of violence. Battering takes place in a cyclic fashion through three phases:

1. In the *tension-building phase*, the batterer demonstrates power and control. This phase is characterized by anger, arguing, blaming the woman for external problems, and possibly minor battering incidents. The woman may blame herself and believe she can prevent the escalation of the batterer's anger by her own actions.

2. The *acute battering incident* is typically triggered by some external event or internal state of the batterer. It is an episode of acute violence distinguished by lack of control, lack of predictability, and major destructiveness. The cycle of violence can be interrupted before the acute battering incident if proper interventions take place.

3. The *tranquil phase* is sometimes termed the honeymoon period. This phase may be characterized by extremely kind and loving behavior on the part of the batterer as he tries to make up with the woman, or it may simply be manifested as an absence of tension and violence. Without intervention, this phase will end and the cycle of violence will continue. Over time the violence increases in severity and frequency.

CHARACTERISTICS OF BATTERED WOMEN

Battered women often hold traditional views of sex roles. Many were raised to be submissive, passive, and dependent and to seek approval from male figures. Some battered women were exposed to violence between their parents, whereas others first experienced it from their partners. Many battered women do not work outside the home. As part of the manipulation of batterers, they are isolated from family and friends and totally dependent on their partners for their financial and emotional needs.

Women with physically abusive partners nearly always experience psychologic abuse as well and have been told repeatedly by their batterers that the family's problems are all their fault. Many believe their batterers' insults and accusations. As these women become more isolated, they find it harder to judge who is right. Eventually they fully believe in their inadequacy, and their low self-esteem reinforces their belief that they deserve to be beaten. Battered women often feel a pervasive sense of guilt, fear, and depression. Their sense of hopelessness and helplessness reduces their problem-solving ability. Battered women may also experience a lack of support from family, friends, and their religious community.

CHARACTERISTICS OF BATTERERS

Batterers come from all backgrounds, professions, religious groups, and socioeconomic levels. Batterers often have feelings of insecurity, socioeconomic inferiority, powerlessness, and helplessness that conflict with their assumptions of male supremacy. Emotionally immature and aggressive men have a tendency to express these overwhelming feelings of inadequacy through violence. Many batterers feel undeserving of their partners, yet they blame and punish the very women they value.

Battered women often describe their husbands or partners as lacking respect toward women in general, having come from homes where they witnessed abuse of their mothers or were themselves abused as children, and having a hidden rage that erupts occasionally. Batterers accept traditional macho values, yet when they are not angry or aggressive, they appear childlike, dependent, seductive, manipulative, and in need of nurturing. They may be well respected in the community. This dual personality of batterers reflects the conflict between their belief that they must live up to their macho image and their feelings of inadequacy in the role of husband or provider. Combined with low frustration tolerance and poor impulse control, their pervasive sense of powerlessness leads them to strike out at life's inequities by abusing women.

Nursing Management

Nurses in various healthcare settings often come in contact with abused women but fail to recognize them, especially if their bruises are not visible. Women who are at high risk of battering often have a history of alcohol or drug abuse, child abuse, or abuse in the previous or present relationship. Other possible signs of abuse include expressions of helplessness and powerlessness; low self-esteem revealed by the woman's dress, her appearance, and the way she relates to healthcare providers; signs of depression evidenced by fatigue, hopelessness, and somatic problems such as headache, insomnia, chest pain, back pain, or pelvic pain; and possible suicide attempts. In addition, the abused woman may have a history of missed or frequently changed appointments, perhaps because she had signs of abuse that kept her from coming in or her partner prevented it.

Because domestic violence is so prevalent, many healthcare providers now advocate *universal screening of all female clients at every healthcare encounter*. Screening should be done privately, with only the nurse and client present, in a safe and quiet place. Specific language leads to higher disclosure rates. Possible screening questions include the following:

1. During the past year, have you been slapped, kicked, hit, choked, or hurt physically by someone?

2. Has your partner or anyone else ever forced you to have sex?

3. Are you afraid of an ex-partner or of anyone at home?

During the screening assure the woman that her privacy will be respected (Figure 5–14). It is essential to remain nonjudgmental. Create a warm, caring climate conducive to sharing and demonstrate a willingness to talk about violence. A battered woman may interpret your willingness to discuss violence as permission for her to discuss it as well.

It is important to consider cultural and religious factors that may impact a woman's willingness to disclose abuse. See *Developing Cultural Competence: Supporting Immigrant Women Who Suffer Abuse.*

When a woman seeks care for an injury, be alert to the following cues of abuse:

- Hesitation in providing detailed information about the injury and how it occurred

- Inappropriate affect for the situation

- Delayed reporting of symptoms

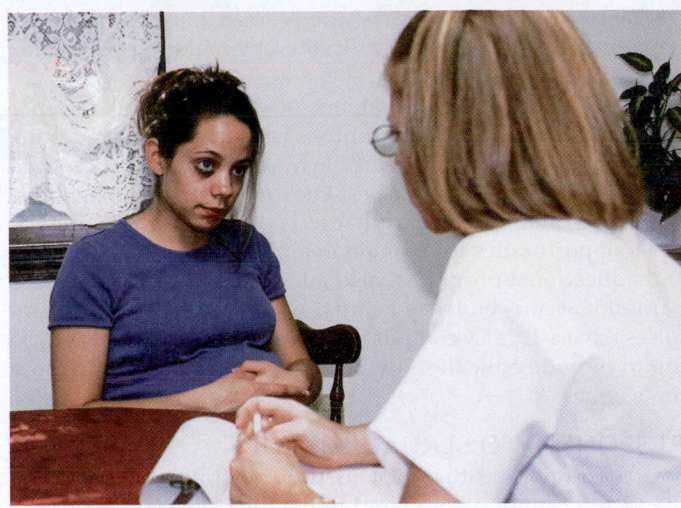

Figure 5–14 Screening for domestic violence should be done privately.

SOURCE: Al Dodge/Pearson Education, Inc.

Developing Cultural Competence Supporting Immigrant Women Who Suffer Abuse

Immigrant women who experience intimate partner violence (IPV) may be reluctant to report it for fear of deportation. Nurses need to be aware that the "U" Nonimmigrant Visa permits immigrants who have been victims of IPV or other crimes to remain in the United States legally if it is justified on humanitarian grounds, is in the public interest, or ensures family unity (ACOG, 2012b).

- Pattern of injury consistent with abuse, including multiple injury sites involving bruises, abrasions, and contusions to the head (eyes and back of the neck), throat, chest, abdomen, or genitals
- Inappropriate explanation for the injuries
- Lack of eye contact
- Signs of increased anxiety in the presence of the possible batterer, who frequently does much of the talking

When a woman who has been battered comes in for treatment, she needs to feel safe physically and secure in talking about her injuries and problems. If a man is with her, ask or tell him to remain in the waiting room while the woman is examined. A battered woman also needs to reestablish a feeling of control over her world. She needs to regain a sense of predictability by knowing what to expect and how she can interact. Provide sufficient information about what to expect in terms the woman can understand.

In providing care let the woman work through her story, problems, and situation at her own pace. Reassure the woman that she is believed and that her feelings are reasonable and normal. Anticipate the woman's ambivalence (because of her fear and possible love–hate relationship with her batterer) but also respect the woman's capacity to change and grow when she is ready. Thus any assessment should include information about a woman's strengths and support system. The woman may require assistance in identifying specific problems and in developing realistic ideas for reducing or eliminating those problems. In all interactions stress

---

Women With Special Needs Intimate Partner Assessment

Women with disabilities are at greater risk of being victimized and of suffering intimate partner violence. Women who rely on their partner for assistance with activities of daily living are at risk for having care withheld and neglect, in addition to physical and mental abuse. They are also at risk for financial abuse. The nurse should provide an extensive intimate partner assessment with the woman without the partner present to determine if abuse is occurring.

---

that no one should be abused and that the abuse is not the woman's fault.

Community-Based Nursing Care

Inform any woman suspected of being in an abusive situation of the services available in the community. A battered woman may need the following:

- Medical treatment for injuries
- Temporary shelter to provide a safe environment for her and her children
- Counseling to raise her self-esteem and help her understand the dynamics of family violence
- Legal assistance for protection or prosecution of the batterer
- Financial assistance to obtain shelter, food, and clothing
- Job training or employment counseling

If the woman returns to an abusive situation, encourage her to develop an exit plan for herself and her children. As part of the plan, she should:

- Pack a change of clothes for herself and the children, including toilet articles and an extra set of car and house keys, stored away from her house with a friend or neighbor
- Ask a neighbor to call the police if violence begins
- Have money, identification papers (driver's license, social security cards), checkbook, bank account information, other financial records (such as mortgage papers, rent and utility receipts, automobile title, insurance policies and numbers), and information about the children to help her enroll them in school
- Have a plan for where she will go, regardless of the day or time

---

Professionalism In Practice Patient Advocacy

Patient advocacy is a nursing responsibility that extends beyond individual nurse–patient relationships. Nurses can follow and become involved in legislative advocacy for issues related to domestic violence and other issues related to women's health through participation in their local and state chapters of the American Nurses Association, by being aware of current issues, by following the progress of specific bills online, by writing to their legislators, and by exercising their right to vote.

- Identify friends and family who know about the situation and will help her. Ask that she establish a code word for danger with those family and friends
- Have a planned escape route and emergency telephone numbers she can call, including personal numbers, the local police, a phone hotline, and a women's shelter if one is available in the community

Working with battered women is challenging, and many healthcare providers feel frustrated and impotent when women repeatedly return to their abusive situations. You must realize that you cannot rescue battered women; a battered woman must decide on her own how to handle her situation. Provide battered women with information that empowers them in decision making and supports their decisions, knowing that incremental assistance over the years may be the only alternative until the woman is ready to explore other options.

Sexual Assault and Rape

Broadly, **sexual assault** is involuntary sexual contact with another person. **Rape** is forced sexual intercourse as a result of physical force or psychologic coercion. Forced sexual intercourse refers to vaginal, oral, or anal penetration by a body part or by an object.

Sexual assault remains one of the most underreported violent crimes in the United States. In 2012, only an estimated 28% of rapes or sexual assaults were reported to the police, making the actual number of victims significantly higher (Truman, Langton, & Planty, 2013). Over 78% of victims know their offender; about 40% of assailants had been drinking or using drugs prior to the assault. Although both men and women can be sexually assaulted, research indicates that 91% or approximately 9 out of every 10 rape or sexual assault victims are female (Planty, Langton, Krebs, et al., 2013).

No woman of any age, cultural or ethnic background, or socioeconomic status is immune, but statistics indicate that young, unmarried women; women who are unemployed or have a low family income; and students have the highest incidence of sexual assault or attempted assault.

Why do men rape? Of the many theories put forth, none provides a completely satisfactory explanation. So few assailants are actually caught and convicted that a clear characteristic of the assailant has not been developed. However, rapists tend to be emotionally weak and insecure and may have difficulty maintaining interpersonal relationships. Many assailants also have trouble dealing with the stresses of daily life. Such men may become angry and overcome by feelings of powerlessness. They then commit a sexual assault as an expression of power or anger.

Acquaintance rape, which occurs when the assailant is someone with whom the victim has had previous nonviolent interaction, is the most common form of rape. One type of acquaintance rape, **date rape**, which occurs between a dating couple, is an increasing problem on high school and college campuses. In some cases an assailant uses alcohol or other drugs to sedate his intended victim. One drug, flunitrazepam (Rohypnol), has gained notoriety as a date rape drug. Gamma hydroxybutyrate (GHB), ketamine, MDMA (Ecstasy), clonazepam, and scopolamine have also been identified as date rape drugs that are used to incapacitate a woman. More recently, prescription drugs have been used in combination with alcohol to facilitate many sexual assaults. Because these drugs frequently produce amnesia, the woman may be unable to remember details of her assault, thereby making prosecution more difficult.

Awareness of the prevalence of date rape and violence against women on college campuses has increased significantly in the wake of several high-profile rape cases at American universities. Title IX legislation, best known for its requirement that all colleges and universities that receive federal funds provide equal opportunities for women in athletic programs, facilities, and educational programs, also addresses the issue of sexual harassment and violence against women. Today, most campuses have a Title IX compliance officer and are actively working to provide education to students, faculty, and staff about these issues.

RESPONSES TO SEXUAL ASSAULT

Sexual assault is a situational crisis. It is a traumatic event that the victim cannot be prepared to handle because it is unforeseen. Following the assault, the victim generally experiences a cluster of symptoms, described by Burgess and Holmstrom (1979) as the *rape trauma syndrome*, that last far beyond the rape itself. These phases are described in Table 5–5. Although the phases of response are listed individually, they often overlap, and individual responses and their duration may vary. A fourth phase—integration and recovery—was later suggested (Holmes, 1998).

Research also suggests that survivors of sexual assault may exhibit high levels of posttraumatic stress disorder (PTSD), the same disorder that develops in many combat veterans. PTSD is marked by varying degrees of intensity. Assault victims with this disorder often require lengthy, intensive therapy to regain a sense of trust and feeling of personal control.

TABLE 5–5 Phases of Recovery Following Sexual Assault

PHASE	RESPONSE
Acute (disorganization) phase	Fear, shock, disbelief, desire for revenge, anger, anxiety, guilt, denial, embarrassment, humiliation, helplessness, dependence, self-blame, wide variety of physical reactions, lost or distorted coping mechanisms
Outward adjustment (denial) phase	Survivor appears outwardly composed, denying and repressing feelings (e.g., she returns to work, buys a weapon); refuses to discuss the assault; denies need for counseling
Reorganization	Survivor makes many life adjustments, such as moving to a new residence or changing her phone number; uses emotional distancing; may engage in risky sexual behaviors; may experience sexual dysfunction, phobias, flashbacks, sleep disorders, nightmares, anxiety; has a strong urge to talk about or resolve feelings; may seek counseling or remain silent
Integration and recovery	Time of resolution; survivor begins to feel safe and be comfortable trusting others; places blame on assailant; may become an advocate for others

Nursing Management

Survivors of sexual assault often enter the healthcare system by way of the emergency department (ED). Thus the ED nurse is often the first person to counsel them. Because the values, attitudes, and beliefs of the caregiver will necessarily affect the competence and focus of the care, it is essential that nurses clearly understand their feelings about sexual assault and assault survivors and resolve any conflicts that may exist. In many communities, specially trained sexual assault nurse examiners coordinate the care of survivors of sexual assault, gather necessary forensic evidence, and are then available as expert witnesses when assailants are tried for the crime.

The first priority in caring for a survivor of a sexual assault is to create a safe, secure milieu. Admission information is gathered in a quiet, private room. Assure the woman that she is safe and not alone. Assess her appearance, demeanor, and ways of communicating for the purpose of planning care. Initially, the woman is evaluated to determine the need for emergency care. Obtaining a careful, detailed history is essential. After the woman has received any necessary emergency care, a forensic chart and kit are completed.

Give the woman a thorough explanation of the procedures to be carried out and have her sign a consent form for the forensic examination and collection of materials. Sexual assault kits contain all the necessary supplies for collecting and labeling evidence. The woman's clothing is collected and bagged, swabs of stains and secretions are taken, hair samples and any fingernail scrapings are collected, blood samples are drawn, tissue swabs are obtained, and photographs are taken. Vaginal and rectal examinations are performed, along with a complete physical examination for trauma. If possible photographs are taken of any injuries.

The woman is offered prophylactic treatment for sexually transmitted infections. If the assailant's HIV status is not known, the woman may be offered postexposure prophylaxis with HIV antiviral medications. In such cases, consultation with an HIV specialist is advised. Question the woman about her menstrual cycle and contraceptive practices. If she could become pregnant as a result of the rape, she should be offered postcoital contraceptive therapy.

The family members and friends on whom the survivor calls will also need nursing care. The reactions of the family will depend on the values to which they ascribe. Many families or partners blame the survivor for the assault and feel angry with her for not having been more careful. They may also incorrectly view the assault as a sexual act rather than an act of violence. They may feel personally wronged and see the survivor as devalued or unclean. Their reactions may compound the survivor's crisis. By spending some time with family members before their first interaction with the survivor, the nurse may be able to reduce their anxiety and absorb some of their frustrations, sparing the woman further trauma.

EDUCATION AND COUNSELING

Sexual assault education and counseling, provided by qualified nurses or other counselors, is a valuable tool in helping the survivor come to terms with her assault and its impact on her life. In counseling, the woman is encouraged to explore and identify her feelings and determine appropriate actions to resolve her problems and concerns. It is important for the counselor to avoid reinforcing the prevalent myth that the assault was somehow the woman's fault. The fault lies with the assailant. The counselor also plays an important role in emphasizing that the loss of control the woman experienced during the rape was temporary and that the woman can regain a feeling of control over life.

PROSECUTION OF THE ASSAILANT

Legally, sexual assault is considered a crime against the state, and prosecution of the assailant is a community responsibility. The survivor, however, must begin the process by reporting the assault and pressing charges against her assailant. In the past, the police and the judicial system were notoriously insensitive in dealing with survivors. However, many communities now have classes designed to help officers work effectively with sexual assault survivors or have special teams to carry out this important task.

Many women who have sought to use the judicial process have had such a traumatic experience that they refer to it as a second assault. The woman may be asked repeatedly to describe the experience in intimate detail, and her reputation and testimony will be attacked by the defense attorney. In addition, publicity may intensify her feelings of humiliation, and, if her assailant is released on bail or found not guilty, she may fear retaliation.

The nurse acting as a counselor needs to be aware of the judicial sequence to anticipate rising tension and frustration in the survivor and her support system. She will need consistent, effective support at this crucial time.

Focus Your Study

- Nurses should provide girls and women with clear information about menstrual issues, such as use of tampons (deodorant type and absorbency); vaginal spray and douching practices; and self-care comfort measures during menstruation, such as maintaining good nutrition, exercising, and using heat and massage.

- Dysmenorrhea usually begins at, or a day before, onset of menses and disappears by the end of menstruation. Hormone therapy (e.g., combined oral contraceptives), nonsteroidal anti-inflammatory drugs, or prostaglandin inhibitors can ease symptoms. Self-care measures include improved nutrition, exercise, applications of heat, and extra rest.

- Premenstrual syndrome occurs most often in women over age 30. Symptoms occur 2 to 3 days before onset of menstruation and subside as menstruation starts, with or without treatment. Medical management usually includes prostaglandin inhibitors and calcium supplementation. Self-care measures include improving nutrition (vitamins B complex and E supplementation and avoiding methylxanthines, which are found in chocolate and caffeine), a program of aerobic exercise, and participation in self-care support groups. In some cases medications such as selective serotonin reuptake inhibitors may be indicated.

- Fertility awareness–based (FAB) methods of natural family planning (NFP) are natural, noninvasive methods of contraception often used by people whose religious beliefs prevent their using other methods.

- Barrier contraceptives such as the diaphragm, cervical cap, and condom act as barriers to prevent the transport of sperm. These methods are used in conjunction with a spermicide.

- N-9, the spermicide available in the United States, is more effective in preventing pregnancy when it is used with a barrier method.

- The Mirena and Skyla levonorgestrel-releasing IUCs (LNg-IUCs) are both hormonal and mechanical contraceptives. Their action is similar to that of the Copper IUC, but they also secrete a progestin, levonorgestrel, that helps the endometrium to become atrophic, the cervical secretions to become thick, and the menstrual flow to be decreased.

- Combined oral contraceptives (the pill) are combinations of estrogen and progesterone. When taken correctly, they are one of the most effective reversible methods of fertility control. They also provide noncontraceptive benefits such as less acne and decreased scheduled bleeding.

- The progestin-only subdermal implant, Nexplanon, is an excellent choice for women desiring long-term contraception who cannot take estrogen.

- Other combined hormonal options (estrogen and progestin) such as the patch (Ortho Evra) and the vaginal ring (NuvaRing) have broadened the range of contraceptive options available.

- The long-acting progestin-only injection, Depo-Provera IM 150 mg or Depo-Provera SC 104 mg, is available for lactating women, or those who cannot take estrogen.

- Permanent sterilization is accomplished by tubal ligation for women and vasectomy for men. Although they are theoretically reversible, clients are advised that these methods should be considered irreversible.

- The termination of pregnancy through abortion may now be achieved by either medical or surgical means.

- A mammogram is a soft tissue X-ray examination of the breast taken without the injection of a contrast medium. Currently both ACS and ACOG recommend that all women over age 40 have an annual mammogram.

- Preconception counseling can be used to identify risk factors and unhealthy behaviors before a pregnancy occurs. Healthful lifestyle changes can be employed.

- Pap smear screening is recommended for all women 21 years of age and older. Several factors put a woman at high risk for an abnormal Pap: intercourse at a young age, multiple partners, history of immunotherapy, long-term combined oral contraceptive (COC) use, smoking, and previous history of dysplasia. Human papilloma virus (HPV) is highly associated with abnormal Pap smears.

- Menopause is a physiologic, maturational change in a woman's life. Physiologic changes include the cessation of menses and decrease in circulating hormones. Hormonal changes sometimes bring unsettling emotional responses. The most common physiologic symptoms are hot flashes, palpitations, dizziness, and increased perspiration at night. The woman's anatomy also undergoes changes, such as atrophy of the vagina, reduction in size and pigmentation of the labia, and myometrial atrophy. Osteoporosis becomes an increasing concern.

- Current management of menopause centers around menopausal hormone therapy (MHT), complementary therapies, and client healthcare education. Decisions about the use of MHT should be made individually based on each woman's symptoms and risks, and the woman should be advised about the known risks.

- Osteoporosis is becoming a significant health problem in the United States. Prevention is the preferred approach to addressing the issue. This includes adequate calcium intake and regular weight-bearing exercise. For women who have already developed osteoporosis, medications are available as a treatment option.

- Batterers use physical, psychologic, and sexual abuse to maintain power and control in a sexual relationship. Battering occurs in a cyclic pattern called the "cycle of violence" and increases in frequency and severity over time.

- Nurses are in an excellent position to intervene and assist battered women by recognizing their cues, diagnosing their problems appropriately, and understanding the complex dynamics of the battering family. Nurses provide information about available community resources, medical attention, and community support.

- Women in abusive relationships who belong to cultural and linguistic minority communities and immigrant women face additional barriers when attempting to access services. The nurse must work to provide culturally aware and competent care.

- Estimates suggest that the majority of sexual assaults are not reported to the police. Rapes and sexual assaults committed by strangers are more likely to be reported to the police than rapes or sexual assaults committed by nonstrangers, including intimate partners, other relatives, and friends or acquaintances.

- Rape is a form of violence acted out sexually. Most sexual assaults are expressions of anger or power. However, estimates suggest that the majority of sexual assaults are not reported to the police.

- Following sexual assault, the survivor will usually experience an assortment of symptoms known as the rape trauma syndrome. Research also links the effects of rape to posttraumatic stress disorder.

Clinical Reasoning in Action

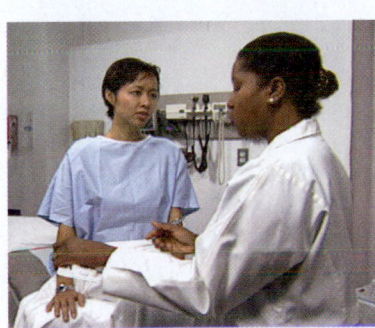

You are working at a local clinic when Joy Lang, age 20, presents for her first pelvic exam. You obtain the following GYN history: menarche age 12, menstrual cycle 28–30 days lasting 4–5 days, heavy one day, then lighter. She tells you that she needs to use superabsorbent tampons on the first day of her period and then she switches to a regular absorbency tampon for the remaining days. She confirms that she changes the tampon every 6 to 8 hours, never leaving it in overnight. She denies premenstrual syndrome, dysmenorrhea, or medical problems and says that she is not taking any medication on a regular schedule. She tells you that she recently got married, but would like to wait before getting pregnant. She'd like to discuss birth control methods. Joy tells you that doctors make her nervous and she admits to being anxious about her first pelvic exam.

1. What steps would you take to reduce Joy's anxiety relating to the pelvic exam?

2. What precaution should be taken when obtaining a Pap smear?

3. Explain the purpose of the Pap smear.

4. What factors do you include in a discussion of the type of birth control that Joy could practice?

References

Alzheimer's Association. (2013). *2013 Alzheimer's disease facts and figures.* Retrieved from http://www.alz.org/downloads/facts_figures_2013.pdf

American Cancer Society (ACS). (2014). American Cancer Society recommendations for early breast cancer detection in women without breast symptoms. Retrieved from http://www.cancer.org/cancer/breastcancer/moreinformation/breastcancerearlydetection/breast-cancer-early-detection-acs-recs

American College of Obstetricians and Gynecologists (ACOG). (2009, reaffirmed 2011). *Medical management of abortion* (ACOG Practice Bulletin No. 67). Washington, DC: Author.

American College of Obstetricians and Gynecologists (ACOG). (2010, reaffirmed 2012a). *Noncontraceptive uses of hormonal contraceptives* (ACOG Practice Bulletin No. 110). Washington, DC: Author.

American College of Obstetricians and Gynecologists (ACOG). (2012b). *Intimate partner violence.* (ACOG Committee Opinion No. 518). Washington, DC: Author.

American College of Obstetricians and Gynecologists (ACOG). (2012c). *The breast self-exam.* Retrieved from http://www.acog.org/~/media/For%20Patients/pfs002.pdf?dmc=1&ts=20120526T1441263798

American College of Obstetricians and Gynecologists (ACOG). (2014). *Breast cancer screening.* (ACOG Practice Bulletin No. 122. Reaffirmed 2014). Washington, DC: Author.

Breiding, M. J., Smith, S. G., Basile, K. C., Walters, M. L., Chen, J., & Merrick, M. T. (2014). Prevalence and characteristics of sexual violence, stalking, and intimate partner violence victimization—National Intimate Partner and Sexual Violence Survey, United States, 2011. *Morbidity and Mortality Weekly Report (MMWR), 63*(SS08), 1–18.

Burgess, A. W., & Holmstrom, L. L. (1979). *Rape: Crisis and recovery.* Englewood Cliffs, NJ: Prentice Hall.

Centers for Disease Control and Prevention (CDC). (2012). *Folic acid: Recommendations.* Retrieved from http://www.cdc.gov/ncbddd/folicacid/recommendations.html

Chen, M-N, Lin, C-C., & Liu, C-F. (2014). Efficacy of phytoestrogens for menopausal symptoms: A meta-analysis and systematic review. *Climacteric, 17,* 1–10.

Cheng, S. J., & Van Leuven, K. A. (2015). Intrauterine contraception and the facts for college health. *The Journal for Nurse Practitioners, 11*(4), 417–424.

Cunningham, F. G., Leveno, K. J., Bloom, S. L., Spong, C. Y., Dashe, J. S., Hoffman, B. L., . . . & Sheffield, J. S. (2014). *Williams obstetrics* (24th ed.). New York, NY: McGraw-Hill.

Deal, M., Moore, A., & Sutton, C. (2014). Individualizing contraception. *Women's Healthcare: A Clinical Journal for NPs, 2*(2), 8–16.

de Villiers, T. J., Gass, M. L. S., Haines, C. J., Hall, J. E., Lobo, R. A., Pierroz, D. D., & Rees, M. (2013). Global consensus statement on menopausal hormone therapy. *Climacteric, 16,* 203–204.

Garza-Cavazos, A., & Loret de Mola, J. R. (2012). Abnormal uterine bleeding: New definitions and contemporary terminology. *The Female Patient, 37*(7), 27–36.

Guttmacher Institute. (2014). *UNFPA Fact Sheet: Adding it up: Investing in sexual and reproductive health.* Retrieved from http://www.unfpa.org/sites/default/files/resource-pdf/383%20AIU3%20Global%20Fact%20sheet%20ENG%2011.20.14%20FINAL_1.pdf

Holmes, M. M. (1998). The clinical management of rape in adolescents. *Contemporary OB/GYN, 43*(5), 62–78.

Kelderhouse, K., & Taylor, J. S. (2013). A review of treatment and management modalities for premenstrual dysphoric disorder. *Nursing for Women's Health, 17*(4), 294–305.

Kridli, S. (2011). Health beliefs and practices of Muslim women during Ramadan. *MCN, the American Journal of Maternal/Child Nursing, 36*(4), 216–221.

Lentz, G., Lobo, R. A., Gersenson, D. M., & Katz, V. L. (2012). *Comprehensive Gynecology* (6th ed.). Philadelphia, PA: Elsevier.

Levy, D. P., Jager, M., Kapp, N., & Abitbol, J. (2014). Ulipristal acetate for emergency contraception: Postmarketing experience after use by more than 1 million women. *Contraception, 89*(5), 431–433.

Matsumoto, T., Asakura, H., & Hayashi, T. (2013). Biopsychosocial aspects of premenstrual syndrome and premenstrual dysphoric disorder. *Gynecological Endocrinology, 29*(1), 67–73.

Myrisk, K., Reinn, R., & Harkins, M. (2014). The prevalence of and attitudes toward oligomenorrhea and amenorrhea in Division I female athletes. *International Journal of Athletic Therapy & Training, 19*(6), 41–17.

National Center for Complementary and Alternative Medicine (NCCAM). (2012). *Get the facts: Menopausal symptoms and complementary health practices*. Retrieved from http://nccam.nih.gov/health/menopause/menopausesymptoms#hed2

National Osteoporosis Foundation (NOF). (2013). *Clinician's guide to prevention and treatment of osteoporosis*. Washington, DC: Author.

Oeffinger, K.C., Fontham, E.T.H., Etzioni, R., Herzig, A., Michaelson, J.S., Shih, Y.T . . . & Walter, L. (2015). Breast cancer screening for women at average risk: 2015 guideline update from the American cancer society. *Journal of the American Medical Society (JAMA), 314*(15), 1599–1614.

Planty, M., Langton, L., Krebs, C., Berzofsky, M., & Smiley-McDonald, H. (2013). *Female victims of sexual violence, 1994–2010*. Retrieved from http://www.bjs.gov/content/pub/pdf/fvsv9410.pdf

Rost, M., Jacobsson, J., Dahlstrom, O., Hammar, M., & Timpka, T. (2014). Amenorrhea in elite athletics athletes: Prevalence and associations to athletics injury. *British Journal of Sports Medicine, 48*(7), 560–674.

Rutkowski, K., Sowa, P., Rutkowski-Talipska, J., Kuryliszyn-Moskal, A., & Rutkowski, R. (2014). Dehydroepiandrosterone (DHEA): Hypes and hopes. *Drugs, 74*(11), 1195–1207.

Santoro, N., & Sutton-Tyrrel, K. (2011). The SWAN song: Study of women's health across the nation. *Obstetric & Gynecologic Clinics of North America, 38*(3), 417–423.

Truman, J., Langton, L., & Planty, M. (2013). *Criminal victimization, 2012*. Retrieved from http://www.bjs.gov/content/pub/pdf/cv12.pdf

U.S. Food and Drug Administration (FDA). (2015). Ortho Evra (norelgestromin/ethinyl estradiol) information. Retrieved from http://www.fda.gov/drugs/drugsafety/postmarketdrugsafetyinformationforpatientsandproviders/ucm110402.htm

U.S. Food and Drug Administration (FDA). (2016). Mifeprex (mifepristone) Information. Retrieved from http://www.fda.gov/Drugs/DrugSafety/PostmarketDrugSafetyInformationforPatientsandProviders/ucm111323.htm

U.S. Preventive Services Task Force (USPSTF). (2012). Screening for cervical cancer. Retrieved from http://www.uspreventiveservicestaskforce.org/uspstf/uspscerv.htm

Walker, L. (1984). *The battered woman syndrome*. New York, NY: Springer.

World Health Organization. (WHO). (2013). Global and regional estimates of violence against women: Prevalence and health effects of intimate partner violence and non-partner sexual violence. Retrieved from http://apps.who.int/iris/bitstream/10665/85239/1/9789241564625_eng.pdf

Zieman, M., Hatcher, R. A., & Allen, A. Z. (2015). *Managing Contraception 2015–2016*. Tiger, GA: Bridging the Gap Foundation.

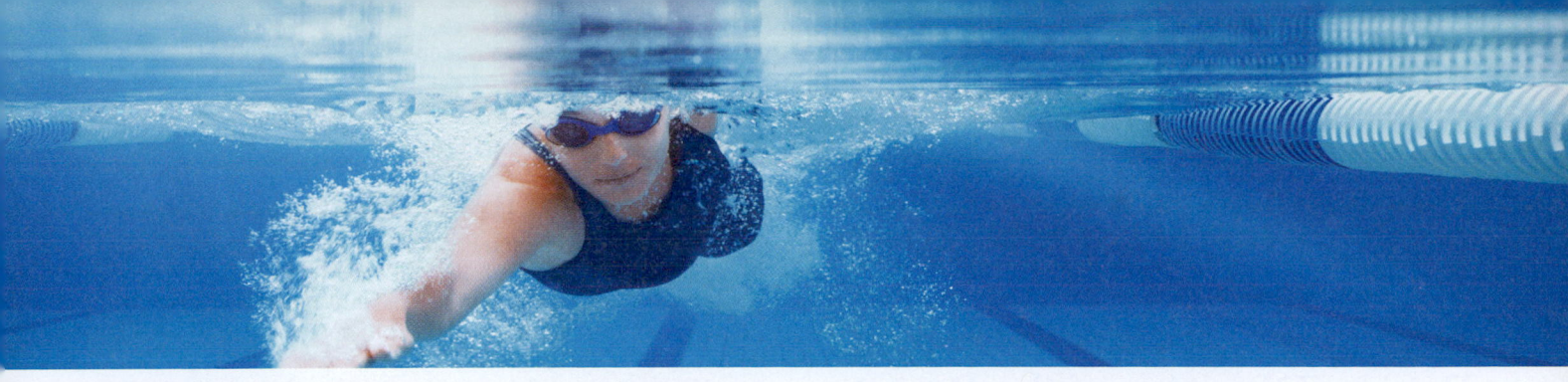

Chapter 6
Common Gynecologic Problems

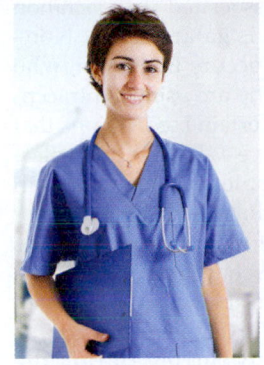

© Minerva Studio/Fotolia.

When I first started working here I was stunned by how little young women knew about sexually transmitted infections. They would come to the clinic devastated to have an infection or worried about AIDS without being aware of the long-term implications of infections such as herpes or genital warts. I decided that I had to do something to try to prevent infection, not just treat it, so now I am working with three of our local high schools offering classes on prevention. Judging from what several of the students have told me, I am making a difference. I'm proud of that.

—Nurse Working at a Sexually Transmitted Infection Clinic in a Major Urban Area

⌄ Learning Outcomes

6.1 Contrast the contributing factors, signs and symptoms, treatment options, and nursing care management of women with common benign breast disorders.

6.2 Explain the signs and symptoms, medical therapy, and implications for fertility of endometriosis.

6.3 Summarize the risk factors, treatment options, and nursing interventions for a woman with toxic shock syndrome.

6.4 Discuss the signs and symptoms, diagnosis criteria, treatment options, and health implications of polycystic ovarian syndrome (POS).

6.5 Compare the causes, signs and symptoms, treatment options, and nursing care for women with vulvovaginal candidiasis versus bacterial vaginosis.

6.6 Compare the common sexually transmitted infections with regard to their etiology, signs and symptoms, treatment options, nursing care, and methods of prevention.

6.7 Summarize the pathology, signs and symptoms, treatment, nursing care, and implications for future fertility of pelvic inflammatory disease (PID).

6.8 Identify the implications of an abnormal finding during a pelvic examination in the provision of nursing care.

6.9 Contrast the causes, signs and symptoms, treatment options, and nursing care for women with cystitis versus pyelonephritis.

6.10 Compare the signs and symptoms and treatment options of the three forms of pelvic relaxation—cystocele, rectocele, and uterine relaxation.

6.11 Contrast laparoscope-assisted vaginal hysterectomy and abdominal hysterectomy with regard to indications for use and the advantages and disadvantages of each procedure.

Throughout her lifetime, a woman is likely to face a variety of gynecologic or urinary tract problems. Some of these problems may be minor and easily treated, whereas others may be more serious. This chapter provides information about a variety of gynecologic conditions with an emphasis on problems commonly addressed in community-based settings.

Care of the Woman With a Benign Disorder of the Breast

This section discusses the most common benign breast disorders women encounter. For information on breast cancer, readers should refer to a medical–surgical nursing textbook.

Fibrocystic Breast Changes

Benign breast disease (BBD), commonly called **fibrocystic breast changes**, is the most common of the benign breast disorders. It is most prevalent in women 20 to 50 years of age. *Fibrosis* is a thickening of the normal breast tissue. Cyst formation that may accompany fibrosis is considered a later change in the condition. The exact etiology of fibrocystic breast changes is unclear. Generally fibrocystic changes are not a risk factor for breast cancer. In some rare cases, if the change is proliferative and results in hyperplasia or buildup of the cells of the breast ducts, atypia may occur.

The woman with fibrocystic breast changes often reports pain, tenderness, and swelling that occur cyclically and are most pronounced just before menses. Physical examination may reveal only mild signs of irregularity, or the breasts may feel dense, with areas of irregularity and nodularity. Women often refer to this irregularity as "lumpiness." Some women may also have expressible nipple discharge. Although unilateral discharge and serosanguineous discharge are the most worrisome findings, all significant nipple discharge should be investigated further.

If the woman has a large, fluid-filled cyst, she may experience a localized painful area as the capsule containing the accumulated fluid distends coincident with her cycle. If small cysts form, however, the woman may experience not a solitary tender lump but a diffuse tenderness. A cyst may often be differentiated from a malignancy because a cyst is more mobile (easily moved with palpation) and tender, whereas a cancer may be fixed (not movable) and may be associated with skin retraction (pulling) in the surrounding tissue.

Mammography, sonography, magnetic resonance imaging (MRI), palpation, and fine-needle aspiration may be used to confirm fibrocystic breast changes and rule out malignancy. Often, fine-needle aspiration is the treatment as well, affording relief from the tenderness or pain. Treatment of palpable cysts is conservative; invasive procedures such as biopsy are used only if the diagnosis is questionable.

Women with mild symptoms may benefit from restricting sodium intake and taking a mild diuretic during the week before the onset of menses. This counteracts fluid retention, relieves pressure in the breast, and helps decrease the pain. In other cases, a mild analgesic is necessary. In severe cases, the hormone inhibitor danazol is often helpful because it suppresses follicle-stimulating hormone (FSH) and luteinizing hormone (LH), resulting in anovulation. However, it can cause undesirable side effects, including masculinization. Women who do not respond to other treatment approaches may be given a trial of bromocriptine, a prolactin inhibitor.

Some researchers suggest that methylxanthines (found in caffeine products, such as coffee, tea, colas, and chocolate, and in some medications) may contribute to the development of fibrocystic breast changes and that limiting intake of these substances will help decrease fibrocystic changes.

Other Benign Breast Disorders

Fibroadenoma is a common benign tumor seen in women in their teens and early twenties. It has not been significantly associated with breast cancer. Fibroadenomas are freely movable, solid tumors that are well defined, sharply delineated, and rounded, with a rubbery texture.

Ultrasound is the best method for imaging women under age 30 with a palpable mass because of the density of their breast tissue. Most women can be observed and followed regularly to detect any changes in the size or appearance of the lump. Surgical removal may be recommended if any findings from the clinical breast examination, ultrasound, or biopsy are abnormal (Mayo Clinic, 2014).

The term for nipple discharge not associated with lactation (production of milk for breastfeeding) is **galactorrhea**. Non–clinically significant nipple discharge occurs in women who have fibrocystic changes in the breast, who are using contraceptives, or who are on hormone therapy. Certain medications that are used to treat psychiatric disorders have a side effect of galactorrhea. The most common types of nipple discharge occur in both breasts, are secreted from several ducts, and vary in color from white to brown. The likelihood of malignancy increases with the presence of a spontaneous discharge arising from a single duct in one breast that is watery or bloody in nature; all unexplained nipple discharge warrants further investigation.

Intraductal papillomas, most often occurring during the menopausal years, are tumors growing in the terminal portion of a duct or, sometimes, throughout the duct system within a section of the breast. Symptoms may include a unilateral mass or a spontaneous, and often bloody, nipple discharge.

The majority of papillomas are present as solitary nodules. These small, ball-like lesions may be detected on mammography but often are nonpalpable. The presence of a papilloma is often frightening to the woman, because her primary symptom is a discharge from the nipple that may be serosanguineous or brownish green because of old blood. The location of the papilloma within the duct system and its pattern of growth determine whether nipple discharge will be present. They are typically benign but are generally excised to rule out the possibility of cancer.

Duct ectasis (comedomastitis), an inflammation of the ducts behind the nipple, commonly occurs during or near the onset of menopause and is not associated with malignancy. The condition typically occurs in women who have borne and nursed children. It results because of an increase in maternal glandular secretions with the resulting production of an irritating lipid fluid that can produce nipple discharge. Duct ectasis is characterized by a thick, sticky nipple discharge and by burning pain, pruritus, and inflammation. Nipple retraction may also be noted, especially in postmenopausal women. Treatment is conservative, with drug therapy aimed at symptomatic relief. The major central ducts of the breast occasionally have to be excised.

Nursing Management

For the Woman With a Breast Disorder

Nursing Assessment and Diagnosis

During the period of diagnosis of any breast disorder, the woman may be anxious about a possible change in body image or a diagnosis of cancer. Use therapeutic communication to assess the significance the woman places on her breasts; her current emotional status, coping mechanisms used during periods of stress, and knowledge and beliefs about cancer; and other variables that may influence her coping and adjustment.

Nursing diagnoses that may apply to a woman with a benign disorder of the breast include the following (NANDA-I © 2014):

- *Knowledge, Readiness for Enhanced,* about diagnostic procedures for breast disorders related to an expressed desire for further information
- *Anxiety* related to threat to body image

Nursing Plan and Implementation

During the prediagnosis period clarify misconceptions and encourage the woman to express her anxiety. Once a diagnosis is made, ensure that the woman clearly understands her condition, its association to breast malignancy, and the treatment options.

Point out that frequent professional breast examinations and regular mammograms are tools that help detect any abnormalities. Although recommendations about the importance of monthly breast self-examination (BSE) have been modified (see Chapter 5), most professionals agree that women should be familiar with their own breasts so that they are able to note changes should they occur.

Evaluation

Expected outcomes of nursing care include the following:

- The woman is able to discuss her fears, concerns, and questions during the period of diagnosis.
- The diagnosis is made quickly and accurately, and treatment is initiated if indicated.

Care of the Woman With Endometriosis

Endometriosis, a condition characterized by the presence of endometrial tissue outside the uterine cavity, occurs in about 10% of reproductive-age women and about 50% of women with infertility (Coleman & Overton, 2015). Endometriosis

has been found almost everywhere in the body, including the vagina, lungs, cervix, central nervous system, and gastrointestinal tract. The most common location, however, is the pelvic cavity. Endometrial tissue bleeds cyclically in response to the hormonal changes of the menstrual cycle. The bleeding results in inflammation, scarring of the peritoneum, and formation of adhesions.

Endometriosis may occur at any age after puberty, although it is most common in women between ages 20 and 45. The exact cause is unknown. Proposed theories include retrograde menstrual flow, hereditary tendency, gene mutations, and a possible immunologic defect (American College of Obstetricians & Gynecologists [ACOG], 2014).

The most common symptom of endometriosis is pelvic pain, which is often dull or cramping. Because the pain is usually related to menstruation, the woman typically assumes it is dysmenorrhea. **Dyspareunia** (painful intercourse) and abnormal uterine bleeding are other common signs. The condition is often diagnosed when the woman seeks evaluation for infertility. Bimanual examination may reveal a fixed, tender, retroverted uterus and palpable nodules in the cul-de-sac. Diagnosis is confirmed by laparoscopy.

Endometriosis has no permanent cure. Treatment may be medical, surgical, or a combination of the two. In women with minimal disease and symptoms, treatment includes observation, analgesics, and nonsteroidal anti-inflammatory drugs (NSAIDs). See *Medications Used to Treat: Endometriosis* for a list of medications used to treat endometriosis.

The Mirena Intrauterine System (IUS) has also been used. It thickens cervical mucus and results in atrophy of the endometrium. Pain scores for pelvic pain and dysmenorrhea show significant improvement in many women. It has fewer side effects than oral progestins and lasts 5 years (Hogg & Vyas, 2015).

In more advanced cases, surgery may be done to remove endometrial implants and break up adhesions. If severe dyspareunia or dysmenorrhea are symptoms, the surgeon may perform a presacral neurectomy to relieve the pain. In advanced cases in which childbearing is not an issue, treatment may be a hysterectomy with bilateral salpingo-oophorectomy (removal of fallopian tubes and ovaries).

Medications Used To Treat: Endometriosis

- **Combined oral contraceptives (COCs)**, which suppress menstruation, can be used in women who do not desire fertility.
- **Progestins** such as medroxyprogesterone acetate (MPA) and Dienogest exert an antiendometriotic effect and ultimate atrophy. The medication is administered intramuscularly every 3 months; the effectiveness of the treatment is evaluated every 3 to 6 months. Side effects may include nausea, weight gain, fluid retention, and breakthrough bleeding.
- **Danazol** is a testosterone derivative that suppresses ovulation and causes amenorrhea. It is intended for short-term therapy. Because of adverse effects on lipid metabolism and significant side effects such as weight gain, hirsutism, acne, oily skin, vaginal dryness, hot flushes, reduced libido, voice changes, clitoral enlargement, and decreased breast size, many clinicians have moved away from danazol to other treatment options.
- **Gonadotropin-releasing hormone (GnRH) analogs** such as *nafarelin acetate* (given as a metered nasal spray twice daily) and *leuprolide acetate* (Lupron, given once a month as an intramuscular injection), are gaining popularity because many women tolerate them better than danazol and their results in treating endometriosis are comparable. GnRH analogs suppress the menstrual cycle through estrogen antagonism. This may result in the hypoestrogen side effects of hot flashes, vaginal dryness, headache, breast reduction, and loss of bone density. Consequently, the use of GnRH agonists should be limited to 6 months (Hogg & Vyas, 2015).

Clinical Question

What interventions are effective for relief of pain among women diagnosed with endometriosis? What treatment options for subfertility are available and effective for these women?

The Evidence

Women with diagnosed endometriosis often experience pain and difficulty becoming pregnant. A team of Cochrane reviewers summarized the evidence from 17 published systematic reviews of the effectiveness of interventions for both conditions. Systematic reviews, particularly those published in the scientifically rigorous Cochrane Reviews, form the highest quality of evidence, and this meta-synthesis of these reviews is the strongest available evidence.

Suppression of menstrual cycles with gonadotrophin-releasing hormone (GnRH), a levonorgestrel-releasing intrauterine device (LNG-IUD), and danazol were all beneficial interventions. Laparoscope treatment and excision of endometriomata were also effective in relieving pain. Non-steroidal anti-inflammatory medications did not provide conclusive relief, and there was no evidence of benefit from long-term hormonal treatment after surgery (Brown, 2014). None of the alternative medical treatments (acupuncture, herbal medicines, vitamins) were effective in pain relief.

Treatment with GnRH-agonists for 3 months improved pregnancy rates, but no other medical treatments were found to be effective. Excisional surgery and laparoscopic removal of excess tissue resulted in improved spontaneous pregnancy rates 9 to 12 months after surgery. Ablative surgery was not effective in improving pregnancy rates and neither were diagnostic laparoscopic procedures. None of the alternative medical treatments had any effect on pregnancy rates in these women.

Best Practice

Medical and surgical treatments can be effective in reducing the pain associated with endometriosis and can enhance fertility within 9 to 12 months. Women can be counseled that fertility after surgical removal of endometriomata is possible. Medical treatment after surgery is not helpful and is unnecessary. Over-the-counter and alternative treatments are not effective; effective medical treatment is focused on the suppression of menstrual cycles through hormonal treatments.

Clinical Reasoning

Why does menstrual suppression affect the pain of endometriosis? Why would surgical removal improve fertility among these women?

Nursing Management

For the Woman With Endometriosis

Nursing Assessment and Diagnosis

Be aware of the common symptoms of endometriosis and elicit an accurate history if a woman mentions these symptoms. If a woman is being treated for endometriosis, assess the woman's understanding of the condition, its implications, and the treatment alternatives.

Nursing diagnoses that may apply to a woman with endometriosis include the following (NANDA-I © 2014):

- *Pain, Acute,* related to peritoneal irritation secondary to endometriosis
- *Coping: Family, Compromised,* related to depression secondary to infertility

Nursing Plan and Implementation

Be available to explain the condition, its symptoms, treatment alternatives, and prognosis. Help the woman evaluate treatment options and make appropriate choices. If the woman begins taking medication, review the dosage, schedule, possible side effects, and any warning signs. A woman with endometriosis is often advised not to delay pregnancy because of the increased risk of infertility that women with endometriosis face. The woman may wish to discuss the implications of this decision on her life choices, relationship with her partner, and personal preferences. Act as a nonjudgmental listener and help the woman consider her options.

Evaluation

Expected outcomes of nursing care include the following:

- The woman is able to discuss her condition, its implications for fertility, and her treatment options.
- After considering the alternatives, the woman chooses appropriate treatment options.

Care of the Woman With Polycystic Ovarian Syndrome

Polycystic ovarian syndrome (PCOS) is a complex endocrine disorder of ovarian dysfunction that is evidenced by menstrual dysfunction, signs of androgen excess (typically hirsutism, acne), and infertility.

The most common clinical signs and symptoms of PCOS include:

- *Menstrual dysfunction.* Irregular menses, ranging from total absence of periods (amenorrhea) to intermittent or infrequent periods (oligomenorrhea) are the hallmarks of PCOS. Anovulation is usually a chronic problem with PCOS and may present as a history of menstrual irregularities.
- *Hyperandrogenism.* Women with PCOS consistently have elevated serum androgen levels. These elevated androgen levels often lead to clinical manifestations such as hirsutism (excessive hair growth), acne, deepening voice, and increased muscle mass.

- *Obesity.* Between 30% and 75% of women who have PCOS are clinically obese (Gateva & Kamenov, 2012). The obesity is generally of the android type, with an increased hip-to-waist ratio.

- *Hyperinsulinemia.* Women with PCOS may be insulin resistant. This insulin resistance, characterized by the failure of insulin to enter the cells appropriately, places these women at increased risk for impaired glucose tolerance and type 2 diabetes mellitus (ACOG, 2014).

- *Infertility.* The majority of women who have been diagnosed with PCOS struggle with some degree of infertility related to anovulation (see Chapter 7).

Clinical Therapy

If a woman presents with complaints of hirsutism, menstrual irregularities, acne, difficulty conceiving, and unexplained weight gain, several other disorders must be ruled out. Important disorders to consider include thyroid disease, congenital adrenal hyperplasia, Cushing syndrome, hyperprolactinemia, primary ovarian failure, and androgen-producing tumors (ACOG, 2014). The diagnostic process is fourfold: history, physical examination, laboratory studies, and imaging.

Once PCOS is diagnosed, the goals for treatment include:

- Decrease the effects of hyperandrogenism (hirsutism, acne, etc.)

- Restore reproductive functioning for women desiring pregnancy

- Protect the endometrium (increased risk for uterine cancer)

- Reduce long-term risks, specifically type 2 diabetes and cardiovascular disease.

If pregnancy is not an immediate goal, menstrual irregularities can be treated with a combined oral contraceptive (COC) or cyclic progesterone. COCs help to regulate menstrual cycles; provide a balance between estrogen and progesterone, thereby protecting the endometrium and decreasing the risk of uterine cancer; and may improve acne by inhibiting ovarian androgen production.

Antiandrogens such as spironolactone (Aldactone) may be used to decrease symptoms of androgen excess. Metformin (Glucophage) inhibits glucose production in the liver and improves glucose uptake by fat and muscle cells. It improves ovarian function, reduces the degree of hyperandrogenism, restores normal ovulation in women with PCOS, and is associated with an improved ability to lose weight. In addition, lifestyle changes should also be a major component in the treatment of PCOS. Modifications should include weight loss, regular exercise, balanced diet, and smoking cessation.

If initial approaches to helping a woman with PCOS become pregnant fail, assisted reproductive technology (ART) may be recommended using in vitro fertilization, intrauterine insemination, or intracytoplasmic sperm injection. This may be combined with gonadotropin therapy (McFarland, 2012).

Long-term, PCOS may increase a woman's risk for developing type 2 diabetes, hypertension, cardiovascular disease, endometrial cancer, breast cancer, and ovarian cancer. Additionally, the woman with PCOS may struggle with significant emotional responses to this chronic disorder. She likely will face issues related to body image, infertility, problematic menses, and depression.

Nursing Care Management

You can play a vital role in the identification of PCOS and its evaluation, management, and follow-up. The signs of PCOS, especially hirsutism, negatively impact women's feelings of femininity, and they may feel physically inferior and lack self-confidence. You can help women recognize these feelings and find ways to develop a more positive body image. You also have an important role in providing accurate information, education, and counseling for a woman diagnosed with PCOS. Finally, because the woman with PCOS is at risk for developing long-term complications, you and subsequent nurses can play a key role in follow-up and continuity of care throughout the life of a woman facing this challenging disorder.

Care of the Woman With Toxic Shock Syndrome

Toxic shock syndrome (TSS) is primarily a disease of women often occurring at or near menses or during the postpartum period. The causative organism is a toxin released by a strain of *Staphylococcus aureus*. The use of superabsorbent tampons has been widely related to the incidence of TSS. However, occluding the cervical os with a contraceptive device such as a diaphragm or cervical cap during menses may also increase the risk of TSS.

Early diagnosis and treatment are important in preventing death. For a diagnosis of TSS to be made, certain criteria must be met, including:

- Fever (often greater than 38.9°C [102°F])

- Hypotension (systolic BP less than 90 mm Hg)

- Rash

- Multisystem involvement

The fever and rash on the trunk present initially followed by desquamation of the skin, especially the palms and soles, which usually occurs 1 to 2 weeks after the onset of symptoms; hypotension; and dizziness. Systemic symptoms often include vomiting, diarrhea, severe myalgia, and inflamed mucous membranes (oropharyngeal, conjunctival, or vaginal). Disorders of the central nervous system, including alterations in consciousness, disorientation, and coma, may also occur. Laboratory findings reveal elevated blood urea nitrogen (BUN), creatinine, aspartate aminotransferase (AST), alanine aminotransferase (ALT), and total bilirubin levels, whereas platelets are often less than $100,000/mm^3$.

Women with TSS are generally hospitalized and given supportive therapy, including oxygen, intravenous fluids to maintain blood pressure, and antibiotics. Severe cases may require renal dialysis, administration of vasopressors, and intubation.

Nursing Care Management

You can play a major role in helping educate women about ways to prevent the development of TSS. Women should understand the importance of avoiding prolonged use of tampons. Women who choose to continue using tampons may reduce their risk of TSS by alternating them with napkins and avoiding overnight use of tampons.

SAFETY ALERT!
Warn women about the danger of using a diaphragm or cervical cap to trap menstrual flow for prolonged periods because of the increased risk of TSS.

Women should avoid the use of tampons for 6 to 8 weeks after childbirth. Women with a history of TSS should never use tampons. Women who use diaphragms or cervical caps should not use them during the postpartum period. Help make women aware of the signs and symptoms of TSS so that they will seek treatment promptly if symptoms occur.

Care of the Woman With a Vaginal Infection

Vaginitis is the most common reason women seek gynecologic care. Symptoms of vaginitis or vulvovaginitis may include increased vaginal discharge, vulvar irritation, pruritus, foul odor, dyspareunia (painful sexual intercourse), bleeding with intercourse, and pain when urine touches irritated vulvar tissue. It may be caused directly by an infection or it may result from an alteration of normal flora, as in the case of bacterial vaginosis or *Candida albicans*.

Bacterial Vaginosis

Bacterial vaginosis (BV) is more prevalent among sexually active women, but it is not considered a sexually transmitted infection because it has also been detected in virginal women. BV is an alteration of normal vaginal bacterial flora that results in the loss of hydrogen peroxide–producing lactobacilli, which are normally the main vaginal flora. With the loss of this natural defense, bacteria such as *Gardnerella vaginalis*, mycoplasmas, and anaerobes overgrow in large numbers, causing vaginitis. The cause of this overgrowth is not clear, although trauma from douching, frequent sexual intercourse without condom use, and an upset in normal vaginal flora are predisposing factors. BV during pregnancy may be a factor in premature rupture of the membranes and preterm birth.

The infected woman often notices an excessive amount of thin, watery, white or gray vaginal discharge with a foul odor described as "fishy." The characteristic "clue" cell is seen on a wet-mount preparation (Figure 6–1). The addition of 10% potassium hydroxide (KOH) solution to the vaginal secretions, called a "whiff" test, releases a strong, fishy odor. The vaginal pH is usually greater than 4.5.

The symptomatic woman, whether nonpregnant or pregnant, is generally treated with metronidazole (Flagyl) orally or as a vaginal cream. Alternately, tinidazole orally or clindamycin (Cleocin) orally or as vaginal cream may be used (Centers for Disease Control and Prevention [CDC], 2015). Women should either avoid intercourse or use condoms during the treatment period.

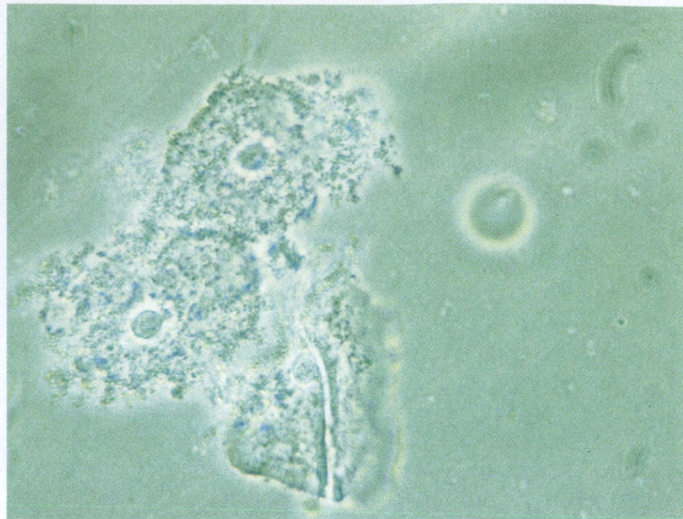

Figure 6–1 The characteristic "clue cells" seen in bacterial vaginosis. Unlike normal epithelial cells, which appear translucent and have a clear border, clue cells are desquamated epithelial cells with bacteria adhering to them. The presence of the bacteria makes the cell appear to be speckled with black dots. The borders are also obscured because of the bacteria.

SOURCE: Centers for Disease Control and Prevention.

Metronidazole is an antimicrobial working in an anaerobic environment. It is an antiprotozoal and antibacterial agent. See *Medications Used to Treat: Bacterial Vaginosis* for a comparison of medication regimens for treating BV.

SAFETY ALERT!
Alcohol should be avoided when taking either metronidazole or tinidazole. When combined with alcohol, both metronidazole and tinidazole can produce effects similar to that of alcohol and disulfiram (Antabuse)—abdominal pain, flushing, and tremors.

Vulvovaginal Candidiasis

Vulvovaginal candidiasis (VVC), also called moniliasis or yeast infection, is one of the most common forms of vaginitis that women experience. Estimates suggest that, in their lifetime, 75% of women will have at least one episode of VVC (CDC, 2015). Recurrences are frequent for some women. *Candida albicans* is

---

Medications Used To Treat: Bacterial Vaginosis

NONPREGNANT AND SYMPTOMATIC PREGNANT WOMEN

- Metronidazole (Flagyl): 500 mg orally twice a day for 7 days
  OR
- Metronidazole gel (0.75%): One full applicator intravaginally, once daily for 5 days
  OR
- Clindamycin (Cleocin) 2% vaginal cream: One full applicator at bedtime for 7 days
- Alternative regimens: Tinidazole or clindamycin

Source: Data from Centers for Disease Control and Prevention (CDC). (2015). Sexually transmitted disease treatment guidelines, 2015. Retrieved from http://www.cdc.gov/mmwr/preview/mmwrhtml/rr6403a1.htm

the fungal species responsible for most vaginal yeast infections. Factors that contribute to the occurrence of this infection are the use of oral contraceptives, immunosuppressants, and antibiotics, which destroy populations of normal bacteria that usually keep the yeast cells in check. Other factors are frequent douching, pregnancy, and diabetes mellitus.

The woman with VVC often complains of thick, curdy vaginal discharge, severe itching, dysuria, and dyspareunia. A male sexual partner may experience a rash or excoriation of the skin of the penis and possibly pruritus. The male may be symptomatic and the female asymptomatic.

On physical examination, the woman's labia may be swollen and excoriated if pruritus has been severe. A speculum examination reveals thick, white, tenacious cheeselike patches adhering to the vaginal mucosa. Diagnosis is confirmed by microscopic examination of the vaginal discharge; hyphae and spores are usually seen on a wet-mount preparation (Figure 6–2). Other diagnostic tests include DNA probe and culture, although cultures are not used for routine diagnosis. The pH of the vagina remains 4.0 to 4.5 or less (the normal pH of the vagina is about 3.8 to 4.2). This vaginal pH level is in contrast to the pH noted with BV or *Trichomonas*.

Medical treatment of VVC includes intravaginal clotrimazole or miconazole cream or suppositories or tioconazole intravaginal ointment, which are available over the counter (OTC). Butoconazole cream, terconazole cream or suppositories, and fluconazole in a single oral dose are available by prescription (CDC, 2015). Single-dose and short-course (3 days) approaches are effective for 80% to 90% of women with uncomplicated VVC. Women who continue to have symptoms after using an OTC preparation and women who have a recurrence of symptoms within 2 months should be evaluated during an office visit because inappropriate use of OTC preparations can lead to a delay in treatment (CDC, 2015).

Treatment of the male partner is generally not necessary unless candidal balanitis (inflammation of the glans penis) is present. Then treatment with a topical antifungal medication is indicated (CDC, 2015).

If a woman experiences recurrent VVC (four or more symptomatic episodes in a year), she should be tested for an elevated blood glucose level to determine whether a diabetic or prediabetic condition is present. Women at high risk for sexually transmitted infections should also be tested for HIV. Recurrent infection is then treated with an intensive regimen of oral and local agents for 7 to 14 days followed by maintenance antifungal

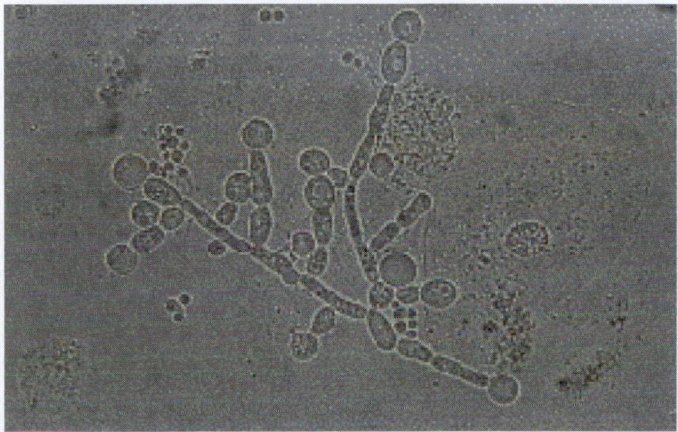

Figure 6–2 Hyphae and spores of *Candida albicans*, the fungus responsible for vulvovaginal candidiasis.

SOURCE: Centers for Disease Control and Prevention.

therapy. Pregnant women with VVC are treated only with topical azole preparations applied for 7 days (CDC, 2014). Infection at the time of birth may cause thrush (a mouth infection) in the newborn.

Nursing Management

For the Woman With Vulvovaginal Candidiasis

Nursing Assessment and Diagnosis

Suspect VVC if a woman complains of intense vulvar itching and a curdy, white discharge. Because pregnant women with diabetes mellitus are especially susceptible to this infection, be alert for symptoms in these women. In some areas nurses are trained to do speculum examinations and wet-mount preparations and can confirm the diagnosis themselves. In most cases, however, if you suspect a vaginal infection, report it to the woman's healthcare provider.

Nursing diagnoses that might apply to the woman with VVC include the following (NANDA-I © 2014):

- *Skin Integrity, Impaired,* related to scratching secondary to discomfort of the infection
- *Knowledge, Readiness for Enhanced,* about yeast infection related to an expressed desire to learn about ways of preventing the development of VVC

Nursing Plan and Implementation

If the woman is experiencing discomfort because of pruritus, recommend gentle bathing of the vulva with a weak sodium bicarbonate solution. If a topical treatment is being used, the woman will need to bathe the area before applying the medication.

Discuss with the woman the factors that contribute to the development of VVC and suggest ways to prevent recurrences, such as wearing cotton underwear and avoiding vaginal powders or sprays that may irritate the vulva. Some women report that the addition of yogurt to the diet or the use of activated culture of plain yogurt as a vaginal douche helps prevent recurrence by maintaining high levels of lactobacilli. For the same reason, some clinicians recommend that women who are taking antibiotics consume yogurt or probiotic supplements (containing acidophilus and other helpful bacteria) simultaneously.

Evaluation

Expected outcomes of nursing care include the following:

- The woman's symptoms are relieved and the infection is cured.
- The woman is able to identify self-care measures to prevent further episodes of VVC.

Care of the Woman with a Sexually Transmitted Infection

The occurrence of **sexually transmitted infection (STI)**, or *sexually transmitted disease (STD)*, has increased during the past few decades. In fact, vaginitis and STIs are the most common reasons for outpatient, community-based treatment of women.

KEY FACTS TO REMEMBER
Vaginitis

To distinguish among the common types of vaginitis and their treatments, it is useful to remember the following:

Vulvovaginal Candidiasis (Moniliasis)

Cause: *Candida albicans*

Appearance of discharge: Thick, curdy, like cottage cheese

Diagnostic test: Slide of vaginal discharge (treated with potassium hydroxide [KOH]) shows characteristic hyphae and spores

Treatment: Azole vaginal cream or suppositories

Bacterial Vaginosis (*Gardnerella Vaginalis* Vaginitis)

Cause: *Gardnerella vaginalis*

Appearance of discharge: Gray, milky

Diagnostic test: Slide of vaginal discharge shows characteristic "clue" cells

Treatment: Metronidazole or clindamycin

Trichomoniasis

Cause: *Trichomonas vaginalis*

Appearance of discharge: Greenish white and frothy

Diagnostic test: Saline slide of vaginal discharge shows motile flagellated organisms, OSOM Trichomoniasis Rapid Test, or Affirm VP III test

Treatment: Metronidazole or tinidazole

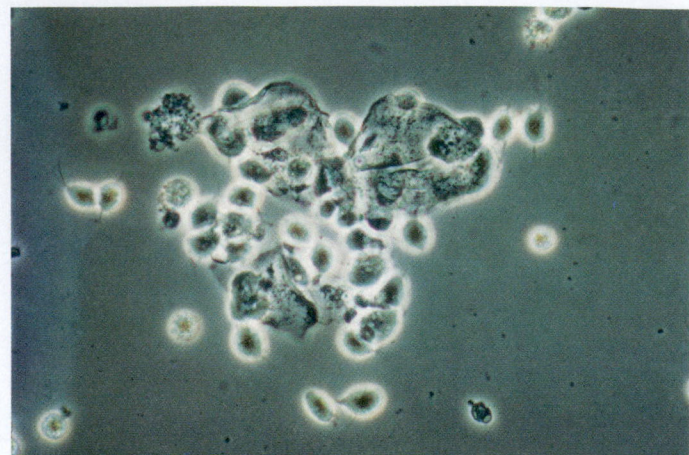

Figure 6–3 Microscopic appearance of *Trichomonas vaginalis*.

SOURCE: Centers for Disease Control and Prevention.

Developing Cultural Competence Racial Disparity in STIs

Racial disparities exist in all STIs, with the highest rates found among African Americans. In 2012, African Americans accounted for 63% of reported gonorrhea cases with known race/ethnicity and almost 40% (39.7%) of the cases of syphilis (CDC, 2014). Though less marked, disparities also exist among Hispanics. These disparities may result, in part, because people from minority populations are more likely to seek care in public health clinics, which report STIs more accurately than private providers do. However, socioeconomic barriers to high-quality health care and to STI prevention and treatment play a role. It is essential that these barriers be addressed if such disparities are to be eliminated.

Trichomoniasis

Trichomoniasis, the most prevalent nonviral STI in the United States, is an infection caused by *Trichomonas vaginalis*, a microscopic motile protozoan that thrives in an alkaline environment. Almost all infections are acquired through sexual intimacy. Transmission by shared bath facilities, wet towels, or wet swimsuits—though possible—is unlikely. Pregnant women with trichomoniasis may be at increased risk for premature

rupture of the membranes, preterm birth, and a low-birth-weight newborn.

Symptoms of trichomoniasis include a yellow-green, frothy, odorous discharge frequently accompanied by inflammation of the vagina and cervix, vulvar itching, dysuria, and dyspareunia. Vaginal pH is 5.0 or higher.

Microscopic visualization of mobile trichomonads and increased leukocytes (Figure 6–3) is commonly used to detect trichomoniasis because it is convenient and relatively inexpensive. However, its sensitivity is low. Thus the use of highly sensitive, specific tests performed on vaginal secretions such as the OSOM Trichomonas Rapid Test (results available in 10 minutes) and the Affirm VP III (results available in 45 minutes) is recommended. Other FDA-approved tests include the APTIMA *T. vaginalis* assay and the BD Probe Tec TV Q amplified DNA assay (CDC, 2015).

Recommended treatment for trichomoniasis is metronidazole (Flagyl) administered in a single 2-g dose or tinidazole in a single 2-g oral dose or, alternatively, metronidazole 500 mg twice daily for 7 days for both male and female sexual partners. Tinidazole has fewer gastrointestinal side effects but is more costly (CDC, 2015). Partners should avoid intercourse until both are cured (therapy is completed and both are symptom free). Symptomatic pregnant women can be considered for treatment with a single 2-gm dose of metronidazole to relieve symptoms of vaginal discharge and decrease risk of transmission to sexual partners (CDC, 2015).

Clinical Reasoning Sexually Transmitted Infections

Ella Matlosz is a 21-year-old, single woman, never pregnant, who comes to the office complaining of excessive, odorous vaginal discharge. She uses an intrauterine device (IUD) for contraception and has several sex partners. She states that she douches with a medicated douche after intercourse.

What should you tell Ella about feminine hygiene? What would you tell Ella about the relationship between contraceptives and sexually transmitted infections?

Chlamydial Infection

Chlamydial infection, caused by *Chlamydia trachomatis*, is the most commonly reported infectious disease in the United States and is most prevalent in people under age 25 (CDC, 2015). Transmission commonly occurs through vaginal sex. A strain of chlamydia is responsible for trachoma, the world's leading cause of preventable blindness.

Healthy People 2020

(STD-2) Reduce chlamydia rates among females aged 15 to 44 years

---

Chlamydia is a major cause of nongonococcal urethritis (NGU) in men. In women it can cause infections similar to those that occur with gonorrhea. Pelvic inflammatory disease, infertility, and ectopic pregnancy are associated with chlamydia. In addition, chlamydia infection is associated with an increased risk of acquiring and transmitting HIV infection. The newborn of a woman with untreated chlamydia is at risk of developing ophthalmia neonatorum (neonatal conjunctivitis), which responds to erythromycin ophthalmic ointment but not to silver nitrate eye prophylaxis at birth. The newborn may also develop chlamydia pneumonia.

In females, signs of chlamydia include a thin or purulent discharge, burning and frequency of urination, a friable cervix (bleeds easily), and lower abdominal pain. Women, however, are often asymptomatic. Diagnosis frequently is made after treatment of a male partner for NGU or in a symptomatic woman with a negative gonorrhea culture. Nucleic acid amplification testing (NAAT) is the recommended test for detecting *C. trachomatis* infection (CDC, 2015). The recommended treatment is a single 1-g dose of azithromycin orally or doxycycline 100 mg orally twice daily for 7 days. Sexual partners should be treated, and couples should abstain from intercourse for 7 days (CDC, 2015). Doxycycline is contraindicated in pregnancy. The CDC (2015) recommends that pregnant women be treated with azithromycin or amoxicillin and that a test of cure be done 3 to 4 weeks after therapy is completed.

Because so many people with chlamydia are asymptomatic, screening of the following groups is recommended as a primary method of decreasing the incidence (CDC, 2015):

- Annual screening for sexually active adolescent females and women under age 25
- Annual screening for women over age 25 who are at risk for chlamydia (history of STIs, multiple sexual partners, new sexual partner, inconsistent use of barrier contraceptives)
- Screening of all pregnant women under age 25 and older women at risk for chlamydia at their first prenatal visit and again during the third trimester of pregnancy. (Note: Many practitioners routinely screen all pregnant women.)

Gonorrhea

Gonorrhea is an infection caused by the bacterium *Neisseria gonorrhoeae*. If a nonpregnant woman contracts the disease, she is at risk of developing pelvic inflammatory disease (PID). If a woman becomes infected after the third month of pregnancy, the mucous plug in the cervix will prevent the infection from ascending, and it will remain localized in the urethra, cervix, and Bartholin glands until the membranes rupture. Then it can spread upward. A newborn exposed to a gonococci-infected birth canal is at risk of developing neonatal conjunctivitis. Eye prophylaxis, generally with erythromycin, is indicated for all newborns to prevent this complication.

Because the majority of women with gonorrhea are asymptomatic, it is accepted practice to screen for this infection by doing a cervical culture during the initial prenatal examination. For women at high risk, the culture may be repeated during the last month of pregnancy. Cultures of the urethra, throat, and rectum may also be required for diagnosis, depending on the body orifices used for intercourse.

The most common symptoms of gonorrheal infection include a purulent, greenish yellow vaginal discharge, dysuria, and urinary frequency. Some women also develop inflammation and swelling of the vulva. The cervix may appear swollen and eroded and may secrete a foul-smelling discharge in which gonococci are present. Diagnosis is confirmed by culture of swab specimens or NAAT.

The preferred treatment for both nonpregnant and pregnant women consists of antibiotic therapy with a single dose of ceftriaxone 250 mg intramuscularly plus a single 1-g dose of azithromycin orally. This dual treatment is used to address the risk of coinfection with chlamydia because gonorrhea and chlamydia often occur together (CDC, 2015). All sexual partners must also be treated or the woman may become reinfected.

Healthy People 2020

(STD-6-1) Reduce gonorrhea rates among females aged 15 to 44 years

---

A test of cure is not needed if the recommended treatment is followed unless symptoms persist. However, retesting 3 months after treatment is recommended because of the risk of reinfection (CDC, 2015).

Herpes Genitalis

Herpes infections are caused by the herpes simplex virus (HSV). Two types of herpes infections can occur: HSV-1 (the cold sore), which can cause genital herpes through oral–genital contact, and HSV-2, which is usually associated with genital infections. The clinical symptoms and treatment of both types are the same. At least 50 million people in the United States have been diagnosed with genital HSV-2 infection—**herpes genitalis**. Even so, many people infected with genital herpes have not been diagnosed because they have mild or unrecognized infections but shed the virus intermittently (CDC, 2015).

The primary episode of herpes genitalis is characterized by the development of single or multiple blisterlike vesicles, which usually occur in the genital area and sometimes affect the vaginal walls, cervix, urethra, and anus. The vesicles may appear within a few hours to 20 days after exposure and rupture spontaneously to form very painful, open, ulcerated lesions. Inflammation and pain secondary to the presence of herpes lesions can cause difficult urination and urinary retention. Inguinal lymph node enlargement may be present. Flulike symptoms and genital pruritus or tingling also may be noticed. Primary episodes usually last the longest and are the most severe. Lesions heal spontaneously in 2 to 4 weeks.

After the lesions heal, the virus enters a dormant phase, residing in the nerve ganglia of the affected area. Some individuals never have a recurrence, whereas others have regular recurrences. Such recurrences are usually less severe than the initial episode and seem to be triggered by emotional stress, menstruation, ovulation, pregnancy, frequent or vigorous intercourse, poor health status or a generally run-down physical condition, tight clothing, or overheating. Diagnosis is made on the basis of the clinical appearance of the lesions, culture of the lesions, polymerase chain reaction (PCR) assays for HSV DNA, and HSV-specific glycoprotein G2 and glycoprotein G1 assays (CDC, 2015).

No known cure for herpes exists. Medications are available to provide relief from pain and prevent complications from secondary infection. The recommended treatment of the first clinical episode of genital herpes is oral acyclovir, valacyclovir, or famciclovir. These same medications, in somewhat different dosages, are also recommended for recurrent herpes infection and for daily suppression therapy for people who have frequent recurrences. Acyclovir or valacyclovir can be administered orally to pregnant women with the first-episode genital herpes or severe recurrent herpes. Its use in the third trimester may reduce the frequency of cesarean births by decreasing the incidence of recurrences at term (CDC, 2015).

Sometimes 2% lidocaine (Xylocaine) is used to decrease intense pain at the site of the lesions. Keeping the genital area clean and dry, wearing loose clothing, and wearing cotton underwear or none at all will promote healing. Primary and recurrent lesions will heal without prescriptive therapies.

If herpes is present in the genital tract of a woman during childbirth, it can have a devastating, even fatal, effect on the newborn. Women with herpetic lesions when labor begins should give birth by cesarean to prevent neonatal herpes.

Syphilis

Syphilis, which is acquired through vaginal, oral, or anal sex, is a chronic infection caused by the spirochete *Treponema pallidum*. Syphilis can be acquired congenitally through transplacental inoculation and can result from maternal exposure to infected exudate during sexual contact or from contact with open wounds or infected blood. The incubation period varies from 10 to 90 days, and even though no symptoms or lesions are noted during this time, the woman's blood contains spirochetes and is infectious.

Syphilis is divided into early and late stages. During the early stage (primary), a chancre appears at the site where the *T. pallidum* organism entered the body. Symptoms include slight fever, weight loss, and malaise. The chancre persists for about 4 weeks and then disappears. In 6 weeks to 6 months, secondary symptoms appear. Skin eruptions called condylomata lata, which resemble wartlike plaques and are highly infectious, may appear on the vulva. Other secondary symptoms are a rash on the palms of the hands and soles of the feet, acute arthritis, enlargement of the liver and spleen, nontender enlarged lymph nodes, iritis, and a chronic sore throat with hoarseness. When infected in utero, the newborn exhibits secondary-stage symptoms of syphilis. Transplacentally transmitted syphilis may cause intrauterine growth restriction, preterm birth, and stillbirth.

As a result of the disease's impact on the fetus in utero, serologic testing of every pregnant woman is recommended; some state laws require it. Testing is done at the initial prenatal screening and may be repeated in the third trimester. Blood studies in early pregnancy may be negative if the woman has only recently contracted the infection. Diagnosis is made by dark-field examination for spirochetes. Blood tests such as the Venereal Disease Research Laboratory (VDRL) test, rapid plasma reagin (RPR) test, or the more specific fluorescent treponemal antibody-absorption (FTA-ABS) test are commonly done.

For pregnant and nonpregnant women with syphilis of less than a year's duration (early latent syphilis), the CDC (2015) recommends 2.4 million units of benzathine penicillin G administered intramuscularly in a single dose. If syphilis is of long (more than a year) or unknown duration, 2.4 million units of benzathine penicillin G is given intramuscularly once a week for 3 weeks. If a woman is allergic to penicillin and nonpregnant, doxycycline or tetracycline can be given. The pregnant woman who is allergic to penicillin should be desensitized to it and then treated with it (CDC, 2015). Maternal serologic testing may remain positive for 8 months, and the newborn may have a positive test for 3 months.

Human Papillomavirus/Condylomata Acuminata

Condylomata acuminata, also called genital or *venereal warts*, is a common sexually transmitted condition caused by the human papillomavirus (HPV). Transmission can occur through vaginal, oral, or anal sex. The infection has received considerable attention because HPV is almost always the cause of cervical cancer.

Over 100 HPV subtypes have been identified. Of these about 40 can infect the genital tract. HPV types 6 and 11 account for most of the visible genital warts whereas high-risk HPV types such as 16 and 18 cause most incidences of cervical cancer (CDC, 2015).

Often a woman seeks medical care after noticing single or multiple soft, grayish pink, cauliflowerlike lesions in her genital area (Figure 6–4). The moist, warm environment of the genital area is conducive to the growth of the warts, which may be present on the vulva, vagina, cervix, and anus. The incubation period following exposure is 3 weeks to 3 years, with the average being about 3 months.

Because condylomata sometimes resemble other lesions and malignant transformation is possible, all atypical, pigmented, and persistent warts should be biopsied and treatment

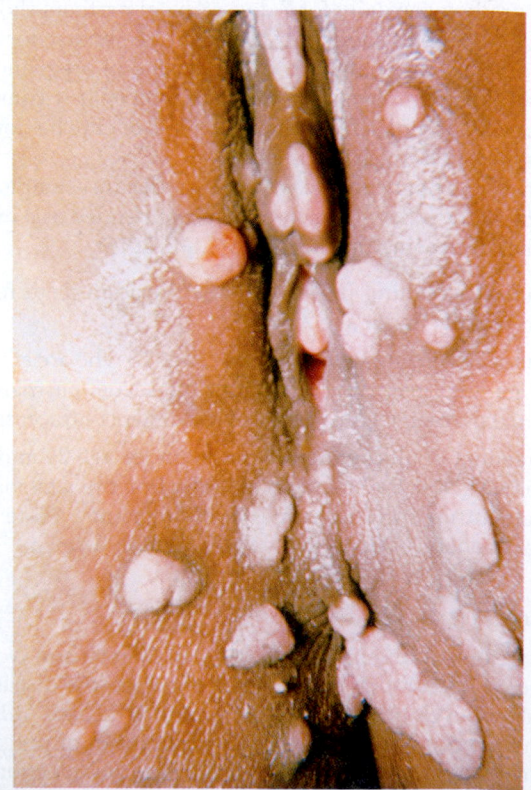

Figure 6–4 Condylomata acuminata on the vulva.
SOURCE: Centers for Disease Control and Prevention.

should be instituted promptly. The CDC (2015) does not specify a treatment of choice for genital warts but recommends that treatment be determined based on client preference, available resources, and experience of the healthcare provider. Provider-administered therapies include cryotherapy with liquid nitrogen or cryoprobe; trichloroacetic acid (TCA); bichloroacetic acid (BCA); surgical removal by tangential scissor excision, shave excision, curettage, or electrocautery; or laser surgery (CDC, 2015). Client-applied therapies include imiquimod cream, podofilox solution or gel, or sinecatechin ointment. These preparations are not used during pregnancy (CDC, 2015).

SAFETY ALERT!

If a client-applied therapy is prescribed, the client must understand exactly how to apply the medication and must be able to identify and reach all warts. These regimens have specific directions for application, frequency, and length of use, which the nurse should review carefully. Both imiquimod and sinecatechin ointment must be washed off after specified time periods.

Three HPV vaccines are now available against herpes simplex virus (HSV) types 16 and 18, which cause 66% of cervical cancers. Gardasil, the first vaccine to receive Food and Drug Administration (FDA) approval, is a quadrivalent vaccine and also provides protection against types 6 and 11, which cause 90% of genital warts. Cervarix is bivalent, and offers protection against only HSV types 16 and 18. Either vaccine is recommended for girls ages 11 to 12 (preferably before they are sexually active) and for 13- to 26-year-old females who did not receive or complete the 3-dose vaccine series. A 9-valent vaccine is also available. The CDC (2015) now recommends that either the quadrivalent or the 9-valent HPV vaccine be routinely given to boys ages 11 to 12 to protect against HPV and also to help provide indirect protection of women by reducing HPV transmission (CDC, 2015). All the vaccines are given as a 3-dose series of IM injections with the second dose given 1 to 2 months and the third dose given 6 months after the initial dose.

Women who have received the vaccine should receive regular Papanicolaou (Pap) smears as recommended. Sex partners of infected females are probably also infected but do not require treatment unless large lesions are present. The use of male or female condoms may reduce the risk of transmitting the virus to an uninfected partner.

Acquired Immunodeficiency Syndrome

Acquired immunodeficiency syndrome (AIDS) is a fatal disorder caused by the *human immunodeficiency virus (HIV)*. Medical–surgical texts more fully describe care of individuals with HIV and AIDS. However, because the diagnosis of HIV/AIDS or the presence of the HIV antibody has profound implications for a fetus if the woman is pregnant, AIDS is discussed in more detail in Chapter 14.

Nursing Management

For the Woman With a Sexually Transmitted Infection

Nursing Assessment and Diagnosis

When you are working with female clients you must become adept at taking a thorough history and identifying women at risk for STIs. Risk factors include multiple sexual partners, a partner's involvement with other partners, high-risk sexual behaviors such as intercourse without barrier contraception or anal intercourse, partners with high-risk behaviors, treatment with antibiotics while taking oral contraceptives, and young age at onset of sexual activity. Be alert for signs and symptoms of STIs and be familiar with diagnostic procedures if an STI is suspected.

Although each STI has certain distinctive characteristics, the following complaints suggest the possibility of infection and warrant further investigation:

- Presence of a sore or lesion on the vulva
- Increased vaginal discharge or malodorous vaginal discharge
- Burning with urination
- Vulvar/vaginal itching or irritation
- Dyspareunia
- Bleeding after intercourse
- Pelvic pain.

In many instances the woman is asymptomatic but may report symptoms in her partner, especially painful urination or urethral discharge. It is often helpful to ask the woman whether her partner is experiencing any symptoms.

Nursing diagnoses that may apply when a woman has an STI include the following (NANDA-I © 2014):

- *Family Processes, Interrupted,* related to the effects of a diagnosis of STI on the couple's relationship
- *Knowledge, Readiness for Enhanced,* about preventing STIs related to an expressed desire to prevent infection

Nursing Plan and Implementation

Some STIs, such as trichomoniasis or chlamydia, may cause a woman concern but, once diagnosed, are rather simply treated. Other STIs may also be fairly simple to treat medically but may carry a stigma and be emotionally devastating for the woman. Thus you should stress prevention with all women and encourage them to require partners, especially new partners, to use condoms. While condoms offer protection from many STIs, they do not protect against infections like herpes and HPV, which are transmitted by direct skin-to-skin contact. It is important to emphasize that, to be effective, condoms must remain in place during each and every act of intercourse.

Encourage the woman to explore her feelings about the diagnosis. She may experience anger or feel betrayed by a partner, she may feel guilt or see her diagnosis as a form of punishment, or she may feel concern about the long-term implications for future childbearing or ongoing intimate relationships. She may experience a myriad of emotions that she never expected. Opportunities to discuss her feelings in a nonjudgmental environment can be very helpful. Offer suggestions about support groups, if indicated.

Professionalism in Practice **Attitudes About STIs**

Many women deal matter-of-factly with an STI diagnosis; other women find it embarrassing and possibly even shameful. The nurse's attitude of straightforward acceptance conveys to the woman that she is still a respectable person who happens to have an infection and can help the woman deal effectively with her diagnosis and its implications.

In a supportive, nonjudgmental way, provide the woman who has an STI with information about the infection, methods of transmission, implications for pregnancy or future fertility, and importance of thorough treatment. If treatment of her partner is indicated, the woman must understand that it is necessary to prevent a cycle of reinfection. She should also understand the need to abstain from sexual activity, if necessary, during treatment.

STIs that can have an impact on pregnancy or the fetus/newborn are discussed in Chapter 15. For basic information to share with women who have STIs or who are at risk for infections, see *Teaching Highlights: Preventing STIs and Their Consequences.*

Evaluation

Expected outcomes of nursing care include the following:

- The infection is identified and cured, if possible. If not, supportive therapy is provided.
- The woman and her partner can describe the infection, its method of transmission, its implications, and the therapy.
- The woman copes successfully with the impact of the diagnosis on her self-concept.

Care of the Woman With Pelvic Inflammatory Disease

Pelvic inflammatory disease (PID) is a clinical syndrome of inflammatory disorders of the upper female genital tract that includes any combination of endometritis, salpingitis (tubal infection), tubo-ovarian abscess, pelvic abscess, and pelvic peritonitis (CDC, 2015). The disease is more common in women who have had multiple sexual partners, a history of PID, early onset of sexual activity, or recent insertion of an intrauterine device (IUD) (at which time organisms can be introduced), and in women who douche regularly. Perhaps the greatest problem of PID is postinfection tubal damage, which is closely associated with infertility.

The organisms most frequently identified with PID include *Chlamydia trachomatis* and *Neisseria gonorrhoeae*, although other organisms such as *G. vaginalis, Haemophilus influenza,* and *Streptococcus agalactiae* have also been implicated (CDC, 2015). Signs and symptoms of PID include bilateral sharp, cramping pain in the lower quadrants, fever greater than 101°F, chills, purulent vaginal discharge, irregular bleeding, malaise, nausea, and vomiting. However, it is also possible to be asymptomatic and have normal laboratory values.

Diagnosis of PID may be difficult because of the wide variety of signs and symptoms that may present. Diagnosis consists of a clinical examination to define symptoms, plus cultures for gonorrhea and chlamydia, a complete blood count (CBC) with differential, and a rapid plasma reagin (RPR) or Venereal Disease Research Laboratory (VDRL) test to check for syphilis. Often the woman with PID has an elevated C-reactive protein and elevated sedimentation rate. Physical examination usually reveals direct abdominal tenderness with palpation, adnexal tenderness, and cervical and uterine tenderness with movement (chandelier sign). A palpable mass is evaluated with ultrasound. Laparoscopy may be used to confirm the diagnosis and to enable the examiner to obtain cultures from the fimbriated ends of the fallopian tubes.

Oral outpatient therapy is comparable to inpatient intravenous (IV) therapy in women with PID of mild to moderate severity (CDC, 2015). The decision to hospitalize is based on clinical judgment and severity of symptoms. Inpatient treatment includes IV fluids, pain medications, and IV antibiotics—often either cefotetan or cefoxitin, plus doxycycline or clindamycin plus gentamicin. Outpatient therapy usually includes ceftriaxone IM plus doxycycline with or without metronidazole (CDC, 2015). Other antibiotic combinations may also be used. In addition, supportive therapy is often indicated for severe symptoms. The sexual partner should be treated. If the woman has an IUD, it is generally removed 24 to 48 hours after antibiotic therapy is started.

Nursing Management

For the Woman With Pelvic Inflammatory Disease

Nursing Assessment and Diagnosis

Be alert to factors in a woman's history that put her at risk for PID. Even though fewer types of IUDs are available, many women still have them, and you should question the woman about possible symptoms, such as aching pain in the lower abdomen, foul-smelling discharge, malaise, and the like. The woman who is acutely ill will have obvious symptoms, but a low-grade infection is more difficult to detect.

Nursing diagnoses that may apply to a woman with PID include the following (NANDA-I © 2014):

- *Pain, Acute*, related to peritoneal irritation
- *Knowledge, Deficient*, related to a lack of information about the possible effects of PID on fertility

Nursing Plan and Implementation

You can play a vital role in helping to prevent or detect PID. Accordingly, spend time discussing risk factors related to this infection. The woman who uses an IUD for contraception and has multiple sexual partners needs to understand clearly the risk she faces. Discuss signs and symptoms of PID and stress the importance of early detection.

Counsel the woman who develops PID on the importance of completing her antibiotic treatment and of returning for follow-up evaluation. She should also understand the possibility of decreased fertility following the infection.

Evaluation

Expected outcomes of nursing care include the following:

- The woman describes her condition, her therapy, and the possible long-term implications of PID on her fertility.
- The woman completes her course of therapy and the PID is cured.

Care of the Woman With an Abnormal Finding During Pelvic Examination

Abnormal Pap Smear Results

As discussed in Chapter 5, a Papanicolaou (Pap) smear is a cervical cytology test done to screen for the presence of cellular abnormalities. Although the Pap smear is useful in detecting a variety of abnormalities, it has had its greatest impact on *cervical cancer*. Cervical cancer is now considered a preventable disease because it is slow growing, has a lengthy preinvasive state, has inexpensive and readily available screening programs, and has effective treatment approaches for preinvasive lesions. The *Bethesda system* (Table 6–1) has become the most widely used system in the United States for reporting Pap smear results. Early detection of abnormalities allows changes to be treated before cells reach the precancerous or cancerous stage. Notification of an abnormal Pap smear usually causes anxiety for a woman, so it is important that she be told in a caring way. The woman needs accurate, complete information about the

meaning of the results and the next steps to be taken. She should also be given time to ask questions and express her concerns.

Colposcopy, the direct, detailed visualization and examination of the cervix, has become an appropriate second step in many cases of abnormal Pap results. The examination, done in an office or clinic, permits more detailed visualization of the cervix in bright light, using a high-power microscope. The cervix can be visualized directly and again following application of acetic acid. The acetic acid causes abnormal epithelium to assume a characteristic white appearance. The colposcope can be used to localize and obtain a directed biopsy.

Endocervical curettage (ECC) may also be done at this time to evaluate for extension into the cervical canal. This involves scraping the endocervix from the internal os to the external os to obtain endocervical cells for cytology. Histologic evaluation of tissue biopsies and ECC samples is necessary for a definitive diagnosis.

Loop electrosurgical excision procedure (LEEP) can be used to treat cervical, vaginal, and vulvar intraepithelial neoplasia. When an abnormal Pap smear and a colposcopic evaluation indicate a premalignant lesion, a small electrically hot wire loop can be used to excise the entire lesion, squamocolumnar junction, and transformation zone. The cutting effect is created by a steam envelope that develops between the wire loop and the water-laden tissue. This procedure can be performed on an outpatient basis, often in the gynecologic office, under local anesthesia. Women who have a LEEP procedure and subsequently become pregnant have a slightly increased risk of preterm birth.

Ovarian Masses

Ovarian masses may be palpated during the pelvic exam. Between 70% and 80% of ovarian masses are benign. More than 50% are functional cysts (cysts that develop from ovarian follicles, from the corpus luteum, or from the theca luteum), occurring most commonly in women 20 to 40 years of age. Functional cysts are associated with abnormal hormone production and are rare in women who take oral contraceptives.

Ovarian cysts usually represent physiologic variations in the menstrual cycle. Dermoid cysts (cystic teratomas) comprise 10% of all benign ovarian masses. Cartilage, bone, teeth, skin, or hair can be observed in these cysts. Endometriomas, or "chocolate cysts," are another common type of ovarian mass.

No relationship exists between the presence of benign ovarian masses and the subsequent development of ovarian cancer. However, ovarian cancer is the most fatal of all cancers in women because it is difficult to diagnose and often has spread throughout the pelvis before it is detected. Refer to medical-surgical nursing texts for an in-depth discussion of ovarian cancer.

Many women with a benign ovarian mass are asymptomatic; the mass may be noted on a routine pelvic examination. Others experience a sensation of fullness or cramping in the lower abdomen (often unilateral), dyspareunia, irregular bleeding, or delayed menstruation.

Diagnosis is made on the basis of a palpable mass with or without tenderness and other related symptoms. Radiography or ultrasonography may be used to assist in the diagnosis.

The woman is frequently kept under observation for a month or two because most cysts will resolve on their own and are harmless. Oral contraceptives may be prescribed for 1 to 2 months to suppress ovarian function. If this regimen is effective, a repeat pelvic examination should be normal. If the mass is still present after 60 days of observation and oral contraceptive

TABLE 6–1 The Bethesda System for Classifying Pap Smears

SPECIMEN TYPE	OTHER
Indicate conventional smear (Pap smear) vs. liquid based vs. other	Endometrial cells (in a woman ≥ 40 years of age) (Specify if negative for squamous intraepithelial lesion)
Specimen Adequacy	*Epithelial cell abnormalities*
Satisfactory for evaluation *(describe presence or absence of endocervical/transformation zone component and any other quality indicators, e.g., partially obscuring blood inflammation, etc.)*	SQUAMOUS CELL
	Atypical squamous cells
	—of undetermined significance (ASC-US)
Unsatisfactory for evaluation . . . *(specify reason)*	—cannot exclude HSIL (ASC-H)
Specimen rejected/not processed *(specify reason)*	Low-grade squamous intraepithelial lesion (LSIL)
Specimen processed and examined, but unsatisfactory for evaluation of epithelial abnormality because of *(specify reason)*	—encompassing HPV/mild dysplasia/CIN-1
	High-grade squamous intraepithelial lesion (HSIL)
General Categorization (optional)	—encompassing moderate and severe dysplasia CIS/CIN-2 and CIN-3
Negative for intraepithelial lesion or malignancy.	—with features suspicious for invasion *(if invasion is suspected)*
Epithelial cell abnormality. See Interpretation/Result *(specify squamous or glandular as appropriate).*	Squamous cell carcinoma
Other: See Interpretation/Result *(e.g., endometrial cells in a woman ≥40 years of age).*	GLANDULAR CELL
	Atypical
Automated Review	—endocervical cells *(NOS or specify in comments)*
If case examined by automated device, specify device and result.	—endometrial cells *(NOS or specify in comments)*
	—glandular cells *(NOS or specify in comments)*
Ancillary Testing	Atypical
Provide a brief description of the test methods and report the result so that it is easily understood by the clinician.	—endocervical cells, favor neoplastic
	—glandular cells, favor neoplastic
Interpretation/Result	Endocervical adenocarcinoma in situ
Negative for intraepithelial lesion or malignancy (when there is no cellular evidence of neoplasia, state this in the General Categorization above and/or in the Interpretation/Result section of the report, whether or not there are organisms or other nonneoplastic findings)	Adenocarcinoma
	—endocervical
	—endometrial
ORGANISMS:	—extrauterine
Trichomonas vaginalis	—not otherwise specified (NOS)
Fungal organisms morphologically consistent with *Candida* spp.	*Other malignant neoplasms (specify)*
Shift in flora suggestive of bacterial vaginosis	
Bacteria morphologically consistent with *Actinomyces* spp.	**Educational Notes and Suggestions (optional)**
Cellular changes associated with herpes simplex virus	Suggestions should be concise and consistent with clinical follow-up guidelines published by professional organizations (references to relevant publications may be included).
OTHER NONNEOPLASTIC FINDINGS *(Optional to report list not inclusive)*	
Reactive cellular changes associated with	
—inflammation (includes typical repair)	
—radiation	
—intrauterine contraceptive device (IUD)	
Glandular cells status post-hysterectomy	
Atrophy	

Source: Courtesy of National Cancer Institute.

therapy, a diagnostic laparoscopy or laparotomy may be considered. Tubal or ovarian lesions, ectopic pregnancy, cancer, infection, or appendicitis also must be ruled out before a diagnosis can be confirmed.

Surgery is not always necessary but will be considered if the mass is larger than 6 to 7 cm in circumference; if the woman is over 40 years of age with an adnexal mass, a persistent mass, or continuous pain; or if the woman is taking oral contraceptives. Surgical exploration is also indicated when a palpable mass is found in an infant, a young girl, or a postmenopausal woman.

Women may need clear explanations about why the initial therapy is observation. A discussion of the origin and resolution of ovarian cysts may clarify this treatment plan. If a surgical treatment removes or impairs the function of one ovary, the woman needs to be assured that the remaining ovary can be expected to take over ovarian functioning and that pregnancy is still possible.

Uterine Abnormalities

Endometrial polyps are pedunculated (growing on a stalk) overgrowths of the endometrium. They can occur as single or multiple growths. Polyps are common and are often accompanied by symptoms of mid-cycle bleeding or spotting, bleeding or spotting after intercourse, or prolonged bleeding or spotting with menstrual cycles. Polyps are generally benign, but they can occasionally coexist with carcinoma of the endometrium. Treatment is dilation and curettage (D&C) using a hysteroscope for visualization.

Fibroid tumors, or *leiomyomas*, are among the most common benign disease entities in women and are the most common reason for gynecologic surgery. By the age of 50, 70% of White women and 80% of Black women have fibroids (Rice, Secrist, Woodrow, et al., 2012).

Most uterine fibroid tumors are asymptomatic and require no treatment. The most common symptoms include pelvic pain, menstrual irregularities, and infertility. Women most often seek treatment for bleeding and pain. On pelvic examination the woman may have an irregularly shaped, enlarged uterus. Diagnosis is most often made using pelvic ultrasound and magnetic resonance imaging (MRI). Occasionally hysterosonography is used for further evaluation (Rice et al., 2012). Treatment for uterine fibroids varies and may include the following:

- Combined oral contraceptives to control heavy menstrual bleeding
- GnRH analogs such as Lupron to reduce the size and subsequent bleeding; GnRH analogs also may be used before surgery to reduce the size of the fibroid and decrease complications (Rice et al., 2012)
- Levonorgestrel intrauterine system (LNG-IUS) for contraception and control of excessive menstrual bleeding by suppression of endometrial growth
- MRI-guided ultrasound, which focuses high-intensity sound waves on the fibroids, resulting in clotting, necrosis, and shrinkage of the tumor
- *Myomectomy*, a surgical procedure to remove the fibroid without removing the uterus, which can preserve or improve fertility
- Uterine artery embolization (UAE), an interventional radiologic procedure in which the uterine arteries are blocked, resulting in diminished blood flow to the uterus and the necrosis of the fibroids
- Hysterectomy may be indicated and can be performed laparoscopically or abdominally depending on the size of the uterus.

Endometrial cancer is the most common female genital tract malignancy, occurring in about 1 of every 45 women. Fortunately it has a high rate of cure if detected early. Although endometrial cancer can occur in younger women, the hallmark sign is vaginal bleeding in postmenopausal women not treated with hormone replacement therapy. Diagnosis is made by endometrial biopsy, by transvaginal ultrasound, or by posthysterectomy pathology examination of the uterus. The treatment is total abdominal hysterectomy (TAH) and bilateral salpingo-oophorectomy (BSO). Radiation therapy may also be indicated, depending on the stage of the cancer.

Nursing Management

Pelvic examinations and Pap smears are not done by nurses unless they have special training. In most cases, nursing assessment is directed toward an evaluation of the woman's understanding of the findings and their implications and her psychosocial response.

The woman needs accurate information on etiology, symptomatology, and treatment options. Encourage her to report symptoms and keep appointments for follow-up examination and evaluation. The woman needs realistic reassurance if her condition is benign; she may require counseling and effective emotional support if a malignancy is likely. If the management plan includes surgery, she may need your support in obtaining a second opinion and making her decision.

Care of the Woman With a Urinary Tract Infection

A **urinary tract infection (UTI)**, defined as significant bacteriuria in the presence of symptoms, is one of the most common problems women experience. Bacteria usually enter the urinary tract by way of the urethra. The organisms are capable of migrating against the downward flow of urine. The shortness of the female urethra facilitates the passage of bacteria into the bladder. Other conditions that are associated with bacterial entry are relative incompetence of the urinary sphincter, frequent enuresis (bedwetting) before adolescence, and urinary catheterization. Wiping from back to front after urination may transfer bacteria from the anorectal area to the urethra.

Voluntarily suppressing the desire to urinate is a predisposing factor. Retention overdistends the bladder and can lead to an infection. Sexual activity is a strong risk factor for UTI, especially in younger women. General poor health or lowered resistance to infection can increase a woman's susceptibility to UTI.

Asymptomatic bacteriuria (ASB) (bacteria in the urine actively multiplying without accompanying clinical symptoms) is a condition that becomes significant if a woman is pregnant because, if untreated, ASB can lead to pyelonephritis in the pregnant woman and low birth weight in the newborn (Cunningham et al., 2014). ASB is almost always caused by a single organism, typically *Escherichia coli*. If more than one type of bacteria is cultured, the possibility of urine-culture contamination must be considered.

A woman who has had a UTI is susceptible to recurrent infection. If a pregnant woman develops an acute UTI, especially with a high temperature, amniotic fluid infection may develop and retard the growth of the placenta.

Lower Urinary Tract Infection

Because urinary tract infections are ascending, it is important to recognize and diagnose a lower UTI early to avoid the sequelae associated with upper UTI. **Cystitis**, or inflammation of the bladder, usually occurs secondary to an ascending infection. *E. coli* is present in the majority of cases. Other common causative organisms include *Klebsiella pneumonia*, *Proteus mirabilis*, *Enterococcus* species, and *Staphylococcus saprophyticus*.

When cystitis develops, the initial symptom is often dysuria, specifically at the end of urination. Urgency and frequency also occur. Cystitis is usually accompanied by a low-grade fever (38.3°C [101°F] or lower), and hematuria is occasionally seen. Urine specimens usually contain an abnormal number of leukocytes and bacteria. Diagnosis is made with a urine culture.

Treatment depends on the causative organism. Nitrofurantoin has reemerged as an effective first-line therapy and is given twice daily for 5 days. A 3-day, twice-daily course of oral trimethoprim may also be used. Fluoroquinolones (FQ) such as ciprofloxacin, levofloxacin, gatifloxacin, or norfloxacin should be reserved for treatment failures and for women with suspected upper UTI infection (Haddock, 2015). (For treatment options during pregnancy, see Table 15–1.)

Upper Urinary Tract Infection (Pyelonephritis)

Pyelonephritis (inflammatory disease of the kidneys) is less common but more serious than cystitis and is often preceded by lower UTI. It is more common during the latter part of pregnancy or early postpartum and poses a serious threat to maternal and fetal well-being. Women with symptoms of pyelonephritis during pregnancy have an increased risk of preterm birth and of intrauterine growth restriction.

Acute pyelonephritis has a sudden onset, with chills, high temperature of 39.6° to 40.6°C (103° to 105°F), and flank pain (either unilateral or bilateral). The right side is almost always involved if the woman is pregnant because the large bulk of intestines to the left pushes the uterus to the right, putting pressure on the right ureter and kidney. Nausea, vomiting, and general malaise may ensue. With accompanying cystitis, the woman may experience frequency, urgency, and burning with urination.

Edema of the renal parenchyma or ureteritis with blockage and swelling of the ureter may lead to temporary suppression of urinary output. This is accompanied by severe colicky (spastic, intense) pain, vomiting, dehydration, and ileus of the large bowel. Women with acute pyelonephritis generally have increased diastolic blood pressure, positive fluorescent antibody (FA) titer, low creatinine clearance, significant bacteremia in urine culture, pyuria, and the presence of white blood cell casts.

Many women can be treated as outpatients or given IV fluids and one IV dose of antibiotics, then discharged on oral medications. Fluoroquinolones (FQs) are the first-line treatment in communities where FQ resistance is low, specifically ciprofloxacin, extended-release ciprofloxacin, or levofloxacin. If local FQ resistance is high, an initial dose of ceftriaxone or gentamicin is given followed by an oral FQ regimen (Colgan, Williams, & Johnson, 2011).

Women with acute pyelonephritis should have a urine culture and sensitivity done to determine the appropriate antibiotic. A woman who is severely ill or has complications may require hospitalization. She should be started on broad-spectrum intravenous (IV) antibiotics until the results of the culture and sensitivity are obtained. This treatment should be followed with an appropriate antibiotic. Therapy also includes IV hydration, urinary analgesics such as phenazopyridine (Pyridium), pain management, and medication to manage fever. In the case of obstructive pyelonephritis, a blood culture is necessary. The woman is kept on bed rest. After the sensitivity report is received, the antibiotic is changed as necessary. If signs of urinary obstruction occur or continue, the ureter may be catheterized to establish adequate drainage.

With appropriate drug therapy, the woman's temperature should return to normal. The pain subsides and the urine shows no bacteria within 2 to 3 days. Follow-up urinary cultures are needed to determine that the infection has been eliminated completely.

Nursing Management

For the Woman With a Urinary Tract Infection

Nursing Assessment and Diagnosis

During the client's visit, obtain a sexual and medical history to identify whether the woman is at risk for UTI. A clean-catch urine specimen is evaluated for evidence of ASB.

Nursing diagnoses that may apply to a woman with an upper UTI include the following (NANDA-I © 2014):

- *Pain, Acute,* related to dysuria, systemic discomforts, or renal pain secondary to upper UTI
- *Fear* related to the possible long-term effects of the disease

Nursing Plan and Implementation

Provide the woman with information to help her recognize the signs of UTI, so she can contact her caregiver as soon as possible. Discuss hygiene practices, the advantages of wearing cotton underwear, and the need to void frequently to prevent urinary stasis.

Stress the importance of maintaining a good fluid intake. Also reinforce instructions and answer any questions the woman may have. UTIs usually respond quickly to treatment, but follow-up clinical evaluation and urine cultures are important.

KEY FACTS TO REMEMBER
Information for Women About Ways to Avoid Cystitis

- If you use a diaphragm for contraception, try changing methods or using another size of diaphragm.
- Avoid bladder irritants such as alcohol, caffeine products, and carbonated beverages.
- Increase fluid intake, especially water, to a minimum of six to eight glasses per day.
- Make regular urination a habit; avoid long waits.
- Practice good genital hygiene, including wiping from front to back after urination and bowel movements.
- Be aware that vigorous or frequent sexual activity may contribute to urinary tract infection.
- Urinate before and after intercourse to empty the bladder and cleanse the urethra.
- Complete medication regimens even if symptoms decrease.
- Do not use medication left over from previous infections.
- Drink cranberry juice to acidify the urine. This has been found to relieve symptoms in some cases.

Evaluation

Expected outcomes of nursing care include the following:

- The woman completes her prescribed course of antibiotic therapy.
- The woman's infection is cured.
- The woman incorporates preventive self-care measures into her daily regimen.

Care of the Woman With Pelvic Relaxation

A **cystocele** is the downward displacement of the bladder, which appears as a bulge in the anterior vaginal wall. Arbitrary classifications of mild to severe are frequently given. Genetic predisposition, childbearing, obesity, and increased age are factors that may contribute to cystocele.

Symptoms of stress urinary incontinence (SUI) are most common, including loss of urine with coughing, sneezing, laughing, or sudden exertion. Vaginal fullness, a bulging out of the vaginal wall, or a dragging sensation may also be noticeable.

If pelvic relaxation is mild, Kegel exercises are helpful in restoring tone. The exercises involve contraction and relaxation of the pubococcygeal muscle (see Chapter 10). Women have found these exercises helpful before and after childbirth for maintaining vaginal muscle tone. Estrogen may improve the condition of vaginal mucous membranes, especially in menopausal women.

Duloxetine, a balanced serotonin and norepinephrine reuptake inhibitor used to treat major depressive disorders and the pain of fibromyalgia or diabetic neuropathy, is the only medication shown to help decrease SUI. Although approved for the treatment of SUI in the European Union, it is not approved for that purpose in the United States, and its administration would be an off-label use (Testa, 2015). Vaginal pessaries or rings may be used if surgery is undesirable or impossible or until surgery can be scheduled. Surgery may be considered for cystoceles considered moderate to severe.

The nurse can instruct the woman in the use of Kegel exercises. Information on causes and contributing factors and discussion of possible alternative therapies will greatly assist the woman.

A **rectocele** may develop when the posterior vaginal wall is weakened. The anterior wall of the rectum can then sag forward, ballooning into the vagina, pushing the weakened posterior wall of the vagina in front of it. When the woman strains to have a bowel movement, a pocket of rectum develops that traps stool, and constipation results. To defecate, a woman with a rectocele may find it necessary to press the tissue between the vagina and rectum, which elevates the rectocele.

Diagnosis is based on history and physical examination. Decisions about treatment are based on the size of the rectocele, the presence and severity of symptoms, and the woman's individual situation, including her overall health. Surgery is often indicated.

Uterine prolapse occurs when the uterus protrudes downward (drops) into the upper vagina, pulling the vagina with it. The extent of the prolapse is determined by the location of the cervix in the vagina. In severe cases the uterus may prolapse below the vaginal introitus. The woman may report a "dragging" sensation in her groin and a backache over the sacrum, which is caused by pulling on the uterosacral ligaments. Typically these symptoms are relieved when the woman lies down. As with cystocele, conservative treatment includes the use of topical or systemic estrogen and vaginal pessaries. Surgery for uterine prolapse often involves hysterectomy and repair of the prolapsed vaginal walls.

Care of the Woman Requiring a Hysterectomy

Hysterectomy is the surgical removal of the uterus. In the United States it is the most common non–pregnancy-related surgical procedure that women undergo. Removal of the uterus through a surgical incision is called a *total abdominal hysterectomy (TAH)* and removal of both fallopian tubes and ovaries is called a *bilateral salpingo-oophorectomy (BSO)*. When both procedures are performed at the same time it is called a TAH-BSO. When the uterus is removed through the vagina it is termed a *total vaginal hysterectomy (TVH)*.

A *laparoscopic-assisted vaginal hysterectomy (LAVH)* may also be used. In this technique, the surgeon inserts a laparoscope through an incision near the umbilicus and uses it to assist with visualization and dissection to facilitate vaginal removal of the uterus. The benefit is that the surgeon can achieve results similar to those of a TAH without a large abdominal incision.

Abdominal hysterectomy is the usual treatment for several conditions including cancer of the cervix, endometrium, or ovary; large fibroids; severe endometriosis; chronic pelvic inflammatory

disease (PID); and adenomyosis. TAH is preferred when cancer is expected because it permits easier exploration of the abdomen. It is also helpful when large uterine masses are present.

Vaginal hysterectomy is generally done for pelvic relaxation, abnormal uterine bleeding, or small fibroids. Advantages of vaginal hysterectomy include earlier ambulation, less postoperative pain, less anesthesia and operative time, less blood loss, no visible scar, and a shorter hospital stay. The major disadvantage is the increased risk of trauma to the bladder.

Nursing Management

For the Woman Requiring a Hysterectomy

Nursing Assessment and Diagnosis

Preoperatively you need to identify the woman's physiologic and psychologic needs as she approaches surgery. Additionally it is important to evaluate her learning needs in relation to the surgery and its implications postoperatively. In assessing the woman, it is important to consider her age, her culture and educational level, the attitudes of her partner and family, her preoperative status, and whether the hysterectomy is being performed because of a cancer diagnosis. The significance of her reproductive health to her self-image is also a consideration.

Nursing diagnoses that may apply to a woman having a hysterectomy include the following (NANDA-I © 2014):

- *Knowledge, Deficient,* related to a lack of information about preoperative routines, postoperative activities, and expected postoperative changes
- *Fear* related to the risk of possible surgical complications

Nursing Plan and Implementation

Preoperative teaching should include information about the procedure, expected preparation, effects of the anesthesia to be used, possible risks and complications, postoperative care routines, and expected recovery time. See Figure 6–5.

Routine postoperative care includes monitoring of physiologic and emotional responses and implementation of nursing interventions to ensure physical well-being and comfort. The woman should be aware of possible complications and when to follow up with her surgeon. Additionally it is important to

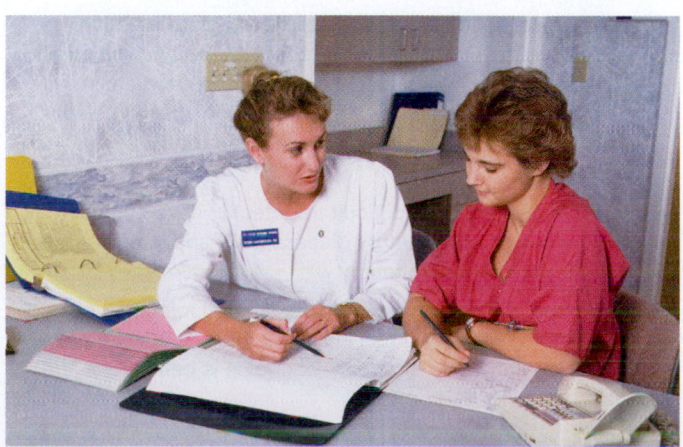

Figure 6–5 The nurse provides information for the woman during preoperative teaching.

SOURCE: George Dodson/Pearson Education, Inc.

follow up with the woman regarding any psychosocial implications discussed preoperatively, such as support at home and potential for sadness or depression related to perception of changed sexuality or self-image.

Evaluation

Expected outcomes of nursing care include the following:

- The woman can discuss the reasons for her hysterectomy and the type of procedure performed, the alternatives, and aspects of self-care following surgery.

- The woman has an uneventful recovery without complications.
- The woman participates in decision making about her care.
- The woman can identify available resources if she has physical or emotional concerns in the postoperative period.

Focus Your Study

- In fibrocystic breast changes, the cysts tend to be round, mobile, and well delineated. The woman generally experiences increased discomfort premenstrually.

- Because of the increased risk of breast cancer, women with fibrocystic breast changes should understand the importance of monthly breast self-examination.

- Endometriosis is a condition in which endometrial tissue occurs outside the endometrial cavity. This tissue bleeds in a cyclic fashion in response to the menstrual cycle. The bleeding leads to inflammation, scarring, and adhesions. The primary symptoms include dysmenorrhea, dyspareunia, and infertility.

- Treatment of endometriosis may be medical, surgical, or a combination. For the woman not desiring pregnancy at present, oral contraceptives are used. Women desiring pregnancy are treated with danazol or GnRH analogs.

- Toxic shock syndrome, caused by a toxin of *Staphylococcus aureus*, is most common in women of childbearing age. There is an increased incidence in women who use tampons or barrier methods of contraception, such as the diaphragm and cervical cap.

- Bacterial vaginosis, a common vaginal infection, is diagnosed by its characteristic fishy odor and by the presence of "clue" cells on a vaginal smear. It is treated with metronidazole.

- Vulvovaginal candidiasis (moniliasis), a vaginal infection caused by *Candida albicans*, is most common in women who use oral contraceptives, are on antibiotics, are currently pregnant, or have diabetes mellitus. It is generally treated with intravaginal miconazole or clotrimazole suppositories or fluconazole orally.

- Chlamydial infection is difficult to detect in a woman but may result in pelvic inflammatory disease (PID) and infertility. It is treated with antibiotic therapy.

- Gonorrhea, a common sexually transmitted infection, may be asymptomatic in women initially but may cause PID if not diagnosed early. The treatment of choice is ceftriaxone and doxycycline or azithromycin.

- Herpes genitalis, caused by the herpes simplex virus, is a recurrent infection with no known cure. Acyclovir (Zovirax), valacyclovir, or famciclovir may reduce the symptoms and decrease the length of viral shedding.

- Syphilis, caused by *Treponema pallidum*, is a sexually transmitted infection that is treatable if diagnosed. The characteristic lesion is the chancre. Syphilis can also be transmitted in utero to the fetus of an infected woman. The treatment of choice is penicillin.

- Condylomata acuminata (venereal or genital warts) are transmitted by the human papillomavirus (HPV). Treatment is indicated, because research suggests a link between certain strains of HPV and the development of cervical cancer. The treatment chosen depends on the size and location of the warts.

- Pelvic inflammatory disease may be life threatening and may lead to infertility. *C. trachomatis* and *N. gonorrhoeae* are the organisms that cause PID most frequently.

- Women with an abnormal finding on a pelvic examination need a careful explanation of the finding and techniques of diagnosis and emotional support during the diagnostic period.

- The classic symptoms of a lower urinary tract infection (UTI) are dysuria, urgency, frequency, and sometimes hematuria.

- An upper UTI is a serious infection that can permanently damage the kidneys if untreated. Generally the woman is acutely ill and requires supportive therapy as well as antibiotics.

- Three common forms of pelvic relaxation exist: A cystocele is a downward displacement of the bladder into the vagina. Often it is accompanied by stress incontinence. Kegel exercises may help restore tone in mild cases. A rectocele is displacement of the rectum into the vagina. Prolapse of the uterus is downward displacement of the cervix into the vagina.

- Hysterectomy is the most common non–pregnancy-related surgery performed in the United States. It may be done vaginally or abdominally and is sometimes accompanied by removal of the ovaries and fallopian tubes.

Clinical Reasoning In Action

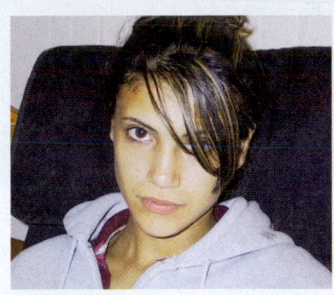

Cherelle Latkowski, age 18, was just diagnosed with gonorrhea by the nurse practitioner at the clinic where you work. Although she had been asymptomatic, she had come in for evaluation after her boyfriend was diagnosed with gonorrhea and started on antibiotics. Cherelle is treated with ceftriaxone administered intramuscularly plus doxycycline by mouth.

1. Cherelle asks you why she received two medications. How would you reply?
2. Cherelle asks you whether she is now immune to gonorrhea. Is she?
3. Cherelle asks whether she can now have sex with her boyfriend. Can she do so?

References

American College of Obstetricians and Gynecologists (ACOG). (2014). *Guidelines for women's health care* (4th ed.). Washington, DC: Author.

Brown, J., & Farquhar, C. (2014). Endometriosis: An overview of Cochrane Reviews. *Cochrane Database of Systematic Reviews 2014*, Issue 3. Art. No.:CD009590.

Centers for Disease Control and Prevention (CDC). (2014). STDs in racial and ethnic minorities. Retrieved from http://www.cdc.gov/std/stats12/minorities.htm

Centers for Disease Control and Prevention (CDC). (2015). Sexually transmitted diseases treatment guidelines, 2015. *Morbidity and Mortality Weekly Report*, *64*(RR#), 1–137.

Coleman, L., & Overton, C. (2015). GPs have a role in the early diagnosis of endometriosis. *Practitioner*, *259*(1780), 13–17.

Colgan, R., Williams, M., & Johnson, J. R. (2011). Diagnosis and treatment of acute pyelonephritis in women. *American Family Physician*, *84*(5), 519–526.

Cunningham, F. G., Leveno, K. J., Bloom, S. L., Spong, C. Y., Dashe, J. S., Hoffman, B. L., . . . & Sheffield, J. S. (2014). *Williams obstetrics* (24th ed.). New York, NY: McGraw-Hill.

Gateva, A. T., & Kamenov, Z. A. (2012). Markers of visceral obesity and cardiovascular risk in patients with polycystic ovarian syndrome. *European Journal of Obstetrics & Gynecology and Reproductive Biology*, *164*(2), 161–166.

Haddock, G. (2015). Improving the management of urinary tract infection. *Nursing and Residential Care*, *17*(1), 22–25.

Hogg, S., & Vyas, S. (2015). Endometriosis. *Obstetrics, Gynaecology & Reproductive Medicine*, *25*(5), 133–141.

Mayo Clinic. (2014). Fibroadenoma. Retrieved from http://www.mayoclinic.org/diseases-conditions/fibroadenoma/basics/definition/con-20032223

McFarland, C. (2012). Treating polycystic ovary syndrome and infertility. *American Journal of Maternal/Child Nursing*, *37*(2), 116–121.

Rice, K. E., Secrist, J. R., Woodrow, E. L., Hallock, L. M., & Neal, J. L. (2012). Etiology, diagnosis, and management of uterine leiomyomas. *Journal of Midwifery & Women's Health*, *57*, 241–247.

Testa, A. (2015). Understanding urinary incontinence in adults. *Urologic Nursing*, *35*(2), 82–86.

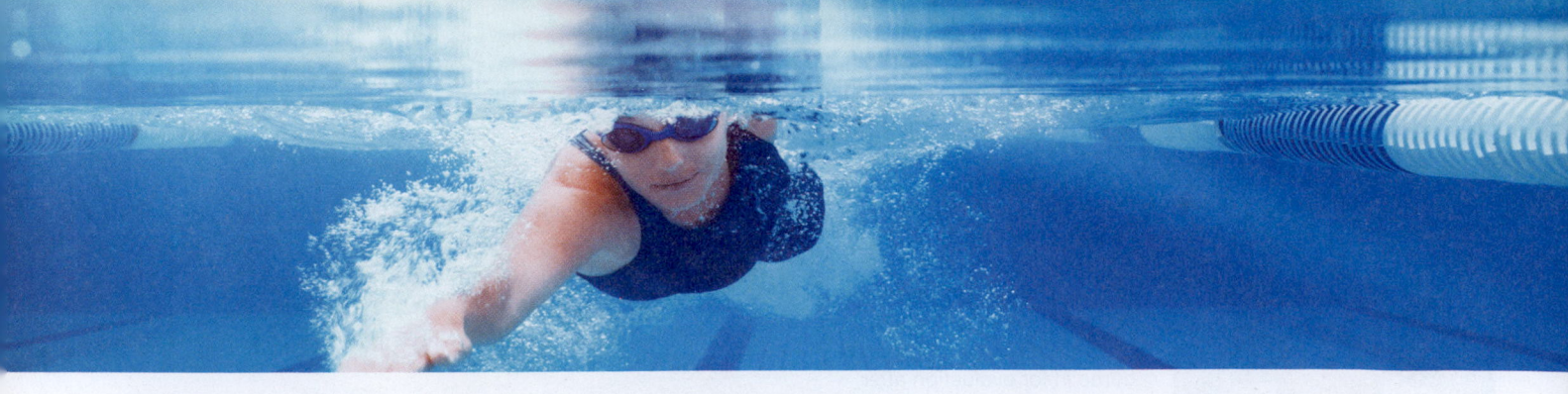

Chapter 7
Families with Special Reproductive Concerns

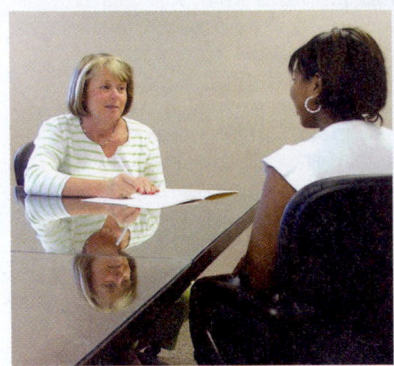

When I first began working in genetics I focused primarily on the science of it, on the odds, on the disorders. Now I recognize the courage of those with known genetic disorders who must decide whether to risk childbirth, the commitment of those who care for and love children with profound disabilities, and the constant sorrow of those who lose a child because of a previously undetected genetic problem. This work is about people—not genes, not DNA, but people.

—A Nurse Genetic Counselor

∨ Learning Outcomes

7.1 Compare the essential components of fertility with the possible causes of infertility.

7.2 Describe the elements of the preliminary investigation of infertility and the nurse's role in supporting/teaching clients during this phase.

7.3 Compare the indications for the tests and associated treatments, including assisted reproductive technologies, that are done in an infertility workup.

7.4 Explain the physiologic and psychologic effects of infertility on a couple in relation to the nursing management of the couple.

7.5 Describe the nurse's role as counselor, educator, and advocate for couples during infertility evaluation and treatment.

7.6 Identify couples who may benefit from preconceptual chromosomal analysis and prenatal testing when providing care to couples with special reproductive concerns.

7.7 Identify the characteristics of autosomal dominant, autosomal recessive, and X-linked (sex-linked) recessive disorders.

7.8 Compare prenatal and postnatal diagnostic procedures used to determine the presence of genetic disorders and the nursing considerations for each.

7.9 Examine the emotional impact on a couple undergoing genetic testing or coping with the birth of a baby with a genetic disorder.

7.10 Explain the nurse's role in supporting the family undergoing genetic counseling.

Most couples who want children are able to conceive them with little difficulty. Pregnancy and childbirth usually take their normal course, and a healthy baby is born. But some less fortunate couples are unable to fulfill their dream of having a baby because of infertility or genetic problems.

This chapter explores two particularly troubling reproductive problems facing some couples: the inability to conceive and the risk of bearing babies with genetic problems.

Infertility

Infertility is defined as the failure to achieve a successful pregnancy after 12 months or more of regular unprotected intercourse (American Society for Reproductive Medicine [ASRM], 2012a). It has a profound emotional, psychologic, and economic impact on affected couples and society. *Sterility* is a term applied when there is an absolute factor preventing reproduction. **Subfertility** is used to describe a couple who have difficulty conceiving because both partners have reduced fertility. **Primary infertility** refers to a woman with no prior pregnancies; **secondary infertility** refers to couples who have been unable to conceive after one or more successful pregnancies or who cannot sustain a pregnancy.

In the United States, approximately 15% of couples in their reproductive years are infertile (ASRM, 2012c). Public perception is that the incidence of infertility is increasing, but in fact there has been no significant change in the proportion of infertile couples in the United States. What has changed is the composition of the infertile population; the infertility diagnosis has increased in the age group 25 to 44 because of delayed childbearing. The perception that infertility is on the rise may be related to the following factors (Fritz & Speroff, 2011):

- Increase in the use of assisted reproductive techniques, which has improved the prognosis for many infertile couples
- The increase in availability and use of infertility services
- The increase in insurance coverage of some socioeconomic groups for diagnosis of and treatment for infertility
- The increased number of childless women over age 35 seeking medical attention for infertility.

Essential Components of Fertility

Understanding the elements essential for normal fertility can help the nurse identify the many factors that may cause infertility. The components necessary for normal fertility are correlated with possible causes of deviation in Table 7–1. Infertility can be due to a male factor (20%), a female factor (40%), or either an unknown cause (unexplained infertility) or a problem with both partners (30% to 40%) (ASRM, 2012b). Professional intervention can help approximately 65% of infertile couples achieve pregnancy.

Young couples with no history that is suggestive of reproductive disorders should be referred for infertility evaluation if they have been unable to conceive after at least 1 year of attempting to achieve pregnancy. An earlier workup is indicated in couples with positive histories of fertility-lowering disease or advancing maternal age. If the woman is over age 35, it may be appropriate to refer the couple after only 6 months of unprotected intercourse without conception or earlier if clinically indicated (ASRM, 2015a). The most important determinant of a couple's fertility is the age of the woman.

TABLE 7–1 Possible Causes of Infertility

NECESSARY NORMS	DEVIATIONS FROM NORMAL
Female	
Favorable cervical mucus	Cervicitis, cervical stenosis, use of coital lubricants, antisperm antibodies (immunologic response)
Clear passage between cervix and tubes	Myomas, adhesions, adenomyosis, polyps, endometritis, cervical stenosis, endometriosis, congenital anomalies (e.g., septate uterus, diethylstilbestrol [DES] exposure)
Patent tubes with normal motility	Pelvic inflammatory disease (PID), peritubal adhesions, endometriosis, intrauterine device (IUD), salpingitis (e.g., chlamydia, recurrent STIs), neoplasm, ectopic pregnancy, tubal ligation
Ovulation and release of ova	Primary ovarian failure, polycystic ovarian disease, hypothyroidism, pituitary tumor, lactation, periovarian adhesions, endometriosis, premature ovarian failure, hyperprolactinemia, Turner syndrome
No obstruction between ovary and tubes	Adhesions, endometriosis, PID
Endometrial preparation	Anovulation, luteal phase defect, malformation, uterine infection, Asherman syndrome
Male	
Normal semen analysis	Abnormalities of sperm or semen, polyspermia, congenital defect in testicular development, mumps after adolescence, cryptorchidism, infections, gonadal exposure to X-rays, chemotherapy, smoking, alcohol abuse, malnutrition, chronic or acute metabolic disease, medications (e.g., morphine, aspirin, ibuprofen), cocaine, marijuana use, constrictive underclothing, heat
Unobstructed genital tract	Infections, tumors, congenital anomalies, vasectomy, strictures, trauma, varicocele
Normal genital tract secretions	Infections, autoimmunity to semen, tumors
Ejaculate deposited at the cervix	Premature ejaculation, impotence, hypospadias, retrograde ejaculation (e.g., as can occur with diabetes), neurologic cord lesions, obesity (inhibiting adequate penetration)

Initial Investigation: Physical and Psychosocial Issues

The easiest and least intrusive infertility testing approach is used first. Extensive testing for infertility is avoided until data confirm that the timing of intercourse and length of coital exposure have been adequate. The nurse provides information about the most fertile times to have intercourse during the menstrual cycle. Teaching the couple the signs and timing of ovulation, the most effective times for intercourse within the cycle, and other fertility awareness behaviors may solve the problem (see *Teaching Highlights: Suggestions for Improving Fertility*). Primary assessment, including a comprehensive history (with a discussion of genetic conditions) and physical examination for any obvious causes of infertility, is done before a costly, time-consuming, and emotionally trying investigation is initiated.

The initial infertility evaluation offers nurses a unique opportunity to initiate preconception counseling, thereby helping infertile couples maximize their chances of delivering a healthy baby. Prenatal vitamins are often one of the earliest recommendations for women planning to conceive.

Preconception is the optimal time to review the importance of rubella and varicella immunity and the risk of congenital anomalies associated with exposure. It also provides the opportunity to address risks associated with alcohol, tobacco, and medications. Women may need a change in medications or stricter management of chronic illnesses.

The mutual desire to have children is a cornerstone of many marriages. A fertility problem is a deeply personal, emotion-laden area in a couple's life. The self-esteem of one or both partners may be threatened if the inability to conceive is perceived as a lack of virility or femininity. It is never easy to discuss one's sexual activity, especially when potentially irreversible problems with fertility exist. The nurse can provide comfort to couples by offering a sympathetic ear, a nonjudgmental approach, and appropriate information and instructions throughout the diagnostic and therapeutic process (Barbieri, 2014). Because counseling includes discussion of very personal matters, nurses who are comfortable with their own sexuality are able to establish rapport and elicit relevant information from couples with fertility problems.

The first interview should involve both partners and include a comprehensive history and physical examination. Table 7–2 lists the items in a complete infertility physical workup and laboratory evaluation for both partners. Because at least 20% of infertility is related to a male factor, a semen analysis should be one of the first diagnostic tests done before moving on to more invasive diagnostic procedures involving the woman. Figure 7–1 outlines the historical database, diagnostic tests usually performed, and healthcare interventions used in cases of infertility.

Assessment of the Woman's Fertility

After a thorough history and physical examination, both partners may undergo tests to identify causes of infertility. A thorough female evaluation includes assessment of the hypothalamic–pituitary axis in terms of ovulatory function, as well as structure and function of the cervix, uterus, fallopian tubes, and ovaries. See Chapter 3 for an in-depth discussion of the fertility cycle and *Key Facts to Remember: Summary of Female Reproductive Cycle* also in Chapter 3.

EVALUATION OF OVULATORY AND CERVICAL FACTORS

Ovulation problems are a common cause of infertility.

Testing for Ovulation. There have been significant changes in ovulation testing as a result of evidence-based studies (ASRM, 2015a). Basal body temperature recording is the least expensive method for detecting ovulation, but interpretation of these charts can be complex and have wide variations depending on who is reading them; however, it is still commonly used by women. Several other tests have limited clinical utility including endometrial biopsy, postcoital testing, and evaluation of cervical factors (e.g., mucus elasticity [see Figure 5–4A] and ferning [see Figure 5–4B]) and are not considered to be the preferred methods in the evaluation of the infertile female.

TEACHING HIGHLIGHTS | Suggestions for Improving Fertility

- Avoid douching and artificial lubricants (gels, oils, saliva) that can alter sperm motility. Prevent alteration of pH of vagina and introduction of spermicidal agents.
- Promote retention of sperm. The male superior position with female remaining recumbent for at least 20 to 30 minutes after intercourse maximizes the number of sperm reaching the cervix.
- Avoid leakage of sperm. Have the woman elevate her hips with a pillow after intercourse for 20 to 30 minutes to allow liquefaction of seminal fluid and motility of the sperm toward the egg. Avoid getting up to urinate or shower for 1 hour after intercourse.
- Maximize the potential for fertilization. Instruct the couple that it is optimal if sexual intercourse occurs every other day during the fertile period. Because each woman's menstrual cycle varies in length, the fertile period can extend from cycle day (CD) 7 through CD 17. Note CD 1 is considered the first day of actual menstrual flow.
- Avoid emphasizing conception during sexual encounters to decrease anxiety and potential sexual dysfunction.
- Maintain adequate nutrition and reduce stress. Stress reduction techniques and good nutritional habits increase sperm production.
- Explore other methods to increase fertility awareness, such as home assessment of cervical mucus and basal body temperature (BBT) recordings, and use of a home ovulation predictor kit (tests LH surge to time intercourse).
- Consider incorporating culturally appropriate methods to enhance fertility.

TABLE 7–2 Initial Infertility Physical Workup and Laboratory Evaluations

FEMALE	MALE
Physical Examination	**Physical Examination**
Assessment of height, weight, blood pressure, temperature, and general health status	General health (assessment of height, weight, blood pressure)
Endocrine evaluation of thyroid for exophthalmos, lid lag, tremor, or palpable gland	Endocrine evaluation (e.g., presence of gynecomastia)
Optic fundi evaluation for presence of increased intracranial pressure, especially in oligomenorrheal or amenorrheal women (possible pituitary tumor)	Visual fields evaluation for bitemporal hemianopia (blindness in one half of the visual field)
Reproductive features (including breast and external genital area)	Abnormal hair patterns
Physical ability to tolerate pregnancy	**Urologic Examination**
Pelvic Examination	Presence or absence of phimosis (narrowing of the preputial orifice)
Papanicolaou (Pap) smear	Location of urethral meatus
Culture for gonorrhea if indicated and possibly chlamydia or mycoplasma culture (opinions vary)	Size and consistency of each testis, vas deferens, and epididymis
Signs of vaginal infections (see Chapter 6)	Presence of varicocele (enlargement of spermatic cord veins above testicles)
Shape of escutcheon (e.g., does pubic hair distribution resemble that of a male?)	**Rectal Examination**
Size of clitoris (enlargement caused by endocrine disorders)	Size and consistency of prostate, with microscopic evaluation of prostate fluid for signs of infection
Evaluation of cervix: old lacerations, tears, erosion, polyps, condition and shape of os, signs of infections, cervical mucus (evaluate for estrogen effect of spinnbarkeit and cervical ferning)	Size and consistency of seminal vesicles
Bimanual Examination	**Laboratory Examination**
Size, shape, position, and motility of uterus	Complete blood count
Presence of congenital anomalies	Sedimentation rate, if indicated
Evaluation for endometriosis	Serology
Evaluation of adnexa: ovarian size, cysts, fixations, or tumors	Urinalysis
Rectovaginal Examination	Rh factor and blood grouping
Presence of retroflexed or retroverted uterus	Semen analysis
Presence of rectouterine pouch masses	If indicated, testicular biopsy, buccal smear (to determine number of Barr bodies)
Presence of possible endometriosis	Hormonal assays, FSH, LH, prolactin
Laboratory Examination	
Complete blood count	
Sedimentation rate, if indicated	
Serology	
Urinalysis	
Rh factor and blood grouping	
Rubella IgG	
Follicle-stimulating hormone (FSH) level regardless of age and regularity of menstrual cycles	
If indicated depending on age and regularity of menstrual cycles: thyroid-stimulating hormone (TSH), prolactin levels (PRL), glucose tolerance test, hormonal assays including estradiol (E_2), luteinizing hormone (LH), midluteal progesterone (MLP), dehydroepiandrosterone (DHEA), androstenedione, testosterone, 17 alpha-hydroxy progesterone (17–OHP).	

Note: Adequate reproductive hormones must be present in both the female and the male.

Serum testing is generally used for assessment of ovulatory function in women with irregular menstrual cycles. A mid-luteal phase serum progesterone level should be obtained approximately 1 week before expected menstruation to document ovulation. A progesterone level greater than 3 ng/mL collected on or about day 21 for a typical 28-day cycle is evidence of recent ovulation. If the progesterone level is less than 3 ng/mL, an evaluation of anovulation is warranted. This includes measurement of serum prolactin, thyroid-stimulating hormone (TSH), FSH, and assessment for PCOS.

Over-the-counter urinary ovulation prediction kits are also available. These kits detect LH and predict the timing of the LH surge, which reliably predicts ovulation. However, they have false-positive and false-negative rates. Serum confirmation may be useful for clients unable to detect urinary LH surge. See *Teaching Highlights: Methods of Determining Ovulation.*

Ovarian Insufficiency. Diminished ovarian reserve should be evaluated during the initial infertility evaluation. Reduced oocyte quality or quantity can impact female fertility, especially for women

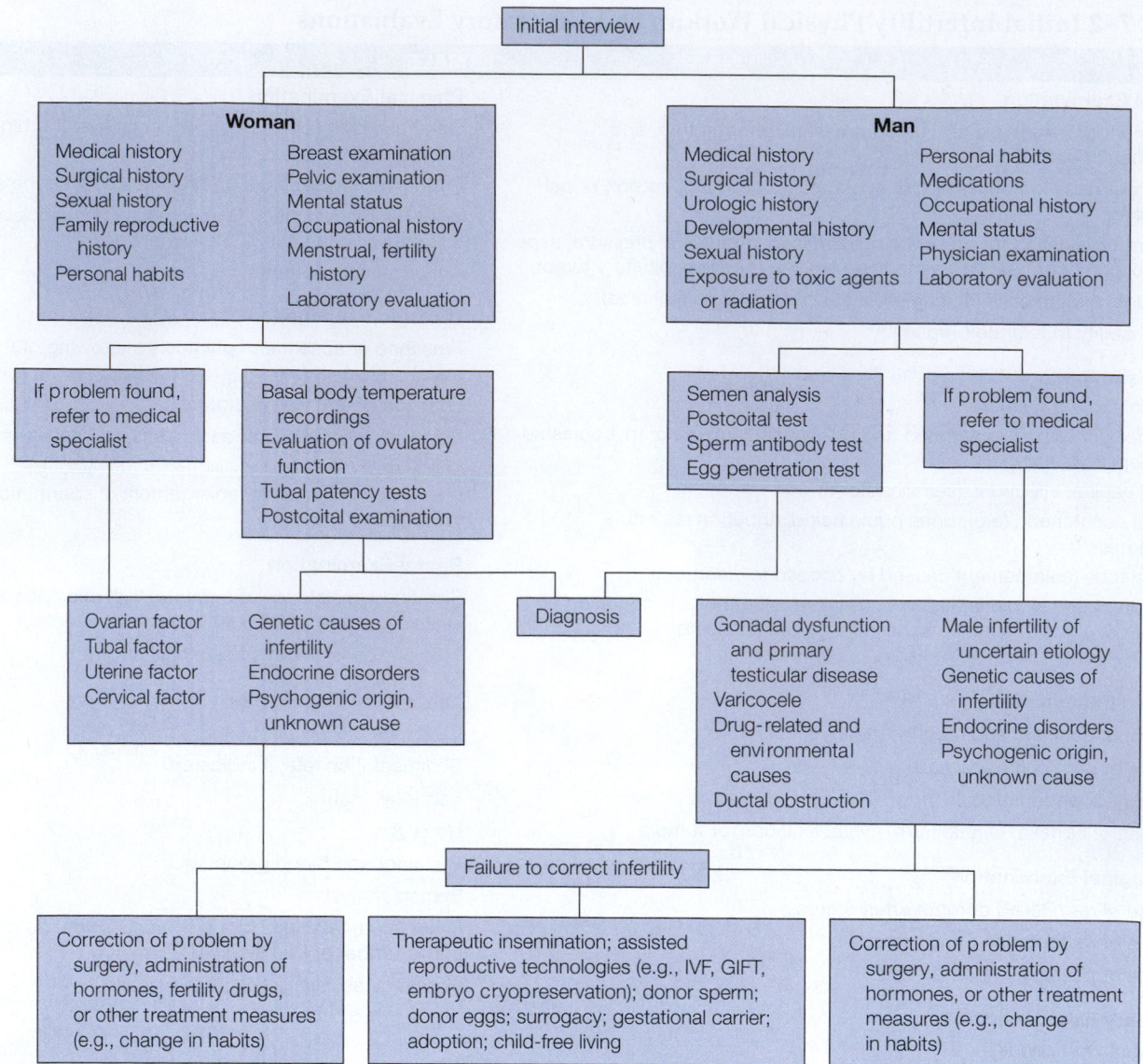

Figure 7–1 Flowchart for management of the infertile couple.

TEACHING HIGHLIGHTS | Methods of Determining Ovulation

Basal Body Temperature Method

The basal body temperature (BBT) method relies on assessing the woman's temperature pattern.

Describe the expected findings with an ovulatory (biphasic) cycle and stress the need to monitor BBT for 3 to 4 months to establish a pattern. BBT can be used to time intercourse if pregnancy is desired or as a method of natural family planning. Describe the timing of intercourse to achieve or avoid pregnancy.

Procedure for Measuring BBT

- Using a BBT thermometer, the woman chooses one site (oral, vaginal, or rectal), which she uses consistently.
- The woman takes her temperature every day before arising and before starting any activity, including

smoking. Any activity can produce an increase in body temperature.

Note: Read and follow manufacturers' instructions for each type of BBT thermometer in regard to the amount of time needed for an accurate reading.

- The result is then recorded immediately on a BBT chart, and the temperature dots for each day are connected to form a graph (Figure 7–2).
- The woman then shakes the thermometer down and cleans it in preparation for use the next day.

Explain that certain situations can disturb body temperature, such as large alcohol intake, sleeplessness, fever, warm climate, jet lag, shift work, the use of an electric blanket, or use of a heated waterbed.

Cervical Mucus Method

Explain that cervical mucus changes throughout a woman's menstrual cycle and that the quality of the mucus can be used to predict ovulation.

Procedure for Assessing Cervical Mucus Changes

- Every day when she uses the bathroom the woman checks her vagina, either by dabbing the vaginal opening with toilet paper or by putting a finger in the opening.
- She notes the wetness (presence of mucus), collects some mucus, determines its color and consistency, and records her findings on a chart.
- She washes her hands before and after the procedure.

LH Predictor Kit Method

Explain that LH kits are a good predictor of ovulation for a woman with a history of regular menstrual cycles.

Procedure for Using an LH Predictor Kit

- Determine the length of the woman's menstrual cycle. Use a calendar to determine the cycle day the woman will initiate testing.
- Testing must occur at the same time daily. The morning is recommended, because the LH concentration is highest upon wakening.
- Begin testing with the first morning urine void and examine the test strips for color changes that indicate if ovulation has occurred or is close to occurring.

Mittelschmerz

Explain that mittelschmerz (midcycle pain) located in the lower pelvis is a common symptom of ovulation.

Encourage the woman to document this occurrence (or absence) on her BBT chart.

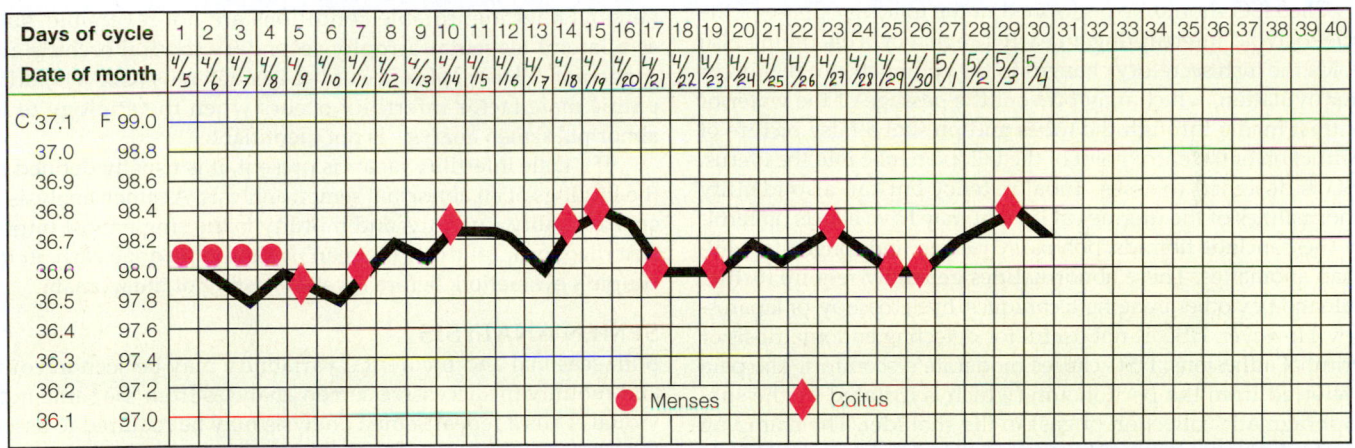

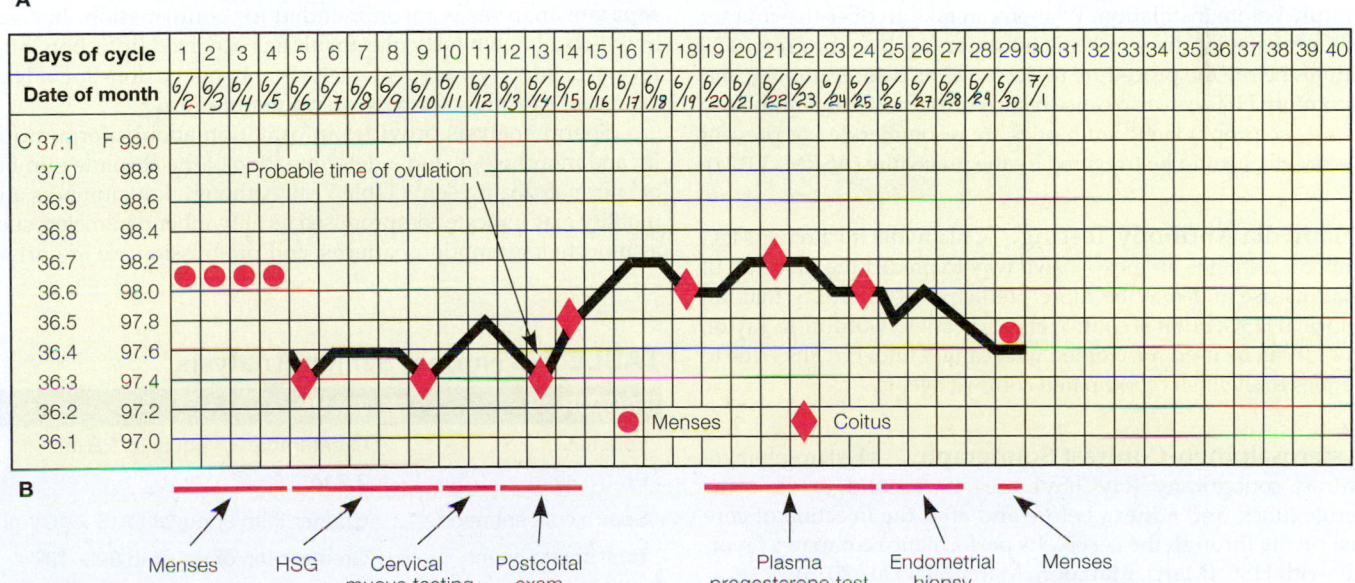

Figure 7–2 A. Monophasic, anovulatory basal body temperature (BBT) chart. B. Biphasic BBT chart illustrating probable time of ovulation, the different types of testing, and the time in the cycle that each would be performed.

over 35 years of age and younger women with risk factors for premature ovarian failure. Ovarian reserve can be tested with a day 3 FSH level or, in some cases, a clomiphene citrate challenge test (CCCT), antral follicle count (AFC), or anti-Müllerian hormone (AMH) level (Mutlu, Erdem, Erdem, et al., 2013).

EVALUATION OF UTERINE STRUCTURES AND TUBAL PATENCY

Uterine abnormalities are a relatively uncommon cause of infertility, but should be considered. Tubal patency and uterine structure are usually evaluated by hysterosalpingography or laparoscopy. Other invasive tests used to evaluate only the uterine cavity are hysteroscopy and sonohysterography. Hysteroscopy may be performed earlier in the evaluation if the woman's history suggests potential for adhesive disease or uterine abnormalities.

Hysterosalpingography.   Hysterosalpingography (HSG), or *hysterogram*, involves an instillation of either water or a lipid-soluble contrast media into the uterine cavity. In addition, HSG may have a therapeutic effect. This effect may be caused by the flushing of debris, breaking of adhesions, or induction of peristalsis produced by the instillation.

The HSG should be performed in the follicular phase of the cycle to avoid interrupting an early pregnancy. This timing also avoids the lush secretory changes in the endometrium that occur after ovulation, which may prevent the passage of the water or contrast media through the tubes and present a false picture of obstruction of the entry point of the fallopian tube into the uterus. HSG is designed to assess tubal patency but can also identify abnormalities of the uterine cavity that may have effects on fertility. These include fibroids, polyps, synechiae, and congenital Müllerian anomalies. These abnormalities generally require further evaluation by other imaging techniques, hysteroscopy, or laparoscopy. However, HSG is not useful for detecting endometriosis or peritubal adhesions. HSG causes moderate discomfort. The pain is referred from the peritoneum (which is irritated by the subdiaphragmatic collection of gas) to the shoulder. The cramping may be decreased if the radiopaque dye is warmed to body temperature before instillation. Women can take an over-the-counter (OTC) prostaglandin synthesis inhibitor (such as ibuprofen) 30 minutes before the procedure to decrease the pain, cramping, and discomfort. HSG can also cause recurrence of pelvic inflammatory disease, so prophylactic antibiotics are recommended to prevent infection that could be triggered by the procedure (ASRM, 2012a).

Chlamydia Antibody Testing.   Chlamydia trachomatis IgG antibody testing is an inexpensive way to predict the presence of tubal disease and may be more predictive of infertility than an abnormal HSG; but it is controversial (Lebovic, Gordon, & Taylor, 2014). It can be used for women who cannot undergo HSG due to allergies to shellfish or iodinated contrast agents.

Hysterosalpingo-Contrast Sonography.   Hysterosalpingo-contrast sonography (HyCoSy) uses ultrasound to view the uterus, tubes, and adnexa before and after the injection of contrast media through the cervix. Its performance compares favorably with HSG (Marci, Marcucci, Marcucci, et al., 2013).

Hysteroscopy and Laparoscopy.   *Hysteroscopy* is the definitive method for both diagnosis and treatment of intrauterine pathology (ASRM, 2015a). Hysteroscopy permits evaluation of any areas of suspicion within the uterine cavity or fallopian tubes revealed by the HSG. It can be done in conjunction with a laparoscopy or independently in the office and does not require general anesthesia.

A fiberoptic instrument called a *hysteroscope* is placed into the uterus for further evaluation of polyps, fibroids, or structural variations. The newest generation hysteroscope allows for minor operative procedures to be performed in the office setting.

Laparoscopy enables direct visualization of the pelvic organs to evaluate endometriosis and pelvic adhesions. It is used only if there is strong clinical suspicion of these conditions or before considering more aggressive treatments with higher risks and/or costs (ASRM, 2012a). Diagnostic laparoscopy is an outpatient procedure requiring the use of general anesthesia. In routine preanesthesia instructions, the nurse should tell the woman that she may have some discomfort from organ displacement and shoulder and chest pain caused by gas in the abdomen. The woman should be informed that she can resume normal activities as tolerated after 24 hours. Using postoperative pain medication and assuming a supine position may help relieve discomfort caused by any remaining gas.

Assessment of the Man's Fertility

Male infertility can be caused by numerous factors, some of which can be identified and are reversible, such as ductal obstruction and varicocele (an abnormal dilation of scrotal veins). Other identifiable conditions are not reversible, such as bilateral testicular atrophy secondary to viral orchitis and congenital bilateral absence of the vas deferens (CBAVD). Idiopathic male factor infertility occurs when the etiology of an abnormal semen analysis is not identifiable.

If a male infertility factor is present, it is usually defined by the findings of an abnormal semen analysis. A semen analysis of sperm quality, quantity, and motility is the single most important diagnostic study of the man. It should be done early in the couple's evaluation, before invasive testing of the woman.

SEMEN ANALYSIS

Both seasonal and incidental variability may be seen in count and motility in successive semen analyses from the same individual. Thus a repeat semen analysis may be required to assess the man's fertility potential adequately; a minimum of two separate analyses is recommended for confirmation. In cases in which a known testicular insult has occurred (infection, high fevers, or surgery), a repeat analysis may not be done for at least 2.5 months to allow for new sperm maturation.

Sperm analysis provides information about sperm motility and morphology and a determination of the absolute number of spermatozoa present (Table 7–3). Although low numbers and motility may indicate compromised fertility, other parameters such as morphology, motion patterns, and progression are important

TABLE 7–3 Normal Semen Analysis

FACTOR	VALUE
Volume	Greater than or equal to 1.5 ml
Ph	7.2 to 7.8
Sperm concentration	Greater than or equal to 15×10^6/ml
Total sperm count	Greater than or equal to 39×10^6
Progressive motility	Greater than or equal to 32%
Total motility	Greater than or equal to 40%
Normal morphology (strict criteria)	Greater than or equal to 4%
Vitality	Greater than or equal to 58%

Source: Cooper, T., Noonan, E., von Eckardstein, S., et al. (2010). World Health Organization reference values for human semen characteristics. *Human Reproduction Update, 16*(3), 231–45.

prognostic indicators. The quality of sperm decreases with increasing paternal age and may result in chromosomal damage. For example, fathers older than 40 years may be at an increased risk for offspring with chromosomal abnormalities or new gene mutations.

Genetic factors may affect male fertility. Men with oligospermia (semen with a low concentration of sperm) and nonobstructive azoospermia (impaired or nonexistent sperm production) have an increased risk for chromosomal abnormalities and Y chromosome deletions (ASRM, 2015b). Spermatozoa have been shown to possess intrinsic antigens that can provoke male immunologic infertility. Any disruption in the blood–testes barrier, such as vasectomy reversals, or genital trauma, such as testicular torsion, can lead to the production of antisperm antibodies (ASA) (Garolla, Pizzol, Bertoldo, et al., 2013). Treatment for antisperm antibodies is directed toward preventing the formation of antibodies or arresting the underlying mechanism that compromises sperm function. The treatment of choice for clinically significant antisperm antibodies is intracytoplasmic sperm injection (ICSI) in conjunction with in vitro fertilization (IVF). If the man's history indicates, he may be referred to an urologist for further testing.

Methods of Infertility Management

Methods of managing infertility include pharmacologic agents, therapeutic insemination, IVF, and other assisted reproductive techniques. In addition, many couples choose adoption as their preferred response to infertility.

PHARMACOLOGIC AGENTS

The pharmacologic treatment chosen depends on the specific cause of infertility.

Clomiphene Citrate. Oral clomiphene citrate (Clomid, Serophene) is often used as first-line therapy to induce ovulation in women with normal ovaries, a normal prolactin level, and an intact pituitary gland. It works by binding to estrogen receptors in the hypothalamus and pituitary gland. This blocks the negative feedback of circulating estrogen and stimulates a release of GnRH, LH, and FSH, thereby inducing ovulation. The antiestrogenic effects of clomiphene may cause a decrease in cervical mucus production and endometrial lining development.

For the first course of clomiphene citrate the woman usually takes 50 mg/day orally for 5 days from cycle day (CD) 3 to day 7 or CD 5 to day 9. Ovulation should be confirmed to ensure that if continued doses are needed, they are at the lowest possible dose. In nonresponders, the dose may be increased to 100 mg/day to a maximum of 250 mg/day, although doses in excess of 100 mg/day are not approved by the FDA. The woman is informed that if ovulation occurs, it is expected to occur 5 to 9 days after the last dose. The nurse determines if the couple has been advised to have sexual intercourse every other day for 1 week, beginning 5 days after the last day of medications. Most women who conceive do so within the first 6 cycles, although the medication can be continued for 12 cycles (Propst & Wright Bates, 2012).

Women can assess the presence of ovulation and possible response to clomiphene therapy by doing BBT and urinary LH tests. The woman should be knowledgeable about side effects and call her healthcare provider if they occur. When visual disturbances (flashes, blurring, or spots) occur, bright lighting should be avoided. This side effect disappears within a few days or weeks after discontinuation of therapy. The occurrence of hot flashes may be because of the antiestrogenic properties of clomiphene citrate. The woman can obtain some relief by increasing intake of fluids and using fans. Other side effects include pain,

soreness, breast discomfort, nausea and vomiting, headaches, dryness or loss of hair, and multiple pregnancies.

After the first treatment cycle, a pelvic ultrasound should be done to rule out ovarian enlargement, ovarian cysts, or hyperstimulation. Ovarian enlargement and abdominal discomfort (bloating) may result from follicular growth and formation of multiple corpora lutea. Persistence of ovarian cysts is a contraindication for further treatment regimens. Failure to conceive after clomiphene induction is an indication to expand the diagnostic evaluation or to change the overall treatment plan if evaluation is complete.

Gonadotropins. *Human menopausal gonadotropins (hMGs)* are indicated as a first line of therapy for anovulatory infertile women with low to normal levels of gonadotropins (FSH and LH). It is a second line of therapy in women who fail to ovulate or conceive with clomiphene citrate therapy and in women undergoing controlled ovarian stimulation with assisted reproduction.

Gonadotropin therapy requires close observation with serum estradiol levels and ultrasound. Follicle development must be monitored to minimize the risk of multiple pregnancies and to avoid ovarian hyperstimulation syndrome.

SAFETY ALERT!

Ovarian hyperstimulation syndrome (OHSS) is a potentially life-threatening complication of ovulation induction and can, in its most severe form, result in massive ovarian enlargement and multiple cysts, hemoconcentration, and third-space accumulation of fluid. This can lead to renal failure, hypovolemic shock, thromboembolism, acute respiratory distress syndrome, and death.

The daily dose of medication given is titrated based on serum estradiol and ultrasound findings, but usually starts with a dose of 50 to 100 IU daily. Human chorionic gonadotropin (hCG) is used to trigger ovulation once ovarian follicles are mature. The couple is advised to have intercourse 24 to 36 hours after hCG administration and each day for the next 2 days. Women who elect to undergo ovarian stimulation with gonadotropins have usually passed through all other forms of management without conceiving. Strong emotional support and thorough education are needed because of the numerous office visits and injections that are required. Often the partner is instructed, with return demonstration, to administer the daily injections. The risk of multiple gestations is higher with gonadotropin therapy than with clomiphene citrate therapy (ASRM, 2012b).

Letrozole. Originally developed for the treatment of advanced breast cancer in postmenopausal women, letrozole is more commonly being used off-label for ovulation induction (Pavone & Bulun, 2013). This aromatase inhibitor blocks the conversion of androgens to estrogens. When estradiol levels are low, there are less negative feedback on the hypothalamus and pituitary and increased levels of GnRH and FSH to stimulate follicular development. Letrozole can be used in women who experience side effects from or do not respond to clomiphene. Like clomiphene, it is given for 5 consecutive days starting as early as day 3 of the cycle. Data suggest that letrozole has a lower incidence of multiple gestation pregnancies compared to clomiphene and gonadotropins (ASRM, 2012b; Propst & Wright Bates, 2012).

Bromocriptine. High prolactin levels may impair the glandular production of FSH and LH or block their action on the ovaries. When hyperprolactinemia accompanies anovulation, the infertility may be treated with bromocriptine (Parlodel).

This medication acts directly on the prolactin-secreting cells in the anterior pituitary. It inhibits the pituitary's secretion of prolactin, thus preventing suppression of the secretion of FSH and LH. This restores normal menstrual cycles and induces ovulation by allowing FSH and LH production.

Gonadatropin-Releasing Hormone (GnRH). *GnRH* is a therapeutic tool for inducing ovulation, but its use is limited to women who have insufficient endogenous release of GnRH or it is used adjunctively with gonadotropin therapy. Pulsatile GnRH therapy is administered by continuous intravenous infusion with a portable infusion pump. With this method, GnRH is released intravenously every 60 to 90 minutes at a dose of 2.5 to 10.0 mcg per pulse. Pulsatile GnRH is available in the United States but is used more widely in other parts of the world.

Insulin-Sensitizing Agents. Approximately 80% of anovulatory women have polycystic ovary syndrome (PCOS), causing insulin resistance and hyperinsulinemia. Strategies to induce ovulation include weight loss followed by oral treatment with clomiphene, aromatase inhibitors including letrozole, or gonadotropin therapy. However, hyperinsulinemia may cause these clients to be more resistant to treatment. Recently, studies have shown that oral hypoglycemia agents (e.g., metformin and rosiglitazone) can induce ovulation in women with PCOS. Clinical trials are underway to determine the appropriateness of oral hypoglycemic agents with and without clomiphene in the infertility setting but so far have shown little improvement in outcomes (Balen, 2013). For this reason, oral hypoglycemia agents are not prescribed unless the client has impairment in glucose tolerance.

Complementary Therapies. Couples experiencing infertility may seek out alternative treatments. Some common complementary therapies include pelvic physical therapy, hypnosis, yoga, homeopathy, spiritual healing, acupuncture, and herbal therapy. Data suggest that the two most common types of complementary or alternative therapies are acupuncture and herbal remedies.

Acupuncture is a therapy used in traditional Chinese medicine (TCM) and involves inserting sterile needles into specific points on the body to control the flow of chi, or life energy. Acupuncture treatment focuses on balancing the flow of chi in the kidneys and adrenal glands. It has been shown to be effective by inhibiting uterine motility during embryo transfer and improving the endometrial environment for embryo implantation. Several studies have shown that acupuncture can increase the clinical pregnancy rate and live birth rate among women undergoing in vitro fertilization (Smith, de Lacey, Chapman, et al., 2012).

Herbs frequently recommended to treat infertility include ginseng and astragalus. Herbalists cite the healing and hormone-balancing effects of these herbs. Ginseng has historically been used in TCM to enhance male virility and fertility.

The nurse should be alert for signs that the couple is pursuing complementary therapies. A sensitive, nonjudgmental approach will go a long way toward comforting a couple and assuring them that many complementary therapies are helpful and not harmful.

THERAPEUTIC INSEMINATION
Therapeutic insemination has replaced the previously used term *artificial insemination* and involves the depositing of semen at the cervical os or in the uterus by mechanical means. *Therapeutic donor insemination (TDI)* is the current term for use of donor semen, and *therapeutic husband insemination (THI)* is the current term for use of the husband's semen.

THI is generally indicated for the following:

- Seminal deficiencies such as oligospermia (low sperm count), asthenospermia (decreased motility), and teratospermia (low percentage, abnormal morphology)
- Anatomic defects accompanied by inadequate deposition of semen such as hypospadia (a congenital abnormal male urethral opening on the underside of the penis)
- Ejaculatory dysfunction (such as retrograde ejaculation)
- Some cases of female factor infertility, such as scant or inhospitable mucus, persistent cervicitis, or cervical stenosis
- Cases of unexplained infertility

The couple undergoing genetic counseling may consider therapeutic donor insemination. This alternative is appropriate in several instances; for example, if the man has an autosomal dominant disease, TDI would decrease to zero the risk of having an affected child (if the sperm donor is not at risk), because the child would not inherit any genes from the affected parent. If the man is affected with an X-linked disorder and does not wish to continue the gene in the family (all his daughters will be carriers), TDI would be an alternative to terminating all pregnancies with a female fetus. If the man is a carrier for a balanced translocation and if termination of pregnancy is against family ethics, TDI is an appropriate alternative. If both parents are carriers of an autosomal recessive disorder, TDI lowers the risk to a very low level or to zero if a carrier test is available. Finally, TDI may be appropriate if the family is at high risk for a multifactorial disorder.

TDI is considered in cases of azoospermia (absence of sperm), severe oligospermia or asthenospermia, inherited male sex-linked disorders, and autosomal dominant disorders. In the past several years, indications for donor insemination have expanded to include single women or lesbians desirous of pregnancy. Some states have specified the parental rights of single women and donors, but most are silent on this issue.

TDI has become more complicated and expensive in the past decade because of the need for strict screening and processing procedures to prevent transmission of a genetic defect or sexually transmitted infection to the offspring or recipient. Guidelines have been established and updated by the American Society for Reproductive Medicine (ASRM, 2013a) that include mandatory medical (genetic) and infectious disease screening of both donor and recipient, the need for informed consent from all parties, the need to limit the number of pregnancies per donor, and the need for accurate means of record keeping. Finally, because of the risk of transmitting infectious diseases, donated sperm must be frozen and quarantined for 6 months from the time of acquisition, and the donor must be retested before sperm can be released for use.

Numerous factors need to be evaluated before TDI is performed. Has every possible effort been made to diagnose and treat the cause of the male infertility? Do tests indicate normal fertility and sperm–ovum transport in the woman? Has the couple had an opportunity to discuss this option with an infertility counselor to explore the issues of secrecy, disclosure, and potential feelings of loss the couple (particularly the male partner) may feel about not having a genetic child? Are there any religious constraints? After making the decision, the couple should allow themselves time to further assess their concerns and explore their feelings individually and together to ensure that this option is acceptable to both.

IN VITRO FERTILIZATION
In vitro fertilization (IVF) is selectively used in cases when infertility has resulted from tubal factors, mucous abnormalities, male infertility, unexplained infertility, male and female immunologic

Developing Cultural Competence Infertility Treatments

The acceptance of infertility treatments varies widely around the world. Some belief systems do not allow various treatments because using a fertility treatment is considered interfering with God's design or because the treatment itself is seen as tainted or sinful. For example, artificial reproductive technology in predominantly Muslim countries is accepted and encouraged because adoption is not an accepted solution. However, the approved methods for treating infertility are limited to use of therapeutic insemination using the husband's sperm or IVF involving the fertilization of the wife's ovum by the husband's sperm because the use of donor sperm, egg, or embryo is condemned by Islamic law (Obeisat, Gharaibeh, Owis, et al., 2012).

In Jewish cultures, infertile couples are encouraged to try all possible means to have children, including egg and sperm donation. However, owing to the *Niddah* laws of separation, Orthodox Jewish women are forbidden from engaging in sexual intercourse from the start of their menstruation until 7 days after the end of menses, when they immerse themselves in a ritual bath (*mikveh*). Women with unexpected spotting or bleeding must seek the advice of a rabbi or physician, and if uterine bleeding is diagnosed, she may not participate in intercourse for 7 days thereafter (Haimov-Kochman, Adler, Ein-Mor, et al., 2012). For this reason, Jewish law has a significant impact on fertility, particularly for women with irregular and unpredictable cycles. If the infertility is because of a male factor, artificial insemination with sperm from a non-Jewish sperm donor is acceptable because "Jewishness" is conferred through the matriline. IVF and embryo transfer (ET) are also acceptable therapeutic insemination methods because they do not involve putting sperm into another's wife.

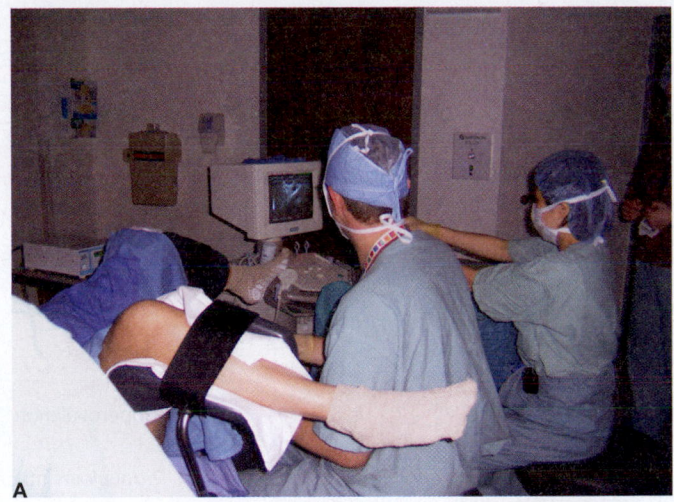

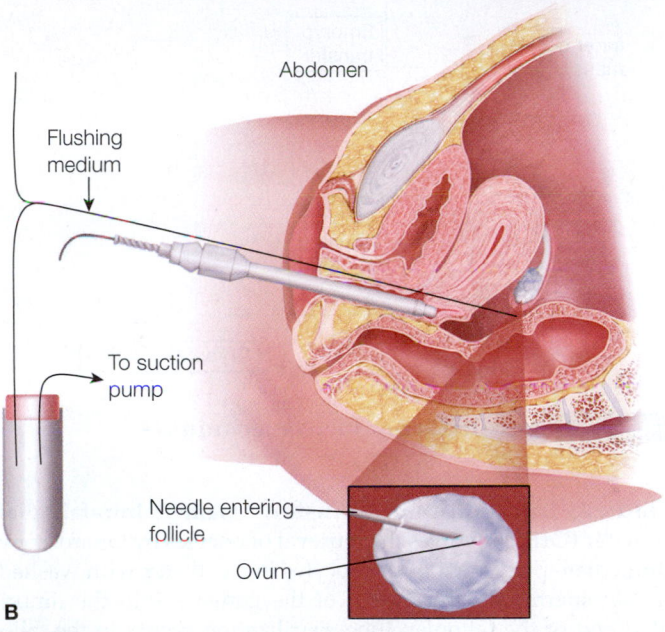

Figure 7–3 **A. Operating room setup for ultrasound-guided oocyte retrieval. B. Transvaginal ultrasound-guided oocyte retrieval.**

infertility, and cervical factors. In IVF a woman's eggs are collected from her ovaries, fertilized in the laboratory, and placed into her uterus after normal embryo development has begun. These steps occur over a 2-week period of time, known as an *IVF cycle*. If the procedure is successful, the embryo continues to develop in the uterus, and pregnancy proceeds naturally.

Fertility drugs are used to induce ovulation before the process of IVF begins. Follicular development and oocyte maturity are monitored frequently with ultrasound and hormonal assays. Monitoring usually begins around cycle day 5, and medications are titrated according to individual response. When follicles appear mature, hCG is given to stimulate final egg maturation and control the induction of ovulation. Egg retrieval is performed approximately 34 to 36 hours later, before ovulation occurs.

In the majority of cases, egg retrieval is performed by a transvaginal approach under ultrasound guidance (Figure 7–3). It is an outpatient procedure performed with intravenous sedation and a cervical block for anesthesia. A needle guide that helps direct the aspiring needle through the posterior vaginal wall into the follicle is attached to the vaginal ultrasound probe. Many follicles can be aspirated with only one puncture, and the procedure generally lasts no more than 30 minutes. Many physicians use prophylactic antibiotics to reduce the risk of infection from the procedure.

Oocytes are then mixed with spermatozoa in culture medium and fertilization is confirmed about 17 hours later by observing two pronuclei within the zygote. After

fertilization, the cells will continue to divide exponentially every 12 to 14 hours so that the embryo is approximately eight cells about 72 hours after retrieval. Many programs will transfer these *cleavage stage* embryos at this time. Some programs wait until day 5 when the embryo is at the *blastocyst stage*, with the theory that better quality embryos can be transferred at a time when natural implantation would be occurring. After the procedure, the woman is advised to engage in only minimal activity for 12 to 24 hours. To optimize endometrial receptivity, progesterone supplementation is prescribed at the time of oocyte retrieval or embryo transfer to promote implantation and support the early pregnancy (Hill, Whitcomb, Lewis, et al., 2013).

OTHER ASSISTED REPRODUCTIVE TECHNIQUES

Other assisted reproductive techniques (Figure 7–4) include procedures for transfer of gametes, zygotes, or embryos; cryopreservation of embryos; IVF using donor oocytes; assisted hatching (AH); and use of a gestational carrier (surrogate).

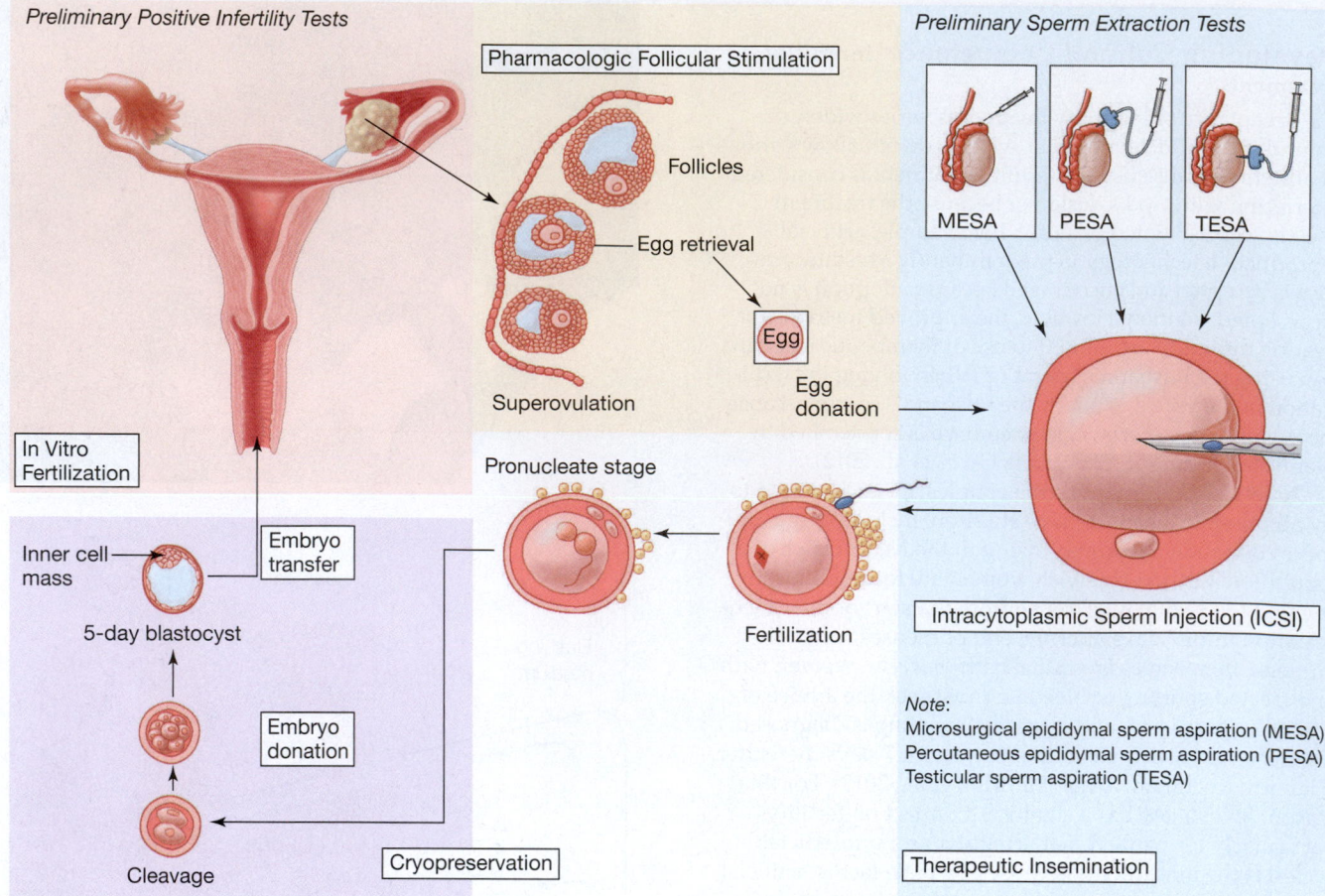

Figure 7–4 Assisted reproductive techniques.

Gamete Intrafallopian Transfer. **Gamete intrafallopian transfer (GIFT)** involves the retrieval of oocytes by laparoscopy; immediate placement of the oocytes in a catheter with washed, motile sperm; and placement of the gametes into the fimbriated end of the fallopian tube. Fertilization occurs in the fallopian tube as with normal conception (in vivo) rather than in the laboratory (in vitro). The fertilized egg then travels through the fallopian tube to the uterus for implantation as in normal reproduction. GIFT may be more acceptable than other procedures such as zygote intrafallopian transfer to adherents of some religions (e.g., Roman Catholic), because fertilization does not occur outside the woman's body.

From the GIFT technology evolved procedures such as **zygote intrafallopian transfer (ZIFT)** and **tubal embryo transfer (TET)**. In these procedures eggs are retrieved and incubated with the man's sperm. However, the eggs are transferred back to the woman's body at a much earlier stage of cell division than in IVF and, as in GIFT, are placed in the fallopian tube or tubes and not the uterus. In TET the placement is done at the embryo stage. These procedures allow fertilization to be documented, which is not possible with GIFT, and the pregnancy rate is theoretically increased when the fertilized ovum is placed in the fallopian tube.

A micromanipulation procedure called *assisted embryo hatching (AH)* has proved to be an effective adjunct therapy in IVF. IVF using a *gestational carrier* allows infertile women who are genetically sound but unable to carry a pregnancy to exercise the option of having their own biologic child. Other technologies involve oocyte donation and cryopreservation of the embryo (embryos are frozen and then thawed at a later date) (Michalakis, DeCherney, & Penzias, 2013).

Clinical Tip

If the woman and her husband have chosen to use cryopreservation to store unused embryos, it will be helpful for the nurse to remind the couple that they need to consider the following issues: Who has legal custody of the embryos? How long will they be frozen? What options does the couple have in the event of divorce, if one or both partners die, or if they do not wish to use the embryos at a later date?

Preimplantation Genetic Diagnosis. Recent advances in micromanipulation allow a single cell to be removed from the embryo for genetic study. Couples at risk for having a detectable single gene or chromosomal anomaly may wish to undergo such preimplantation genetic testing, called *blastomere analysis* or, more recently, *preimplantation genetic diagnosis (PGD)*. PGD is a term used when one or both genetic parents carry a gene mutation or balanced chromosome rearrangement and testing is performed to determine whether that mutation or unbalanced chromosomal complement has been passed to the oocyte or embryo. *Preimplantation genetic screening (PGS)* is a term used when the genetic parents are known or presumed to have normal chromosomes, and their embryos are screened for aneuploidy with the purpose of increasing the likelihood of a viable pregnancy with normal chromosomes. Results of genetic screening or testing on the preimplantation embryos are available in 4 to 24 hours, so unaffected embryos may still be transferred during the required biologic window of time without the need for cryopreservation. Both PGD and PCS can produce false positive and false negative results. Prenatal diagnostic testing to confirm the results is recommended.

The diagnosis of genetic disorders before implantation provides couples with the option of foregoing the attempt to establish a pregnancy and thereby avoiding a difficult decision about terminating an affected pregnancy (Kalfoglou, Kammersell, Philpott, et al., 2013). This technology raises several other ethical issues, including the following:

- Identification of couples at risk. There is a need for criteria that identify couples at risk for diseases that constitute significant hardship and suffering so that "wrongful birth" cases can be avoided.

- Availability of and access to centers providing PGD. Should society provide access for those at risk for genetic transfer of disease but without the financial resources to pay for the services?

- Analysis of blastomeres for sex chromosome testing when a genetic disorder carried on the sex chromosomes is suspected. In X-linked diseases, the only way to prevent the disorder is to select against the blastomere with the Y chromosome.

- Identification of late-onset diseases. The Human Genome Project has aided in the identification of genetic markers for late-onset disease. Couples may wish to choose to implant blastomeres that do not carry these markers.

- Effect on the offspring as a result of removing cells from the embryo.

- Selection for nonmedical reasons and potential concern of eugenics "designer babies."

Sperm Sorting. Sperm sorting is a technology designed to separate sperm that primarily produce females or those that primarily produce males. Sorted sperm enriched with male- or female-producing sperm is then used for IUI or IVF. The accuracy depends on the laboratory that performs the sorting and the technology it uses. Study data indicate that 9 out of 10 clients sorting for a girl will conceive a female. Approximately 3 out of 4 clients that sort for a boy will conceive a male. This technology is used to increase the likelihood of having a child of a particular gender in couples at risk for an X-linked genetic disorder or for couples interested in family balancing (gender selection when a couple has two or more children of the same gender) (Kalfoglou et al., 2013).

ADOPTION

Infertile couples consider various alternatives for resolving their infertility; adoption is one option that will be considered at several points during the treatment process. The adoption of a baby in the United States can be difficult and frustrating, often involving long waiting periods, continual setbacks, and high costs. Thus many couples seek international adoption, or consider adopting older children or children with handicaps, because the adoption process in such cases is quicker and more children are available. Nurses in the community can assist couples considering adoption by providing information on community resources for adoption and support through the adoption process. Informational books, websites such as Childless by Choice, and support groups such as San Francisco RESOLVE's "living without children" are available for couples who remain childless by choice or circumstance.

PREGNANCY AFTER INFERTILITY

The feeling of being infertile does not necessarily disappear with pregnancy. Although there may be initial ecstasy when the pregnancy is confirmed, couples may face a whole new arena of fear and anxiety, and the parents-to-be often do not know where they

"fit in." They may feel a great sense of isolation because those who have had no trouble conceiving cannot relate to the physical and emotional pain they endured to achieve the pregnancy. Contact with their past support system of other infertile couples may vanish when peers learn the couple has resolved their infertility. Although the desperation to become pregnant may have superseded the couple's ability to acknowledge their concerns about undergoing various treatments or procedures, questions about the repeated cycle of fertility drugs or the achievement of pregnancy through IVF technology or cryopreservation may now arise.

Couples may need reassurance throughout the pregnancy to allay these anxieties. The nurse can assist couples who conceive after infertility by acknowledging their past experiences of infertility treatment; validating their fears and anxieties as they face childbirth classes, birth, and parenting issues; and providing support and education about what to anticipate physically and emotionally throughout the pregnancy. The nurse can also counsel couples that infertility because of nonstructural causes may correct itself following a successful pregnancy and birth; therefore, postchildbirth contraception counseling may be warranted. These interventions will go a long way toward normalizing the experience for the couple.

> ### Women With Special Needs Down Syndrome and Fertility
>
> Women with Down syndrome have reduced fertility but can become pregnant. When one partner has Down syndrome, the risk of the baby having Down syndrome is 50%. If both parents have Down syndrome, the risk is higher. Most men with Down syndrome cannot conceive children. When a woman with Down syndrome does conceive, there is a high incidence of spontaneous abortions. These women also have higher rates of premature labor and cesarean birth.

RECURRENT PREGNANCY LOSS

Recurrent pregnancy loss (RPL) is a disease distinct from infertility, defined by two or more failed pregnancies (ASRM, 2013b). There are several etiologies, including maternal medical complications, chromosomal abnormalities and other genetic conditions, autoimmune disorders, and thrombotic causes. However, in up to 50% of couples with RPL, an etiology will not be identified (ASRM, 2013b).

Nursing Management

Infertility therapy taxes a couple's financial, physical, and emotional resources. Treatment can be costly, and insurance coverage is limited. Years of effort and numerous evaluations and examinations may take place before conception occurs, if it occurs at all. In a society that values children and considers them to be the natural result of marriage, infertile couples face a myriad of tensions and discrimination.

You will need to be constantly aware of the emotional needs of the couple confronting infertility evaluation and treatment. Often an intact marriage will become stressed with intrusive infertility procedures and treatments. Paying constant attention to temperature charts and following instructions about their sex life that came from a person outside the relationship understandably affect the spontaneity of a couple's interactions. Tests and treatments may heighten feelings of frustration or anger between partners. The need to share this intimate area of a relationship, especially when one or the other is identified as "the cause" of infertility, may precipitate feelings of guilt or shame. Many men report receiving less social support than women, leading to a sense of isolation (Fisher & Hammarberg, 2012; Agostini, Monti, Pascalis, et al., 2011).

The couple may experience feelings of loss of control, feelings of reduced competency and defectiveness, loss of status and ambiguity as a couple, a sense of social stigma, stress on the marital and sexual relationship, and a strained relationship with healthcare providers. The couple will need to recognize and express how infertility affects their lives and grieve the loss of potential children. They then can decide on a plan to manage their infertility (Sawatzky, 1981). Your roles can be summarized as those of counselor, educator, and advocate.

Your ability to assess and respond to emotional and educational needs is essential to give infertile couples a sense of control and help them negotiate the treatment process. It is important to use a nursing framework that recognizes the multidimensional needs of the infertile individual or couple within physical, social, psychologic, spiritual, and environmental contexts.

Infertility may be perceived as a loss by one or both partners. Affected individuals have described this as the loss of their relationships with spouses, family, or friends; their health; their status or prestige; their self-esteem and self-confidence; their security; and the potential child. Any one of these losses may lead to depression, but in many cases the crisis of infertility evokes feelings similar to those associated with all these losses (Barbieri, 2014). Each couple passes through several stages of feelings: surprise, denial, anger, isolation, guilt, grief, and resolution. The impact of these feelings on the couple and how fast they move into resolution, if ever, may depend on the cause and on the duration of treatment. Each partner may progress through the stages at different rates.

Nonjudgmental acceptance and a professional, caring attitude on your part can go far in dissipating the negative emotions the couple may experience while going through these stages. This is also a time when you may assess the couple's relationship: Are both partners able and willing to communicate verbally and share feelings? Are the partners mutually supportive? The answers to such questions may help to identify areas of strength and weakness and to construct an appropriate plan of care.

Referral to mental health professionals is helpful when the emotional issues become too disruptive in the couple's relationship or life. The couple should be aware of infertility support and education organizations that can help meet some of their needs and validate their feelings. Finally, individual or group counseling with other infertile couples can help the couple resolve feelings brought about by their own difficult situation.

Genetic Disorders

Even when conception has been achieved, families can have special reproductive concerns. The desired and expected outcome of any pregnancy is the birth of a healthy, "perfect" baby. Parents experience grief, fear, and anger when they discover that their baby has been born with a defect or a genetic disease. Such an abnormality may be evident at birth or may not appear for some time. The baby may have inherited a disorder from one parent or both, creating guilt and strife within the family.

Regardless of the type or scope of the problem, parents will have many questions: "What did I do?" "What caused it?" "How do I cope with it?" "Will it happen again?" The nurse must anticipate the couple's questions and concerns and guide, direct, and support the family. To do so, the nurse must have a basic knowledge of genetics and genetic counseling. Professional nurses can help expedite this process if they understand the principles involved and can direct the family to the appropriate resources.

Chromosomes and Chromosomal Analysis

All hereditary material is carried on tightly coiled strands of DNA known as **chromosomes**. The chromosomes carry the *genes*, the smallest units of inheritance, as discussed in greater detail in Chapter 4. The Human Genome Project has made remarkable advances toward determining the exact DNA sequence of human genes and the precise genes that are associated with certain abnormalities such as fragile X syndrome and cystic fibrosis, as discussed in greater detail later in the chapter (National Human Genome Research Institute, 2015).

All *somatic (body) cells* contain 46 chromosomes, which is the *diploid* number; the sperm and the egg each contain half as many (23) chromosomes, or the *haploid* number. There are 23 pairs of homologous chromosomes (a matched pair of chromosomes, one inherited from each parent). Twenty-two of the pairs are **autosomes** (nonsex chromosomes), and one pair is made up of the sex chromosomes, X and Y. A normal female has a 46, XX chromosome constitution; the normal male, 46, XY (Figures 7–5 and 7–6).

The **karyotype**, or pictorial analysis of these chromosomes, is usually obtained from specially treated and stained peripheral blood lymphocytes. Placental tissue or amniotic fluid can be obtained prenatally and sent for karyotyping of the fetus.

Chromosomal abnormalities can occur in either the autosomes or the sex chromosomes and can be divided into two categories: abnormalities of number and abnormalities of structure. Even small alterations in chromosomes can cause problems, especially those associated with delayed growth and

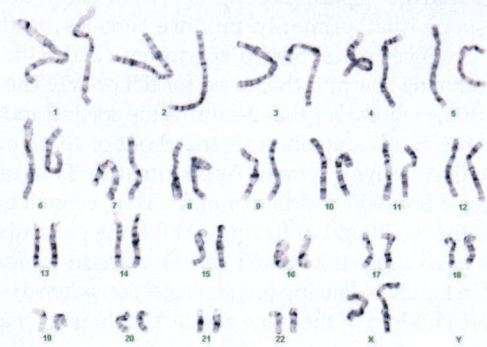

Figure 7–5 Normal female karyotype.

SOURCE: Susan Olson, PhD, Oregon Health & Science University Knight Diagnostic Laboratory.

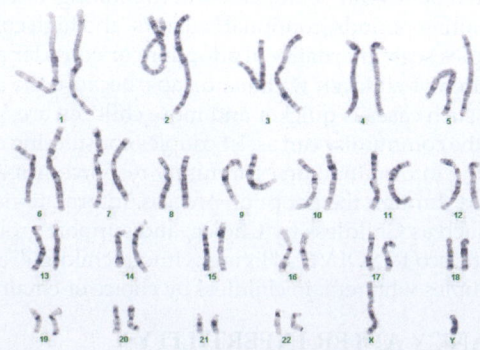

Figure 7–6 Normal male karyotype.

SOURCE: Susan Olson, PhD, Oregon Health & Science University Knight Diagnostic Laboratory.

development. Some of these abnormalities can be passed on to other offspring. Thus in some cases chromosomal analysis is appropriate even if clinical manifestations are mild.

ABNORMALITIES OF CHROMOSOMAL NUMBER

Abnormalities of chromosomal number are most commonly seen as trisomies, monosomies, and mosaicism. In all three cases, the abnormality is most often caused by *nondisjunction*, a failure of paired chromosomes to separate during cell division. If nondisjunction occurs in either the sperm or the egg before fertilization, the resulting zygote (fertilized egg) will have an abnormal chromosome makeup in all of the cells (trisomy or monosomy).

If nondisjunction occurs after fertilization, the developing zygote will have cells with two or more different chromosome makeups, evolving into two or more different cell lines (mosaicism).

Trisomies are the product of the union of a normal gamete (egg or sperm) with a gamete that contains an extra chromosome. The individual will have 47 chromosomes and be trisomic (i.e., will have three copies of the same chromosome) for whichever chromosome is extra (Table 7–4). Down syndrome (formerly called mongolism) is the most common trisomy abnormality seen in children (see Figure 7–7). The presence of the extra chromosome 21 produces distinctive clinical features (see Table 7–4 and Figure 7–8). Although children born with

TABLE 7–4 Chromosomal Syndromes

Altered Chromosome: 21	Characteristics
Genetic defect: trisomy 21 (Down syndrome) (secondary nondisjunction or 14/21 unbalanced translocation) Incidence: average 1 in 700 live births, incidence variable with age of woman	CNS: mild to moderate intellectual disability; hypotonia at birth Head: flattened occiput; depressed nasal bridge; almond-shaped eyes that slant up; prominent epicanthal folds; white specking of the iris (Brushfield spots); protrusion of the tongue; high, arched palate; low-set ears Hands: broad, short fingers; abnormalities of finger and foot; dermal ridge patterns (dermatoglyphics); transverse palmar crease (simian line) Other: congenital heart disease
Altered Chromosome: 18	**Characteristics**
Genetic defect: trisomy 18 Incidence: 1 in 3000 live births	CNS: intellectual disability; severe hypotonia Head: prominent occiput; low-set ears; corneal opacities; ptosis (drooping eyelids) Hands: third and fourth fingers overlapped by second and fifth fingers; abnormal dermatoglyphics; syndactyly (webbing of fingers) Other: congenital heart defects (>90%); renal abnormalities; single umbilical artery; gastrointestinal tract abnormalities; rocker-bottom feet; cryptorchidism; various malformations of other organs
Altered Chromosome: 13	**Characteristics**
Genetic defect: trisomy 13 Incidence: 1 in 5000 live births	CNS: intellectual disability; severe hypotonia; seizures; anatomic defects of the brain (holoprosencephaly) in 60% Head: microcephaly; microphthalmia, and/or coloboma (keyhole-shaped pupil); malformed ears; aplasia of external auditory canal; micrognathia (abnormally small lower jaw); cleft lip and palate Hands: polydactyly (extra digits); abnormal posturing of fingers; abnormal dermatoglyphics Other: congenital heart defects; hemangiomas; gastrointestinal tract defects; various malformations of other organs
Altered Chromosome: 5P	**Characteristics**
Genetic defect: deletion of short arm of chromosome 5 (cri du chat, or cat-cry syndrome) Incidence: 1 in 20,000 live births	CNS: severe intellectual disability; a catlike cry in infancy Head: microcephaly; hypertelorism (widely spaced eyes); epicanthal folds; low-set ears Other: failure to thrive; various organ malformations
Altered Chromosome: X (Sex Chromosome)	**Characteristics**
Genetic defect: only one X chromosome or partially missing second X chromosome in female (Turner syndrome) Incidence: 1 in 300 to 7000 live female births (see Figure 7–11)	CNS: no intellectual impairment; some perceptual difficulties Head: low hairline; webbed neck Trunk: short stature; cubitus valgus (increased carrying angle of arm); excessive nevi (congenital discoloration of skin because of pigmentation); broad, shieldlike chest with widely spaced nipples; puffy feet; no toenails Other: fibrous streaks in ovaries; underdeveloped secondary sex characteristics; primary amenorrhea; usually infertile; renal anomalies; coarctation of the aorta
Altered Chromosome: XXY (Sex Chromosome)	**Characteristics**
Genetic defect: extra X chromosome in male (Klinefelter syndrome) Incidence: 1 in 1000 live male births	CNS: mild intellectual disability Trunk: occasional gynecomastia (abnormally large male breasts); abnormal body proportions (long legs, short trunk, shoulder equal to hip size) Other: small, soft testes; underdeveloped secondary sex characteristics; reduced fertility

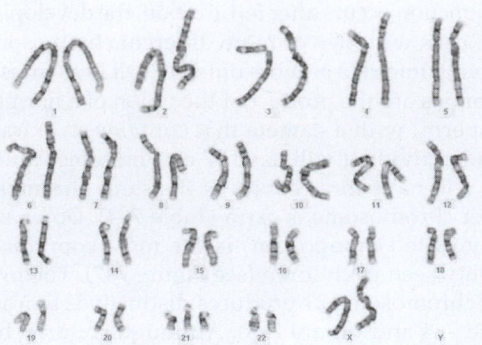

Figure 7–7 Karyotype of a female who has trisomy 21 (Down syndrome). Note the extra chromosome 21.

SOURCE: Susan Olson, PhD, Oregon Health & Science University Knight Diagnostic Laboratory.

Down syndrome have a variety of physical ailments, advances in medical science have extended their life expectancy.

Two other common trisomies are trisomy 18 and trisomy 13 (refer to Table 7–4 and Figures 7–9 and 7–10). The prognosis for both trisomies 13 and 18 is extremely poor. Most children (70%) die within the first 3 months of life secondary to complications related to respiratory and cardiac abnormalities. However, 10% survive the first year of life; therefore, the family needs to plan for the possibility of long-term care of a severely affected infant and for family support.

Monosomies occur when a normal gamete unites with a gamete that is missing a chromosome. In this case, the individual has only 45 chromosomes and is said to be monosomic. Most monosomies of an entire autosomal chromosome are incompatible with life. The only monosomy of an entire chromosome that is compatible with life is 45, X (Turner syndrome).

Mosaicism occurs after fertilization and results in an individual who has two different cell lines, each with a different chromosomal number. Mosaicism tends to be more common in the sex chromosomes than in the autosomes; when it occurs in the autosomes, it is most common in Down syndrome.

ABNORMALITIES OF CHROMOSOME STRUCTURE

Abnormalities of chromosome structure involve only parts of the chromosome and occur in two forms: translocation and deletions or duplications. Most (>95%) children born with Down syndrome

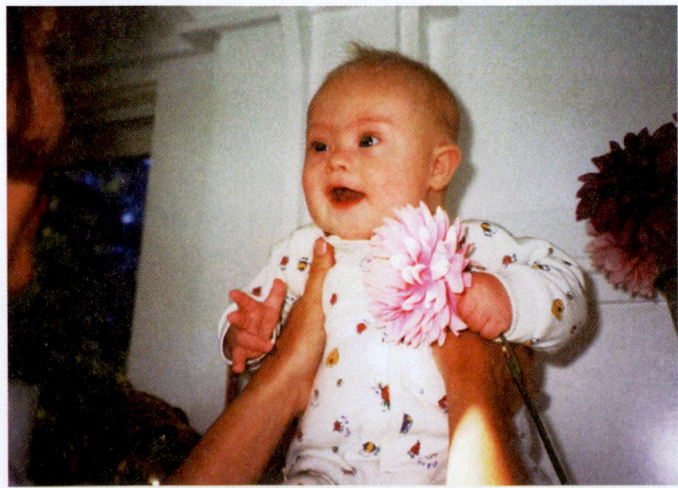

Figure 7–8 A boy with Down syndrome.

SOURCE: Joni Hofmann/Fotolia.

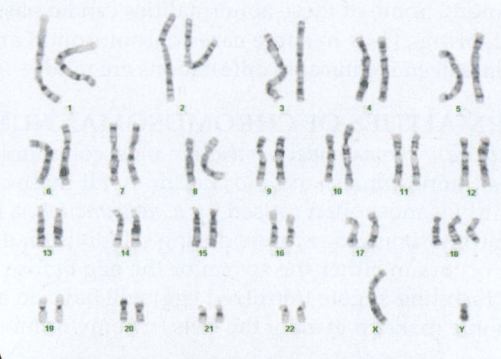

A

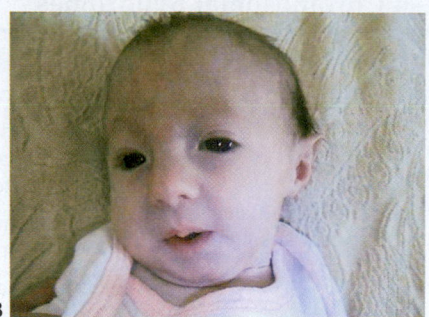

B

Figure 7–9 A. Karyotype of a male who has trisomy 18. B. Infant girl with trisomy 18.

SOURCE: A, Susan Olson, PhD, Oregon Health & Science University Knight Diagnostic Laboratory. B, OHSU Department of Obstetrics & Gynecology.

have trisomy 21, whereas some (<5%) have an abnormal rearrangement of chromosomal material known as a *translocation*. Clinically the two types of Down syndrome are indistinguishable; the only way to distinguish them is to do a chromosomal analysis.

The translocation occurs when the carrier parent has 45 chromosomes, usually with one chromosome fused to another. For example, a common translocation is one in which a particle of chromosome 14 breaks and fuses to chromosome 21. The parent has one normal 14, one normal 21, and one 14/21 chromosome. Because all the chromosomal material is present and functioning normally, the parent is clinically normal. This individual is known as a *balanced translocation carrier*. When a person who is a balanced translocation carrier has a child with a partner who has a structurally normal chromosome constitution, the child can have a normal number of chromosomes, be a carrier, or have an extra chromosome 21. Such a child has an *unbalanced translocation* and has Down syndrome.

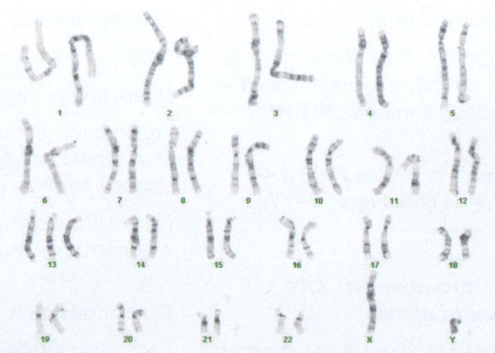

Figure 7–10 Karyotype of male with trisomy 13.

SOURCE: Susan Olson, PhD, Oregon Health & Science University Knight Diagnostic Laboratory.

Structure abnormality is also caused by *duplications* or *deletions* of chromosomal material. Any portion of a chromosome may be lost or added, generally leading to some adverse effect. Depending on how much chromosomal material is involved, the clinical effects may be mild or severe. Many types of duplications and deletions have been described, such as the deletion of the short arm of chromosome 5 (*cri du chat*, or cat-cry syndrome) or the deletion of the long arm of chromosome 18 (Edwards syndrome). Table 7–4 lists other chromosomal syndromes.

ABNORMALITIES OF THE SEX CHROMOSOME

To better understand abnormalities of the sex chromosomes, the nurse should know that in a female, at an early embryonic stage, one of the two normal X chromosomes becomes inactive. The inactive X chromosome forms a dark staining area known as a *Barr body*. The typical female has one Barr body, because one of her two X chromosomes has been inactivated. The typical male has no Barr bodies because he has only one X chromosome.

The most common sex chromosomal abnormalities are Turner syndrome in females (45, X with no Barr bodies present; Figure 7–11); and Klinefelter syndrome in males (47, XXY with one Barr body present). See Table 7–4 for clinical descriptions of these abnormalities.

Modes of Inheritance

Many inherited diseases are produced by an abnormality in a single gene or pair of genes. In such instances, the chromosomes are grossly normal. The defect is at the gene level. Some of these gene defects can be detected by technologies such as DNA sequencing and other biochemical assays.

The two major categories of inheritance are **Mendelian (single-gene) inheritance** and **non-Mendelian (multifactorial) inheritance**. Each single-gene trait is determined by a pair of genes working together. These genes are responsible for the observable expression of the traits (e.g., brown eyes, dark skin), referred to as the **phenotype**. The total genetic makeup of an individual is referred to as the **genotype** (pattern of the genes on the chromosomes).

One of the genes for a trait is inherited from the mother, the other is from the father. An individual who has two identical genes at a given locus is considered to be *homozygous* for that trait. Individuals are considered to be *heterozygous* for a particular trait when they have two different alleles (alternate forms of the same gene) at a given locus on a pair of homologous chromosomes.

The best-known modes of single-gene inheritance are autosomal dominant, autosomal recessive, and X linked (sex linked).

AUTOSOMAL DOMINANT INHERITANCE

A person is said to have an autosomal dominant inherited disorder if the disease trait is heterozygous—that is, the abnormal gene overshadows the normal gene of the pair to produce the trait. The genetic condition may be familial, meaning it was passed to an individual from one of his or her parents; or it may be the result of a *de novo* (new) mutation that occurred during meiosis of the egg or sperm that created the individual, and he or she is the first and only affected person in the family. It is essential to remember that in autosomal dominant inheritance, the following occurs:

- An affected individual generally has an affected parent. Thus the family **pedigree** (graphic representation of a family tree) usually shows multiple generations with the disorder.

- Affected individuals have a 50% chance of passing on the abnormal gene to each of their children (Figure 7–12).

- Males and females are equally affected, and a father can pass the abnormal gene on to his son. This is an important principle when distinguishing autosomal dominant disorders from X-linked disorders.

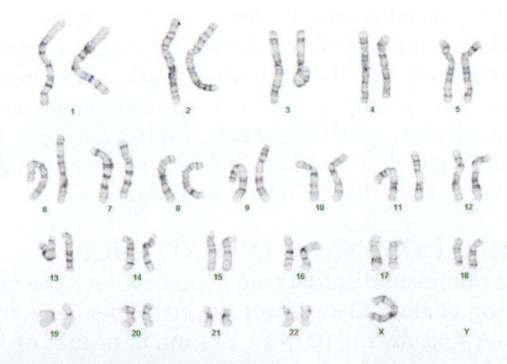

A

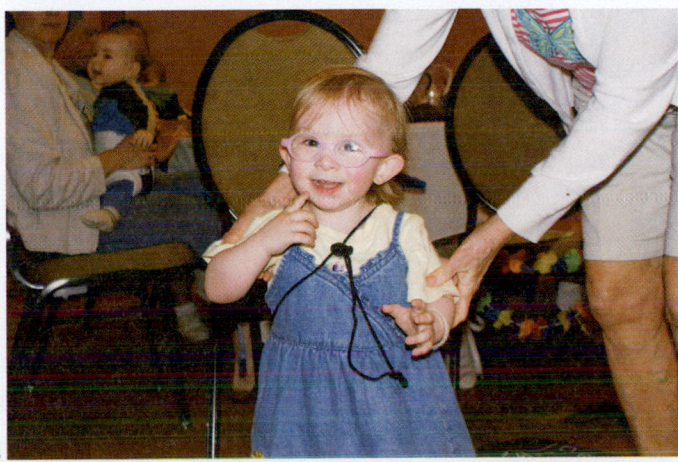

B

Figure 7–11 **A. Karyotype of a female with Turner syndrome. B. Toddler girl with Turner syndrome.**

SOURCE: A, Susan Olson, PhD, Oregon Health & Science University Knight Diagnostic Laboratory. B, Turner Syndrome Society. Copyright © by Cindy Scurlock. Used by permission of Cindy Scurlock.

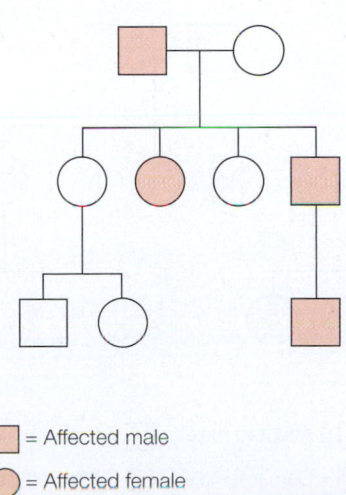

◼ = Affected male

● = Affected female

Figure 7–12 **Autosomal dominant pedigree. One parent is affected. Statistically 50% of offspring will be affected regardless of sex.**

- Autosomal dominant inherited disorders have varying degrees of presentation. This is an important factor when counseling families concerning autosomal dominant disorders. Although a parent may have a mild form of the disease, the child may have a more severe form.

Autosomal dominant conditions such as phocomelia (a developmental anomaly characterized by the absence of the upper portion of the limbs) can have minimal expression in a parent but severe effects in a child. Other common autosomal dominant disorders are Huntington disease, myotonic dystrophy, and fragile X syndrome (an X-linked disorder).

AUTOSOMAL RECESSIVE INHERITANCE

In an autosomal recessive inherited disorder, the individual must have two abnormal genes to be affected. A *carrier* is an individual who is heterozygous for the abnormal gene and clinically normal. It is not until two individuals mate and pass on the same abnormal gene that affected children may appear. It is essential to remember that in autosomal recessive inheritance the following occurs:

- An affected individual may have clinically normal parents, but both parents generally are carriers of the abnormal gene (Figure 7–13).
- In the case where both parents are carriers, there is a 25% chance that the abnormal gene will be passed on to any of their offspring. Each pregnancy has a 25% chance of resulting in an affected child.
- If a child of two carrier parents is clinically normal, there is a two-thirds chance that the child is a carrier of the gene.
- Both males and females are equally affected.
- There is an increased history of consanguineous mating (mating of blood relatives).

Some common autosomal recessive inherited disorders are cystic fibrosis, phenylketonuria (PKU), galactosemia, sickle cell disease, Tay–Sachs disease, and most metabolic disorders.

X-LINKED RECESSIVE INHERITANCE

X-linked, or sex-linked, disorders are those for which the abnormal gene is carried on the X chromosome. Thus an X-linked disorder is manifested in a male who carries the abnormal gene

on his only X chromosome and is considered *hemizygous* for the condition. Approximately two thirds of the time, the mother of a male with an X-linked disorder will be a carrier. Most carrier females (known as *heterozygous females*) do not have symptoms of the condition. It is essential to remember that in X-linked recessive inheritance, the following occurs:

- There is no male-to-male transmission. Affected males are related through the female line (see Figure 7–14).
- There is a 50% chance that a carrier mother will pass the abnormal gene to each of her sons, who will thus be affected.
- There is a 50% chance that a carrier mother will pass the normal gene to each of her sons, who will thus be unaffected.
- There is a 50% chance that a carrier mother will pass the abnormal gene to each of her daughters, who become carriers.
- Fathers affected with an X-linked disorder cannot pass the disorder to their sons, but all their daughters become carriers of the disorder. They are known as *obligate carriers*.

Common X-linked recessive disorders are hemophilia, Duchenne muscular dystrophy, and some forms of color blindness.

Fragile X syndrome is an X-linked recessive disorder that exhibits anticipation. This condition is a common form of inherited intellectual disability second only to Down syndrome. It is caused by an increased number of CGG trinucleotide repeats in the *FMR1* gene, located at a "fragile site" on the long arm of the X chromosome. The normal number of CGG repeats is up to 60. Individuals with a repeat number ranging between 60 and 200 have a *premutation* allele, meaning that the copy number can increase during maternal (but not paternal) meiosis. If the CGG repeat number increases to over 200, the individual (particularly hemizygous males) can have fragile X syndrome. Approximately one third of females with over 200 CGG repeats will be affected with fragile X syndrome, one third will have mild developmental or learning disabilities, and one third will have no symptoms at all.

X-LINKED DOMINANT INHERITANCE

X-linked dominant disorders are extremely rare, the most common being vitamin D–resistant rickets. When X-linked dominance does occur, the pattern is similar to that of X-linked

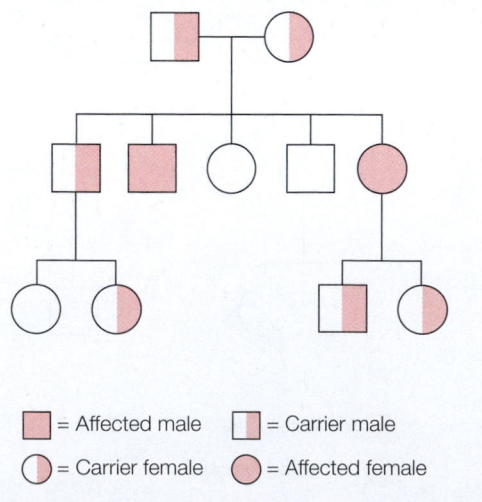

= Affected male   = Carrier male
= Carrier female   = Affected female

Figure 7–13 Autosomal recessive pedigree. Both parents are carriers. Statistically 25% of offspring are affected regardless of sex.

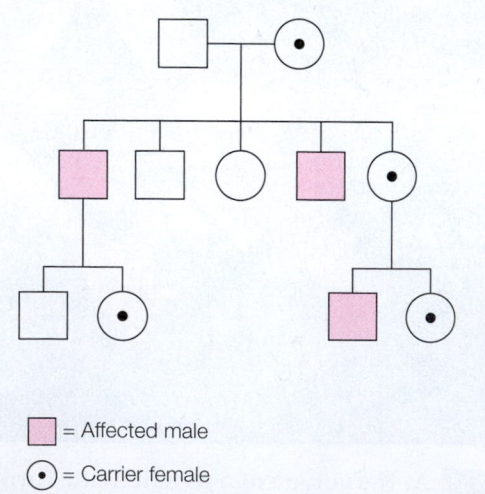

= Affected male
= Carrier female

Figure 7–14 X-linked recessive pedigree. The mother is the carrier. Statistically 50% of male offspring are affected, and 50% of female offspring are carriers.

recessive inheritance except that heterozygous females are affected. It is essential to remember that in X-linked dominant inheritance there is no male-to-male transmission. Affected fathers will have affected daughters; however, because they pass only the Y chromosome to male offspring, any sons will not be affected.

MULTIFACTORIAL INHERITANCE

Many common congenital malformations such as cleft palate, heart defects, spina bifida, dislocated hips, clubfoot, and pyloric stenosis do not follow a clear pattern of Mendelian inheritance. They are generally caused by an interaction of many genes and environmental factors and are considered to have "multifactorial" inheritance. In multifactorial inheritance the following occurs:

- The malformations may vary from mild to severe. For example, spina bifida may range in severity from mild (spina bifida occulta) to more severe (myelomeningocele). The more severe the defect, the greater the number of genes present for that defect.
- There is often a gender bias, and the risk is higher for relatives of a person of the gender in which the condition is less common. For example, pyloric stenosis is more common in males, whereas cleft palate is more common in females. When a member of the less commonly affected gender shows the condition, a greater number of genes must usually be present to cause the defect.
- Not only is increased risk greatest among closest relatives and decreased with distance of relationship, but the risk is increased when multiple family members are affected.

Although most congenital malformations are multifactorial, a careful family history should always be taken, because cleft lip and palate, certain congenital heart defects, and other malformations occasionally can be inherited as autosomal dominant or recessive traits. Other disorders thought to be within the multifactorial inheritance group are diabetes, hypertension, some heart diseases, and mental illness.

Prenatal Diagnostic Tests

Parent–child and family-planning counseling has become a major responsibility of professional nurses. To be effective counselors, nurses must have the most up-to-date information about prenatal diagnostic testing. Appropriate counseling should occur before prenatal screening or diagnostic testing is done. It is essential that couples be completely informed about the known and potential risks of each of the genetic diagnostic procedures. The prescreening counseling should include the conditions detectable by the screening, what diagnostic tests are available if the screening is positive, risk to the mother and child of the test performed, accuracy of the test, and limitations of the test. The nurse needs to recognize the emotional impact on the family of a decision to undergo or not to undergo a genetic diagnostic procedure.

Screening and invasive diagnostic testing for chromosome abnormalities should be available to all women who present for prenatal care before 20 weeks of pregnancy regardless of maternal age (American College of Obstetricians and Gynecologists Committee on Genetics and the Society for Maternal Fetal Medicine Publications Committee [ACOG/SMFM], 2012). Women should be counseled regarding the differences between screening and invasive diagnostic testing. Screening tests, such as nuchal translucency ultrasound and maternal serum screening, are designed to gather information about the risk that the pregnancy could have chromosome abnormalities or open spina bifida. If the risk is increased above a specific cutoff, the woman is offered invasive prenatal diagnosis. Prenatal diagnostic techniques, such as amniocentesis and chorionic villus sampling (CVS), obtain cells from the pregnancy to rule out or diagnose a chromosome abnormality or certain genetic disorders. They are associated with a small risk of pregnancy complications, including miscarriage.

GENETIC ULTRASOUND

Ultrasound may be used to assess the fetus for genetic or congenital problems. With ultrasound, one can visualize the fetal head for fetal abnormalities in size, shape, and structure. (For a detailed discussion of ultrasound technology, see Chapter 13.) Craniospinal defects (anencephalus, microcephaly, hydrocephalus), thoracic malformations (diaphragmatic hernia), gastrointestinal malformations (omphalocele, gastroschisis), renal malformations (dysplasia or obstruction), and skeletal malformations (caudal regression, conjoined twins) are only some of the disorders that can be diagnosed in utero by ultrasound.

Screening by ultrasound for congenital anomalies is best done at 16 to 20 weeks, when fetal structures have developed completely. First trimester screening for chromosome abnormalities is widely available by measuring the fetal nuchal translucency between 11 and 13 weeks. The nuchal translucency is a fluid-filled space at the back of the fetal neck. An increased amount of fluid is associated with an increased risk for chromosomal abnormalities, birth defects, genetic syndromes, and poor pregnancy outcome—the larger the nuchal translucency, the higher the risk for abnormalities. The nuchal translucency should be measured only by a specifically trained sonographer or physician. There is no information documenting harm to the fetus or long-term effects with exposure to ultrasound. However, there is no guarantee of complete safety; therefore, the practitioner and the parents must evaluate the risks versus the benefits on an individual basis.

MATERNAL SERUM SCREENING

Measuring specific hormones and proteins in the maternal serum during the first and/or second trimester can determine the risk for Down syndrome, trisomy 18, or open spina bifida. In the first trimester, the nuchal translucency measurement is often added to improve the detection rate for Down syndrome and trisomy 18. Detection and false-positive rates differ depending on the type of screening test that is performed and may also differ depending on the laboratory that performs the screening.

NONINVASIVE PRENATAL TESTING THROUGH CELL-FREE FETAL DNA

Noninvasive prenatal testing (NIPT) for chromosome abnormalities is now available by measuring circulating *cell-free fetal DNA (cffDNA)* in maternal serum. Approximately 3% to 13% of the circulating DNA in a woman's plasma is derived from the placenta (ACOG/SMFM, 2012). Several laboratories have developed techniques to quantify the amount of these DNA fragments as early as 9 to 10 weeks of gestation in order to detect some of the common trisomies (including Down syndrome, trisomy 18, and trisomy 13) at higher sensitivity and specificity than traditional maternal serum screening. However, NIPT is not meant to replace diagnostic testing such as chorionic villus sampling (CVS) or amniocentesis, and it has its limitations, including limited data on low-risk pregnancies, twin gestations, and pregnancies with a vanishing twin as well as concerns about false-positive results due to maternal or placental mosaicism (ACOG/SMFM, 2012). At this time, cffDNA screening is recommended only for women of advanced maternal age and women with fetal ultrasound findings suggestive of aneuploidy, history of prior pregnancy with trisomy 21, trisomy 18, or trisomy 13, or positive first or second trimester serum screening. Clients with abnormal NIPT results, or those with other factors suggestive of a chromosome abnormality, should receive genetic counseling and be given the option of standard confirmatory diagnostic testing (Devers, Cronister, Ormond, et al., 2013).

GENETIC AMNIOCENTESIS

A major method of prenatal diagnosis is genetic amniocentesis (Figure 7–15). The procedure is described in Chapter 13. The risk for pregnancy complications, including infection and miscarriage, are thought to be less than 0.5%. The indications for genetic amniocentesis include the following:

1. *Maternal age 35 or older.* Women age 35 or older are at greater risk for having children with chromosomal abnormalities. Chromosomal abnormalities because of maternal age include trisomy 21, trisomy 13, trisomy 18, XXX, or XXY. The risk of having a live-born baby with a chromosome problem is 1 in 200 for a 35-year-old woman; the risk for trisomy 21 is 1 in 385. At age 44, the risks are 1 in 20 and 1 in 37, respectively (Harper, 2010).

2. *Previous child born with a chromosomal abnormality.* Young couples who have had a child with a trisomy 21, 18, or 13 have an approximately 1% risk or their age-related risk, whichever is higher, of a future child having a chromosomal abnormality.

3. *Parent carrying a chromosomal abnormality (balanced translocation).* These couples are at an increased risk to have conceptions with an unbalanced translocation. Depending on the chromosomes involved in the translocation, there may be an increased risk for pregnancy loss or a viable offspring with congenital anomalies and/or intellectual disability. A woman who carries a balanced 14/21 translocation has a risk of approximately 10% to 15% that her children will be affected with the unbalanced translocation of Down syndrome; if the father is the carrier, there is a 2% to 5% risk.

4. *Mother carrying an X-linked disease.* In families in which the woman is a known or possible carrier of an X-linked disorder such as hemophilia A or B or Duchenne muscular dystrophy, the risk of an affected male fetus is 25%. Now DNA testing may make it possible to distinguish affected males from nonaffected males in some disorders.

5. *Both parents carrying an autosomal recessive disease.* When both parents are carriers of an autosomal recessive

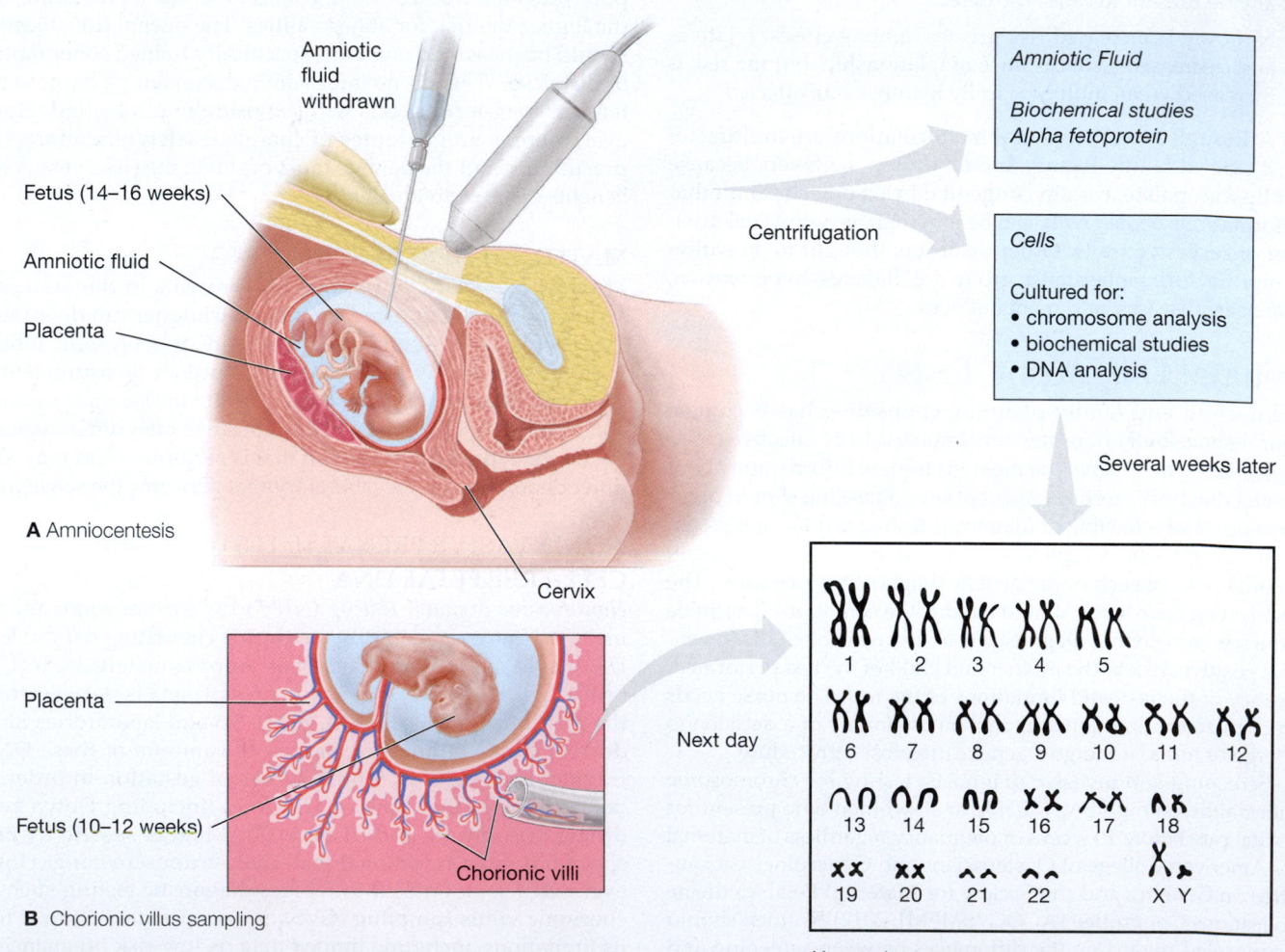

Figure 7–15 A. Genetic amniocentesis for prenatal diagnosis is done at 15 to 21 weeks' gestation. B. Chorionic villus sampling is done at 10 to 13 weeks, and the cells are cultured and karyotyped. Results generally take 7 to 14 days.

disease, there is a 25% risk for *each pregnancy* that the fetus will be affected. Autosomal recessive diseases identified by amniocentesis are hemoglobinopathies such as sickle cell anemia, thalassemia, and cystic fibrosis.

6. *Family history of neural tube defects.* Genetic amniocentesis is available to couples who have had a child with neural tube defects or who have a family history of these conditions, which include anencephaly, spina bifida, and myelomeningocele. The diagnosis is made by measuring amniotic fluid alpha-fetoprotein (AFP) and a neurotransmitter called acetylcholinesterase. Neural tube defects are usually multifactorial traits.

7. *Fetus with major or minor anomalies on ultrasound.*

8. *Women with positive serum screening results, including NIPT.*

PERCUTANEOUS UMBILICAL BLOOD SAMPLING AND CHORIONIC VILLUS SAMPLING

Percutaneous umbilical blood sampling (PUBS) is a technique used for obtaining blood that allows for rapid chromosome diagnosis, genetic studies, or transfusion for Rh isoimmunization or hydrops fetalis. However, the risk for pregnancy complications is thought to be considerably higher than with chorionic villus sampling and amniocentesis.

Chorionic villus sampling (CVS) is a technique that obtains chorionic villi tissue from the placenta either transabdominally or transcervically. Its diagnostic capability is similar to that of amniocentesis. Its advantages are that diagnostic information is available at 10 to 12 weeks' gestation. The risk for pregnancy complications, including infection and pregnancy loss, is estimated to be around 1%. For further discussion of CVS, see Chapter 13.

Nursing Management

Nurses are on the front line of client care and need to be competent in genetic- and genomic-related health care. They need to know how to find reliable genetic information and where to refer clients and families for further genetic information and counseling (Consensus Panel on Genetic/Genomic Nursing Competencies, 2009). In both prospective and retrospective genetic counseling, timely nursing intervention is a crucial factor. During annual examinations and other clinical appointments, interview all women of childbearing age to determine any family history or other risk factors for genetic disorders. If the woman is planning to conceive, encourage genetic counseling before discontinuation of contraception.

Nursing Implications of Prenatal Diagnostic Testing

It is imperative that counseling precede any procedure for prenatal diagnosis. Many questions and points must be considered if the family is to reach a satisfactory decision. See *Key Facts to Remember: Couples Who May Benefit from Prenatal Diagnosis.*

With the advent of diagnostic techniques such as amniocentesis and CVS, at-risk couples who would not otherwise have a first child or additional children can decide to conceive. Following prenatal diagnosis a couple may decide to interrupt the pregnancy. Even when termination is not an option, prenatal diagnosis can give parents an opportunity to prepare for the birth of a child with special needs, to contact other families with children with similar problems, or to contact support services before the birth.

Every pregnancy has a 3% to 4% risk of resulting in a newborn with a birth defect. When an abnormality is detected or

---

KEY FACTS TO REMEMBER
Couples Who May Benefit from Prenatal Diagnosis

- Women age 35 or over at time of birth
- Couples with a balanced translocation (chromosomal abnormality)
- Family history of known or suspected Mendelian genetic disorder (e.g., cystic fibrosis, hemophilia A and B, Duchenne muscular dystrophy)
- Couples with a previous child with chromosomal abnormality
- Couples in which either partner or a previous child is affected with, or in which both partners are carriers for, a diagnosable metabolic disorder
- Family history of birth defects and/or intellectual disability (e.g., neural tube defects, congenital heart disease, cleft lip and/or palate)
- Ethnic groups at increased risk for specific disorders (see *Developing Cultural Competence: Genetic Screening Recommendations for Various Ethnic and Age Groups*)
- Couples with history of two or more first-trimester spontaneous abortions
- Women with an abnormal maternal serum alpha-fetoprotein (MSAFP or AFP) test
- Women with a teratogenic risk secondary to an exposure or maternal health condition (e.g., diabetes).

Clinical Tip

- Remember that prenatal screening and diagnosis are an optional part of routine prenatal care.
- Present options to clients using a nondirective manner. *Nondirective counseling* is a technique designed to allow clients to talk about their problems or emotional difficulties and reach the decision that is best for themselves or their families with a minimum of direction from the person serving as their counselor.
- Give clients accurate, up-to-date information about the various prenatal screening and diagnostic testing options, but remain impartial and do not recommend any specific course of action.
- Be aware of the language you use when discussing these options with clients. For example, in discussing prenatal screening for Down syndrome, terms such as *handicapped* or *retarded* should be replaced with *disabled* and/or *developmentally/cognitively/intellectually disabled*. Also consider using the terms *risk for*, *chance of*, or *possibility of*.

---

suspected before birth, an attempt is made to determine the diagnosis by assessing the family health history (via the pedigree) and the pregnancy history and by evaluating the fetal anomaly or anomalies via ultrasound. After experts on a specific disorder are consulted, healthcare professionals can then present the parents with options. Treatment of prenatally diagnosed disorders may begin during the pregnancy, thus possibly preventing irreversible damage. In light of the philosophy of preventive health care, information that can be obtained prenatally should be made available to all couples who are expecting a baby or who are contemplating pregnancy.

Newborn Screening

The United States has implemented newborn screening for hearing loss, congenital heart disease, hemoglobinopathies, certain endocrine disorders, and several metabolic and other inherited genetic diseases. A uniform panel of approximately 30 disorders is currently recommended. Newborn screening is generally a state-level program (Kuehn, 2013). It is the nurse's responsibility to know what conditions are screened for in her or his state and what methods are used. To find out more about newborn screening in your state, visit the website of *Baby's First Test*, which is funded by the Health Resource and Service Administration (HRSA).

Postnatal Diagnosis

Questions concerning genetic disorders (cause, treatment, and prognosis) are most often first discussed in the newborn nursery or during the baby's first few months of life. When a child is born with anomalies, has a stormy newborn period, or does not progress as expected, a genetic evaluation may be warranted. An accurate diagnosis and an optimal treatment plan incorporate the following:

- Complete detailed history to determine whether the problem is prenatal (congenital), postnatal, or familial in origin
- Thorough physical and dermorphology examination by a trained clinical geneticist
- Laboratory analysis, which includes chromosome analysis; enzyme assay for inborn errors of metabolism (see Chapter 26 for further discussion of these tests); DNA studies (both direct and by linkage); and antibody titers for infectious teratogens, such as toxoplasmosis, rubella, cytomegalovirus, and herpes virus (TORCH syndrome) (see Chapter 15 for more information on infections that threaten the fetus).

Professionalism in Practice 2008 Prenatally and Postnatally Diagnosed Conditions Act

The Prenatally and Postnatally Diagnosed Conditions Act was signed into law in 2008. This law requires that medical providers give parents accurate, updated, and scientific information regarding their child's diagnosis, prognosis, treatment, and life expectancy. Nurses are often an important source of information and support when a prenatal or postnatal diagnosis of a genetic condition or birth defect is made. Nurses also need support groups that push to be sure that the annual government appropriations are funded.

To make an accurate diagnosis, the geneticist consults with other specialists and reviews the current literature, evaluating all the available information before arriving at a diagnosis and plan of action.

The Human Genome Project has significant implications for the identification and management of inherited disorders. Once genes have been identified, it will be possible to detect their presence in carriers and lead to better genetic counseling. However, concerns have been voiced about ethical considerations with genetic research. What guidelines are needed to protect children and families so that genetic testing does not lead to discrimination in future employment or health insurance? Who should be tested for genetic diseases, and who should have access to the results? Because children cannot yet give informed consent for genetic testing (see Chapter 1 for discussion of informed consent), parents and guardians should be informed about the risks and benefits of testing, their permission should be obtained and, if appropriate, the assent of the child should be obtained.

Genetic Counseling

Genetic counseling is a communication process in which a genetic counselor, physician, or specially trained and certified nurse helps a family or individuals understand and adapt to the medical, psychologic, and familial implications of genetic contributions to disease (National Society of Genetic Counselors [NSGC], 2015).

REFERRAL

Genetic counseling referral is advised for any of the following categories:

- *Congenital abnormalities, including intellectual disability.* Any couple who has a child or a relative with a congenital malformation may be at increased risk and should be so informed. If a developmental/cognitive/intellectual disability of unidentified cause has occurred in a family, there may be an increased risk of recurrence. In some cases, the genetic counselor will identify the cause of a malformation as a teratogen (see Chapter 10). The family should be aware of teratogenic substances so they can avoid exposure to them during any subsequent pregnancy.
- *Familial disorders.* Families should be told that certain diseases may have a genetic component and that the risk of their occurrence in a particular family may be higher than that in the general population. Such disorders as diabetes, heart disease, cancer, and mental illness fall into this category.
- *Known inherited diseases.* Families may know that a disease is inherited but not know the mechanism or the specific risk for them. An important point to remember is that family members who are not at risk for passing on a disorder should be as well informed as family members who are at risk.
- *Metabolic disorders.* Any families at risk for having a child with a metabolic disorder or biochemical defect should be referred for genetic counseling. Because most inborn errors of metabolism are autosomal recessively inherited, a family may not be identified as being at risk until the birth of an affected child. Carriers of the sickle cell trait can be identified before pregnancy is begun and the risk of having an affected child can be determined.
- *Chromosomal abnormalities.* As discussed previously, any couple who has had a child with a chromosomal abnormality may be at increased risk of having another child similarly affected. This group includes families in which there is concern about a possible translocation.

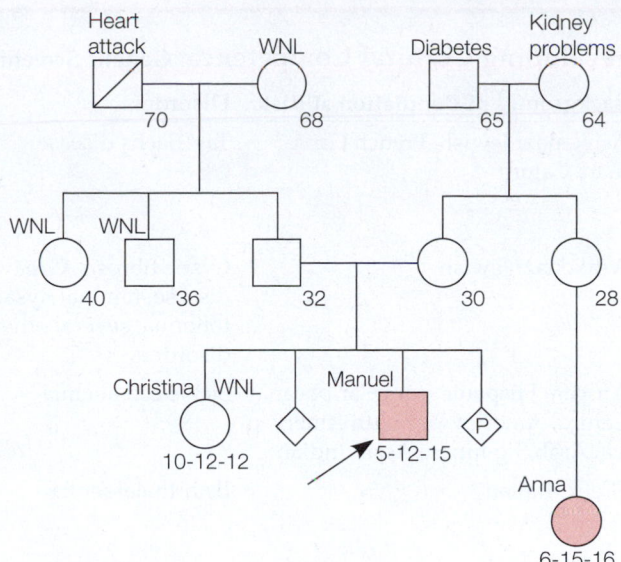

In the United States, marriage between related individuals is generally taboo. In Western medicine, there is a concern that a child conceived by people who are related by blood may have an increased risk for autosomal recessive disorders. This has not, however, been supported by recent research unless the relationship is closer than first cousins. In many other cultures, marriage of first cousins and others who are related by blood is acceptable and even common. In several Middle Eastern cultures, consanguineous marriage, generally between cousins, is common. Reasons for consanguineous marriage include "increase family links," "they knew each other and everything would be clear before marriage," "customs and traditions," and "less cost."

After a couple has been referred to the genetics clinic, they are sent a form requesting information on the health status of various family members. This information assists the genetic counselor in creating the family's pedigree. The pedigree and history facilitate identification of other family members who might also be at risk for the same disorder (Figure 7–16). The couple being counseled may wish to notify relatives at risk so that they, too, can begin genetic counseling. When done correctly, the family history and pedigree can be powerful tools for determining a family's risk.

INITIAL SESSION

During the initial session, the counselor gathers additional information about the pregnancy, the affected child's growth and development, and the family's understanding of the problem. The counselor also elicits information concerning ethnic background and family origin. Many genetic disorders are more common among certain ethnic groups or in particular geographic areas. (See *Developing Cultural Competence: Genetic Screening Recommendations for Various Ethnic and Age Groups*.)

Generally the child undergoes a physical examination. Other family members may also be examined. If laboratory tests such as chromosomal analyses, metabolic studies, or viral titers are indicated, they are performed at this time. The genetic counselor may then give the parents some preliminary information based on the data at hand.

FOLLOW-UP COUNSELING

After all the data have been carefully examined and analyzed, the couple returns for a follow-up visit. At this time, the genetic counselor gives the parents all the information available, including the following:

- Medical facts
- Diagnosis
- Probable course of the disorder and any available management
- Inheritance pattern for this particular family
- Risk of recurrence and the options or alternatives for dealing with recurrence.

The remainder of the counseling session is spent discussing the course of action that seems appropriate to the family in view

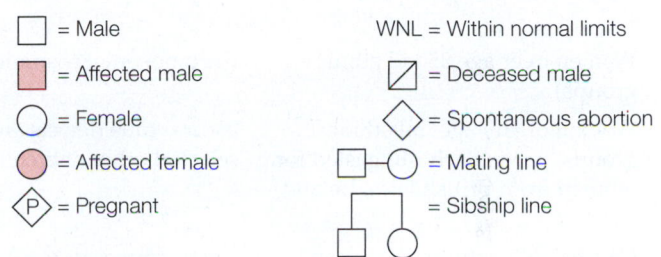

Figure 7–16 Screening pedigree. Arrow indicates the nearest family member affected with the disorder being investigated. Numbers refer to the ages of the family members.

of the risk and family goals. For couples who desire to become parents or who want a subsequent child, options include prenatal diagnosis, early detection and treatment, preimplantation genetic diagnosis or other assisted reproductive therapies, and delayed childbearing until prenatal diagnosis is available or a disease can be detected and treated early to prevent irreversible damage, or, in some cases, adoption. When the parents have completed the counseling sessions, the counselor sends them and their certified nurse-midwife or physician a letter detailing the contents of the sessions. The family keeps this document for reference.

Nursing Management

The nurse has a key role in preventing recurrence. One cannot expect a couple who has just learned that their child has a birth defect or Down syndrome to take in any information concerning future risks. However, the couple should never be "put off" from genetic counseling for so long that they conceive another affected child because of lack of information. The perinatal nursing team frequently has the first contact with the family who has a newborn with a congenital abnormality. At the birth of an affected child, inform the parents that before they attempt having another child, genetic counseling is available.

After genetic counseling, the nurse with the appropriate knowledge of genetics is in an ideal position to help families review what has been discussed during the sessions and to answer any additional questions they might have. As the family returns to the daily aspects of living, provide helpful

Developing Cultural Competence Genetic Screening Recommendations for Various Ethnic and Age Groups

Background of Population at Risk	Disorder	Screening Test	Definitive Test
Ashkenazi Jewish, French Canadian, Cajun	Tay–Sachs disease	Decreased serum hexosaminidase-A or DNA mutation analysis	Chorionic villus sampling (CVS) or amniocentesis for hexosaminidase-A assay or DNA mutation analysis
Ashkenazi Jewish	Cystic fibrosis, Canavan disease, familial dysautonomia, several other disorders	DNA mutation analysis	CVS or amniocentesis for DNA mutation analysis
African; Hispanic from Caribbean, Central America, or South America; Arab, Egyptian; Asian Indian	Sickle cell anemia	Presence of sickle cell hemoglobin; confirmatory hemoglobin electrophoresis	CVS or amniocentesis for DNA mutation analysis
Greek, Italian	Beta-thalassemia	Mean corpuscular volume less than 80%; confirmatory hemoglobin electrophoresis	CVS or amniocentesis for DNA mutation analysis
Southeast Asian (Vietnamese, Laotian, Cambodian), Filipino	Alpha-thalassemia	Mean corpuscular volume less than 80%; confirmatory hemoglobin electrophoresis	CVS or amniocentesis for DNA mutation analysis or gene deletion studies
Women over age 35 (all ethnic groups)	Chromosomal trisomies	Prenatal serum and/or ultrasound screening	CVS or amniocentesis for cytogenetic analysis
Women of any age (all ethnic groups; particularly suggested for women from British Isles, Ireland)	Neural tube defects and selected other anomalies	Maternal serum alpha-fetoprotein (MSAFP)	Amniocentesis for amniotic fluid alpha-fetoprotein (AFP) and acetylcholinesterase assays
Caucasian (northern European, Celtic population), Ashkenazi Jewish	Cystic fibrosis	DNA mutation analysis of the cystic fibrosis transmembrane regulation (CFTR) gene	CVS or amniocentesis for DNA mutation analysis

information on the day-to-day aspects of caring for the child, answer questions as they arise, support parents in their decisions, and refer the family to other health and community agencies. The family may return to the genetic counselor a number of times to air their questions and concerns, especially if the couple is considering having more children or if siblings want information about their affected brother or sister. It is most desirable, when working with a family undergoing genetic counseling, for you to attend many or all of these counseling sessions. Because you have already established a rapport with the couple, you can act as a liaison between the family and the genetic counselor. Hearing directly what the genetic counselor says helps you clarify issues for the family, which in turn helps them formulate questions. Many genetic centers have found the public health nurse to be the ideal health professional to provide such follow-up care. See *Key Facts to Remember: Nursing Responsibilities in Genetic Counseling.*

KEY FACTS TO REMEMBER
Nursing Responsibilities in Genetic Counseling

- Identify families at risk for genetic problems.
- Determine how the genetic problem is perceived and what information is desired before proceeding.
- Assist families in acquiring accurate information about the specific problem.
- Act as a liaison between the family and genetic counselor.
- Assist the family in understanding and dealing with information received.
- Provide information on support groups.
- Aid families in coping with this crisis.
- Provide information about known genetic factors.
- Ensure continuity of nursing care to the family.

Focus Your Study

- Couples are considered infertile when they do not conceive after 1 year of unprotected coitus.

- A thorough history and a physical examination of both partners are essential as a basis for infertility investigation.

- General fertility investigations include evaluation of ovarian function, cervical mucus adequacy and receptivity to sperm, sperm number and function, tubal patency, general condition of the pelvic organs, and certain laboratory tests.

- Among cases of infertility, 20% involve male factors, 40% involve female factors, and 30% to 40% involve either unidentifiable cause (unexplained infertility) or a problem with both partners.

- Medications may be prescribed to induce ovulation, facilitate cervical mucus formation, reduce antibody concentration, increase sperm count and motility, and suppress endometriosis.

- The emotional aspects of infertility may be more difficult for the couple than the testing and therapy.

- The nurse needs to be prepared to provide accurate information about infertility and dispel myths.

- The nurse assesses coping responses and initiates counseling referrals as indicated.

- In autosomal dominant inherited disorders, an affected parent has a 50% chance of having an affected child. Such disorders equally affect males and females. The characteristic presentation varies in each individual with the gene. Some of the common autosomal dominant inherited disorders are Huntington disease, polycystic kidney disease, and neurofibromatosis (von Recklinghausen disease).

- Autosomal recessive inherited disorders are characterized by both parents being carriers; each offspring having a 25% chance of having the disease, a 25% chance of not being affected, and a 50% chance of being a carrier; and males and females being equally affected. Some common autosomal recessive inherited disorders are cystic fibrosis, phenylketonuria, galactosemia, sickle cell disease, Tay–Sachs disease, and most metabolic disorders.

- X-linked recessive disorders are characterized by no male-to-male transmission, effects limited to males, a 50% chance that a carrier mother will pass the abnormal gene to her son, a 50% chance that a carrier mother will not transmit the abnormal gene to her son; a 50% chance that the daughter of a carrier mother will be a carrier; and a 100% chance that daughters of affected fathers will be carriers. Common X-linked recessive disorders are hemophilia, some forms of color blindness, and Duchenne muscular dystrophy.

- Multifactorial inheritance disorders include cleft lip and palate, spina bifida, developmental dysplasia of the hips, clubfoot, and pyloric stenosis.

- Some genetic conditions that can currently be diagnosed prenatally are neural tube and craniospinal defects, renal malformations, hemophilia, fragile X syndrome, thalassemia, cystic fibrosis, and many inborn errors of metabolism such as Tay–Sachs disease. This list expands daily as new technology allows more conditions to be detected.

- The chief tools of prenatal diagnosis are ultrasound, serum alpha-fetoprotein testing, amniocentesis, chorionic villus sampling, and percutaneous umbilical blood sampling.

- Based on sound knowledge about common genetic problems, the nurse should prepare the family for genetic counseling and act as a resource person during and after the counseling sessions. Many nurses with advanced training are entering the field of genetic counseling.

Clinical Reasoning In Action

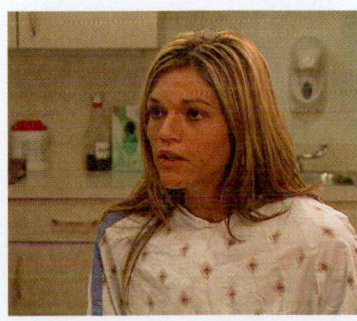

Marie Neives, age 19, presents while you are working at a Planned Parenthood clinic. She is there for a GYN exam and tells you that she is sexually active with her boyfriend but doesn't want to become pregnant. Since she lives at home with her parents, she does not want to use "the pill" because her mother might find out. Marie tells you she has a family history of cystic fibrosis (CF) and is concerned that she will pass the disease on. Marie asks you for information concerning fertility awareness. You obtain a menstrual history as follows: menarche age 12, cycle every 28 days for 5 days, dysmenorrhea the first 2 days with moderate flow. She has had one sexual partner. She states her boyfriend, also 19 years of age and of Northern European ancestry, doesn't like to use condoms and that she has been lucky so far in not getting pregnant. You assist the nurse practitioner with a physical and pelvic examination. The results show that Marie is essentially healthy. The nurse practitioner asks you to review with Marie fertility awareness and discuss her risk of having a child with CF.

1. Explore with Marie "natural family planning." How would you explain this to her?

2. What is the chance that Marie is a carrier for CF? Given that her boyfriend does not have a family history of CF, could the couple still have an affected child if Marie were a carrier and were to become pregnant?

3. After figuring out her menstruation cycle, to avoid conception when would you tell Marie to abstain from unprotected intercourse?

4. Explain carrier screening for CF to Marie. In what circumstances would you refer Marie and her boyfriend to genetic counseling?

References

Agostini, F., Monti, F., Pascalis, L., Paterlini, M., Battista La Sala, G., & Blickstein, I. (2011). Psychosocial support for infertile couples during assisted reproductive technology treatment. *Fertility & Sterility, 95*(2), 707–710.

American College of Obstetricians and Gynecologists Committee on Genetics and the Society for Maternal Fetal Medicine Publications Committee (ACOG/SMFM). (2012). Noninvasive prenatal testing for fetal aneuploidy. Committee Opinion No. 545. *Obstetrics and Gynecology, 120,* 1532 –1534.

American Society for Reproductive Medicine (ASRM). (2012a). *Medications for inducing ovulation—A guide for patients.* Retrieved from https://www .asrm.org/uploadedFiles/ASRM_Content/Resources/Patient_Resources/Fact_Sheets_and_Info_Booklets/ovulation_drugs.pdf

American Society for Reproductive Medicine (ASRM). (2012b). Multiple gestation associated with infertility therapy: An American Society for Reproductive Medicine Practice Committee opinion. *Fertility and Sterility, 97*(4), 825–834. doi:10.1016/j.fertnstert.2011.11.048

American Society for Reproductive Medicine (ASRM). (2012c). Smoking and infertility: A committee opinion. *Fertility and Sterility, 98*(6), 1400–1406. doi:10.1016/j.fertnstert.2012.07.1146

American Society for Reproductive Medicine (ASRM). (2013a). Criteria for number of embryos to transfer: A committee opinion. *Fertility & Sterility, 99*(1), 44–46. doi:10.1016/j.fertnstert.2012.09.038

American Society for Reproductive Medicine. (2013b). Definitions of infertility and recurrent pregnancy loss: A committee opinion. *Fertility & Sterility, 99*(1), 63. doi:10.1016/j.fertnstert.2012.09.023

American Society for Reproductive Medicine (ASRM). (2015a). Diagnostic evaluation of the infertile female: A committee opinion. *Fertility and Sterility, 103*(6), e44–50.

American Society for Reproductive Medicine (ASRM). (2015b). Diagnostic evaluation of the infertile male: A committee opinion. *Fertility and Sterility, 103*(3), e18–25.

Balen, A. H. (2013). Ovulation induction in the management of anovulatory polycystic ovary syndrome. *Molecular and Cellular Endocrinology, 373,* 77–82.

Barbieri, R. L. (2014). Female infertility. In J. F. Strauss III & R. L. Barbieri (Eds). *Yen & Jaffe's reproductive endocrinology: Physiology, pathophysiology, and clinical management* (7th ed., pp. 512–537). Philadelphia, PA: Elsevier/Saunders.

Consensus Panel on Genetic/Genomic Nursing Competencies. (2009). *Essentials of genetic and genomic nursing: Competencies, curricula guidelines, and outcome indicators* (2nd ed.). Silver Springs, MD: American Nurses Association.

Devers, P. L., Cronister, A., Ormond, K. E., Facio, F., Brasington, C. K., & Flodman, P. (2013). Noninvasive prenatal testing/noninvasive prenatal diagnosis: The position of the National Society of Genetic Counselors. *Journal of Genetic Counseling, 22*(3), 291–295. doi:10.1007/s10897-012-9564-0

Fisher, J., & Hammarberg, K. (2012). Psychological and social aspects of infertility in men: An overview of the evidence and implications for psychologically informed clinical care and future research. *Asian Journal of Andrology, 14*(1), 121–129.

Fritz, M. A., & Speroff, L. (2011). *Clinical gynecologic endocrinology and infertility* (8th ed.). Philadelphia, PA: Lippincott Williams & Wilkins.

Garolla, A., Pizzol, D., Bertoldo, A., De Toni, L., Barzon, L., & Foresta, C. (2013). Association, prevalence, and clearance of human papillomavirus and antisperm antibodies in infected semen samples from infertile patients. *Fertility and Sterility, 99*(1), 125–131.

Haimov-Kochman, R., Adler, C., Ein-Mor, E., Rosenak, D., & Hurwitz, A. (2012). Infertility associated with pre-coital ovulation in observant Jewish couples: Prevalence, treatment, efficacy and side effects. *Israel Medical Association Journal (IMAJ), 14,* 100–103.

Harper, P. S. (2010). *Practical genetic counseling* (7th ed.) London, UK: Hodder Arnold.

Hill, M. J., Whitcomb, W., Lewis, T. D., Wu, M., Terry, N., Decherney, A. H., Levens, E. D., & Propst, A. M. (2013). Progesterone luteal support after ovulation induction and intrauterine insemination: A systematic review and meta-analysis. *Fertility and Sterility, 100*(5), 1373–1380.

Kalfoglou, A., Kammersell, M., Philpott, S., & Dahl, E. (2013). Ethical arguments for and against sperm sorting for non-medical sex selection: A review. *Reproductive BioMedicine Online 26*(3), 231–239. doi:10.1016/j.rbmo.2012.11.007

Kuehn, B. M. (2013). After 50 years, newborn screening continues to yield public health gains. *Journal of the American Medical Association (JAMA), 309*(12), 1215–1217.

Lebovic, D. I., Gordon, J. D., & Taylor, R. N. (2014). *Reproductive endocrinology and infertility: Handbook for clinicians* (2nd ed.). Arlington, VA: Scrub Hill Press, Inc.

Marci, R., Marcucci, I., Marcucci, A. A., Pacini, N., et al. (2013). Hysterosalpingocontrast sonography (HyCoSy): Evaluation of the pain perception, side effects and complications. *BMC Medical Imaging, 13*(28). doi:10.1186/1471-2342-13-28

Michalakis, K. G., DeCherney, A. H., & Penzias, A. S. (2013). Assisted reproductive technologies: In vitro fertilization & related techniques. In A. H. DeCherney, L. Nathan, N. Laufer, & A. S. Roman (Eds.), *Current diagnosis & treatment: Obstetrics & gynecology* (11th ed., pp. 920–947). New York, NY: McGraw-Hill.

Mutlu, M. F., Erdem, M., Erdem, A., Yildiz, I., Mutlu, I., Arisoy, O., & Oktem, M. (2013). Antral follicle count determines poor ovarian response better than anti-Müllerian hormone but age is the only predictor for live birth in in vitro fertilization cycles. *Journal of Assisted Reproduction and Genetics 30*(5), 657–665.

National Human Genome Research Institute. (2015). *Frequently asked questions about genetic disorders.* Retrieved from http://www.genome.gov/19016930

National Society of Genetic Counselors (NSGC). (2015). *Students and prospective genetic counselors: What is genetic counseling?* Retrieved from http:/www.nsgc.org/p/cm/d/fid=43

Obeisat, S., Gharaibeh, M. K., Owis, A., & Gharaibeh, H. (2012). Adversities of being infertile: The experience of Jordanian women. *Fertility and Sterility, 98*(2), 444–449. doi:10.1016/j.fertnstert.2012.04.036

Pavone, M. E., & Bulun, S. E. (2013). The use of aromatase inhibitors for ovulation induction and superovulation. *Journal of Clinical Endocrinology & Metabolism, 98*(5), 1838–1844.

Propst, A., & Wright Bates, G. (2012). Evaluation and treatment of anovulatory and unexplained infertility. *Obstetrics & Gynecology Clinics of North America, 39,* 507–519.

Sawatzky, M. (1981). Tasks of the infertile couple. *Journal of Obstetric, Gynecologic, and Neonatal Nursing, 10,* 132.

Smith, C. A., de Lacey, S., Chapman, M., Ratcliffe, J., Norman, R. J., Johnson, N., Sacks, G., Lyttleton, J., & Boothroyd, C. (2012). Acupuncture to improve live birth rates for women undergoing in vitro fertilization: A protocol for a randomized controlled trial. *Trials, 13*(60).

Chapter 8

Physical and Psychologic Changes of Pregnancy

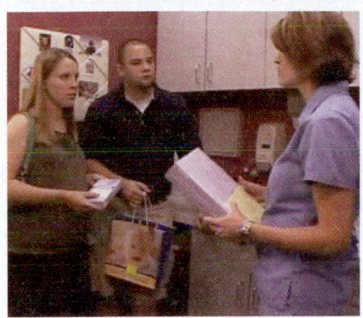

In my experience, few women are ever really prepared for all the changes they experience during pregnancy, especially a first pregnancy. That is why early prenatal care is important. Yes, starting care early gives us a better chance to identify risk factors, but it also enables us to do a better job of prenatal education. I am constantly amazed by what a difference it makes for a woman when she has a good idea of what to expect and why.

—A Nurse Working with an Obstetrician in Private Practice

∨ Learning Outcomes

8.1 Identify the anatomic and physiologic changes that occur during pregnancy.

8.2 Relate the physiologic and anatomic changes that occur in the body systems during pregnancy to the signs and symptoms that develop in the woman.

8.3 Compare subjective (presumptive), objective (probable), and diagnostic (positive) changes of pregnancy.

8.4 Contrast the various types of pregnancy tests.

8.5 Examine the emotional and psychologic changes that commonly occur in a woman, her partner, and her family during pregnancy.

8.6 Summarize cultural factors that may influence a family's response to pregnancy.

No matter how much we learn about pregnancy and the changes that occur in the woman and the developing fetus, we never cease to be amazed. First, it is nothing short of a miracle that the union of two microscopic entities—an ovum and a sperm—can produce a living being. Second, the woman's body must undergo extraordinary physical changes to maintain a pregnancy.

Pregnancy is divided into three trimesters, each approximately a 3-month period. Each trimester brings predictable changes for both the mother and the fetus. This chapter describes these physical and psychologic changes. It also presents the various cultural factors that can affect a pregnant woman's well-being. Subsequent chapters build on this information in describing effective approaches to planning and providing care.

Anatomy and Physiology of Pregnancy

The changes that occur in the pregnant woman's body may result from hormonal influences, the growth of the fetus, or the mother's physiologic adaptation to the pregnancy.

Reproductive System

Some of the most dramatic changes of pregnancy occur in the reproductive organs.

UTERUS

The changes in the uterus during pregnancy are amazing. Before pregnancy, the uterus is a small, semisolid, pear-shaped organ measuring approximately 7.5 × 5 × 2.5 cm (3 × 2 × 1 in.) and weighing about 60 g (2 oz). At the end of pregnancy it measures about 28 × 24 × 21 cm (11 × 9.5 × 8.25 in.) and weighs approximately 1100 g (2.4 lb); its capacity has also increased from about 10 mL to 5000 mL (5 L) or more (Cunningham et al., 2014).

The enlargement of the uterus is primarily because of the enlargement (hypertrophy) of the preexisting myometrial cells as a result of the stimulating influence of estrogen and the distention caused by the growing fetus. Only a limited increase in cell number (hyperplasia) occurs. The fibrous tissue between the muscle bands increases markedly, which adds to the strength and elasticity of the muscle wall. The enlarging uterus, developing placenta, and growing fetus require additional blood flow to the uterus. By the end of pregnancy, one sixth of the total maternal blood volume is contained within the vascular system of the uterus.

Braxton Hicks contractions, which are irregular, generally painless contractions of the uterus, occur intermittently throughout pregnancy. They may be felt through the abdominal wall beginning about the fourth month of pregnancy. In later months, these contractions become uncomfortable and may be confused with true labor contractions.

Clinical Tip

Beginning after the first trimester, have the woman feel her uterus periodically so that she becomes familiar with its size and the way it feels. As her pregnancy progresses she then will be more likely to identify Braxton Hicks contractions and preterm labor, if it occurs.

CERVIX

Estrogen stimulates the glandular tissue of the cervix, which increases in cell number and becomes hyperactive. The endocervical glands secrete a thick, sticky mucus that accumulates and forms a **mucous plug**, which seals the endocervical canal and prevents the ascent of microorganisms into the uterus. This plug is expelled when cervical dilatation begins. The hyperactivity of the glandular tissue also increases the normal physiologic mucorrhea, at times resulting in profuse discharge. Increased cervical vascularity also causes both the softening of the cervix (**Goodell sign**) and its bluish discoloration (**Chadwick sign**).

OVARIES

The ovaries stop producing ova during pregnancy, but the corpus luteum continues to produce hormones until about weeks 6 to 8. It secretes progesterone until about the seventh week of pregnancy to maintain the endometrium until the placenta assumes the task. The corpus luteum then begins to disintegrate slowly.

VAGINA

Estrogen causes a thickening of the vaginal mucosa, a loosening of the connective tissue, and an increase in vaginal secretions. These secretions are thick, white, and acidic (pH 3.5 to 6.0). The acid pH helps prevent bacterial infection but favors the growth of yeast organisms. Thus the pregnant woman is more susceptible to *Candida* infection than usual.

The supportive connective tissue of the vagina loosens throughout pregnancy. By the end of pregnancy, the vagina and perineal body are sufficiently relaxed to permit passage of the baby. Because blood flow to the vagina is increased, the vagina may show the same bluish-purple color (Chadwick sign) as the cervix.

Breasts

Estrogen and progesterone cause many changes in the mammary glands. The breasts enlarge and become more nodular as the glands increase in size and number in preparation for lactation. Superficial veins become more prominent, the nipples become more erectile, and the areolas darken. Montgomery's follicles (sebaceous glands) enlarge, and **striae** (reddish stretch marks that slowly turn silver after childbirth) may develop.

Colostrum, an antibody-rich yellow secretion, may leak or be expressed from the breasts during the last trimester. Colostrum gradually converts to mature milk during the first few days after childbirth.

Respiratory System

Many respiratory changes occur to meet the increased oxygen requirements of a pregnant woman. The volume of air breathed each minute increases 30% to 40% (Gordon, 2012). In addition, progesterone decreases airway resistance, permitting a 15% to 20% increase in oxygen consumption, as well as increases in carbon dioxide production and in the respiratory functional reserve.

As the uterus enlarges, it presses upward and elevates the diaphragm. The subcostal angle increases, so that the rib cage flares. The anteroposterior diameter increases, and the chest circumference expands by as much as 6 cm; as a result, there is no significant loss of intrathoracic volume. Breathing changes from abdominal to thoracic as pregnancy progresses, and descent of the diaphragm on inspiration becomes less possible. Some hyperventilation and difficulty in breathing may occur.

Nasal stuffiness and epistaxis (nosebleeds) may also occur because of estrogen-induced edema and vascular congestion of the nasal mucosa.

Cardiovascular System

Blood volume progressively increases beginning in the first trimester, increases rapidly until about 30 to 34 weeks, and then plateaus until birth at about 40% to 50% above nonpregnant levels. This increase is a result of increases in both erythrocytes and plasma (Gordon, 2012).

During pregnancy, blood flow increases to organ systems with an increased workload. Thus blood flow increases to the uterus, placenta, and breasts, whereas hepatic and cerebral flow remains unchanged. Cardiac output begins to increase early in pregnancy and peaks at 25 to 30 weeks' gestation at 30% to 50% above pre-pregnant levels. It generally remains elevated in the third trimester.

The pulse may increase by as many as 10 to 15 beats per minute at term. The blood pressure decreases slightly, reaching its lowest point during the second trimester. It gradually increases to near pre-pregnant levels by the end of the third trimester.

The enlarging uterus puts pressure on pelvic and femoral vessels, interfering with returning blood flow and causing stasis of blood in the lower extremities. This condition may lead to dependent edema and varicosity of the veins in the legs, vulva, and rectum (hemorrhoids) in late pregnancy. This increased blood volume in the lower legs may also make the pregnant woman prone to postural hypotension.

When the pregnant woman lies supine, the enlarging uterus may press on the vena cava, thus reducing blood flow to the right atrium, lowering blood pressure, and causing dizziness, pallor, and clamminess. Research indicates that the enlarging uterus may also press on the aorta and its collateral circulation (Cunningham et al., 2014). This condition is called **supine hypotensive syndrome**. It may also be referred to as *vena caval*

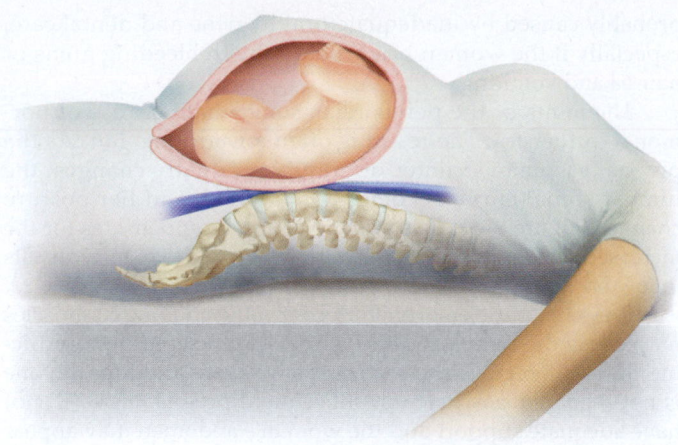

Figure 8–1 Supine hypotensive syndrome (vena caval syndrome). The gravid uterus compresses the vena cava when the woman is supine. This reduces the blood flow returning to the heart and may cause maternal hypotension.

syndrome or *aortocaval compression* (Figure 8–1). It can be corrected by having the woman lie on her left side or by placing a pillow or wedge under her right hip as she lies in a supine position.

The total erythrocyte (red blood cell [RBC]) volume increases by about 30% in women who receive iron supplementation; it increases only about 18% without iron supplementation. This increase in erythrocytes is necessary to transport the additional oxygen required during pregnancy. However, the increase in plasma volume during pregnancy averages about 50%. Because the plasma volume increase (50%) is greater than the erythrocyte increase (25%), the hematocrit, which measures the concentration of RBCs in the plasma, decreases slightly (Cao & O'Brien, 2013). This decrease is referred to as the **physiologic anemia of pregnancy** (*pseudoanemia*).

Iron is necessary for hemoglobin formation, and hemoglobin is the oxygen-carrying component of erythrocytes. Thus the increase in erythrocyte levels results in an increased need for iron by the pregnant woman. The American College of Obstetricians and Gynecologists (ACOG, 2013a) recommendation for an iron supplement during pregnancy is 27 mg of iron daily. This can be found in most prenatal supplements. Women who were diagnosed with anemia prior to pregnancy may require more iron supplementation.

Leukocyte production increases slightly to an average of 8500 mm^3 with a range of 5600 to 12,200 mm^3. During labor and the early postpartum period, these levels may reach 25,000/mm^3 or higher. Although the exact cause of the leukocytosis is not known, this increase is a normal finding (Cunningham et al., 2014).

Both the fibrin and the plasma fibrinogen levels increase during pregnancy. Although the blood-clotting time of the pregnant woman does not differ significantly from that of the non-pregnant woman, clotting factors VII, VIII, IX, and X increase; thus pregnancy is a somewhat hypercoagulable state. These changes, coupled with venous stasis in late pregnancy, increase the pregnant woman's risk of developing venous thrombosis.

Gastrointestinal System

Nausea and vomiting are common during the first trimester because of elevated human chorionic gonadotropin levels and changed carbohydrate metabolism. Gum tissue may soften and bleed easily. The secretion of saliva may increase and even become excessive (ptyalism).

Elevated progesterone levels cause smooth muscle relaxation, resulting in delayed gastric emptying and decreased peristalsis. As a result, the pregnant woman may complain of bloating and constipation. These symptoms are aggravated as the enlarging uterus displaces the stomach upward and the intestines are moved laterally and posteriorly. The cardiac sphincter also relaxes, and heartburn (pyrosis) may occur because of reflux of acidic secretions into the lower esophagus. Hemorrhoids frequently develop in late pregnancy from constipation and from pressure on vessels below the level of the uterus.

Only minor liver changes occur with pregnancy. Plasma albumin concentrations and serum cholinesterase activity decrease with normal pregnancy, as with certain liver diseases.

The emptying time of the gallbladder is prolonged during pregnancy as a result of smooth muscle relaxation from progesterone. This, coupled with the elevated levels of cholesterol in the bile, can predispose the woman to gallstone formation. Pruritus (itching) caused by retained bile salts may also occur (Cunningham et al., 2014).

Urinary Tract

During the first trimester, the enlarging uterus is still a pelvic organ and presses against the bladder, producing urinary frequency. This symptom decreases during the second trimester, when the uterus becomes an abdominal organ and pressure against the bladder lessens. Frequency reappears during the third trimester, when the presenting part descends into the pelvis and again presses on the bladder, reducing bladder capacity, contributing to hyperemia, and irritating the bladder.

The ureters (especially the right ureter) elongate and dilate above the pelvic brim. The glomerular filtration rate (GFR) rises by as much as 50% beginning in the second trimester and remains elevated until birth. To compensate for this increase, renal tubular reabsorption also increases. However, glycosuria is seen sometimes during pregnancy because of the kidneys' inability to reabsorb all the glucose filtered by the glomeruli. Glycosuria may be normal or may indicate gestational diabetes, so it always warrants further testing.

Skin and Hair

Changes in skin pigmentation commonly occur during pregnancy. They are thought to be stimulated by increased estrogen, progesterone, and α-melanocytic-stimulating hormone levels. Pigmentation of the skin increases primarily in areas that are already hyperpigmented: the areola, the nipples, the vulva, and the perianal area. The skin in the middle of the abdomen may develop a pigmented line, the **linea nigra**, which usually extends from the umbilicus or above to the pubic area (Figure 8–2). Facial **chloasma** or **melasma gravidarum** (also known as the "mask of pregnancy"), a darkening of the skin over the cheeks, nose, and forehead, may develop. Chloasma or melasma is more prominent in dark-haired women and is aggravated by exposure to the sun. Fortunately, the condition fades or becomes less prominent soon after childbirth when the hormonal influence of pregnancy subsides. In addition, the sweat and sebaceous glands are often hyperactive during pregnancy, and may cause heavy perspiration, night sweats, and the development of acne.

Striae, or stretch marks, may appear on the abdomen, thighs, buttocks, and breasts. They result from reduced connective tissue strength because of elevated adrenal steroid levels.

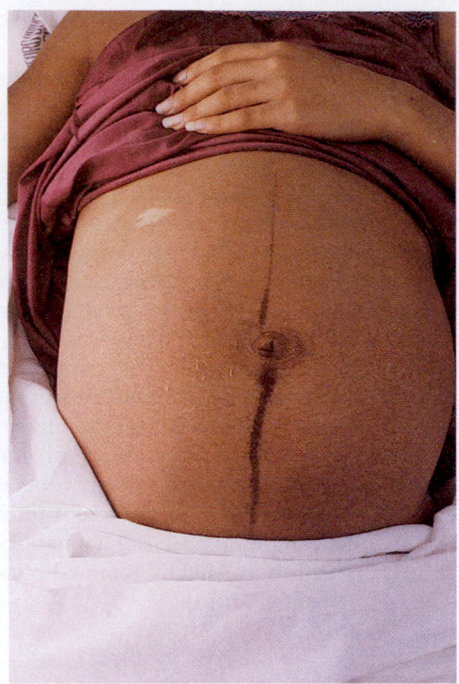

Figure 8–2 Linea nigra.

Vascular spider nevi—small, bright red elevations of the skin radiating from a central body—may develop on the chest, neck, face, arms, and legs. They may be caused by increased subcutaneous blood flow in response to elevated estrogen levels.

The rate of hair growth may decrease during pregnancy; the number of hair follicles in the resting or dormant phase also decreases. After birth, the number of hair follicles in the resting phase increases sharply and the woman may notice increased hair shedding for 1 to 4 months. However, practically all hair is replaced within 6 to 12 months (Cunningham et al., 2014).

Musculoskeletal System

No demonstrable changes occur in the teeth of pregnant women. The dental caries that sometimes accompany pregnancy are probably caused by inadequate oral hygiene and dental care, especially if the woman has problems with bleeding gums or nausea and vomiting.

The joints of the pelvis relax somewhat because of hormonal influences. The result is often a waddling gait. As the pregnant woman's center of gravity gradually changes, the lumbar spinal curve becomes accentuated, and her posture changes (Figure 8–3). This posture change compensates for the increased weight of the uterus anteriorly and frequently results in low backache.

Pressure of the enlarging uterus on the abdominal muscles may cause the rectus abdominis muscle to separate, producing **diastasis recti**. If the separation is severe and muscle tone is not regained postpartum, subsequent pregnancies will not have adequate support and the woman's abdomen may appear pendulous.

Central Nervous System

Pregnant women frequently describe decreased attention, concentration, and memory during and shortly after pregnancy, but few studies have explored this phenomenon. One study did compare a group of pregnant women against a control group, finding a decline in memory that could not be attributed to depression, anxiety, sleep deprivation, or other physical changes of pregnancy. This memory loss disappears soon after childbirth (Cunningham et al., 2014).

Eyes

During pregnancy, intraocular pressure decreases, probably because of increased vitreous outflow, and the cornea thickens slightly because of fluid retention. As a result, some pregnant women experience difficulty wearing previously comfortable contact lenses (Cunningham et al., 2014). These changes usually disappear by 6 weeks postpartum.

Metabolism

Most metabolic functions increase during pregnancy because of the increased demands of the growing fetus and its support system. For a detailed discussion of nutrient, vitamin, and mineral metabolism, see Chapter 11.

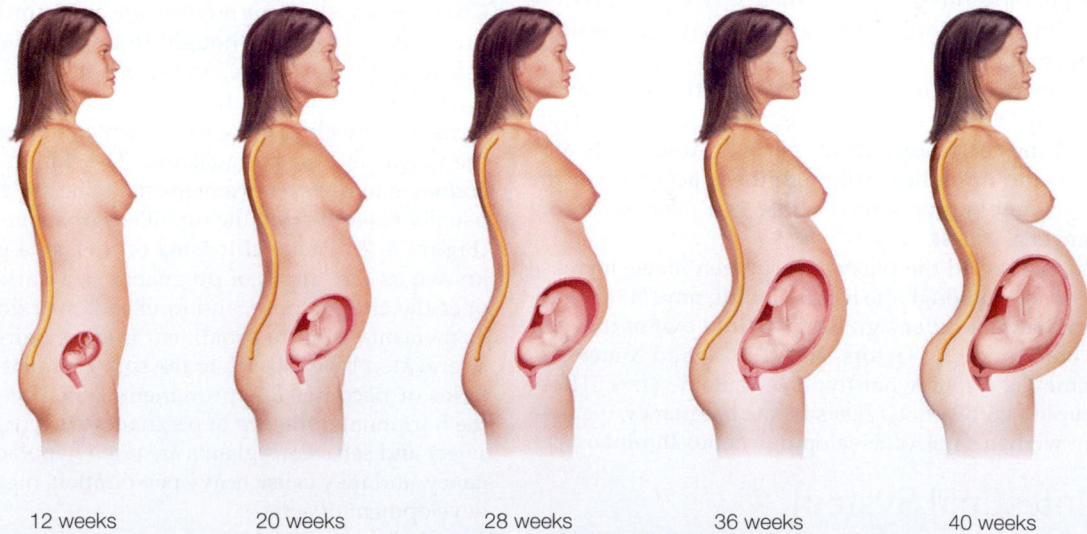

| 12 weeks | 20 weeks | 28 weeks | 36 weeks | 40 weeks |

Figure 8–3 Postural changes during pregnancy. Note the increasing lordosis of the lumbosacral spine and the increasing curvature of the thoracic area.

WEIGHT GAIN

The recommended total weight gain during pregnancy for a woman of normal weight before pregnancy is 11.5 to 16 kg (25 to 35 lb); for women who were overweight before becoming pregnant, the recommended gain is 6.8 to 11.5 kg (15 to 25 lb). Women who are obese are advised to limit weight gain to 5 to 9 kg (11 to 20 lb). Underweight women are advised to gain 12.7 to 18.1 kg (28 to 40 lb) (Institute of Medicine [IOM], 2009). A woman of normal weight should gain about 0.5 to 2 kg (1.1 to 4.4 lb) during the first trimester, followed by an average gain of about 0.45 kg (1 lb) per week during the last two trimesters (IOM, 2009).

ACOG (2013b) supports the IOM recommendations and recommends that healthcare providers determine a woman's body mass index (BMI) at the initial prenatal visit. Individualized care and clinical judgment should then be used to determine the appropriate weight gain.

WATER METABOLISM

Increased water retention, a basic alteration of pregnancy, is caused by several interrelated factors. The increased level of steroid sex hormones affects sodium and fluid retention. The lowered serum protein also influences fluid balance, as do increased intracapillary pressure and permeability. The extra water is needed for the fetus, placenta, and amniotic fluid and the mother's increased blood volume, interstitial fluids, and enlarged organs.

NUTRIENT METABOLISM

The fetus makes its greatest protein and fat demands during the second half of pregnancy, doubling in weight during the last 6 to 8 weeks. Protein (contributing nitrogen) must be stored during pregnancy to maintain a constant level within the breast milk and to avoid depletion of maternal tissues. Carbohydrate needs also increase, especially during the second and third trimesters.

Fats are more completely absorbed during pregnancy, and the level of free fatty acids increases in response to human placental lactogen. The levels of lipoproteins and cholesterol also increase. Because of these changes, increased levels of dietary fat or reduced carbohydrate production may lead to ketonuria in the pregnant woman. See Chapter 11 for a complete discussion of the mother's nutritional requirements.

Endocrine System

THYROID GLAND

The thyroid gland often enlarges slightly during pregnancy because of increased vascularity and hyperplasia of glandular tissue. Its capacity to bind thyroxine is greater, resulting in an increase in serum protein-bound iodine. These changes are a result of higher blood levels of estrogen during pregnancy.

The basal metabolic rate increases by as much as 20% to 25% during pregnancy. The increased oxygen consumption is primarily because of fetal metabolic activity. Within a few weeks after birth all thyroid function returns to normal limits.

PITUITARY GLAND

Pregnancy is made possible by the hypothalamic stimulation of the anterior pituitary gland. The anterior pituitary produces follicle-stimulating hormone (FSH), which stimulates ovum growth, and luteinizing hormone (LH), which brings about ovulation. Stimulation of the pituitary also prolongs the ovary's corpus luteal phase, which maintains the endometrium in case conception occurs. Prolactin, another anterior pituitary hormone, is responsible for lactation.

The posterior pituitary secretes vasopressin (antidiuretic hormone) and oxytocin. Vasopressin causes vasoconstriction, which results in increased blood pressure; it also helps regulate water balance. Oxytocin promotes uterine contractility and stimulates ejection of milk from the breasts (the letdown reflex) in the postpartum period.

ADRENAL GLANDS

During pregnancy circulating cortisol, which regulates carbohydrate and protein metabolism, increases in response to increased estrogen levels. Cortisol blood levels return to normal within 1 to 6 weeks postpartum. The adrenal glands secrete increased levels of aldosterone by the early part of the second trimester. This increase in aldosterone in a normal pregnancy may be the body's protective response to the increased sodium excretion associated with progesterone (Cunningham et al., 2014).

PANCREAS

The pregnant woman has increased insulin needs, and the pancreatic islets of Langerhans, which secrete insulin, are stressed to meet this increased demand. Any marginal pancreatic function quickly becomes apparent, and the woman may show signs of gestational diabetes (see Chapter 14).

HORMONES IN PREGNANCY

Human Chorionic Gonadotropin. The trophoblast secretes human chorionic gonadotropin (hCG) in early pregnancy. This hormone stimulates progesterone and estrogen production by the corpus luteum to maintain the pregnancy until the placenta has developed sufficiently to assume that function.

Human Placental Lactogen. Also called *human chorionic somatomammotropin*, human placental lactogen (hPL) is produced by the syncytiotrophoblast. Human placental lactogen is an antagonist of insulin; it increases the amount of circulating free fatty acids for maternal metabolic needs and decreases maternal metabolism of glucose to favor fetal growth.

Estrogen. Estrogen, secreted originally by the corpus luteum, is produced primarily by the placenta as early as the seventh week of pregnancy. Estrogen stimulates uterine development to provide a suitable environment for the fetus. It also helps develop the ductal system of the breasts in preparation for lactation.

Progesterone. Progesterone, also produced initially by the corpus luteum and then by the placenta, plays the greatest role in maintaining pregnancy. It maintains the endometrium and inhibits spontaneous uterine contractility, thus preventing early spontaneous abortion. Progesterone also helps develop the acini and lobules of the breasts in preparation for lactation.

Relaxin. Relaxin is detectable in the serum of a pregnant woman by the time of the first missed menstrual period. Relaxin inhibits uterine activity, diminishes the strength of uterine contractions, aids in the softening of the cervix, and has the long-term effect of remodeling collagen. Its primary source is the corpus luteum, but small amounts are believed to be produced by the placenta and uterine decidua.

PROSTAGLANDINS IN PREGNANCY

Prostaglandins (PGs) are lipid substances that can arise from most body tissues but occur in high concentrations in the female reproductive tract and are present in the decidua during pregnancy. The exact functions of PGs during pregnancy are still unknown, although it has been proposed that they are responsible for maintaining reduced placental vascular resistance. Decreased prostaglandin levels may contribute to hypertension and preeclampsia. Prostaglandins are also believed to play a role in the complex biochemistry that initiates labor.

Signs of Pregnancy

Many of the changes women experience during pregnancy are used to diagnose the pregnancy itself. They are called the subjective, or presumptive, changes; the objective, or probable, changes; and the diagnostic, or positive, changes of pregnancy.

Subjective (Presumptive) Changes

The subjective changes of pregnancy are the symptoms the woman experiences and reports. Because they can be caused by other conditions, they cannot be considered proof of pregnancy (Table 8–1). The following subjective signs can be diagnostic clues when other signs and symptoms of pregnancy are also present:

- *Amenorrhea,* or the absence of menses, is the earliest symptom of pregnancy. The missing of more than one menstrual period, especially in a woman whose cycle is ordinarily regular, is an especially useful diagnostic clue.
- *Nausea and vomiting of pregnancy (NVP)* occur frequently during the first trimester and may be the result of elevated human chorionic gonadotropin (hCG) levels and changed carbohydrate metabolism. Because these symptoms often occur in the early part of the day, they are commonly referred to as **morning sickness**. In reality, the symptoms may occur at any time and can range from a mere distaste for food to severe vomiting.

- *Excessive fatigue* may be noted within a few weeks after the first missed menstrual period and may persist throughout the first trimester.
- *Urinary frequency* is experienced during the first trimester as the enlarging uterus presses on the bladder.
- *Changes in the breasts* are frequently noted in early pregnancy. These changes include tenderness and tingling sensations, increased pigmentation of the areola and nipple, and changes in Montgomery glands. The veins also become more visible and form a bluish pattern beneath the skin.
- **Quickening,** or the mother's perception of fetal movement, occurs about 18 to 20 weeks after the last menstrual period in a woman pregnant for the first time but may occur as early as 16 weeks in a woman who has been pregnant before. Quickening is a fluttering sensation in the abdomen that gradually increases in intensity and frequency.

Clinical Tip

Some women suggest that it is easiest to imagine the fluttering associated with quickening by letting the outer tips of the eyelashes brush a finger and then imagining that same sensation deep inside the abdomen.

Objective (Probable) Changes

An examiner can perceive the objective changes that occur in pregnancy. Because these changes can also have other causes, they do not confirm pregnancy (Table 8–2).

- *Changes in the pelvic organs*—the only physical changes detectable during the first 3 months of pregnancy—are

TABLE 8–1 Differential Diagnosis of Pregnancy—Subjective Changes

SUBJECTIVE CHANGES	POSSIBLE ALTERNATIVE CAUSES
Amenorrhea	Endocrine factors: early menopause; lactation; thyroid, pituitary, adrenal, ovarian dysfunction
	Metabolic factors: malnutrition, anemia, climatic changes, diabetes mellitus, degenerative disorders, long-distance running
	Psychologic factors: emotional shock, fear of pregnancy or sexually transmitted infection, intense desire for pregnancy (pseudocyesis), stress
	Obliteration of endometrial cavity by infection or curettage
	Systemic disease (acute or chronic), such as tuberculosis or malignancy
Nausea and vomiting	Gastrointestinal disorders
	Acute infections such as encephalitis
	Emotional disorders such as pseudocyesis or anorexia nervosa
Urinary frequency	Urinary tract infection
	Cystocele
	Pelvic tumors
	Urethral diverticula
	Emotional tension
Breast tenderness	Premenstrual tension
	Chronic cystic mastitis
	Pseudocyesis
	Hyperestrogenism
Quickening	Increased peristalsis
	Flatus ("gas")
	Abdominal muscle contractions
	Shifting of abdominal contents

TABLE 8–2 Differential Diagnosis of Pregnancy—Objective Changes

OBJECTIVE CHANGES	POSSIBLE ALTERNATIVE CAUSES
Changes in pelvic organs	Increased vascular congestion
Goodell sign	Estrogen–progestin oral contraceptives
Chadwick sign	Vulvar, vaginal, cervical hyperemia
Hegar sign	Excessively soft walls of nonpregnant uterus
Uterine enlargement	Uterine tumors
Braun von Fernwald sign	Uterine tumors
Enlargement of abdomen	Obesity, ascites, pelvic tumors
Braxton Hicks contractions	Hematometra, pedunculated, submucous, and soft myomas
Uterine souffle	Large uterine myomas, large ovarian tumors, or any condition with greatly increased uterine blood flow
Pigmentation of skin	Estrogen–progestin oral contraceptives
Chloasma (melasma)	Melanocyte hormonal stimulation
Linea nigra	
Nipples/areola	
Abdominal striae	Obesity, pelvic tumor
Ballottement	Uterine tumors/polyps, ascites
Positive pregnancy tests	Increased pituitary gonadotropins at menopause, choriocarcinoma, hydatidiform mole
Palpation for fetal outline	Uterine myomas

caused by increased vascular congestion. These changes are noted on pelvic examination. As noted earlier, there is a softening of the cervix called Goodell sign. Chadwick sign is a bluish, purple, or deep red discoloration of the mucous membranes of the cervix, vagina, and vulva (some sources consider this a presumptive sign). **Hegar sign** is a softening of the isthmus of the uterus, the area between the cervix and the body of the uterus (Figure 8–4). **McDonald sign** is an ease in flexing the body of the uterus against the cervix. General enlargement and softening of the body of the uterus can be noted after the eighth week of pregnancy. The fundus of the uterus is palpable just above the symphysis pubis at about 10 to 12 weeks' gestation and at the level of the umbilicus at 20 to 22 weeks' gestation (Figure 8–5).

- *Enlargement of the abdomen* during the childbearing years is usually regarded as evidence of pregnancy, especially if it is continuous and accompanied by amenorrhea.

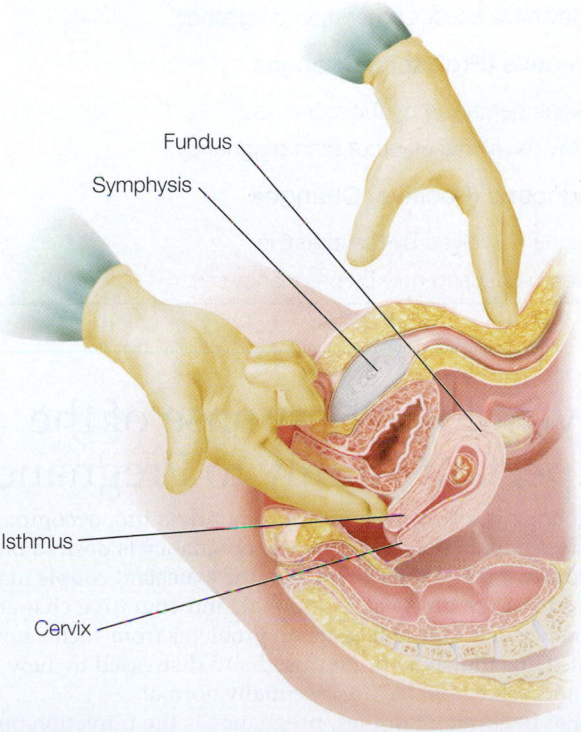

Figure 8–4 Hegar sign, a softening of the isthmus of the uterus, can be determined by the examiner during a vaginal examination.

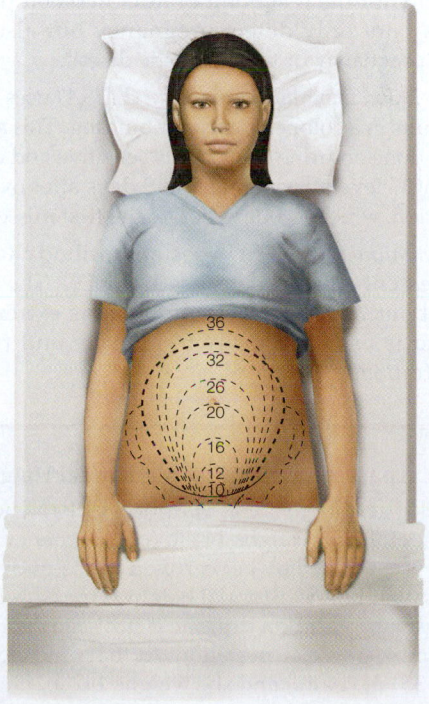

Figure 8–5 Approximate height of the fundus at various weeks of pregnancy.

- *Braxton Hicks contractions* can be palpated most commonly after 28 weeks. As the woman approaches the end of pregnancy, these contractions may become uncomfortable. They are then often called false labor.

- *Uterine souffle* may be heard when the examiner auscultates the abdomen over the uterus. It is a soft, blowing sound that occurs at the same rate as the maternal pulse and is caused by the increased uterine blood flow and blood pulsating through the placenta. It is sometimes confused with the *funic souffle,* a soft, blowing sound of blood pulsating through the umbilical cord. The funic souffle occurs at the same rate as the fetal heart rate.

- *Changes in pigmentation of the skin* are common in pregnancy. The nipples and areola may darken, and the linea nigra may develop. Facial melasma (chloasma) may become noticeable, and striae may appear.

- The *fetal outline* may be identified by palpation in many pregnant women after 24 weeks' gestation. **Ballottement** is the passive fetal movement elicited when the examiner inserts two gloved fingers into the vagina and pushes against the cervix. This action pushes the fetal body up, and, as it falls back, the examiner feels a rebound.

- *Pregnancy tests* detect the presence of hCG in the maternal blood or urine. These are not considered a positive sign of pregnancy because other conditions can cause elevated hCG levels.

CLINICAL PREGNANCY TESTS

A variety of assay techniques are available to detect hCG in either blood or urine during early pregnancy. Most healthcare providers use urine screening tests because the results are immediate, the cost is minimal, the tests are reasonably accurate, and no invasive procedure (blood draw) is required (Levin, Hopkins, & Tiffany, 2011).

- *β-Subunit radioimmunoassay (RIA)* uses an antiserum with specificity for the β-subunit of hCG in blood plasma. This test may not only detect pregnancy but also detect an ectopic pregnancy or trophoblastic disease.

- *Enzyme-linked immunosorbent assay (ELISA)* uses a substance that results in a color change after binding. This assay, which may be done on urine or blood, is sensitive and quick. It can detect hCG levels as early as 7 to 9 days after ovulation and conception, which is 5 days before the first missed period.

- *Fluoroimmunoassay (FIA)* uses an antibody tagged with a fluorescent label to detect serum hCG. The test, which takes about 2 to 3 hours to perform, is extremely sensitive and is used primarily to identify and follow hCG concentrations.

Clinical Reasoning Evaluating Fundal Height

At 33 weeks' gestation, Elena Martinez, G2P1, who is 5 feet 4 inches tall and weighs 144 lb (prepregnancy weight of 120 lb), is examined by her certified nurse-midwife (CNM). At that time her fundal height is measured as 33 cm. Because of a vacation trip, she is not seen again by her midwife until 36 weeks' gestation. At that time, her fundus measures 35 cm (14 in.) and she weighs 147 lb. Elena asks if there is something wrong with her baby's growth.

What is your assessment?

OVER-THE-COUNTER PREGNANCY TESTS

Home pregnancy tests (HPTs) are available over the counter at a reasonable cost. These ELISA tests, performed on urine, detect even low levels of hCG. HPT instructions should be followed carefully for optimal results. If the results are negative, the woman should repeat the test in 1 week if she has not started her period.

Diagnostic (Positive) Changes

The positive signs of pregnancy are completely objective, cannot be confused with a pathologic state, and offer conclusive proof of pregnancy:

- *Fetal heartbeat* can be detected with an electronic Doppler device as early as weeks 10 to 12. The heartbeat can be detected with a fetoscope by weeks 17 to 20.

- *Fetal movement* is actively palpable by a trained examiner after about week 20 of pregnancy.

- *Visualization of the fetus* by ultrasound examination confirms a pregnancy. The gestational sac can be observed by 4 to 5 weeks' gestation (2 to 3 weeks after conception). Fetal parts and fetal heart movement can be seen as early as 8 weeks' gestation. More recently, ultrasound using a vaginal probe has been used to detect a gestational sac as early as 10 days after implantation (Cunningham et al., 2014).

KEY FACTS TO REMEMBER
Differentiating the Signs of Pregnancy

These guidelines help differentiate among the presumptive, probable, and positive changes of pregnancy.

Subjective (Presumptive) Changes

- Symptoms the woman experiences and reports
- May have causes other than pregnancy

Objective (Probable) Changes

- Signs perceived by the examiner
- May have causes other than pregnancy

Diagnostic (Positive) Changes

- Signs perceived by the examiner
- Can be caused only by pregnancy

Psychologic Response of the Expectant Family to Pregnancy

Pregnancy is a turning point in a family's life, accompanied by stress and anxiety, whether the pregnancy is desired or not. Especially if this is their first child, the expectant couple may be unaware of the physical, emotional, and cognitive changes of pregnancy and may anticipate no problems from such a normal event. Thus they may be confused and distressed by new feelings and behaviors that are essentially normal.

For beginning families, pregnancy is the transition period from childlessness to parenthood. If the expectant woman is married or has a stable partner, she no longer is only a mate but must also assume the role of mother. Her partner, whether male or female, will become a parent, too. The anticipation of parenthood brings significant role changes for them. Career goals and mobility may be affected, and the couple's relationship takes on a different meaning to them and their families and community. If the pregnancy results in the birth of a child, the couple enters a new, irreversible stage of their life together. With each subsequent pregnancy, routines and family dynamics are again altered, requiring readjustment and realignment.

In most pregnancies, finances are an important consideration. Traditional lore relegates to the father the role of primary breadwinner, and indeed finances are often a very real concern for fathers. In today's society, however, there are many types of families (see Chapter 2) and even pregnant women with stable partners recognize the financial impact of a child and may feel concern about financial issues. Decisions about financial matters need to be made at this time. Will the woman work during her pregnancy and return to work after her child is born? If so, who will provide child care? Couples may also need to decide about the division of domestic tasks. Any differences of opinion must be discussed openly and resolved so that the family can meet the needs of its members.

If the pregnant woman has no stable partner, she must deal alone with the role changes, fears, and adjustments of pregnancy or seek support from family or friends. She also faces the reality of planning for the future as a single parent. Finances may be a major source of concern. Even if the pregnant woman plans to relinquish her baby, she must still deal with the adjustments of pregnancy. These adjustments can be especially difficult without a good support system.

Developmental Tasks of the Expectant Couple

Pregnancy can be viewed as a developmental stage with its own distinct developmental tasks. For a couple, it can be a time of support or conflict, depending on the amount of adjustment each is willing to make to maintain the family's equilibrium.

During a first pregnancy, the woman and her partner plan together for the child's arrival, collecting information on how to be parents. At the same time, each continues to participate in some separate activities with friends or family members. The availability of social support is an important factor in psychosocial well-being during pregnancy. Most pregnant women find their partners are their greatest source of support, followed by family and friends (Widarsson, Kerstis, Sundquist, et al., 2012). In addition, the broader social network is often a major source of advice for the pregnant woman; however, both sound and unsound information may be conveyed.

During pregnancy, the expectant parents both face significant changes and must deal with major psychosocial adjustments (Table 8–3). Other family members, especially other children of the woman or couple and the grandparents-to-be, must also adjust to the pregnancy.

For some, pregnancy is more than a developmental stage; it is a crisis. *Crisis* can be defined as a disturbance or conflict in which the individual cannot maintain a state of equilibrium. Pregnancy can be considered a *maturational crisis*, as it is a

TABLE 8–3 Parental Reactions to Pregnancy

FIRST TRIMESTER	SECOND TRIMESTER	THIRD TRIMESTER
Mother's Reactions	*Mother's Reactions*	*Mother's Reactions*
Informs father secretively or openly	Remains regressive and introspective, projects all problems with authority figures onto partner, may become angry if she perceives his lack of interest as a sign of weakness in him	Experiences more anxiety and tension, with physical awkwardness
Feels ambivalent toward pregnancy, anxious about labor and responsibility of child	Continues to deal with feelings as a mother; shops for nursery furniture as something concrete to do	Feels much discomfort and insomnia from physical condition
Is aware of physical changes, daydreams of possible miscarriage	May experience anxiety or, alternately, may be very lackadaisical and wait until ninth month to look for furniture and clothes for baby	Prepares for birth, assembles layette, picks out names
Develops special feelings for and renewed interest in her own mother, with formation of a personal identity	Feels movement and is aware of fetus and incorporates it into herself	Dreams often about misplacing baby or not being able to give birth, fears birth of deformed baby
	Dreams that partner will be killed, telephones him often for reassurance	Feels ecstasy and excitement, has spurt of energy during last month
	Experiences more distinct physical changes; sexual desires may increase or decrease	
Father's Reactions	*Father's Reactions*	*Father's Reactions*
Differ according to age, parity, desire for child, economic stability	If he can cope, will give her extra attention she needs; if he cannot cope, will develop a new time-consuming interest outside of home	Adapts to alternative methods of sexual contact
Acceptance of pregnant woman's attitude or complete rejection and lack of communication	May develop a creative feeling and a "closeness to nature"	Becomes concerned over financial responsibility
Is aware of his sexual feelings, may develop more or less sexual arousal	May become involved in pregnancy and buy or make furniture	May show new sense of tenderness and concern, treat partner like doll
Accepts, rejects, or resents mother-in-law	Feels for movement of baby, listens to heartbeat, or remains aloof, with no physical contact	Daydreams about child as if older and not newborn, dreams of losing partner
May develop new hobby outside of family as sign of stress	May have fears and fantasies about himself being pregnant, may become uneasy with this feminine aspect in himself	Renewed sexual attraction to partner
	May react negatively if partner is too demanding; may become jealous of physician and of physician's importance to partner and her pregnancy	Feels he is ultimately responsible for whatever happens

common event in the normal growth and development of the family. If the crisis is not resolved, it will result in maladaptive behaviors in one or more family members and possible disintegration of the family. Families that are able to resolve a maturational crisis will return successfully to normal functioning and can even strengthen the bonds in the family relationship.

The Mother

Pregnancy is a condition that alters body image and necessitates a reordering of social relationships and changes in the roles of family members. The way each woman meets the stresses of pregnancy is influenced by her emotional makeup, her sociologic and cultural background, and her acceptance or rejection of the pregnancy. However, many women manifest similar psychologic and emotional responses during pregnancy, including ambivalence, acceptance, introversion, mood swings, and changes in body image.

A woman's attitude toward her pregnancy can be a significant factor in its outcome. Even if the pregnancy is planned, there is an element of surprise at first. Many women commonly experience feelings of ambivalence during early pregnancy. This ambivalence may be related to feelings that the timing is somehow wrong; worries about the need to modify existing relationships or career plans; fears about assuming a new role; unresolved emotional conflicts with the woman's own mother; and fears about pregnancy, labor, and birth. These feelings may be more pronounced if the pregnancy is unplanned or unwanted. Research indicates that women who are ambivalent about pregnancy are generally younger, less likely to have been pregnant previously, and more likely to have been a victim of sexual violence, to have experienced pregnancy coercion, to have unhealthy behaviors such as smoking, and to have psychologic risk factors. They are also more likely to experience stress and depression during pregnancy (Patel, Laz, & Berenson, 2015). Indirect expressions of ambivalence include complaints about considerable physical discomfort, prolonged or frequent depression, significant dissatisfaction with changing body shape, excessive mood swings, and difficulty in accepting the life changes resulting from the pregnancy.

Many pregnancies are unintended, but not all unintended pregnancies are unwanted. A pregnancy can be unintended and wanted at the same time. For some women, an unintended pregnancy has more psychologic and social advantages than disadvantages. It provides purpose and direction to life and allows a woman to test the devotion and love of her partner and family. However, an unintended pregnancy can be a risk factor for depression. Higher levels of depression were found in women who reported more negative responses to pregnancy, who believed that their pregnancies had greater consequences, and who experienced more symptoms, especially in the third trimester (Jessop, Craig, & Ayers, 2014).

Acceptance of pregnancy is influenced by many factors. Lower acceptance tends to be related to an unplanned pregnancy and greater evidence of fear and conflict. The woman carrying an unplanned pregnancy tends to experience more physical discomfort and depression. When a pregnancy is well accepted, the woman demonstrates feelings of happiness and pleasure in the pregnancy. She experiences less physical discomfort and shows a high degree of tolerance for the discomforts associated with the third trimester.

Conflicts about adapting to pregnancy are no more pronounced for older pregnant women (age 35 and over) than for younger ones. Moreover, older pregnant women tend to be less concerned about the normal physical changes of pregnancy and are confident about handling issues that arise during pregnancy and parenting. This difference may result because mature pregnant women have more experience with problem solving.

Pregnancy produces marked changes in a woman's body within a relatively short period of time. Pregnant women experience changes in body image because of physical alterations and may feel a loss of control over their bodies during pregnancy and later during childbirth. Although changes in body image are normal, they can be very stressful for the woman. Explanation and discussion of the changes may help both the woman and her partner deal with the stress associated with this aspect of pregnancy.

FIRST TRIMESTER

During the first trimester, feelings of disbelief and ambivalence are paramount. The woman's baby does not seem real, and she focuses on herself and her pregnancy. She may experience one or more of the early symptoms of pregnancy, such as breast tenderness or morning sickness, which are unsettling and at times unpleasant.

At this time, the expectant mother also begins to exhibit some characteristic behavioral changes. She may become increasingly introspective and passive. She may be emotionally labile, with characteristic mood swings from joy to despair. She may fantasize about a miscarriage and feel guilty because of these fantasies. She may worry that these thoughts will harm the baby in some way.

SECOND TRIMESTER

During the second trimester, quickening occurs. This perception of fetal movement helps the woman think of her baby as a separate person, and she generally becomes excited about the pregnancy even if earlier she was not. The woman becomes increasingly introspective as she evaluates her life, her plans, and her child's future. This introspection helps the woman prepare for her new mothering role. Emotional lability, which may be unsettling to her partner, persists. In some instances, the partner may react by withdrawing. This withdrawal is especially distressing to the woman, because she needs increased love and affection. Once the couple understands that these behaviors are characteristic of pregnancy, it is easier for the couple to deal with them effectively, although they may be sources of stress to some extent throughout pregnancy.

As pregnancy becomes more noticeable, the woman's body image changes. She may feel great pride, embarrassment, or concern. Generally, women feel best during the second trimester, which is a relatively tranquil time.

THIRD TRIMESTER

In the third trimester, the woman feels both pride about her pregnancy and anxiety about labor and birth. Physical discomforts increase, and the woman is eager for the pregnancy to end. She experiences increased fatigue, her body movements are more awkward, and her interest in sexual activity may decrease. During this time, the woman tends to be concerned about the health and safety of her unborn child and may worry that she will not cope well during childbirth. Toward the end of this period, there is often a surge of energy as the woman prepares a "nest" for the baby. Many women report bursts of energy, during which they vigorously clean and organize their homes.

PSYCHOLOGIC TASKS OF THE MOTHER

Rubin (1984) identified four major tasks that the pregnant woman undertakes to maintain her intactness and that of her family and at the same time incorporate her new child into the family system. These tasks form the foundation for a mutually gratifying relationship with her baby:

1. *Ensuring safe passage through pregnancy, labor, and birth.* The pregnant woman feels concern for both her unborn

child and herself. She looks for competent maternity care to provide a sense of control. She may seek information from literature, observation of other pregnant women and new mothers, and discussion with others. She often engages in self-care activities related to diet, exercise, and alcohol consumption. In the third trimester she becomes more aware of external threats in the environment—a toy on the stairs, the awkwardness of an escalator—that pose a threat to her well-being. Sleep becomes more difficult and she longs for birth even though it, too, is frightening.

2. *Seeking acceptance of this child by others.* The birth of a child alters a woman's primary support group (her family) and her secondary affiliative groups. The woman slowly and subtly alters her network to meet the needs of her pregnancy. In this adjustment, the woman's partner is the most important figure. The partner's support and acceptance help form a maternal identity. If there are other children in the home, the mother also works to ensure their acceptance of the coming child. The woman without a partner looks to others such as a family member or friend for this support.

3. *Seeking commitment and acceptance of herself as mother to the child (binding in).* During the first trimester, the child remains a rather abstract concept. With quickening, however, the child begins to become a real person, and the mother begins to develop bonds of attachment. The mother experiences the movement of the child within her in an intimate, exclusive way, and bonds of love form. This binding-in process, characterized by its strong emotional component, motivates the pregnant woman to become competent in her role and provides satisfaction for her in the role of mother.

4. *Learning to give of herself on behalf of her child.* Childbirth involves many acts of giving. The man "gives" a child to the woman; she in turn "gives" a child to him. Life is given to a baby; a sibling is given to older children of the family. The woman begins to develop a capacity for self-denial and learns to delay immediate personal gratification to meet the needs of another. Baby showers and gifts are acts of giving that increase the mother's self-esteem and help her recognize the separateness and needs of the coming baby.

Accomplishment of these tasks helps the expectant woman develop her self-concept as mother. The expectant woman who was well nurtured by her own mother may view her mother as a role model and emulate her; the woman who views her mother as a "poor mother" may worry that she will make similar mistakes. A woman's self-concept as a mother expands with actual experience and continues to grow through subsequent childbearing and childrearing.

The Father

For the expectant father, pregnancy is a psychologically stressful time because he, too, must make the transition from nonparent to parent or from parent of one or more to parent of two or more. Most men handle the transition to fatherhood well, and in general, any anxieties they feel resolve over time. Fathers' feelings of anxiety often stem from inadequate preparation and can be addressed by recognizing paternal needs and including fathers more in antepartum education.

Initially, expectant fathers may feel pride in their virility, which pregnancy confirms, but they also have many of the same ambivalent feelings as expectant mothers (Kowlessar, Fox, & Wittkowski, 2015). The extent of ambivalence depends on many factors, including the father's relationship with his partner, his previous experience with pregnancy, his age, his economic stability, and whether the pregnancy was planned.

In adjusting to his role, the expectant father must first deal with the reality of the pregnancy and then struggle to gain recognition as a parent from his partner, family, friends, coworkers, and society—and from his baby as well. The expectant mother can help her partner be a participant and not merely a helpmate to her if she has a definite sense of the experience as *their* pregnancy and *their* baby and not *her* pregnancy and *her* baby.

The expectant father must establish a fatherhood role, just as the woman develops a motherhood role. Fathers who are most successful at this task generally like children, are excited about the prospect of fatherhood, are eager to nurture a child, and have confidence in their ability to be a parent. Fathers may have a lack of understanding of their role if they came from a dysfunctional family, if they lacked positive role models, or if there was a general lack of education available (Alio, Lewis, Scarborough, et al., 2013).

FIRST TRIMESTER

During the first trimester feelings of worry or anxiety are common among men, especially as related to the health of their partner and unborn baby. Men also worry about their ability to fulfill the expectations of this new role (Kowlessar et al., 2015).

After the initial excitement attending the announcement of the pregnancy, an expectant father may begin to feel left out and may have a sense that he is "on the outside looking in" at the pregnancy (Kowlessar et al., 2015). He may be confused by his partner's mood changes. He might resent the attention she receives and her need to modify their relationship as she experiences fatigue and possibly a decreased interest in sex. In addition, he might be concerned about what kind of father he will be. During this time, his child is a "potential" baby. Fathers often picture interacting with a child of 5 or 6 years, not a newborn. The pregnancy itself may seem unreal until the woman shows more physical signs.

SECOND TRIMESTER

The second trimester is a time of growing acceptance as the man sees evidence of pregnancy in his partner's bodily changes. He begins to develop an emotional attachment to their baby and to feel part of the pregnancy process (Kowlessar et al., 2015). His involvement may increase as he watches and feels fetal movement and listens to the fetal heartbeat during a prenatal visit. For many men, seeing the fetus during an ultrasound is an important experience in accepting the reality of pregnancy. Like expectant mothers, expectant fathers need to confront and resolve some of their conflicts about the parenting they received. A father needs to sort out which behaviors of his own father he wants to imitate and which he wants to avoid (Kowlessar et al., 2015).

The anxiety of the father-to-be is lessened if both parents agree on the paternal role the man is to assume. For example, if both see his role as that of breadwinner, the man's stress is low. However, if the man views his role as that of breadwinner and the woman expects him to be actively involved in child care, his stress increases. An open, honest discussion about the expectations the parents have about their roles will help the father-to-be in his transition to fatherhood.

As the woman's appearance begins to change, her partner may have several reactions. Her changed appearance may decrease his sexual interest, or it may have the opposite effect. Because of the variety of emotions both partners may feel, continued communication and acceptance are important.

THIRD TRIMESTER

During the third trimester, the man redefines himself as a father and begins to visualize doing things with his child. In essence he recognizes that he is leaving his old life behind and needs to rethink his own values and priorities (Kowlessar et al., 2015).

If the couple's relationship has grown through effective communication of their concerns and feelings, the third trimester is often a rewarding time. They may attend childbirth classes and make concrete preparations for the arrival of the baby. If the father has developed a detached attitude about the pregnancy, however, it is unlikely he will become a willing participant, even though his role becomes more obvious.

Concerns and fears may recur. The father may worry about hurting the unborn baby during intercourse or become concerned about labor and birth. Also, he may wonder what kind of parents he and his partner will be.

COUVADE

Couvade has traditionally referred to the observance of certain rituals and taboos by the male to signify the transition to fatherhood. This observance affirms his psychosocial and biophysical relationship to the woman and child. More recently, the term has been used to describe the unintentional development of physical symptoms such as fatigue, increased appetite, difficulty sleeping, depression, headache, or backache by the partner of a pregnant woman. The frequency of symptoms seems to be related to male empathy or emotional sensitivity to the reactions of his partner (Kazmierczak, Kielbratowska, & Pastwa-Wojciechowska, 2013). Men who demonstrate couvade syndrome tend to have a higher degree of paternal role preparation and be involved in more activities related to this preparation.

Siblings

Bringing a new baby home often marks the beginning of sibling rivalry. The siblings view the baby as a threat to the security of their relationships with their parents. Parents who recognize this potential problem early in pregnancy and begin constructive actions can minimize the problem of sibling rivalry.

Preparation of the young child begins several weeks before the anticipated birth. Because they do not have a clear concept of time, young children should not be told too early about the pregnancy. From the toddler's point of view, several weeks is a very long time. The mother may let the child feel the baby moving in her uterus, explaining that the uterus is "a special place where babies grow." The child can help the parents put the baby clothes in drawers or prepare the nursery.

Consistency is important in dealing with young children. They need reassurance that certain people, special things, and familiar places will continue to exist after the new baby arrives. The crib is an important, although transient, object in a child's life. If it is to be given to the new baby, the parents should thoughtfully help the child adjust to this change. Any move from crib to bed or from one room to another should precede the baby's birth by several weeks or more. If the new baby is to share a room with siblings, the parents must discuss this with the older child or children.

Some parents advocate *cosleeping* or bed sharing (one or both parents sleeping with their baby or young child), and so the crib is less of an issue. Cosleeping, which is common in many non-Western cultures, is on the increase in the United States. It is discussed further in Chapter 29.

Pregnant women may find it helpful to bring their children on a prenatal visit to the physician/CNM to give them an opportunity to listen to the fetal heartbeat. Such a visit helps make the baby more real to the children.

If siblings are school-age children, pregnancy should be viewed as a family affair. Teaching should be suitable to the child's level of understanding and may be supplemented with appropriate books. Taking part in family discussions, attending sibling preparation classes, feeling fetal movement, and listening to the fetal heartbeat help the school-age child take part in the experience of pregnancy and not feel like an outsider.

Older children or adolescents may appear to have sophisticated knowledge but may have many misconceptions about pregnancy and birth. The parents should make opportunities to discuss their concerns and involve the children in preparations for the new baby.

Sibling preparation is essential, but other factors are equally important. These include the amount of parental attention the new arrival receives, the amount of attention the older child receives after the baby comes home, and parental skill in dealing with regressive or aggressive behavior. See the discussion of sibling preparation in Chapter 10.

Grandparents

The first relatives told about a pregnancy are usually the grandparents. Often, the expectant grandparents become increasingly supportive of the couple, even if conflicts previously existed. But it can be difficult for even sensitive grandparents to know how deeply to become involved in the childrearing process.

Because grandparenting can occur over a wide expanse of years, people's response to this role can vary considerably. Younger grandparents leading active lives may not demonstrate as much interest as the young couple would like. In other cases, expectant grandparents may give advice and gifts unsparingly. For grandparents, conflict may be related to the expectant couple's need to feel in control of their lives, or it may stem from events signaling changing roles in the grandparents' own lives (e.g., retirement, financial concerns, menopause, or death of a friend). Some parents of expectant couples may already be grandparents with a developed style of grandparenting. This influences their response to the pregnancy.

Because childbearing and childrearing practices have changed, family cohesiveness is promoted by effective communication and frank discussion between young couples and interested grandparents about the changes and the reasons for them. Clarifying the role of the helping grandparent ensures a comfortable situation for all.

Cultural Values and Pregnancy

A universal tendency exists to create ceremonial rituals or rites around important life events. Thus pregnancy, childbirth, marriage, and death are often tied to ritual. The rituals and customs of a group are a reflection of the group's values. In many developed countries such as the United States, Canada, England, Germany, and so forth, populations are becoming more and more ethnically diverse as the number of immigrants continues to grow. Research indicates that the experiences they have had in their country of origin shape their expectations of pregnancy and birth (Benza & Liamputtong, 2014). Thus, it is not realistic or appropriate to assume that people who are new to a country or area will automatically abandon their ways and adopt the practices of the dominant culture. Consequently, the identification of cultural values is useful in planning and providing culturally sensitive care.

The *National Standards for Culturally and Linguistically Appropriate Services in Health and Health Care,* the CLAS Standards, developed in 2000 by the Office of Minority Health within the U.S. Department of Health & Human Services, provided a blueprint for advancing and sustaining culturally and linguistically appropriate services. Revised and updated, the national CLAS standards also provide tools for health professionals including nurses (U.S. Department of Health & Human Services, Office of Minority Health, 2013). Additional guidelines and resources are available from the Joint Commission and from professional organizations such as the American Nurses Association and the Transcultural Nursing Society.

Developing Cultural Competence: Providing Effective Prenatal Care to Families of Different Cultures summarizes the key actions a nurse can take to become more culturally aware.

Developing Cultural Competence Providing Effective Prenatal Care to Families of Different Cultures

In interacting with expectant families from different cultures or ethnic groups, you can provide more effective, culturally sensitive nursing care by incorporating the following:

- Develop an understanding of your own cultural healthcare beliefs and practices as well as your own cultural values and biases.
- Learn the rituals, customs, and practices of the major cultural and ethnic groups with whom you have contact.
- Determine the client's level of English proficiency; provide a qualified interpreter if needed.
- Include cultural assessment and assessment of the family's expectations of the healthcare system as a routine part of prenatal nursing care.
- Avoid gestures or body language that may be misunderstood or seen as offensive.
- Allow the client to choose the amount of eye contact used; many cultures consider it impolite to make frequent eye contact.
- Incorporate the family's cultural and spiritual practices into prenatal care as much as possible.
- Foster an attitude of respect for and cooperation with alternative healers and caregivers whenever possible.
- Learn the language (or at least several key phrases) of at least one of the cultural groups with whom you interact.
- Evaluate whether the woman's healthcare beliefs have any potential negative consequences for her health.

Source: Adapted from Spector, R. (2013). *Cultural diversity in health and illness.* 8th ed. Upper Saddle River, NJ: Pearson.

Focus Your Study

- Virtually all systems of a woman's body are altered in some way during pregnancy.

- Blood pressure decreases slightly during pregnancy. It reaches its lowest point in the second trimester and gradually increases to near normal levels in the third trimester.

- The enlarging uterus may cause pressure on the vena cava when the woman lies supine, causing supine hypotensive syndrome.

- A physiologic anemia may occur during pregnancy because the total plasma volume increases more than the total number of erythrocytes. This difference produces a drop in the hematocrit.

- The glomerular filtration rate increases somewhat during pregnancy. Glycosuria may be caused by the body's inability to reabsorb all the glucose filtered by the glomeruli.

- Changes in the skin include the development of chloasma; linea nigra; darkened nipples, areola, and vulva; striae; and spider nevi.

- Insulin needs increase during pregnancy. A woman with a latent deficiency state may respond to the increased stress on the islets of Langerhans by developing gestational diabetes.

- The subjective (presumptive) signs of pregnancy are symptoms experienced and reported by the woman, such as amenorrhea, nausea and vomiting, fatigue, urinary frequency, breast changes, and quickening.

- The objective (probable) signs of pregnancy can be perceived by the examiner but may be caused by conditions other than pregnancy.

- The diagnostic (positive) signs of pregnancy can be perceived by the examiner and can be caused only by pregnancy.

- During pregnancy, the expectant mother may experience ambivalence, acceptance, introversion, emotional lability, and changes in body image.

- Rubin (1984) identified four developmental tasks for the pregnant woman: (1) ensuring safe passage through pregnancy, labor, and birth; (2) seeking acceptance of this child by others; (3) seeking commitment and acceptance of herself as mother to the child; and (4) learning to give of herself on behalf of her child.

- The father faces a series of adjustments as he accepts his new role. The father must deal with the reality of pregnancy, gain recognition as a parent, and confront and resolve any personal conflicts about the fathering he himself received.

- Siblings of all ages require assistance in dealing with the birth of a new baby.

- Cultural values, beliefs, and behaviors influence a family's response to childbearing and the healthcare system.

Clinical Reasoning In Action

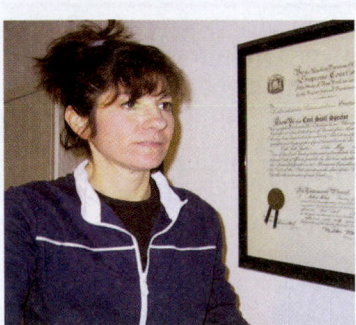

Twenty-two-year-old Jean Simmons is an aerobics instructor, G0P0 in her first trimester of pregnancy. She presents to you at the local clinic complaining of frequent nausea, urinary frequency, and fatigue. You obtain her vital signs as: BP 108/60, temperature 97°F, pulse 68, respirations 12, weight 125 lb, height 64 inches. Her urine tests negative for ketones, albumin, leukocytes, and sugar. You note that Jean has lost 3 lb since her last visit. You assist the CNM with a physical examination, the findings of which are essentially normal. Jean says that while she knows it could become an issue, she would like to continue working as an aerobics instructor for as long as she possibly can during the pregnancy. You identify Jean's complaints as normal discomforts of pregnancy, and proceed with prenatal education.

1. What advice would you suggest to cope with the nausea of pregnancy?

2. What advice might you suggest to cope with urinary frequency?

3. What teaching would be important relating to exercise in pregnancy?

4. What symptoms related to exercise should Jean report to her physician?

References

Alio, A. P., Lewis, C. A., Scarborough, K., Harris, K., & Fiscella, K. (2013). A community perspective on the role of fathers during pregnancy: A qualitative study. *BMC Pregnancy and Childbirth, 13*(60), 1–11.

American College of Obstetricians and Gynecologists (ACOG). (2013a). Nutrition during pregnancy [frequently asked questions faq001 pregnancy]. Retrieved from http://www.acog.org/~/media/For%20Patients/faq001.pdf?dmc=1&ts=20130711T1116342432

American College of Obstetricians and Gynecologists (ACOG). (2013b). *Weight gain during pregnancy* (ACOG Committee Opinion no. 548]. Washington, D. C.: Author.

Benza, S., & Liamputtong, P. (2014). Pregnancy, childbirth and motherhood: A meta-analysis of the lived experiences of immigrant women. *Midwifery, 30,* 575–584.

Cao, C., & O'Brien, K. O. (2013). Pregnancy and iron homeostasis: An update. *Nutrition Reviews, 71*(1), 35–51.

Cunningham, F. G., Leveno, K. J., Bloom, S. L., Spong, C. Y., Dashe, J. S., Hoffman, B. L., . . . & Sheffield, J. S. (2014). *Williams obstetrics* (24th ed.). New York, NY: McGraw-Hill.

Gordon, M. C. (2012). Maternal physiology. In S. G. Gabbe, J. R. Niebyl, J. L. Simpson, M. B. Landon, H. L. Galan, E. R. M. Jauniaux, & D. A. Driscoll (Eds.), *Obstetrics: Normal and problem pregnancies* (6th ed.). Philadelphia, PA: Churchill Livingstone.

Institute of Medicine (IOM). (2009). *Weight gain during pregnancy: Reexamining the guidelines.* Washington, DC: National Academies Press.

Jessop, D. C., Craig, L., & Ayers, S. (2014). Applying Leventhal's self-regulatory model to pregnancy: Evidence that pregnancy-related beliefs and emotional responses are associated with maternal health outcomes. *Journal of Health Psychology, 19*(9), 1091–1102.

Kazmierczak, M., Kielbratowska, B., & Pastwa-Wojciechowska, B. (2013). Couvade syndrome among Polish expectant fathers. *Medical Science Monitor: International Medical Journal of Experimental and Clinical Research, 19,* 132–138.

Kowlessar, O., Fox, J. R., & Wittkowski, A. (2015). The pregnant male: A metasynthesis of first-time fathers' experiences of pregnancy. *Journal of Reproductive & Infant Psychology, 33*(2), 106–127.

Levin, L., Hopkins, P., & Tiffany, D. (2011). Experts weigh in on hCG testing. *Medical Laboratory Observer, 43*(2), 22–24.

Patel, P. R., Laz, T. H., & Berenson, A. B. (2015). Patient characteristics associated with pregnancy ambivalence. *Journal of Women's Health, 24*(1), 37–41.

Rubin, R. (1984). *Maternal identity and the maternal experience.* New York, NY: Springer.

Spector, R. E. (2013). *Cultural diversity in health and illness,* 8th ed. Upper Saddle River, NJ: Pearson.

U.S. Department of Health & Human Services, Office of Minority Health. (2013). The National CLAS Standards. Retrieved from https://www.thinkculturalhealth.hhs.gov/pdfs/EnhancedCLASStandardsBlueprint.pdf

Widarsson, M., Kerstis, B., Sundquist, K., Engstrom, G., & Sarkadi, A. (2012). Support needs of expectant mothers and fathers: A qualitative study. *Journal of Perinatal Education, 21*(1), 36–44.

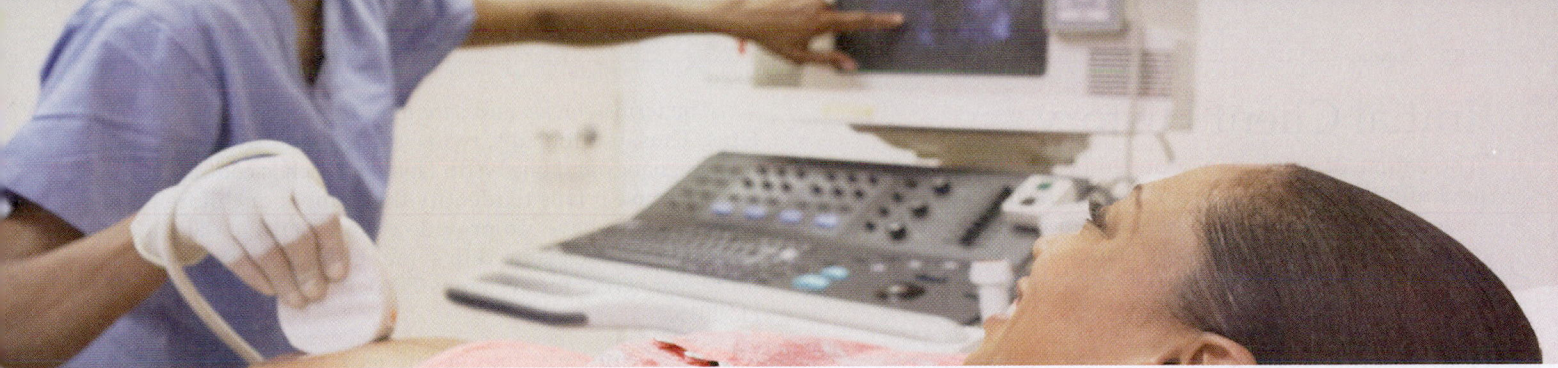

Chapter 9
Antepartum Nursing Assessment

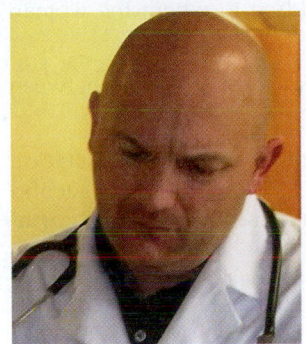

When I work the prenatal clinic I constantly remind myself to look past stereotypes about people of different cultures and ethnic groups to see each woman and family as unique. It has helped me tremendously to do some reading about various cultural groups and their common practices—that way I don't make glaring mistakes during my initial contact with a family. However, I have found it most useful simply to ask people about their preferences in a respectful, accepting way. Almost always they tell me gladly because their childbearing experience is important to them and they sense that I am sincere.

—A Nurse Working in a Large County Health Department

⌄ Learning Outcomes

9.1 Summarize the essential components of a prenatal history.

9.2 Define common obstetric terminology found in the history of maternity clients.

9.3 Predict the normal physiologic changes a nurse would expect to find when performing a physical assessment of a pregnant woman.

9.4 Calculate the estimated date of birth using the common methods.

9.5 Describe the essential measurements that can be determined by clinical pelvimetry.

9.6 Summarize the results of the major screening tests used during the prenatal period in the assessment of the prenatal client.

9.7 Relate the danger signs of pregnancy to their possible causes.

9.8 Relate the components of the subsequent prenatal history and assessment to the progress of pregnancy and the nursing care of the prenatal client.

The primary roles of a nurse in an office or prenatal clinic are to counsel, to educate, to meet the psychologic needs of the expectant family, and to perform other nursing care assessments and functions. The registered nurse caring for a woman who is pregnant establishes an environment of comfort and open communication at each antepartum visit. Advanced practice nurses such as certified nurse-midwives (CNMs) and nurse practitioners have the education and skill to perform full and complete antepartum assessments.

This chapter focuses on the prenatal assessments completed initially and at subsequent visits to provide optimum care for the childbearing family.

Healthy People 2020

(MICH-1) Reduce the rate of fetal and infant deaths

(MICH-5) Reduce the rate of maternal mortality

(MICH-6) Reduce maternal illness and complications due to pregnancy (complications during hospitalized labor and delivery)

(MICH-10) Increase the proportion of pregnant women who receive early and adequate prenatal care

Initial Client History

The course of a pregnancy depends on a number of factors, including the woman's prepregnancy health, presence of disease/illness states, family history, emotional status, and past health care. A thorough history is useful in determining the status of a woman's prepregnancy health.

Definition of Terms

The following terms are used in recording the history of maternity clients:

Gestation: the number of weeks since the first day of the last menstrual period

Abortion: birth that occurs before the end of 20 weeks' gestation or the birth of a fetus/newborn who weighs less than 500 g (Cunningham, Leveno, Bloom, et al., 2014)

Term: a word that was formerly used to identify the normal duration of pregnancy. The stand-alone use of this word is now discouraged because it represents such a wide range of time and related risk (Spong, 2013). The American College of Obstetrics and Gynecology (ACOG, 2013a) recommends that the following definitions be used:

- **Early term:** births occurring between 37 weeks 0 days and 38 weeks 6 days
- **Full term:** births occurring between 39 weeks 0 days and 40 weeks 6 days
- **Late term:** births occurring between 41 weeks 0 days through 41 weeks 6 days
- **Postterm:** births occurring after 42 weeks

Antepartum: time between conception and the onset of labor; often used to describe the period during which a woman is pregnant; used interchangeably with *prenatal*

Intrapartum: time from the onset of true labor until the birth of the baby and placenta

Postpartum: time from birth until the woman's body returns to an essentially prepregnant condition

Preterm labor: labor that occurs after 20 weeks' but before completion of 37 weeks' gestation

Late preterm: births that occur between 34 0/7 through 36 6/7 weeks' gestation (ACOG, 2013c)

Postterm labor: labor that occurs after 42 weeks' gestation

Gravida: any pregnancy, regardless of duration, including present pregnancy

Nulligravida: a woman who has never been pregnant

Primigravida: a woman who is pregnant for the first time

Multigravida: a woman who is in her second or any subsequent pregnancy

Para: birth after 20 weeks' gestation regardless of whether the baby is born alive or dead

Nullipara: a woman who has had no births at more than 20 weeks' gestation

Primipara: a woman who has had one birth at more than 20 weeks' gestation, regardless of whether the baby was born alive or dead

Multipara: a woman who has had two or more births at more than 20 weeks' gestation

Stillbirth: a baby born dead after 20 weeks' gestation

The terms *gravida* and *para* refer to pregnancies, not to the fetus. Thus, traditionally, twins, triplets, and so forth count as one pregnancy and one birth. This approach is confusing, however, because it fails to identify the number of children that a woman might have. To provide comprehensive data, a more detailed approach is used in some settings. A useful acronym for remembering the system is TPAL (King, Brucker, Kriebs, et al., 2015).

T: number of early, full, or late term births the woman has experienced (number of babies born at 37 0/7 weeks' gestation or beyond)

P: number of *preterm* births (births after 20 weeks' but before 37 0/7 weeks' gestation, whether living or stillborn)

A: number of pregnancies ending in either spontaneous or therapeutic *abortion* (before 20 weeks' gestation)

L: number of currently *living* children to whom the woman has given birth

The following examples delineate the differences between the two systems.

1. Jean Sanchez has one child born at 39 weeks' gestation and became pregnant for a second time. The second pregnancy ended in a miscarriage at 15 weeks' gestation. Using the *traditional approach* her obstetric history would be recorded as "gravida 2 para 1 ab 1." Using the *detailed approach,* her obstetric history would be recorded as "gravida 2 para 1011."

2. Tracy Hopkins is pregnant for the fourth time. At home she has a child who was born at full term. Her second pregnancy ended at 10 weeks' gestation. She then gave birth to twins at 35 weeks. Using the *traditional approach* her obstetric history would be recorded as gravida 4 para 2 ab 1. Using the *detailed approach* her obstetric history would be recorded as "gravida 4 para 1113."

To avoid confusion, practicing nurses should clarify the recording system used at their facilities.

Clinical Tip

In general, it is best to avoid an initial discussion of a woman's gravida and para in front of her partner. It is possible that the woman had a previous pregnancy that she has not mentioned to her partner, and revealing the information could violate her right to privacy.

Client Profile

The history is essentially a screening tool that identifies factors that may place the mother or fetus at risk during the pregnancy. The following information is obtained for each pregnant woman at the first prenatal assessment.

1. Current pregnancy:
   - First day of last normal menstrual period (LMP). Is she sure of the date or uncertain? Do her cycles normally occur every 28 days, or do her cycles tend to be longer or shorter? Was her last LMP normal in duration and amount?
   - Presence of cramping, bleeding, or spotting since LMP
   - Woman's opinion about the time when conception occurred and when baby is due

- Woman's attitude toward pregnancy. (Is this pregnancy planned or unplanned? Wanted?)
- Results of pregnancy tests, if completed
- Any pregnancy discomforts since LMP, such as nausea, vomiting, urinary frequency, fatigue, or breast tenderness

2. Past pregnancies:
   - Number of pregnancies
   - Number of abortions, spontaneous or induced
   - Number of living children
   - History of previous pregnancies, length of pregnancy, length of labor and birth, type of birth (vaginal, forceps-assisted or vacuum-assisted birth, or cesarean), location of birth, type of anesthesia used (if any), woman's perception of the experience, and complications (antepartum, intrapartum, and postpartum)
   - Neonatal status of previous children: Apgar scores, birth weights, general development, complications, and feeding patterns (breast milk, formula, or both). If breastfed, for how long?
   - Loss of a child (miscarriage, elective or medically indicated abortion, stillbirth, neonatal death, relinquishment, or death after the neonatal period). Cause of loss? What was the experience like for her? What coping skills helped? How did her partner, if involved, respond?
   - Blood type and Rh factor. (If Rh negative, was Rh immune globulin received after birth/miscarriage/abortion?)
   - Prenatal education classes and resources (books, websites)

3. Gynecologic history:
   - Date of last Papanicolaou (Pap) smear; result? Any history of abnormal Pap smear; any follow-up therapy completed?
   - Previous infections: vaginal, cervical, pelvic inflammatory disease (PID), sexually transmitted infections (STIs)
   - Previous surgery (uterine, ovarian)
   - Age at menarche
   - Regularity, frequency, and duration of menstrual flow
   - History of dysmenorrhea
   - History of infertility
   - Sexual history
   - Contraceptive history. (If hormonal method used, did pregnancy occur immediately following cessation of method? If not, how long after? When was contraception last used?)
   - Any issues related to infertility or fertility treatments

4. Current medical history:
   - Weight (prepregnancy and current), height, body mass index (BMI) (determine recommended weight gain)
   - Blood type and Rh factor, if known
   - General health including nutrition (dietary practices such as vegetarianism; lactose intolerance; food allergies), regular exercise program (type, frequency, and duration); information on the benefits and limitations of monthly breast self-examinations; eye examination; date of last dental examination
   - Any medications presently being taken (including nonprescription, homeopathic, or herbal medications) or taken since the onset of pregnancy
   - Previous or present use of alcohol, tobacco, or caffeine. (Ask specifically about the amounts of alcohol, cigarettes, and caffeine [specify coffee, tea, colas, or chocolate] consumed each day.)
   - Illicit drug use or abuse. (Ask about specific drugs such as cocaine, crack, methamphetamines, and marijuana; planning cessation?)
   - Drug allergies and other allergies. (Ask about latex allergies or sensitivities.)
   - Potential teratogenic insults to this pregnancy such as viral infections, medications, x-ray examinations, surgery, or cats in the home (source of toxoplasmosis)
   - Presence of chronic disease conditions such as diabetes, hypertension, cardiovascular disease, renal problems, or thyroid disorder
   - Infections or illnesses since LMP (flu, measles)
   - Record of immunizations (especially rubella); up to date?
   - Presence of any abnormal signs/symptoms

5. Past medical history:
   - Childhood diseases
   - Past treatment for any disease condition. (Any hospitalizations? Major accidents?)
   - Surgical procedures
   - Presence of any bleeding disorders or bleeding tendencies. (Has she received blood transfusions? Will she accept blood transfusions?)

6. Family medical history:
   - Presence of diabetes, cardiovascular disease, cancer, hypertension, hematologic disorders, tuberculosis, thyroid disease
   - Occurrence of multiple births
   - History of congenital diseases or deformities
   - History of mental illness
   - Causes of death of deceased parents or siblings
   - Occurrence of cesarean births and cause, if known

7. Genetic history (woman, father of the child [FOC], and both families):
   - Birth defects
   - Recurrent pregnancy loss
   - Stillbirth
   - Down syndrome, intellectual disability, developmental delay, chromosomal abnormalities
   - Ethnic background (Mediterranean descent, Jewish, Asian, etc.)
   - Genetic disorders (cystic fibrosis, sickle cell disease/trait, muscular dystrophy)

8. Religious, spiritual, and cultural history:
   - Does the woman wish to specify a religious preference in her medical record? Does she have any spiritual beliefs or practices that might influence her health care or that of her child, such as prohibition against receiving blood products, dietary considerations, or circumcision rites?
   - What practices are important to maintain her spiritual well-being?
   - Might practices in her culture or that of her partner influence her care or that of her child?

9. Occupational history:
   - Occupation
   - Physical demands. (Does she stand all day, or are there opportunities to sit and elevate her legs? Any heavy lifting?)

- Exposure to chemicals or other harmful substances
- Opportunity for regular meals and breaks for nutritious snacks
- Provision for maternity or family leave

10. Birth father's history:
   - Age
   - Significant health problems
   - Blood type and Rh factor
   - Presence of genetic conditions or diseases in him or in his family history

11. Father's/partner's social history:
   - Occupation
   - Educational level; methods by which he or she learns best
   - Current tobacco use, drug use, and alcohol intake
   - Thoughts/feelings about the pregnancy

12. Personal information about the pregnant woman (social history):
   - Age
   - Relationship status. (Married? Birth father involved? Partner's level of involvement [if partner is not the father of the child]?)
   - Educational level; methods by which she learns best
   - Race or ethnic group (to identify need for prenatal genetic screening and racially or ethnically related risk factors)
   - Housing; stability of living conditions; neighborhood safety; animals in the home
   - Economic level: ability to pay bills, purchase nutritious food; use of supplemental government programs
   - Acceptance of pregnancy, whether intended or unintended
   - Any history of emotional or physical deprivation or abuse of herself or children or any abuse in her current relationship. Has she been hit, slapped, kicked, or hurt within the past year or since she has been pregnant? Is she afraid of her partner or anyone else? If yes, of whom is she afraid? (Note: Ask these questions when you are alone with the woman.)
   - History of emotional/mental health problems (depression in general, postpartum depression, anxiety, bipolar disorder)
   - Support systems
   - Personal preferences about the birth (expectations of both the woman and her partner, presence of others, and so on). (See Chapter 10 for information about childbearing decisions.)
   - Plans for care of child following birth; plans for circumcision if the baby is male
   - Feeding preference for the baby (breast milk or formula?)

Obtaining Data

A questionnaire is used in many settings to obtain information. The woman should complete the questionnaire in a quiet place with a minimum of distractions. The nurse can obtain further information in an interview, which allows the pregnant woman to clarify her responses to questions and gives the nurse and client the opportunity to begin developing rapport.

SAFETY ALERT!
Because some medications may pose a risk to the fetus if taken during pregnancy, it is crucial to develop a list of all the medications the pregnant woman is currently taking as well as those she had been taking before she learned she was pregnant. This list should be given to the client's primary healthcare provider. (See discussion of a classification system for medications taken during pregnancy in Chapter 10.)

The expectant father or partner can be encouraged to attend the prenatal examinations. He or she is often able to contribute to the history and may use the opportunity to ask questions or express concerns that are important to him or her.

Prenatal Risk Factor Screening

Risk factors are any findings that suggest the pregnancy may have a negative outcome, for either the woman or her unborn child. Screening for risk factors is an important part of the prenatal assessment. Many risk factors can be identified during the initial assessment; others may be detected during subsequent prenatal visits. It is important to identify high-risk pregnancies early so that appropriate interventions can be started promptly. Not all risk factors threaten a pregnancy equally, so many agencies use a scoring sheet to determine the degree of risk. Information must be updated throughout the pregnancy as necessary. Any pregnancy may begin as low risk and change to high risk because of complications.

Clinical Reasoning Hot Tub Use in Pregnancy
Karen Blade, a 23-year-old woman, G1P0, is 10 weeks pregnant when she sees you for her first prenatal examination. She has been experiencing some mild nausea and fatigue but otherwise is feeling well. She asks you about continuing with her routine exercises (walking 3 miles a day and lifting light weights). She also asks about using the heated pool and a hot tub.
What should you tell her?

Table 9–1 identifies the major prenatal risk factors currently recognized. The table also identifies maternal and fetal or newborn implications if the risk is present in the pregnancy.

Initial Prenatal Assessment

The initial prenatal assessment focuses on the woman holistically by considering physical, cultural, and psychosocial factors that influence her health. The establishment of the nurse–client relationship is a chance to develop an atmosphere that is conducive to interviewing, support, and education. Because many women are excited and anxious at the first antepartum visit, the initial psychosocial–cultural assessment is general.

As part of the initial psychosocial–cultural assessment, the nurse discusses with the woman any religious or spiritual, cultural, or socioeconomic factors that may influence the woman's expectations of the childbearing experience. It is especially

TABLE 9–1 Prenatal High-Risk Factors

FACTOR	MATERNAL IMPLICATIONS	FETAL/NEONATAL IMPLICATIONS
Social–Personal		
Low income level and/or low educational level	Insufficient antenatal care or late antenatal care ↑ risk preterm birth Poor nutrition ↑ risk of preeclampsia	Low birth weight Prematurity Intrauterine growth restriction (IUGR)/small for gestational age (SGA)
Poor diet	Inadequate nutrition/inadequate weight gain ↑ risk preterm birth ↑ risk anemia ↑ risk preeclampsia	Fetal malnutrition Prematurity IUGR/SGA
Living at high altitude	↑ hemoglobin	Prematurity IUGR ↑ hemoglobin (polycythemia)
Multiparity greater than 3	↑ risk antepartum or postpartum hemorrhage	Anemia Fetal death
Weight less than 45.5 kg (100 lb)	Poor nutrition Cephalopelvic disproportion Prolonged labor	IUGR Hypoxia associated with difficult labor and birth
Weight greater than 91 kg (200 lb)	↑ risk hypertension ↑ risk cephalopelvic disproportion ↑ risk diabetes	↓ fetal nutrition ↑ risk macrosomia
Age less than 16	Poor nutrition Insufficient antenatal care ↑ risk preeclampsia ↑ risk cephalopelvic disproportion	Low birth weight ↑ fetal demise
Age over 35	↑ risk preeclampsia ↑ risk cesarean birth Psychosocial issues	↑ risk congenital anomalies ↑ chromosomal abnormalities
Smoking one pack/day or more	↑ risk hypertension ↑ risk cancer	↓ placental perfusion → ↓ O_2 and nutrients available Low birth weight; IUGR/SGA; preterm birth
Use of addictive drugs	↑ risk poor nutrition ↑ risk of infection with intravenous (IV) drugs ↑ risk HIV, hepatitis C ↑ risk abruptio placentae	↑ risk congenital anomalies ↑ risk low birth weight Neonatal withdrawal Lower serum bilirubin
Excessive alcohol consumption	↑ risk poor nutrition Possible hepatic effects with long-term consumption	↑ risk fetal alcohol syndrome
Preexisting Medical Disorders		
Diabetes mellitus	↑ risk preeclampsia, hypertension Episodes of hypoglycemia and hyperglycemia ↑ risk cesarean birth	Low birth weight Macrosomia Neonatal hypoglycemia ↑ risk congenital anomalies ↑ risk respiratory distress syndrome

(continued)

TABLE 9–1 Prenatal High-Risk Factors *(continued)*

FACTOR	MATERNAL IMPLICATIONS	FETAL/NEONATAL IMPLICATIONS
Preexisting Medical Disorders (*continued*)		
Cardiac disease	Cardiac decompensation Further strain on mother's body ↑ maternal death rate	↑ risk fetal demise ↑ perinatal mortality
Anemia: hemoglobin less than 11 g/dL or less than 32% hematocrit	Iron deficiency anemia Low energy level Decreased oxygen-carrying capacity	Fetal death Prematurity Low birth weight
Hypertension	↑ vasospasm ↑ risk central nervous system (CNS) irritability → convulsions ↑ risk cerebrovascular accident (CVA) ↑ risk renal damage	↑ placental perfusion → low birth weight Preterm birth
Thyroid disorder	↑ infertility	↑ spontaneous abortion
Hypothyroidism	↓ basal metabolic rate (BMR), goiter, myxedema ↑ risk miscarriage, preterm labor/birth ↑ risk preeclampsia	↑ risk congenital goiter ↑ risk IUGR/SGA ↑ risk stillbirth
Hyperthyroidism	↑ risk postpartum hemorrhage ↑ risk preeclampsia Danger of thyroid storm	↑ risk of intellectual disability → cretinism ↑ incidence congenital anomalies ↑ incidence preterm birth, IUGR/SGA ↑ neonatal hyperthyroidism
Renal disease (moderate to severe)	↑ risk renal failure	↑ risk IUGR/SGA ↑ risk preterm birth
DES exposure	↑ infertility, spontaneous abortion ↑ cervical insufficiency ↑ risk breech presentation	↑ risk preterm birth
Obstetric Considerations		
Previous Pregnancy		
Stillborn	↑ emotional/psychologic distress	↑ risk IUGR/SGA ↑ risk preterm birth
Recurrent abortion	↑ emotional/psychologic distress	↑ risk abortion
Cesarean birth	↑ possibility repeat cesarean birth Risk of uterine rupture	↑ risk preterm birth ↑ risk respiratory distress
Rh or blood group sensitization		Hydrops fetalis Icterus gravis Neonatal anemia Kernicterus Hypoglycemia
Large baby	↑ risk cesarean birth ↑ risk gestational diabetes ↑ risk instrument-assisted birth	Birth injury Hypoglycemia
Current Pregnancy		
Rubella (first trimester)		Congenital heart disease Cataracts Nerve deafness Bone lesions Prolonged virus shedding
Rubella (second trimester)		Hepatitis Thrombocytopenia

FACTOR	MATERNAL IMPLICATIONS	FETAL/NEONATAL IMPLICATIONS
Current Pregnancy (**continued**)		
Cytomegalovirus		IUGR
		Encephalopathy
Herpes virus type 2	Severe discomfort	Neonatal herpes virus type 2
	Concern about possibility of cesarean birth, fetal infection	Hepatitis with jaundice
		Neurologic abnormalities
Syphilis	↑ incidence abortion	↑ fetal demise
		Congenital syphilis
Urinary tract infection	↑ risk preterm labor	↑ risk preterm birth
	Uterine irritability	
Abruptio placentae and placenta previa	↑ risk hemorrhage	Fetal/neonatal anemia
	Bed rest	Intrauterine hemorrhage
	Extended hospitalization	↑ fetal demise
Preeclampsia/eclampsia	See hypertension	↑ placental perfusion
		→ low birth weight
Multiple gestation	↑ risk postpartum hemorrhage	↑ risk preterm labor/birth
	↑ risk gestational diabetes mellitus	↑ risk fetal demise
	↑ risk placenta previa	↑ risk IUGR/SGA
	↑ risk preeclampsia	↑ risk malpresentation
		↑ risk stillbirth
Elevated hematocrit Greater than 41% (White mothers) Greater than 38% (Black mothers)	Increased viscosity of blood	Fetal death rate five times normal rate
Spontaneous premature rupture of membranes	↑ uterine infection	Preterm birth
		Fetal demise

Note: This table is not inclusive of all potential outcomes.

helpful if the nurse is familiar with common practices of the members of various religious and cultural groups who reside in the community.

Women With Special Needs Assessing Care Needs During Pregnancy

During the initial assessment, the woman with a disability should be questioned to determine her current level of functioning and the degree of assistance she normally requires in her everyday routine. This assists the healthcare team in planning care and interventions that may be needed. Care needs may change during pregnancy and warrant ongoing assessments of the woman's level of functioning.

After obtaining the history, the nurse prepares the woman for the physical examination. The physical examination begins with assessment of vital signs; then the woman's body is examined. The pelvic examination is performed last.

Before the examination, the woman should provide a clean urine specimen for screening. When her bladder is empty, the client is more comfortable during the pelvic examination and the examiner can palpate the pelvic organs more easily. After the woman has emptied her bladder, the nurse asks her to disrobe and gives her a gown and sheet or some other protective covering.

Thoroughness and a systematic procedure are the most important considerations when performing the physical portion of an antepartum examination. To promote completeness, *Assessment Guide: Initial Prenatal Assessment* is organized in three columns that address the areas to be assessed (and normal findings), the variations or alterations that may be observed, and nursing responses to the data. Certain organs and systems are

Professionalism in Practice Physical Examinations and Scope of Practice

Increasing numbers of nurses, such as CNMs, nurse practitioners, and other nurses in advanced practice, are educationally prepared to perform complete physical examinations. The nurse who is not an advanced practitioner assesses the woman's vital signs, explains the procedures to allay apprehension, positions her for examination, and assists the examiner as necessary. Each nurse is responsible for operating at expected professional standards within his or her skill level, educational preparation, and knowledge base.

assessed concurrently with others during the physical portion of the examination.

Nursing interventions based on assessment of the normal physical and psychosocial changes of pregnancy, evaluation of the cultural influences associated with pregnancy, and client teaching and counseling needs that have been mutually defined are discussed further in Chapter 10.

Determination of Due Date

Childbearing families generally want to know the "due date," or the date around which childbirth will occur. Historically the due date has been called the *estimated date of confinement (EDC)*. The concept of confinement is, however, rather negative, and many caregivers avoid it by referring to the due date as the EDD or estimated date of delivery. Childbirth educators often stress that babies are not "delivered" like a package; they are born. In keeping with a view that emphasizes the normalcy of the process, this text refers to the due date as the **estimated date of birth (EDB)**.

To calculate the EDB, it is crucial to know the first day of the last menstrual period (LMP). However, some women have episodes of irregular bleeding or fail to keep track of menstrual cycles. Thus other techniques also help to determine how far along a woman is in her pregnancy—that is, at how many weeks' gestation she is. Techniques that can be used include evaluating uterine size, determining when quickening occurs (or occurred), using early ultrasound, and auscultating fetal heart rate with a Doppler device or ultrasound and later a fetoscope. An early ultrasound should be obtained if an accurate LMP is not available to help establish an accurate EDB.

ASSESSMENT GUIDE | Initial Prenatal Assessment

Physical Assessment/Normal Findings	Alterations and Possible Causes*	Nursing Responses to Data†
Vital Signs		
Blood Pressure (BP): Less than or equal to 120/80 mmHg	High BP (essential hypertension; renal disease; pregestational hypertension, apprehension; preeclampsia if initial assessment not done until after 20 weeks' gestation)	BP of 120–139/80–89 is considered prehypertensive. BP greater than 140/90 requires immediate consideration; establish woman's BP; refer to healthcare provider if necessary. Assess woman's knowledge about high BP; counsel on self-care and medical management.
Pulse: 60–100 beats/min; rate may increase 10 beats/min during pregnancy	Increased pulse rate (excitement or anxiety, dehydration, infection, cardiac disorders)	Count for 1 full minute; note irregularities. Evaluate temperature, increase fluids.
Respirations: 12–20 breaths/min (or pulse rate divided by four); pregnancy may induce a degree of hyperventilation; thoracic breathing predominant	Marked tachypnea or abnormal patterns	Assess for respiratory disease.
Temperature: 36.2°–37.6°C (97°–99.6°F)	Elevated temperature (infection)	Assess for infection process or disease state if temperature is elevated; refer to healthcare provider.
Weight		
Gain depends on body build Underweight: 12.5–18.0 kg (28–40 lb) Normal weight: 11.5–16.0 kg (25–35 lb) Overweight: 7.0–11.5 kg (15–25 lb) Obese: 5.0–9.1 kg (11–20 lb)	Weight less than 45.4 kg (100 lb) or greater than 91.1 kg (200 lb); rapid, sudden weight gain (preeclampsia)	Evaluate need for nutritional counseling; obtain information on eating habits, cooking practices, food regularly eaten, food allergies, income limitations, need for food supplements, pica and other abnormal food habits. Note initial weight to establish baseline for weight gain throughout pregnancy. Determine body mass index (BMI) and recommend weight gain for pregnancy.

Physical Assessment/Normal Findings	Alterations and Possible Causes*	Nursing Responses to Data†
Skin		
Color: Consistent with racial background; pink nail beds	Pallor (anemia); bronze, yellow (hepatic disease; other causes of jaundice) Bluish, reddish, mottled; dusky appearance or pallor of palms and nail beds in dark-skinned women (anemia)	The following tests should be performed: complete blood count (CBC), bilirubin level, urinalysis, and blood urea nitrogen (BUN). If abnormal, refer to healthcare provider.
Condition: Absence of edema (slight edema of lower extremities is normal during pregnancy)	Edema (preeclampsia, normal pregnancy changes); rashes, dermatitis (allergic response)	Counsel on relief measures for slight edema. Initiate preeclampsia assessment; refer to healthcare provider.
Lesions: Absence of lesions	Ulceration (varicose veins, decreased circulation)	Further assess circulatory status; refer to healthcare provider if lesion is severe.
Spider nevi common in pregnancy	Petechiae, multiple bruises, ecchymosis (hemorrhagic disorders; abuse)	Evaluate for bleeding or clotting disorder. Provide opportunities to discuss abuse if suspected.
Moles		
Pigmentation: Pigmentation changes of pregnancy include linea nigra, striae gravidarum, melasma	Change in size or color (carcinoma)	Refer to healthcare provider. Assure woman that these are normal manifestations of pregnancy and explain the physiologic basis for the changes.
Café-au-lait spots	Six or more (Albright syndrome or neurofibromatosis)	Consult with healthcare provider.
Nose		
Character of Mucosa: Redder than oral mucosa; in pregnancy nasal mucosa is edematous in response to increased estrogen, resulting in nasal stuffiness (rhinitis of pregnancy) and nosebleeds	Olfactory loss (first cranial nerve deficit)	Counsel woman about possible relief measures for nasal stuffiness and nosebleeds (epistaxis); refer to healthcare provider for olfactory loss.
Mouth		
May note hypertrophy of gingival tissue because of estrogen	Edema, inflammation (infection); pale in color (anemia)	Assess hematocrit for anemia; counsel regarding dental hygiene habits. Refer to healthcare provider or dentist if necessary. Routine dental care appropriate during pregnancy.
Neck		
Nodes: Small, mobile, nontender nodes	Tender, hard, fixed, or prominent nodes (infection, carcinoma)	Examine for local infection; refer to healthcare provider.
Thyroid: Small, smooth, lateral lobes palpable on either side of trachea; slight hyperplasia by third month of pregnancy	Enlargement or nodule tenderness (hyperthyroidism)	Test to perform: thyroid-stimulating hormone (TSH). Listen over thyroid for bruits, which may indicate hyperthyroidism. Question woman about dietary habits (iodine intake). Ascertain history of thyroid problems; refer to healthcare provider.
Chest and Lungs		
Chest: Symmetric, elliptic, smaller anteroposterior (AP) than transverse diameter	Increased AP diameter, funnel chest, pigeon chest (emphysema, asthma, pulmonary disease)	Evaluate for emphysema, asthma, pulmonary disease.
Ribs: Slope downward from nipple line	More horizontal (pulmonary disease); angular bumps sometimes called rachitic rosary (vitamin C deficiency)	Evaluate for pulmonary disease. Evaluate for fractures. Consult healthcare provider. Consult nutritionist.
Inspection and Palpation: No retraction or bulging of intercostal spaces (ICS) during inspiration or expiration; symmetric expansion.	ICS retractions with inspirations, bulging with expiration; unequal expansion (respiratory disease)	Do thorough initial assessment. Refer to healthcare provider.

(continued)

Physical Assessment/Normal Findings	Alterations and Possible Causes*	Nursing Responses to Data†
Tactile fremitus	Tachypnea, hyperpnea (respiratory disease)	Refer to healthcare provider.
Percussion: Bilateral symmetry in tone	Flatness of percussion, which may be affected by chest wall thickness	Evaluate for pleural effusions, consolidations, or tumor.
Low-pitched resonance of moderate intensity	High diaphragm (atelectasis or paralysis), pleural effusion	Refer to healthcare provider.
Auscultation: Upper lobes: bronchovesicular sounds above sternum and scapulas; equal expiratory and inspiratory phases	Abnormal if heard over any other area of chest	Refer to healthcare provider.
Remainder of chest: Vesicular breath sounds heard; inspiratory phase longer (3:1)	Rales, rhonchi, wheezes; pleural friction rub; absence of breath sounds; bronchophony, egophony, whispered pectoriloquy	Refer to healthcare provider.

Breasts

Supple: Symmetric in size and contour; darker pigmentation of nipple and areola; may have supernumerary nipples, usually 5–6 cm (2.0 to 2.4 in.) below normal nipple line	"Pigskin" or orange-peel appearance, nipple retractions, swelling, hardness (carcinoma); redness, heat, tenderness, cracked or fissured nipple (infection)	Discuss risks and benefits of monthly self-examination; instruct woman on how to examine her own breasts if she elects to do so.
Axillary nodes nonpalpable or pellet sized	Tenderness, enlargement, hard node (carcinoma); may be visible bump (infection)	Refer to healthcare provider for evaluation of abnormal breast findings. Plan ultrasound/mammogram/MRI of breasts.

Pregnancy Changes:

1. Size increase noted primarily in first 20 weeks.
2. Become nodular.
3. Tingling sensation may be felt during first and third trimester; woman may report feeling of heaviness.
4. Pigmentation of nipples and areolae darkens.
5. Superficial veins dilate and become more prominent.
6. Striae seen in multiparas.
7. Tubercles of Montgomery enlarge.
8. Colostrum may be present after 12th week.
9. Secondary areola appears at 20 weeks, characterized by series of washed-out spots surrounding primary areola.
10. Breasts less firm, old striae may be present in multiparas.

Discuss normalcy of changes and their meaning with the woman. Teach and/or institute appropriate relief measures. Encourage use of supportive, well-fitting brassiere.

Heart

Normal rate, rhythm, and heart sounds	Enlargement, thrills, thrusts, gross irregularity or skipped beats, gallop rhythm or extra sounds (cardiac disease)	Complete an initial assessment. Explain normal pregnancy-induced changes. Refer to healthcare provider if indicated.

Pregnancy Changes:

1. Palpitations may occur due to sympathetic nervous system disturbance.
2. Short systolic murmurs that increase in held expiration are normal due to increased volume.

Physical Assessment/Normal Findings	Alterations and Possible Causes*	Nursing Responses to Data†
Abdomen Normal appearance, skin texture, and hair distribution; liver nonpalpable; abdomen nontender	Muscle guarding (anxiety, acute tenderness); tenderness, mass (ectopic pregnancy, inflammation, carcinoma)	Assure woman of normalcy of diastasis. Provide initial information about appropriate prenatal and postpartum exercises. Evaluate woman's anxiety level. Refer to healthcare provider if indicated.
Pregnancy Changes:		
1. Purple striae may be present (or silver striae on a multipara) as well as linea nigra.		
2. Diastasis of the rectus muscles late in pregnancy.	Size of uterus inconsistent with length of gestation (intrauterine growth restriction [IUGR], multiple pregnancy, fetal demise, incorrect estimated date of birth [EDB], abnormal amniotic fluid, hydatidiform mole)	Reassess menstrual history regarding pregnancy dating. Evaluate increase in size using McDonald method. Use ultrasound to establish diagnosis.
3. Size: Flat or rotund abdomen; progressive enlargement of uterus due to pregnancy. 10–12 weeks: Fundus slightly above symphysis pubis. 16 weeks: Fundus halfway between symphysis and umbilicus. 20–22 weeks: Fundus at umbilicus. 28 weeks: Fundus three fingerbreadths above umbilicus. 36 weeks: Fundus just below ensiform cartilage.		
4. Fetal heart rate: 110–160 beats/min; may be heard with Doppler at 10–12 weeks' gestation; may be heard with fetoscope at 17–20 weeks.	Failure to hear fetal heartbeat with Doppler (fetal demise, hydatidiform mole)	Refer to healthcare provider. Administer pregnancy tests. Use ultrasound to establish diagnosis.
5. Fetal movement palpable by a trained examiner after the 18th week.	Failure to feel fetal movements after 20 weeks' gestation (fetal demise, hydatidiform mole)	Refer to healthcare provider.
6. Ballottement: During fourth to fifth month, fetus rises and then rebounds to original position when uterus is tapped sharply.	No ballottement (oligohydramnios)	Refer to healthcare provider.
Extremities Skin warm, pulses palpable, full range of motion; may be some edema of hands and ankles in late pregnancy; varicose veins may become more pronounced; palmar erythema may be present	Unpalpable or diminished pulses (arterial insufficiency); marked edema (preeclampsia)	Evaluate for other symptoms of heart disease; initiate follow-up if woman mentions that her rings feel tight on her fingers. Discuss prevention and self-treatment measures for varicose veins; refer to healthcare provider if indicated.
Spine **Normal Spinal Curves:** Concave cervical, convex thoracic, concave lumbar	Abnormal spinal curves; flatness, kyphosis, lordosis	Refer to healthcare provider if indicated.
In pregnancy, lumbar spinal curve may be accentuated	Backache	May have implications for administration of spinal anesthetics.
Shoulders and iliac crests should be even	Uneven shoulders and iliac crests (scoliosis)	Refer very young women to healthcare provider; discuss back-stretching exercise with older women.
Reflexes Normal and symmetric	Hyperactivity, clonus (preeclampsia)	Evaluate for other symptoms of preeclampsia.

(continued)

ASSESSMENT GUIDE	Initial Prenatal Assessment (*continued*)

Physical Assessment/Normal Findings	Alterations and Possible Causes*	Nursing Responses to Data†
Pelvic Area		
External Female Genitals: Normally formed with female hair distribution; in multiparas, labia majora loose and pigmented; urinary and vaginal orifices visible and appropriately located	Lesions, hematomas, varicosities, inflammation of Bartholin glands; clitoral hypertrophy (masculinization)	Explain pelvic examination procedure. Encourage woman to minimize her discomfort by relaxing her hips. Provide privacy.
Vagina: Pink or dark pink, vaginal discharge odorless, nonirritating; in multiparas, vaginal folds smooth and flattened; may have episiotomy scar	Abnormal discharge associated with vaginal infections	Obtain vaginal smear. Provide understandable verbal and written instructions about treatment for woman and partner, if indicated.
Cervix: Pink color; os closed except in multiparas, in whom os admits fingertip	Eversion, reddish erosion, nabothian or retention cysts, cervical polyp; granular area that bleeds (carcinoma of cervix); lesions (herpes, human papilloma virus [HPV]); presence of string or plastic tip from cervix (intrauterine device [IUD] in uterus)	Provide woman with a hand mirror and identify genital structures for her; encourage her to view her cervix if she wishes. Refer to healthcare provider if indicated. Advise woman of potential serious risks of leaving an IUD in place during pregnancy; refer to healthcare provider for removal.
Pregnancy Changes:		
1–4 weeks' gestation: Enlargement in anteroposterior diameter		
4–6 weeks' gestation: Softening of cervix (Goodell sign); softening of isthmus of uterus (Hegar sign); cervix takes on bluish coloring (Chadwick sign)	Absence of Goodell sign (inflammatory conditions, carcinoma)	Refer to healthcare provider.
8–12 weeks' gestation: Vagina and cervix appear bluish violet in color (Chadwick sign)	Fixed (pelvic inflammatory disease [PID]); nodular surface (fibromas)	Refer to healthcare provider.
Uterus: Pear shaped, mobile; smooth surface		
Ovaries: Small, walnut shaped, nontender (ovaries and Fallopian tubes are located in the adnexal areas)	Pain on movement of cervix (PID); enlarged or nodular ovaries (cyst, tumor, tubal pregnancy, corpus luteum of pregnancy)	Evaluate adnexal areas; refer to healthcare provider.
Pelvic Measurements		
Internal Measurements:		
1. Diagonal conjugate at least 11.5 cm (4.5 in.) (see Figure 9–4A)	Measurement below normal	Vaginal birth may not be possible if deviations are present.
2. Obstetric conjugate estimated by subtracting 1.5–2 cm (0.6–0.8 in.) from diagonal conjugate	Disproportion of pubic arch	
3. Inclination of sacrum	Abnormal curvature of sacrum	
4. Motility of coccyx; external intertuberosity diameter greater than 8 cm (3.2 in.)	Fixed or malposition of coccyx	
Anus and Rectum		
No lumps, rashes, excoriation, tenderness; cervix may be felt through rectal wall	Hemorrhoids, rectal prolapse; nodular lesion (carcinoma)	Counsel about appropriate prevention and relief measures; refer to healthcare provider for further evaluation.
Laboratory Evaluation		
Hemoglobin: 12–16 g/dL; women residing in areas of high altitude may have higher levels of hemoglobin	Less than 11 g/dL in the first trimester, less than 10.5 g/dL in the second trimester, and less than 11 g/dL in the third trimester (anemia) (King et al., 2015)	Hemoglobin less than 12 g/dL requires nutritional counseling; less than 11 g/dL requires iron supplementation.

Physical Assessment/Normal Findings	Alterations and Possible Causes*	Nursing Responses to Data†
ABO and Rh Typing: Normal distribution of blood types	Rh negative	If Rh negative, check for presence of anti-Rh antibodies. Check partner's blood type; if partner is Rh positive, discuss with woman the need for Rh immune globulin administration at 28 weeks, management during the intrapartum period, and possible need for Rh immune globulin after childbirth. (See Chapter 15.)
Complete Blood Count (CBC)		
Hematocrit: 38%–47% physiologic anemia (pseudoanemia) may occur	Marked anemia or blood dyscrasias	Perform CBC and Schilling differential cell count.
Red Blood Cells (RBC): 4.2–5.4 million/mcL		
White Blood Cells (WBC): 5,000–12,000/mcL	Presence of infection; may be elevated in pregnancy and with labor	Evaluate for other signs of infection.
Differential		
Neutrophils: 40%–60%		
Bands: up to 5%		
Eosinophils: 1%–3%		
Basophils: up to 1%		
Lymphocytes: 20%–40%		
Monocytes: 4%–8%		
First-Trimester Aneuploidy Screening (testing to detect conditions related to abnormal chromosome number); if nuchal translucency (NT) testing is available, offer first-trimester screening for Down syndrome using nuchal translucency and serum markers (PAPP-A and free β-hCG). Normal range.	Increased nuchal translucency, elevated β-hCG, and reduced pregnancy-associated plasma protein A (PAPP-A) (Down syndrome, trisomy 18, trisomy 13, Turner syndrome)	If findings are positive, genetic counseling and diagnostic testing using chorionic villus sampling (CVS) or second-trimester amniocentesis are offered.
Integrated Screening: Combines first-trimester aneuploidy screening results with second-trimester quadruple (quad) screen to detect aneuploidy and neural tube defects; may be used in areas in which NT testing is not available. (See discussion in *Assessment Guide: Subsequent Prenatal Assessment* later in the chapter.)		
Syphilis Tests: Serologic tests for syphilis (STS), complement fixation test, Venereal Disease Research Laboratory (VDRL) test—nonreactive	Positive reaction STS—tests may have 25%–45% incidence of biologic false-positive results; false results may occur in individuals who have acute viral or bacterial infections, hypersensitivity reactions, recent vaccinations, collagen disease, malaria, or tuberculosis	Positive results may be confirmed with the fluorescent treponemal antibody-absorption (FTA-ABS) test; all tests for syphilis give positive results in the secondary stage of the disease; antibiotics may cause negative test results. Refer to healthcare provider for treatment.
Gonorrhea Culture: Negative	Positive	Refer for treatment.
Urinalysis (u/a): Normal color, specific gravity; pH 4.6–8	Cloudy appearance (infection; pus or tissue)	Repeat u/a; refer to healthcare provider.
	Abnormal color (porphyria, hemoglobinuria, bilirubinemia): alkaline urine (metabolic alkalemia, *Proteus* infection, old specimen)	

(continued)

Physical Assessment/Normal Findings	Alterations and Possible Causes*	Nursing Responses to Data†
Negative for protein, red blood cells, white blood cells, casts	Positive findings (contaminated specimen, urinary tract infection [UTI], kidney disease)	Repeat u/a; urine culture with sensitivities if bacteria detected; refer to healthcare provider.
Glucose: Negative (small degree of glycosuria may occur in pregnancy)	Glycosuria (low renal threshold for glucose, diabetes mellitus)	Assess blood glucose level; test urine for ketones.
Rubella Titer: Hemagglutination-inhibition (HAI) test—result of 1:10 or above indicates woman is immune	HAI titer less than 1:10	Immunization will be given postpartum. Instruct woman whose titers are less than 1:10 to avoid children who have rubella.
Hepatitis B Screen for hepatitis B surface antigen (HBsAg): negative	Positive	If positive, refer to physician. Babies born to women who test positive are given hepatitis B immune globulin soon after birth followed by first dose of hepatitis B vaccine.
HIV Screen: Completed unless woman specifically opts out of screening	Positive	Refer to healthcare provider.
Illicit Drug Screen: Offered to all women; negative	Positive	Refer to healthcare provider.
Sickle Cell Screen for Clients of African or Hispanic descent: Negative	Positive; test results would include a description of cells	Refer to healthcare provider.
Pap Smear: If indicated because the woman is due for the test; negative	Test results that show abnormal cells with negative or positive high-risk human papilloma virus (HPV)	Refer to healthcare provider. Discuss with the woman the meaning of the findings and the importance of follow-up. Plan colposcopy if indicated by results.

Cultural Assessment	Variations to Consider*	Nursing Responses to Data†
Determine the woman's fluency in written and oral English.	Woman may be fluent in language other than English.	Work with a knowledgeable translator to provide information and answer questions.
Ask the woman how she prefers to be addressed. Nickname?	Some women prefer informality; others prefer to use titles.	Address the woman according to her preference. Maintain formality in introducing oneself if that seems preferred.
Determine customs and practices regarding prenatal care:	Practices are influenced by individual preference, cultural expectations, or religious beliefs.	Honor a woman's practices and provide for specific preferences unless they are contraindicated because of safety.
• Ask the woman if there are certain practices she expects to follow when she is pregnant.	Some women believe that they should perform certain acts related to sleep, activity, or clothing.	Have information printed in the languages of different cultural groups that live in the area.
• Ask the woman if there are any activities she cannot do while she is pregnant.	Some women have restrictions or taboos they follow related to work, activity, or sexual, environmental, or emotional factors.	
• Ask the woman whether there are certain foods she is expected to eat or avoid while she is pregnant. Determine whether she has lactose intolerance or food allergies.	Foods are an important cultural factor. Some women may have certain foods they must eat or avoid; many women have lactose intolerance and have difficulty consuming sufficient calcium.	Respect the woman's food preferences, help her plan an adequate prenatal diet within the framework of her preferences, and refer to a dietitian if necessary.
• Ask the woman whether the gender of her caregiver is of concern.	Some women are comfortable only with a female caregiver.	Arrange for a female caregiver if it is the woman's preference.
• Ask the woman about the degree of involvement in her pregnancy that she expects or wants from her support person, mother, and other significant people.	A woman may not want her partner involved in the pregnancy. For some the role falls to the woman's mother or a female relative or friend.	Respect the woman's preferences about her partner or husband's involvement; avoid imposing personal values or expectations.
• Ask the woman about her sources of support and counseling during pregnancy.	Some women seek advice from a family member, *curandera*, tribal healer, and so forth.	Respect and honor the woman's sources of support.

Cultural Assessment	Variations to Consider*	Nursing Responses to Data†
Psychologic Status Excitement and/or apprehension, ambivalence	Marked anxiety (fear of pregnancy diagnosis, fear of medical facility)	Establish lines of communication. Active listening is useful. Establish trusting relationship. Encourage woman to take active part in her care.
	Apathy; display of anger with pregnancy diagnosis	Establish communication and begin counseling. Use active listening techniques.
Educational Needs May have questions about pregnancy or may need time to adjust to reality of pregnancy		Establish educational, supporting environment that can be expanded throughout pregnancy.
Support System Can identify at least two or three individuals with whom woman is emotionally intimate (partner, parent, sibling, friend)	Isolated (no telephone, unlisted number); cannot name a neighbor or friend whom she can call on in an emergency; does not perceive parents as part of her support system	Institute support system through community groups. Help woman to develop trusting relationship with healthcare professionals.
Family Functioning Emotionally supportive Communications adequate Mutually satisfying Cohesiveness in times of trouble	Long-term problems or specific problems related to this pregnancy, potential stressors within the family, pessimistic attitudes, unilateral decision making, unrealistic expectations of this pregnancy or child	Help identify the problems and stressors, encourage communication, and discuss role changes and adaptations. Refer to counseling if indicated.
Economic Status Source of income is stable and sufficient to meet basic needs of daily living and medical needs	Limited prenatal care; poor physical health; limited use of healthcare system; unstable economic status	Discuss available resources for health maintenance and the birth. Institute appropriate referral for meeting expanding family's needs—food stamps, WIC (Women, Infants, and Children, a federally funded nutrition program), and so forth.
Stability of Living Conditions Adequate, stable housing for expanding family's needs	Crowded living conditions; questionable supportive environment for newborn	Refer to appropriate community agency. Work with family on self-help ways to improve situation.

*Possible causes of alterations are identified in parentheses.
†This column provides guidelines for further assessment and initial intervention.

Clinical Tip

Gloves are worn for procedures that involve contact with body fluids such as drawing blood for lab work, handling urine specimens, and conducting pelvic examinations. Because of the increased incidence of latex allergies, it is becoming more common for nonlatex gloves to be used. It is important to inquire about latex allergies with any client before beginning the examination.

NÄGELE'S RULE

The most common method of determining the EDB is **Nägele's rule**. To use this method, one begins with the first day of the last menstrual period, subtracts 3 months, and adds 7 days. For example:

First day of LMP	November 21
Subtract 3 months	− 3 months
	August 21
Add 7 days	+ 7 days
EDB	August 28

It is simpler to change the months to numeric terms:

November 21 becomes	11–21
Subtract 3 months	− 3
	8–21
Add 7 days	+ 7
EDB	August 28

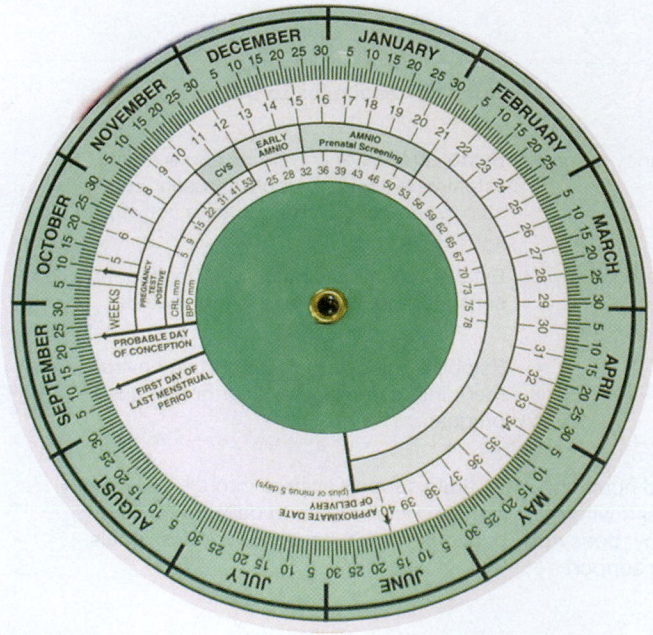

Figure 9–1 The EDB wheel can be used to calculate the due date. To use it, place the arrow labeled "First day of last period" on the date of the woman's LMP. Then read the EDB at the arrow labeled 40. In this case the LMP is September 8 and the EDB is June 15.

A gestation calculator or wheel permits the caregiver to calculate the EDB even more quickly (Figure 9–1). In addition to the wheel, a computer application is now available that reconciles discrepancies that might occur between the dates of the LMP and the first ultrasound, leading to a more accurate EDB calculation.

Nägele's rule may be a fairly accurate determiner of the EDB if the woman has a history of menses every 28 days, remembers her LMP, and was not taking oral contraceptives before becoming pregnant. However, *ovulation usually occurs 14 days before the onset of the next menses, not 14 days after the previous menses.* Consequently, if a woman's cycle is irregular, or more than 28 days long, the time of ovulation may be delayed. If a woman has been using oral contraceptives, ovulation may be delayed several weeks following her last menses. Then, too, a postpartum woman who is breastfeeding may resume ovulating but be amenorrheic for a time, making calculation impossible. Thus Nägele's rule, although helpful, is not foolproof and, in such cases, an ultrasound is done to visualize the gestational sac and obtain measurements of the embryo/fetus to determine EDB.

Uterine Assessment

PHYSICAL EXAMINATION

When a woman is examined in the first 10 to 12 weeks of her pregnancy and her uterine size is compatible with her menstrual history, uterine size may be the single most important clinical method for dating her pregnancy. In many cases, however, women do not seek maternity care until well into their second trimester, when it becomes much more difficult to evaluate specific uterine size. In obese women it is difficult to determine uterine size early in a pregnancy because the uterus is more difficult to palpate.

FUNDAL HEIGHT

Fundal height may be used as an indicator of uterine size, although this method is less accurate late in pregnancy. A tape measure is

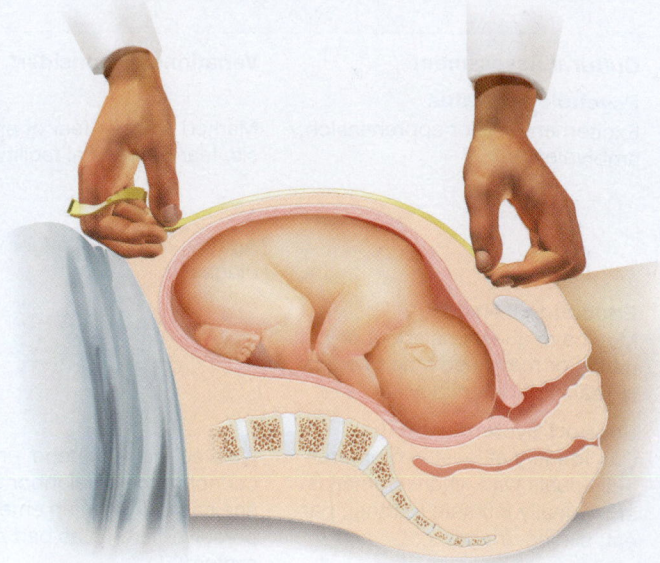

Figure 9–2 A cross-sectional view of fetal position when McDonald method is used to assess the fundal height.

used to measure the distance in centimeters from the top of the symphysis pubis to the top of the uterine fundus (McDonald method) (Figure 9–2). Fundal height in centimeters correlates well with weeks of gestation between 22 and 34 weeks. At 26 weeks' gestation, for example, fundal height is probably about 26 cm (10.24 in.). If the woman is very tall or very short, fundal height will differ. To be most accurate, fundal height should be measured by the same examiner each time. The woman should have voided within 30 minutes of the examination and should lie in the same position each time. In the third trimester, variations in fetal weight decrease the accuracy of fundal height measurements.

A lag in progression of measurements of fundal height from month to month and week to week may signal intrauterine growth restriction (IUGR). A sudden increase in fundal height may indicate twins or hydramnios (excessive amount of amniotic fluid).

Assessment of Fetal Development

QUICKENING

Fetal movements felt by the mother, called *quickening*, may indicate that the fetus is nearing 20 weeks' gestation. However, quickening may be experienced between 16 and 22 weeks' gestation, so this method is not completely accurate.

FETAL HEARTBEAT

The ultrasonic Doppler device (Figure 9–3) is the primary tool for assessing fetal heartbeat. It can detect fetal heartbeat, on average, at 8 to 12 weeks' gestation. The normal range for fetal heart tones (FHT) is 110 to 160. An ultrasound should be completed if the nurse is unable to auscultate between 10 and 12 weeks because there may be a discrepancy of EDB, twins, or a missed abortion. In the case of twins or the obese woman, it may be later before the fetal heartbeat can be detected.

ULTRASOUND

Transvaginal ultrasound is often used in early pregnancy; after about 10 weeks, transabdominal ultrasound is indicated (ACOG, 2013d). In the first trimester, ultrasound can detect a gestational sac as early as 4 to 5 weeks after the LMP, fetal

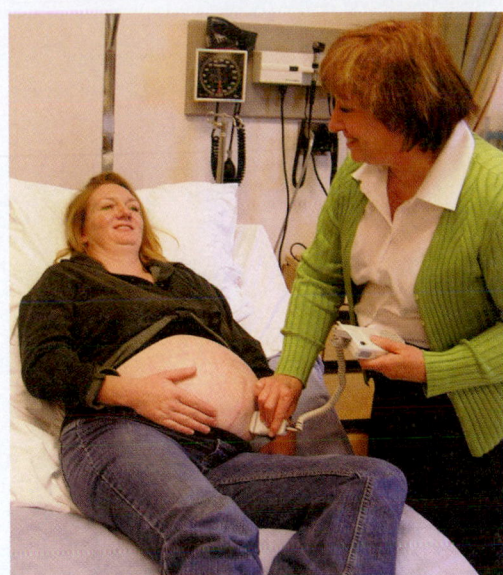

Figure 9–3 **Listening to the fetal heartbeat with a Doppler device.**

SOURCE: Michele Davidson.

heart activity by 6 to 7 weeks, and fetal breathing movements by 10 to 11 weeks of pregnancy. Crown–rump length (CRL) measurements can be made to assess fetal age from 4 days up to about 12 weeks (until the fetal head can be visualized clearly). Biparietal diameter (BPD), which is the widest transverse diameter of the fetal head, can then be used. BPD measurements can be made by approximately 12 to 13 weeks and are most accurate between 14 and 26 weeks, when rapid growth in the biparietal diameter occurs. (See Chapter 15 for discussion of fetal ultrasound scanning.)

Assessment of Pelvic Adequacy (Clinical Pelvimetry)

The pelvis can be assessed vaginally to determine whether its size is adequate for a vaginal birth. This procedure, *clinical pelvimetry*, is typically performed by physicians or by advanced practice nurses. For a detailed description of clinical pelvimetry, readers are referred to a nurse-midwifery text. This section provides basic information about the assessment of the inlet and outlet, which were described in Chapter 3.

1. Pelvic inlet (see Figure 9–4)
   - **Diagonal conjugate** (the distance from the lower posterior border of the symphysis pubis to the sacral promontory), at least 11.5 cm (4.5 in.)
   - **Obstetric conjugate** (a measurement approximately 1.5 cm (0.6 in.) smaller than the diagonal conjugate), 10 cm (3.9 in.) or more
2. Pelvic outlet (see Figures 9–4 and 9–5)
   - Anteroposterior diameter, 9.5 to 11.5 cm (3.75 to 4.5 in.)
   - Transverse diameter (bi-ischial or intertuberous diameter), 8 to 10 cm (3.15 to 3.9 in.)

The pelvic cavity (midpelvis) cannot be accurately measured by clinical examination. Examiners estimate its adequacy. However, that discussion is beyond the scope of this text.

Screening Tests

Many screening tests are routinely performed and/or offered either at the initial prenatal visit or at a specified time during pregnancy. These tests include a Pap smear if indicated, a complete blood count, HIV screening, urine culture, rubella titer, ABO and Rh typing, and a hepatitis B screen, as well as testing

---

EVIDENCE-BASED PRACTICE | Determination of Gestational Age Using Ultrasound

Clinical Question

Is ultrasound biometry an accurate way of determining the gestational age of a fetus?

The Evidence

Accurate gestational dating is an important part of prenatal care. Assessment of fetal growth and development, timely screening tests, and maternal preparation for birth depend on having an accurate prediction of fetal maturity. In addition, accurate assignment of gestational age may reduce the rate of labor induction for postdate pregnancy. Three Canadian obstetricians and a consulting committee of diagnostic radiologists used strict review criteria to evaluate a dozen research studies relative to the safety and effectiveness of ultrasound for gestational dating. The resulting guideline forms the strongest level of evidence for clinical practice.

The strongest evidence supports first trimester crown–rump length as the best parameter for determining gestational age (Butt & Lim, 2014). Between the 12th and 14th weeks, crown–rump length and biparietal diameter are similar in accuracy. Abdominal ultrasound is as accurate as transvaginal ultrasonography, although the latter is more accurate for visualizing early embryonic structures. If ultrasound is used in the second or third trimester, gestational age is best

determined by a combination of multiple biometric parameters, including biparietal diameter, head circumference, abdominal circumference, and femur length. During the second and third trimesters, no single measure best predicts gestational age. The most difficult time to determine a due date is during the third trimester. When performed accurately and precisely, ultrasound is more accurate than even a "certain" missed menstrual date for determining gestational age in spontaneous conceptions. It is the best method for estimating the birth date.

Best Practice

Ideally, every pregnant woman should be offered a first trimester ultrasound to determine gestational age. Abdominal ultrasound is as accurate as transvaginal ultrasound and is more comfortable for the mother. Dating can still be accomplished later in the pregnancy, but ultrasound becomes a less accurate predictor as gestation progresses through the second and third trimesters.

Clinical Reasoning

What are some of the reasons that an accurate gestational age is important to prenatal care? Can a case be made for the cost-effectiveness of early ultrasound to determine an accurate birth due date?

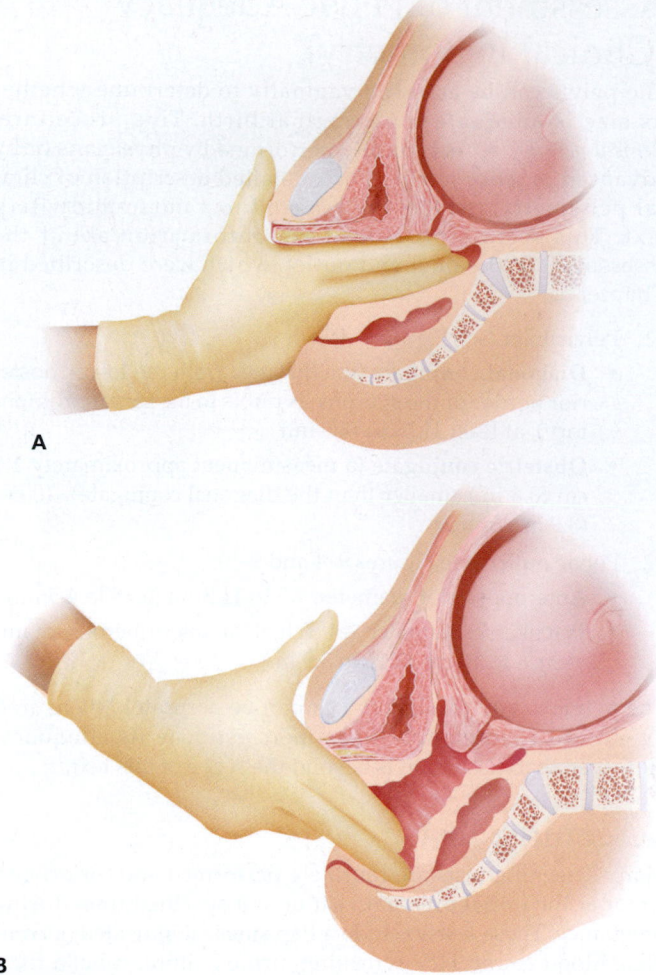

A

B

Figure 9–4 Manual measurement of inlet and outlet. A. Estimation of the diagonal conjugate, which extends from the lower border of the symphysis pubis to the sacral promontory. B. Estimation of the anteroposterior diameter of the outlet, which extends from the lower border of the symphysis pubis to the tip of the sacrum.

for sexually transmitted infections such as syphilis, chlamydia, and gonorrhea. The urine is screened for abnormal findings initially and at each prenatal visit.

Hemoglobin electrophoresis should be performed in women of African, Southeast Asian, and Mediterranean descent to evaluate for sickle cell disease and thalassemias. Prenatal screening for cystic fibrosis has been a routine screening test for all pregnant women for over a decade. To avoid redundant testing, caregivers should determine whether the woman was screened for cystic fibrosis during a previous pregnancy (ACOG, 2011).

A tuberculin test (either purified protein derivative [PPD] or Quantiferon Gold) should also be completed on women who are considered to be high risk. High-risk populations include women born outside of the United States, those who have a known exposure to tuberculosis, and healthcare workers who care for clients with tuberculosis.

All pregnant women, regardless of age, should be offered screening for fetal chromosome anomalies *(aneuploidy)* including Down syndrome, trisomy 18, trisomy 13, and Turner syndrome. First-trimester screening is available at many centers using ultrasound assessment of the thickness of the fetal nuchal

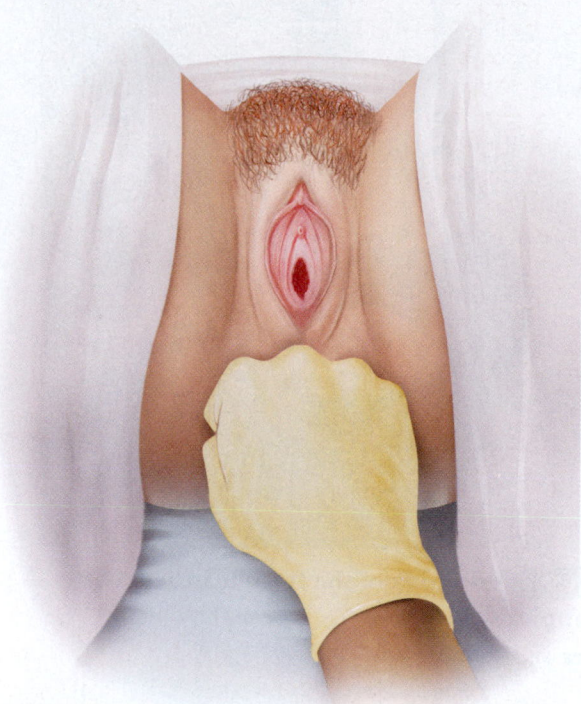

Figure 9–5 Use of a closed fist to measure the outlet. Most examiners know the distance between their first and last proximal knuckles. If they don't, they can use a measuring device.

fold (called *nuchal translucency [NT]*) combined with serum screening for free β-hCG and for pregnancy-associated plasma protein A (PAPP-A). Increased NT, elevated free β-hCG, and reduced PAPP-A suggest aneuploidy. Women with these findings are offered genetic counseling and chorionic villus sampling or second-trimester amniocentesis for diagnosis. If these tests are all negative, no further testing is indicated. Instead, during the second trimester, the woman is simply offered a test for maternal serum alpha-fetoprotein to detect the risk of neural tube defects.

The *quadruple screen* (quad screen) is a safe, useful screening test performed on the mother's serum between weeks 15 and 20 of pregnancy. The test is used to detect levels of specific serum markers—alpha-fetoprotein (AFP), human chorionic gonadotropin (hCG), unconjugated estriol (UE), and inhibin-A (a placental hormone). Test results that reveal higher than normal AFP levels might indicate an increased risk of a fetal neural tube defect, a multiple gestation, or a pregnancy that is farther along than believed. Lower than normal AFP could indicate that the woman is at risk for Down syndrome or trisomy 18. Higher than normal levels of hCG and inhibin-A and lower than normal UE may also indicate that a woman is at increased risk of having a baby with Down syndrome. NT evaluation requires a skilled ultrasonographer and specialized training. In areas where NT is not available, first-trimester free β-hCG screening and PAPP-A screening may be combined with second-trimester quad screening in an integrated approach to detection of aneuploidy.

Noninvasive prenatal testing for fetal aneuploidy (trisomy), specifically trisomy 13, trisomy 18, and trisomy 21, is also available using *cell free fetal DNA* (cffDNA) from the blood of pregnant women. Cell free fetal DNA is thought to be derived from the placenta and can be collected as early as 10 weeks' gestation. Currently ACOG (2012) does not recommend this testing as routine screening for all women, but it can serve as a primary screening test for women at high risk of a trisomy.

It is important for healthcare professionals to provide parents with factual information about the results of tests that detect chromosomal defects or fetal anomalies including the false-positive and detection rates and the implications of the findings. Parents then need to decide on any course of action based on their own spiritual and cultural beliefs.

Screening for gestational diabetes mellitus (GDM) is typically completed between 24 and 28 weeks' gestation. ACOG (2013b) recommends that the testing be done using a 50-g 1-hour glucose screen. If results are abnormal, diagnostic testing using a 100-g 3-hour oral glucose tolerance test is indicated (for a discussion of GDM, see Chapter 14). The American Diabetes Association (2015) recommends that pregnant women at average risk should be screened using either the two-step approach recommended by ACOG or a one-step diagnostic approach using a 75-g 2-hour oral glucose tolerance test (OGTT). A hemoglobin or hematocrit is also completed at this time to evaluate for iron deficiency anemia.

Group B streptococcus (GBS) can cause serious problems for a newborn. Consequently, rectal and vaginal swabs of the mother are obtained at 35 to 37 weeks' gestation to screen for the infection. Women with GBS in the urine at any time during the pregnancy are considered to be positive and do not need a culture completed.

Additional tests are completed in the event of pathologic findings or known disease states. For example, a woman with known chronic hypertension should have a 24-hour urine, metabolic panel, and uric acid completed.

Subsequent Client History

At subsequent prenatal visits the nurse continues to gather data about the course of the pregnancy to date and the woman's responses to it. The nurse also asks about:

- Adjustment of the support person and of other children, if any, in the family
- Preparations the family has made for the new baby
- Discomfort, especially the kinds of discomfort that are often seen at specific times during a pregnancy
- Physical changes that relate directly to the pregnancy, such as fetal movement
- Exposure to contagious illnesses
- Medical treatments and therapies prescribed for nonpregnancy problems since the last visit
- Consumption of prescription or over-the-counter medications or herbal supplements that were not prescribed as part of the woman's prenatal care
- Use of complementary and alternative therapies
- Danger signs of pregnancy (Figure 9–6) (*Note:* Many of the danger signs indicate conditions that are potential complications.)

Periodic prenatal examinations offer the nurse an opportunity to assess the childbearing woman's psychologic needs and emotional status. If the woman's partner attends the antepartum visits, the nurse can also identify the partner's needs and concerns. The woman should have sufficient time to ask

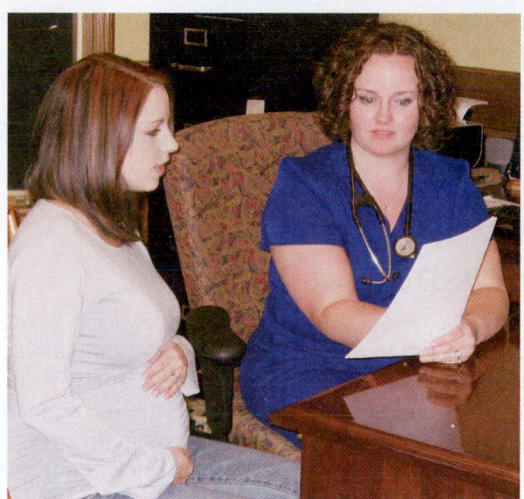

Figure 9–6 The nurse reviews the danger signs in pregnancy at the initial prenatal visit and at each subsequent visit.

KEY FACTS TO REMEMBER
Danger Signs in Pregnancy

The woman should report the following danger signs in pregnancy immediately:

Danger Sign	Possible Cause
Sudden gush of fluid from vagina	Premature rupture of membranes
Vaginal bleeding	Abruptio placentae, placenta previa
	Lesions of cervix or vagina, "bloody show"
Abdominal pain	Premature labor, abruptio placentae
Temperature above 38.3°C (101°F) and chills	Infection
Dizziness, blurring of vision, double vision, spots before eyes	Hypertension, preeclampsia
Persistent vomiting	Hyperemesis gravidarum
Severe headache	Hypertension, preeclampsia
Edema of hands, face, legs, and feet	Preeclampsia
Muscular irritability, convulsions	Preeclampsia, eclampsia
Epigastric pain	Preeclampsia, ischemia in major abdominal vessel
Oliguria	Renal impairment, decreased fluid intake
Dysuria	Urinary tract infection
Absence of fetal movement	Maternal medication, obesity, fetal death

questions and air concerns. If the nurse provides the time and demonstrates genuine interest, the woman will be more at ease bringing up questions that she may believe are silly or has been afraid to verbalize.

The nurse should also be sensitive to religious or spiritual, cultural, and socioeconomic factors that may influence a family's response to pregnancy, as well as the woman's expectations of the healthcare system. The nurse can avoid stereotyping clients simply by asking each woman about her expectations for the antepartum period. Although many women's responses may reflect what are thought to be traditional norms, other women will have decidedly different views or expectations that represent a blending of beliefs or cultures.

During the antepartum period, it is essential to begin assessing the readiness of the woman and her partner (if possible) to assume their responsibilities as parents successfully.

Subsequent Prenatal Assessment

Assessment Guide: Subsequent Prenatal Assessment provides a systematic approach to the regular physical examinations the pregnant woman should undergo for optimal antepartum care and also provides a model for evaluating both the pregnant woman and the expectant father, if he is involved in the pregnancy.

Generally the recommended frequency of antepartum visits is as follows:

Clinical Tip

When assessing blood pressure, have the pregnant woman sit up with her arm resting on a table so that her arm is at the level of her heart. Expect a decrease in her blood pressure from baseline during the second trimester because of normal physiologic changes.

- Every 4 weeks for the first 28 weeks' gestation
- Every 2 weeks until 36 weeks' gestation
- After week 36, every week until childbirth

During the subsequent antepartum assessments, most women demonstrate ongoing psychologic adjustment to pregnancy. However, some women may exhibit signs of possible psychologic problems such as the following:

- Increasing anxiety
- Inability to establish communication
- Inappropriate responses or actions
- Denial of pregnancy
- Inability to cope with stress
- Intense preoccupation with the sex of the baby
- Failure to acknowledge quickening
- Failure to plan and prepare for the baby (e.g., living arrangements, clothing, and feeding methods)
- Indications of substance abuse

If the woman's behavior indicates possible psychologic problems, the nurse can provide ongoing support and counseling and also refer the woman to appropriate professionals as indicated.

ASSESSMENT GUIDE | Subsequent Prenatal Assessment

Physical Assessment/Normal Findings	Alterations and Possible Causes*	Nursing Responses to Data†
Vital Signs		
Temperature: 36.2°–37.6°C (97°–99.6°F)	Elevated temperature (infection)	Evaluate for signs of infection. Refer to healthcare provider.
Pulse: 60–100 beats/min	Increased pulse rate (anxiety, cardiac disorders)	Note irregularities. Assess for anxiety and stress.
Rate may increase 10 beats/min during pregnancy		
Respiration: 12–20 breaths/min	Marked tachypnea or abnormal patterns (respiratory disease)	Refer to healthcare provider.
Blood Pressure: Less than or equal to 120/80 (falls in second trimester)	BP of 120–139/80–89 is considered prehypertensive. Greater than 140/90 or increase of 30 mm systolic and 15 mm diastolic (preeclampsia)	Assess for edema, proteinuria, and hyperreflexia. Refer to healthcare provider.
		Schedule appointments more frequently.
Weight Gain		
Prepregnant weight based on body mass index (BMI): Normal BMI: Total recommended weight gain 11.5–16.0 kg (25–35 lb)		
First Trimester: 1.6–2.3 kg (3.5–5.0 lb)	Inadequate weight gain (poor nutrition, nausea, IUGR)	Discuss appropriate weight gain.
Second Trimester: 5.5–6.8 kg (12–15 lb) **Third Trimester:** 5.5–6.8 kg (12–15 lb)	Excessive weight gain (excessive caloric intake, edema, preeclampsia)	Provide nutritional counseling. Assess for presence of edema or anemia. Refer to a dietitian as needed.
Edema		
Small amount of dependent edema, especially in last weeks of pregnancy	Marked edema in hands, face, legs, and feet (preeclampsia)	Identify any correlation between edema and activities, blood pressure, or proteinuria. Refer to healthcare provider if indicated.

Physical Assessment/Normal Findings	Alterations and Possible Causes*	Nursing Responses to Data†
Uterine Size		
See *Assessment Guide: Initial Prenatal Assessment* for normal changes during pregnancy	Unusually rapid growth (multiple gestation, hydatidiform mole, hydramnios, miscalculation of EDB)	Evaluate fetal status. Determine height of fundus. Use diagnostic ultrasound.
Fetal Heartbeat		
120–160 beats/min Funic souffle	Absence of fetal heartbeat after 20 weeks' gestation (maternal obesity, fetal demise)	Evaluate fetal status.
Laboratory Evaluation		
Hemoglobin: 12–16 g/dL, pseudoanemia of pregnancy	Less than 11 g/dL (anemia)	Provide nutritional counseling. Hemoglobin is repeated at 7 months' gestation. Women of Mediterranean heritage need a close check on hemoglobin because of possibility of thalassemia.
Quad Marker Screen: Blood test performed at 15–21 weeks' gestation but best performed between 16–18 weeks' gestation. Evaluates four factors: maternal serum alpha-fetoprotein (MSAFP), unconjugated estriol (UE), hCG, and inhibin-A: normal levels	Elevated MSAFP (neural tube defect, underestimated gestational age, multiple gestation). Lower than normal MSAFP (Down syndrome, trisomy 18). Higher than normal hCG and inhibin-A (Down syndrome). Lower than normal UE (Down syndrome).	Offered to all pregnant women. If quad screen abnormal, further testing such as ultrasound or amniocentesis may be indicated.
Indirect Coombs Test done on Rh negative women: Negative (done at 28 weeks' gestation)	Rh antibodies present (maternal sensitization has occurred)	If Rh negative and unsensitized, Rh immune globulin given (see Chapter 15). If Rh antibodies present, Rh immune globulin not given; fetus monitored closely for isoimmune hemolytic disease.
50-g 1-hour glucose screen (done between 24 and 28 weeks' gestation) (ACOG, 2013b) or as an alternative, the one-step diagnostic approach using a 75-g 2-hour oral glucose tolerance test (OGTT) (ADA, 2015)	Plasma glucose level greater than 130–140 mg/dL depending on the facility (gestational diabetes mellitus [GDM])	Discuss implications of GDM. Refer for a diagnostic 100-g oral glucose tolerance test. Refer to healthcare provider.
Urinalysis: See *Assessment Guide: Initial Prenatal Assessment* for normal findings	See *Assessment Guide: Initial Prenatal Assessment* for deviations	Urinalysis and culture is completed at initial visit and at subsequent visits as indicated.
Protein: Negative	Proteinuria, albuminuria (contamination by vaginal discharge, urinary tract infection, preeclampsia)	Obtain dipstick urine sample. Refer to healthcare provider if deviations are present.
Glucose: Negative	Persistent glycosuria (diabetes mellitus)	Refer to healthcare provider.
Note: Glycosuria may be present due to physiologic alterations in glomerular filtration rate and renal threshold.		
Screening for Group B Streptococcus (GBS):	Positive culture (maternal infection)	Explain maternal and fetal/neonatal risks. (See Chapter 15.)
Rectal and vaginal swabs obtained at 35–37 weeks' gestation for all pregnant women		Refer to healthcare provider for therapy.

Cultural Assessment	Variations to Consider*	Nursing Responses to Data†
Determine the mother's (and family's) attitudes about the sex of the unborn child.	Some women have no preference about the sex of the child; others do. In many cultures, boys are especially valued as firstborn children.	Provide opportunities to discuss preferences and expectations; avoid a judgmental attitude to the response.
Ask about the woman's expectations of childbirth. Will she want someone with her for the birth? Whom does she choose? What is the role of her partner?	Some women want their partner present for labor and birth; others prefer a female relative or friend. Some women expect to be separated from their partners once labor begins.	Provide information on birth options but accept the woman's decision about who will attend.

(continued)

ASSESSMENT GUIDE | Subsequent Prenatal Assessment (*continued*)

Cultural Assessment	Variations to Consider*	Nursing Responses to Data†
Ask about preparations for the baby. Determine what is customary for the woman.	Some women may have a fully prepared nursery; others may not have a separate room for the baby.	Explore reasons for not preparing for the baby. Support the mother's preferences and provide information about possible sources of assistance if the decision is related to a lack of resources.

Expectant Mother

Psychologic Status	Increased stress and anxiety	Encourage woman to take an active part in her care.
First Trimester (*Period of Adjustment*): Incorporates idea of pregnancy; may feel ambivalent or anxious, especially if she must give up desired role; usually looks for signs of verification of pregnancy, such as increase in abdominal size or fetal movement	Inability to establish communication; inability to accept pregnancy; inappropriate response or actions; denial of pregnancy; inability to cope	Establish lines of communication. Discuss and provide anticipatory guidance regarding normalcy of feelings and actions. Establish a trusting relationship. Counsel as necessary. Refer to appropriate professional as needed.
Second Trimester (*Period of Radiant Health*): Baby becomes more real to woman as abdominal size increases and she feels movement; she begins to turn inward, becoming more introspective		
Third Trimester (*Period of Watchful Waiting*): Begins to think of baby as separate being; may feel restless, uneasy, and may feel that time of labor will never come; remains self-centered and concentrates on preparing place for baby. Fears for her well-being and that of her baby.		

Educational Needs: **Self-care measures and knowledge about the following:**
  Health promotion
  Breast care
  Hygiene
  Rest
  Exercise
  Nutrition
  Relief measures for common discomforts of pregnancy
  Danger signs in pregnancy (see Key Facts to Remember)
	Inadequate information	Provide information and counseling.

Sexual Activity: Woman knows how pregnancy affects sexual activity	Lack of information about effects of pregnancy and/or alternative positions during sexual intercourse	Provide counseling.
Preparation for Parenting: Appropriate preparation	Lack of preparation (denial, failure to adjust to baby, unwanted child)	Counsel. If lack of preparation is due to inadequacy of information, provide information.
Preparation for Childbirth: Client aware of the following:		
1. Prepared childbirth techniques		If couple chooses particular technique, refer to classes. (See Chapter 10 for description of childbirth preparation techniques.)
2. Normal processes and changes during childbirth		Encourage prenatal class attendance. Educate woman during visits based on current physical status. Provide reading list for more specific information.
3. Problems that may occur as a result of drug and alcohol use and of smoking	Continued abuse of drugs and alcohol; denial of possible effect on self and baby	Review danger signs that were presented on initial visit.

Cultural Assessment	Variations to Consider*	Nursing Responses to Data†
Woman has met other physician or nurse-midwife who may be attending her birth in the absence of primary caregiver	Introduction of new individual at birth may increase stress and anxiety for woman and partner	Introduce woman to all members of group practice.
Impending Labor: Client knows signs of impending labor: 1. Uterine contractions that increase in frequency, duration, and intensity 2. Bloody show 3. Expulsion of mucous plug 4. Rupture of membranes	Lack of information	Provide appropriate teaching, stressing importance of seeking appropriate medical assistance.
Expectant Father		
Psychologic Status		
First Trimester: May express excitement over confirmation of pregnancy and of his virility; concerns move toward providing for financial needs; energetic, may identify with some discomforts of pregnancy and may even exhibit symptoms	Increasing stress and anxiety; inability to establish communication; inability to accept pregnancy diagnosis; withdrawal of support; abandonment of the mother	Encourage partner to come to prenatal visits. Establish line of communication. Establish trusting relationship.
Second Trimester: May feel more confident and be less concerned with financial matters; may have concerns about the woman's changing size and shape, her increasing introspection		Counsel. Let expectant partner know that it is normal for him to experience these feelings.
Third Trimester: May have feelings of rivalry with fetus, especially during sexual activity; may make changes in his physical appearance and exhibit more interest in himself; may become more energetic; fantasizes about child but usually imagines older child; fears mutilation and death of woman and child		Include expectant partner in pregnancy activities as he desires. Provide education, information, and support. Increasing numbers of expectant partners are demonstrating desire to be involved in many or all aspects of prenatal care, education, and preparation.

*Possible causes of alterations are identified in parentheses.
†This column provides guidelines for further assessment and initial intervention.

Focus Your Study

- A complete history forms the basis of prenatal care and is re-evaluated and updated as necessary throughout the pregnancy.

- The initial prenatal assessment is a careful and thorough physical examination and cultural and psychosocial assessment designed to identify variations and potential risk factors.

- Laboratory tests completed at the initial visit, such as a complete blood count, ABO and Rh typing, urinalysis/culture, Pap smear, chlamydia culture, testing for syphilis (Venereal Disease Research Laboratory [VDRL], rapid plasma regain [RPR], or other serology test), gonorrhea culture, rubella titer, various blood screens, and tuberculin test (PPD) for women

in high-risk groups with no known history of a positive test, provide information about the woman's health during early pregnancy and also help detect potential problems.

- The estimated date of birth (EDB) can be calculated by using Nägele's rule. Using this approach, one begins with the first day of the last menstrual period, subtracts 3 months, and adds 7 days. A gestational calculator or wheel may also be used to calculate the EDB.

- Accuracy of the EDB may be evaluated by physical examination to assess uterine size, measurement of fundal height, and ultrasound. Perception of quickening and auscultation of fetal heartbeat are also helpful in confirming the gestation of a pregnancy.

- The diagonal conjugate is the distance from the lower posterior border of the symphysis pubis to the sacral promontory. The obstetric conjugate is estimated by subtracting 1.5 cm from the length of the diagonal conjugate.

- As part of the assessment of the pelvic cavity (midpelvis), the prominence of the ischial spines is assessed, the sacrosciatic notch and the length of the sacrospinous ligament are measured, and the shape of the pelvic side walls is evaluated. Finally, the hollowness of the sacrum is determined.

- The anteroposterior diameter of the pelvic outlet is determined, the mobility of the coccyx is assessed, the suprapubic angle is estimated, and the contour of the pubic arch is evaluated to assess the adequacy of the pelvic outlet.

- The nurse begins evaluating the woman psychosocially during the initial prenatal assessment. This assessment continues and is modified throughout the pregnancy.

- Religious, cultural, and ethnic beliefs may strongly influence the woman's attitudes and apparent cooperation with care during pregnancy.

Clinical Reasoning In Action

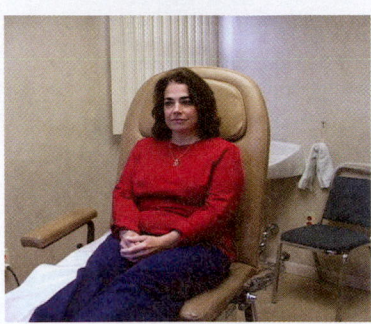

Wendy Stodard, age 40, G3P0020 comes to the obstetrician's office where you are working for a prenatal visit. Wendy has experienced two spontaneous abortions followed by a D & C at 14 and 15 weeks' gestation during the previous year. She has a history of *Chlamydia trachomatis* infection 3 years ago, which was treated with azithromycin. She is at 10 weeks' gestation. Wendy tells you that she is afraid of losing this pregnancy as she did previously. She says that she has been experiencing some mild nausea, breast tenderness, and fatigue, which did not occur with her other pregnancies. You assist the obstetrician with an ultrasound. The gestational sac is clearly seen, fetal heartbeat is observed, and crown–rump measurements are consistent with gestational age of 10 weeks. The pelvic examination demonstrates a closed cervix, and positive Goodell, Hegar, and Chadwick signs. You discuss with Wendy the signs of a healthy pregnancy.

1. What signs are reassuring with this pregnancy?

2. What symptoms should be reported to the obstetrician immediately?

3. What is the frequency of antepartal visits?

References

American College of Obstetricians and Gynecologists (ACOG). (2011). *Update on carrier screening for cystic fibrosis.* (ACOG Committee Opinion No. 486), Washington, DC: Author.

American College of Obstetricians and Gynecologists (ACOG). (2012). *Noninvasive prenatal testing for fetal aneuploidy.* (ACOG Committee Opinion No. 545), Washington, DC: Author.

American College of Obstetricians and Gynecologists (ACOG). (2013a). *Definition of term pregnancy.* (ACOG Committee Opinion No. 579), Washington, DC: Author.

American College of Obstetricians and Gynecologists (ACOG). (2013b). *Gestational diabetes mellitus.* (ACOG Practice Bulletin No. 137), Washington, DC: Author.

American College of Obstetricians and Gynecologists (ACOG). (2013c). *Medically indicated late-preterm and early-term deliveries.* (ACOG Committee Opinion No. 560), Washington, DC: Author.

American College of Obstetricians and Gynecologists (ACOG). (2013d). *Ultrasound exams.* (ACOG Patient Education Pamphlet No. APO25), Washington, DC: Author.

American Diabetes Association (ADA). (2015). Position statement: Standards of medical care in diabetes—2015. *Diabetes Care, 38*(Suppl. 1), S1–87.

Butt, K., & Lim, K. (2014). Determination of gestational age by ultrasound. *Journal of Obstetrics and Gynaecology Canada, 36*(2), 171–181.

Cunningham, F. G., Leveno, K. J., Bloom, S. L., Spong, C. Y., Dashe, J. S., Hoffman, B. L., . . . Sheffield, J. S. (2014). *Williams obstetrics* (24th ed.). New York, NY: McGraw-Hill.

King, T. L., Brucker, M. C., Kriebs, J. M., Fahey, J. O., Gegor, C. L., & Varney, H. (2015). *Varney's midwifery* (5th ed.). Burlington, MA: Jones & Bartlett Learning.

Spong, C. Y. (2013). Defining "term" pregnancy: Recommendations from the defining "term" pregnancy workgroup. Published online May 3, 2013. doi:10.1001/jama.2013.6235

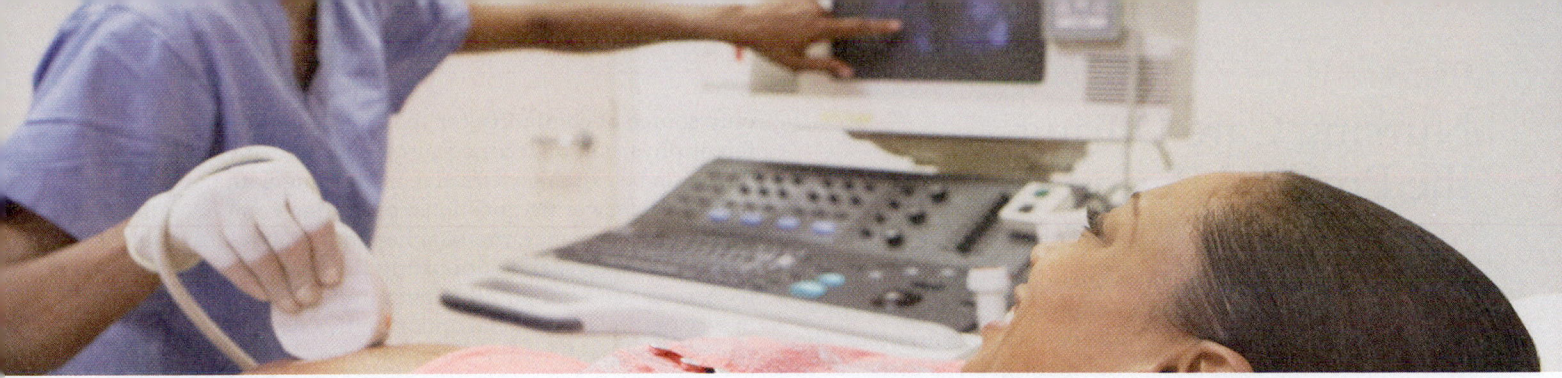

Chapter 10
The Expectant Family: Needs and Care

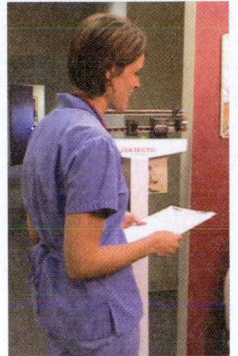

In my role, I have a very special opportunity to help women and their loved ones prepare for their new baby. I give them information about what to expect and answer their questions so that they can make more informed decisions. Sometimes I have to stop and remind myself to be clear about information that is important for any pregnant woman. Otherwise I might make the mistake of trying to impose my values. It is all too easy to view my way as the only way. When I do that, I fail them and I fail myself.

—A Registered Nurse Working in a Prenatal Clinic at an Inner-City Hospital

∨ Learning Outcomes

10.1 Describe the significance of using the nursing process to promote health in the woman and her family during pregnancy.

10.2 Describe actions the nurse can take to help maintain the well-being of the expectant father and siblings during a family's pregnancy.

10.3 Discuss the significance of cultural considerations in managing nursing care during pregnancy.

10.4 Identify information that expectant parents may need to assist them in making the best decisions possible about issues related to pregnancy, labor, and birth.

10.5 Explain the basic goals of childbirth education in providing care to expectant couples and their families.

10.6 Identify the common discomforts of pregnancy and their causes.

10.7 Summarize appropriate measures to alleviate the common discomforts of pregnancy.

10.8 Delineate self-care actions a pregnant woman and her family can take to maintain and promote well-being during each trimester of pregnancy.

10.9 Identify some of the concerns that an expectant couple may have about sexual activity.

From the moment a woman finds out she is pregnant, she faces a future marked by dramatic changes— changes in her appearance, in her relationships, and in her psychologic state. In coping with these changes, she and her loved ones need to make adjustments in their daily lives.

Nurses caring for pregnant women need an up-to-date understanding of pregnancy to be effective in implementing the nursing process as they plan and provide care. With this in mind, Chapter 8 provides a database for the nurse by presenting material related to the normal physical, psychologic, social, and cultural changes of pregnancy. Chapter 9 then uses that database to begin discussing nursing management by focusing on assessment. This chapter further addresses nursing management as it relates to the needs of the expectant woman and her loved ones.

Nursing Care During the Prenatal Period

Nursing Diagnoses During Pregnancy

The nurse may see a pregnant woman only once every 3 to 4 weeks during the first several months of her pregnancy. Therefore, a written care plan or clinical path that incorporates the database, nursing diagnoses, and client goals is essential to ensure continuity of care.

The nurse can anticipate that, for many women with a low-risk pregnancy, certain nursing diagnoses will be made more frequently than others. The diagnoses will, of course, vary from woman to woman and according to the time in the pregnancy. After formulating an appropriate diagnosis, the nurse and woman establish related goals to guide the nursing plan and interventions.

Planning and Implementation During Pregnancy

Once nursing diagnoses have been identified, the next step is to establish priorities of nursing care. Sometimes priorities of care are based on the most immediate needs or concerns expressed by the woman. For example, during the first trimester, when she is experiencing nausea or is concerned about sexual intimacy with her partner, the woman is not likely to want to hear about labor and birth. At other times, priorities may develop from findings during a prenatal examination. For example, a woman who is showing signs of preeclampsia (a pregnancy complication discussed in Chapter 14) may feel physically well and find it hard to accept the nurse's emphasis on the need for frequent rest periods. It then becomes the responsibility of medical and nursing professionals to help the woman and her family to understand the significance of a problem and to plan interventions to deal with it.

HEALTHY PEOPLE 2020

(MICH-10) Increase the proportion of pregnant women who receive early and adequate prenatal care

---

Health Promotion   Anticipatory Guidance for the Postpartum Period

Throughout the prenatal period, the nurse shares information with the family, both verbally and through written materials. Anticipatory guidance helps the expectant couple identify and discuss issues that could be sources of postpartum stress. Issues to be addressed beforehand may include the sharing of baby and household chores, help in the first few days after childbirth, options for babysitting to allow the mother (and couple) some free time, the mother's return to work after the baby's birth, and sibling rivalry. Couples resolve these issues in different ways, but postpartum adjustment tends to be easier for couples who agree on the issues beforehand than for couples who do not confront and resolve these issues.

NURSING CARE IN THE COMMUNITY

Prenatal care, especially for women with low-risk pregnancies, is community based, typically in a clinic or a private office. The nurse in a clinic or health maintenance organization may be the only source of continuity for the woman, who may see a different physician or certified nurse-midwife at each visit. The nurse can be extremely effective in working with the expectant family by answering questions; providing complete information about pregnancy, prenatal healthcare activities, and community resources; and supporting the healthcare activities of the woman and her family. Communities often have a wealth of services and educational opportunities available for pregnant women and their families, and the knowledgeable nurse can help expectant mothers to assess and access these services.

Home Care. Home care can be of benefit to any pregnant woman, but it is especially effective in removing barriers for women who have difficulty accessing healthcare. These barriers may include lack of locally available healthcare facilities, problems with transportation to the facility, or schedule conflicts with available appointment times because of employment hours or family responsibilities.

In-home nursing assessments vary according to the experience and preparation of the nurse and include current history, vital signs, weight, urine screen, physical activity, dietary intake, reflexes, tests of fetal well-being, and cervical examinations, if indicated. Once the assessments are completed, the nurse can determine the level of follow-up home care or telephone contact needed. See Chapter 29 for further discussion of home care of the childbearing family.

Currently, home care is not routinely used because of the cost, but when home care is available, it is most often used for women with prenatal complications that can be managed without hospitalization if effective nursing assessment and care are provided in the home.

Care of the Pregnant Woman's Family

The well-being of the pregnant woman is intertwined with the well-being of those to whom she is closest. Thus the nurse also addresses the needs of the woman's family. Although the expectant father is often involved in the pregnancy, his presence cannot be assumed. If he is not part of the family structure, it is important to assess the woman's support system to determine which significant people in her life will play a major role during this childbearing experience. This may be a spouse or a same-sex partner. The following information still applies.

Anticipatory guidance of the expectant father, if he is involved in the pregnancy, is a necessary part of any plan of care. He may need information about the anatomic, physiologic, and emotional changes that occur for the expectant mother and father during and after pregnancy; the couple's sexuality and sexual response; and the reactions that he is experiencing. He may wish to express his feelings about the sex of the child, his ability to parent, and other topics.

If it is culturally acceptable to the couple and personally acceptable to the expectant father, refer the couple to expectant parents' classes. These classes provide valuable information about pregnancy and childbirth, using a variety of teaching strategies such as discussion, films, demonstrations with educational models, and written handouts. Some classes even give the father the opportunity to get a "feel" for pregnancy by wearing a pregnancy simulator (Figure 10–1). Such classes also offer the couple an opportunity to gain support from other couples.

The nurse assesses the father's intended degree of participation during labor and birth and his knowledge of what to expect.

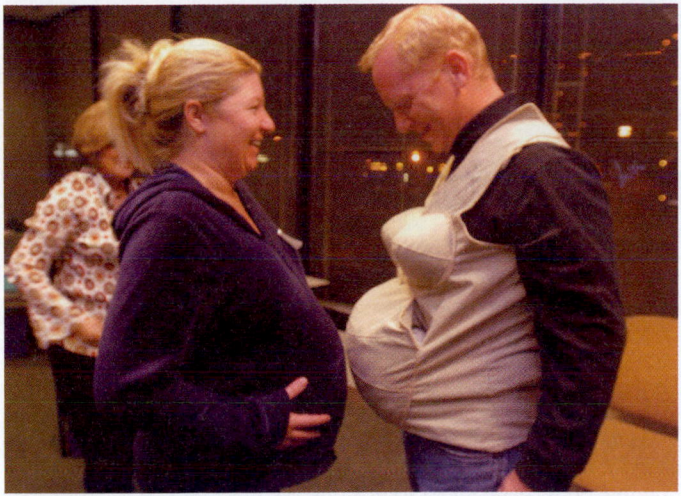

Figure 10–1 The Empathy Belly® is a pregnancy simulator that allows men and women to experience some of the symptoms of pregnancy. The "belly," which weighs 33 lb, produces symptoms such as shortness of breath, bladder pressure, shift in the center of gravity with resulting waddling gait, increased lordosis and backache, and fatigue. It also can simulate fetal kicking movements.

SOURCE: ZUMA Press/Alamy.

If the couple prefers that his participation be minimal or restricted, support their decision. Research indicates that increased focus on the father's needs during prenatal care aids his transition to fatherhood and also improves the mother's stress levels and prenatal health behavior. Assessing and fostering progress in the father's journey to becoming a parent has significant long-term benefits for the man, his partner, and their child (Alio, Lewis, Scarborough, et al., 2013). In the plan for prenatal care, the nurse also incorporates a discussion about the negative feelings older children may develop. Parents may be distressed to see an older child regress to "babyish" behavior or become aggressive toward the newborn. Parents who are unprepared for an older child's feelings of anger, jealousy, and rejection may respond inappropriately in their confusion and surprise. The nurse emphasizes that open communication between parents and children (or acting out feelings with a doll if the child is too young to verbalize) helps children master their feelings. Children may feel less neglected and more secure if they know that their parents are willing to help with their anger and aggressiveness.

The nurse can encourage the couple to address relationship changes with in-laws as well as the woman's or couple's expectations of the grandparents. Although some grandparents are eager to assist with child care by babysitting, others are not (Figure 10–2). The parents should also give some thought to the best ways of dealing with possible conflicts with the grandparents over childrearing approaches. However, postpartum adjustment is easiest for couples who acknowledge potential problems and develop strategies to address them beforehand.

Cultural Considerations in Pregnancy

As discussed in Chapter 2, actions taken during pregnancy are often determined by cultural beliefs. Table 10–1 presents activities encouraged or forbidden by some specific cultures.

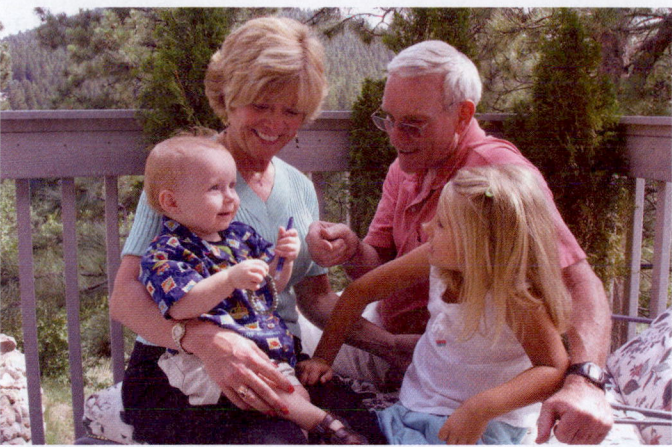

Figure 10–2 Grandparents can offer nurturing and guidance to their grandchildren, not to mention lots of fun.

The table is not meant to be all-inclusive, nor is it meant to imply that all members of a given culture hold these beliefs. Rather, it offers a few examples of cultural activities that may be important to some women during the prenatal period.

In working with clients of other cultures, health professionals should be open to and respectful of others' beliefs. Effective nurses recognize that each childbearing family, shaped by culture and life experience, has expectations of both its members and the healthcare system during pregnancy and birth.

Language barriers often pose a challenge in providing effective prenatal nursing care. When possible, it is important to have an interpreter—family member, friend, or staff person—present at prenatal visits so that the nurse can provide basic information about pregnancy and prenatal care. It is essential to have printed material available in the woman's language. (See *Nursing Care Plan: Language Barriers at First Prenatal Visit*.)

Childbearing Decisions

Childbearing decisions are decisions parents face about their childbirth preferences and experiences. A method that has assisted many couples in making these choices is called a birth plan. In the birth plan, prospective parents identify aspects of the childbearing experience that are most important to them. (A sample birth plan is presented in Figure 10–3.) The birth plan helps identify available options and becomes a tool for communication among the expectant parents, the healthcare providers, and the healthcare professionals at the birth setting.

The birth plan also helps pregnant women and couples set priorities. Using the plan, they identify areas that they want to incorporate in their own birth experience. Then they can take the birth plan to a visit with their physician/certified nurse-midwife (CNM) or other healthcare provider and use it in discussing and comparing their wishes with the philosophy and beliefs of the provider. It is imperative that the couple discuss their preferences at a prenatal visit before labor. Sometimes couples may include requests that need clarification. For example, if the couple states they do not want any external monitoring, the provider needs to explain that intermittent monitoring could be provided but that eliminating all monitoring during labor could jeopardize both the mother and the fetus. Possible obstetric interventions that may be needed should also be part of the birth plan. They can also take the birth plan to the birth setting and use it as a basis for communicating their wishes during the childbirth experience.

TABLE 10–1 Cultural Beliefs and Practices During Pregnancy

These are a few examples of cultural beliefs and practices related to pregnancy. It is important not to make assumptions about a client's beliefs, because cultural norms vary greatly within a culture and from generation to generation. The nurse should observe the client carefully and take the time to ask questions. Clients will benefit greatly from the nurse's increased awareness of their cultural beliefs and practices.

BELIEF OR PRACTICE	NURSING CONSIDERATION
Home Remedies	
Pregnant women of Native American background may use herbal remedies. An example is the dandelion, which contains a milky juice in its stem believed to increase breast milk flow in mothers who choose to breastfeed (Spector, 2013). Clients of Chinese descent may drink ginseng tea for faintness after childbirth or as a sedative when mixed with bamboo leaves. Some people of African heritage may use self-medication for pregnancy discomforts—for example, laxatives to prevent or treat constipation (Purnell, 2014).	Find out what medications and home remedies your client is using, and counsel your client regarding overall effects. It is common for individuals to avoid telling healthcare workers about home remedies; the client may feel this will be judged unfavorably. Phrase your questions in a sensitive, accepting way. In some cases, you might want to suggest remedies that may be more effective—for example, eating high-fiber foods to reduce constipation. If the home remedy is not harmful, there is no reason to ask a client to discontinue this practice.
Nutrition	
Some women of Italian background may believe that it is necessary to satisfy desires for certain foods in order to prevent congenital anomalies. Also, they may believe that they must eat food that they smell, or else the fetus will move "inside," which will result in a miscarriage. So, too, people of Ethiopian descent may believe that unfulfilled cravings may cause miscarriage (Spector, 2013). Pregnant women of Vietnamese descent are considered to be in a weak, cold state and must correct this by eating and drinking hot foods during the first trimester (Purnell, 2014).	Discuss the client's beliefs and practices in regard to nutrition during pregnancy. Obtain a diet history from the client. Discuss the importance of a well-balanced diet during pregnancy with consideration of the client's cultural beliefs and practices.
Alternative Healthcare Providers	
Pregnant women of Mexican background may choose to seek out the care of a *partera* (midwife) for prenatal and intrapartum care. A partera speaks their language, shares a similar culture, and can care for pregnant women at home or in a birthing center instead of a hospital. Some people in Hispanic American communities may use the *curandero,* the holistic folk healer. The curanderos are believed to have received their gift from God and may use herbs or prescribe over-the-counter medications (Spector, 2013).	Discuss the variety of choices of healthcare providers available to the pregnant woman. Contrast the benefits and risks of different settings for prenatal care and birth. Provide reassurance that the goal of healthcare during pregnancy and birth is a healthy outcome for mother and baby with respect for the specific cultural beliefs and practices of the client.
Exercise	
Pregnant women of Korean descent may work hard toward the end of pregnancy to increase the chances of giving birth to a small baby (Purnell, 2014). Some people of European, African, and Mexican descent believe that reaching over the head during pregnancy can harm the baby.	Ask your client whether there are any activities she is afraid to do because of the pregnancy. Assure her that reaching over her head will not harm the baby, and evaluate other activities as to their effect on the pregnancy.
Spirituality	
Navajo Indians are aware of the mind–soul connection and may try to follow certain practices to have a healthy pregnancy and birth. Practices could include focus on peace and positive thoughts as well as certain types of prayers and ceremonies. A traditional healer may assist them (Purnell, 2014). Some people of European background may tend to pay more attention to spirituality in their life to alleviate fears and ensure a safe birth.	Encourage the use of support systems and spiritual aids that provide comfort for the mother.
Birth Rituals	
In certain countries such as Algeria, Brazil, China, and Korea, the father is not present at birth. In Japan, a new mother may be confined for up to 100 days, whereas in Bangladesh the new mother remains indoors for up to 40 days. In Iran, Iraq, and Greece, amulets may be placed on the baby or crib (Spector, 2013)	Recognize the importance of birth practices that are part of a family's tradition and honor these practices when possible.

Nursing Care Plan: Language Barriers at First Prenatal Visit

Nursing Diagnosis: *Health Maintenance, Ineffective*, related to alteration in verbal and written communication skills (NANDA-I ©2014)

GOAL: Client will demonstrate understanding of health information received during prenatal visits.

INTERVENTION	RATIONALE
• If no interpreter is available, refer to posters with pictures to explain routine care and procedures during the prenatal examination.	• Posters put words into verbal images and are helpful in communicating information.
• Provide handouts and brochures about prenatal care in the woman's native language.	• Translated handouts provide information that the client can refer to at home. This reinforces information discussed during the visit and helps the family understand what the woman will experience during the pregnancy and at each visit.
• Use teaching models to demonstrate procedures. Teaching models may include plastic pelvis, knitted uterus, fetal model, breast model, birth control devices, ultrasound equipment, and so forth.	• Visual aids help to communicate information during the examination.
• Schedule an interpreter for subsequent prenatal visits.	• If a family member cannot translate the health information to the client, an independent translator is essential to ensure that information is accurately provided. When an interpreter is used (especially a family member), the nurse should be sure that the interpreter is translating information received from the woman and not simply answering the questions for her.
• Refer the woman to prenatal classes taught in her own language, if available.	• Prenatal classes taught in the woman's language enable her to receive health information that is easily understood, which will provide a better understanding of what she should expect during pregnancy, birth, and postpartum. Prenatal classes may also provide a social outlet for clients.
• Involve other members of the healthcare team in planning and providing care.	• Cultures vary in language, nonverbal expression, dietary habits, use of time, spatial expectations, and so forth. Use of medication and blood products may also be influenced by cultural beliefs. Social workers who are familiar with the client's cultural beliefs, for example, may help the client adjust to different healthcare practices while providing suggestions to ensure prenatal care that is more in line with the woman's cultural beliefs. Dietitians may help the woman plan meals that are aligned with her cultural practices while meeting the nutritional needs of pregnancy.

EXPECTED OUTCOME: Effective communication occurs. The client will gain an understanding of basic prenatal information as evidenced by using hand gestures, by pointing to pictures on posters and translated phrases on handouts, and through an interpreter, if one is available.

Today, there are many more choices that pregnant women and couples make. Some of these are explored in Table 10–2. Although most birth experiences are close to those presented in the birth plan, at times expectations cannot be met. This may be because of the unavailability of some choices in the community or unexpected problems during pregnancy or birth. While research indicates maternal satisfaction is highest when a planned cesarean section or vaginal birth is achieved, it is important for nurses to help expectant parents keep sight of what is realistic for their situation (Bloomquist, Quiroz, MacMillan, et al., 2011).

Healthcare Provider

One of the first decisions facing expectant parents is the selection of a healthcare provider. The nurse assists them by explaining the various options and outlining what can be expected from each. A thorough understanding of the differences of educational preparation, skill level, practice style, and general philosophy and characteristics of practice of certified nurse-midwives, obstetricians, family practice physicians, and lay midwives is essential. The nurse can encourage expectant parents to investigate the healthcare provider's credentials, basic and special education and

Developing Cultural Competence Pregnant Women of African American Heritage

In caring for pregnant women of African American heritage, it is helpful to consider the following general points (Purnell, 2014):

- Pregnant African American women may be guided by their extended family into common practices such as geophagia, the ingestion of dirt or clay, which is believed to reduce mineral deficiencies. This practice has implications for the focus of teaching a nurse will offer.

- Many African American families are matriarchal. Women are respected and heeded in decision making and often stress good behavior and firm parenting with their children, especially to keep them safe in dangerous situations.

- Three-generation extended families are common, and the grandmother is often highly respected for her wisdom. She may play a critical role in the care of the children.

- Certain taboos may exist, such as the belief in the need to avoid taking pictures during pregnancy to prevent stillbirths. Some women of African American descent may also believe that the purchase of baby clothing or supplies can result in a stillbirth. Thus they may appear to be unprepared for the arrival of the baby.

Professionalism in Practice Providing Culturally Sensitive Care

In providing effective, culturally sensitive care, nurses can use the following strategies (University of South Carolina, 2011):

- Take actions that help break down language barriers.
- Ask the client what she or he believes caused the illness.
- Integrate folk treatments and Western medicine as much as possible.
- Enlist the family caretaker and others as needed.
- Respect the client's beliefs.
- Provide printed materials in the client's language.

training, fee schedule, and availability to new clients; this is often accomplished by telephoning the healthcare provider's office.

The nurse can also help the woman/couple develop a list of interview questions for their first visit to a healthcare provider. These could include the following:

- Who is in practice with you, or who covers for you when you are unavailable?
- At what point after admission do you come to the hospital or birth setting to provide support?
- How do your partners' philosophies compare to yours?
- How do you feel about my partner, other support person, or other children coming to the prenatal visits?
- Do you offer centering (group care) or individual prenatal care visits?

Sample Birth Plan

Choice	Choice
Care provider:	Position during birth:
Certified nurse-midwife	On side
Obstetrician	Hands and knees
Family physician	Kneeling
Lay midwife	Squatting
Birth setting:	Birthing chair
Hospital:	Birthing bed
Birthing room	Other:
Delivery room	Family present (sibs)
Birth center	Filming of birth (videotaping)
Home	Photography of birth
Support during labor and birth:	Leboyer
Partner present	Episiotomy
Doula present	No sterile drapes
During labor:	Partner to cut umbilical cord
Ambulate as desired	Hold baby immediately after birth
Shower if desired	Breastfeed immediately after birth
Wear own clothes	No separation after birth
Use hot tub	Save the placenta
Use own rocking chair	Collect cord blood for banking
Have perineal prep	Newborn care:
Have enema	Eye treatment for the baby
Water birth	Vitamin K injection
Electronic fetal monitor	Heptovac injection
Membranes:	Breastfeeding
Rupture naturally	Formula feeding
Amniotomy if needed	Pacifier use
Labor stimulation if needed	Glucose water
Medication:	Circumcision
Identify type desired	Postpartum care:
Fluids or ice as desired	Short stay
Music during labor and birth	48-hour stay after vaginal birth
Massage	Home visits after discharge
Therapeutic touch	Home doula
Healing touch	Other:

Figure 10–3 Birth plan for childbirth choices. The columns list various choices that the couple may consider during their childbirth experience. Once the couple has considered each of the choices, they can circle the items they desire.

SOURCE: Based on Davidson et al., Olds' Maternal-Newborn Nursing & Women's Health, 10e, p. 276.

- What weight gain do you recommend and why?
- What are your feelings about (fill in special desires for the birth event, such as different positions assumed during labor, avoidance of an episiotomy, induction of labor, other people present during the birth, pain control measures, breastfeeding immediately after the birth, no separation of newborn and parents following birth, and so on)?
- If a cesarean is necessary, can my partner be present?
- What are your feelings regarding complementary treatments during labor (herbs to augment labor, use of acupressure/massage/hypnosis, use of oils for perineal massage, and so on)?

Expectant parents also need to discuss the qualities they want in a healthcare provider for the newborn. They may want to visit several pediatric healthcare providers before the birth to select someone who will meet their needs and those of their child.

Prenatal Care Services

The nurse can assist expectant parents in obtaining the type of prenatal care services that are most appropriate for their personal needs. Most practitioners offer individual prenatal care services in which the woman or the woman and her family attend a clinic or office visit on a regular basis depending on her stage of pregnancy.

TABLE 10–2 Benefits and Risks of Some Consumer and Medical Decisions During Pregnancy, Labor, and Birth

ISSUE	BENEFITS	RISKS
Breastfeeding	• No additional expense • Contains maternal antibodies • Decreases incidence of infant otitis media, vomiting, and diarrhea, hospitalizations during the first year of life, and allergies • Easier to digest than formula • Immediately after birth, promotes uterine contractions and decreases incidence of postpartum hemorrhage • Promotes maternal–newborn bonding	• Transmission of maternal infections to newborn, such as HIV • Irregular ovulation and menses can cause false sense of security and nonuse of hormonal contraceptives • Increased nutritional requirement in mother

Ambulation during labor	• Comfort for laboring woman
	• May assist in labor progression by
	  • Stimulating contractions
	  • Allowing gravity to help descent of fetus
	  • Giving sense of independence and control
		• Cord prolapse with rupture of membranes unless engagement has occurred
		• Birth of baby in undesirable locations (hallways, outdoors, waiting area)
		• Inability to monitor fetal heart rate (FHR) unless telemetry unit available

Electronic fetal monitoring	• Helps evaluate fetal well-being • Helps identify fetal stress • Useful in diagnostic testing • Helps evaluate labor progress	• Supine postural hypotension • Intrauterine perforation (with internal uterine pressure device) • Infection (with internal monitoring) • Decreases personal interaction with mother because of attention paid to the machine • Mother is unable to ambulate or change her position freely
Whirlpool (jet hydrotherapy)	• Increased relaxation • Decreased anxiety • Stimulation of labor • Provides pain relief • Slight decrease in blood pressure (BP) • Increased diuresis • Decreased incidence of vacuum and forceps deliveries • Increased pain threshold • Higher satisfaction with birth • Decreased use of pain medication (Avery, 2013)	• May slow contractions if used before active labor is established • Possible risk of infection if membranes are ruptured • Slight increase in maternal temperature and pulse in tub • Hypothermia • Increases fetal heart rate (FHR) by 10–20 beats/min
Analgesia	• Maternal relaxation facilitates labor	• All drugs reach the fetus in varying degrees and with varying effects
Episiotomy	• Decreases irregular tearing of perineum • Easier to repair for practitioner	• Increased pain after birth and for 1–3 months following birth • Dyspareunia • Infection • Increased frequency of third- and fourth-degree lacerations (Cunningham et al., 2014)

CENTERINGPREGNANCY®

When empowering women to choose health-promoting behaviors, it may be helpful to consider an innovative model for prenatal care called *CenteringPregnancy®*. CenteringPregnancy® integrates two main components of care—*assessment* and *education*—into a unified program providing complete prenatal care to women within a group setting, thereby providing the added benefit of support (DeCesare & Jackson, 2015). This model replaces the traditional one-on-one visits in an examination room with a healthcare provider. Instead, group meetings are held where mothers-to-be and their partners receive care and education and form a sense of community with other group members.

Clients begin meeting in small groups of women with similar due dates at 12 to 16 weeks' gestation and continue to meet monthly for the first 4 months and biweekly as their due dates approach. Each group session begins with the expectant mothers taking their own blood pressure, monitoring weight gain, checking urine samples, and recording data on medical records under their provider or nurse's guidance. The provider then reviews each group member's information privately and completes any further assessments that are indicated. After all assessments are completed, the group members convene in a circle to discuss topics such as nutrition, fetal development, common discomforts of pregnancy and possible remedies, exercise, relaxation, labor and birth procedures, parenting and relationship issues, contraception, and baby care (Bell, 2012). Both mothers and fathers report an increased investment in the pregnancy and self-care after attending group sessions. Additional positive outcomes of centering pregnancy include (DeCesare & Jackson, 2015):

• Increased maternal satisfaction and cooperation with care
• Increased knowledge about pregnancy

- Increased healthcare provider satisfaction
- Reduced incidence of preterm birth
- Lower no-show rate among pregnant teens

Birth Setting

The nurse can help expectant parents choose a birth setting by suggesting they tour facilities and talk with nurses there as well as talk with friends or acquaintances who are recent parents. Questions that may be asked of new parents include the following:

- What kind of support did you receive during labor? Was it what you wanted?
- Were you allowed to take an active role in decision making throughout the birth process?
- If you had a doula, was her role respected? Was she welcome in the birth setting?
- Was your birth plan respected? Did you share it with the facility before the birth? If something did not work, why do you think there were problems?
- Did the nurse offer suggestions regarding comfort measures?
- Did the healthcare team provide emotional support?
- How were medications handled during labor? Were you comfortable with this?
- Were siblings welcomed in the birth setting? At the birth? After the birth?
- Did you feel you were given ample time to spend with your baby immediately after childbirth?
- Was the nursing staff helpful after the baby was born? Did you receive self-care and baby care information? Was it in a usable form? Did you have a choice about what information you got? Did they let you decide what information you needed?
- Did you feel your choice of feeding method was supported?

The nurse helps expectant parents understand the array of choices available to them. The nurse can encourage them to consider options early in the pregnancy to allow time for talking with other parents and touring facilities.

Nurses involved in childbirth education need to include the concept of individuality when providing information to expectant parents about the process of childbirth and their own pattern of coping. The wave of the future in childbirth education is to encourage women to incorporate their natural responses into coping with the pain of labor and birth. Alternative self-care activities should be explored with the expectant couple to identify preferences.

Nurses should encourage expectant women and couples to personalize the birth setting. The woman might plan, for example, to bring items from home to enhance relaxation and comfort, such as warm socks, slippers, bath powder, lotion, or a favorite blanket. She may wish to bring photographs of children, parents, or friends who cannot be there to share the birth experience. Many expectant parents enjoy listening to tapes of favorite music or watching home videos or favorite films. Such personalization of the birth setting may give expectant parents feelings of increased serenity and empowerment.

Clinical Tip

Call the birthing facilities in your community and inquire about what choices are available in each facility so that you can answer expectant parents' questions.

Labor Support Person

Some of the first formal childbirth preparation classes were patterned after a book titled *Husband Coached Childbirth* by Dr. Robert Bradley, which was published in 1965. Since that time, husbands and other partners of expectant women have been very involved in acting as "coaches" or support persons during childbirth classes, labor, and birth. Although some men

---

EVIDENCE-BASED PRACTICE | Interventions to Reduce Childbirth Fear in Pregnant Women

Clinical Question
Can education and psychological support reduce the fear of childbirth in healthy pregnant women?

The Evidence
Fear of the process of childbirth has been linked to adverse maternal outcomes, including high rates of surgical birth, mental health issues, and increased postpartum depression. Many women with childbirth fear may request surgical birth if they perceive their fears have not been addressed. These researchers used a randomized trial to test an antenatal intervention of psychological support and education delivered by nurse-midwives. More than 1,400 women were included in the study population. Randomized trials with large sample sizes form a strong level of evidence.

The intervention was a telephone education counseling intervention that reviewed the woman's current expectations and feelings regarding fear of childbirth. The nurse supported the expression of feelings, and provided a framework for women to identify and work through the elements of childbirth that they found frightening. The intervention focused on

helping the mother develop situational supports for the birth and a plan for dealing with the childbirth experience that gave the mother control over her birth process. The women who received the intervention reported lower levels of fear and higher levels of self-efficacy and sense of control (Toohill et al., 2014). These mothers also had fewer depression symptoms and requested surgical birth with less frequency.

Best Practice
Prenatal psychological support and education may reduce the fear of childbirth among women. Improving antenatal emotional well-being has a myriad of positive benefits and may result in an optimal childbirth experience. Providing this support leads to fewer requests for surgical births.

Clinical Reasoning
What are some of the ways that the nurse can help the mother gain a sense of control over the birth process? What might be some of the benefits of reduced childbirth fear for the mother and for the provider?

or support persons welcome the role and look forward to providing emotional and physical support, others do not. Some men may become anxious and fearful. These feelings can be related to past experiences and/or cultural factors. In these situations, the nurse provides encouragement and support to both the woman and her support person.

Continuous labor support facilitates birth; enhances the mother's memory of the experience; strengthens mother–newborn bonding; increases breastfeeding success; and significantly reduces many forms of medical intervention, including cesarean birth and the use of analgesia, anesthesia, vacuum extraction, and forceps (Donna, 2011). A woman's satisfaction with childbirth is directly affected by the relationship with the healthcare provider, the support she received from healthcare providers, personal expectations, and her involvement with decision making. Clearly, the role of the nurse cannot be overestimated.

For centuries, women have been serving and assisting other women in childbirth. Out of this need for companionship and special support in the birthing journey, the role of the doula has evolved. The doula is specially trained to assist with births and to provide continuous labor support, which includes emotional, physical, and informational support. The doula does not perform clinical tasks but she acts as an advocate for the woman and her family by verbalizing their wishes to the nurses and physicians/CNMs. A doula may also be trained to provide support and care during the postpartum period. Later postpartum benefits for the mother include increased bonding/interaction with the baby and decreased symptoms of depression. The doula may accompany the childbearing couple on a volunteer basis or may be paid a fee by the family.

Siblings at Birth

Some couples decide to have their other children present at the birth. Children who will attend a birth can be prepared through books, audiovisual materials, models, discussion, and sibling classes.

It is imperative that the child has his or her own support person or coach whose sole responsibility is tending to the needs of that child during the labor and birth experience. The support person should be familiar to the child, warm, sensitive, flexible, knowledgeable about the birth process, and comfortable with sexuality and birth. This person must be prepared to interpret to the child what is happening and to intervene when necessary. The support person should be prepared and willing to leave the birthing room at any time, should that be the child's desire. The support person for the child should assume responsibility for providing distractions such as trips to the cafeteria, visits to the nursery window, outdoor walks, and other age-appropriate activities.

Children should be given the option of relating to the birth in whatever manner they choose as long as it is not disruptive. Children should understand that it is their own choice to be there and that they may stay or leave the room as they choose. To help children recognize their needs and desires, the nurse may wish to elicit exactly what they expect from the experience. Children need to feel free to ask questions and express feelings.

Allowing children to participate in the arrival of their sibling engenders the desire to nurture "our" baby, as opposed to jealousy and rivalry directed at "Mom's" baby. The mother does not disappear mysteriously into the hospital and return with a demanding outsider. Instead, the family attending the birth together finds a new opportunity for closeness and growth by sharing in the birth of a new member.

Developing Cultural Competence Female Relatives as Caregivers

In most Middle Eastern countries, childbirth is exclusively attended to by women. A woman in labor is most commonly surrounded by female relatives and friends. Most Arab Muslim women prefer to have a female healthcare provider attend the labor and birth (Abushaikha & Massah, 2013).

Classes for Family Members During Pregnancy

Childbirth classes are routinely taught by certified childbirth educators (CBEs or CCEs). These are individuals who have received specific educational preparation related to pregnancy, labor, birth, and postpartum/newborn care and issues. Many CBEs are also registered nurses; however, nursing training is not required. The majority of the certification programs do, however, require witnessing a minimum number of births.

CBEs should consider elements developed by authoritative organizations such as the Coalition for Improving Maternity Services (CIMS) when developing their own Philosophy of Childbirth for their classes. The "Mother-Friendly Childbirth Initiative" was created in 1996 by the Coalition for Improving Maternity Services (CIMS), a national alliance of more than 50 childbirth organizations and many prominent individuals. The coalition's mission is to promote a wellness model of maternity care that will improve birth outcomes and substantially reduce costs. The philosophic cornerstones of mother-friendly care are: (1) normalcy of the birthing process, (2) empowerment, (3) autonomy, (4) do no harm, and (5) responsibility (Coalition for Improving Maternity Services [CIMS], 2013).

Prenatal education programs provide important opportunities to share information about pregnancy, childbirth, coping mechanisms, and choices available for the woman and her support person. Studies have shown that prepared childbirth education programs can have a beneficial effect on performance in labor and birth. The prenatal period should be used to expose the prospective parents to up-to-date, evidence-based information about the following topics:

- Labor and birth
- Pain relief
- Obstetric complications and procedures
- Breastfeeding
- Normal newborn care
- Postpartum adjustment

The content of each class is generally directed by the overall goals of the program. For example, specific classes may address the following subjects:

- Gestational changes and fetal development
- Childbirth choices available today
- Preparation of the mother for pregnancy and birth
- Preparation for cesarean birth or for vaginal birth after cesarean
- Preparation for couples who desire an unmedicated birth
- Preparation of the grandparents or siblings for the birth

- Newborn care and safety
- Self-care during the postpartum period

The nurse who knows the types of prenatal programs available in the community can direct expectant parents to programs that meet their special needs and learning goals.

From the expectant parents' point of view, class content is best presented in chronology with the pregnancy. It is important that the classes begin by identifying the parents' needs, goals, and learning styles. Although both parents expect to learn breathing and relaxation techniques and baby care, fathers usually expect facts and mothers expect coping strategies. Women's goals commonly include gaining information, reducing anxiety/increasing confidence, having their partner present and involved, and having a positive emotional experience in childbirth. Classes that provide an environment supportive of practicing newly learned techniques and the freedom to ask questions and receive explanations are beneficial in helping class participants obtain these goals (Figure 10–4). By the end of the class, parents should feel that they will be able to make appropriate and informed decisions by participating in a class where information is given in a nonjudgmental, nonthreatening environment. Classes may be divided into early and late classes so specific needs can be addressed.

Education of the Family Having Cesarean Birth

Cesarean birth is an alternative method of birth that now accounts for 32.7% of births in the United States (Martin, Hamilton, & Osterman, 2014). Consequently, although the need for a cesarean birth is not often known in advance, more and more childbirth preparation classes are integrating content on cesarean birth into the curriculum.

Class content should cover what the parents can expect to happen during a cesarean birth, what they might feel, and what choices are available. All pregnant women and couples should be encouraged to discuss with their physician/CNM the progression of events if a cesarean birth becomes necessary. Cesarean birth and repeat cesarean birth are discussed in detail in Chapter 22.

When expectant parents are anticipating a repeat cesarean birth, they have time to plan and prepare. Many birthing units provide preparation classes for repeat cesarean birth. Parents who have had previous negative experiences need an opportunity

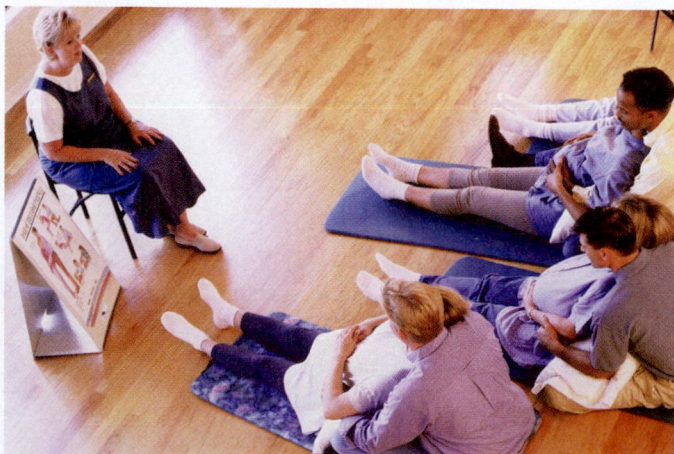

Figure 10–4 In a group setting with a nurse-instructor, expectant parents share information about pregnancy and childbirth.

SOURCE: Jiang Jin/Alamy.

to describe what contributed to their feelings. They should be encouraged to identify what they would like to change and to list interventions that would make the experience more positive. Those who have had positive experiences require reassurance that their needs and desires will be met in a similar manner. All parents should be encouraged to air any fears or anxieties.

Often, a woman facing a repeat cesarean birth is concerned about postoperative pain. She needs reassurance that subsequent cesarean births are often less painful than the first. In addition, planned cesarean births involve less fatigue than unplanned procedures because they are not preceded by a long, strenuous labor. Providing this information will help the woman cope more effectively with stressful stimuli, including pain.

Preparation for Parents Desiring Trial of Labor after Cesarean Birth

Trial of labor after cesarean birth (TOLAC) was previously termed *vaginal birth after cesarean (VBAC)* and is discussed in detail in Chapter 22. Parents who have had a cesarean birth and are now anticipating a vaginal birth have unique needs. Because they may have unresolved questions and concerns about the last birth, it is helpful to begin the series of classes with an informational session. The nurse can supply information about the criteria necessary to attempt a trial of labor and identify decisions to be made regarding the birth experience. Some childbirth educators suggest that parents prepare two birth plans: one for vaginal birth and one for cesarean birth. Preparing birth plans seems to give parents some sense of control over the birth experience and tends to increase the positive aspects of the experience.

Breastfeeding Programs

Programs offering information on breastfeeding are increasing. For decades, a primary source of information has been the La Leche League. Information can also be obtained from lactation consultants, peer counselors, labor and postpartum nurses, birthing centers, hospitals, and health clinics. Online support groups can also be an important resource for breastfeeding mothers.

Healthy People 2020

(MICH-21) Increase the proportion of infants who are breastfed

Rates of breastfeeding in the United States are well below the *Healthy People 2020* objective of 81.9% (U.S. Department of Health and Human Services [HHS], 2013). *Healthy People 2020* has set goals not only for increasing the rate of breastfed infants, but also for increasing the availability of worksite lactation support programs to encourage mothers to continue breastfeeding following their return to work.

Classes and support groups typically include information about the following topics:

- Advantages and challenges of breastfeeding
- Techniques and positioning
- Methods of breast pumping and milk storage
- How to involve the father or partner in the feeding process, such as having him or her bring the baby to the mother for feedings, burp the baby between or after feedings, or rock the baby back to sleep
- Ways of successfully breastfeeding and returning to work

Sibling Preparation: Adjustment to a Newborn

The birth of a new sibling is a significant event in a child's life. Positive adjustment can be enhanced by attendance at formal sibling preparation classes (Figure 10–5). Typically, the classes are attended by children ages 3 to 12 years. Children younger than 3 tend to have shorter attention spans and may have difficulty participating in the class; however, many facilities will allow younger children to attend, especially if an older sibling is enrolled in the class. These classes can assist with decreasing sibling rivalry and reducing children's anxiety. They help children feel that they are part of the birthing process. The classes also enable parents to identify children's concerns related to the new baby. They provide a means to facilitate communication and explore children's feelings. They also provide basic information about pregnancy, childbirth, and the characteristics and behavior of newborns. The classes usually focus on:

- Reducing anxiety in the child
- Providing opportunities for the child to express feelings and concerns
- Encouraging realistic expectations of the newborn
- Teaching the older child to be an active participant in the baby's care by showing how to safely hold the newborn, feed and burp the baby, or even change diapers

Typically, parents and their children attend the class together. Many activities are devised to help each child feel special. Time is usually allotted at the end of the class for talking with parents about coping skills and providing hints about dealing with sibling jealousy. Class content typically includes care and behavior of new babies, a practice session holding anatomically correct dolls, changing diapers, and a tour of the "bedroom" and the nursery where Mom and baby will stay. Many times, a newborn is held up at the nursery window so the children can see a "real baby." Some facilities give the children a special gift for attendance or a trip to the cafeteria for a special treat. In addition, parents may wish to take advantage of books and videos designed to help children prepare for a new sibling.

Classes for Grandparents

Grandparents are an important source of support and information for prospective and new parents. They are now being included in the birthing process more frequently. Prenatal programs for grandparents can address current roles, transitioning to a new role, beliefs regarding childbirth, and ways to support the new family unit. Grandparents can also benefit from educational information, such as the benefits of breastfeeding, and updates on baby care, such as proper baby sleep positions and when to introduce foods. If they plan to be integral members of the labor and birth team, they will need information about being coaches.

Common Discomforts of Pregnancy

The common discomforts of pregnancy result from physiologic and anatomic changes and are fairly specific to each of the three trimesters. See *Health Promotion: Self-Care Measures for Common Discomforts of Pregnancy* at the end of this section for an at-a-glance summary of the common discomforts of pregnancy, their possible causes, and self-care measures that often help relieve the discomfort.

First Trimester

NAUSEA AND VOMITING

Nausea and vomiting of pregnancy (NVP) are early, common symptoms occurring in up to 80% of pregnant women (Fantasia, 2014). These symptoms appear sometime after the first missed menstrual period and usually cease by the fourth missed menstrual period. Some women develop an aversion to specific foods, many experience nausea when they get up in the morning, and others experience nausea throughout the day or in the evening.

The exact cause of NVP is unknown, but it is thought to be multifactorial. An elevated human chorionic gonadotropin (hCG) level is believed to be a major factor, but relaxation of the smooth muscle of the stomach, changes in carbohydrate metabolism, fluctuating hormone levels, fatigue, and emotional factors may also play a role.

In addition to common self-care measures for NVP, certain complementary or alternative therapies such as the use of acupressure wristbands (Figure 10–6) or the ingestion of ginger

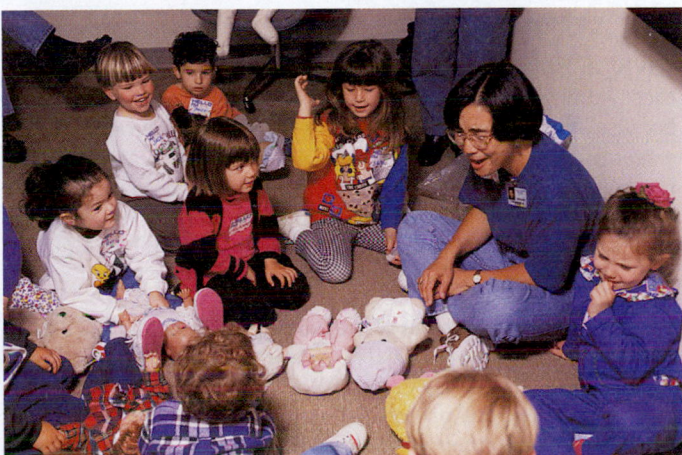

Figure 10–5 It is especially important that siblings be well prepared when they are going to be present at the birth. However, even siblings who will not be present at the birth can benefit from information about childbirth and the new baby ahead of time.

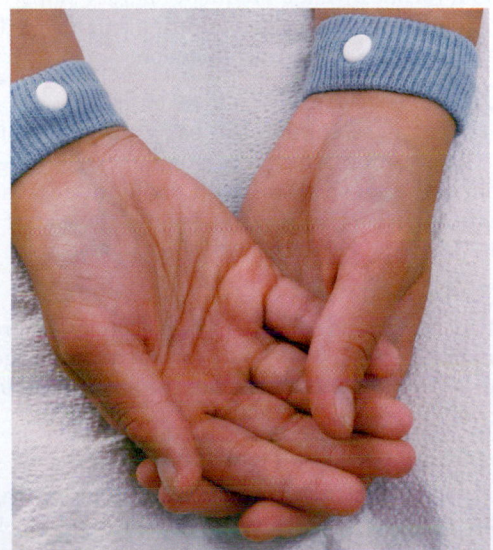

Figure 10–6 Morning sickness relief. Acupressure wristbands are sometimes used to help relieve nausea during early pregnancy.

may be helpful for some women. Ginger has long been used as a traditional remedy for treating nausea and vomiting associated with early pregnancy. Ginger is available in a variety of forms, including fresh or dried root, capsules, tea, candy, cookies, crystals, inhaled powdered ginger, and sugared ginger. It has few side effects when taken in small doses (National Center for Complementary and Integrative Health [NCCIH], 2015). Some women find pyridoxine (vitamin B_6) helpful. Diclegis, a combination of pyridoxine 10 mg plus doxylamine succinate 10 mg, was approved by the Food and Drug Administration (FDA) in 2013 specifically for the treatment of NVP (Fantasia, 2014). Antihistamine H_1-receptor blockers, benzamines, and phenothiazines are considered to be safe and effective for treating refractory cases. In very severe cases, methylprednisolone, a steroid, may be used but strictly as a last resort because it poses a potential risk to the fetus (American College of Obstetricians and Gynecologists [ACOG], 2015a).

The nurse should advise a woman to contact her healthcare provider if she vomits more than once a day or shows signs of dehydration such as dry mouth and concentrated urine. In such cases the physician/CNM might order an antiemetic. However, antiemetics should be avoided if possible during this time because of possible harmful effects on embryo development.

Nausea and vomiting symptoms generally decrease by the 16th week of pregnancy. If they do not, hyperemesis gravidarum, which occurs in 0.3% to 2% of pregnancies, must be considered. Hyperemesis symptoms include weight loss, dehydration, and nutrition imbalance (Johnson, Hallock, Bienstock, et al., 2015).

URINARY FREQUENCY

Urinary frequency, a common discomfort of pregnancy, occurs early in pregnancy and again during the third trimester because the enlarging uterus puts pressure on the bladder. Although frequency is considered normal during the first and third trimesters, advise the woman to tell her healthcare provider about signs of bladder infection such as pain, burning with voiding, or blood in the urine. Fluid intake should never be decreased to prevent frequency. The woman needs to maintain an adequate fluid intake—at least 2,000 mL (eight to ten 8-oz glasses) per day. Also, encourage her to empty her bladder frequently (about every 2 hours while awake). Frequent bladder emptying helps decrease the incidence of leakage of urine and also reduces the risk of developing a urinary tract infection.

FATIGUE

Marked fatigue is so common in early pregnancy that it is considered a presumptive sign of pregnancy. It is aggravated if the woman cannot sleep through the night because of urinary frequency. Typically, it resolves after the end of the first trimester.

BREAST TENDERNESS

Sensitivity of the breasts occurs early and continues throughout the pregnancy. Increased levels of estrogen and progesterone contribute to soreness and tingling of the breasts and increased sensitivity of the nipples.

INCREASED VAGINAL DISCHARGE

Increased whitish vaginal discharge, called **leukorrhea**, is common in pregnancy. It occurs as a result of hyperplasia of the vaginal mucosa and increased mucus production by the endocervical glands. The increased acidity of the secretions encourages the growth of *Candida albicans*, so the woman is more susceptible to monilial vaginitis.

NASAL STUFFINESS AND EPISTAXIS

Once pregnancy has progressed somewhat, elevated estrogen levels may produce edema of the nasal mucosa, which results in nasal stuffiness, nasal discharge, and obstruction. *Epistaxis* (nosebleeds) may also result. Cool air vaporizers and normal saline nasal sprays may help, but the problem is often unresponsive to treatment. Women experiencing these problems find it difficult to sleep and may resort to using medicated nasal sprays and decongestants. Such interventions may provide initial relief but can actually increase nasal stuffiness over time.

PTYALISM

Ptyalism is a rare discomfort of pregnancy in which excessive, often bitter, saliva is produced. The cause is unknown, and effective treatments are limited (King, Brucker, Kriebs, et al., 2015).

Second and Third Trimesters

The discomforts discussed in this section usually do not appear until the third trimester in primigravidas but may occur earlier with each succeeding pregnancy.

HEARTBURN (PYROSIS)

Heartburn is the regurgitation of acidic gastric contents into the esophagus. It creates a burning sensation in the esophagus and sometimes leaves a bad taste in the mouth. As many as 80% of women experience heartburn in the third trimester (King et al., 2015). Heartburn during pregnancy appears to be primarily a result of the displacement of the stomach by the enlarging uterus. The increased production of progesterone in pregnancy, decreased gastrointestinal motility, and relaxation of the cardiac (esophageal) sphincter also contribute to heartburn.

Liquid forms of low-sodium antacids are often most effective in providing relief. However, many women prefer chewable over-the-counter antacid tablets. The nurse should advise women that antacids containing aluminum may cause constipation, and antacids containing magnesium can cause diarrhea. The nurse should also let women know that they should avoid sodium bicarbonate (baking soda) and Alka-Seltzer because they may lead to electrolyte imbalance.

If maternal heartburn is severe, not relieved by antacids, and accompanied by gastrointestinal reflux, an antisecretory agent (H_2 blocker) such as ranitidine (Zantac), cimetidine (Tagamet), or omeprazole (Losec) may be helpful. To date they have not been linked with an excessive risk of birth defects.

ANKLE EDEMA

Most women experience ankle edema in the last part of pregnancy because of the increasing difficulty of venous return from the lower extremities. Prolonged standing or sitting and warm weather increase the edema. It is also associated with varicose veins. Ankle edema becomes a concern only when accompanied by hypertension or proteinuria or when the edema is not postural in origin.

VARICOSE VEINS

Varicose veins are a result of weakening of the walls of veins or faulty functioning of the valves. Poor circulation in the lower extremities predisposes people to varicose veins in the legs and thighs, as does prolonged standing or sitting. The pregnant uterus puts pressure on the pelvic veins, preventing good venous return, so it may aggravate existing problems or contribute to obvious changes in the veins of the legs (Figure 10–7).

Surgical correction of varicose veins is not generally recommended during pregnancy. The nurse should advise the woman that treatment may be needed after she gives birth because the problem will be aggravated by a succeeding pregnancy.

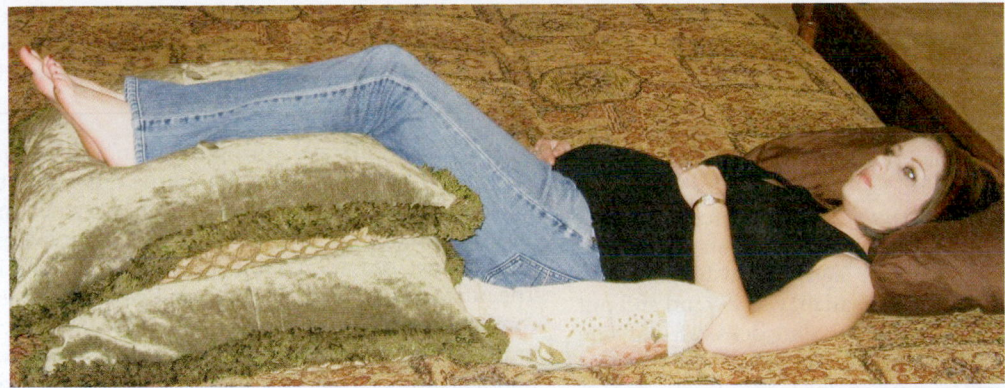

Figure 10–7 Swelling and discomfort from varicosities can be decreased by lying down with the legs and one hip elevated (to avoid compression of the vena cava).

Although less common, varicosities in the vulva and perineum may also develop. They produce aching and a sense of heaviness. Wearing a foam rubber commercial product that is placed across the perineum and held in place by a sanitary pad–type belt can provide support for vulvar varicosities (Cunningham et al., 2014). It is important that the pelvic area be elevated to promote venous drainage into the trunk of the body. The woman may best relieve uterine pressure on the pelvic veins by resting on her side. Blocks may also be placed under the foot of her bed to elevate it slightly.

FLATULENCE

Flatulence results from decreased gastrointestinal motility, leading to delayed emptying, and from pressure on the large intestine by the growing uterus. Air swallowing may also contribute to the problem.

HEMORRHOIDS

Hemorrhoids are varicosities of the veins in the lower rectum and the anus. During pregnancy the gravid uterus presses on the veins and interferes with venous circulation. In addition, the straining that accompanies constipation is frequently a contributing cause of hemorrhoids.

Some women may not be bothered by hemorrhoids until the second stage of labor, when the hemorrhoids appear as they push. These hemorrhoids usually become asymptomatic a few days after childbirth. Symptoms of hemorrhoids include itching, swelling, pain, and bleeding. Women who have had hemorrhoids before pregnancy will probably experience difficulties with them during pregnancy.

Some women find relief by gently reinserting the hemorrhoid. The woman lies on her side, places some lubricant on her finger, and presses against the hemorrhoid, pushing it inside the rectum. She holds the hemorrhoid in place for 1 to 2 minutes and then gently withdraws her finger. The anal sphincter should then hold it inside the rectum. The woman will find it especially helpful if she can maintain a side-lying (Sims) position for a time, so this method is best done before bed or prior to a daily rest period.

The woman should contact her healthcare provider if the hemorrhoid(s) becomes hardened and noticeably tender to touch. Rectal bleeding that is more than spotting following defecation should also be reported.

CONSTIPATION

Conditions that predispose the pregnant woman to constipation include general bowel sluggishness caused by increased progesterone and steroid metabolism; displacement of the intestines, which increases with growth of the fetus; and the oral iron supplements most pregnant women need. In severe or preexisting cases of constipation, the woman may need stool softeners, mild laxatives, or suppositories as recommended by her healthcare provider.

BACKACHE

Nearly 70% of women experience lower backache during pregnancy (King et al., 2015) primarily caused by exaggeration of the lumbosacral curve that occurs as the uterus enlarges and becomes heavier. Maintaining good posture and using proper body mechanics throughout pregnancy can help prevent backache. Advise the pregnant woman to avoid bending over at the waist to pick up objects and to bend from the knees instead (Figure 10–8). She should place her feet 12 to 18 inches apart to maintain body balance. If the woman uses work surfaces that require her to bend, advise her to adjust the height of the surfaces.

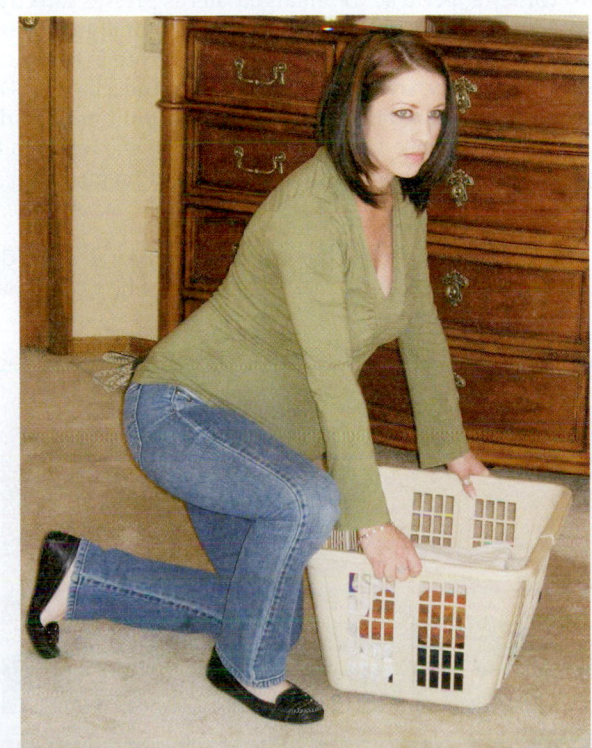

Figure 10–8 Body mechanics in pregnancy. When picking up objects from floor level or lifting objects, the pregnant woman must use proper body mechanics.

LEG CRAMPS

Leg cramps are painful muscle spasms in the gastrocnemius muscles. They occur most often after the woman has gone to bed at night but may occur at other times. Extension of the foot can often cause leg cramps. The nurse should warn the pregnant woman not to extend the foot during childbirth preparation exercises or during rest periods.

Stretching provides immediate relief of the muscle spasm. With the woman lying on her back, another person presses the woman's knee down to straighten her leg while pushing her foot toward her leg (Figure 10–9). The woman may also stand and put her foot flat on the floor. Massage and warm packs can alleviate the discomfort of leg cramps. A diet that includes daily portions of both calcium and phosphorus may help prevent leg cramps.

FAINTNESS

Many pregnant women occasionally feel faint, especially in warm, crowded areas. Faintness is caused by a combination of changes in the blood volume and postural hypotension due to pooling of blood in the dependent veins. Sudden change of position or standing for prolonged periods can also cause this sensation, and the woman may faint.

If a woman begins to feel faint from prolonged standing or from being in a stuffy room, she should sit down and lower her head between her knees. If this procedure does not help, she should ask someone to help her to an area where she can lie down and get fresh air. The nurse should advise the woman that when getting up from a resting position, it is important to move slowly. Women whose jobs require standing in one place for long periods should march in place regularly to increase venous return from the legs.

SHORTNESS OF BREATH (DYSPNEA)

Shortness of breath occurs as the uterus rises into the abdomen and causes pressure on the diaphragm. This problem worsens in the last trimester because the enlarged uterus presses directly on the diaphragm, decreasing vital capacity. The primigravida experiences considerable relief from shortness of breath in the last few weeks of pregnancy, when **lightening** occurs, and the fetus and uterus move down in the pelvis. Because the multigravida does not usually experience lightening until labor, she tends to feel short of breath throughout the latter part of her pregnancy.

DIFFICULTY SLEEPING

Many physical factors in late pregnancy may make sleeping difficult. The enlarged uterus may make it difficult to find a comfortable

position for sleep, and an active fetus may aggravate the problem. Other discomforts of pregnancy such as urinary frequency, shortness of breath, and leg cramps may also make it hard to sleep.

ROUND LIGAMENT PAIN

As the uterus enlarges during pregnancy, the round ligaments stretch and hypertrophy as the uterus rises up in the abdomen, causing pain. The woman may feel concern when she first experiences round ligament pain because it is often intense and causes a "grabbing" sensation in the lower abdomen and inguinal area. The nurse should warn the pregnant woman of this possible discomfort. Once it has been determined that the cause of the pain is not a medical complication such as appendicitis, the woman may find that applying a heating pad to the abdomen brings relief.

CARPAL TUNNEL SYNDROME

Carpal tunnel syndrome, characterized by numbness and tingling of the hand near the thumb, occurs in about 25% to 50% of pregnant women (Kimberly, Niebyl, & Johnson, 2012). It is caused by compression of the median nerve in the carpal tunnel of the wrist. The syndrome is aggravated by repetitive hand movements such as typing and may disappear following childbirth. Fluid retention during pregnancy and high weight gain may aggravate the condition (Gregory, Niebyl, & Johnson, 2012). Treatment usually involves splinting and avoiding aggravating movements, but surgery may be needed in severe cases if more conservative approaches are not effective.

Health Promotion During Pregnancy

Fetal Activity Monitoring

Many healthcare providers encourage pregnant women to monitor their unborn child's well-being by regularly assessing fetal activity beginning at 28 weeks' gestation. Vigorous activity generally provides reassurance of fetal well-being, but a marked decrease in activity or cessation of movement may indicate a problem that needs immediate evaluation. Fetal activity is affected by fetal sleep, sound, time of day, blood glucose levels, cigarette smoking, and some illicit drugs such as crack and cocaine. At times a healthy fetus may be minimally active or inactive. See Chapter 13 for an in-depth discussion of maternal–fetal activity monitoring and *Teaching Highlights: What to Tell the Pregnant Woman About Assessing Fetal Activity*.

Breast Care

Whether the pregnant woman plans to formula-feed or breast-feed her baby, support of the breasts is important to promote comfort, retain breast shape, and prevent back strain, particularly if the breasts become large and pendulous. The sensitivity of the breasts in pregnancy is often relieved by good support.

A well-fitting, supportive bra has the following qualities:

- The straps are wide and do not stretch (elastic straps soon lose their tautness with the weight of the breasts and frequent washing).
- The cups hold all breast tissue comfortably.
- The bra has tucks or other devices that allow it to expand and accommodate the enlarging chest circumference.
- The bra supports the nipple line approximately midway between the elbow and shoulder but is not pulled up in the back by the weight of the breasts.

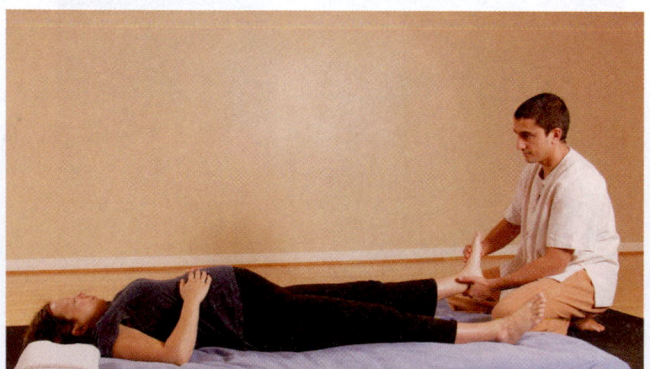

Figure 10–9 Leg cramp relief. The expectant father can help relieve the woman's painful leg cramps by flexing her foot and straightening her leg.

SOURCE: Yanik Chauvin/Fotolia.

Health Promotion Self-Care Measures for Common Discomforts of Pregnancy

Discomfort	Influencing Factors	Self-Care Measures
FIRST TRIMESTER		
Nausea and vomiting	Increased levels of human chorionic gonadotropin	Avoid odors or causative factors.
	Changes in carbohydrate metabolism	Eat dry crackers or toast before arising in morning.
	Emotional factors	Have small but frequent meals.
	Fatigue	Avoid greasy or highly seasoned foods.
		Take dry meals with fluids between meals.
		Drink carbonated beverages.
		Avoid lying supine for 2 hours after eating.
Urinary frequency	Pressure of uterus on bladder in both first and third trimesters	Void when urge is felt.
		Increase fluid intake during the day.
		Decrease fluid intake only in the evening to decrease nocturia.
Fatigue	Specific causative factors unknown	Plan time for a nap or rest period daily.
	May be aggravated by nocturia due to urinary frequency	Go to bed earlier.
		Seek family support and assistance with responsibilities so that more time is available to rest.
Breast tenderness	Increased levels of estrogen and progesterone	Wear well-fitting, supportive bra.
Increased vaginal discharge	Hyperplasia of vaginal mucosa and increased production of mucus by the endocervical glands due to the increase in estrogen levels	Promote cleanliness by daily bathing.
		Avoid douching, nylon underpants, and pantyhose; use cotton underpants, which are more absorbent; can use powder to maintain dryness, if not allowed to cake.
Nasal stuffiness and nosebleed (epistaxis)	Elevated estrogen levels	May be unresponsive, but cool air vaporizer may help; avoid use of nasal sprays and decongestants.
Ptyalism (excessive, often bitter salivation)	Specific causative factors unknown	Use astringent mouthwashes, chew gum, or suck hard candy.
SECOND AND THIRD TRIMESTERS		
Heartburn (pyrosis)	Increased production of progesterone, decreasing gastrointestinal motility and increasing relaxation of cardiac sphincter	Eat small and more frequent meals.
		Use low-sodium antacids.
	Displacement of stomach by enlarging uterus, thus regurgitation of acidic gastric contents into the esophagus	Avoid overeating, fatty and fried foods, lying down after eating, and sodium bicarbonate.
Ankle edema	Prolonged standing or sitting	Practice frequent dorsiflexion of feet when prolonged sitting or standing is necessary.
	Increased levels of sodium due to hormonal influences	Elevate legs when sitting or resting.
	Circulatory congestion of lower extremities	Avoid tight garters or restrictive bands around legs.
	Increased capillary permeability	
	Varicose veins	
Varicose veins	Venous congestion in the lower veins that increases with pregnancy	Elevate legs frequently.
		Wear supportive hose.
	Hereditary factors (weakening of walls of veins, faulty valves)	Avoid crossing legs at the knees, standing for long periods, garters, and hosiery with constrictive bands.
	Increased age and weight gain	

(continued)

Health Promotion Self-Care Measures for Common Discomforts of Pregnancy (continued)

Discomfort	Influencing Factors	Self-Care Measures
Hemorrhoids	Constipation (see following discussion)	Avoid constipation.
	Increased pressure from gravid uterus on hemorrhoidal veins	Apply ice packs, topical ointments, anesthetic agents, warm soaks, or sitz baths; gently reinsert into rectum as necessary.
Constipation	Increased levels of progesterone, which cause general bowel sluggishness	Increase fluid intake, fiber in the diet, and exercise.
	Pressure of enlarging uterus on intestine	Develop regular bowel habits.
	Iron supplements	Use stool softeners as recommended by physician.
	Diet, lack of exercise, and decreased fluids	
Backache	Increased curvature of the lumbosacral vertebrae as the uterus enlarges	Use proper body mechanics.
		Practice the pelvic tilt exercise.
	Increased levels of hormones, which cause softening of cartilage in body joints	Avoid uncomfortable working heights, high-heeled shoes, lifting of heavy loads, and fatigue.
	Fatigue	
	Poor body mechanics	
Leg cramps	Imbalance of calcium/phosphorus ratio	Practice dorsiflexion of feet to stretch affected muscle.
	Increased pressure of uterus on nerves	Evaluate diet.
	Fatigue	Apply heat to affected muscles.
	Poor circulation to lower extremities	Rise slowly from resting position.
	Pointing the toes	
Faintness	Postural hypotension	Avoid prolonged standing in warm or stuffy environments.
	Sudden change of position causing venous pooling in dependent veins	Evaluate hematocrit and hemoglobin.
	Standing for long periods in warm area	
	Anemia	
Dyspnea	Decreased vital capacity from pressure of enlarging uterus on the diaphragm	Use proper posture when sitting and standing.
		Sleep propped up with pillows for relief if problem occurs at night.
Flatulence	Decreased gastrointestinal motility leading to delayed emptying time	Avoid gas-forming foods.
		Chew food thoroughly.
	Pressure of growing uterus on large intestine	Get regular daily exercise.
		Maintain normal bowel habits.
	Air swallowing	
Carpal tunnel syndrome	Compression of median nerve in carpal tunnel of wrist	Avoid aggravating hand movements.
		Use splint as prescribed.
	Aggravated by repetitive hand movements	Elevate affected arm.

Cleanliness of the breasts is important, especially as the woman begins producing colostrum. Colostrum that crusts on the nipples can be removed with warm water. The nurse should advise the woman planning to breastfeed not to use soap on her nipples because of its drying effect.

Some women have flat or inverted nipples. True nipple inversion, which is rare, is usually diagnosed during the initial prenatal assessment. Breast shields designed to correct inverted nipples are effective for some women but others gain no benefit from them. Information on breastfeeding can be found on the websites of the La Leche League, the American Academy of Pediatrics, the National Organization of Mothers of Twins Club, and other breastfeeding-focused sites.

Clothing

Traditionally maternity clothes have been constructed with fuller lines to allow for the increase in abdominal size that occurs during pregnancy. However, in recent years maternity clothing has changed and now also includes more clothes that are fitted with little attempt to hide the pregnant abdomen. Maternity clothing can be expensive and is worn for a relatively short time, so women can economize by sharing clothes with friends, sewing their own garments, or buying used maternity clothes.

High-heeled shoes tend to aggravate back discomfort by increasing the curvature of the lower back. Women who experience backache or have problems with balance do best to avoid them. Shoes should fit properly and feel comfortable.

Bathing

Hygiene is important because perspiration and mucoid vaginal discharge increase during pregnancy. Keep in mind, however, that cultural norms often influence bathing and cleansing practices. A pregnant woman may choose to cleanse only some portions of her body regularly or may elect to take showers or tub baths. Advise women to be careful in the tub because balance becomes a problem in late pregnancy. Rubber mats and hand grips are important safety devices. Vasodilation due to warm water may cause the woman to feel faint when she gets out of the tub, so she may need assistance, especially during the last trimester.

Employment

Pregnant women who have no complications can usually continue to work until they go into labor (American Academy of Pediatrics [AAP] & ACOG, 2012). Although pregnant women who are employed in jobs that require prolonged standing (more than 3 hours) do have a higher incidence of preterm birth, this has no effect on fetal growth. However, the workplace environment can affect maternal well-being as well as birth outcomes (Katz, 2012). Overfatigue, prolonged standing, excessive physical strain, fetotoxic hazards in the environment, and medical or obstetric complications are the major deterrents to certain types of employment during pregnancy. In the second half of pregnancy, women whose occupations involve balance should make adjustments as needed.

Fetotoxic hazards are always a concern to the expectant couple. The pregnant woman (or the woman contemplating pregnancy) who works in industry should contact her company physician or nurse about possible hazards in her work environment and should do her own reading and research on environmental hazards as well. Her partner can also find out how hazards in his workplace might affect his sperm.

Travel

Pregnant women without complications can travel as usual. Pregnant women should avoid travel if they have a history of preterm birth, bleeding, or preeclampsia or if multiple births are anticipated.

Travel by automobile can be tiring, aggravating many of the discomforts of pregnancy. The pregnant woman needs frequent opportunities to get out of the car and walk. (A good pattern is to stop every 2 hours and walk around for about 10 minutes.) She should wear both lap and shoulder belts. The lap belt should fit snugly and be positioned under the abdomen and across the upper thighs; the shoulder strap should rest comfortably between the woman's breasts. Seat belts play an important role in preventing fetal and maternal injury and death (Cunningham et al., 2014). Fetal death in car accidents is sometimes caused by placental separation (abruptio placentae) as a result of uterine distortion. Shoulder belts decrease the risk of traumatic flexion of the woman's body, making placental separation less likely.

As pregnancy progresses, long-distance trips are best taken by plane or train. Currently, occasional flying is considered safe in the absence of any obstetric or medical complications (AAP & ACOG, 2012). Before flying the woman should check with her airline to see if they have any travel restrictions because many prohibit flying after 36 weeks' gestation. To avoid the development of phlebitis or blood clots, pregnant women should drink plenty of fluid to avoid dehydration and hemoconcentration. They should also walk about the plane at regular intervals and change position frequently. Air travel is not recommended during pregnancy for women who have obstetric or medical conditions that could require emergency care or that might be exacerbated by flight (AAP & ACOG, 2012). Remind near-term women who travel to think about the availability of medical care at the destination.

Activity and Rest

Exercise during pregnancy helps maintain maternal fitness and muscle tone, leads to improved self-image, promotes regular bowel function, improves cardiovascular function, increases energy, improves sleep, relieves tension, helps control weight gain, and is associated with improved postpartum recovery. Exercise also improves symptoms of depression during pregnancy (Shivakumar, 2015). Regular maternal exercise is associated with a reduced incidence of preterm birth when compared to those who didn't exercise. Preliminary findings suggest that women who exercised during pregnancy had a reduced risk of both small-for-gestational age (SGA) and large-for-gestational-age (LGA) newborns but further research is needed (Kuhrt, Hezelgrave, & Shennan, 2015). Normal participation in exercise can continue throughout an uncomplicated pregnancy and is encouraged.

Exercise may play a role in the prevention of maternal and fetal complications (Kuhrt et al., 2015). For women who are morbidly obese, exercise may assist in the prevention of gestational diabetes. Exercise is also recommended by the American Diabetes Association (2013) to assist in glycemic control for women with gestational diabetes.

The woman can check with her certified nurse-midwife or physician about taking part in strenuous sports. ACOG (2015b) recommends that women avoid sky diving; scuba diving; "hot yoga"; activities with a high risk for falling, such as downhill skiing, water skiing, gymnastics, off-road cycling, surfing, and horseback riding; and those activities that have a high risk of blunt trauma, such as ice hockey, soccer, boxing, and basketball. Certain conditions do contraindicate exercise. Absolute contraindications to exercise include the following (ACOG, 2015b):

- Rupture of the membranes
- Preeclampsia-eclampsia
- Cervical insufficiency (cerclage)
- Persistent vaginal bleeding in the second or third trimesters
- Multiple gestation at risk for preterm labor
- Preterm labor in the current pregnancy
- Placenta previa after 26 weeks' gestation
- Chronic medical conditions that might be negatively impacted by vigorous exercise such as significant heart disease, restrictive lung disease, or severe anemia.

Before beginning an exercise program, the woman should have a thorough evaluation to be sure no medical contraindications exist.

The following guidelines are helpful in counseling pregnant women about exercise.

- Moderate intensity exercise for at least 20 to 30 minutes per day on most, if not all, days of the week (ACOG, 2015b).

- A moderate, rhythmic exercise routine involving large muscle groups such as swimming, cycling, or brisk walking is best. Other safe exercises include low impact aerobics and modified yoga or Pilates (ACOG, 2015b).

- Women who were regular exercisers before pregnancy and who have uncomplicated pregnancies should be able to continue high intensity programs such as running, jogging, racquet sports, and strength training without untoward effects while women who were sedentary before pregnancy should begin a gradually increasing exercise program (ACOG, 2015b).

- After the first trimester, women should avoid exercising in the supine position. In most pregnant women, the supine position is associated with decreased cardiac output. Because uterine blood flow is reduced during exercise as blood is shunted from the visceral organs to the muscles, the remaining cardiac output is further decreased. Similarly, women should also avoid standing motionless for prolonged periods (Katz, 2012).

- Light muscle strength training using lighter weights (or resistance bands) and more repetitions done once or twice per week helps improve overall fitness and does not negatively affect the fetus.

- Because decreased oxygen is available for aerobic exercise during pregnancy, women should modify the intensity of their exercise based on their symptoms, should stop when they become fatigued, and should avoid exercising to the point of exhaustion.

- A normal pregnancy requires an additional 300 kcal per day. Women who exercise regularly at high intensity or for prolonged periods during pregnancy should be careful to ensure that their diet is adequate (ACOG, 2015b).

- To augment heat dissipation, especially during the first trimester, pregnant women who exercise should wear appropriate clothing that is comfortable and loose, ensure adequate hydration, and avoid prolonged overheating.

- As a result of the cardiovascular changes of pregnancy, heart rate is not an accurate indicator of the intensity of exercise for pregnant women. If a pregnant, exercising woman is unable to maintain a conversation, then the exercise effort is too high.

The woman should wear a supportive bra and appropriate shoes when exercising. She should also warm up and stretch to help prepare the joints for activity and cool down with a period of mild activity to help restore circulation and avoid pooling of blood.

Warning signs to discontinue exercising include the following (ACOG, 2015b):

- Chest pain
- Vaginal bleeding
- Regular, painful uterine contractions
- Leakage of amniotic fluid
- Calf pain or swelling
- Dizziness, headache, dyspnea before exertion, and muscle weakness affecting balance.

The woman should stop exercising if any of these symptoms occur and modify her exercise program. If the symptoms persist, the woman should contact her healthcare provider.

Clinical Reasoning Counseling About Strenuous Physical Activity

Ana Gonzalez, a 24-year-old, G1P0, is 11 weeks pregnant when she presents for her first prenatal examination. She has been a long-distance runner for 6 years. Because of her low body fat, her menses have always been irregular, and it had not occurred to Ana that she might be pregnant. Ana says she has been told that it is fine to continue any physical activity at which one is proficient and says that she would like to continue running long distances while pregnant.

What should you tell Ana about running long distances?

Adequate rest is important for both physical and emotional health. Pregnant women need more sleep, particularly in the first and last trimesters, when they tire easily. Without enough rest, pregnant women have less resilience. Finding time to rest during the day may be difficult for women who work outside the home or who have small children. The nurse can help the expectant mother examine her daily schedule to develop a realistic plan for short periods of rest and relaxation.

Sleeping becomes more difficult during the last trimester because of the enlarged abdomen, increased frequency of urination, and greater activity of the fetus. Finding a comfortable position becomes difficult. Figure 10–10 shows a position most pregnant women find comfortable. Women can also prepare for sleep with progressive relaxation techniques similar to those taught in prepared childbirth classes.

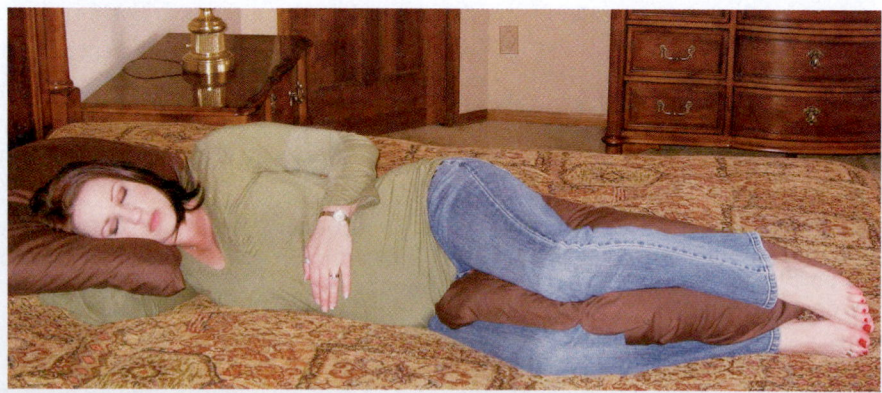

Figure 10–10 Position for relaxation and rest as pregnancy progresses.

Exercises to Prepare for Childbirth

Certain exercises help strengthen muscle tone in preparation for birth and promote more rapid restoration of muscle tone after birth. A few of the more common body-conditioning exercises for pregnancy are discussed here.

The **pelvic tilt**, or pelvic rocking, helps maintain pelvic flexibility and prevent or reduce back strain as it helps strengthen abdominal muscles. To do the pelvic tilt in early pregnancy, the pregnant woman lies on her back and puts her feet flat on the floor. This flexes the knees and helps prevent strain or discomfort. She decreases the curvature in her back by pressing her spine toward the floor. With her back pressed to the floor, the woman tightens her abdominal muscles as she tightens and tucks in her buttocks. In the second and third trimesters, the woman can also do the pelvic tilt on her hands and knees (Figure 10–11), while sitting in a chair, or while standing with her back against a wall. The woman should maintain the body alignment that results when the pelvic tilt is done correctly as much as possible throughout the day.

Clinical Tip

Doing the pelvic tilt on hands and knees may aggravate back strain. Teach women with a history of minor back problems to do the pelvic tilt only in the standing position.

ABDOMINAL EXERCISES

A basic exercise to increase abdominal muscle tone is tightening abdominal muscles with each breath. It can be done in any position, but it is best learned while lying supine. With knees flexed and feet flat on the floor, the woman expands her abdomen and slowly takes a deep breath. Exhaling slowly, she gradually pulls in

her abdominal muscles until they are fully contracted. She relaxes for a few seconds and then repeats the exercise. The pregnant woman should avoid the supine position after the first trimester.

Partial sit-ups strengthen abdominal muscle tone and are done according to individual comfort levels. In early pregnancy, partial sit-ups may be done with the knees flexed and the feet flat on the floor to avoid strain on the lower back. The woman stretches her arms toward her knees as she slowly pulls her head and shoulders off the floor to a comfortable level (if she has poor abdominal muscle tone, she may not be able to pull up very far). She then slowly returns to the starting position, takes a deep breath, and repeats the exercise. To strengthen the oblique abdominal muscles, she repeats the process but stretches the left arm to the side of her right knee, returns to the floor, takes a deep breath, and then reaches with the right arm to the left knee. During the second and third trimesters, these exercises can be done on a large exercise ball.

Women can do these exercises approximately 5 times in a sequence and repeat the sequence at other times during the day as desired. It is important to do the exercises slowly to prevent muscle strain and overtiring.

PERINEAL EXERCISES

Pelvic floor muscle tightening, also called **Kegel exercises**, strengthens the pubococcygeus muscle and increases its elasticity (Figure 10–12). Research indicates that Kegel exercises performed during pregnancy and postpartum increase pelvic floor muscle strength and help prevent symptoms associated with childbirth such as urinary incontinence, pelvic organ prolapse, and fecal impaction (Sut & Kaplan, 2015).

The woman can identify the specific muscle group to be exercised by stopping urination midstream. Doing Kegel exercises while urinating is discouraged, however, because this practice has been associated with urinary stasis and urinary

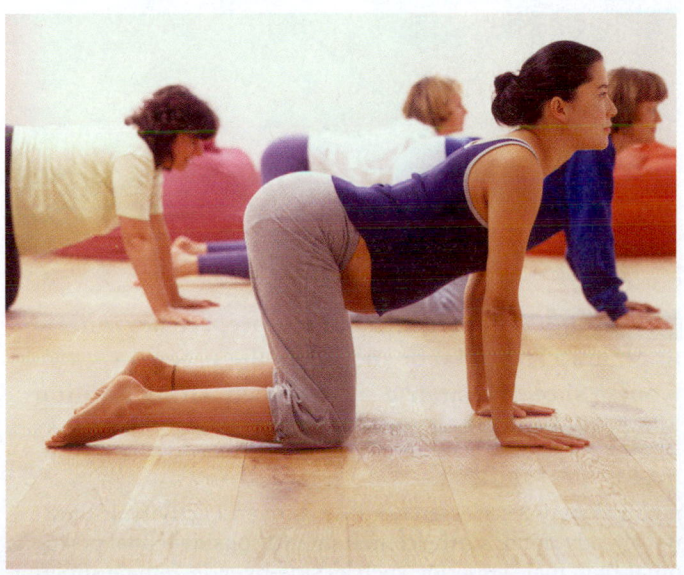

A

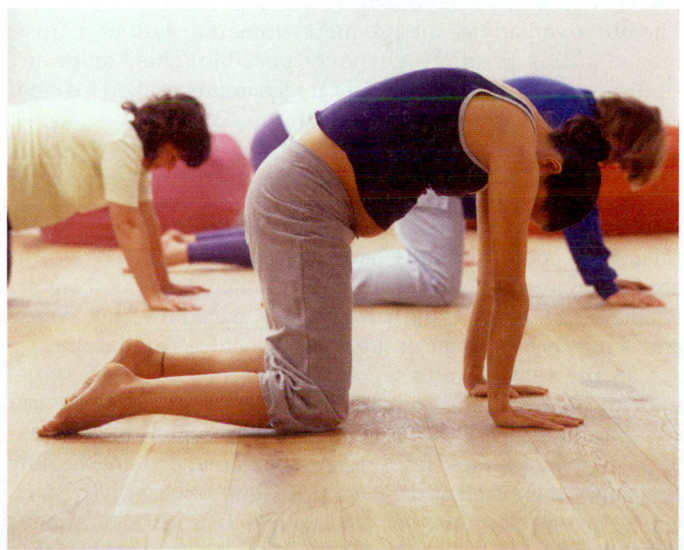

B

Figure 10–11 When the pelvic tilt is done on hands and knees, the starting position is back flat and parallel to the floor, hands below the head, and knees directly below the buttocks. A. For the first part of the tilt, head is up, neck is long and separated from the shoulders, buttocks are up, and pelvis is thrust back, allowing the back to drop and release on an inhaled breath. B. The next part of the tilt is done on a long exhalation, allowing the pregnant woman to arch her back, drop her head loosely, push away from her hands, and draw in the muscles of her abdomen to strengthen them. Note that in this position the pelvis and buttocks are tucked under, and the buttock muscles are tightened.

SOURCE: Moose Azim/Alamy.

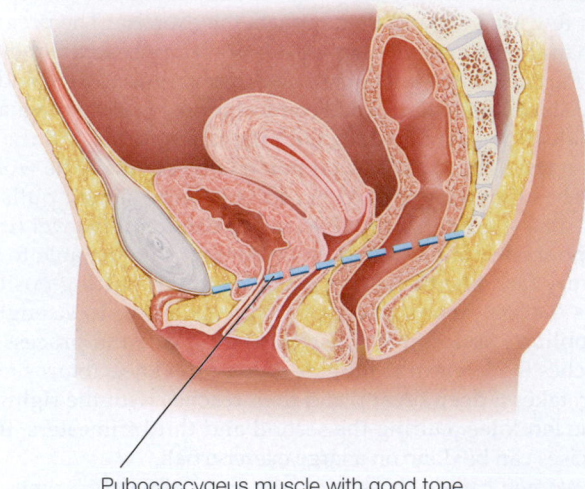
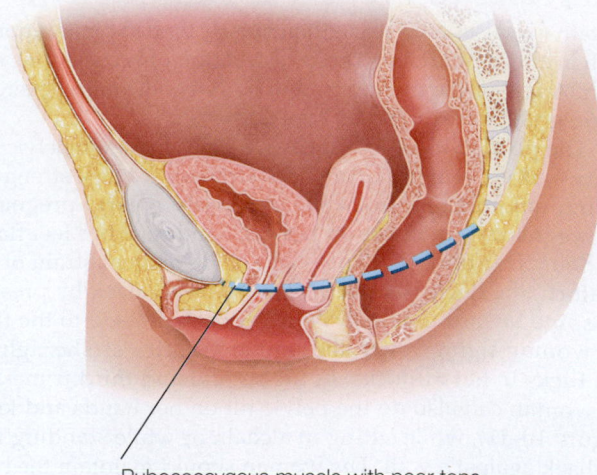

Pubococcygeus muscle with good tone

Pubococcygeus muscle with poor tone

Figure 10–12 Kegel exercises. The woman learns to tighten the pubococcygeus muscle, which improves support to the pelvic organs.

tract infection. Childbirth educators sometimes use the following technique to teach Kegel exercises. They tell the woman to think of her perineal muscles as an elevator. When she relaxes, the elevator is on the first floor. To do the exercises, she contracts, bringing the elevator to the second, third, and fourth floors. She keeps the elevator on the fourth floor for a few seconds, and then gradually relaxes the area. If the exercise is properly done, the woman does not contract the muscles of the buttocks and thighs. Kegel exercises can be done at almost any time. Some women use ordinary events—for instance, stopping at a red light or talking on the telephone—as a cue to remember to do the exercise.

INNER THIGH EXERCISES

The nurse can advise the pregnant woman to assume a cross-legged sitting position whenever possible. This "tailor sit" stretches the muscles of the inner thighs in preparation for labor and birth. See Figure 10–13.

Sexual Activity

Because of the physiologic, anatomic, and emotional changes of pregnancy, couples usually have many questions and concerns about sexual activity during pregnancy. Often these questions are about possible injury to the baby or the woman during intercourse and about changes in the desire each partner feels for the other.

In the past, couples were often warned to avoid sexual intercourse during the last 6 to 8 weeks of pregnancy to prevent complications such as infection or premature rupture of the membranes. However, these fears seem to be unfounded. In a healthy pregnancy, there is no medical reason to limit sexual activity. Intercourse is contraindicated for medical reasons such as threatened miscarriage or risk of preterm labor (Cunningham et al., 2014).

The expectant mother may experience changes in sexual desire and response. Often these changes are related to the various discomforts that occur throughout pregnancy. For instance, during the first trimester, fatigue or nausea and vomiting may decrease sexual desire. During the second trimester, many of these discomforts are lessened and sexual satisfaction increases. During the third trimester, interest in sex may again decrease as the woman becomes more uncomfortable and tired. Shortness of breath, urinary frequency, leg cramps, and decreased

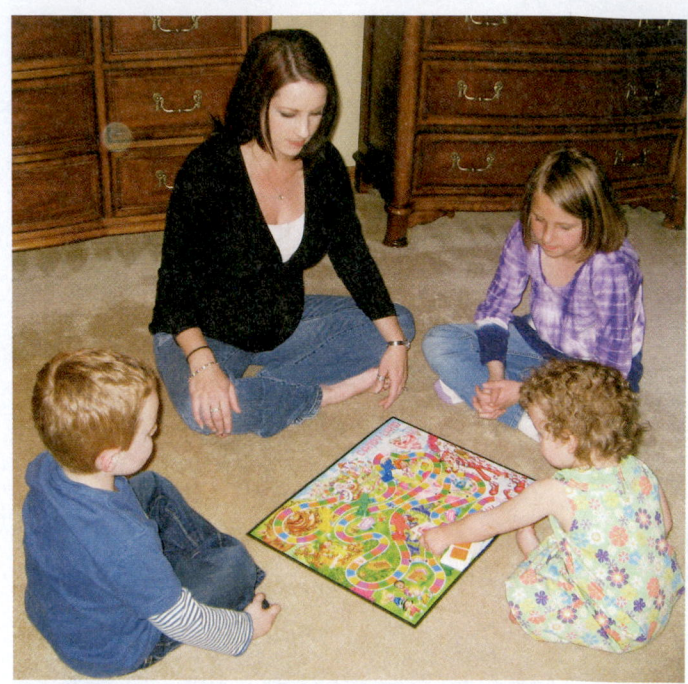

Figure 10–13 Tailor sitting. To help prepare her inner thigh muscles for labor and birth, the pregnant woman should assume a cross-legged sitting position whenever possible during the day.

mobility may also lessen sexual desire and activity. If they are not already doing so, the couple should consider coital positions other than male superior, such as side-by-side, female superior, and vaginal rear entry.

Sexual activity does not have to include intercourse. Many of the nurturing and sexual needs of the pregnant woman can be satisfied by cuddling, kissing, and being held. The warm, sensual feelings that accompany these activities can be an end in themselves. Her partner, however, may choose to masturbate for satisfaction.

Many factors in pregnancy also affect the sexual desires of men. The man's previous relationship with the partner,

TEACHING HIGHLIGHTS | Sexual Activity During Pregnancy

In starting a discussion about sexual activity during pregnancy, universal statements that give permission, such as "Many couples experience changes in sexual desire during pregnancy. What kind of changes have you experienced?" are often effective.

In your teaching, explain the following points to the woman and her partner:

- The pregnant woman may experience changes in desire during the course of pregnancy. During the first trimester, discomforts such as nausea, fatigue, and breast tenderness may make intercourse less desirable for many women. In the second trimester, as symptoms decrease, desire may increase. In the third trimester, discomfort and fatigue may lead to decreased desire in the woman.

- Men may notice changes in their level of desire, too. This may be related to feelings about their partner's changing appearance, their belief about the acceptability of sexual activity with a pregnant woman, or concern about hurting the woman or fetus. Some men find the changes of pregnancy erotic; others must adjust to the notion of their partners as mothers.

- The woman may notice that orgasms are much more intense during the last weeks of pregnancy and may be followed by cramping.

- Because of the pressure of the enlarging uterus on the vena cava, the woman should not lie flat on her back for intercourse after about the fourth month. If the couple prefer that position, a pillow should be placed under her right hip to displace the uterus. Alternative positions such as side-by-side, female superior, or vaginal rear entry may become necessary as her uterus enlarges.

- Sexual activities that both partners enjoy are generally acceptable. It is not advisable for couples who favor anal sex to go from anal penetration to vaginal penetration because of the risk of introducing *Escherichia coli* into the vagina.

- Alternative methods of expressing intimacy and affection such as cuddling, holding and stroking each other, and kissing may help maintain the couple's feelings of warmth and closeness. If the man feels desire for further sexual release, his partner may help him masturbate to ejaculation, or he may prefer to masturbate in private.

- Sexual intercourse is contraindicated once the membranes are ruptured or if bleeding is present. Women with a history of preterm labor may be advised to avoid intercourse because the oxytocin that is released with orgasm stimulates uterine contractions and may trigger preterm labor. Because oxytocin is also released with nipple stimulation, fondling the breasts may also be contraindicated in those cases.

Stress the importance of open communication so that the couple feels comfortable expressing their feelings, preferences, and concerns. Deal with any specific questions about the physical and psychologic changes that the couple may have.

---

acceptance of the pregnancy, attitudes toward the partner's change of appearance, and concern about hurting the expectant mother or baby can all play a role. Some men find it difficult to view their partners as sexually appealing while they are adjusting to the concept of them as mothers. Other men find their partners' pregnancies arousing and experience feelings of increased happiness, intimacy, and closeness.

The expectant couple should be aware of their changing sexual desires, the normality of these changes, and the importance of communicating these changes to each other so that they can make nurturing adaptations. It is important that the couple feel free to express concerns about sexual activity. Use a relaxed manner when responding to questions and giving anticipatory guidance. (See *Teaching Highlights: Sexual Activity During Pregnancy*.)

Dental Care

Proper dental hygiene is important in pregnancy because ensuring a healthy oral environment is essential to overall health. In spite of such discomforts as nausea and vomiting, gum hypertrophy, and heartburn, it is important for pregnant women to maintain regular oral hygiene by brushing at least twice a day and flossing daily. Dental treatment is safe throughout pregnancy; however, the second trimester is considered the most appropriate time for dental treatment because the risk of pregnancy loss tends to be lower and the woman tends to be more comfortable. It is important to encourage the woman to have a dental checkup early in pregnancy. She should inform her dentist that she is pregnant so that she is not exposed to teratogenic substances.

Immunizations

Immunizations with attenuated live viruses, such as rubella vaccine, should not be given in pregnancy because of the teratogenic effect of the live viruses on the developing embryo or fetus. The most current recommendations on vaccines during pregnancy should be obtained from the Centers for Disease Control and Prevention website.

Women should be assessed during the preconception stage for varicella, rubella, hepatitis B, and HIV. Women anticipating global travel should pay careful attention to vaccinations that are required. There are multiple vaccinations that can be given during pregnancy; however, others are contraindicated and should not be administered (Centers for Disease Control and Prevention [CDC], 2014).

Complementary Health Approaches

As discussed in Chapter 2, many women use complementary health approaches such as homeopathy, herbal medicine, acupressure and acupuncture, biofeedback, therapeutic touch, massage, and chiropractic as part of a holistic approach to their healthcare. Thus the nurse should inquire about the use of complementary therapies as part of routine antepartum assessment. Nurses working with pregnant women and childbearing families need to develop a general understanding of the more commonly used therapies to be able to answer basic questions and to provide resources as needed.

It is important for the pregnant woman to understand that herbs are considered to be dietary supplements and are not regulated as prescription or over-the-counter drugs are through the FDA. In general, it is best to advise pregnant women not to ingest any herbs, except ginger, during the first trimester of pregnancy. The website of the National Center for Complementary and Integrative Health (NCCIH) is a reliable source of information about herbs, homeopathic remedies, and other alternative options.

Teratogenic Substances

Substances that adversely affect the normal growth and development of the fetus are called *teratogens*. Many substances are known or suspected teratogens, including certain medications, psychotropic drugs, and alcohol. The harmful effects of other substances, such as some pesticides or exposure to x-rays in the first trimester of pregnancy, have also been documented. It is essential to provide pregnant women with information about recognized teratogens and environmental risks.

MEDICATIONS

The use of medications during pregnancy, including prescriptions, over-the-counter drugs, and herbal remedies, is of great concern because maternal drug exposure is associated with birth defects. Many pregnant women need medication to treat infections, allergies, or other pathologic processes. In these situations the problem can be complex. Even when a woman is highly motivated to avoid taking any medications, she may have taken potentially teratogenic medications before her pregnancy was confirmed, especially if she has an irregular menstrual cycle.

The fetus is at highest risk for gross abnormalities during the first trimester of pregnancy, when fetal organs are first developing. The classic period of teratogenesis in a woman with a 28-day cycle extends from day 31 after the last menstrual period (17 days after fertilization) to day 71 (57 days after fertilization) (Niebyl & Simpson, 2012). Many factors influence teratogenic effects, including the type of teratogen and the dose, the stage of embryo development, and the genetic sensitivity of the mother and the fetus. For example, the commonly prescribed acne medication isotretinoin (Accutane) is associated with a high incidence of spontaneous abortion and congenital malformations if taken early in pregnancy.

Formerly drugs were classified in categories A, B, C, D, and X, with category X indicating that the demonstrated fetal risks clearly outweigh any possible benefit. In 2014, the FDA amended its regulations governing the labeling of prescription drugs and biologic products for women who are pregnant or lactating. These regulations became effective in June 2015. According to the new requirements, three categories have been specified (FDA, 2014):

- *Pregnancy.* If the drug is absorbed systemically, labeling must include a risk summary of adverse developmental outcomes that includes data from all relevant sources including human, animal, and/or pharmacologic information. The labeling must also contain relevant information to help healthcare providers counsel women about the use of the drug during pregnancy. In addition, if there is a pregnancy exposure registry for the drug, the labeling should include a specific statement to that effect followed by contact information needed to obtain information about the registry or to enroll.
- *Lactation.* For drugs that are absorbed systemically labeling must include a summary of the risks of using a drug when the woman is lactating. To the extent that information is available, the summary should include relevant information about the drug's presence in human milk, the effects of the drug on milk production, and the effects of the drug on the breastfed child.

- *Females and males of reproductive potential.* This section must include information when human or animal data suggest drug-associated effects on fertility. It should also specify when contraception or pregnancy testing is required or recommended, such as before, during, or after the drug therapy.

Although the first trimester is the critical period for teratogenesis, some medications are known to have a teratogenic effect when taken in the second and third trimesters. For example, tetracycline taken in late pregnancy is commonly associated with staining of teeth in children and has been shown to depress skeletal growth, especially in premature babies. Sulfonamides taken in the last few weeks of pregnancy are known to compete with bilirubin attachment of protein-binding sites, increasing the risk of jaundice in the newborn (Niebyl & Simpson, 2012).

Pregnant women need to avoid all medications—prescribed, homeopathic, or over-the-counter—if possible. If no alternative exists, it is wisest to select a well-known medication rather than a newer drug whose potential teratogenic effects may not be known. When possible, the oral form of a drug should be used, and it should be prescribed in the lowest possible therapeutic dose for the shortest time possible. Caution is the watchword for pregnant women who have been taking medications. The advantage of using a particular medication must outweigh the risks. Any medication with possible teratogenic effects is best avoided.

SAFETY ALERT!

It is essential that pregnant women check with their healthcare provider about any herbs or medications they were taking when pregnancy began and about any nonprescription drugs they are thinking of using. (See Chapter 14 for a discussion of the use of alcohol and illicit drugs during pregnancy.)

TOBACCO

In the United States, smoking during pregnancy is one of the most significant, modifiable causes of poor pregnancy outcomes. It is associated with an increased risk of spontaneous abortion, intrauterine growth restriction, low birth weight, preterm birth, premature rupture of the membranes, perinatal mortality, placenta previa, abruptio placentae, and premature rupture of membranes (Cunningham et al., 2014). Research also links maternal smoking, both during pregnancy and afterward, with an increased risk of sudden infant death syndrome (SIDS) (Van Nguyen & Abenhaim, 2013). Maternal smoking also exposes young children to other risks of secondhand smoke including middle ear infections; acute and chronic respiratory tract illnesses such as asthma, bronchitis, and pneumonia; inflammatory bowel disease; sleep disturbances; and learning disabilities and conduct disorders (Al-Sayed & Ibrahim, 2014).

The ingredients in cigarette smoke, such as carbon monoxide, nicotine, lead, and cotinine, are toxic to the fetus and decrease the availability of oxygen to maternal and fetal tissues (Cunningham et al., 2014).

In response to public health education campaigns in the United States, smoking during pregnancy has decreased significantly. In fact, approximately 46% of women who smoke quit during pregnancy. Unfortunately, about 50% to 60% of women who quit smoking during their pregnancy resume smoking within a year after giving birth (ACOG, 2013a). This finding suggests that although women are aware of the potential impact of smoking on the fetus, they may be less knowledgeable about the effects of passive smoke on the baby.

Any decrease in smoking during pregnancy most likely improves fetal outcome, and researchers continue to explore approaches designed to help women quit smoking. Pregnancy may be a difficult time for a woman to stop smoking, but the nurse should encourage her to reduce the number of cigarettes she smokes daily. The perceived need to protect her unborn child may increase her motivation. Many educational resources are available for healthcare providers and consumers on smoking cessation programs through organizations such as the American Lung Association, the March of Dimes, and Healthy Mothers, Healthy Babies.

ALCOHOL

Fetuses of women who drink heavily are at increased risk of developing **fetal alcohol syndrome (FAS)**. This syndrome, which is characterized by growth restriction, facial anomalies, and central nervous system (CNS) dysfunction of varying severity, is a major cause of intellectual disability in the United States (Cunningham et al., 2014). (Chapter 26 discusses the neonate exposed to alcohol in utero.)

The effects of moderate drinking during pregnancy are unclear. Research indicates an increased incidence of lowered birth weight and some neurologic effects, such as attention deficit disorder. Evidence suggests that the risk of teratogenic effects increases proportionately with increased average daily intake of alcohol. Although an occasional drink during pregnancy does not carry any known risk, no safe level of drinking during pregnancy has been identified; thus healthcare providers recommend that pregnant women abstain from all alcohol during pregnancy. In most cases, once a woman becomes aware of her pregnancy, she decreases her consumption of alcohol. However, the alcohol consumed after conception and before pregnancy is diagnosed remains a cause for concern. For this reason and for their general well-being, women of childbearing age—and indeed all women—should be counseled to avoid heavy or binge drinking.

Assessment of alcohol intake is a major part of every woman's medical history. The nurse should ask questions in a direct, nonjudgmental manner. All women need to be counseled about the role of alcohol in pregnancy. If heavy consumption is involved, the nurse should refer the pregnant woman immediately to an alcohol treatment program. Counselors in these programs need to know about a woman's pregnancy before drug therapy is suggested, since certain drugs may be harmful to the developing fetus. For example, the drug disulfiram (Antabuse), often used in conjunction with alcohol treatment, is contraindicated during pregnancy because it potentiates the teratogenic effect of alcohol (Wisner et al., 2012).

CAFFEINE

While studies continue, current research reveals no evidence that moderate levels of caffeine are linked to birth defects, spontaneous abortion, or preterm birth, nor is there any clear evidence of a link between caffeine intake and intrauterine growth restriction (ACOG, 2013b). Until more definitive data are available, nurses can advise women about common sources of caffeine, including coffee, tea, colas, and chocolate, and suggest that they limit their caffeine intake to less than 200 mg/day (Cunningham et al., 2014). The average cup of brewed coffee has 100 mg, a cup of tea has 50 mg, a regular cola drink has up to 40 mg, and a normal-sized chocolate bar has up to 50 mg of caffeine.

Evaluation

Throughout the antepartum period, evaluation is an ongoing and essential part of effective nursing care. In evaluating the effectiveness of the interactions, the nurse should try creative solutions that are logical and carefully thought out. Creative solutions are especially important in dealing with families from other cultures. If a practice is important to a woman and not harmful, the culturally competent nurse will not discourage it.

The nurse needs to be alert for situations that require referral for further evaluation. For example, a woman who has gained 4 lb in a single week does not require counseling about nutrition; she needs further assessment for preeclampsia. The nurse who has a sound knowledge of theory will recognize this need and act immediately.

Throughout the course of pregnancy, certain criteria determine the quality of care. In essence, nursing care has been effective if the following occur:

- The common discomforts of pregnancy are quickly identified and are relieved or lessened effectively.
- The woman is able to discuss the physiologic and psychologic changes of pregnancy.
- The woman uses self-care measures, if needed, during pregnancy.
- The woman avoids substances and situations that pose a risk to her or her child's well-being.
- The woman seeks regular prenatal care.

Focus Your Study

- Providing anticipatory guidance about childbirth, the postpartum period, and childrearing is a primary responsibility of the nurse caring for women in an antepartal setting.
- The nurse assesses the expectant father's knowledge level and intended degree of participation and then works with the couple to help ensure a satisfying experience.
- Culturally based practices and taboos may have a major impact on the childbearing family.

- Childbearing decisions include the healthcare provider, birth setting, support persons, and whether to include siblings in the birth experience.
- Prenatal classes may be offered early or late in the pregnancy. The class content varies depending on the type of class and the individual offering it. Expectant parents tend to want information in chronologic sequence with the pregnancy.

- Breastfeeding programs in the prenatal period offer encouragement, practical instruction, and resources for the breastfeeding family.

- Siblings are now included in the whole birthing process, and classes for them are available from many sources.

- Grandparents have unique information needs that are addressed in grandparents' classes.

- The common discomforts of pregnancy occur as a result of physiologic and anatomic changes. The nurse provides the woman with information about self-care activities aimed at reducing or relieving discomfort.

- To make appropriate self-care choices and ensure healthful habits, a pregnant woman requires accurate information about a range of subjects from exercise to sexual activity, from bathing to immunization.

- Maternal assessment of fetal activity keeps the woman "in touch" with her fetus and provides ongoing assessment of fetal status.

- Teratogenic substances are substances that adversely affect the normal growth and development of the fetus.

- A pregnant woman should avoid taking nonessential medications or using over-the-counter preparations during pregnancy.

- Evidence confirms that smoking or consuming alcohol during pregnancy may be harmful to the fetus.

Clinical Reasoning in Action

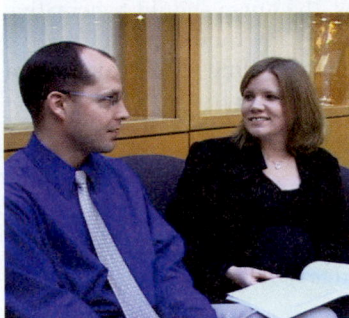

Thirty-seven-year-old Cathy Sommers, G1P0, presents to you, with her husband, at the OB physician's office at 32 weeks' gestation. Cathy tells you that she and her husband are practicing lawyers with their own firm. The couple delayed starting a family because it has been important to them to advance their careers and establish their firm. Cathy had an amniocentesis at 18 weeks' gestation because of her advanced maternal age, and the results ruled out chromosomal abnormalities. The couple knows that the baby is a boy, and they are anticipating a vaginal birth. Cathy tells you that she is experiencing more fatigue, leg cramps, and shortness of breath when climbing stairs. The physical examination, including a negative Homans sign, is within normal limits with the exception of slight ankle edema. Her weight is 150 lb, temperature 98.6°F (37.0°C), pulse 88, respirations 16, BP 126/70. You discuss pregnancy discomforts in the third trimester with Cathy and her husband.

1. What measures can you suggest to cope with fatigue?
2. Discuss measures to decrease leg cramps.
3. Discuss the physiologic changes underlying dyspnea.
4. Review Braxton Hicks contractions.

References

Abushaikha, L., & Massah, R. (2013). Perceptions of barriers to paternal presence and contribution during childbirth: An exploratory study from Syria. *Birth: Issues in Perinatal care, 40*(1), 61–66.

Alio, A. P., Lewis, C. A., Scarborough, K., Harris, K., & Fiscella, K. (2013). A community perspective on the role of fathers during pregnancy: A qualitative study. *Pregnancy and Childbirth, 13*(2), 1–11.

Al-Sayed, E. M., & Ibrahim, K. S. (2014). Second-hand tobacco smoke in children. *Toxicology and Industrial Health, 30*(7), 635–644.

American Academy of Pediatrics (AAP) and the American College of Obstetricians and Gynecologists (ACOG). (2012). *Guidelines for perinatal care* (7th ed.). Elk Grove Village, IL: Author.

American College of Obstetricians and Gynecologists (ACOG). (2013a). *Smoking cessation during pregnancy*. (Committee Opinion No. 471, reaffirmed 2013). Washington, DC: Author.

American College of Obstetricians and Gynecologists (ACOG). (2013b). *Moderate caffeine consumption during pregnancy*. (Committee Opinion No. 462). Washington, DC: Author.

American College of Obstetricians and Gynecologists (ACOG). (2015a). *Nausea and vomiting of pregnancy*. (ACOG Practice Bulletin No. 153). Washington, DC: Author.

American College of Obstetricians and Gynecologists (ACOG). (2015b). *Physical activity and exercise during pregnancy and the postpartum period*. (ACOG Committee Opinion No. 267). Washington, DC: Author.

American Diabetes Association. (2013). *How to treat gestational diabetes*. Retrieved from http://www.diabetes.org/diabetes-basics/gestational/how-to-treat-gestational.html

Avery, M. D. (2013). *Supporting a physiologic approach to pregnancy and birth: A practical guide*. Ames, IA: Wiley & Sons, Inc.

Bell, K. M. (2012). Centering Pregnancy: Changing the system, empowering women and strengthening families. *International Journal of Childbirth Education, 27*(12), 70–76.

Bloomquist, J. L., Quiroz, L. H., MacMillan, D., Mccullough, A., & Handa, V. L. (2011). Mothers' satisfaction with planned vaginal and planned cesarean birth. *American Journal of Perinatology, 28*(5), 383–388.

Centers for Disease Control and Prevention (CDC). (2014). *Vaccines for pregnant women*. Retrieved from http://www.cdc.gov/vaccines/adults/rec-vac/pregnant.html

Coalition for Improving Maternity Services (CIMS). (2013). *Mother-friendly childbirth initiative*. Retrieved from http://www.motherfriendly.org/MFCI

Cunningham, F. G., Leveno, K. J., Bloom, S. L., Spong, C. Y., Dashe, J. S., Hoffman, B. L., . . . Sheffield, J. S. (2014). *Williams obstetrics* (24th ed.). New York, NY: McGraw-Hill.

DeCesare, J. Z., & Jackson, J. R. (2015). Centering Pregnancy: Practical tips for your practice. *Archives of Gynecology and Obstetrics, 291*, 499–507.

Donna, S. (2011). *Promoting normal birth: Research, reflections and guidelines*. United Kingdom: Fresh Heart Publishing.

Fantasia, H. C. (2014). A new pharmacologic treatment for nausea and vomiting of pregnancy. *Nursing for Women's Health, 18*(1), 73–77.

Food and Drug Administration (FDA). (2014). *Content and format of labeling for human prescription drug and biological products: Requirements for pregnancy and lactation labeling*. Retrieved from https://s3.amazonaws.com/public-inspection.federalregister.gov/2014-28241.pdf

Gregory, K. D., Niebyl, J. R., & Johnson, T. R. B. (2012). Preconception and prenatal care: Part of the continuum. In S. G. Gabbe, J. R. Niebyl, J. L. Simpson, M. B. Landon, H. L. Galan, E. R. M. Jauniaux, & D. A. Driscoll (Eds.), *Obstetrics: Normal and problem pregnancies* (6th ed.). Philadelphia, PA: Elsevier Saunders.

Johnson, C. T., Hallock, J. L., Bienstock, J. L., Fox, H. E., & Wallach, E. E. (2015). *The John Hopkins manual of gynecology and obstetrics* (5th ed.). Philadelphia, PA: Wolters Kluwer.

Katz, V. (2012). Work and work-related stress in pregnancy. *Clinical Obstetrics and Gynecology, 55*(3), 765–773.

Kimberly, D. G., Niebyl, J. R., & Johnson, T. R. B. (2012). Preconception and prenatal care: Part of the continuum. In S. G. Gabbe, J. R. Niebyl, J. L. Simpson, M. B. Landon, H. L. Galan, E. R. M. Jauniaux, & D. A. Driscoll (Eds.), *Obstetrics: Normal and problem pregnancies* (6th ed.). Philadelphia, PA: Elsevier Saunders.

King, T. L., Brucker, M. C., Kriebs, J. M., Fahey, J. O., Gegor, C. L., & Varney, H. (2015). *Varney's midwifery* (5th ed.). Burlington, MA: Jones & Bartlett Learning.

Kuhrt, K., Hezelgrave, N. L., & Shennan, A. H. (2015). Exercise in pregnancy. *The Obstetrician & Gynaecologist, 17,* 281–287.

Martin, J. A., Hamilton, B. E., & Osterman, M. J. K. (2014). Births in the United States, 2013. *NCHS Data Brief.* Retrieved from http://www.cdc.gov/nchs/data/databriefs/db175.htm

National Center for Complementary and Integrative Health (NCCIH). (2015). *Herbs at a glance: Ginger.* Retrieved from http://nccih.nih.gov/health/ginger

Niebyl, J. R., & Simpson, J. L. (2012). Drugs and environmental agents in pregnancy and lactation: Embryology, teratology, epidemiology. In S. G. Gabbe, J. R. Niebyl, J. L. Simpson, M. B. Landon, H. L. Galan, E. R. M. Jauniaux, & D. A. Driscoll (Eds.), *Obstetrics: Normal and problem pregnancies* (6th ed.). Philadelphia, PA: Elsevier Saunders.

Purnell, L. D. (2014). *Guide to culturally competent health care.* (3rd ed.). Philadelphia, PA: F. A. Davis.

Shivakumar, G. (2015). Exercise improves depressive symptoms during pregnancy. *BJOG: An International Journal of Obstetrics and Gynaecology, 122*(1), 63.

Spector, R. E. (2013). *Cultural diversity in health and illness* (8th ed.). Upper Saddle River, NJ: Prentice Hall Health.

Sut, H. K., & Kaplan, P.B. (2015). Effect of pelvic muscle floor exercise on pelvic floor muscle activity and voiding functions during pregnancy and the postpartum period. *Neurourology and Urodynamics.* doi:10.1002/nau.22728

Toohill, J., Fenwick, J., Gamble, J., Creedy, D., Bulst, A., Turkstra, E., & Ryding, E. (2014). A randomized controlled trial of a psycho-education intervention by midwives in reducing childbirth fear in pregnancy women. *Birth, 41*(4), 384–395.

United States Department of Health and Human Services (HHS). (2013). *Healthy People 2020.* Retrieved from http://www.healthypeople.gov/2020

University of South Carolina. (2011). *Cultural knowledge.* Retrieved from http://www.usc.edu/hsc/ebnet/Cc/knowledge/ccknow.htm

Van Nguyen, J. M., & Abenhaim, H. A. (2013). Sudden infant death syndrome: Review for the obstetric care provider. *American Journal of Perinatology, 30*(9), 703–714.

Wisner, K. L., Sit, D. K. Y., Altemus, M., Bogen, D. L., Famy, C. S., Pearlstein, T. B., . . . Perel, J. M. (2012). Mental health and behavioral disorders in pregnancy. In S. G. Gabbe, J. R. Niebyl, J. L. Simpson, M. B. Landon, H. L. Galan, E. R. M. Jauniaux, & D. A. Driscoll (Eds.), *Obstetrics: Normal and problem pregnancies* (6th ed.). Philadelphia, PA: Elsevier Saunders.

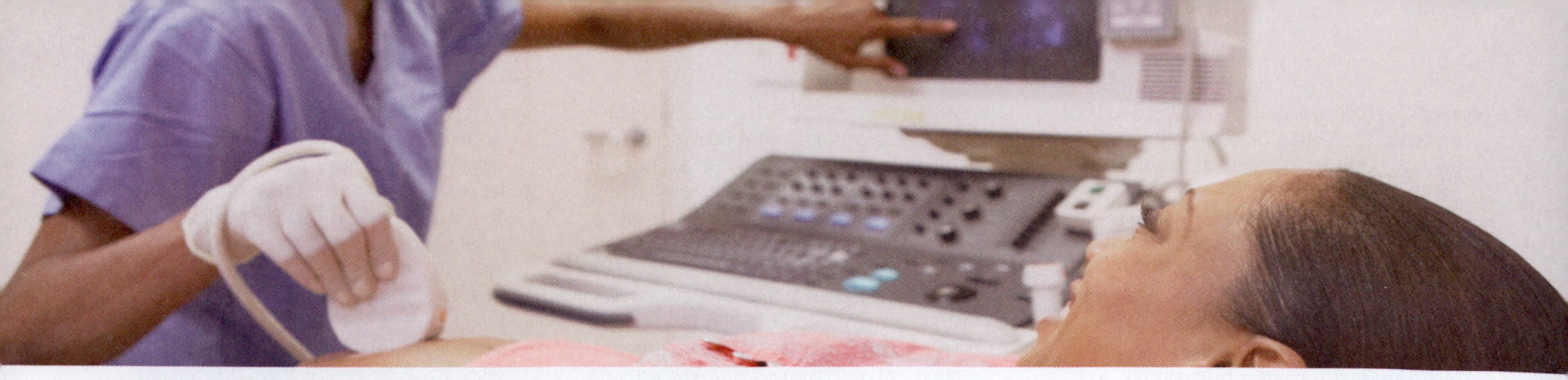

Chapter 11
Maternal Nutrition

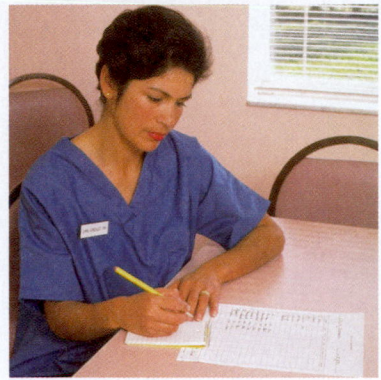

When I was a nursing student I thought nutrition was boring—was I wrong! Now I know how important good nutrition is to every aspect of life, but especially to pregnancy, and I find it endlessly fascinating. When my enthusiasm sparks a response in a pregnant woman I am meeting with, I feel that I am having a long-term impact on the woman's life and hopefully on her family, too.

—A Nurse Working as a Client Educator

⌄ Learning Outcomes

11.1 Describe the recommended levels of weight gain during pregnancy when providing nursing care for pregnant women.

11.2 Explain the significance of specific nutrients in the diet of a pregnant woman.

11.3 Compare nutritional needs during pregnancy, the postpartum period, and lactation with nonpregnant requirements.

11.4 Plan adequate prenatal vegetarian diets based on the nutritional requirements of pregnancy.

11.5 Explain the ways in which various physical, psychosocial, and cultural factors can affect

nutritional intake and status in the nursing management of pregnant women.

11.6 Compare recommendations for weight gain and nutrient intakes in the pregnant adolescent with those for the mature pregnant adult.

11.7 Describe basic factors a nurse should consider when offering nutritional counseling to a pregnant adolescent.

11.8 Compare nutritional counseling issues for breastfeeding and formula-feeding mothers.

A woman's nutritional status before and during pregnancy can significantly influence her health and that of her fetus. In most prenatal clinics and offices, nurses offer nutritional counseling directly or work closely with the nutritionist in providing nutritional assessment and teaching.

This chapter focuses on the nutritional needs of a pregnant woman. Special sections consider the nutritional needs of the pregnant adolescent and the woman after giving birth.

Fetal growth occurs in three overlapping stages:

1. Growth by increase in cell number
2. Growth by increases in cell number and cell size
3. Growth by increase in cell size alone.

Nutritional problems that interfere with cell division may have permanent consequences. If the nutritional insult occurs when cells are mainly enlarging, the changes are usually reversible when normal nutrition resumes.

Growth of fetal and maternal tissues requires increased quantities of nutrients. These are listed in the **dietary reference intakes (DRIs)**, a broad array of dietary reference values developed jointly by the United States and Canada. The DRIs are subdivided into the **recommended dietary allowance (RDA)** and **adequate intake (AI)**. An RDA is the daily dietary intake that is considered sufficient to meet the nutritional requirements of nearly all individuals in a specific life stage and gender group. An AI is a value cited for a nutrient when there are insufficient data to calculate an estimated average requirement. Most of the recommended nutrients can be obtained by eating a well-balanced diet each day. The basic food groups, nutrients provided, food sources, and recommended amounts during pregnancy and lactation are presented in Table 11–1.

Maternal Weight Gain

Maternal weight gain is an important factor in fetal growth and newborn birth weight. The optimal weight gain depends on the woman's weight for height (body mass index [BMI]) and her prepregnant nutritional state. An adequate weight gain indicates an adequate caloric intake. It does not, however, ensure that the woman has a sufficient nutrient intake. The pregnant woman must maintain the nutritional quality of her diet as her weight gain progresses.

The Institute of Medicine (IOM) (2009) recommends weight gains in terms of optimum ranges based on pre-pregnant BMI, and the American College of Obstetricians and Gynecologists

TABLE 11–1 Daily Food Plan for Pregnancy and Lactation

FOOD GROUP	NUTRIENTS PROVIDED	FOOD SOURCE	RECOMMENDED DAILY AMOUNT DURING PREGNANCY	RECOMMENDED DAILY AMOUNT DURING LACTATION
Dairy products	Protein; riboflavin; vitamins A, D, and others; calcium; phosphorus; zinc; magnesium	Milk—whole, 2%, skim, dry, buttermilk. Cheeses—hard, semisoft, cottage. Yogurt—plain, low-fat. Soybean milk—canned, dry	Four (8 oz) cups (five for teenagers) used plain or with flavoring, in shakes, soups, puddings, custards, cocoa. Calcium in 1 cup milk equivalent to 1½ cups cottage cheese, 1½ oz hard or semisoft cheese, 1 cup yogurt, 1½ cups ice cream (high in fat and sugar)	Four (8 oz) cups (five for teenagers); equivalent amount of cheese, yogurt, and other dairy products
Meat and meat alternatives	Protein; iron; thiamine, niacin, and other vitamins; minerals	Beef, pork, veal, lamb, poultry, animal organ meats, fish, eggs; legumes; nuts, seeds, peanut butter, grains in proper vegetarian combination (vitamin B₁₂ supplement needed)	Three servings (one serving = 2 oz), combination in amounts necessary for same nutrient equivalent (varies greatly)	Two servings
Grain products, whole grain or enriched	B vitamins; iron; whole grain also has zinc, magnesium, and other trace elements; provides fiber	Breads and bread products such as cornbread, muffins, waffles, hotcakes, biscuits, dumplings, cereals, pastas, rice	Six to 11 servings daily: one serving = one slice bread, ¾ cup or 1 oz dry cereal, ½ cup rice or pasta	Same as for pregnancy
Fruits and fruit juices	Vitamins A and C; minerals; raw fruits for roughage	Citrus fruits and juices, melons, berries, all other fruits and juices	Two to four servings (one serving for vitamin C): one serving = one medium fruit, ½–1 cup fruit, 4 oz orange or grapefruit juice	Same as for pregnancy
Vegetables and vegetable juices	Vitamins A and C; minerals; provides roughage	Leafy green vegetables; deep yellow or orange vegetables such as carrots, sweet potatoes, squash, tomatoes; green vegetables such as peas, green beans, broccoli; other vegetables such as beets, cabbage, potatoes, corn, lima beans	Three to five servings (one serving of dark green or deep yellow vegetable for vitamin A): one serving = ½–1 cup vegetable, two tomatoes, one medium potato	Same as for pregnancy
Fats	Vitamins A and D; linoleic acid	Butter, cream cheese, fortified table spreads; cream, whipped cream, whipped toppings; avocado, mayonnaise, oil, nuts	As desired in moderation (high in calories): one serving = 1 tbsp butter or enriched margarine	Same as for pregnancy
Sugar and sweets		Sugar, brown sugar, honey, molasses	Occasionally, if desired	Same as for pregnancy

(continued)

TABLE 11–1 Daily Food Plan for Pregnancy and Lactation (*continued*)

FOOD GROUP	NUTRIENTS PROVIDED	FOOD SOURCE	RECOMMENDED DAILY AMOUNT DURING PREGNANCY	RECOMMENDED DAILY AMOUNT DURING LACTATION
Desserts		Nutritious desserts such as puddings, custards, fruit whips, and crisps; other rich, sweet desserts and pastries	Occasionally, if desired	Same as for pregnancy
Beverages	Fluid	Coffee, decaffeinated beverages, tea, bouillon, carbonated drinks	As desired, in moderation	Same as for pregnancy
Miscellaneous		Iodized salt, herbs, spices, condiments	As desired	Same as for pregnancy

Note: The pregnant woman should eat regularly, three meals a day, with nutritious snacks of fruit, cheese, milk, or other foods between meals if desired. (More frequent but smaller meals are also recommended.) Between 4 to 6 (8 oz) glasses of water and a total of 8 to 10 (8 oz) cups total fluid intake should be consumed daily. Water is an essential nutrient.

Healthy People 2020

(MICH-16.5) Increase the proportion of women delivering a live birth who had a healthy weight prior to pregnancy

(ACOG) (2013a) supports these recommendations. The IOM recommendations are as follows:

- Underweight woman: BMI less than 18.5: 12.5–18 kg (28–40 lb)
- Normal-weight woman: BMI 18.5–24.9: 11.5–16 kg (25–35 lb)
- Overweight woman: BMI 25–29.9: 7–11.5 kg (15–25 lb)
- Obese woman: BMI over 30: 5–9.1kg (11–20 lb).

The average maternal weight gain is distributed as follows:

5.0 kg (11 lb)	Fetus, placenta, amniotic fluid
0.9 kg (2 lb)	Uterus
1.8 kg (4 lb)	Increased blood volume
1.4 kg (3 lb)	Breast tissue
2.3–4.5 kg (5–10 lb)	Maternal stores

The pattern of weight gain is important. For women of normal weight, assuming a gain of 0.5 to 2 kg (1.1 to 4.4 lb) during the first trimester, the recommended gain during the second and third trimesters is 0.45 kg (1 lb) per week. The rate of weight gain in the second and third trimesters needs to be slightly higher for underweight women and slightly lower for overweight (0.6 lb) and obese (0.5 lb) women (IOM, 2009). A normal-weight woman who is expecting twins is advised to gain about 1.5 lb (0.7 kg) per week during the second half of her pregnancy.

The prevalence of obesity in the United States has increased dramatically over the past 25 years. The recent National Health and Nutrition Examination Survey found that in the United States more than one third of women are obese and 8% of reproductive-aged women are extremely obese (ACOG, 2013a). Pregnant women who are obese are at risk for many pregnancy complications including gestational diabetes mellitus, preeclampsia, and cesarean birth. Their fetuses are at increased risk for congenital anomalies, stillbirth, prematurity, macrosomia,

and childhood obesity. Thus it is recommended that these women receive counseling on strategies to move toward and to remain at a healthful weight prior to conceiving (ACOG, 2013b).

The incidence of bariatric surgery among obese reproductive-aged women is increasing (ACOG, 2013a). Women who lose weight after weight loss surgery are less likely to have complications during pregnancy. The need for vitamin supplementation should be evaluated as these women are at risk for deficiencies in iron, vitamin B_{12}, folate, vitamin D, and calcium. Women who have undergone gastric band surgery should be referred to their general surgeon to evaluate the need for a band adjustment.

Clinical Tip

Weight varies with time of day, amount of clothing, inaccurate scale adjustment, or weighing error. Do not overemphasize a single weight, but pay attention to the overall pattern of weight gain.

Because of the association between maternal weight gain and pregnancy outcome, most caregivers pay close attention to weight gain during pregnancy (Figure 11–1). Weight gain charts can be useful in monitoring the rate and pattern of weight gain over time.

All pregnant women should include a variety of nutrient-rich foods each day to ensure they are meeting the nutritional needs of both themselves and their babies. The U.S. Department of Agriculture offers an online tool (choosemyplate.gov) that can help expectant women customize an eating plan based on age, weight, height, physical activity, and gestation stage (Figure 11–2).

Nutritional Requirements

The recommended dietary allowance (RDA) for almost all nutrients increases during pregnancy, although the amount of increase varies with each nutrient. These increases reflect the additional requirements of both the mother and the developing fetus.

Calories

The term **calorie (cal)** designates the amount of heat required to raise the temperature of 1 g of water 1°C (33.8°F). The **kilocalorie (kcal)** is equivalent to 1000 cal and is the unit used to express the energy value of food.

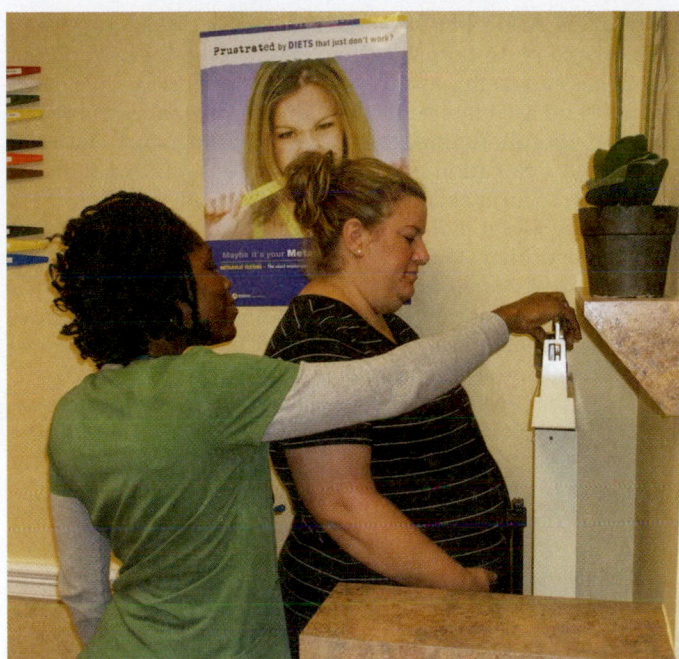

Figure 11–1 It is important to monitor a pregnant woman's weight over time.

SOURCE: Michele Davidson.

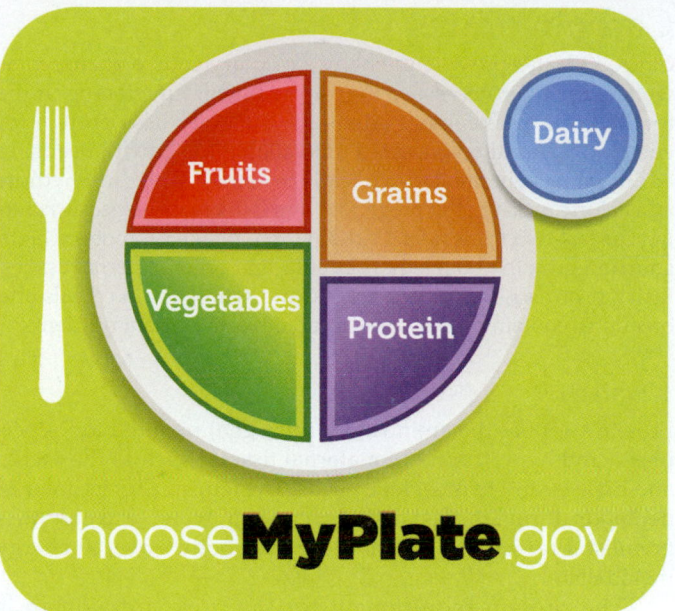

Figure 11–2 MyPlate is part of an initiative to encourage healthy eating. It illustrates the five food groups and encourages people to fill half their plates with fruits and vegetables.

SOURCE: U.S. Department of Agriculture; U.S. Department of Health and Human Services.

The dietary reference intakes (DRIs) for energy do not change during the first trimester. During the second and third trimesters, pregnant women should consume an extra 300 kcal per day. Prepregnant weight, height, maternal age, health status, and activity level all influence caloric needs, and weight should be monitored regularly during the pregnancy. See *Teaching Highlights: Adding 300 Kcal During Pregnancy.*

TEACHING HIGHLIGHTS | Adding 300 kcal During Pregnancy

- The notion of "eating for two" may result in overeating. Emphasize the relatively small increase in calories necessary during pregnancy.
- The additional 300 kcal/day recommended during pregnancy can be achieved by adding two milk servings and one serving of meat or alternative.
- MyPlate is designed to represent the food groups needed to make a balanced diet. Following MyPlate recommendations, women should aim to have half their plate consist of fruits and vegetables, make at least half their grains whole grains, and switch to fat-free or low-fat (1%) milk. Women are encouraged to drink water rather than sugary drinks and to compare the sodium content of foods and choose foods that are lower in sodium (USDA, 2012a). A balanced diet includes the following:
  - *Grains:* Six to eleven servings (one serving = 1 slice bread, ½ hamburger roll, 1 oz dry cereal, 1 tortilla, ½ cup pasta, rice, grits)
  - *Fruits:* Two to four servings; one should be a good source of vitamin C (one serving = 1 medium-sized piece of fruit, ½ cup juice)
  - *Vegetables:* Three to five servings (one serving = 1 cup raw vegetable, 1 cup green leafy vegetable, ½ cup cooked vegetable)
  - *Dairy:* Two to three servings (one serving = 1 cup milk or yogurt, 1.5 oz hard cheese, 2 cups cottage cheese, 1 cup pudding made with milk)
  - *Meats and alternatives:* Two to three servings (one serving = 2 oz cooked lean meat, poultry, or fish; 2 eggs; ½ cup cottage cheese; 1 cup cooked legumes [kidney, lima, garbanzo, or soybeans, split peas]; 6 oz tofu; 2 oz nuts or seeds; 4 tbsp peanut butter)
- Not all foods that are nutritionally equivalent have the same number of calories; it is important to consider that when making food choices.
- Consider using low-fat milk, lean cuts of meat, or fish broiled or baked instead of fried.
- Foods can be combined. For example, 1 cup spaghetti with a 2-oz meatball would count as 1 serving meat, ¾ cup spaghetti = 1 grain, and ¼ cup tomato sauce = ½ serving vegetable.
- Use a calorie-counting guide to compare the calories in a variety of foods that are equivalent, such as 2 oz beef and 2 oz fish or 1 cup low-fat milk and 1 cup whole milk.

Carbohydrates

Carbohydrates provide the body's primary source of energy as well as the fiber necessary for proper bowel functioning. If the total caloric intake is not adequate, the body uses protein for energy. Protein then becomes unavailable for growth needs. In addition, protein breakdown leads to ketosis. The carbohydrate and caloric needs of the pregnant woman increase, especially during the last two trimesters. Carbohydrate intake promotes weight gain and growth of the fetus, placenta, and other maternal tissues. Dairy products, fruits, vegetables, and whole-grain cereals and breads all contain carbohydrates and other important nutrients.

Protein

Protein supplies the amino acids (nitrogen) required for hyperplasia and hypertrophy of maternal tissues, such as the uterus and breasts, and to meet fetal needs. The fetus makes its greatest demands during the last half of pregnancy, when fetal growth is greatest. Protein also contributes to the body's overall energy metabolism.

The protein requirement for the pregnant woman is 60 g/day, an increase of 14 g over nonpregnant levels. Animal products such as meat, fish, poultry, and eggs are sources of high-quality protein. Dairy products are also important protein sources. A quart of milk supplies 32 g of protein, more than half the average daily protein requirement. Milk can be incorporated into the diet in a variety of dishes, including soups, puddings, custards, sauces, and yogurt. Beverages such as hot chocolate and milk-and-fruit drinks can also be included, but they are high in calories. Various kinds of hard and soft cheeses and cottage cheese are excellent protein sources, although cream cheese is categorized as a fat source only.

Women who have allergies to milk, are lactose intolerant, or practice vegetarianism may find soy milk acceptable. Soy milk can be used in cooked dishes or as a beverage. Tofu, or soybean curd, can replace cottage cheese.

Fat

Fats are valuable sources of energy for the body. Fats are more completely absorbed during pregnancy, resulting in a marked increase in serum lipids, lipoproteins, and cholesterol and decreased elimination of fat through the bowel. Fat deposits in the fetus increase from about 2% at midpregnancy to almost 12% at term. However, fat requirements are unchanged during pregnancy and should account for about 20% to 35% of daily caloric intake, of which 10% or less should be saturated fat.

Essential fatty acids are important for the development of the central nervous system of the fetus. Of particular interest are the omega-3 fatty acids and their derivative, docosahexaenoic acid (DHA). Maternal dietary intake of DHA during pregnancy may reduce the risk of preterm birth and low birth weight, and enhance fetal and neonatal brain development (Carlson, Colombo, Gajewski, et al., 2013). Oily fish provide the best source of DHA (however, see the *Mercury in Fish* section later in this chapter); other sources include fortified dairy products, and even some fortified soymilk. Plant sources of omega-3 fatty acids include soybean oil, canola oil, flaxseeds and their oil, and walnuts.

Minerals

Increased minerals needed for the growth of new tissue during pregnancy are obtained by improved mineral absorption and an increase in mineral allowances.

CALCIUM AND PHOSPHORUS

Calcium and phosphorus are involved in the mineralization of fetal bones and teeth as well as acid–base buffering. Calcium is absorbed and used more efficiently during pregnancy. Some calcium and phosphorus are required early in pregnancy, but most fetal bone calcification occurs during the last 2 to 3 months. Teeth begin to form at about 8 weeks' gestation and are formed by birth. The 6-year molars begin to calcify just before birth.

The identified AI for calcium for the pregnant or lactating woman 19 years of age or older is 1000 mg per day. It is 1300 mg per day for pregnant women under age 19. If calcium intake is low, fetal needs will be met at the mother's expense by demineralization of maternal bone.

A diet that includes 4 cups of milk or an equivalent alternative (such as calcium-fortified soy milk or orange juice) and a variety of other foods will provide sufficient calcium. Smaller amounts of calcium are supplied by legumes, nuts, dried fruits, and dark green leafy vegetables (such as kale, cabbage, collards, and turnip greens).

The RDA for phosphorus does not change from that of the nonpregnant woman age 19 or older: 700 mg per day. Similarly for females age 18 and younger it remains stable at 1250 mg per day. Phosphorus is readily supplied through calcium- and protein-rich foods.

IODINE

Iodine is an essential part of the thyroid hormone thyroxine. Inorganic iodine is excreted in the urine during pregnancy. Enlargement of the thyroid gland may occur if iodine is not replaced by adequate dietary intake or an additional supplement. Moreover, cretinism may occur in the baby if the mother has a severe iodine deficiency. The iodine requirement of 220 mcg per day can be met by using iodized salt. When sodium is restricted, the healthcare provider may prescribe an iodine supplement.

SODIUM

The sodium ion is essential for proper metabolism and the regulation of fluid balance. Sodium intake in the form of salt is never entirely curtailed during pregnancy, even when hypertension or preeclampsia is present. The pregnant woman may lightly season food to taste during cooking but should avoid using extra salt at the table. She can avoid excessive intake by eliminating salty foods such as potato chips, ham, sausages, and sodium-based seasonings.

ZINC

Zinc is involved in protein metabolism and the synthesis of deoxyribonucleic acid (DNA) and ribonucleic acid (RNA). It is essential for normal fetal growth and development as well as milk production during lactation. The RDA during pregnancy for women age 19 and older is 11 mg per day. This increases to 12 mg during lactation. Sources include meats, shellfish, poultry, whole grains, and legumes.

MAGNESIUM

Magnesium is essential for cellular metabolism and structural growth. The RDA for pregnant women is 350 mg/day for women ages 19 to 30 and 360 mg for women 31 to 50 years of age. Good sources include milk, whole grains, dark green vegetables, nuts, and legumes.

IRON

Iron requirements increase during pregnancy because of the growth of the fetus and placenta and the expansion of maternal blood volume. Anemia in pregnancy is mainly caused by low iron stores, although it may also be caused by inadequate intake of other nutrients such as vitamins B_6 and B_{12}, folic acid, ascorbic acid, copper, and zinc. Iron deficiency anemia is defined as a decrease in the oxygen-carrying capacity of the blood. Anemia leads to a significant reduction in hemoglobin in the volume of packed red cells per deciliter of blood (hematocrit) or in the number of erythrocytes. Iron deficiency anemia in pregnancy is associated with an increased incidence of low-birth-weight babies and preterm birth (Cunningham, Leveno, Bloom, et al., 2014).

Fetal demands for iron further contribute to symptoms of anemia in the pregnant woman. The fetal liver stores iron, especially during the third trimester. The baby needs this stored iron during the first 4 months of life to compensate for the normally inadequate levels of iron in breast milk and non–iron-fortified formulas.

To prevent anemia, the woman must balance iron requirements and intake. Adequate iron intake is a problem for nonpregnant women and a greater one for pregnant women. By carefully selecting foods high in iron, the woman can increase her daily iron intake considerably. Lean meats, dark green leafy vegetables, eggs, and whole-grain and enriched breads and cereals are the usual food sources of iron. Other iron sources include dried fruits, legumes, shellfish, and molasses.

Iron absorption is generally higher for animal products than for vegetable products. However, the woman can enhance absorption of iron from nonmeat sources by combining them with meat or a food rich in vitamin C. The RDA for iron during pregnancy is 27 mg per day, but this intake is almost impossible to achieve through diet alone. Thus, in the second and third trimesters the pregnant woman should take a daily supplement of 30 mg elemental iron (Hark & Catalano, 2012). Unfortunately iron supplements often cause gastrointestinal discomfort, especially if taken on an empty stomach. Iron supplements may also cause constipation, so an adequate intake of fluid and fiber is especially important in pregnancy.

Vitamins

Vitamins are organic substances necessary for life and growth. They are found in small amounts in specific foods and generally cannot be synthesized by the body in adequate amounts.

Vitamins are grouped according to solubility. Vitamins that dissolve in fat are A, D, E, and K; those soluble in water include vitamin C and the B complex. An adequate intake of all vitamins is essential during pregnancy; however, several are required in larger amounts to fulfill specific needs.

FAT-SOLUBLE VITAMINS

Fat-soluble vitamins A, D, E, and K are stored in the liver and thus are available if the dietary intake becomes inadequate. They are not excreted in the urine, so excessive consumption of these vitamins, particularly vitamins A and D, can lead to toxicity. Symptoms of vitamin toxicity include nausea, gastrointestinal upset, dryness and cracking of the skin, and loss of hair.

Vitamin A.   Vitamin A is involved in the growth of epithelial cells, which line the entire gastrointestinal tract and compose the skin. Vitamin A plays a role in the metabolism of carbohydrates and fats. In the absence of vitamin A, the body cannot synthesize glycogen, and the body's ability to handle cholesterol is also affected. The protective layer of tissue surrounding nerve fibers does not form properly if vitamin A is lacking.

Probably the best known function of vitamin A is its effect on vision in dim light. A person's ability to see in the dark depends on the eye's supply of retinol, a form of vitamin A. In this manner, vitamin A prevents night blindness. Vitamin A is associated with the formation and development of healthy eyes in the fetus. The RDA for vitamin A is 770 mcg/day for pregnant women ages 19 and older.

Although routine supplementation with vitamin A is not recommended, supplementation with 5000 International Units is indicated for women whose dietary intake may be inadequate, specifically strict vegetarians and recent emigrants from countries where deficiency of vitamin A is endemic.

Rich plant sources of vitamin A include deep green, deep orange, and yellow vegetables. Animal sources include egg yolk, cream, butter, and fortified margarine and milk.

Vitamin D.   Vitamin D is critical for the absorption and use of calcium and phosphorus in skeletal development. To supply the needs of the developing fetus, the pregnant woman should have a vitamin D intake of 15 mcg (600 International Units) per day. Main food sources of vitamin D include fortified milk, margarine, butter, liver, and egg yolks. Drinking a quart of milk daily provides the vitamin D needed during pregnancy. Vitamin D is also obtained through the synthesis of sunlight on the skin. However, during the winter months women who live in northern latitudes are at risk for limited sun exposure, as are women who routinely wear sun protection, including high sun protection factor (SPF) products and protective clothing.

Vitamin D deficiency is more common than previously recognized. Although universal screening for vitamin D deficiency is not currently recommended, women at risk (vegetarians, women with limited sun exposure, ethnic and racial groups with dark skin) may be screened. If a deficiency is identified, a daily dose of 1000 to 2000 International Units is safe (ACOG, 2011).

Excessive intake of vitamin D usually comes from taking high-potency vitamin preparations, not from diet. Overdoses during pregnancy can cause hypercalcemia, or high blood calcium levels, because of withdrawal of calcium from the skeletal tissue. Symptoms of toxicity are excessive thirst, loss of appetite, vomiting, weight loss, irritability, and high blood calcium levels.

Vitamin E.   The major function of vitamin E, or tocopherol, is antioxidation. Antioxidants such as vitamin E protect the body's cells from the destructive effects of free radicals. Vitamin E takes on oxygen, thus preventing another substance from combining with the oxygen in a process called *oxidation*. For example, vitamin E helps spare vitamin A by preventing its oxidation in the intestinal tract and in the tissues. It decreases the oxidation of polyunsaturated fats, thus helping to retain the flexibility and health of the cell membrane. In protecting the cell membrane, vitamin E affects the health of all cells in the body.

Vitamin E is also involved in certain enzymatic and metabolic reactions. It is an essential nutrient for the synthesis of nucleic acids required in the formation of red blood cells in the bone marrow. Vitamin E is beneficial in treating certain types of muscular pain and intermittent claudication, in surface healing of wounds and burns, and in protecting lung tissue from the damaging effects of smog. These functions may help explain the abundant claims and cures attributed to vitamin E, many of which have not been scientifically proved.

The recommended intake of vitamin E is unchanged at 15 mg per day. Vitamin E is widely distributed in foodstuffs, especially vegetable fats and oils, whole grains, greens, and eggs. Excessive intake of vitamin E has been associated with abnormal coagulation in the newborn.

Vitamin K.   Vitamin K, or menadione (as used synthetically in medicine), is an essential factor for the synthesis of prothrombin, so its function is related to normal blood clotting. It is synthesized in the intestinal tract by the *Escherichia coli* bacterium normally inhabiting the large intestine. However, the body's need for vitamin K is not totally met by synthesis. Green leafy vegetables are excellent sources. The RDA for vitamin K, 90 mcg per day, does not increase during pregnancy.

Intake of vitamin K is usually adequate in a well-balanced prenatal diet. Secondary problems may arise if an illness is present that results in malabsorption of fats or if antibiotics are used for an extended period, which would inhibit vitamin K synthesis by destroying intestinal *E. coli*.

WATER-SOLUBLE VITAMINS

Water-soluble vitamins are excreted in the urine. Because only small amounts are stored, there is little protection from dietary inadequacies. Thus adequate amounts must be ingested daily. During pregnancy, the concentration of water-soluble vitamins in the maternal serum falls, whereas high concentrations are found in the fetus.

Vitamin C. The requirement for vitamin C (ascorbic acid) increases in pregnancy from 75 to 85 mg per day. The major function of vitamin C is to aid in the formation and development of connective tissue and the vascular system. Ascorbic acid is essential to the formation of collagen, which binds cells together. If the collagen begins to disintegrate because of a lack of ascorbic acid, cell functioning is disturbed and cell structure breaks down, resulting in muscular weakness, capillary hemorrhage, and eventual death. These are symptoms of scurvy, the disease caused by vitamin C deficiency. Newborns of women who have taken megadoses of vitamin C may experience a rebound form of scurvy.

Maternal plasma levels of vitamin C progressively decline during pregnancy, with values at term being about half those at midpregnancy. It appears that ascorbic acid concentrates in the placenta; levels in the fetus are 50% or more above maternal levels.

A nutritious diet should meet the pregnant woman's needs for vitamin C without additional supplementation. Common food sources of vitamin C include citrus fruit, tomatoes, cantaloupe, strawberries, potatoes, broccoli, and other leafy greens. Ascorbic acid is readily destroyed by water and oxidation. Therefore, foods containing vitamin C must be stored and cooked properly.

The B Vitamins. The B vitamins include thiamine (B_1), riboflavin (B_2), niacin, folic acid, pantothenic acid, vitamin B_6, and vitamin B_{12}. These vitamins serve as vital coenzyme factors in many reactions such as cell respiration, glucose oxidation, and energy metabolism. Consequently, the quantities needed invariably increase as caloric intake increases to meet the metabolic and growth needs of the pregnant woman.

- *Thiamine.* Required amount increases from the prepregnant level of 1.1 mg/day to 1.4 mg/day. Sources: pork, liver, milk, potatoes, and enriched breads and cereals.

- *Riboflavin.* Deficiency is manifested by *cheilosis* (fissures and cracks of the lips and corners of the mouth) and other skin lesions. During pregnancy women may excrete less riboflavin and still require more because of increased energy and protein needs. An additional 0.3 mg/day, to 1.4 mg/day, is recommended for pregnant women age 19 and older. Sources: milk, liver, eggs, enriched breads, and cereals.

- *Niacin.* Intake should increase 4 mg/day during pregnancy to 18 mg. Sources: meat, fish, poultry, liver, whole grains, enriched breads, cereals, and peanuts.

- *Folic acid (folate).* Required for normal growth, reproduction, and lactation, **folic acid** prevents the macrocytic, megaloblastic anemia of pregnancy, which is rarely found in the United States, but does occur. Inadequate intake of folic acid has been associated with neural tube defects (NTDs) (spina bifida, meningomyelocele) in the fetus or newborn. Although these defects are considered multifactorial, research indicates that most of these birth defects could be prevented if folic acid supplementation recommendations were followed. Specifically the CDC and the U. S. Public Health Service recommend that all women of childbearing age (15 to 45 years) consume 400 mcg of folic acid daily because half of all U.S. pregnancies are unplanned and NTDs occur very early in pregnancy (3 to 4 weeks after conception), before most women realize they are pregnant (CDC, 2015). Folic acid can be made inactive by oxidation, ultraviolet light, and heating. To prevent unnecessary loss, foods should be stored covered to protect them from light, cooked with only a small amount of water, and not overcooked. Sources: fresh green leafy vegetables, liver, peanuts, and whole-grain breads and cereals.

Healthy People 2020

(MICH-14) Increase the proportion of women of childbearing potential with intake of at least 400 mcg of folic acid from fortified foods or dietary supplements

- *Pantothenic acid.* No allowance has been set during pregnancy, but 5 mg/day is considered a safe, adequate intake. Sources: meats, egg yolk, legumes, and whole-grain cereals and breads.

- *Vitamin B_6 (pyridoxine).* Associated with amino acid metabolism, thus a higher-than-average protein intake requires increased pyridoxine intake. The RDA during pregnancy is 1.9 mg/day, an increase of 0.6 mg over the allowance for nonpregnant women. Generally, the slightly increased need can be supplied by diet. Sources: wheat germ, yeast, fish, liver, pork, potatoes, and lentils.

- *Vitamin B_{12} (cobalamin).* Plays a role in the synthesis of DNA and red blood cells, and is important in maintaining the myelin sheath of nerve cells. Vitamin B_{12} is the cobalt-containing vitamin found only in animal sources. Women of reproductive age rarely have a B_{12} deficiency. Vegetarians/vegans (see later discussion on vegetarianism) can develop a deficiency, however, so it is essential that their dietary intake be supplemented with this vitamin. Occasionally vitamin B_{12} levels decrease during pregnancy but increase again after childbirth. The RDA during pregnancy is 2.6 mcg/day, an increase of 0.2 mcg. A deficiency may be because of a congenital inability to absorb vitamin B_{12}, resulting in pernicious anemia. Infertility is a complication of this type of anemia. Sources: foods that come from animals.

Clinical Tip

More women are consuming over-the-counter (OTC) vitamin, mineral, and food supplements today than in the past. Ask about the use of any OTC supplements to help avoid potentially harmful excess intakes.

Fluid

Water is essential for life, and it is found in all body tissues. Water is necessary for many biochemical reactions. It also serves as a lubricant, as a medium of transport for carrying

Clinical Question

Can prenatal counseling improve the nutritional intake of pregnant women? Are these interventions effective across cultures?

The Evidence

Lack of sound nutritional intake can lead to a host of problems during pregnancy. Excessive weight gain has been linked to significant morbidity for both mother and baby. Even when weight is controlled, many pregnant women do not get adequate dietary intake of fruits, vegetables, and fiber in particular. Current practice guidelines recommend aggressive management of maternal weight before, during, and after pregnancy, and it is widely supported that nutritional counseling can be effective in preventing excessive weight gain. Two studies focused on nutritional counseling as a part of prenatal care, and its effectiveness in affecting eating behavior. In one study, researchers measured whether a relationship existed between healthcare providers discussing diet with their pregnant clients and subsequent changes in dietary intake. A second study reviewed a community-based, healthcare provider–led lifestyle intervention exclusively aimed at Spanish-speaking mothers. Taken together, more than 600 mothers were included in these studies; this yields a strong level of evidence.

The researchers found that healthcare providers can influence maternal nutritional intake when they counsel mothers about its importance during routine prenatal care (May, Suminski, Berry, et al., 2014). Mothers who were provided information in the context of healthy behaviors were more likely to engage in healthy dietary practices during pregnancy than mothers who did not receive counseling from their healthcare providers. Similar findings were yielded in the Spanish-speaking population. When mothers received culturally appropriate interventions about lifestyle modifications in the prenatal period, they were more likely to reduce daily consumption of sugar, saturated fat, and caloric intake, and to increase vegetable and fiber intake (Kieffer, Welmerink, Sinco, et al., 2014).

Best Practice

The healthcare provider can have an impact on prenatal nutrition simply by addressing healthy lifestyle issues during pregnancy. This type of prenatal counseling is effective across other cultures when provided in an appropriate language and in a culturally sensitive way.

Clinical Reasoning

What are some cultural influences on nutrition that should be considered in prenatal counseling? What are other lifestyle behaviors that should be addressed alongside nutritional counseling in prenatal support services?

---

substances in and out of the body, and as an aid in temperature control. A pregnant woman should consume at least eight to ten 8-oz glasses of fluid each day, of which four to six glasses should be water. Because of their sodium content, diet sodas should be consumed in moderation. Caffeinated beverages have a diuretic effect, which is counterproductive to increasing fluid intake.

Vegetarianism

Vegetarianism is the dietary choice of many people for religious, health, or ethical reasons. There are several types of vegetarians. **Lacto-ovovegetarians** include milk, dairy products, and eggs in their diets. **Lactovegetarians** include dairy products but no eggs in their diets. **Vegans** are "pure" vegetarians who will not eat any food from animal sources.

The expectant woman who is vegetarian must eat the proper combination of foods to obtain adequate nutrients. If her diet allows, a woman can obtain ample and complete proteins from dairy products and eggs. An adequate, pure vegan diet contains protein from unrefined grains (brown rice, whole wheat), legumes (beans, split peas, lentils), nuts in large quantities, and a variety of cooked and fresh vegetables and fruits. Complete proteins can be obtained by eating different types of plant-based proteins such as beans and rice, peanut butter on whole-grain bread, and whole-grain cereal with soy milk, either in the same meal or over the day. Seeds may provide adequate protein in the vegan diet if the quantity is large enough. Obtaining sufficient calories to ensure adequate weight gain may be difficult because vegan diets tend to be high in fiber and

therefore filling. Because vegans use no animal products, a daily supplement of 4 mg of vitamin B_{12} is necessary. If soy milk is used, only partial supplementation may be needed. If no soy milk is taken, daily supplements of 1200 mg of calcium and 10 mg of vitamin D are needed.

A vegan diet may be low in iron and zinc because the best sources of these minerals are found in animal products. In addition, a high-fiber intake may reduce mineral (calcium, iron, and zinc) bioavailability. The nurse should emphasize the use of foods containing these nutrients.

A guide to vegetarian food groups is provided in Table 11–2.

Factors Influencing Nutrition

It is important to consider the many factors that affect a client's nutrition. What environmental risks should the woman consider? What are the age, lifestyle, and culture of the pregnant woman? What food beliefs and habits does she have? What a person eats is determined by availability, economics, and symbolism. These factors and others influence the expectant mother's acceptance of dietary recommendations.

Common Discomforts of Pregnancy

Gastrointestinal functioning can be altered at various times throughout pregnancy, resulting in discomforts such as nausea, vomiting, heartburn, and constipation. Although these changes can be uncomfortable for the woman, they are seldom a major problem. These discomforts, as well as dietary modifications that may provide relief, are discussed in Chapter 10.

TABLE 11–2 Vegetarian Food Groups

FOOD GROUP	MIXED DIET	LACTO-OVOVEGETARIAN	LACTOVEGETARIAN	VEGAN
Grain	Bread, cereal, rice, pasta	Bread, cereal, rice, pasta	Bread, cereal, rice, pasta	Bread, cereal, rice, pasta
Fruit	Fruit, fruit juices	Fruit, fruit juices	Fruit, fruit juices	Fruit, fruit juices
Vegetable	Vegetables, vegetable juices	Vegetables, vegetable juices	Vegetables, vegetable juices	Vegetables, vegetable juices
Dairy and dairy alternatives	Milk, yogurt, cheese	Milk, yogurt, cheese	Milk, yogurt, cheese	Fortified soy milk, rice milk
Meat and meat alternatives	Meat, fish, poultry, eggs, legumes, tofu, nuts, nut butters	Eggs, legumes, tofu, nuts, nut butters	Legumes, tofu, nuts, nut butters	Legumes, tofu, nuts, nut butters

Complementary Health Approaches

While the use of complementary health approaches, such as herbal, botanical, and alternative therapies, may seem like a natural and safe alternative to some individuals, the pregnant consumer should take caution. Very few clinical trials exist that have examined the safety of supplements and herbs during pregnancy. Many herbs, such as black haw, chamomile, dandelion, ginger, nettle leaf, and red raspberry are considered safe for use in pregnancy. Other herbs could pose a risk (Shinde, Patil, & Bairagi, 2012). Pregnant women should be advised to consult reputable sources such as the National Center for Complementary and Integrative Health website about these therapies and should also speak with their healthcare providers to determine the safety of such products or therapies.

Use of Artificial Sweeteners

Foods and beverages that contain artificial sweeteners are increasingly available. Sweeteners classified as generally recognized as safe (GRAS) by the U.S. Food and Drug Administration (FDA) are acceptable for use during pregnancy and include acesulfame potassium (Sweet One), aspartame (NutraSweet, Equal), saccharin (Sweet'N Low, Sugar Twin), sucralose (Splenda), and stevia (Truvia, PureVia, SunCrystals). As with other foods, moderation should be exercised in using artificial sweeteners.

Energy Drinks

Energy drinks, such as Monster Energy, Red Bull, and 5-Hour Energy, used to boost performance and delay fatigue have become increasingly popular in recent years. These beverages are soft drinks with ingredients such as caffeine, ginseng, guarana, taurine, and sugar added to provide stimulation and increase energy. Because they are classified as dietary supplements and not food, they are not subject to the same regulations and monitoring as food (Guilbeau, 2012). The caffeine content of energy drinks can be as high as 300 mg (equivalent to about three average cups of brewed coffee). Excessive intake of energy drinks can cause a variety of symptoms including anxiety, headache, agitation, tremors, seizures, psychosis, and altered mental state (Rath, 2012).

Energy drinks have come under scrutiny for the general public because of concerns about workplace safety when drinks are used to counter the effects of inadequate sleep and reports of deaths following excessive use (Meier, 2012). Research on the effects of caffeine on pregnancy are mixed; therefore, pregnant women are advised to use energy drinks cautiously and include the drink's caffeine content in calculating daily caffeine intake in order to stay within recommended levels.

Mercury in Fish

Fish and shellfish are important parts of a healthy diet, but nearly all contain traces of mercury. Although this is not a concern for most people, some fish and shellfish contain higher levels of methyl mercury than others, and methyl mercury can pose a threat to the developing nervous system of a fetus or young child.

SAFETY ALERT!

Women who are pregnant or who may become pregnant, breast-feeding mothers, and young children should not eat swordfish, shark, tilefish, or king mackerel because these fish contain high levels of methyl mercury.

Many pregnant women are aware of the mercury warning, but far less aware of the important nutritional value of fish, especially fish high in DHA. Consequently fish consumption has declined but a strong body of evidence supports the nutritional value of fish during pregnancy (Carlson et al., 2013). Thus, pregnant women need to be encouraged to eat at least 8 oz and up to 12 oz/week (two average meals) of a variety of shellfish and fish that are lower in mercury (USDA, 2012b). Commonly eaten fish that are lower in mercury include canned light tuna, shrimp, salmon, trout, sardines, and pollack. Albacore (white) tuna has more mercury than canned light tuna; therefore only 6 oz/week of albacore tuna is recommended.

Foodborne Illnesses

Because of the risk of *Salmonella* contamination in raw eggs, pregnant women are advised to avoid eating or tasting foods that may contain raw or lightly cooked eggs. These foods include, for example, cake batter, homemade eggnog, sauces made with raw eggs such as Caesar salad dressing, and homemade ice cream.

Listeria monocytogenes is another bacterium that poses a threat to an expectant mother and her fetus. Listeria organisms are especially challenging because they can be found in refrigerated, ready-to-eat foods such as unpasteurized milk and dairy products, meat, poultry, and seafood. To prevent listerial infection (listeriosis), pregnant women should be advised to do the following (U.S. Food and Drug Administration [FDA], 2015):

- Maintain refrigerator temperature at 4°C (40°F) or below and the freezer at –18°C (0°F).
- Refrigerate or freeze prepared foods, leftovers, and perishables within 2 hours after eating or preparation.
- Do not eat hot dogs, deli meats, or luncheon meats unless they are reheated until they are steaming hot or 165°F.
- Avoid soft cheeses such as feta, brie, Camembert, blue veined cheeses, queso fresco, or queso blanco unless the label clearly states that they are made with pasteurized milk.
- Do not eat refrigerated pâtés or meat spreads or foods that contain raw (unpasteurized) milk or drink unpasteurized milk.
- Avoid eating refrigerated smoked seafood such as salmon, trout, cod, tuna, or mackerel unless it is in a cooked dish such as a casserole. Canned or shelf-stable pâtés, meat spreads, and smoked seafood are considered safe to eat.

Lactase Deficiency (Lactose Intolerance)

Some individuals have difficulty digesting milk and milk products. This condition, known as **lactase deficiency** or **lactose intolerance**, results from an inadequate amount of the enzyme lactase, which breaks down the milk sugar lactose into smaller digestible substances.

Lactase deficiency is found in many adults of African, Mexican, Native American, Ashkenazi Jewish, and Asian descent and, indeed, in many other adults worldwide. People who are not affected are mainly of northern European heritage. Symptoms may include abdominal distention, discomfort, nausea, vomiting, loose stools, and cramps.

In counseling pregnant women who might be intolerant of milk and milk products, the nurse should be aware that tolerances vary among individuals and even one glass of milk can produce symptoms. Milk in cooked form, such as custards, is sometimes tolerated, as are cultured or fermented dairy products such as buttermilk, some cheeses, kefir, and yogurt. Lactase deficiency need not be a problem for pregnant women because the enzyme is available over the counter in tablets or drops. Lactase-treated milk is also available commercially in most large grocery stores.

Cultural, Ethnic, and Religious Influences

Cultural, ethnic, and occasionally religious backgrounds determine one's experiences with food and influence food preferences and habits (Figure 11–3). People of different nationalities are accustomed to eating different foods because of the kinds of foodstuffs available in their countries of origin. The way food is prepared varies, depending on the customs and traditions of the ethnic and cultural group. In addition, the laws of certain religions sanction particular foods, prohibit others, and direct the preparation and serving of meals (see *Developing Cultural Competence: Dietary Practices to Protect Health*).

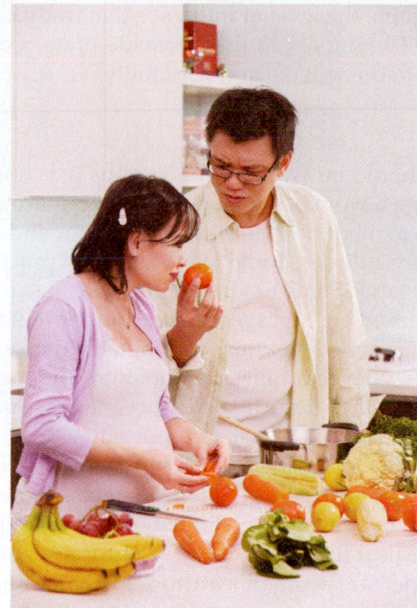

Figure 11–3 Cultural factors affect food preferences and habits.

SOURCE: © Arto / Fotolia.

Developing Cultural Competence Dietary Practices to Protect Health

Dietary practices to protect health vary across the world but many are practiced to maintain health and prevent illness. Following are a few examples (Spector, 2013):

- The kosher diet followed by many Jewish people forbids the eating of pork products and shellfish. In addition, according to kosher dietary rules, meat and dairy products should not be mixed and eaten at the same meal.
- Many Muslims also avoid pork products and the meats that are eaten must be *halel* or approved by Islamic law.
- Among some traditional Chinese people thousand-year old-eggs are viewed as health promoting and are eaten with rice.
- In some Italian, Greek, or Native American homes garlic or onions may be eaten, worn on the body, or hung in the home to prevent illness.
- In some Hispanic homes foods must be balanced between those that are considered to be *hot* and those that are considered to be *cold*.

In each culture, certain foods have symbolic significance. Generally these symbolic foods are related to major life experiences such as birth, death, or developmental milestones. Although generalizations have been made about the food practices of ethnic and religious groups, there are many variations. The extent to which individuals continue to consume traditional ethnic foods and follow food-related ethnic customs is affected by the extent of exposure to other cultures; the availability, quality, and cost of traditional foods; and the recency of immigration.

When working with pregnant women from any ethnic background, it is important for the nurse to understand the impact of the woman's cultural and spiritual beliefs on her eating habits and to identify any beliefs the woman may have about food and pregnancy. Talking with the client can help the nurse determine the level of influence that traditional food customs exert. The nurse can then provide dietary advice that is meaningful to the woman and her family.

Psychosocial Factors

The nurse should be aware of the various psychosocial factors that influence a woman's food choices. The sharing of food has long been a symbol of friendliness, warmth, and social acceptance in many cultures. Some foods and food practices are associated with status. Some foods are prepared "just for company"; others are served only on special occasions or holidays.

Socioeconomic level may be a determinant of nutritional status. Poverty-level families cannot afford the same foods that higher-income families can. Thus pregnant women with low incomes are frequently at risk for poor nutrition.

Knowledge about the basic components of a balanced diet is essential. Often educational level is related to economic status, but even people on very limited incomes can prepare well-balanced meals if their knowledge of nutrition is adequate.

The expectant woman's attitudes and feelings about her pregnancy influence her nutritional status. For example, foods may be used as a substitute for the expression of emotions, such as anger or frustration, or as a way of expressing feelings of joy. The woman who is depressed or does not wish to be pregnant may manifest these feelings in loss of appetite or overindulgence in certain foods.

Eating Disorders

Two serious eating disorders, *anorexia nervosa* and *bulimia nervosa* (or simply *bulimia*), develop most commonly in adolescent girls and young women. Both conditions are psychiatric disorders that can have a major impact on physiologic well-being.

Anorexia nervosa is an eating disorder characterized by an extreme fear of weight gain and fat. People with this problem have distorted body images and perceive themselves as fat even when they are extremely underweight. Their dietary intake is very restrictive in both variety and quantity. They may also engage in excessive exercise to prevent weight gain. Bulimia is characterized by binge eating (secretly consuming large amounts of food in a short time) and purging. Self-induced vomiting is the most common method of purging; laxatives and/or diuretics may also be used. Individuals with bulimia nervosa often maintain normal or near-normal weight for their height, so it is difficult to know whether bingeing and purging occur.

Women with anorexia nervosa do not often become pregnant because of the physiologic changes that affect their reproductive systems. Women with bulimia can become pregnant. Their self-induced vomiting may produce many of the same complications as hyperemesis gravidarum (see Chapter 15). The consequences of the restricting, bingeing, and purging behaviors characteristic of eating disorders can result in a lack of nutrients available for the fetus. When working with a pregnant woman with an eating disorder, education and individualized meal plans can help the woman increase her dietary intake while maintaining a sense of control. In both anorexia nervosa and bulimia, a multidisciplinary approach to treatment involving medical, nursing, psychiatric, and dietetic practitioners is indicated. Pregnant women with eating disorders need to be closely monitored and supported throughout their pregnancies.

Pica

Pica is the craving for and persistent eating of nonnutritive substances, such as soil or clay (geophagia), powdered

---

Clinical Reasoning **Weight Gain in Pregnancy**

Jaya Singh, a 28-year-old G1P0, is 14 weeks pregnant. The rate and total amount of her weight gain during the first trimester have been consistent with recommendations. She has gained an average of 0.5 kg (1 lb) per week during both of the past 2 weeks. Her appetite is good, and she consumes three meals per day and snacks between meals on occasion.

Jaya has altered her diet because she is concerned about excessive weight gain. She told you that she has decreased her intake from the bread and dairy groups in order to limit her caloric intake. Because she has omitted most dairy products, she has increased her consumption of salads and broccoli to provide calcium sources.

A diet history revealed the following:

Grain	3–4 servings, mainly cereal and rice
Fruit	2–4 servings, fresh fruit
Vegetables	3–5 servings, salads, peas, corn, broccoli
Meat	4–5 servings, beef, pork, chicken
Dairy	Occasionally cheese, ice cream, pudding
Fats, oils, sweets	Occasionally salad dressings, margarine, desserts
Beverages	8–10 servings, soda, juices, water

After assessing her diet history, what is your evaluation of Jaya's diet? How would you counsel her?

---

laundry starch or corn starch (amylophagia), soap, baking powder, freezer frost, ice (pagophagia), charcoal, burnt matches, paint, or ashes, that are not ordinarily considered edible or nutritionally valuable. Most women who eat such substances do so only during pregnancy.

Iron deficiency anemia is the most common concern in pica. The ingestion of laundry starch or certain types of clay may contribute to iron deficiency by replacing iron-containing foods from the diet or by interfering with iron absorption. Women with pica that involves eating ice or freezer frost often have poor weight gain because of lack of appetite, whereas the ingestion of starch may be associated with excessive weight gain. The ingestion of large quantities of clay could fill the intestine and cause fecal impaction.

Assessment for pica is an important part of a nutritional history. However, a woman may be embarrassed about her cravings or reluctant to discuss them for fear of criticism. Using a nonjudgmental approach, the nurse can provide the woman with information that is useful in helping her to decrease or eliminate this practice. Some women are able to switch to eating nonfat powdered milk instead of powdered laundry starch and frozen fruit juice instead of ice. Others find that sucking on hard lemon or mint candies helps decrease the craving.

Nutritional Care of the Pregnant Adolescent

Nutritional care of the pregnant adolescent is of particular concern to healthcare professionals. Many adolescents are nutritionally at risk because of a variety of complex and interrelated emotional, social, and economic factors. Important nutrition-related factors to assess in pregnant adolescents include low prepregnant weight, low weight gain during pregnancy, young age at menarche, smoking, excessive prepregnant weight, anemia, unhealthy lifestyle (drugs or alcohol use), chronic disease, and history of an eating disorder.

The nutritional needs of adolescents are generally determined by using the dietary references intakes (DRI) for nonpregnant teenagers (ages 11 to 14 or 15 to 18) and adding nutrient amounts recommended for all pregnant women. If she is mature (more than 4 years since menarche), the pregnant adolescent's nutritional needs approach those reported for pregnant adults. However, adolescents who become pregnant less than 4 years after menarche are at high biologic risk because of their physiologic and anatomic immaturity. They are more likely than older adolescents to still be growing, which can impact the fetus's development. Thus young adolescents (age 14 and under) need to gain more weight than older adolescents (18 years and older) to produce babies of equal size.

In determining the optimal weight gain for the pregnant adolescent, the nurse adds the recommended weight gain for an adult pregnancy to that expected during the postmenarchal year in which the pregnancy occurs. If the teenager is underweight, additional weight gain is recommended to bring her to a normal weight for her height.

Specific Nutrient Concerns

Caloric needs of pregnant adolescents vary widely. Major factors in determining caloric needs include whether growth has been completed and the physical activity level of the individual. Figures as high as 50 kcal/kg have been suggested for young, pregnant adolescents who are very active physically. A satisfactory weight gain usually confirms an adequate caloric intake.

An inadequate iron intake is a major concern with the adolescent diet. Iron needs are high for the pregnant teen because of the requirement for iron by the enlarging maternal muscle mass and blood volume. Iron supplements—providing between 30 and 60 mg of elemental iron—are definitely indicated.

Calcium is another nutrient that demands special attention from pregnant adolescents. Inadequate intake of calcium is frequently a problem in this age group. Adequate calcium intake is necessary to support normal growth and development of the fetus as well as growth and maintenance of calcium stores in the adolescent. An extra serving of dairy products is usually suggested for teenagers. Calcium supplementation is indicated for teens who dislike milk, unless they consume enough other dairy products or significant calcium sources.

Because folic acid plays a role in cell reproduction, it is also an important nutrient for pregnant teens. As previously indicated, a supplement is usually recommended for all pregnant females, whether adult or teenager.

Other nutrients and vitamins must be considered when evaluating the overall nutritional quality of the teenager's diet. Nutrients that have frequently been found to be deficient in this age group include zinc and vitamins A, D, and B_6. Inclusion of a wide variety of foods—especially fresh and lightly processed foods—is helpful in obtaining adequate amounts of trace minerals, fiber, and other vitamins.

Dietary Patterns

Healthy adolescents often have irregular eating patterns. Many skip breakfast, and most tend to be frequent snackers. Teens rarely follow the traditional three-meals-a-day pattern. Their day-to-day intake often varies drastically, and they eat food combinations that may seem bizarre to adults. Despite these practices, adolescents usually achieve a better nutritional balance than most adults would expect.

In assessing the diet of the pregnant adolescent, the nurse should consider the eating pattern over time, not simply a single day's intake. Once the pattern is identified, counseling can be directed toward correcting deficiencies.

Counseling Issues

Counseling about nutrition and healthy eating practices is an important element of care for pregnant teenagers that nurses can effectively provide in a community setting. If an adolescent's family member does most of the meal preparation, it may be useful to include that person in the discussion if the adolescent agrees. Involving the expectant father in counseling may also be beneficial. Clinics and schools often offer classes and focused activities designed to address this topic.

The pregnant teenager will soon become a parent, and her understanding of nutrition will influence not only her well-being but also that of her child. However, teens tend to live in the present, and counseling that stresses long-term changes may be less effective than more concrete approaches. In many cases group classes are effective, especially those with other teens. In a group atmosphere, adolescents often work together to plan adequate meals including foods that are special favorites.

Nursing Management

For the Pregnant Woman Desiring Optimum Nutrition

Nursing Assessment and Diagnosis

To plan an optimal diet with each woman, it is essential to assess nutritional status. The woman's medical record and a client interview provide information about the following:

- Woman's height and weight, as well as her weight gain during pregnancy
- Pertinent laboratory values, especially hemoglobin and hematocrit
- Clinical signs that have possible nutritional implications, such as constipation, anorexia, or heartburn
- Dietary history to evaluate the woman's views on nutrition as well as her specific nutrient intake.

You can obtain a dietary history by asking the woman to complete a 24-hour diet recall, in which she lists everything she has eaten in the past 24 hours, including foods, fluids, and any supplements. At least 3 days of recall should be done to compensate for daily variations. Diet may also be evaluated using a food frequency questionnaire. The questionnaire lists common categories of foods and asks the woman how frequently in a day (or a week) she consumes food from the list. Common categories include vegetables, fruits, milk or cheese, meat or poultry, fish, desserts or sweets, coffee or tea, and alcohol. This method may be less reliable because it requires a person to be accurate about intake.

While gathering data, you have an opportunity to discuss important aspects of nutrition within the context of the family's needs and lifestyle. Seek information about psychologic, cultural, and socioeconomic factors that may influence food intake.

Once the data is obtained, begin to analyze the information, formulate appropriate nursing diagnoses, and, with the woman, develop goals and desired outcomes. For a woman during the first trimester, for example, the diagnosis may be *Nutrition, Imbalanced: Less than Body Requirements* related to nausea and vomiting. In other cases, the diagnosis may be related to excessive weight gain. In such situations the diagnosis might be *Overweight, Risk for,* related to excessive caloric intake. Although these diagnoses are broad, the nurse needs to be specific in addressing issues such as inadequate intake of nutrients including iron, calcium, or folic acid; problems with nutrition because of a limited food budget; problems related to physiologic alterations including anorexia, heartburn, or nausea; and behavioral problems related to excessive dieting, binge eating, and so on. At other times the diagnosis *Knowledge, Readiness for Enhanced,* **related to nutrition** may seem most appropriate, especially if the woman asks for information about nutrition.

Nursing Plan and Implementation

After determining the nursing diagnosis, plan an approach to address any nutritional deficiencies or improve the overall quality of the diet. To be truly effective, this plan must be made in cooperation with the woman. The following example demonstrates ways in which you can plan with the woman based on the nursing diagnosis (NANDA-I © 2014).

- *Diagnosis: Nutrition, Imbalanced: Less than Body Requirements* related to low intake of calcium
- *Client goal:* The woman will increase her daily intake of calcium to the DRI level.
- *Implementation:*

  1. Plan with the woman how to add more milk or dairy products to the diet (specify amounts).
  2. Encourage the use of other calcium sources such as leafy greens and legumes.
  3. Plan for the addition of powdered milk in cooking and baking.
  4. If none of the preceding options is realistic or acceptable, consider the use of calcium supplements.

Health Promotion Optimizing Maternal–Fetal Health

- Achieve appropriate weight gain based on prepregnancy weight and BMI
- Participate in regular physical activity (at least 30 minutes of moderate, safe activity on most, if not all, days)
- Consume a variety of healthy foods that form the basic food groups, including fruits, vegetables, grains, proteins, and dairy using MyPlate as a guideline
- Consume 8 to 12 ounces of fish high in omega-3 fatty acids weekly
- Take appropriate vitamin and mineral supplements
- Consume caffeine in moderation
- Avoid alcohol, tobacco, and other harmful substances
- Follow safe food handling practices.

Source: Data from the American College of Obstetricians and Gynecologists (2013). Nutrition during pregnancy. Patient Education Pamphlet AP001. Washington, DC: Author.

Most families can benefit from guidance about food purchasing and preparation. Women should be advised to plan food purchases thoughtfully by preparing general menus and a list before shopping. It may be helpful to offer clients techniques for keeping food costs down, such as monitoring sales, comparing brands, limiting "convenience" foods, buying food in season, using bulk foods when appropriate, using whole-grain or enriched products, and buying lower-grade eggs (grading has no relation to the egg's nutritional value).

Health Promotion: Optimizing Maternal–Fetal Health summarizes key actions pregnant women can take to optimize maternal health and reduce the risk of birth defects.

Evaluation

Once a plan has been developed and implemented, you and the client may wish to identify ways of evaluating its effectiveness. Evaluation may involve keeping a food journal, writing out weekly menus, returning for weekly weigh-ins, and the like. If anemia is a special problem, periodic hematocrit assessments are indicated.

Refer to a dietitian a woman with serious nutritional deficiencies. You can then work closely with the dietitian and the client to improve the pregnant woman's health by modification of her diet.

KEY FACTS TO REMEMBER
Prenatal Nutrition

- The pregnant woman should eat regularly, three meals a day, and snack on fruits, cheese, milk, or other nutritious foods between meals if desired.
- More frequent but smaller meals are recommended.
- The woman should diet *only* under the guidance of her primary healthcare provider.
- Water is an essential nutrient. The woman should drink 4 to 6 (8-oz) glasses of water and a total of 8 to 10 glasses of fluid daily.
- If the diet is adequate, iron is the only supplement necessary during pregnancy.
- A multivitamin supplement is indicated for women with a poor diet and for those at high nutritional risk.
- To avoid possible deficiencies, many caregivers also recommend a daily vitamin supplement.
- Taking megadoses of vitamins during pregnancy is unnecessary and potentially dangerous.

Postpartum Nutrition

Nutritional needs change following childbirth. Nutrient requirements vary depending on whether the mother decides to breastfeed. An assessment of postpartum nutritional status is necessary before nutritional guidance is given.

Postpartum Nutritional Status

Postpartum nutritional status is determined primarily by assessing the new mother's weight, hemoglobin and hematocrit levels, clinical signs, and dietary history. After birth there is a weight loss of approximately 10 to 12 lb (4.5 kg to 5.4 kg).

Additional weight loss is most rapid during the next few weeks as the body adjusts to the completion of pregnancy. Weight stabilization may take 6 months or longer.

The amount of weight gained during pregnancy is a major determinant of weight loss after childbirth. Generally, women who gain excessive weight during pregnancy are more likely to sustain a weight gain 1 year following childbirth, putting them at increased risk of long-term overweight or obesity.

The mother's weight should be considered in terms of ideal weight, prepregnancy weight, and weight gain during pregnancy. Women who desire information about weight reduction can be referred to a dietitian for individual counseling or to community-based educational programs.

Hemoglobin and erythrocyte levels should return to normal within 2 to 6 weeks after childbirth. Hematocrit levels gradually rise because of hemoconcentration as extracellular fluid is excreted. Iron supplements are generally continued for 2 to 3 months following childbirth to replenish stores depleted by pregnancy.

The nurse assesses clinical symptoms the new mother may be experiencing. Constipation, in particular, is a common problem following birth and can be prevented if the woman maintains a high fluid intake to keep the stool soft. Dietary sources of fiber, such as whole grains, fruits, and vegetables, are also helpful in preventing constipation.

The nurse obtains specific information on dietary intake and eating habits directly from the woman. Visiting the mother during mealtimes provides an opportunity for unobtrusive nutritional assessment. Which foods has the woman selected? Is her diet nutritionally sound? A comment focusing on a positive aspect of her meal selection may initiate a discussion of nutrition.

The nurse needs to notify the dietitian of any woman whose cultural or religious beliefs require specific foods so appropriate meals can be prepared for her. The nurse may also refer women with unusual eating habits or numerous questions about good nutrition to the dietitian. In addition, the nurse provides literature on nutrition so that the woman will have a source of appropriate information at home.

During the childbearing years the risk for obesity becomes especially problematic for women. Consequently it is critical to use the postpartum period to change behaviors and help promote effective weight management in women.

Nutritional Care of Formula-Feeding Mothers

After birth, the formula-feeding mother's dietary requirements return to prepregnancy levels. If the mother has a good understanding of nutritional principles, it is sufficient to advise her to reduce her daily caloric intake by about 300 kcal and to return to prepregnancy levels for other nutrients. If the mother has a limited understanding of nutrition, now is the time to teach her the basic principles and the importance of a well-balanced diet. Her eating habits and dietary practices will eventually be reflected in the diet of her child.

If the mother has gained excessive weight during pregnancy (or perhaps was overweight before pregnancy) and wishes to lose weight, a referral to a dietitian is appropriate. The dietitian can design weight-reduction diets to meet nutritional needs and food preferences. Weight loss goals of 1 to 2 lb (0.45 to 0.9 kg)/week are usually suggested.

In addition to meeting her own nutritional needs, the new mother is usually interested in learning how to provide for her baby's nutritional needs. A discussion of newborn and infant feeding that includes topics such as selecting newborn and infant formulas, formula preparation, and vitamin and mineral supplementation is appropriate and generally well received.

Nutritional Care of Breastfeeding Mothers

Nutrient needs are increased during breastfeeding. Table 11–1 provides a sample daily food guide for lactating women.

It is especially important for the breastfeeding mother to consume sufficient calories, because inadequate caloric intake can reduce milk volume. However, milk quality generally remains unaffected. The breastfeeding mother should increase her calories by about 200 kcal over her pregnancy requirement, or 500 kcal over her prepregnancy requirement. This results in a total of about 2,500 to 2,700 kcal per day for most women.

Because protein is an important ingredient in breast milk, an adequate intake while breastfeeding is essential. An intake of 65 g/day during the first 6 months of breastfeeding and 62 g/day during the second 6 months is recommended. As in pregnancy, it is important to consume adequate nonprotein calories to prevent the use of protein as an energy source.

Calcium is an important ingredient in milk production, and requirements during lactation remain the same as during pregnancy—an increase of 1,000 mg/day. If the intake of calcium from food sources is not adequate, calcium supplements are recommended.

Because iron is not a principal mineral component of milk, the needs of lactating women are not substantially different from those of nonpregnant women. As previously mentioned, however, supplementation for 2 to 3 months after childbirth is advisable to replenish maternal stores depleted by pregnancy.

Clinical Tip

Explain to breastfeeding mothers that liquids are especially important during lactation, because inadequate fluid intake may decrease milk volume. Encourage them to drink at least eight to ten 8-oz glasses of fluid daily, including water, juice, milk, and soups.

In addition to counseling nursing mothers on how to meet their increased nutrient needs during breastfeeding, it is important to discuss a few issues related to newborn and infant feeding. For example, many mothers are concerned about how specific foods they eat will affect their babies during breastfeeding. Generally the nursing mother need not avoid any foods except those to which she might be allergic. Occasionally, however, some nursing mothers find that their babies are affected by certain foods; that is, they may cause the baby to be colicky after nursing, or to develop a skin rash. Onions, turnips, cabbage, chocolate, spices, and seasonings are common offenders. The best advice to give the nursing mother is to avoid those foods she suspects cause distress in her baby. For the most part, however, she should be able to eat any nourishing food she wants without fear that her baby will be affected. For further discussion of successful newborn/infant feeding, see Chapter 25.

Community Resources

Food is a significant portion of a family's budget, and meeting nutritional needs may be a challenge for families on limited incomes. Community-based services offered through clinics, local agencies, schools, and volunteer organizations address these needs. Increasingly nurses play an important role in managing such community-based services, especially services focusing on client education. Most communities offer special assistance to qualifying families to meet their nutritional needs. The Supplemental Nutrition Assistance Program (SNAP), formerly referred to as the Food Stamp Program, provides an Electronic Benefit Transfer or EBT card, which is similar to a debit card, for participating households whose net monthly income is below a specified level. This card can be used to purchase food for the household each month.

The Special Supplemental Nutrition Program for Women, Infants, and Children (WIC) is designed to assist pregnant or breastfeeding women with low incomes and their children under 5 years of age. To be eligible, applicants must meet income guidelines (income at or below 185% of the U.S. poverty level) and state residency requirements, and be individually determined to be nutritionally at risk by a healthcare professional (Food and Nutrition Service, 2013). The program provides food assistance, nutrition education, and referrals to healthcare providers. The food distributed, including dried beans and peas, peanut butter, eggs, cheese, milk, fortified adult and infant cereals, juice, and iron-fortified formula, is designed to provide good sources of iron, protein, and certain vitamins and minerals for people with an inadequate diet.

Focus Your Study

- Maternal weight gains averaging 11.5 to 16.0 kg (25 to 35 lb) for normal-weight women are associated with the best reproductive outcomes.

- If the diet is adequate, folic acid and iron are the only supplements generally recommended during pregnancy.

- Because of the risk of neural tube defects, all women of childbearing age should be encouraged to take a 0.4-mg supplement of folic acid daily.

- Women should not restrict caloric intake to reduce weight during pregnancy.

- It is most healthful for pregnant women to eat regularly and choose a wide variety of foods, especially fresh and lightly processed foods.

- Taking megadoses of vitamins during pregnancy is unnecessary and potentially dangerous.

- Pregnant women who eat vegetarian/vegan diets should place special emphasis on obtaining ample protein, calories, calcium, iron, vitamin D, vitamin B$_{12}$, and zinc through food sources or supplementation if necessary.

- Pregnant women should avoid eating fish that contain high levels of mercury such as swordfish, shark, tilefish, or king mackerel and limit their intake of fish that are lower in mercury.

- Food safety and sanitation should be a priority when preparing and storing food; foods that are known to cause foodborne illness should be avoided during pregnancy.

- Evaluation of physical, psychosocial, and cultural factors that affect food intake is essential before the nurse can determine nutritional status and plan nutritional counseling.

- Adolescents who become pregnant less than 4 years after menarche have higher nutritional needs than older pregnant adolescents and are considered to be at high biologic risk.

- Weight gains during adolescent pregnancy need to accommodate recommended gains for a normal pregnancy plus necessary gains because of maternal growth.

- After giving birth, the formula-feeding mother's dietary requirements return to prepregnancy levels.

- Breastfeeding mothers need an additional 200 kcal above pregnancy intake and increased fluid intake to maintain ample milk volume.

Clinical Reasoning in Action

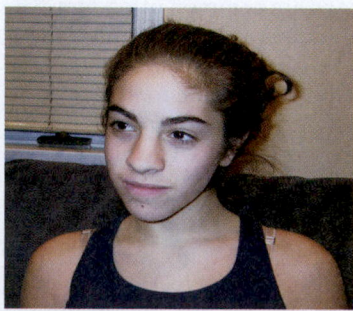

Sandra Hill is a 17-year-old at 19 weeks' gestation with her first pregnancy. She presents to you accompanied by her mother. Her mother tells you that Sandra is an active teenager who plays sports and has been taking dance lessons for 5 years. She maintains a B- average in school. Sandra voices concern about potential weight gain during pregnancy. She tells you that this was not a planned pregnancy and she has ambivalent feelings about it. You become concerned as she tells you that she has reduced her caloric intake over the last few months to try to keep her weight down and camouflage her pregnancy. You do a nutritional assessment and find that she is deficient in calcium, iron, and protein. Sandra seems to have irregular eating patterns and she admits to skipping breakfast often. She asks why she has to gain so much weight when you explain the nutritional needs of her baby during the pregnancy.

1. Discuss weight distribution in pregnancy.

2. Discuss foods that will increase calcium, protein, and iron in her diet.

3. Explain why folate supplementation is important.

4. What criteria will measure adequate caloric intake during pregnancy?

References

American College of Obstetricians and Gynecologists (ACOG). (2011). *Vitamin D: Screening and supplementation during pregnancy*. (Committee Opinion No. 495). Washington, DC: Author.

American College of Obstetricians and Gynecologists (ACOG). (2013a). *Obesity in pregnancy*. (Committee Opinion No. 549). Washington, DC: Author.

American College of Obstetricians and Gynecologists (ACOG). (2013b). *Weight gain during pregnancy*. (Committee Opinion No. 548). Washington, DC: Author.

Carlson, S. E., Colombo, J., Gajewski, B. J., Gustafson, K. M., Mundy, D., Yeast, J., . . . Shaddy, D. J. (2013). DHA supplementation and pregnancy outcomes. *The American Journal of Clinical Nutrition, 97*(4), 808–815.

Centers for Disease Control and Prevention (CDC) and the U. S. Public Health Service. (2015). *Folic acid: Recommendations*. Retrieved from http://www.cdc.gov/ncbddd/folicacid/recommendations.html

Cunningham, F. G., Leveno, K. J., Bloom, S. L., Spong, C. Y., Dashe, J. S., Hoffman, B. L., . . . Sheffield, J. S. (2014). *Williams obstetrics* (24th ed.). New York, NY: McGraw-Hill.

Food and Nutrition Service. (2013). *WIC: The special supplemental nutrition program for women, infants, and children*. Retrieved from http://www.fns.usda.gov/wic/default.htm

Guilbeau, J. R. (2012). Health risks of energy drinks. *Nursing for Women's Health, 16*(5), 423–428.

Hark, L., & Catalano, P. M. (2012). Nutritional management during pregnancy. In S. G. Gabbe, J. R. Niebyl, J. L. Simpson, M. B. Landon, H. L. Galan, E. R. M. Jauniaux, & D. A. Driscoll (Eds.), *Obstetrics: Normal and problem pregnancies* (6th ed.). Philadelphia, PA: Elsevier Saunders.

Institute of Medicine (IOM). (2009). *Weight gain during pregnancy: Reexamining the guidelines*. Retrieved from http://www.iom.edu/Reports/2009/Weight-Gain-During-Pregnancy-reexamining-the-Guidelines.aspx

Kieffer, E., Welmerink, D., Sinco, B., Welch, K., Clayton, E., Schumann, C., & Uhley, V. (2014). Dietary outcomes in a Spanish-language randomized controlled diabetes prevention trial with pregnant Latinas. *American Journal of Public Health, 104*(3), 526–533.

May, L., Suminski, R., Berry, A., Linklater, E., & Jahnke, S. (2014). Diet and pregnancy: Healthcare providers and patient behaviors. *The Journal of Perinatal Education, 23*(1), 50–56.

Meier, B. (2012). F.D.A. may tap experts on energy drinks. *New York Times*. Retrieved from http://www.nytimes.com/2012/11/28/business/fda-may-tap-experts-on-energy-drinks.html?_r=0

Rath, M. (2012). Energy drinks: What is all the hype? The dangers of energy drink consumption. *Journal of the American Academy of Nurse Practitioners, 24*(2), 70–76.

Shinde, P., Patil, P., & Bairagi, V. (2012). Herbs in pregnancy and lactation: A review appraisal. *International Journal of Pharmaceutical Sciences and Research, 3*(9), 3001–3006.

Spector, R. E. (2013). *Cultural diversity in health and illness* (8th ed.). Upper Saddle River, NJ: Pearson.

U.S. Department of Agriculture (USDA). (2012a). *Getting started with MyPlate*. Retrieved from http://www.choosemyplate.gov/downloads/GettingStartedWithMyPlate.pdf

U.S. Department of Agriculture (USDA). (2012b). *Maternal intake of seafood omega-3 fatty acids and infant health: A review of the evidence*. Retrieved from http://www.cnpp.usda.gov/sites/default/files/nutrition_insights_uploads/Insight46.pdf

U.S. Food and Drug Administration (FDA). (2015). *Food safety for pregnant women*. Retrieved from https://wicworks.fns.usda.gov/pregnancy/food-safety

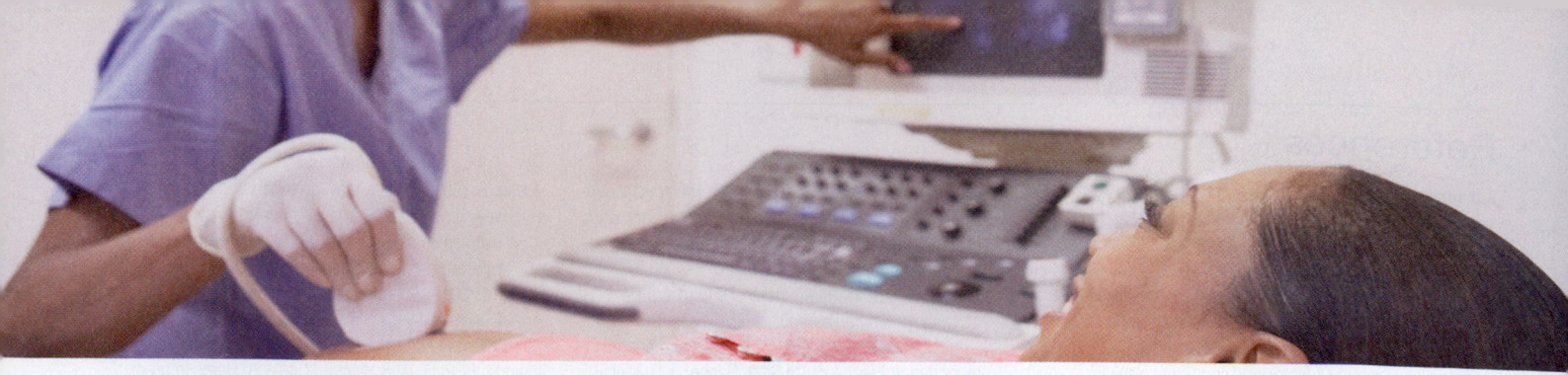

Chapter 12
Pregnancy in Selected Populations

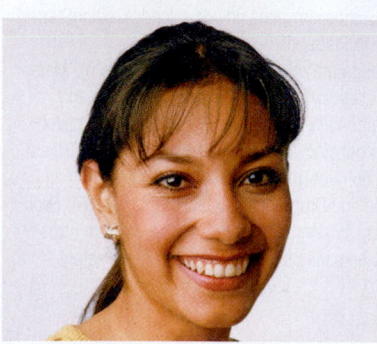

My daughter and I make quite a pair. She is 16 and pregnant with my first grandchild and I am 39 and, quite unexpectedly, pregnant with my third child. I am not sure which of us was more surprised but we are adjusting. As a nurse myself, I know that we both face risks because of our ages but we are doing all we can to ensure that our babies—we are both expecting boys—stay healthy.

—A Registered Nurse and Certified Childbirth Educator

⌄ Learning Outcomes

12.1 Describe the scope of the problem and the impact of adolescent pregnancy.

12.2 Identify the physical, psychologic, and sociologic risks a pregnant adolescent faces.

12.3 Delineate the characteristics of the fathers of children of adolescent mothers.

12.4 Discuss the possible reactions of the adolescent's family and social network to her pregnancy.

12.5 Describe successful community approaches to prevention of adolescent pregnancy.

12.6 Describe factors that have contributed to the increased incidence of pregnancy in women over 35 years of age.

12.7 Summarize the nursing care needs of an expectant woman over age 35.

12.8 Discuss general healthcare risks that a woman with a significant chronic physical disability might face during pregnancy.

12.9 Identify the key needs of a pregnant woman with an intellectual disability.

While pregnancy is a normal process, for certain women it carries increased risk. This is especially true for adolescents, pregnant women over age 35, and women with physical and/or mental disabilities. This chapter focuses on their needs and care.

Adolescent Pregnancy

About 614,000 teenage girls ages 15 to 19 become pregnant each year in the United States (Alan Guttmacher Institute [AGI], 2014). Nevertheless, U.S. teenage childbearing has declined steadily over the last few decades. In 2013, the birth rate (number of births per 1000 women) for adolescents ages 15 to 19 fell to 26.5, a historic low level, specifically the lowest rate reported in over half a century (Martin, Hamilton, Osterman, et al., 2015).

See Figure 12–1. Equally significant, these declines occurred for all race and Hispanic origin groups, although rates for Hispanic teens (46.3) and non-Hispanic black teens (43.9) remain considerably higher than the rates for non-Hispanic white teens (20.5) (Ventura, Hamilton, & Matthews, 2014).

During the past decade there has not been a significant change in the overall proportion of teens who are sexually active. The decline in the birth rate of U.S. teenagers seems to be primarily attributable to improvements in their use of contraceptives. Improved comprehensive sex education programs, messages in the media, the AIDS crisis, and a shift in fertility patterns as more women delay marriage may also be factors (Boonstra, 2014).

Even with this recent decline in adolescent pregnancies, the U.S. teenage birth rate remains one of the highest of any industrialized nation (exceeded only by Bulgaria's [41.7] and

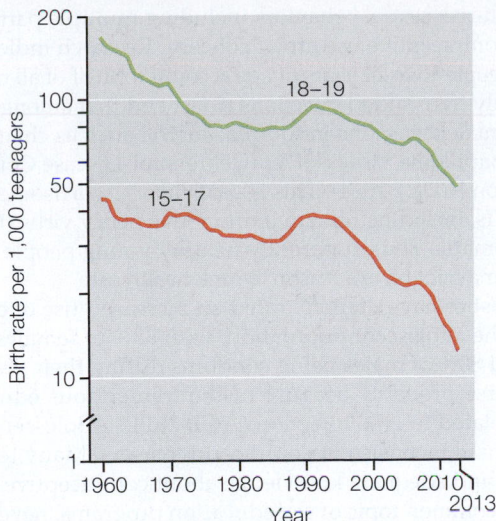

Figure 12–1 Birth rates for teenagers ages 15–17 and 18–19: United States, 1960–2013.

SOURCE: CDC/NCHS National Vital Statistics System. Retrieved from http://www.cdc.gov/nchs/data/nvsr/nvsr63/nvsr63_04.pdf

Romania's [35.2]), almost twice as high as that of Canada (14.1) and 6 times as high as those of the Netherlands (4.8) and Japan (4.5) (Ventura et al., 2014).

Healthy People 2020

(FP-8) Reduce pregnancies among adolescent females

(FP-9) Increase the proportion of adolescents aged 17 years and under who have never had sexual intercourse

(FP-12) Increase the proportion of adolescents who received formal instruction on reproductive health topics before they were 18 years old

Overview of the Adolescent Period

PHYSICAL CHANGES

Puberty—that period during which an individual becomes capable of reproduction—is a maturational process that can last from 1.5 to 6 years. The major physical changes of puberty include a growth spurt, weight change, and the appearance of secondary sexual characteristics. Menarche, or the time of the first menstrual period, usually occurs in the last half of this maturational process, with the average age between 12 and 13. The initial menstrual cycles are usually irregular and often anovulatory, although not always. Thus, contraception is important for all sexually active adolescents.

PSYCHOSOCIAL DEVELOPMENT

Many authorities have described the developmental tasks of adolescence, based on a variety of classic theories. The following are major developmental tasks of this period (Steinberg, 2014):

- Developing a sense of identity
- Gaining autonomy and independence
- Developing intimacy in a relationship
- Developing comfort with one's own sexuality
- Developing a sense of achievement

Resolution of these tasks is a developmental process that occurs over time. Although average ages for the completion of tasks have been identified, these ages are somewhat arbitrary and are affected by many factors, including culture, religion, and socioeconomic status.

In **early adolescence** (ages 14 and under), teens still see authority in their parents. However, they begin the process of gaining independence from the family by spending more time with friends. Conformity to peer group standards is important. Adolescents in this phase are very egocentric and are concrete thinkers, with only a minimal ability to see themselves in the future or to foresee the consequences of their behavior. Teens perceive their locus of control as external; that is, their destinies are controlled by others such as parents and school authorities.

Middle adolescence (ages 15 to 17 years) is the time for challenging; experimenting with drugs, alcohol, and sex are common avenues for rebellion. Middle adolescents seek independence and turn increasingly to their peer groups. They begin to move from concrete thinking to formal operational thought, but they are not yet able to anticipate the long-term implications of all their actions. These years are often a time of great turmoil for the family as the adolescent struggles for independence and challenges the family's values and expectations.

In **late adolescence** (ages 18 to 19 years) teens are more at ease with their individuality and decision-making ability. They can think abstractly and anticipate consequences. Late adolescents are capable of formal operational thought. They learn to solve problems, to conceptualize, and to make decisions. These abilities help them see themselves as having control, which leads to the ability to understand and accept the consequences of their behavior.

Factors Contributing to Adolescent Pregnancy

SOCIOECONOMIC AND CULTURAL FACTORS

Poverty is a major risk factor for adolescent pregnancy. Adolescents who do not have access to middle-class opportunities tend to maintain their pregnancies because they see pregnancy as their only option for adult status. Kearney and Levine (2012) suggest that teens who are on a low economic trajectory are more likely to become pregnant because of the lack of economic opportunity and the social marginalization that comes with poverty. Specifically, these girls are more likely to "drop out" of the economic mainstream and opt for early parenthood instead of investing in their own economic progress because they feel that they have little chance of advancing.

In the United States, the adolescent birth rate is higher among African American teens and Hispanic teens than among White teens. To some degree, the higher teenage pregnancy rate in these groups reflects the impact of poverty because a disproportionately high number of African American and Hispanic youths live in poverty (Yoost, Hertweck, & Barnett, 2014).

Higher levels of competence cognitively, behaviorally, and socially tend to have a protective effect on adolescent sexuality and reproductive health (House, Bates, Markham, et al., 2010). Teens from warm, nurturing families who value future accomplishments and are engaged in academic pursuits are less likely to engage in risky sexual behavior (Kogan, Cho, Allen, et al., 2013). Teens with future goals (i.e., college or job) tend to use birth control more consistently compared with other teens; if they become pregnant, they are also more likely to have abortions.

The younger the teen when she first gets pregnant, the more likely she is to have another pregnancy in her teens. Just over one third (35%) of adolescents who have had an abortion or recent birth become pregnant again within 2 years (Baldwin & Edelman, 2013). Moreover, the likelihood of repeat pregnancies increases when the teen is living with her sexual partner and has dropped out of school.

Internationally, female adolescents who are married are more likely to welcome a pregnancy in countries in which Islam is the predominant religion, where large families are desired, where social change is slow in coming, and where most childbearing occurs within marriage. Early pregnancy is less desired in countries in which the reverse is true.

Developing Cultural Competence Impact of Education on Marriage and Childbearing

Throughout the world, the higher a woman's educational level, the more likely she is to delay marriage and childbirth.

HIGH-RISK BEHAVIORS

Developmentally, adolescents, especially younger ones, are not yet able to foresee the consequences of their actions. As a result, they may have a sense of invulnerability that leads to the mistaken idea that harm will not befall them. This sense of invulnerability may also result in an overly optimistic view of the risks associated with their actions.

Among American adolescents there is great peer pressure to become sexually active during the teen years. Premarital sexual activity is commonplace, and teenage pregnancy is more socially acceptable today than it was in the past. In fact, by age 19, 71% of all teens have had intercourse (AGI, 2014). Sexual innuendo permeates every aspect of the popular media, but issues of sexual responsibility are commonly ignored.

Texting is a form of flirting and social behavior that has become commonplace among teens and young adults. Of particular note is the current blend of "sex and text" called "sexting" in which teens and young adults share semi-nude or nude pictures of themselves or others using cell phones, websites, and social media networks. Sexting is associated with an increased likelihood of being sexually active and of engaging in risky sexual behavior such as using drugs and alcohol before sex and having unprotected sex. Individuals in a romantic relationship are more likely to engage in sexting (Klettke, Hallford, & Mellor, 2014).

High-risk sexual behaviors including multiple partners and lack of contraceptive use are of concern. Research indicates that young people 15 to 24 years of age account for half of all new cases of sexually transmitted infections (STIs) and that among sexually active female teens, one in four has an STI such as chlamydia or human papilloma virus (HPV) (Centers for Disease Control and Prevention [CDC], 2014). This is particularly worrisome because many STIs, including human immunodeficiency virus (HIV), are asymptomatic. Thus apparently healthy young people who are infected may not have a reason to seek health care.

Statistics have demonstrated an increased use of condoms among the adolescent population, with 68% of females ages 15 to 19 and 80% of males using condoms during their first sexual intercourse probably because of the tremendous educational efforts related to HIV infection (AGI, 2014). Adolescents, however, remain inconsistent contraceptive users. Many teens lack accurate and adequate knowledge about contraceptive options. This is a common topic of sex education programs; nevertheless, debate continues about the appropriateness of such programs in schools. Proponents advocate early sex education to provide teens with the knowledge they need to avoid unwanted pregnancy and the risk of STIs. Opponents feel that sex education is the responsibility of parents and worry that sex education in the schools will promote sexual activity. However, a review of research on comprehensive sex education reveals that it does not increase initiation of sexual activity at an earlier age. In fact, it helps delay the start of sexual activity, increases condom or contraceptive use, reduces the number of sexual partners and the frequency of sex, and reduces sexual risk taking (Boonstra, 2014). Other factors affecting the use of contraception include access or availability, cost of supplies, and concern about confidentiality.

PSYCHOSOCIAL FACTORS

Pregnancy desire tends to be higher among teens who are older, who were younger when they became sexually active, who are in a short-term relationship (which may be romanticized and intense), and who have greater perceived stress in their lives (Sipsma, Ickovics, Lewis, et al., 2011).

Family dysfunction and poor self-esteem are also major risk factors for adolescent pregnancy. Some young teenagers

---

EVIDENCE-BASED PRACTICE | Risk Factors for Adolescent Pregnancy

Clinical Question

What are risk factors for adolescent pregnancy in vulnerable populations?

The Evidence

Unplanned pregnancy for an adolescent can result in a host of adverse outcomes for both mother and baby. These risks are even higher among vulnerable populations. Two research studies focused on identifiable risk factors in specific vulnerable populations in an effort to target preventive efforts effectively. Researchers conducted an integrated literature review of 18 research studies that identified risk factors for teen pregnancy among African American adolescents. A second study used a predictive model to study risk factors among nearly 300 adolescents in the child welfare system/foster homes. Taken together, these studies form a strong basis of evidence. Lee, Cintron, & Kocher (2014) found that five major factors contributed to adolescent pregnancy among African American youth: substance use, gender roles, peer influences, parental

involvement, and level of knowledge about sexual health. Of these, substance use was also a predictive factor for teens in the welfare system, but in this population, delinquency was also a risk factor (Helfrich & McWey, 2014). In the latter study, the timing of pregnancy was also identified; pregnancy occurred, on average, within 3 years of a predictive event.

Best Practice

Knowing specific predictive factors for a population enables the development of risk-specific educational programs for the prevention of adolescent pregnancy. These data suggest that supports need to be wide reaching and include reducing substance abuse, encouraging parental involvement, and integration of peer support into interventions.

Clinical Reasoning

How can the nurse determine risk factors of teen pregnancy for a specific population? How can parents and peers be involved in adolescent pregnancy prevention programs?

deliberately plan to get pregnant. A female adolescent may use pregnancy for various subconscious or conscious reasons: to punish her parents, to escape from an undesirable home situation, to gain attention, or to feel that she has someone to love and someone who loves her. Pregnancy may also be an adolescent's form of acting out. For others, pregnancy marks an important milestone that leads to enhanced maturity, better decision making, and healthier behaviors (Herrman & Nandakumar, 2012).

Evidence suggests that teens who have a history of sexual abuse, physical abuse, or neglect are more likely to give birth as a teenager than those who have not been maltreated (Garwood, Gerassi, Johnson-Reid, et al., 2015; Herrman, 2014). Teenage pregnancy also can result from an incestuous relationship. In the very young adolescent, incest or sexual abuse should be suspected as a possible cause of pregnancy. More teens who become pregnant, compared with teens who have not been pregnant, have been physically, emotionally, or sexually abused. In fact, maltreatment of any kind is a high-risk contributor to early teen pregnancy. Teenage pregnancy could also be caused by other nonvoluntary sexual experiences such as acquaintance rape.

Risks to the Adolescent Mother

PHYSIOLOGIC RISKS

Adolescents older than 15 years who receive early, thorough prenatal care are at no greater risk during pregnancy than women older than age 20. Unfortunately, adolescents often begin prenatal care later in pregnancy than other age groups. Thus, risks for pregnant adolescents include preterm births, low-birth-weight newborns, cephalopelvic disproportion, iron deficiency anemia, and preeclampsia and its sequelae. In the adolescent age group, prenatal care is the critical factor that most influences pregnancy outcome.

Teenagers ages 15 to 19 have a high incidence of STIs, including herpes virus, syphilis, and gonorrhea. The incidence of chlamydial infection is also increased in this age group. The presence of such infections during a pregnancy greatly increases the risk to the fetus. Other problems seen in adolescents are cigarette smoking and drug use. By the time pregnancy is confirmed, the fetus may already have been harmed by these substances.

PSYCHOLOGIC RISKS

The major psychologic risk to the pregnant adolescent is the interruption of her developmental tasks. Adding the tasks of pregnancy to her own developmental tasks creates a huge amount of psychologic work, the completion of which will affect the adolescent's and her newborn's futures. Table 12–1 suggests typical behaviors of the adolescent when she becomes aware of her pregnancy. In reviewing these behaviors, the nurse should realize that other factors may influence individual response.

SOCIOLOGIC RISKS

Being forced into adult roles before completing adolescent developmental tasks causes a series of events that may result in prolonged dependence on parents, lack of stable relationships

TABLE 12–1 Initial Reaction to Awareness of Pregnancy

AGE	ADOLESCENT BEHAVIOR	NURSING IMPLICATIONS
Early adolescent (14 years and younger)	Fears rejection by family and peers. Enters healthcare system with an adult, most likely mother (parents still seen as locus of control). Value system closely reflects that of parents, so teen turns to parents for decisions or approval of decisions. Pregnancy probably not a result of intimate relationship. Is self-conscious about normal adolescent changes in body. Self-consciousness and low self-esteem likely to increase with rapid breast enlargement and abdominal enlargement of pregnancy.	Be nonjudgmental in approach to care. Focus on needs and concerns of adolescent, but if parent accompanies daughter, include parent in plan of care. Encourage both to express concerns and feelings regarding pregnancy and options: abortion, maintaining pregnancy, adoption. Be realistic and concrete in discussing implications of each option. During physical exam of adolescent, respect increased sense of modesty. Explain in simple and concrete terms physical changes that are produced by pregnancy versus puberty. Explain each step of physical exam in simple and specific terms.
Middle adolescent (15–17 years)	Fears rejection by peers and parents. Unsure of whom to confide in. May seek confirmation of pregnancy on own with increased awareness of options and services, such as over-the-counter pregnancy kits and Planned Parenthood. If in an ongoing, caring relationship with partner (peer), may choose him as confidant. Economic dependence on parents may determine if and when parents are told. Future educational plans and perception of parental support or lack of support are significant factors in decision regarding termination or maintenance of the pregnancy. Possible conflict between parental and own developing value system.	Be nonjudgmental in approach to care. Reassure the adolescent that confidentiality will be maintained. Help adolescent identify significant individuals in whom she can confide to help make a decision about the pregnancy. Be aware of state laws regarding requirement of parental notification if abortion intended. Also be aware of state laws regarding requirements for marriage: usually, minimum age for both parties is 18; 16- and 17-year-olds are, in most states, allowed to marry only with consent of parents. Encourage adolescent to be realistic about parental response to pregnancy.
Late adolescent (18–19 years)	Most likely to confirm pregnancy on own and at an earlier date due to increased acceptance and awareness of consequences of behavior. Likely to use pregnancy kit for confirmation. Relationship with father of baby, future educational plans, and personal value system are among significant determinants of decision about pregnancy.	Be nonjudgmental in approach to care. Reassure the adolescent that confidentiality will be maintained. Encourage adolescent to identify significant individuals in whom she can confide. Refer to counseling as appropriate. Encourage adolescent to be realistic about parental response to pregnancy.

with the opposite sex, and lack of economic and social stability. Many teenage mothers have their schooling interrupted or drop out of school. Research indicates that teen mothers are less likely to graduate from high school and to enroll in and finish college (Sonfield, Hasstedt, Kavanaugh, et al., 2013). In addition, teenage mothers are more likely to have big families and more likely to be single. Lack of education in turn reduces the quality of jobs available and leads to more tenuous employment and increased poverty (Herrman & Nandakumar, 2012).

Some pregnant adolescents choose to marry the father of the baby, who may also be a teenager. Unfortunately, most adolescent marriages end in divorce. This fact should not be surprising because pregnancy and marriage interrupt the adolescents' childhood and basic education. Lack of maturity in dealing with an intimate relationship also contributes to marital breakdown.

Dating violence is often an issue for teens. When surveyed, 10.3% of adolescents report some level of physical dating violence and 10.4% experienced some form of sexual dating violence ranging from touching and kissing to forced intercourse (Kann, Kinchen, Shanklin, et al., 2014). The violence increases in pregnant teens. However, research suggests that this number is significantly lower than reality because teens are far less likely to report domestic violence than are adults.

The increased incidence of maternal complications, preterm birth, and low-birth-weight babies among teen mothers also affects society because many of these mothers are on welfare. The need for increased financial support for good prenatal care and nutritional programs remains critical.

In the United States, the results of teenage childbearing cost taxpayers $9.4 billion annually (Ventura et al., 2014). Much of this cost comes from Medicaid, state health department maternal care clinics, federal monies for Aid to Families with Dependent Children programs, the Supplemental Nutrition Assistance Program (SNAP), and direct payments to healthcare providers.

Table 12–2 identifies the early adolescent's response to the developmental tasks of pregnancy. Middle and older adolescents respond differently, reflecting their progression through developmental tasks. In addition to her maturational level, the amount of nurturing the pregnant adolescent receives is a critical factor in the way she handles pregnancy and motherhood.

Risks for the Child

Children of adolescent parents are at a disadvantage in many ways because teens are not developmentally or economically prepared to be parents. In general, children of teenage mothers

TABLE 12–2 The Early Adolescent's Response to the Developmental Tasks of Pregnancy

STAGE	DEVELOPMENTAL TASKS OF PREGNANCY	EARLY ADOLESCENT'S RESPONSE TO PREGNANCY	NURSING IMPLICATIONS
First trimester	Pregnancy confirmation. Seeks early prenatal care as a confirmation tool. Begins to evaluate her diet and general health habits. Initial ambivalence common. Usually supportive partner.	May delay confirmation of pregnancy until late first trimester or later. Reasons for delay may include lack of awareness that she is pregnant, fear of confiding in anyone, and/or denial. Rapid enlargement and sensitivity of breasts are embarrassing and frightening to early adolescents—may be perceived as changes of puberty. If confiding in mother, may be experiencing family turmoil in response to pregnancy.	Explain physiologic changes of pregnancy versus those associated with puberty. Explain that ambivalence is normal with any pregnancy, but recognize it as a much greater concern with adolescent pregnancy. Emphasize need for good nutrition as important for her well-being as much as baby's (prevention of preeclampsia and anemia). Use simple explanations and lots of audiovisual aids. Have adolescent listen to fetal heart rate with Doppler.
Second trimester	Changes in physical appearance begin, and fetal movement is experienced, causing pregnancy to be experienced as a reality. Begins wearing maternity clothes to accommodate the physical changes. As a result of quickening, she perceives her fetus as a real baby and begins preparing for the maternal role and new relationships with her partner and members of her family.	Some teenagers may delay validation of pregnancy until now, with family turmoil occurring at this time. Abdominal enlargement and quickening may be perceived as loss of control over body image. May try to maintain prepregnant weight and wear restrictive clothing to control and conceal changing body. Becomes dependent on her own mother for support. Egocentric; unable to develop a maternal role at this time.	Continue to discuss importance of good nutrition and adequate weight gain as noted above. Discuss ways of wearing common teenage clothing (large sweatshirts, blouses) to promote comfort but preserve adolescent image to some degree. Discuss plans being made for baby, continued educational plans, and role of teen's parents. Explain physiologic changes of pregnancy versus those associated with puberty. Explain that ambivalence is normal with any pregnancy, but recognize it as a much greater concern with adolescent pregnancy.
Third trimester	At end of second trimester, begins to view fetus as separate from self. Buys baby clothes and supplies. Prepares a place for the baby. Realistic about what baby is like. Prepares to give birth to baby. Anxiety increases as labor and birth approach and has concerns about well-being of fetus.	May focus on "wanting it to be over." May have trouble individuating fetus. May have fantasies, dreams, or nightmares about childbirth. Natural fears of labor and birth greater than with older primigravida. Probably has not been in a hospital, and may associate this with negative experiences.	Assess whether adolescent is preparing for baby by buying supplies and preparing a place in the home. Childbirth education is important. Provide hospital tour. Assess for discomforts of pregnancy, such as heartburn and constipation. Adolescent may be uncomfortable mentioning these and other problems.

are found to be at a developmental disadvantage compared with children whose mothers were older at the time of their birth. Many factors contribute to these differences, especially the adverse social and economic conditions many teenage mothers face. These factors result in high rates of family instability, disadvantaged neighborhoods, and high rates of behavior problems. In addition, these children do not do as well in school and are less likely to complete high school. Children born to adolescent mothers also have higher rates of abuse and neglect (March of Dimes [MOD], 2012).

Partners of Adolescent Mothers

Approximately half of the fathers of babies born to adolescent mothers are not teens but 20 years of age or older (Herrman, 2010). Teen mothers in poor, recently immigrated populations are especially likely to have older partners. Adolescent males tend to become sexually active at an earlier age than females, and they have more sexual partners in their teenage years. When the father is an adolescent, he too has uncompleted developmental tasks for his age group and is no better prepared psychologically than his female counterpart to deal with the consequences of pregnancy. Teenage fatherhood may lead to a decrease in the years of schooling the male receives, and increases the rate of cohabitation and early marriage. It also is associated with full-time and military employment status (Fletcher & Wolfe, 2012).

In general, adolescent males tend to view an unintended pregnancy as negative because of the impact on their aspirations, life goals, and current freedoms. Attitudes toward teen pregnancy tend to be more favorable among adolescent men of lower socioeconomic status and/or lower educational level (Lohan, Cruise, O'Halloran, et al., 2010).

The adolescent who attempts to assume his responsibility as a father faces many of the same psychologic and sociologic risks as the adolescent mother. The mother and father are generally from similar socioeconomic backgrounds and have similar educational levels.

Although they may not be married, many adolescent couples have meaningful relationships. The male partners may be very involved in the pregnancy and may be present for the birth. In situations in which the adolescent father wants to assume some responsibility, healthcare providers should support him in his decision. It is also important to ensure that the pregnant adolescent has the opportunity to decide for herself whether she wants the father to participate in her health care.

Fathers are included on birth certificates far more frequently today than in the past. This inclusion helps ensure the fathers' rights and encourages them to meet their responsibilities to their children. In addition, legal paternity gives children access to military and Social Security benefits and to medical information about their fathers. In some situations the pregnant adolescent may not want to identify or contact the father of the baby, and the male may not readily acknowledge paternity. Those situations include rape, exploitative sexual relations, incest, and casual sexual relations. If healthcare providers suspect any of the first three causes, further investigation into the situation is important for the well-being of the pregnant adolescent, and referral to other resources should be made as appropriate.

Even if the adolescent father has been included in the health care of the young woman throughout the pregnancy, it is not unusual for her to want her mother as her primary support person during labor and birth. Younger adolescents are especially likely to choose their mothers for this role. It is important to support the pregnant adolescent's wishes and to acknowledge and support the adolescent father's wishes as appropriate.

Father love is an important predictor of a child's well-being. Children whose fathers are involved and loving are more likely to have healthy self-esteem, do well in school, and avoid drug use and criminal activity than those children with fathers who are uninvolved (Kirven, 2014). Therefore, it behooves healthcare professionals to do what they can to support the efforts of adolescent fathers to be effective.

As a part of counseling, the nurse should assess the young man's stressors, his support systems, his plans for involvement in the pregnancy and childbearing, and his future plans. He should be referred to social services for counseling about his educational and vocational future. When the father is involved in the pregnancy, the young mother feels less deserted, more confident in her decision making, and better able to discuss her future.

Reactions of Family and Social Network to Adolescent Pregnancy

The reactions of families and support groups to adolescent pregnancy vary widely. In families that foster children's educational and career goals, adolescent pregnancy is often a shock. Anger, shame, and sorrow are common reactions. The majority of pregnant adolescents from these families are likely to choose abortion, with the exception of teens whose cultural and religious beliefs prevent them from seeking abortions.

In populations in which adolescent pregnancy is more prevalent and more socially acceptable, family and friends may be more supportive of the adolescent parents. In many cases the teen's friends and mother are present at the birth. The expectant parents may also have friends who are already teen parents. Some male partners of these adolescent mothers see pregnancy and the birth of a baby as signs of adult status and increased sexual prowess—a source of pride.

The mother of the pregnant adolescent is usually among the first to be told about the pregnancy. She typically becomes involved with decision making, especially with the young adolescent, about issues such as maintaining the pregnancy, abortion, and dealing with the father-to-be and his family.

Once the pregnant adolescent decides how to proceed, it is often her mother who helps her access health care, and her mother's support is essential if the teen self-image is to grow to include the notion of herself as "mother" (Turnage & Pharris, 2013). If the pregnancy is maintained, the mother may participate in prenatal care and classes and can be an excellent source of support for her daughter. She should be encouraged to participate if the mother–daughter relationship is positive. If the baby's father is involved in the pregnancy, he and the pregnant adolescent's mother may be able to work together to support the teenage mother. The nurse can update the pregnant adolescent's mother on current childbearing practices to clarify any misconceptions she might have. During labor and birth, the mother may be a key figure for her daughter, offering reassurance and instilling confidence in the teen.

The younger the adolescent when she gives birth, the more she needs her mother's support. Children of adolescent parents experience more negative outcomes, including more aggressive behavior at a younger age, when the adolescent is in constant conflict with her mother and becomes less involved in parenting.

Nursing Management

For the Adolescent Mother-to-Be

Nursing Assessment and Diagnosis

In working with adolescents, remember that oftentimes the nurse is the first contact with the healthcare system that the adolescent has. Then, too, many adolescents have never before accessed health care without a parent. Establish a knowledge base to plan interventions for the adolescent mother-to-be and family. Areas of assessment include history of family and personal physical health, developmental level and impact of pregnancy, and emotional and financial support. Also assess the family and social support network and the father's degree of involvement in the pregnancy.

As with all pregnant women, it is important to have information on the teen's general physical health. This may be the first time the adolescent has ever provided a health history. Consequently it may be helpful to ask specific questions and give examples if the young woman appears confused about a question. The teen's mother may be best able to answer questions about family history because the adolescent is often unaware of this information.

The following areas should be assessed:

- Family and personal health history
- Medical history
- Menstrual history
- Obstetric and gynecologic history
- Substance abuse history

It is important to assess the maturational level of each person. The adolescent's development level and the impact of pregnancy are reflected in the degree of recognition of the realities and responsibilities involved in teenage pregnancy and parenting. Also assess the teen mother's self-concept (including body image), her relationship with the significant adults in her life, her attitude toward her pregnancy, and her coping methods in the situation, as well as the teen's knowledge of, attitude toward, and anticipated ability to care for the coming baby. Ask specifically about dating violence. Teens are not likely to reveal dating violence unless they are asked about it.

The socioeconomic status of the pregnant adolescent often places the baby at risk throughout life, beginning with conception. It is essential to assess family and social support systems, as well as the extent of financial support available.

The nursing diagnoses applicable to pregnant women in general apply to the pregnant adolescent. Other nursing diagnoses are influenced by the adolescent's age, support systems, socioeconomic situation, health, and maturity. Examples of nursing diagnoses specific to the pregnant adolescent may include the following (NANDA-I © 2014):

- *Nutrition, Imbalanced: Less than Body Requirements,* related to poor eating habits
- *Self-Esteem, Situational Low, Risk for,* related to unanticipated pregnancy

Planning and Implementation

COMMUNITY-BASED NURSING CARE

Early, thorough prenatal care is the strongest and most critical determinant for reducing risk for the adolescent mother and her newborn. The nurse needs to understand the special needs of the adolescent mother to meet this challenge successfully.

Many new and innovative community-based programs have evolved to provide care for high-risk clients and their partners throughout the childbearing experience and beyond. Nurses in community-based agencies can help adolescents access the healthcare system as well as social services and other support services (e.g., food banks and the Special Supplemental Nutrition Program for Women, Infants, and Children [WIC]). These nurses are also involved extensively in counseling and client teaching.

Teaching adolescents in groups according to their ages is often more effective for learning. In addition, many teens prefer teaching aids that are visual and that they can handle, such as realistic fetal models. Pregnant teens with low reading levels tend to prefer handouts and posters that have visual interest, short sentences, bulleted items, and white space.

Issue of Confidentiality

Most states have passed legislation that confirms the right of some minors to assume the rights of adults; they are then called **emancipated minors**. An adolescent may be considered emancipated if he or she is self-supporting and living away from home, married, pregnant, a parent, or in the military service. Even if a minor has not become formally "emancipated," all 50 states permit confidential testing and treatment for sexually transmitted infections (STIs) but only 26 states and the District of Columbia explicitly permit all minors to consent to contraception without a parent's knowledge or consent; 20 states permit minors to consent to contraception in certain circumstances (AGI, 2015). Currently 36 states and the District of Columbia explicitly allow some minors to consent to prenatal care; of that group, 32 states allow all minors to give consent, whereas 13 states have no relevant law or policy (AGI, 2015). All states either explicitly allow minors to give consent for their children's medical care or have no policy about it (AGI, 2015).

> **Professionalism in Practice** Emancipated Minors
>
> It is important to remember that if a pregnant minor is considered emancipated, she has the right and responsibility to consent to health care for herself and later for her child. She is entitled to respect and confidentiality in her dealings with healthcare providers. Only with her consent can other adults, including her parents, be included in communication.

Development of a Trusting Relationship With the Pregnant Adolescent

The first visit to the clinic or caregiver's office may make the young woman feel anxious and vulnerable. Making this first experience as positive as possible for the young woman will encourage the adolescent to return for follow-up care and to cooperate with her healthcare providers and will help her recognize the importance of health care for her and her baby. Developing a trusting relationship with the pregnant adolescent is essential. Honesty, respect, and a caring attitude promote self-esteem.

Clinical Tip

During the initial pelvic examination, with the consent of the examiner, offer the teen a handheld mirror. A mirror is helpful in enabling the young woman to see her cervix, thus educating her about her anatomy. It also gives her an active role in the examination if she so desires.

Depending on the adolescent's age, this may be her first pelvic examination, an anxiety-provoking experience for any woman. Provide explanations during the procedure. A gentle and thoughtful examination technique will help the young woman to relax.

Promotion of Self-Esteem and Problem-Solving Skills

Assist the adolescent in her decision-making and problem-solving skills so that she can proceed with her developmental tasks and begin to assume responsibility for her life and that of her newborn. Many adolescents are not aware of the legally available options for handling an unplanned pregnancy. In an open, nonjudgmental way, without imposing personal values, educate the teen about her alternatives: terminating the pregnancy, maintaining the pregnancy and parenting the baby, or relinquishing the baby for adoption. The nurse can also provide information about community resources available to help with each alternative. Once the teen has decided on a course of action, healthcare providers should respect her decision and support her efforts to achieve her goals.

Adolescents who choose to terminate a pregnancy cite reasons such as economic hardship or interference with school or a career. Teens most often involve their parents and their partners in the decision. Their involvement does not always indicate that they support the adolescent's decision. Research, however, indicates that a significant portion of pregnant teens report pressure from their mother, partner, or other family member to consider terminating the pregnancy. Teens are similar to adults in how they experience abortion. They expect to feel a range of emotions and believe they are prepared to cope with them after the abortion (Ralph, Gould, Baker, et al., 2014).

If the adolescent chooses to continue her pregnancy, describe what she can expect over the prenatal period and provide an explanation and rationale for each procedure as it occurs. This overview fosters the adolescent's understanding and gives her some control.

Early adolescents tend to be egocentric and oriented to the present. They may not think it is important that their health and habits affect the fetus. Thus it is often helpful to emphasize how these practices affect the teens themselves. Early adolescents also need help in problem solving and in visualizing the future so they can plan effectively.

Middle adolescents are developing the ability to think abstractly and can recognize that actions may have long-term consequences. They may not yet have acquired assertive communication skills, however, and may be reluctant to ask questions. Therefore, ask teens directly if they have questions. Middle adolescents can absorb more detailed health teaching and apply it.

Late adolescents can usually think abstractly, plan for the future, and function in a manner comparable to older pregnant women. They can also handle complex information and apply it.

Promotion of Physical Well-Being

Baseline weight and blood pressure measurements are valuable in assessing weight gain and predisposition to preeclampsia (Figure 12–2). Encourage the adolescent to take part in her care by measuring and recording her own weight. Use this time as an opportunity for assisting the young woman in problem solving. Encourage her to ask herself the following questions: "Have I gained too much or too little weight?" "What influence does my diet have on my weight?" "How can I change my eating habits?"

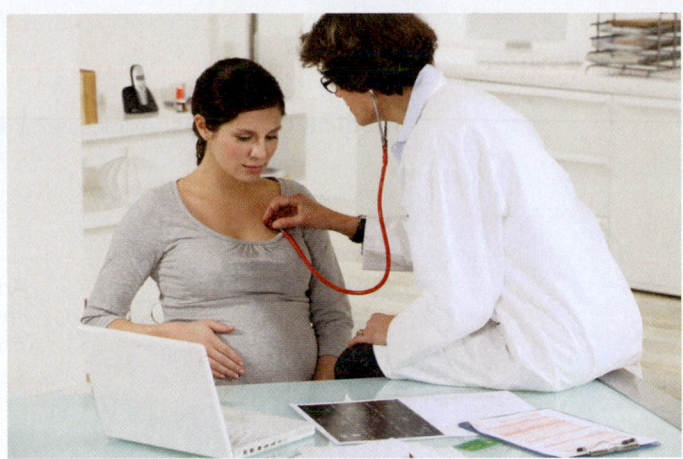

Figure 12–2 The nurse carefully assesses this pregnant teen.
SOURCE: © Auremar/Fotolia.

Introduce the subject of nutrition during measurement of baseline and subsequent hemoglobin and hematocrit values. Because the adolescent is at risk for anemia, she needs education about the importance of iron in her diet. Indeed, basic education about nutrition is a critical component of care for pregnant teens. See *Concept Map: Anemia in Pregnancy*.

Preeclampsia is the most prevalent medical complication of pregnant adolescents. Blood pressure readings of 140/90 mmHg are not acceptable as the determinant of preeclampsia in adolescents. Young women ages 14 to 20 years without evidence of high blood pressure usually have diastolic readings between 50 and 66 mmHg. Gradual increases from the prepregnant diastolic readings, along with excessive weight gain, must be evaluated as precursors to preeclampsia. Establishment of baseline readings is one reason early prenatal care is vital to management of the pregnant adolescent.

Adolescents have an increased incidence of STIs. The initial prenatal examination should include gonococcal and chlamydial cultures; wet-mount prep for *Candida, Trichomonas,* and *Gardnerella;* and tests for syphilis. Although today's teens are knowledgeable about HIV/AIDS, they know much less about other STIs, especially with regard to symptoms and risk reduction, so education is important. If the adolescent's history indicates that she is at increased risk for HIV, she should be given information about it and offered HIV screening.

Discuss substance abuse with the adolescent. It is important to review the risks associated with the use of tobacco, caffeine, drugs, and alcohol. The young woman should be aware of how these substances affect both her and her fetus's development.

Clinical Reasoning   A Mother Considering Adoption

Rachel Kalaras is an 18-year-old G1P0 who is 16 weeks pregnant when she arrives for her prenatal visit. When discussing her plans for the pregnancy, Rachel indicates that she is considering adoption. She has not discussed this plan with anyone but is seeking information about the process of relinquishment.

What should you consider in discussing this issue with Rachel?

Ongoing care should include the same assessments that an older pregnant woman receives. Pay special attention to evaluating fetal growth by determining when quickening occurs

Concept Map

Medical Diagnosis: Adolescent Pregnancy 17 y.o., Iron Deficiency Anemia

Physical Exam
Pallor
Headaches
Palpitations
98.4, 106, 22, 136/84
Skin – pale
Heart RRR, Lungs CTAB
Edema – minimal
Gravid uterus

Labs
Hgb 9
HCt 27
Ferritin 10
MCV 78
WBC 8.0

Anemia in
Pregnancy
Adolescence

Risk Factors
• Teen pregnancy
• G3 P2
• Noncompliance
• Vegan diet
• Closely-spaced pregnancies
• Previous anemia

Noncompliance
• Prevention is key
• Explain etiology of anemia
• Begin ferrous sulfate 325 mg po t.i.d.q.d.
• Reassess anemia status in 4 weeks
• Explain negative outcomes to both mother and fetus

**Nursing
Diagnoses
(NANDA-I © 2014)**

Imbalanced Nutrition: less than body requirements
• Increase green, leafy vegetables, dried fruits, and peanut butter
• Provide nutritional counseling
• Encourage adequate calorie intake
• 72 hour diet recall
• Food diary at each prenatal visit for review

Fatigue
• Frequent rest periods
• Retire at same time each night
• Avoid caffeine prior to bedtime
• Nap during the day
• Avoid television late at night

Deficient Knowledge
• Continue prenatal vitamins and iron
• Begin treatment immediately when first identified
• Take iron on empty stomach with orange juice
• Monitor for gastrointestinal side effects

and by measuring fundal height, fetal heart rate, and fetal movement. If there is a question of size–date discrepancy by 2 cm either way when assessing fundal height, an ultrasound is warranted to establish fetal age so that instances of intrauterine growth restriction can be detected early.

Promotion of Family Adaptation

Assess the family situation during the first prenatal visit and find out the level of involvement the adolescent wants from each of her family members and the father of the child, as well as her perception of their present support. If the mother and daughter agree, the mother should be included in the client's care. Pregnancy may change a teen's relationship with her mother from one of antagonism to one of understanding and empathy. The opportunity to renew or establish a positive relationship with their mothers is welcomed by most teens. Help the teen's mother assess and meet her daughter's needs. Some adolescents become more dependent during pregnancy, and some become more independent. The mother can ease and encourage her daughter's self-growth by understanding how best to respond to and support the adolescent.

The adolescent's relationship with her father is also affected by her pregnancy. Provide information to the adolescent's father and encourage his involvement to whatever degree is acceptable to both daughter and her father.

The father of the adolescent's baby should not be forgotten in promoting the family's adaptation to the pregnancy. He should be included in prenatal visits, classes, health teaching, and the birth itself to the extent that he wishes and that

is acceptable to the teenage mother. He should also have the opportunity to express his feelings and concerns and to have his questions answered.

Most childbirth educators believe that prenatal classes with other teens are best, even though they can be challenging to teach (Figure 12–3). The pregnant teen may be accompanied by her mother, her boyfriend, or her girlfriends. Those who bring

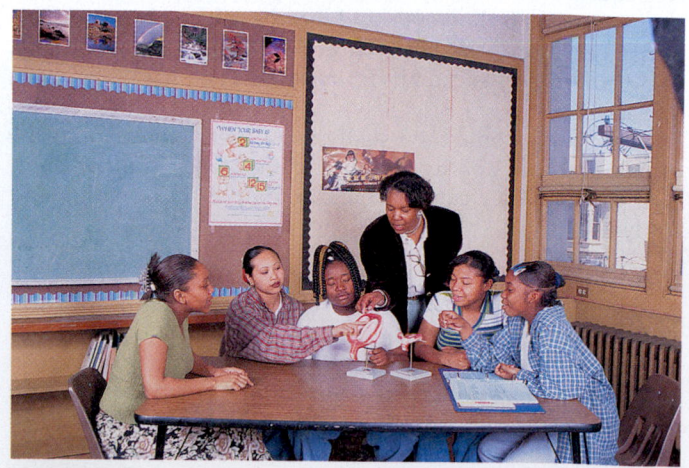

Figure 12–3 Prenatal classes for adolescents. Young adolescents may benefit from prenatal classes designed for them.

girlfriends may bring a different one each time, and giggling and side conversations may occur. Such activity reflects the short attention span of the teen and is fairly typical.

Goals for prenatal classes may include some or all of the following:

- Providing anticipatory guidance about pregnancy
- Preparing participants for labor and birth
- Helping participants identify the problems and conflicts of teenage pregnancy and parenting
- Promoting increased self-esteem
- Providing information about available community resources
- Helping participants develop adaptive coping skills

To keep the attention of adolescent participants in childbirth preparation classes, it is important to use a variety of teaching strategies including audiovisual aids, demonstrations, and games. Although parenting topics are sometimes included in prenatal classes for adolescents, teens may not retain the information because they tend to be present oriented. Parenting skills are crucial, but adolescents generally are not ready to learn about these skills until birth makes the newborn—and thus parenting—a reality.

Health Promotion Education: What Schools Can Do

- School systems attempt to meet prenatal education needs in many ways. The most effective method appears to be mainstreaming the pregnant adolescent in academic classes with her peers and adding classes appropriate to her needs during pregnancy and postpartum.

- Classes about growth and development beginning with the newborn and early infancy periods can help teenage parents to develop realistic expectations of their babies and may help decrease child abuse.

- Vocational guidance in this setting is also beneficial as they plan for their futures.

HOSPITAL-BASED NURSING CARE

As mentioned earlier, the adolescent's mother is often present during the teen's labor and birth. The father of the baby may also be involved. Close girlfriends may arrive soon after the teen is admitted. At admission, ask the teen who will be her primary support person in labor and whom she wants involved in the labor and birth. This information may also be included on her prenatal record. The adolescent in labor has the same care needs as any pregnant woman. However, she may require more sustained care. Be readily available and answer questions simply and honestly, using lay terminology. Also help the adolescent's support people understand their roles in assisting the teen. If the father of the baby is involved, encourage him, at his own level of comfort, to play an active role in all phases of the birth process, perhaps by supporting the teen's relaxation techniques, feeding her ice chips, timing her contractions, and coaching her with her breathing. Recommend hand-holding, back rubs, and supportive touching.

During the postpartum period, most teens do not foresee that they will become sexually active in the near future and are often adamant that they will not become pregnant again for a long time. However, the statistics demonstrate a different reality. Consequently, predischarge teaching should include information about the resumption of ovulation and the importance of contraception.

Several safe and effective contraceptive options are available for adolescents. Condoms are by far the most common method of contraception among teens and, when used consistently and correctly, they offer the added advantage of protection against STIs. Increasingly, experts are recommending a dual approach to prevent pregnancy and STIs—a condom combined with a second method of contraception. The American Academy of Pediatrics (AAP) (2014) has issued a policy statement on contraception for adolescents that advises caregivers to recommend contraceptive methods that require the least individual adherence, specifically, long-acting reversible contraception (LARC) such as progestin implants and intrauterine contraceptives (IUCs), followed by Depo-Provera (DMPA), combined oral contraceptives (COCs), and other hormone-based approaches including the vaginal ring, transdermal patch, and progestin-only pills.

Implanon and Nexplanon are both single-rod implants that may be left in place for 3 years. They are highly effective. DMPA is convenient for teens because it is easy to use. However, it does require an injection every 13 weeks.

IUC is now considered to be a safe, first-line contraceptive choice for adolescents. Research indicates that IUCs do not increase the adolescent's risk of pelvic inflammatory disease (PID) or affect her fertility (American Academy of Pediatrics [AAP], 2014), and the levonorgestrel-releasing intrauterine system (LNG-IUS) can be beneficial in teens by reducing heavy menstrual bleeding and alleviating symptoms of dysmenorrhea (Forcier & Harel, 2011).

COCs are a popular method of contraception among teenage girls, especially long term, and have few contraindications; however, they do require individual adherence. Extended or continuous-cycle pills are an option for teens who prefer amenorrhea.

SAFETY ALERT!

Nurses need to be certain that adolescents who are prescribed combined oral contraceptives (COCs) clearly understand the correct use, possible complications, warning signs, and implications of missed pills. They should also be aware that some medications, such as certain antibiotics, decrease the effectiveness of COCs.

As part of discharge planning, ensure that the teen is aware of community resources available to assist her and her family. Postpartum classes, especially with peers, can be particularly beneficial. Such classes address a variety of topics, including postpartum adaptation, newborn, infant, and child development, and parenting skills.

Evaluation

Expected outcomes of nursing care include the following:

- A trusting relationship is established with the pregnant adolescent.
- The adolescent is able to use her problem-solving abilities to make appropriate choices.

- The adolescent follows the recommendations of the healthcare team and receives effective health care throughout her pregnancy, the birth, and the postpartum period.

- The adolescent, her partner (if he is involved), and their families are able to cope successfully with the effects of the pregnancy.

- The adolescent is able to discuss pregnancy, prenatal care, and childbirth.

- The adolescent develops skill in child care and parenting.

Prevention of Adolescent Pregnancy

At the individual level, balanced and realistic sexual education, which includes information on both abstinence and contraception, can delay teens' onset of sexual activity, increase the use of contraception by sexually active teens, and reduce the number of their sexual partners. The AAP policy statement (2014) on contraception for adolescents addresses the role of healthcare providers in working with adolescents. The statement stresses the importance of encouraging abstinence while also providing counseling on risk-reduction approaches, including the use of latex condoms for every act of sexual intercourse. It points out that latex condoms also help reduce the transmission of STIs. In addition, the statement emphasizes the need to ensure ready access to contraceptive services and appropriate follow-up.

In 2012, AAP issued a policy statement (AAP, 2012) supporting the availability of emergency contraception (EC) and recommending that both male and female teens should be counseled about emergency contraception as part of routine anticipatory guidance about safe sex and family planning. In 2013 the Food and Drug Administration (FDA) approved Plan B One-Step emergency contraceptive for use by all women of childbearing potential without any age restrictions, thereby giving teens access to EC (FDA, 2013).

At the national level, the National Campaign to Prevent Teen and Unplanned Pregnancy (NCPTUP), a private, non-profit organization made up of a broad spectrum of religious, political, social, human services, health, and academic organizations, is working to reduce teenage pregnancy by 20% by 2020 (NCPTUP, 2015). The Association of Women's Health, Obstetric and Neonatal Nurses (AWHONN) is one of the many professional organizations that joined this group and made a commitment to focus on adolescent pregnancy prevention. Not surprisingly, the National Campaign has found that adolescent pregnancy is a multifaceted problem with no easy answers. The best approaches are local ones based on strong, community-wide involvement with a variety of programs directed at the multiple causes of the problem.

A problem in local communities continues to be conflict among different groups about how to approach adolescent pregnancy prevention. Most teens and adults believe that teens should be strongly encouraged to avoid having sex until they have completed high school, but both groups also favor providing young people with information about both abstinence and contraception (Albert, 2012). Nevertheless, some parents favor an abstinence-only approach. No evidence to date supports the effectiveness of this approach and it may have the unintended consequence of deterring teens from using contraceptives, thereby increasing the risk of sexually transmitted infections (STIs) or unintended pregnancy (Boonstra, 2014). Most Americans support providing

TABLE 12–3 Recommendations for Parents to Help Their Teens Avoid Pregnancy

- Parents should be clear about their own sexual attitudes and values in order to communicate clearly with children.

- Parents need to talk with their children about sex early and often and be specific in the discussions.

- Parents should supervise and monitor their children and teens with well-established rules, expectations, curfews, and standards of behavior.

- Parents should know their children's friends and their families.

- Parents need to clearly discourage early dating as well as frequent and steady dating.

- Parents should take a strong stand against allowing a daughter to date a much older boy; similarly, they should not allow a son to develop an intense relationship with a much younger girl.

- Parents need to help children set goals for their future and have options that are more attractive than early pregnancy and childrearing.

- Parents should show their children that they value education and take school performance seriously.

- Parents need to monitor what their children are reading, listening to, and watching.

- It is especially important for parents to build a strong, loving relationship with their children from an early age by showing affection clearly and regularly, spending time with them doing age-appropriate activities, building children's self-esteem, and having meals together as a family often.

Source: National Campaign to Prevent Teen and Unplanned Pregnancy (NCPTUP). (2012). *Ten tips for parents.* Retrieved from http://www.thenationalcampaign.org/parents/ten_tips.aspx

education in junior and senior high schools with information about protection against unplanned pregnancy and STIs. Evidence suggests that comprehensive programs that support both abstinence and the use of contraceptives and condoms have a positive effect in delaying or reducing sexual activity or in increasing the use of condoms or other contraceptives (Boonstra, 2014).

The National Campaign's task forces have identified characteristics shared by all successful programs, regardless of the type of offering or community. Effective adolescent pregnancy prevention programs are long term and intensive. They also involve adolescents in program planning, include good role models from the same cultural and racial backgrounds, and focus on the adolescent male.

The National Campaign has identified a list of recommendations for parents that are designed to help teens avoid pregnancy (see Table 12–3). Nurses can use this information when working with parents (NCPTUP, 2012)

Care of Expectant Parents Over Age 35

Today an increasing number of women are choosing to have their first baby after age 35. In fact, in 2013, birth rates rose for women in their 30s and late 40s and remained unchanged for women in their early 40s (Martin, Hamilton, Osterman, et al., 2015). Many factors have contributed to this trend, including the following:

- The availability of effective birth control methods
- The expanded roles and career options available for women
- The increased number of women getting advanced education, pursuing careers, and delaying parenthood until they are established professionally
- The increased incidence of later marriage and second marriage
- The high cost of living, which causes some young couples to delay childbearing until they are more financially secure
- The increased availability of specialized reproductive technologies, which may help women previously considered infertile

There are advantages to having a first baby after age 35. Single women or couples who delay childbearing until they are older tend to be well educated and financially secure. Usually their decision to have a baby was deliberately and thoughtfully made (Figure 12–4). Because of their greater life experiences, they also are more aware of the realities of having a child and what it means to have a baby at their age. Many of the women have experienced fulfillment in their careers and feel secure enough to take on the added responsibility of a child. Some women are ready to make a change in their lives, wanting to stay home with a new baby. Those who plan to continue working typically can afford good child care.

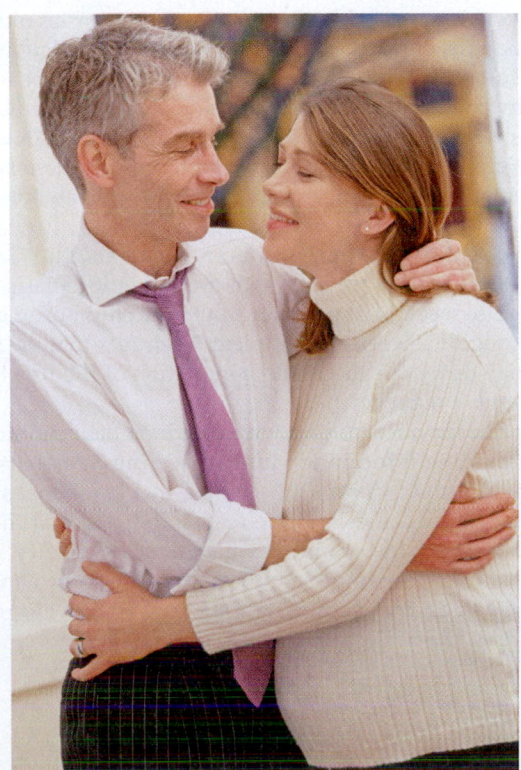

Figure 12–4 For many older couples, the decision to have a child may be very rewarding.

SOURCE: Ruth Jenkinson/DK Images.

Medical Risks

In the United States and Canada, the risk of death has declined dramatically during the past 30 years for women of all ages. However, the risk of maternal death is higher for women over age 35 and even higher for women age 40 and older. These women are more likely to have chronic medical conditions that can complicate a pregnancy. Pre-existing medical conditions such as hypertension or diabetes probably play a more significant role than age in maternal well-being and the outcome of pregnancy. In addition, the rate of miscarriage, stillbirth, preterm birth, low birth weight, and perinatal morbidity and mortality is higher in pregnant women over age 35 (Carolan, 2013). Nevertheless, while the risk of pregnancy complications is higher in women over age 35 who have a chronic condition such as hypertension or diabetes or who are in poor general health, the risks are much lower than previously believed for physically fit women without pre-existing medical problems (Cunningham et al., 2014).

Because of advances in reproductive technology, the number of women over age 45 who give birth is increasing although these women still constitute a very small percentage of overall births. While these women have a higher risk of complications than their younger counterparts, the absolute rate of stillbirth or perinatal death is still low (less than 10 per 1000) if they are healthy and free of pre-existing disease. Thus, for most, the outcome of pregnancy is positive (Carolan, 2013).

The risk of conceiving a child with Down syndrome does increase with age, especially over age 35. ACOG (2013) recommends that all pregnant women, regardless of age, be screened for Down syndrome. A quadruple screening to detect Down syndrome and trisomy 18 is often used. Noninvasive analysis of cell-free fetal DNA (cffDNA) is also available for prenatal diagnosis early in the first trimester and has great potential as a screening method although currently ACOG (2015) recommends conventional screening approaches. Alternatively, first-trimester ultrasound assessment of the thickness of fetal nuchal folds (nuchal translucency [NT]), combined with serum screens of free beta-human chorionic gonadotropin (β-hCG) and pregnancy-associated plasma protein A (PAPP-A), may be used in the detection of Down syndrome, trisomy 18, and trisomy 13. If the screening results are not in the normal range, follow-up testing using ultrasound and amniocentesis is often indicated (ACOG, 2013).

Advanced paternal age is associated with adverse fetal and neonatal outcomes (Wiener-Megnazi, Auslender, & Dirnfeld, 2012). Additionally, advanced paternal age increases the risk for autism spectrum disorders (Lampi, Hinkka-Yli-Salomäki, Lehti, et al., 2013; Ben Itzchak, Lahat, & Zachor, 2011).

Special Concerns of Expectant Parents Over Age 35

No matter what their age, most expectant parents have concerns about the well-being of the fetus and their ability to parent. Expectant parents over age 35 often have additional concerns about their age, especially the closer they are to age 40. Some couples are concerned about whether they will have enough energy to care for a new baby. Of greater concern is their ability to deal with the needs of the child as they age.

The financial concerns of the older couple are usually different from those of the younger couple. The older couple is generally more financially secure, but when their "baby" is ready for college, the older couple may be close to retirement and might not have the means to provide for their child. The older couple may also be forced to face their own mortality. Certainly the realization of one's mortality is not uncommon in midlife, but older expectant parents may confront the issue earlier as they consider what will happen as their child grows.

Older couples facing pregnancy in a late or second marriage or after therapy for infertility may find themselves somewhat isolated socially. They may feel different because they are often the only couple in their peer group expecting their first baby. In fact, many of their peers are likely to be parents of adolescents or young adults and may be grandparents as well.

Older couples who already have children may respond quite differently to learning that the woman is pregnant, depending on whether the pregnancy was planned or unexpected. Other factors influencing their response include their children's, family's, and friends' attitudes toward the pregnancy; the impact on their lifestyle; and the financial implications of having another child. Sometimes couples who had previously been married to other mates will choose to have a child together. *Blended families* are formed when "her" children, "his" children, and "their" children come together as a new family group.

Healthcare professionals may treat older expectant parents differently than they would a younger couple. They may offer older women more medical procedures, such as amniocentesis and ultrasound, than younger women. They may also discourage an older woman from using a birthing room or birthing center even if she is healthy because her age is considered to put her at risk.

The woman who has delayed pregnancy may be concerned about the limited amount of time that she has to bear children. When pregnancy does not occur as quickly as she had hoped, the older woman may become increasingly anxious as time slips away on her "biological clock." When an older woman becomes pregnant but has a spontaneous abortion, her grief for the loss of her unborn child is exacerbated by anxiety about her ability to conceive again in the time remaining to her.

Nursing Management

For the Pregnant Woman Over Age 35

Nursing Assessment and Diagnosis

In working with a woman in her late 30s or 40s who is pregnant, make the same assessments as are indicated in caring for any woman who is pregnant. Assess physical status, the woman's understanding of pregnancy and its changes, the couple's attitudes about the pregnancy and their expectations of the impact a baby will have on their lives, their health teaching needs, the degree of support the woman has, and her knowledge of infant care.

The nursing diagnoses applicable to pregnant women in general apply to pregnant women over age 35. Examples of other nursing diagnoses that may apply include the following (NANDA-I © 2014):

- *Decisional Conflict* related to unexpected pregnancy
- *Anxiety* (moderate) related to uncertainty about fetal well-being

Planning and Implementation

Once an older couple has made the decision to have a child, respect and support the couple in this decision. As with any client, discuss risks, identify concerns, and promote strengths. Do not make the woman's age an issue. It is helpful in promoting a sense of well-being to treat the pregnancy as normal unless the woman has specific health risks.

As the pregnancy continues, identify and discuss concerns the woman may have related to her age or to specific health problems. The older woman who has made a conscious decision to become pregnant often has carefully thought through potential problems and may actually have fewer concerns than a younger woman or one with an unplanned pregnancy.

Childbirth education classes are important in promoting adaptation to the event of childbirth for expectant parents of any age. However, older expectant parents often feel uncomfortable in classes in which most of the participants are much younger. Consequently, classes for expectant parents over age 35 are now available in many communities.

Women who are over age 35 and having their first baby tend to be better educated than other healthcare consumers. These clients frequently know the kind of care and services they want and may be assertive in their interactions with the healthcare system. You should not be intimidated by these individuals and you should not assume that anticipatory guidance and support are not needed. Instead, support the couple's strengths and be sensitive to their individual needs.

In working with older expectant couples or an older single woman, be sensitive to special needs. A particularly difficult issue these couples face is the possibility of bearing an unhealthy child or a child with a genetic disorder. As discussed previously, screening tests are available to assess for Down syndrome. Because of the risk of Down syndrome in these families, amniocentesis is often suggested or may be indicated if screening results are not in the normal range.

For couples who agree to amniocentesis, the first few months of pregnancy are a difficult time. Amniocentesis cannot be done until week 14 of pregnancy, and the chromosomal studies take roughly 2 weeks to complete. Their fear that the fetus is at risk may delay the successful completion of the psychologic tasks of early pregnancy.

You can support couples who decide to have amniocentesis by providing information and answering questions about the procedure and by providing comfort and emotional support during the amniocentesis. If the results indicate that the fetus has Down syndrome or another genetic abnormality, ensure that the couple has complete information about the condition, its range of possible manifestations, and its developmental implications.

Evaluation

Expected outcomes of nursing care include the following:

- The woman and her partner are knowledgeable about the pregnancy and express confidence in their ability to make appropriate healthcare choices.

- The expectant parents (and their children) are able to cope with the pregnancy and its implications for the future.

- The woman receives effective health care throughout her pregnancy and during birth and the postpartum period.

- The woman and her partner develop skills in child care and parenting.

Care of the Pregnant Woman With Special Needs

More than 1 million women of childbearing age report that they have a chronic physical disability (CPD) that causes them to need assistance with activities of daily living (Signore, Spong, Kroloski, et al., 2011). Of this number, approximately 163,700 women with a CPD become pregnant each year (Iezzoni, Yu, Wint, et al., 2014).

Chronic physical disabilities may include mobility difficulties that involve upper or lower extremities, arthritis, vision or hearing problems, disorders such as multiple sclerosis or cerebral palsy, heart or lung problems, and a variety of diseases. These numbers are predicted to increase because dramatic improvements in medical care are enabling women born with a CPD and those who acquire them through accident or illness to live into their childbearing years and beyond. Moreover, changes in societal attitudes have led to a decrease in stigmatization of disability, and civil rights laws such as the Americans with Disabilities Act provide increased support and acceptance for women with disabilities who seek motherhood. In addition, technologically sophisticated maternity and newborn care has made positive pregnancy outcomes more likely (Iezzoni, Yu, Wint, et al., 2013).

Women with an intellectual or developmental disability (IDD) may also become pregnant and have special needs for teaching and support. Among these women there is a high incidence of unplanned pregnancy, and they often seek prenatal care late. Typically they have lower reading and comprehension levels and are at a disadvantage when presented with complex information (Porter, Kidd, Murray, et al., 2012). Healthcare providers may perceive the pregnancy negatively, and the woman may experience social isolation and anxiety.

Women with IDD have a higher incidence of preterm birth and of preeclampsia, longer hospital stays, and a higher rate of caesarean births when compared to other women. In addition, their babies are more likely to have low birth weight (Parish, Mitra, Son, et al., 2015). Women with intellectual disabilities are also at increased risk of intervention by social services, which may result in the removal of the newborns from their custody.

Collectively, women with disabilities have often been discouraged from becoming mothers. Research suggests that these women often perceive themselves as "perennial outsiders" who are automatically categorized as high risk because of their disability (Walsh-Gallagher, Conkey, Sinclair, et al., 2013).

A family-centered approach is designed to optimize the childbearing experience of *all* women by providing a high quality, individualized experience that builds on the strength of each woman rather than perceived limitations. Ideally, this begins with preconception counseling so that the woman is in optimal health before conception. The woman and her family should be advised of potential health concerns and given information about their management.

During pregnancy, professional support and a team effort are essential. The woman needs to have a sense that she is empowered to make her healthcare decisions and that she has a good degree of control over the experience. In many cases, care at a tertiary level facility is important to an optimal outcome.

Women With Special Needs Intimate Partner Violence

Women with disabilities are at greater risk of being victimized and of sustaining intimate partner violence. Women who rely on their partner for assistance with activities of daily living are at risk for having care withheld and being neglected, in addition to physical and mental abuse. They are also at risk for financial abuse. The nurse should provide an extensive intimate partner assessment with the woman without the partner present to determine if abuse is occurring.

Nursing Management
For the Woman With a Disability

Nursing Assessment and Diagnosis

In addition to the assessments made for all pregnant women, nursing assessment of a woman with a disability needs to be condition specific. These assessments will vary depending on the extent of the woman's disability. A discussion of every possible disability is beyond the scope of this text. Some general principles are provided here.

A woman with a mobility disorder, especially if it is extensive, as in the case of a spinal cord injury, needs careful assessment. Be alert for commonly occurring complications associated with her condition such as pressure ulcers, bladder infection, gastroesophageal reflux disease (GERD), deep vein thrombosis, stool impaction, anemia, and autonomic dysreflexia (a rapid increase in blood pressure in response to a noxious stimulus such as catheterization or uterine contractions below the level of the spinal cord lesion) (Camune, 2013). Weight gain and changes in the woman's center of gravity may increase the risk for falls. In addition, the woman may be unaware of preterm labor and thus faces the possibility of an unattended birth.

Assess the woman with an intellectual disability for her level of understanding of instructions and printed materials. Determine her awareness of the signs of complications and of the onset of labor. Also evaluate her level of support from her partner and family members. Nursing diagnoses that may apply include the following (NANDA I © 2014):

- *Dysreflexia, Autonomic,* related to a spinal cord injury
- *Skin Integrity, Risk for Impaired,* related to decreased or absent mobility
- *Knowledge, Deficient,* related to a documented learning disability.

Nursing Plan and Implementation

Women with a disability involving a lower extremity (e.g., amputation, spinal cord injury, and so forth) may need assistance in issues involving mobility such as transferring to an examination table or bed. Typically, they will have adaptive equipment. Women who use wheelchairs may find that additional weight late in pregnancy may interfere with their ability to propel their chairs (Figure 12–5). Thus it is important that the woman avoid excessive weight gain and regularly perform range of motion exercises (Signore et al., 2011).

During labor assist the woman to change position periodically to avoid dependent edema. Be alert for signs of respiratory distress, DVT, and autonomic dysreflexia. Provide necessary adaptive equipment. Women with a loss of sensation in the lower extremities may find it difficult or impossible to push effectively and consequently have an increased incidence of cesarean birth. Women with upper extremity disorders may need assistance with, for example, position change or holding the newborn. Assist with breastfeeding as necessary.

The most important need of pregnant women with intellectual disabilities is for information that is timely, accessible, and understandable. They often find that information available for the general population is too difficult to understand. To address this need, easy-to-understand information should be available. It is also helpful for caregivers to allow extra consultation time and good communication aids. This might include videotaping or audiotaping information so the woman can refer to it as needed (Porter et al., 2012).

Evaluation

Expected outcomes of nursing care include the following:

- The expectant woman is able to cope with the pregnancy and its implications for the future.
- The woman receives effective health care throughout her pregnancy and during birth and the postpartum period.

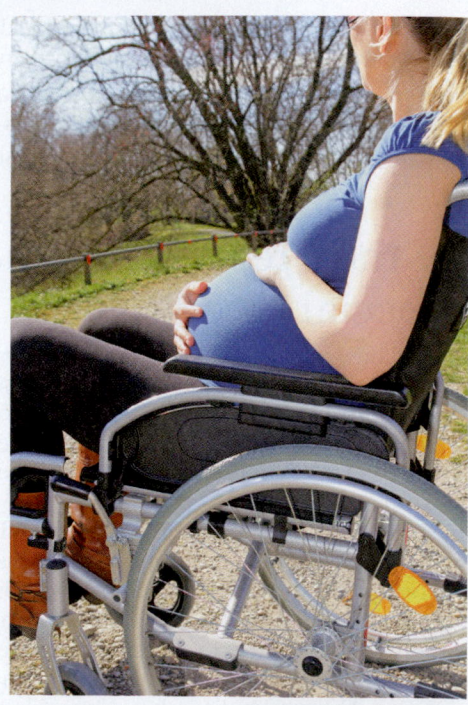

Figure 12–5 Pregnant woman with a lower extremity disability.

SOURCE: RioPatuca Images/Fotolia.

Focus Your Study

- Many factors contribute to the high teenage pregnancy rate, including earlier age of first sexual intercourse, lack of knowledge about conception, lack of easy access to contraception, lessened stigma associated with adolescent pregnancy in some populations, poverty, early school failure, and early childhood sexual abuse.

- Physical risks of adolescent pregnancies include preterm births, low-birth-weight newborns, cephalopelvic disproportion, iron deficiency anemia, and preeclampsia and its sequelae.

- Factors affecting an adolescent's response to pregnancy include her degree of achievement of the developmental tasks of adolescence (which can be closely associated with age) as well as cultural, religious, and socioeconomic factors.

- Nurses working with pregnant adolescents face many challenges, including safeguarding the client's confidentiality, winning her trust, and helping to build her sense of self-esteem.

- Often the adolescent has little understanding of pregnancy, childbirth, or parenting. Consequently, education is a primary responsibility of the nurse.

- Adolescent pregnancy prevention programs should be multifaceted, target males as well as females, and involve community-wide approaches.

- Childbirth among women over 35 is becoming increasingly common. It poses fewer health risks than previously believed and offers advantages for the woman or couple who makes this choice.

- A major risk for the older expectant couple relates to the increased incidence of Down syndrome in children born to women over age 35. Screening tests and amniocentesis can provide information as to whether the fetus has Down syndrome. The couple can then decide whether they wish to continue the pregnancy.

- Common risks of a pregnant woman with a mobility disorder include pressure ulcers, bladder infection, gastroesophageal reflux disease (GERD), deep vein thrombosis, stool impaction, anemia, and autonomic dysreflexia.

- The most pressing needs of a woman with an intellectual disability who becomes pregnant are accurate information appropriate to her level of understanding and consistent emotional support.

Clinical Reasoning in Action

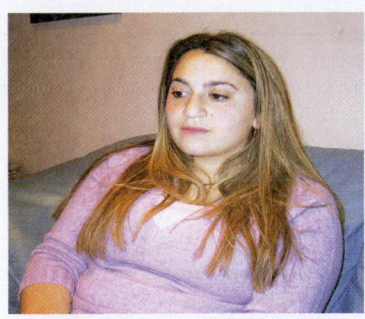

Sixteen-year-old Linda Perez and her mother present to you at the OB clinic for Linda's first prenatal visit. You determine that Linda is 20 weeks pregnant. Her weight is 135 lb, height 5 ft 4 in., T 98°F (36.6°C), P 80, R 14, BP 100/64. You assess that Linda's mother has type 2 diabetes, and that her siblings are healthy. Linda admits to having one sexual partner and says she has never been hospitalized. Her immunizations are up to date and she has never used tobacco or recreational drugs. To date, the father of the baby is not involved. Mrs. Perez is clearly upset that Linda's pregnancy is so far advanced without her knowledge. Linda is quiet and speaks only when questioned directly. You do your best to try to establish a trusting relationship with Linda and her mother by providing an atmosphere where issues can be discussed.

1. What psychologic factors contribute to teenage pregnancy?
2. Explore reasons why teenagers delay prenatal care.
3. Linda's mother asks you what factors facilitate adolescent pregnancies.
4. You assess that Linda has some anxiety concerning the birth process. She states she is not interested in prenatal classes because she is single and does not want to have natural childbirth. What would be your best response?

References

Alan Guttmacher Institute (AGI). (2014). *Fact sheet: American teens' sexual and reproductive health.* Retrieved from https://www.guttmacher.org/pubs/FB-ATSRH.html

Alan Guttmacher Institute (AGI). (2015). An overview of minors' consent laws. *Guttmacher Institute State Policies in Brief.* Washington, DC: Author.

Albert, B. (2012). *With one voice: America's adults and teens sound off about teen pregnancy.* Retrieved from http://thenationalcampaign.org/resource/one-voice-2012

American Academy of Pediatrics (AAP). (2012). Policy statement: Emergency contraception. *Pediatrics, 130*(6), 1174–1180.

American Academy of Pediatrics (AAP). (2014). Policy statement: Contraception for adolescents. *Pediatrics, 134,*(4), e1244–e1256.

American College of Obstetricians and Gynecologists (ACOG). (2013). *Screening for fetal chromosomal abnormalities.* Practice Bulletin No. 77. Washington, DC: Author.

American College of Obstetricians and Gynecologists (ACOG). (2015). *Cell-free DNA screening for fetal aneuploidy.* Committee Opinion No. 640. Washington, DC: Author.

Baldwin, M. K., & Edelman, A. B. (2013). The effect of long-acting reversible contraception on rapid repeat pregnancy in adolescents: A review. *The Journal of Adolescent Health, 52*(4 Suppl), S47–53.

Ben Itzchak, E., Lahat, E., & Zachor, D. A. (2011). Advanced parental ages and low birth weight in autism spectrum disorders—Rates and effect on functioning. *Research in Developmental Disabilities, 32*(5), 1776–1781.

Boonstra, H. D. (2014). What is behind the declines in teen pregnancy rates? *Guttmacher Policy Review, 17*(3), 1–21.

Camune, B. D. (2013). Challenges in the management of the pregnant woman with a spinal cord injury. *Journal of Perinatal and Neonatal Nursing, 27*(3), 225–231.

Carolan, M. (2013). Maternal age ≥ 45 years and maternal and perinatal outcomes: A review of the evidence. *Midwifery, 29,* 479–489.

Centers for Disease Control and Prevention (CDC). (2014). *Sexually transmitted disease surveillance 2013.* Atlanta, GA: U.S. Department of Health and Human Services.

Cunningham, F. G., Leveno, K. J., Bloom, S. L., Spong, C. Y., Dashe, J. S., Hoffman, B. L., . . . Sheffield, J. S. (2014). *Williams obstetrics* (24th ed.). New York, NY: McGraw-Hill.

Fletcher, J. M., & Wolfe, B. L. (2012). The effects of teenage fatherhood on young adult outcomes. *Economic Inquiry, 50*(1), 182–201.

Food and Drug Administration, (FDA). (2013). *FDA approves Plan B One-Step emergency contraceptive for use without prescription for all women of childbearing potential.* Retrieved from http://www.fda.gov/NewsEvents/Newsroom/PressAnnouncements/ucm358082.htm

Forcier, M., & Harel, Z. (2011). Adolescents and the IUD: An underutilized contraception for a high-risk population. *The Female Patient, 36*(6), 22–25.

Garwood, S. K., Gerassi, L., Jonson-Reid, M., Plax, K., & Drake, B. (2015). More than poverty: The effect of abuse and neglect on teen pregnancy risk. *Journal of Adolescent Health, 57*(2), 164–158.

Helfrich, C., & McWey, L. (2014). Substance use and delinquency: High-risk behaviors as predictors of teen pregnancy among adolescents involved with the child welfare system. *Journal of Family Issues, 35*(10), 1322–1338.

Herrman, J. W. (2010). Assessing the teen parent family. *Nursing for Women's Health, 14*(3), 214–224.

Herrman, J. W. (2014). Adolescent girls who experience abuse or neglect are at an increased risk of teen pregnancy. *Evidence Based Nursing, 17*(3), 79.

Herrman, J. W., & Nandakumar, R. (2012). Development of a survey to assess adolescent perceptions of teen parenting. *Journal of Nursing Measurement, 20*(1), 3–20.

House, L., Bates, J., Markham, C., & Lesesne, C. (2010). Competence as a predictor of reproductive health outcomes for youth: A systematic review. *Journal of Adolescent Health, 46*(3, Suppl. 1), S7–S22.

Iezzoni, L. I., Yu, J, Wint, A. J., Smeltzer, S. C., & Eaker, J. L. (2013). Prevalence of current pregnancy among U. S. women with and without chronic physical disabilities. *Medical Care, 51*(6), 555–562.

Iezzoni, L. I., Yu, J, Wint, A. J., Smeltzer, S. C., & Eaker, J. L. (2014). General health, health conditions, and current pregnancy among U. S. women with and without chronic physical disabilities. *Disability and Health Journal, 7,* 181–188.

Kann, L., Kinchen, S., Shanklin, S. L., Flint, K. H., Hawkins, J., Harris, W. A., Lowry, R., . . . Zaza, S. (2014). Youth risk behavior surveillance—United States, 2013. *MMWR Surveillance Summaries, 63*(4), 1–172.

Kearney, M. S., & Levine, P. B. (2012). Why is the teen birth rate in the United States so high and why does it matter? *Journal of Economic Perspectives, 26*(2), 141–166.

Kirven, J. (2014). Helping teen dads obtain and sustain parental success. *International Journal of Childbirth Education, 29*(2), 85–88.

Klettke, B., Hallford, D. J., & Mellor, D. J. (2014). Sexting prevalence and correlates: A systematic literature review. *Clinical Psychology Review, 34*(1), 44–53.

Kogan, S. M., Cho, J., Allen, K., Lei, M., Beach, S. R. H., Gibbons, F. X., Simons, L. G., Simons, R. L., & Brody, G. H. (2013). Avoiding adolescent pregnancy: A longitudinal analysis of African-American youth. *Journal of Adolescent Health, 53,* 14–20.

Lampi, K., Hinkka-Yli-Salomäki, S., Lehti, V., Helenius, H., Gissler, M., Brown, A., & Sourander, A. (2013). Parental age and risk of autism spectrum disorders in a Finnish national birth cohort. *Journal of Autism and Developmental Disorders, 43*(11), 2526–2535.

Lee, Y., Cintron, A., & Kocher, S. (2014). Factors related to risky sexual behaviors and effective STI/HIV and pregnancy intervention programs for African American adolescents. *Public Health Nursing, 31*(5), 414–427.

Lohan, M., Cruise, S., O'Halloran, P., Alderdice, F., & Hyde, A. (2010). Adolescent men's attitudes in relation to pregnancy and pregnancy outcomes: A systematic review of the literature from 1980–2009. *Journal of Adolescent Health, 47,* 327–345.

March of Dimes (MOD). (2012). *Teenage pregnancy.* Retrieved from http://www.marchofdimes.com/materials/teenage-pregnancy.pdf

Martin, J. A., Hamilton, B. E., Osterman, M. J. K., Curtin, S. C., & Mathews, T. J. (2015). Births: Final data for 2013. *National Vital Statistics Reports, 64*(1), 1–65.

National Campaign to Prevent Teen and Unplanned Pregnancy (NCPTUP). (2012). *Ten tips for parents.* Retrieved from http://www.thenationalcampaign.org/parents/ten_tips.aspx

National Campaign to Prevent Teen and Unplanned Pregnancy (NCPTUP). (2015). *Our mission: Goal.* Retrieved from http://thenationalcampaign.org/about

Parish, S. L., Mitra, M., Son, E., Bonardi, A., Swoboda, P. T., & Igdalsky, L. (2015). Pregnancy outcomes among U.S. women with intellectual and developmental disabilities. *American Journal on Intellectual & Developmental Disabilities, 120*(5), 433–443.

Porter, E., Kidd, G., Murray, N., Spink, A., & Anderson, B. (2012). Developing the pregnancy support pack for people who have a learning disability. *British Journal of Learning Disabilities, 40*, 310–317.

Ralph, L., Gould, H., Baker, A., & Foster, D. G. (2014). The role of parents and partners in minors' decisions to have an abortion and anticipated coping after abortion. *Journal of Adolescent Health, 54*, 428–434.

Signore, C., Spong, C. Y., Krotoski, D., Shinowara, N. L., & Blackwell, S. C. (2011). Pregnancy in women with physical disabilities. *Obstetrics & Gynecology, 117*(4), 935–947.

Sipsma, H. L., Ickovics, J. R., Lewis, J. B., Ethier, K. A., & Kershaw, T. S. (2011). Adolescent pregnancy desire and pregnancy incidence. *Women's Health Issues, 21*(2), 110–116.

Sonfield, A., Hasstedt, K., Kavanaugh, M. L., & Anderson, R. (2013). The social and economic benefits of women's ability to determine whether and when to have children. *Guttmacher Institute Report*, May 2013. New York, NY: Guttmacher Institute.

Steinberg, L. (2014). *Adolescence* (10th ed.). New York, NY: McGraw-Hill.

Turnage, B. F., & Pharris, A. D. (2013). Supporting the pregnant adolescent. *International Journal of Childbirth Education, 28*(4), 72–76.

Ventura, S. J., Hamilton, B. E., & Mathews, T. J. (2014). National and state patterns of teen births in the United States, 1940–2013. *National Vital Statistics Reports, 63*(4), 1–34.

Walsh-Gallagher, D., McConkey, R., Sinclair, M., & Clarke, R. (2013). Normalising birth for women with a disability: The challenges facing practitioners. *Midwifery, 29*(4), 294–299.

Wiener-Megnazi, Z., Auslender, R., & Dirnfeld, M. (2012). Advanced paternal age and reproductive outcome. *Asian Journal of Andrology, 14*(1), 69–76.

Yoost, J. L., Hertweck, S. P., & Barnett, S. N. (2014). The effect of an educational approach to pregnancy prevention among high-risk early and late adolescents. *Journal of Adolescent Health, 55*(2), 222–227.

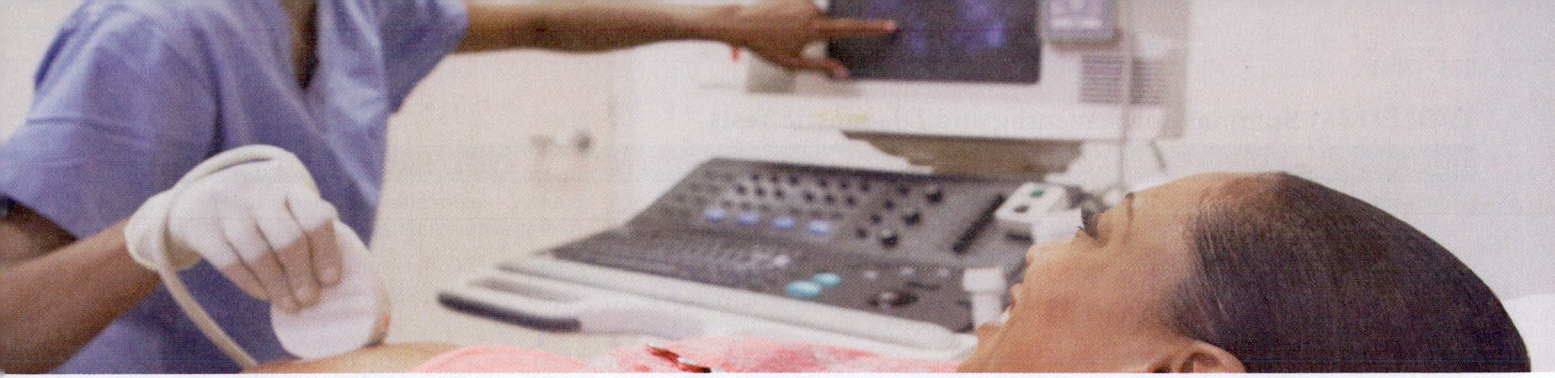

Chapter 13
Assessment of Fetal Well-Being

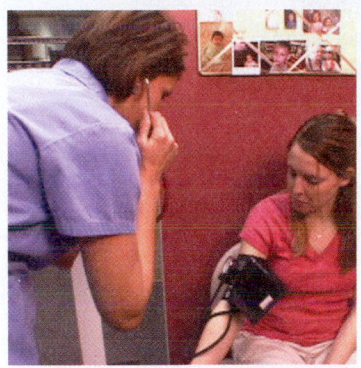

What makes my job special is the relationships I develop with my clients. Many of the expectant mothers I work with begin coming to our office in early pregnancy and continue on a regular basis until they give birth. I know that some of the diagnostic tests we do can be intimidating, and it's my responsibility to help make those tests understandable. I love connecting with my clients, building a personal relationship with them, and explaining things to them when they have questions or fears. I feel a sense of accomplishment and pride when they feel comfortable enough to express those concerns with me.

—A Perinatal and Genetics Office Nurse

∨ Learning Outcomes

13.1 Identify pertinent information to be discussed with the woman regarding her own assessment of fetal activity and methods of recording fetal activity as a means of establishing fetal well-being.

13.2 Describe the methods, clinical applications, and results of ultrasound in the nursing care management of the pregnant woman.

13.3 Explain the different methods used to identify a fetus with an aneuploidy defect.

13.4 Describe the use, procedure, information obtained, and nursing considerations to evaluate fetal well-being when using Doppler

blood flow studies/umbilical velocimetry, non-stress test, contraction stress test, and biophysical profile test.

13.5 Explain the use of amniocentesis as a diagnostic tool.

13.6 Describe the nurse's role and responsibilities in assisting during amniocentesis.

13.7 Compare the advantages and disadvantages of chorionic villus sampling (CVS) versus amniocentesis.

13.8 Identify nursing interventions that are aimed at ensuring the safety of the mother and the fetus during antepartum testing.

The past few decades have produced a notable increase in the number of antenatal techniques used to assess fetal well-being. From the relatively simple maternal assessment of fetal movement to more complex diagnostic tests guided by ultrasound and sophisticated serum screening to detect first-trimester anomalies, each technique is used to obtain accurate and helpful data about the developing fetus. For example, specialized diagnostic tests can provide information about the normal growth of the fetus, the presence of

congenital anomalies, the location of the placenta, and fetal lung maturity. At times just one test is done, and in other circumstances a combination of testing is needed.

Some of these assessment techniques pose risks to the fetus and possibly to the pregnant woman; the risk to both should be considered before deciding to perform the test. The healthcare provider must be certain that the advantages outweigh the potential risks and added expense. In addition, the diagnostic accuracy and applicability of these tests may vary.

233

TABLE 13–1 Summary of Screening and Diagnostic Tests

GOAL	TEST	TIMING
To validate the pregnancy	Ultrasound: gestational sac volume	5 and 6 weeks after last menstrual period (LMP) by transvaginal ultrasound
To determine how advanced is the pregnancy	Ultrasound: crown–rump length	6–10 weeks' gestation
	Ultrasound: biparietal diameter, femur length, abdominal circumference	13–40 weeks' gestation
To identify normal growth of the fetus	Ultrasound: biparietal diameter	Most useful from 20–30 weeks' gestation
	Ultrasound: head/abdomen ratio	13–40 weeks' gestation
	Ultrasound: estimated fetal weight	About 24–40 weeks' gestation
To detect congenital anomalies and problems	Nuchal translucency testing	11–13 weeks' gestation
	Ultrasound	18–40 weeks' gestation
	Chorionic villus sampling	10–12 weeks' gestation
	Amniocentesis	15–20 weeks' gestation
	Fetoscopy	18 weeks' gestation
	First-trimester combined screening test	11–13 weeks' gestation
	Quadruple test	Generally 15–20 weeks' gestation
	Cell-free fetal DNA testing	After 10 weeks' gestation
To localize the placenta	Ultrasound	Usually in third trimester or before amniocentesis
To assess fetal status	Biophysical profile	Approximately 28 weeks to birth
	Maternal assessment of fetal activity	Approximately 28 weeks to birth
	Non-stress test	Approximately 28 weeks to birth
	Contraction stress test	After 28 weeks
To diagnose cardiac problems	Fetal echocardiography	Second and third trimesters
To assess fetal lung maturity	Amniocentesis	33–40 weeks
	L/S ratio	33 weeks to birth
	Phosphatidylglycerol	33 weeks to birth
	Phosphatidylcholine	33 weeks to birth
	Lamellar body counts	33 weeks to birth
To obtain more information about breech presentation	Ultrasound	Just before labor is anticipated or during labor

Rationale for Antenatal Testing

Some tests are for screening purposes, meaning that they indicate the fetus *may* be at risk for a certain disorder or abnormality, others are diagnostic, meaning that they can diagnose the abnormality (Table 13–1). Certainly not all high-risk pregnancies require the same tests. Conditions that indicate a pregnancy at risk include the following:

- Maternal age less than 16 or more than 35 years
- Chronic maternal hypertension, preeclampsia, diabetes mellitus, or heart disease
- Presence of Rh alloimmunization
- A maternal history of unexplained stillbirth
- Suspected intrauterine growth restriction (IUGR)
- Pregnancy prolonged past 42 weeks' gestation
- Multiple gestation
- Maternal history of preterm labor
- Previous cervical insufficiency

See Chapter 14 and Chapter 15 for descriptions of various conditions that may threaten the successful completion of pregnancy.

Nursing care for the woman who is undergoing diagnostic testing focuses on outcomes to ensure that she understands the reasons for the test, understands the test results, and has had support during the test, thus avoiding complications, and ensuring maternal and fetal safety during the test (see Table 13–2).

Clinical Tip

Families undergoing fetal testing experience a wide range of emotions based on personal expectations, past experiences, fears, and cultural norms. Encouraging the family to verbalize concerns, ask questions, and express any apprehensions or fears can help put the family at ease.

Maternal Assessment of Fetal Activity

Vigorous and regular fetal activity is associated with fetal well-being, while marked decreases in activity or cessation of movement may indicate possible fetal compromise (or even death)

TABLE 13–2 Suggested Nursing Approaches to Pretest Teaching

Assess whether the woman knows the reason why the screening or diagnostic test is being recommended.
Examples:

"Has your healthcare provider told you why this test is necessary?"

"Sometimes tests are done for many different reasons. Can you tell me why you are having this test?"

"What is your understanding about what the test will show?"

Provide an opportunity for questions.
Examples:

"What questions do you have about the test?"

"Is there anything that is not clear to you?"

Explain the test procedure, paying particular attention to any preparation the woman needs before the test.
Examples:

"The test that has been ordered for you is designed to _____." (Add specific information about the particular test. Give the explanation in simple language.)

Validate the woman's understanding of the preparation.
Examples:

"Tell me what you will have to do to get ready for this test."

Give permission for the woman to continue to ask questions if needed.
Examples:

"I'll be with you during the test. If you have any questions at any time, please don't hesitate to ask."

Provide information on whether the test is a screening test or a diagnostic test.
Examples:

"Do you understand this test is a screening test, meaning it will not tell you if the baby has a specific problem, but will give us more information to determine if your baby is at risk?"

"Do you understand this is a diagnostic test and will likely determine if your baby is affected with _____?"

and require immediate assessment. Fetal activity monitoring is typically advised to begin at 28 gestational weeks. Decreased fetal movement can be associated with the following (Hofmeyr & Novikova, 2012):

- Previous undiagnosed risk factors
- Fetal hypoxia
- Fetal growth restriction
- Preterm birth
- Fetal death

Although more research is needed to determine if fetal activity assessment improves neonatal outcomes, a Cochrane Review found that Doppler ultrasound studies, computerized cardiotocography, and fetal arousal to facilitate cardiotocography is more likely to identify fetal adverse conditions than maternal fetal movement monitoring. However, because fetal movement monitoring costs nothing and can be performed without risk, the practice is still routinely performed and remains an important tool, particularly when modern technology is not available.

SAFETY ALERT!

Lack of fetal movement can be an indication of an adverse fetal event. The woman should call her healthcare provider and if advised she should come in for testing.

There is no definitive definition of how many movements should occur within a specified time period. To obtain a **fetal movement count (FMC)**, the mother is instructed to count fetal movements at the same time each day. If she experiences less than 10 movements in a 3-hour period or if the amount of movement is significantly less than normal, the woman should immediately notify her healthcare provider. Fetuses spend approximately 10% of their time making gross body movements, which are directly related to their sleep–wake cycles (Blackburn, 2013). Factors that may affect fetal movements include maternal weight, poor placental perfusion, oligohydramnios, impending preterm labor, sound, hemorrhage, cigarette smoking, intrauterine infections, and drugs (Cunningham et al., 2014).

Women With Special Needs Women With Paralysis

Women with paralysis often warrant intermittent fetal surveillance since they are unable to feel fetal movement or premature contractions. These women are at risk for unattended birth since they cannot perceive their contractions. Their partners or healthcare providers should be trained to palpate contractions and observe for fetal movement on a regular basis.

A **fetal movement record (FMR)**, such as the Cardiff Count-to-Ten method (Figure 13–1), is a noninvasive technique. See *Teaching Highlights: What to Tell the Pregnant Woman About Assessing Fetal Activity.*

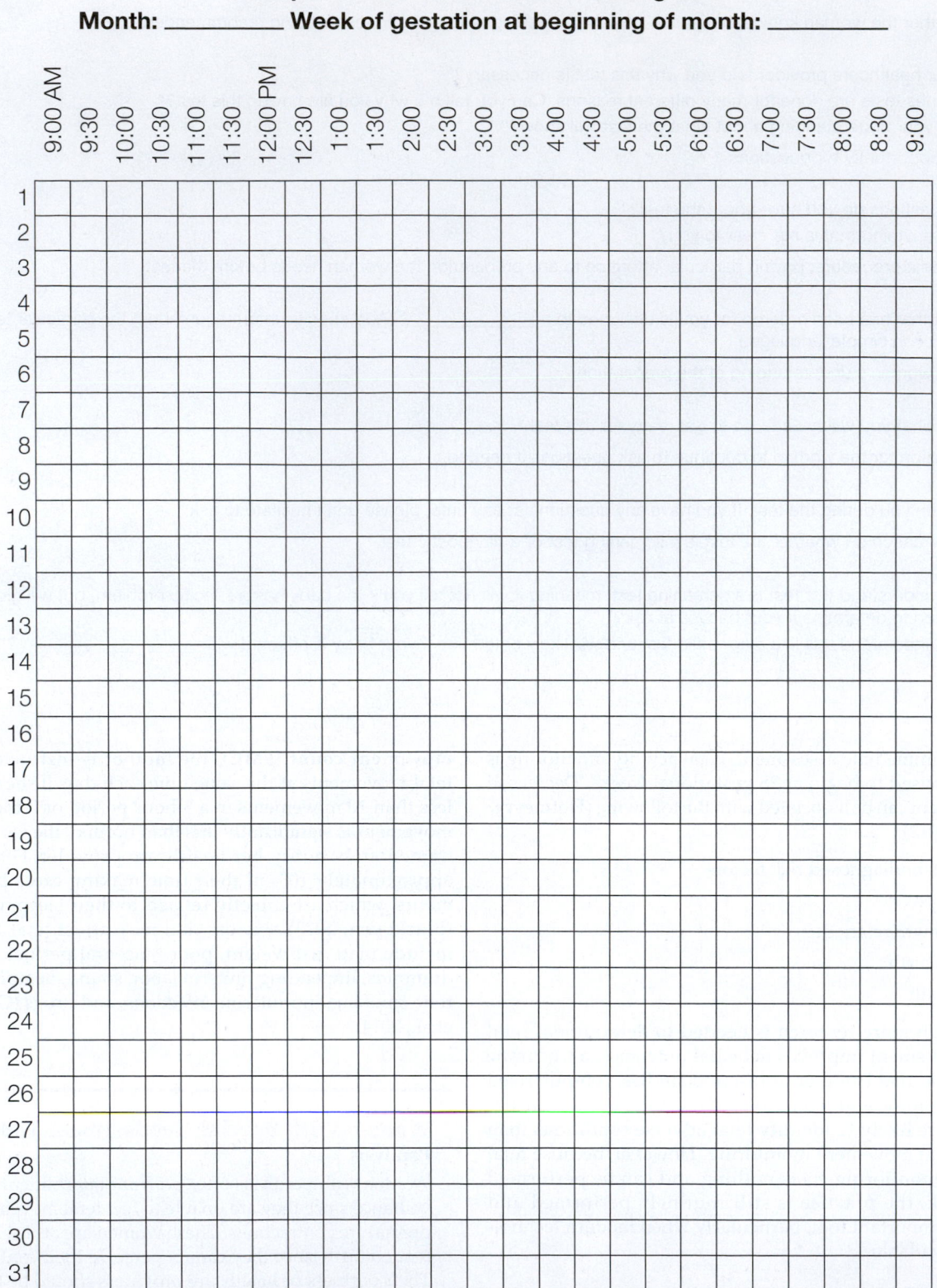

Figure 13–1 An adaptation of the Cardiff Count-to-Ten scoring card for fetal movement assessment.

Ultrasound

Valuable information about the fetus may be obtained from **ultrasound** testing. Intermittent ultrasonic waves (high-frequency sound waves) are transmitted by an alternating current to a transducer, which is applied to the woman's abdomen. The ultrasonic waves deflect off tissues within the woman's abdomen, showing structures of varying densities (Figures 13–2 and 13–3).

Diagnostic ultrasound has several advantages. It is non-invasive, painless, and nonradiating to both the woman and the fetus, and it has no known harmful effects to either.

TEACHING HIGHLIGHTS | What to Tell the Pregnant Woman About Assessing Fetal Activity

CONTENT

- Explain that fetal movements are first felt around 18 weeks' gestation. From that time the fetal movements get stronger and easier to detect. A slowing or stopping of fetal movement may be an indication that the fetus needs some attention and evaluation.

- Explain the procedure for the Cardiff Count-to-Ten method or for the fetal movement record (FMR). For both methods, advise the woman as follows:
  - Beginning at about 28 weeks' gestation, keep a daily record of fetal movement.
  - Try to begin counting at about the same time each day, about 1 hour after a meal if possible.
  - Lie quietly in a side-lying position.

- Using the Cardiff card, have the woman place an X for each fetal movement until she has recorded 10. Movement varies considerably, but most women feel fetal movement at least 10 times in 3 hours.

- Using the FMR, have the woman count three times a day for 20 to 30 minutes each session. If there are fewer than three movements in a session, have the woman count for 1 hour or more.

- Explain when to contact the care provider:
  - If there are fewer than 10 movements in 3 hours.
  - If overall the fetus's movements are slowing, and it takes much longer each day to note 10 movements.
  - If there are no movements in the morning.

TEACHING METHOD

Describe procedures and demonstrate how to assess fetal movement. Sit beside the woman and show her how to place her hand on the fundus to feel fetal movement.

Provide a written teaching sheet for the woman's use at home.

Demonstrate how to record fetal movements on a Cardiff Count-to-Ten scoring card or on an FMR.

Watch the woman fill out the record as examples are provided. Encourage her to complete the record each day and bring it with her to each prenatal visit. Assure her that the record will be discussed at each prenatal visit, and questions may be addressed at that time if desired.

Provide the woman with a name and phone number in case she has further questions.

Serial studies (several ultrasound tests done over a span of time) may be done for assessment and comparison. Soft-tissue masses (such as tumors) can be differentiated, the fetus can be visualized, fetal growth can be followed with serial ultrasound assessments (especially in the presence of multiple gestation), cervical length and impending cervical insufficiency can be detected, and a number of other potential problems can be identified and possibly averted; in addition, results are immediately available (Cunningham et al., 2014).

Future research in fetal well-being will be generated and enhanced by the use of *four-dimensional ultrasound*. Four-dimensional ultrasound combines the components of three-dimensional ultrasound with a fourth dimension, time, because it monitors live action. The technology produces images of photolike quality, allowing healthcare providers to better visualize fetal structures, and providing better guidance during invasive intrauterine procedures such as amniocentesis and chorionic villus sampling (CVS) (discussed later in this chapter). The use of three- and four-dimensional ultrasound has been helpful in identifying facial anomalies, neural tube defects, chromosomal defects, and skeletal malformations (Cunningham et al., 2014).

Ultrasound is a useful tool in monitoring the fetus but does have limitations, and cannot guarantee that a fetus or placenta

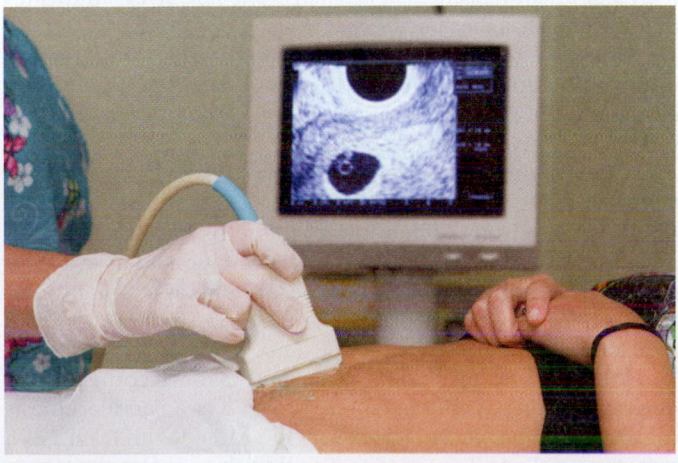

Figure 13–2 Ultrasound scanning permits visualization of the fetus in utero.

SOURCE: Steven Frame/Shutterstock.

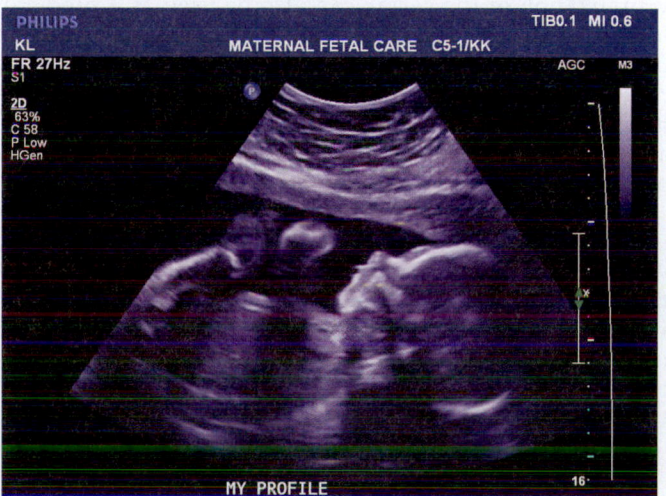

Figure 13–3 Ultrasound of the face and body of a fetus.

does not have certain disorders or defects. Ultrasound is limited by maternal obesity, fetal positioning, and technician or physician skill. Even though fetal problems can be diagnosed via the technology, there are times that abnormalities go unrecognized. A "normal" ultrasound is reassuring for the parents and healthcare team, but it is important that parents realize a normal sonogram is not 100% reliable.

Procedures

The two most common methods of ultrasound scanning are transabdominal and transvaginal.

TRANSABDOMINAL ULTRASOUND

In the transabdominal approach, a transducer is moved across the woman's abdomen. The woman is often scanned with a full bladder. When the bladder is full, the examiner can assess other structures, especially the vagina and cervix, in relation to the bladder. The ability to see the lower portion of the uterus and cervix is particularly important when vaginal bleeding is noted and placenta previa (the placenta implanted over the cervix) is the suspected cause. (See Chapter 20 for a full discussion of placenta previa.) The woman is advised to drink 1 to 1.5 quarts of water approximately 2 hours before the examination, and she is asked to refrain from emptying her bladder. If the bladder is not sufficiently filled, she is asked to drink three to four 8-oz glasses of water and is rescanned 30 to 45 minutes later.

Ultrasound gel is generously spread over the woman's abdomen, and the sonographer slowly moves a transducer over the abdomen to obtain a picture of the uterine contents. The gel can be warmed prior to application to increase comfort. Ultrasound testing takes 20 to 30 minutes. The woman may feel discomfort caused by pressure applied over a full bladder. In addition, if the woman lies on her back during the test, shortness of breath can develop. This may be relieved by elevating her upper body during the test.

TRANSVAGINAL ULTRASOUND

The transvaginal approach uses a transvaginal probe inserted into the vagina after the woman has emptied her bladder. Once inserted, the probe is close to the structures being imaged and produces a clearer, more defined image. The improved images obtained by transvaginal ultrasound have enabled sonographers to identify structures and fetal characteristics earlier in pregnancy (Blackburn, 2013). Internal visualization of the cervix can also be used as a predictor for preterm birth in high-risk cases (Funai, 2014). Use of the ultrasound to detect shortened cervical length or funneling (a cone-shaped indentation in the cervical os) is helpful in predicting preterm labor and provides guidance for additional antepartum surveillance, especially in women with a previous history of preterm labor (Funai, 2014).

After the procedure has been explained to her, the woman is assisted into the lithotomy position and draped for privacy with a female attendant present. Her buttocks should be positioned at the end of the table so the probe can be moved in various directions. A small, lightweight vaginal transducer is covered with a specially fitted sterile sheath, a condom, or one finger of a glove. Ultrasound coupling gel is then applied to both the inside and the outside of the covering, making insertion into the vagina easier and providing a medium for enhancing the ultrasound image. The probe is smaller than a speculum, so insertion is usually completed with ease. The woman may feel the movement of the probe during the examination as various structures are visualized, along with some pelvic pressure. Some women may want to insert the probe themselves to enhance their comfort, whereas others would feel embarrassed even to be asked.

Nuchal Translucency Testing and First-Trimester Combined Screening

Nuchal translucency testing (NTT), also known as *nuchal testing (NT)* or the *nuchal fold test*, is performed at 11 to 13 6/7 gestational weeks to screen for aneuploidies such as trisomies 13, 18, and 21 (Cunningham et al., 2014). An **aneuploidy** is an abnormal number of chromosomes that is often responsible for genetic defects. Although women over the age of 35 have a higher risk of chromosomal disorders, all women should be offered first- and second-trimester screening. The test uses ultrasound to scan the translucent or clear area on the back of the fetal neck, measuring the diameter of the area. Fetuses with certain genetic disorders often have an excess accumulation of fluid that can be seen at the end of the first trimester. The results are computed using the nuchal measurement, exact gestational age, and maternal age.

First-trimester combined screening utilizes NTT and additionally includes serum testing to increase accuracy by testing for pregnancy-associated plasma protein-A (PAPP-A) and free beta human chorionic gonadotropin (βhCG) to determine if a fetus is at risk for trisomies 13, 18, and 21. First-trimester combined screening is more accurate than NTT alone because it provides additional data.

When performing the nuchal translucency ultrasound assessment, the examiner should also assess for the presence of the fetal nasal bone to increase the accuracy in identifying a risk for trisomy 21. Assessing the nasal bone is a valuable tool in assessing for Down syndrome and increases accuracy to 93% to 96%, whereas NTT and serum testing alone yield detection rates of 85% to 95% (Cunningham et al., 2014). Fetuses with abnormal nuchal translucency thickness and lacking a nasal bone should also be screened for accompanying heart defects, including tricuspid flow or ductus venosus flow, because both can occur in fetuses with Down syndrome (Blackburn, 2013).

Fetuses that have a nuchal translucency measurement of greater than 3 mm are at risk for trisomies 13, 18, and 21 and their mothers should be offered a chorionic villus sampling (CVS) or an amniocentesis. The NTT is a *screening test*, meaning it indicates that a fetus is at risk. Diagnostic testing, such as a CVS or an amniocentesis, is a *diagnostic test*, which indicates that the fetus has the specific diagnosis.

The NTT test has several advantages over other testing options, including the ability to screen in the first trimester, elimination of risk of spontaneous abortion, and reduction in parental anxiety.

Disadvantages to testing including a 5% risk of false positives, meaning the test will indicate that the fetus is at risk for Down syndrome when in fact the fetus has normal chromosomes. Combining the methods to include an assessment of maternal age, serum testing, nasal bone assessment, and fetal echocardiogram reduces the false-positive rate to 2.5% (Blackburn, 2013).

Women who receive an abnormal test are counseled to determine if they would like to have a CVS or an amniocentesis for diagnostic purposes. The choice to proceed with testing is a very personal one. Some women will wish to obtain the test so they will be more prepared for the diagnosis; other women will want to discontinue the pregnancy. Some women may decide not to have additional testing.

Because fetuses with an above average nuchal translucency measurement are also at risk for congenital heart disease, a fetal echocardiogram should be performed to determine if a cardiac anomaly is present. Early research suggests that in addition to these markers, increased blood flow to the fetal hepatic artery may be another marker for trisomy 21 (Blackburn, 2013).

Clinical Tip

When advising clients that a screening test, such as the NTT, is abnormal, be sure to explain that this does *not* mean their baby definitely has the disorder, but rather indicates that the baby *may* be at risk. It is imperative for parents to understand that an abnormal NTT, or any type of screening test, is only an indication that more testing is needed to make the actual diagnosis. Advise parents that some women with abnormal test results have normal fetuses and that because the test only screens and does not actually diagnosis the fetus, a fetus that screens within the normal criteria could have an unrecognized anomaly.

Clinical Applications

Ultrasound testing can be of benefit in the following ways:

- *Early identification of pregnancy.* Pregnancy may be detected as early as the fifth or sixth week after the last menstrual period (LMP) by assessing the gestational sac and the presence of a fetal heart rate after 6 gestational weeks.

- *Observation of fetal heartbeat and fetal breathing movements (FBMs).* FBMs have been observed as early as week 11 of gestation.

- *Identification of more than one embryo or fetus.*

- *Measurement of the biparietal diameter of the fetal head or the fetal femur length to assess growth patterns.* These measurements help determine the gestational age of the fetus and identify intrauterine growth restriction (IUGR).

- *Clinical estimations of birth weight.* This assessment helps to identify macrosomia (newborns greater than 4000 g at birth) and low-birth-weight newborns (babies less than 2500 g at birth). Macrosomia has been identified as a predictor of birth-related trauma and is a risk factor for both maternal and fetal morbidity.

- *Detection of fetal anomalies such as anencephaly and hydrocephalus.*

- *Examination of nuchal translucency in the first trimester to assess for Down syndrome, chromosomal disorders, and other fetal structural anomalies.*

- *Examination of fetal cardiac structures (echocardiography).*

- *Measurement of fetal nasal bone.*

- *Identification of amniotic fluid index.* The maternal abdomen is divided into quadrants. The umbilicus is used to divide the upper and lower sections, and the linea nigra divides the right and left sections. The vertical diameter of the largest amniotic fluid pocket in each quadrant is measured. All measurements are totaled to obtain the **amniotic fluid index (AFI)** in centimeters. Women with an AFI of more than 20 cm are considered to have hydramnios (an excess of amniotic fluid), and women with less than 5 cm at term are considered to have oligohydramnios (a decreased amount of amniotic fluid). See *Care of the Woman with Abnormal Amniotic Fluid Volume* in Chapter 20 for detailed information about these conditions. An AFI between 5 and 20 cm is considered normal. After 39 weeks, the amniotic fluid volume begins to decline (Cunningham et al., 2014). Both hydramnios and oligohydramnios are associated with increased risk to the fetus, including nonreassuring fetal status, IUGR, meconium-stained amniotic fluid, and an increase in admissions to the neonatal intensive care unit, and may indicate a maternal high-risk condition, such as gestational diabetes or maternal infection (Cunningham et al., 2014).

- *Location of the placenta.* The placenta is located before amniocentesis to avoid puncturing the placenta. Ultrasound is valuable in identifying and evaluating placenta previa, abruptio placentae, and other placental abnormalities (see Chapter 20 for discussion of these conditions).

- *Placental grading.* As the fetus matures, the placenta calcifies. These changes can be detected by ultrasound and graded according to the degree of calcification. Placenta grading can be used to identify internal placenta vasculature, which can be associated with preeclampsia and chronic hypertension. It can also identify disorders such as fetal growth abnormalities, triploidy, nonimmune hydrops, and infections.

- *Detection of fetal death.* Inability to visualize the fetal heart beating and the separation of the bones in the fetal head are signs of fetal death.

- *Determination of fetal position and presentation.*

- *Accompanying procedures.* Amniocentesis, chorionic villus sampling, intrauterine procedures, external cephalic version, and other procedures, which will be discussed shortly.

Risks of Ultrasound

Ultrasound has been used clinically for over 50 years; to date no clinical studies verify harmful effects to the mother, the fetus, or the newborn.

Nursing Management

It is important to identify if the woman knows why she is having the procedure. Ascertain that the woman understands why the ultrasound is being suggested and ensure that the woman realizes that ultrasound results are not 100% reliable. Provide time for the woman to ask questions and act as her advocate if she does not fully understand the information. The option of fetal evaluation should be offered to all women, regardless of age, and should include noninvasive procedures and invasive testing, such as amniocentesis and chorionic villus sampling (CVS). Explain what will happen and prepare the woman for the examination. After the test is completed, assist with clarifying or interpreting test results for the woman and her partner.

Cell-Free Fetal DNA (cffDNA) Testing

In late 2011, the first **cell-free fetal DNA (cffDNA)** test was introduced as a screening tool that could be used to test for trisomy 13, 18, and 21. The test detects circulating fetal deoxyribonucleic acid (DNA) within the maternal serum, which is as high as 6% to 10%. The test is noninvasive and detects 99% of fetuses affected with Down syndrome (trisomy 21) (Cunningham et al., 2014). In laboratory testing, false positives occurred in only 0.1% of testing samples, making cell-free fetal DNA testing a viable testing option.

Umbilical Velocimetry (Doppler Blood Flow Studies)

Umbilical velocimetry, also known as **Doppler blood flow studies**, is a noninvasive ultrasound test that measures blood flow changes that occur in maternal and fetal circulation in order to assess placental function. An ultrasound beam, like that provided by the pocket Doppler (a handheld ultrasound device), is directed at the umbilical artery (in some cases a maternal vessel such as the arcuate can also be used). The signal is reflected off the red blood cells moving within the vessels, creating a "picture" (waveform) that looks like a series of waves. The highest-velocity peak of the waves is the systolic measurement, and the lowest point is the diastolic velocity. To interpret the waveforms, the systolic (S) peak is divided by the end-diastolic (D) component. This calculation is called the S/D ratio. The normal S/D ratio is approximately 2.0 at 20 weeks' gestation and below 3 after 30 gestational weeks. A decrease in uteroplacental perfusion (because of narrowing of the vessels) causes an increase in placental bed resistance and a decrease in diastolic flow, resulting in an elevated S/D ratio (Cunningham et al., 2014). Elevations above the 95th percentile for the gestational age are considered abnormal. Doppler blood flow studies are helpful in assessing and managing pregnancies with suspected uteroplacental insufficiency before asphyxia occurs (Cunningham et al., 2014). Abnormal Doppler flow studies accompanied by a decrease in amniotic fluid have been associated with small-for-gestational-age (SGA) fetuses, intrauterine growth restriction (IUGR), cesarean section for nonreassuring fetal status, 5-minute Apgar score of less than 7, respiratory distress syndrome (RDS), neonatal intensive care unit (NICU) admission, and perinatal death (Cunningham et al., 2014). In extreme cases of IUGR, end flow may become absent or reversed. It is not uncommon for these fetuses to have a fetal aneuploidy or a major anomaly; thus complete fetal assessment is warranted when an abnormal S/D ratio has been identified (Cunningham et al., 2014). Doppler velocimetry is used primarily for fetuses suspected of having IUGR or other maternal or fetal complications.

Health Promotion **Infants with Down Syndrome**

Healthy People 2020 strives to reduce the mortality of infants with Down syndrome at 1 year of age. Early detection and intensive treatment of identified comorbidities can help reduce infant mortality for this group.

Doppler blood flow studies are relatively easy to obtain. The woman lies supine with a wedge under the right hip (to promote uteroplacental perfusion). Warmed transducer gel is applied to the abdomen, and a pulsed-wave Doppler device is used to ascertain the blood flow. The Doppler flow study takes about 15 to 20 minutes. Doppler flow studies can be initiated at 16 to 18 weeks' gestation and are then scheduled at regular intervals for women at risk.

Non-Stress Test (NST)

The **non-stress test (NST)**, a widely used method of evaluating fetal status, may be used alone or as part of a more comprehensive diagnostic assessment called a *biophysical profile (BPP)*. The non-stress test is based on the knowledge that when the fetus has adequate oxygenation and an intact central nervous system, there are accelerations of the fetal heart rate (FHR) with fetal movement. An NST requires an electronic fetal monitor to observe and record these fetal heart rate accelerations (see discussion of acceleration in Chapter 17). A nonreactive NST is fairly consistent in identifying at-risk fetuses (Cunningham et al., 2014). The advantages of the NST are as follows:

- Quick to perform, permits easy interpretation, and is inexpensive
- Can be done in an office or clinic setting
- No known side effects

The disadvantages of the NST include the following:

- Difficult sometimes to obtain a suitable tracing
- Woman has to remain relatively still for at least 20 minutes
- Has a high false-positive rate due to the fetal sleep cycle

Procedure for NST

The test can be done with the woman in a reclining chair or in bed in a left-tilted, semi-Fowler, or side-lying position. Research has shown that certain maternal positions can help produce more favorable results. Women in left-tilted semi-Fowler, in sitting positions, and in left lateral positions have more fetal movement and are more likely to have a reactive tracing. Women should not be placed in a supine position because it is associated with less fetal movement, maternal back pain, and maternal shortness of breath. An electronic fetal monitor is used to obtain a tracing of the fetal heart rate (FHR) and fetal movement (FM). The nurse places the monitor under the woman's clothing. Privacy should be provided. The examiner puts two elastic belts on the woman's abdomen. One belt holds a device that detects uterine or fetal movement; the other belt holds a device that detects the FHR. As the NST is done, each fetal movement is documented, so that associated or simultaneous FHR changes can be evaluated.

Interpretation of NST Results

Women with a high risk factor will probably begin having NSTs at 30 to 32 weeks' gestation and at frequent intervals for the remainder of the pregnancy. The results of the NST are interpreted as follows:

- *Reactive test.* A reactive NST shows at least two accelerations of FHR with fetal movements of 15 beats per minute (beats/min), lasting 15 seconds or more, over 20 minutes (Figure 13–4). This is the desired result. (See *Key Facts to Remember: Non-Stress Test.*) In preterm fetuses, the rate is 10 beats above baseline for 10 seconds in a 20-minute window. Up to 50% of 28- to 32-week gestational age fetuses have a nonreactive NST (Family Practice Notebook, 2015).
- *Nonreactive test.* In a nonreactive test, the reactive criteria are not met. For example, the accelerations do not meet the requirements of 15 beats/min or do not last 15 seconds (Figure 13–5).
- *Unsatisfactory test.* An NST is unsatisfactory if the data cannot be interpreted or there was inadequate fetal activity.

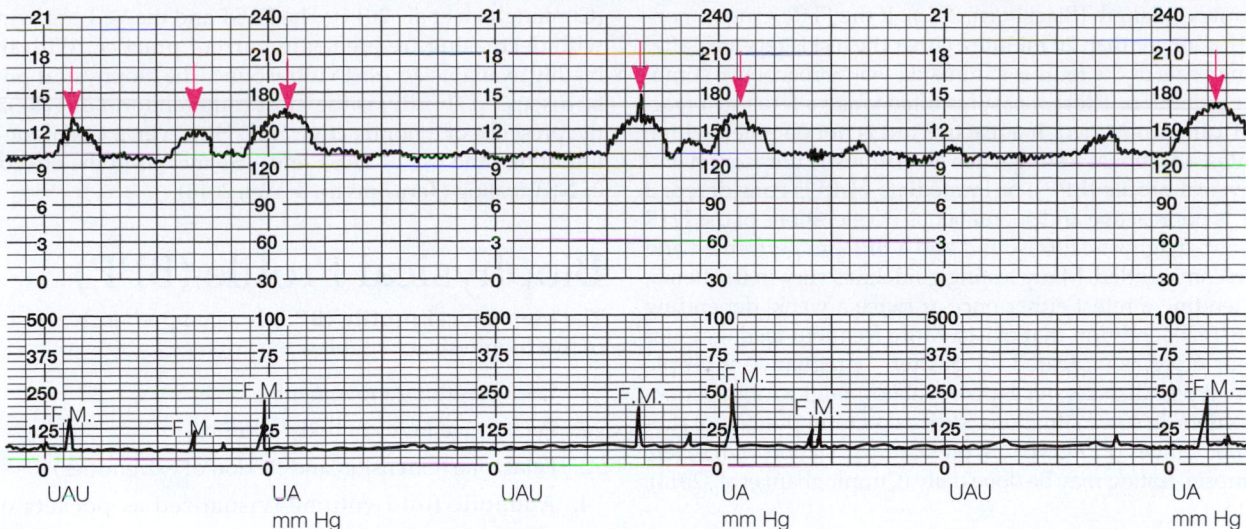

Figure 13–4 Example of a reactive non-stress test (NST). Accelerations of 15 beats/min lasting 15 seconds with each fetal movement (FM). Top of strip shows fetal heart rate (FHR); bottom of strip shows uterine activity tracing. Note that FHR increases (above the baseline) at least 15 beats and remains at that rate for at least 15 seconds before returning to the former baseline.

KEY FACTS TO REMEMBER
Non-Stress Test

Diagnostic value: Demonstrates fetus's ability to respond to its environment by acceleration of FHR with movement.

Results

- **Reactive test:** Accelerations (at least 2) of 15 beats/min above the baseline, lasting 15 seconds or more in a 20-minute window, are present, indicating fetal well-being. In preterm fetuses, the rate is 10 beats above baseline for 10 seconds in a 20-minute window.

- **Nonreactive test:** Accelerations are not present or do not meet the above criteria, indicating that the fetus is at risk or asleep.

- **Unsatisfactory test:** Data cannot be interpreted or there was inadequate fetal activity.

It is important that anyone who performs the NST understand the significance of any decelerations of the FHR during testing. If decelerations are noted, the healthcare provider should be notified for further evaluation of fetal status. (See Chapter 17 for further discussion of FHR decelerations.)

Clinical Management

The clinical management of potential nonreassuring fetal status may vary somewhat among clinicians depending on the clinical judgment of the care provider. One commonly used protocol is as follows: If the NST is reactive in less than 20 minutes, the test is concluded and rescheduled as indicated by the high-risk condition that is present; if it is nonreactive, the test time is extended for 20 minutes until the results are reactive, and then the test is rescheduled as indicated. It is estimated that fetuses between 30 and 40 gestational weeks have typical sleep cycles averaging

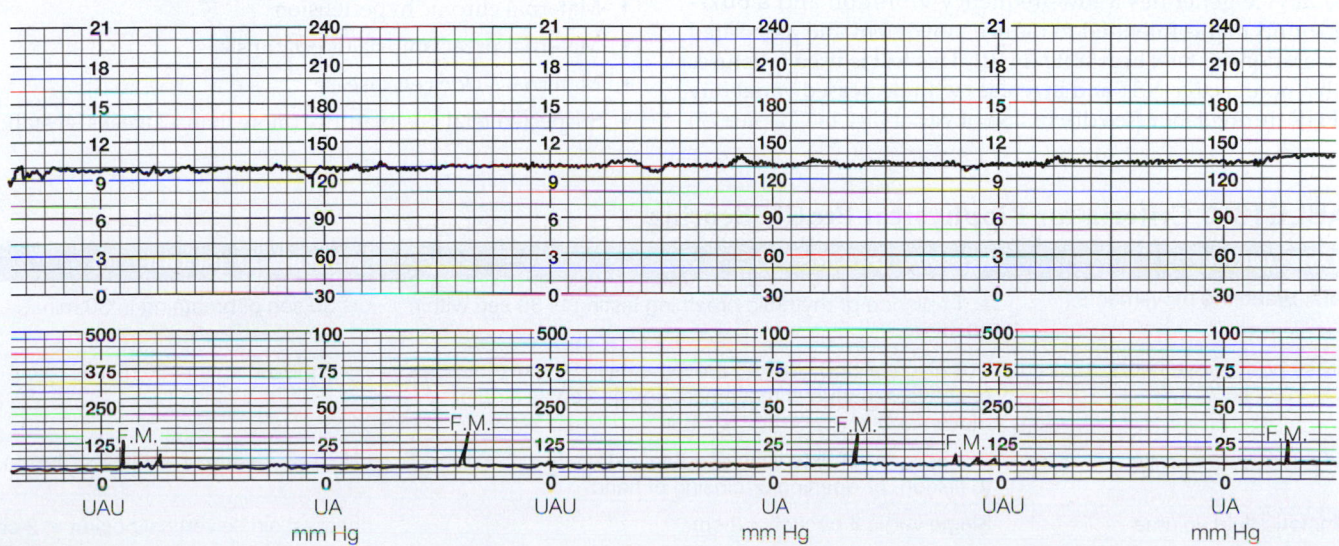

Figure 13–5 Example of a nonreactive non-stress test (NST). There are no accelerations of fetal heart rate (FHR) with fetal movement (FM). Baseline FHR is 130 beats/min. The tracing of uterine activity is on the bottom of the strip.

15.1 minutes in length (Blackburn, 2013). If the FHR remains nonreactive for longer than 20 minutes, either the test is repeated after the woman eats or the fetus is stimulated via vibroacoustic stimulation or palpation. These measures often wake a fetus so a reactive NST can be obtained. If a reactive test is not obtained within 40 minutes, additional testing (such as diagnostic ultrasound and a biophysical profile [BPP]) or immediate birth is considered; if the NST is nonreactive and spontaneous decelerations of the FHR are present, diagnostic ultrasound and a BPP are performed and birth is recommended. Many testing guidelines vary in frequency, recommending a retest either once or twice a week, depending on the at-risk condition that exists. More frequent testing, twice weekly or more, is indicated for postterm pregnancy, multiple gestation, type 1 diabetes, fetal growth abnormalities, or hypertensive disorders. In some situations, such as preterm premature rupture of membranes (PPROM) or a premature gestation with severe preeclampsia, testing may be done daily (Cunningham et al., 2014).

Nursing Management

Evaluate the woman's understanding of the NST and the possible results. Review the reasons for the NST and the procedure before beginning the test. Administer the NST, interpret the results, and report the findings to the healthcare provider and the expectant woman.

Clinical Tip

If a non-stress test fails to become reactive, a 3-minute foot massage has been shown to stimulate the fetus and increase fetal activity. It also helps the woman to relax during the test.

Fetal Acoustic Stimulation Test (FAST) and Vibroacoustic Stimulation Test (VST)

Acoustic (sound) and vibroacoustic (vibration and sound) stimulation of the fetus, in which a handheld, battery-operated device is applied to the woman's abdomen over the area of the fetal head, can be used as an adjunct to the non-stress test (NST). The device generates a low-frequency vibration and a buzzing sound that is intended to induce movement and associated accelerations of fetal heart rate (FHR). This test is used in fetuses with a nonreactive NST and in fetuses with decreased variability of FHR during labor (see discussion of variability in Chapter 17)

(Cunningham et al., 2014). The FAST and the VST are being used with decreasing frequency in current practice. With the now readily available access to ultrasound, the biophysical profile (to be discussed shortly) is the most common form of evaluation in the presence of a nonreactive NST. However, a Cochrane review found that the use of FAST and VST increased the effectiveness of NST testing (Tan, Smyth, & Wei, 2013).

Biophysical Profile (BPP)

The **biophysical profile (BPP)** is a comprehensive assessment of five biophysical variables:

1. Fetal breathing movement
2. Fetal movements of body or limbs
3. Fetal tone (extension and flexion of extremities)
4. Amniotic fluid volume (visualized as pockets of fluid around the fetus)
5. Reactive fetal heart rate (FHR) with activity (reactive non-stress test [NST]).

The first four variables are assessed by ultrasound scanning; FHR reactivity is assessed with the NST. By combining these five assessments, the BPP helps to either identify the compromised fetus or confirm the healthy fetus. It also provides an assessment of placental functioning. Specific criteria for normal and abnormal assessments are presented in Table 13–3. A score of 2 is assigned to each normal finding, and 0 to each abnormal one, for a maximum score of 10. The absence of a specific activity is difficult to interpret, because it may be indicative of central nervous system (CNS) depression or simply the resting state of a healthy fetus. Scores of 8 (with normal amniotic fluid) and 10 are considered normal. Such scores have the least chance of being associated with a compromised fetus unless a decrease in the amount of amniotic fluid is noted, in which case birth may be indicated (Cunningham et al., 2014).

The BPP is indicated when there is risk of placental insufficiency or fetal compromise because of the following:

- Intrauterine growth restriction (IUGR)
- Maternal diabetes mellitus
- Maternal heart disease
- Maternal chronic hypertension
- Maternal preeclampsia or eclampsia
- Maternal sickle cell disease
- Suspected fetal postmaturity (more than 42 weeks' gestation)

TABLE 13–3 Criteria for Biophysical Profile Scoring

COMPONENT	NORMAL (SCORE = 2)	ABNORMAL (SCORE = 0)
Fetal breathing movements	≥ 1 episode of rhythmic breathing lasting ≥ 30 sec within 30 min	≤ 30 sec of breathing in 30 min
Gross body movements	≥ 3 discrete body or limb movements in 30 min (episodes of active continuous movement considered as single movement)	≤ 2 movements in 30 min
Fetal tone	≥ 1 episode of extension of a fetal extremity with return to flexion, or opening or closing of hand	No movements or extension/flexion
Amniotic fluid volume	Single vertical pocket > 2 cm amniotic fluid index (AFI) > 5 cm	Largest single vertical pocket ≤ 2 cm AFI < 5 cm
Non-stress test	≥ 2 accelerations of ≥ 15 beats/min for ≥ 15 sec in 20–40 min	0 or 1 acceleration in 20–40 min

- History of previous stillbirths
- Rh alloimmunization
- Abnormal estriol excretion
- Hyperthyroidism
- Renal disease
- Nonreactive NST

- History of preterm labor (if being done before term)
- Multiple gestation

Contraction Stress Test (CST)

The **contraction stress test (CST)** is a means of evaluating the respiratory function (oxygen and carbon dioxide exchange) of the placenta and identifying the fetus at risk for intrauterine asphyxia by observing the response of the fetal heart rate (FHR) to the stress of uterine contractions (spontaneous or induced). During contractions, intrauterine pressure increases. Blood flow to the intervillous space of the placenta is reduced momentarily, thereby decreasing oxygen transport to the fetus. A healthy fetus usually tolerates this reduction well and maintains a steady heart rate. If the placental reserve is insufficient, fetal hypoxia, depression of the myocardium, and a decrease in FHR occur. Testing has disadvantages in that it is time consuming and yields a high false-positive result or equivocal results.

In many areas, the CST has given way to the biophysical profile (BPP). It is still used in areas where the availability of other technology is reduced (such as during night shifts) or limited (such as at small community hospitals or birthing centers). It may also be used as an adjunct to other forms of fetal assessment.

The CST is contraindicated in the following (Cunningham et al., 2014):

- Third-trimester bleeding from placenta previa
- Marginal abruptio placentae or unexplained vaginal bleeding
- Previous cesarean with classical incision
- Premature rupture of the membranes
- Cervical insufficiency
- Cerclage in place
- Anomalies of the maternal reproductive organs

Procedure

The critical component of the CST is the presence of uterine contractions, which may occur spontaneously or may be stimulated.

An electronic fetal monitor is used to provide continuous data about the fetal heart rate and uterine contractions. After a 15-minute baseline recording of uterine activity and FHR, the tracing is evaluated for evidence of spontaneous contractions. If three spontaneous contractions of good quality and lasting 40 to 60 seconds occur in a 10-minute window, the results are evaluated, and the test is concluded. If no contractions occur or they are insufficient for interpretation, contractions may be stimulated by pitocin administration or application of an electric breast pump to produce contractions of good quality. (See Chapter 22 for more information on nursing management of oxytocin induction.)

SAFETY ALERT!

CST testing should be conducted only in a setting where tocolytic medications are available in case a hypersystole pattern occurs or if labor is stimulated from the test. Prompt administration of a tocolytic agent may be needed to ensure that the fetus and mother maintain a safe and healthy status.

Interpretation of CST Results

The CST is classified as follows:

- *Negative.* A negative CST shows three contractions of good quality lasting 40 or more seconds in 10 minutes without evidence of late decelerations. This is the desired result. It implies that the fetus can handle the hypoxic stress of uterine contractions.
- *Positive.* A positive CST shows repetitive persistent late decelerations with more than 50% of the contractions (Figure 13–6). This is not a desired result. The hypoxic stress

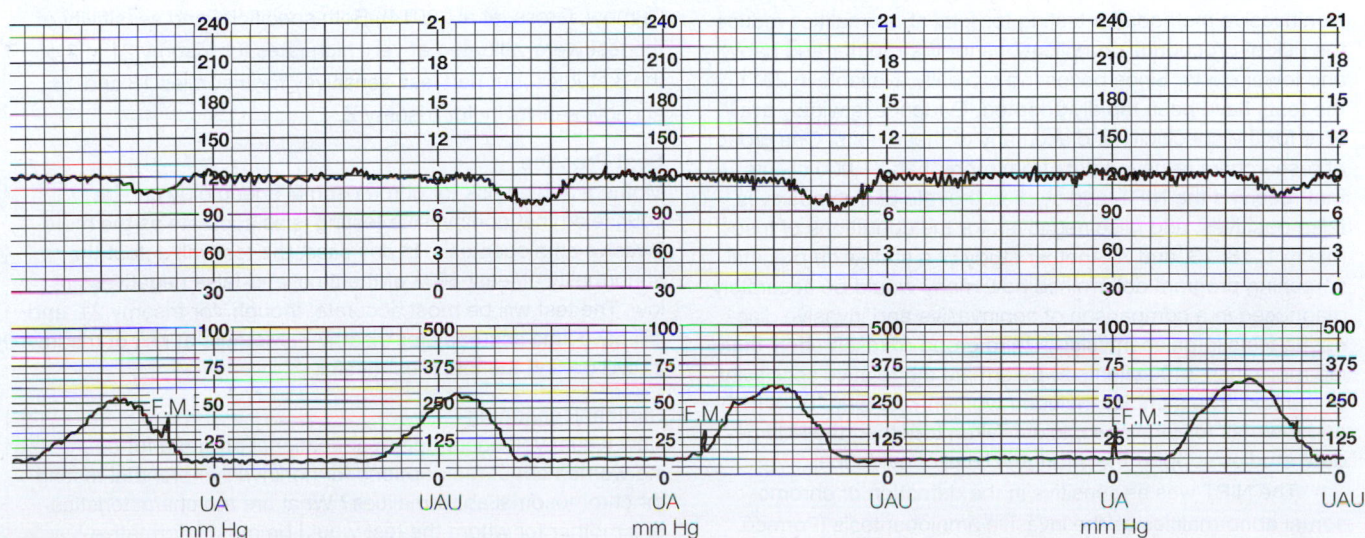

Figure 13–6 Example of a positive contraction stress test (CST). Repetitive late decelerations occur with each contraction. Note that there are no accelerations of fetal heart rate (FHR) with three fetal movements (FM). The baseline FHR is 120 beats/min. Uterine contractions (bottom half of strip) occurred four times in 12 minutes.

of the uterine contraction causes a slowing of the FHR. The pattern will not improve and will most likely get worse with additional contractions. There do not have to be three contractions in 10 minutes if late decelerations are occurring to be considered a positive test.

- *Equivocal.*
  - An equivocal-suspicious test result occurs when intermittent late decelerations occur or when significant variable decelerations occur.
  - An equivocal-hyperstimulation test result occurs when there are uterine contractions occurring every 2 minutes or a contraction lasting greater than 90 seconds with a fetal deceleration occurs. When this test result occurs, more information is needed.
- *Unsatisfactory.* The quality of tracing is too poor to accurately interpret FHR with contractions or the frequency of three contractions lasting 40 to 60 seconds occurring in a 10-minute window of time cannot be obtained for endpoint of the test or the tracing is unreadable.

Clinical Application

A negative CST implies that the placenta is functioning normally, fetal oxygenation is adequate, and the fetus will probably be able to withstand the stress of labor. If labor does not occur in the ensuing week, further testing is done.

A positive CST with a nonreactive NST presents evidence that the fetus will not likely withstand the stress of labor. Although a negative CST is reliable in predicting fetal status, a positive result needs additional testing, such as a biophysical profile.

Nursing Management

Ascertain the woman's understanding of the reasons for the test and the possible results. Have the healthcare provider obtain written consent if required. Administer the CST, interpret the results, and report the findings to the healthcare provider and the expectant woman. The presence of the healthcare provider may be required because there is a risk of initiating labor or hypersystolic uterine contractions.

Key Facts To Remember
Contraction Stress Test

Diagnostic value: Demonstrates reaction of FHR to stress of uterine contraction.

Results

- *Negative test:* Stress of uterine contraction shows three contractions of good quality lasting 40 or more seconds in 10 minutes without evidence of late decelerations.
- *Positive test:* Stress of uterine contraction shows repetitive persistent late deceleration with more than 50% of the uterine contractions even if less than three contractions in a 10-minute period.
- *Equivocal:* Suspicious test shows inconsistent late decelerations or significant variable decelerations. Hyperstimulation test shows uterine contraction frequency of every 2 minutes or contractions lasting greater than 90 seconds with a late deceleration occurring.

EVIDENCE-BASED PRACTICE | Validity of the Noninvasive Prenatal Test for the Detection of Chromosomal Abnormalities

Clinical Question
Does the Noninvasive Prenatal Test (NIPT) detect chromosomal abnormalities with a strong degree of accuracy? Which abnormalities are best detected with the NIPT?

The Evidence
Noninvasive methods for testing for fetal abnormalities reduce the risk of procedural complications for the mother and baby, and lower costs. Since becoming clinically available in 2011, the tests have been rapidly adopted. Evidence is widely available for the specificity and accuracy of these tests. One group of researchers retrieved data from more than 31,000 clients that received the NIPT, and studied the rate of true positives, false positives, and false negatives for the conditions of trisomies 21, 18, 13, and X. Another study of a statewide prenatal screening program determined how many would be accurately diagnosed in a comparison of noninvasive and invasive diagnostic tests (amniocentesis). A third group of researchers studied more than 3400 clients to determine the relative sensitivity of the test. The samples included women who were both high- and low-risk for fetal aneuploidy. Taken together, these large-data studies support the strongest level of evidence.

The NIPT was as sensitive in the detection of chromosomal abnormalities as the invasive amniocentesis (Porreco, Garite, Maurel, et al., 2014). Norton, Currier, & Jeliffe-Pawlowski (2014) determined that 80% of chromosomal abnormalities were detected by NIPT; 17% were missed and were false negatives. In the large-scale report, the predictive value was 83%, with only 2 of 500 false negatives (Dar, Curnow, Gross, et al., 2014). Both specificity and sensitivity of the test were validated at very high rates for trisomy 21 in 2 of the 3 studies, but had less sensitivity for trisomies 18 and 13 and low sensitivity for trisomy X.

Best Practice
Mothers at high risk for chromosomal aneuploidy can be counseled that noninvasive testing is as accurate as the more invasive amniocentesis. In any case, the test will detect the abnormality at least 80% of the time, and false negatives are low. The test will be most accurate, though, for trisomy 21, and will have little accuracy for trisomy X. Mothers at risk of trisomy 21 will be find the test most useful.

Clinical Reasoning
How would you construct an educational program for counseling women about their options for noninvasive prenatal testing for chromosomal abnormalities? What are the characteristics of a mother for whom the test would be most informative?

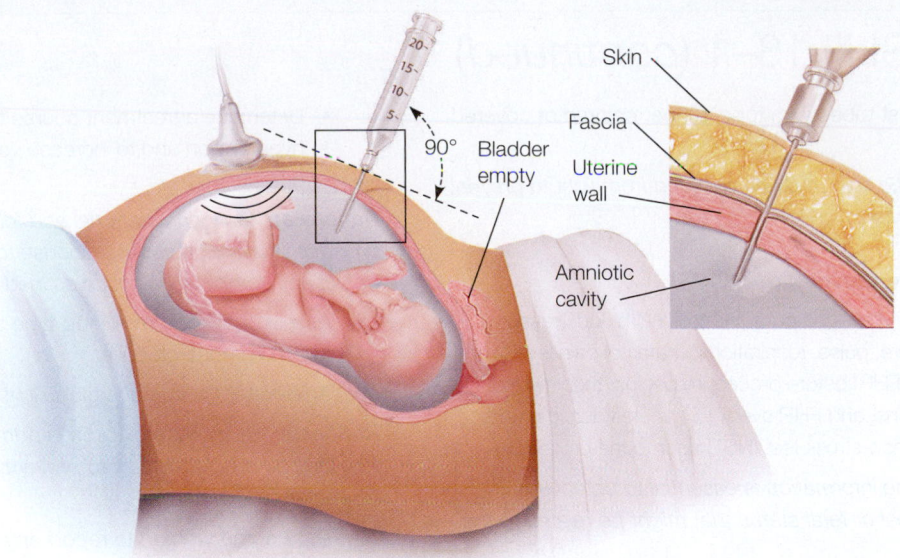

Figure 13–7 Amniocentesis. The woman is usually scanned by ultrasound to determine the placenta site and to locate a pocket of amniotic fluid. As the needle is inserted, three levels of resistance are felt when the needle penetrates the skin, fascia, and uterine wall. When the needle is placed within the amniotic cavity, amniotic fluid is withdrawn.

Amniotic Fluid Analysis

Amniocentesis is a procedure used to obtain amniotic fluid for genetic testing for fetal abnormalities or to determine fetal lung maturity in the third trimester of pregnancy. During an amniocentesis, the healthcare provider scans the uterus using ultrasound to identify the fetal and placental positions and to identify adequate pockets of amniotic fluid. The skin is then cleaned with a Betadine solution. The use of a local anesthesia at the needle insertion site is optional. A 22-gauge needle is then inserted into the uterine cavity to withdraw amniotic fluid (Figure 13–7). After 15 to 20 mL of fluid has been removed, the needle is withdrawn and the site is assessed for streaming (movement of fluid), which is an indication of bleeding. The fetal heart rate and maternal vital signs are then assessed. Rh immune globulin is given to all Rh-negative women. The analysis of amniotic fluid provides valuable information about fetal status. Amniocentesis is a fairly simple procedure, although complications do occur on rare occasions (less than 1% of cases). See *Clinical Skill: Assisting During Amniocentesis* for nursing interventions during amniocentesis.

Diagnostic Uses of Amniocentesis

A number of studies can be performed on amniotic fluid. These tests can provide information about genetic disorders (see Chapter 7), fetal health, and fetal lung maturity.

EVALUATION OF FETAL HEALTH

Concentrations of certain substances in amniotic fluid provide information about the health status of the fetus. The **quadruple screen** is the most widely used test to screen for Down syndrome (trisomy 21), trisomies 13 and 18, and neural tube defects (NTDs). The serum test assesses for appropriate levels of alpha-fetoprotein (AFP), human chorionic gonadotropin (hCG), unconjugated estriol (UE3), and dimeric inhibin-A. The quadruple screen offers the advantage of being noninvasive but is only a screening test and does not actually diagnose genetic abnormalities (see Chapter 7). An amniocentesis is 99% accurate in diagnosing genetic abnormalities.

EVALUATION OF FETAL MATURITY

Because gestational age, birth weight, and the rate of development of organ systems do not necessarily correspond, amniotic fluid may also be analyzed to determine the maturity of the fetal

---

Clinical Skill 13–1
Assisting During Amniocentesis

NURSING ACTION

Preparation

- Explain the procedure and the indications for it, and reassure the woman.

Rationale: Explanation of the procedure decreases anxiety.

- Determine whether an informed consent has been signed. If not, verify that the woman's healthcare provider has explained the procedure and ask her to sign a consent form.

Rationale: It is the healthcare provider's responsibility to obtain informed consent. The woman's signature indicates her awareness of risks and gives her consent to the procedure.

Equipment and Supplies

Prepare and arrange the following items so they are easily accessible:

- 22-gauge spinal needle with stylet
- 10- and 20-mL syringes
- 1% Xylocaine
- Povidone–iodine (Betadine)

(continued)

Clinical Skill 13–1 (*continued*)

- Three 10-mL test tubes with tops (amber colored or covered with tape)

Rationale: *Amniotic fluid must be shielded from light to prevent breakdown of bilirubin.*

Procedure: Sterile Gloves

1. Obtain baseline vital signs data on maternal blood pressure (BP), temperature, pulse, respirations, maternal pain level, and fetal heart rate (FHR) before procedure begins; then monitor BP, pulse, respirations, and FHR every 15 minutes during procedure. Obtain a non-stress test (NST) prior to the procedure.

Rationale: *Baseline information is essential to detect any changes in maternal or fetal status that might be related to the procedure.*

2. Provide gel for the ultrasound and assist with the real-time ultrasound to assess needle insertion during the procedure as needed.

3. Cleanse the woman's abdomen.

Rationale: *Cleansing the woman's abdomen before needle insertion helps decrease the risk of infection.*

4. The healthcare provider dons gloves, inserts the needle into the identified pocket of fluid, and withdraws a sample.

5. Obtain the test tubes from the healthcare provider.

6. Label the tubes with the women's correct identification and adhere client labels and send to the lab with the appropriate lab slips.

7. Monitor the woman and reassess her vital signs:
   - Determine the woman's BP, pulse, respirations, maternal pain level, and FHR.
   - Palpate the woman's fundus to assess for uterine contractions.
   - Monitor the woman with an external fetal monitor. Maintain continuous monitoring and obtain an NST after the procedure.

- Determine a treatment course to counteract any supine hypotension and to increase venous return and cardiac output.

Rationale: *Monitoring maternal and fetal status postprocedure provides information about response to the procedure and helps detect any complications such as inadvertent fetal puncture.*

8. Assess the woman's blood type and determine any need for Rh immune globulin.

9. Administer Rh immune globulin if indicated.

Rationale: *Rh immune globulin is administered prophylactically following an amniocentesis to prevent Rh sensitization in an Rh-negative woman.*

10. Instruct the woman to report any of the following changes or symptoms to her primary caregiver:
    - Unusual fetal hyperactivity or, conversely, any lack of movement
    - Vaginal discharge—clear drainage or bleeding
    - Uterine contractions or abdominal pain
    - Fever or chills

Rationale: *These are signs of potential complications and require further evaluation.*

11. Encourage the woman to engage in only light activity for 24 hours and to increase her fluid intake.

Rationale: *Decreased maternal activity helps decrease uterine irritability and increase uteroplacental circulation. Increased fluid intake helps replace amniotic fluid through the uteroplacental circulation.*

12. Complete the client record.
    - Record the type of procedure, the date and time, name of the healthcare provider who performed the procedure, and the disposition of the specimen.
    - Record the maternal–fetal response such as maternal vital signs, level of discomfort, FHR, NST results, and presence of contractions, bleeding, and fluid leakage, if occurred. Discharge instructions given should be documented.

---

lungs. Fetal lung maturity determination is important when making clinical decisions regarding the timing of birth for women who may have complications, such as preeclampsia or diabetes.

Health Promotion **Reducing the Rate of Preterm Births**

Healthy People 2020 goals include reducing the rate of preterm births. Fetal lung maturity testing can reduce the number of babies born prematurely related to incorrect dating in earlier stages of pregnancy and reduce the rates of late preterm newborns.

Lecithin/Sphingomyelin (L/S) Ratio.   The alveoli of the lungs are lined with a substance called **surfactant**, which is composed of phospholipids. Surfactant lowers the surface tension of the alveoli when the newborn exhales. When a newborn

with mature pulmonary function takes its first breath, a tremendously high pressure is needed to open the lungs. By lowering the alveolar surface tension, surfactant stabilizes the alveoli, and a certain amount of air always remains in the alveoli during expiration. Thus when the baby exhales, the lungs do not collapse. A baby born before synthesis of surfactant is complete is unable to maintain lung stability. Each breath requires the same effort as the first. This results in underinflation of the lungs and the development of respiratory distress syndrome (RDS).

Fetal lung maturity was once commonly ascertained by using the **lecithin/sphingomyelin (L/S) ratio**; lecithin and sphingomyelin are two components of surfactant. Early in pregnancy, the sphingomyelin concentration in amniotic fluid is greater than the concentration of lecithin, and so the L/S ratio is low (lecithin levels are low and sphingomyelin levels are high). At about 32 weeks' gestation, sphingomyelin levels begin to fall and the amount of lecithin begins to increase. By 35 weeks' gestation, an L/S ratio of 2:1 (also reported as 2.0) is usually achieved in the normal fetus. A 2:1 L/S ratio indicates that the risk of RDS is very low. Under certain conditions of stress (a physiologic problem in the mother, placenta, and/or fetus, such as hypertension or placental insufficiency), the fetal lungs mature more rapidly (Cunningham et al., 2014).

Phosphatidylglycerol (PG). Phosphatidylglycerol (PG) is another phospholipid in surfactant. Phosphatidylglycerol is not present in the fetal lung fluid early in gestation. It appears when fetal lung maturity has been attained, at about 35 weeks' gestation. Because the presence of PG is associated with fetal lung maturity, when it is present the risk of RDS is low. Phosphatidylglycerol determination is also useful in blood-contaminated specimens. Because PG is not present in blood or vaginal fluids, its presence is reliable in predicting fetal lung maturity. (See *Key Facts to Remember: Fetal Lung Maturity Values*.)

Lamellar Body Count. *Lamellar body counts (LBC)* are present in amniotic fluid when phosphatidylglycerol (PG) is present (Cunningham et al., 2014). When the LBC is over 50,000 counts/μl, probable lung maturity is assumed. The laboratory analysis for LBC is considerably less costly than the previously discussed tests and can usually be performed at an acute care facility rather than a reference laboratory (Cunningham et al., 2014).

Future Advances in Fetal Lung Maturity Testing Some researchers are now examining the use of Doppler ultrasound as a means of identifying fetuses whose lungs have matured by using the measurement of the fetal pulmonary artery Doppler wave acceleration time/ejection time ratio (PATET) (Schenone, Samson, Suhag, et al., 2012). Although further research is needed, research in noninvasive screening tools continues to evolve and could potentially reduce risk factors for mothers and fetuses.

KEY FACTS TO REMEMBER
Fetal Lung Maturity Values

Diagnostic value: Provides information to help determine fetal lung maturity.

Results

- An L/S ratio of 2:1 and presence of PG correlate with 35 weeks' gestation.
- An L/S ratio lower than 2:1 and/or an absence of PG may indicate underinflation of lungs and an increased risk for development of respiratory distress syndrome.
- An LBC over 50,000 counts/mcL is predictive of fetal lung maturity.

Chorionic Villus Sampling (CVS)

Chorionic villus sampling (CVS) involves obtaining a small sample of chorionic villi from the developing placenta. Chorionic villus sampling is performed in some medical centers for first-trimester diagnosis of genetic and deoxyribonucleic acid (DNA) studies. CVS can be performed either transabdominally or transcervically depending on placenta location. The fetal loss rate is the same regardless of the approach used although vaginal spotting is more common with the transcervical approach.

The use of CVS testing in modern obstetrics has decreased with the increased noninvasive testing options. CVS is mostly utilized for clients at risk, such as those with a family history of a genetic disorder, when parents are known carriers of genetic disorders, or when noninvasive screening tests show an increased risk of a genetic anomaly. The advantages of this procedure are early diagnosis (10 to 13 weeks) and short waiting time for results. Risks of CVS include failure to obtain tissue, rupture of membranes, leakage of amniotic fluid, bleeding, intrauterine infection, maternal tissue contamination of the specimen, and Rh alloimmunization. The spontaneous abortion rate following CVS is based on the method used for the procedure. The transcervical approach has a spontaneous abortion rate 3.5% greater than an amniocentesis, whereas the transabdominal approach carries the same risk as an amniocentesis (Ghidini, 2015).

Because CVS testing is performed so early in the pregnancy, it cannot detect neural tube defects. Women who desire testing for neural tube defects would need a quadruple screening at 15 to 20 weeks' gestation.

Clinical Tip

When explaining genetic testing options to expectant parents, inform the mother that even if a CVS shows no chromosomal abnormality, it cannot screen for neural tube defects. Women who had a normal CVS and an abnormal quadruple screen test would be offered amniocentesis. Women with risk factors for neural tube defects may want to consider amniocentesis instead of CVS because it screens for both types of disorders.

Nursing Management

Assist the healthcare provider during the amniocentesis or CVS and support the woman undergoing the procedure. Generally the healthcare provider has explained the procedure and informed consent has been obtained. Due to anxiety, emotional support of the woman is often needed and includes clarifying the healthcare provider's instructions or explanations, relieving the woman's physical discomfort when possible, and responding verbally and physically to the woman's need for reassurance.

Following the procedure, reiterate explanations given by the healthcare provider, allow opportunities for questions, review the experience with the woman, and present self-care measures. Typically, the woman is monitored for a short time following the procedure to assess for contractions or uterine activity, amniotic fluid leakage, bleeding, or pain. Advise the woman of the warning signs of complications following the procedure.

Following an amniocentesis, approximately 1% to 2% of women develop complications such as amniotic fluid leakage from the puncture site or vaginal spotting. Approximately 1 in 1000 women develop infection. Needle puncture of the fetus rarely occurs during amniocentesis because of the use of ultrasound technology, which allows for continuous visualization of the fetus (Cunningham et al., 2014). Reassure the client that although the complication rates are low, notification of her healthcare provider is necessary if any of these symptoms develop.

Because fetal loss occurs more commonly before 15 weeks, many practitioners theorize that the loss rates associated with CVS are higher than those associated with amniocentesis. Early amniocentesis before 15 weeks is associated with an increased risk of fetal loss when compared with performing the procedure after 15 weeks. When an amniocentesis is performed between 15 and 20 weeks, the risk of fetal loss is 1 in 300 to 1 in 500 (Cunningham et al., 2014).

When an invasive procedure, such as an amniocentesis or a CVS, is performed, administer RhoGAM to the woman if she is Rh negative to prevent alloimmunization. Document in the medical record, which can be provided to the woman for future reference.

Focus Your Study

- Maternal assessment of fetal activity can be used as a screening tool to provide information about fetal well-being.

- Ultrasound offers a valuable means of assessing intrauterine fetal growth because the growth can be followed over a period of time. It is noninvasive and painless, allows the healthcare provider to study the gestation serially, is nonradiating to both the woman and her fetus, and has no known harmful effects.

- Nuchal translucency testing (NTT) is used as a tool to screen for trisomies 13, 18, and 21. It is noninvasive and painless, but is not diagnostic in determining if a fetus has an abnormality.

- First-trimester combined screening includes nuchal translucency testing (NTT), ultrasound detection of the nasal bone, and serum tests; combined screening is more accurate than using only the ultrasound screening.

- Cell-free fetal DNA (cffDNA) testing is a maternal screening blood test that tests for trisomies 13, 18, and 21 by detecting circulating fetal DNA within the maternal serum. It is noninvasive and detects 99% of fetuses affected with Down syndrome (trisomy 21).

- Doppler blood flow studies are used to assess placental function and sufficiency and are routinely performed in fetuses with intrauterine growth restriction (IUGR) and maternal or fetal complications.

- A non-stress test (NST) is based on the knowledge that the fetal heart rate (FHR) normally increases in response to fetal activity and to sound stimulation. The desired result is a reactive test.

- A fetal biophysical profile (BPP) includes five variables to assess the fetus at risk for intrauterine compromise: fetal breathing movement, fetal body movement, fetal tone, amniotic fluid volume, and FHR reactivity.

- A contraction stress test (CST) provides a method for observing the response of the FHR to the stress of uterine contractions. The desired result is a negative test.

- Amniocentesis can be used to obtain amniotic fluid for genetic testing or for evaluating fetal lung maturity.

- The quadruple screen measures substances contained in the amniotic fluid that provide information regarding the presence of fetal anomalies, such as neural tube defects, Down syndrome, and trisomies 13 and 18.

- The lecithin/sphingomyelin (L/S) ratio, presence of phosphatidylglycerol, and level of lamellar body counts (LBC) can be assessed to determine fetal lung maturity.

- Advantages of chorionic villus sampling (CVS) include early detection of certain fetal disorders with a decreased waiting time for results. Disadvantages include an increased risk to the fetus, inability to detect neural tube defects, and the potential for repeated invasive procedures.

Clinical Reasoning in Action

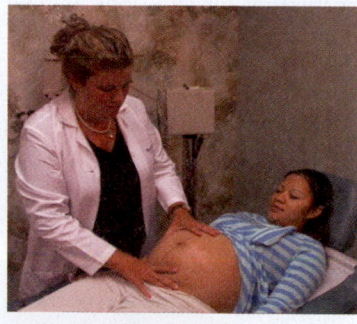

Patricia Adams is a 20-year-old, married, G2 P0010 at 36 weeks' gestation with gestational diabetes. She presents to you during her prenatal visit with a complaint of decreased fetal movement for the "last day or so." Her OB history includes a 13-lb weight gain, hematocrit of 29%, diastolic BP ranging 80–96 mm Hg, and 1+ proteinuria. A 19-week ultrasound demonstrated no fetal anatomic defects. A hemoglobin A1c at 23 weeks was 5.8%. Patricia has had weekly NST since 28 weeks' gestation. You place Patricia on the fetal monitor for an NST. You obtain vital signs of T 97°F, P 88, R 14, BP 130/88. After 30 minutes you observe that the fetal heart rate baseline is 160–165, long-term variability is decreased, and repetitive variable decelerations are occurring. No contractions are noted. The fetus is very active. You notify the healthcare provider of the fetal heart rate baseline and unsatisfactory NST. The healthcare provider orders a biophysical profile (BPP) for fetal well-being. You describe and explain the biophysical profile test to Patricia.

1. How would you describe and explain the biophysical profile test?

2. To heighten Patricia's awareness of fetal movement, how would you instruct her to do a daily fetal movement record (FMR)?

3. Explain when Patricia should contact her healthcare provider.

4. Discuss the significance of fetal movement.

5. Explore factors that decrease fetal movements.

References

Blackburn, S. T. (2013). Maternal, fetal, and neonatal physiology (4th ed.). Saunders: St. Louis, MO.

Cunningham, F. G., Leveno, K. J., Bloom, S. L., Spong, C. Y., Dashe, J. S., Hoffman, B. L., ... Sheffield, J. S. (2014). *Williams obstetrics* (24th ed.). New York, NY: McGraw-Hill.

Dar, P., Curnow, K., Gross, S., Hall, M. P., Stosic, M., Demko, Z., ... Benn, P. (2014). Clinical experience and follow-up with large scale single-nucleotide polymorphism-based noninvasive prenatal aneuploidy testing. *American Journal of Obstetrics and Gynecology, 211*(527), e1–e17.

Family Practice Notebook. (2015). Fetal testing indications. Retrieved from http://www.fpnotebook.com/ob/fetus/FtlTstngIndctns.htm

Funai, E. F. (2014). Preterm labor. Up-to-date. Retrieved from http://www.uptodate.com/contents/preterm-labor-beyond-the-basics

Ghidini, A. (2015). Chorionic villus sampling. Up-to-date. Retrieved from http://www.uptodate.com/contents/chorionic-villus-sampling-beyond-the-basics

Hofmeyr, G. J., & Novikova, N. (2013). Management of reported decreased fetal movements for improving pregnancy outcomes. Cochrane Database. CD009148. doi: 10.1002/14651858.CD009148.pub2

Norton, M., Currier, B., & Jeliffe-Pawlowski, L. (2014). Rare chromosome abnormalities detected by current prenatal screening compared to expected performance using non-invasive prenatal testing (NIPT). *American Journal of Obstetrics and Gynecology, Supplement to January, 2014,* s3–s4.

Porreco, R., Garite, T., Maurel, K., Marusiak, B., Ehrich, M., van den Boom, D., Deciu, C., & Bombard, A. (2014).

Noninvasive prenatal screening for fetal trisomies 21, 18, 13, and the common sex chromosome aneuploidies from maternal blood using massively parallel genomic sequencing of DNA. *American Journal of Obstetrics and Gynecology, 211*(365), e1–12.

Schenone, M., Samson, J., Suhag, A., Jenkins, L., & Mari, G. (2012). *A non-invasive method to predict fetal lung maturity using fetal pulmonary artery Doppler wave acceleration time/ejection time ratio.* Retrieved from http://www.eventkaddy.com/smfm2012/pdfs/363.pdf

Tan, K. H., Smyth, R. M. D., & Wei, X. (2013). Fetal vibroacoustic stimulation for facilitation of tests of the wellbeing of the unborn baby. *Cochrane Database of Systematic Reviews* 2013, Issue 12. Art. No.: CD002963. doi: 10.1002/14651858.CD002963.pub2

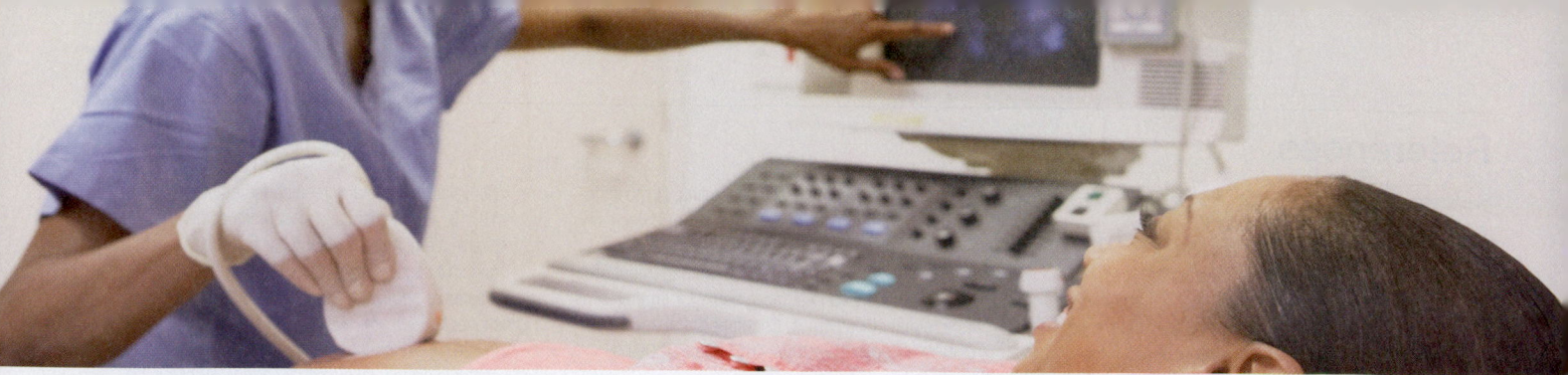

Chapter 14

Pregnancy at Risk: Pregestational Problems

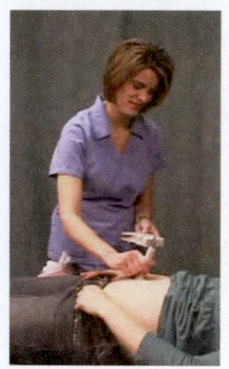

When you work on a high-risk maternity unit, it is sometimes easy to get caught up in technology and procedures, but this area is about families—their fears, their pain, their health, their future. We can never lose sight of that reality and remain effective nurses. Never.

—A Maternity Nurse Working with High-Risk Pregnant Women

⌄ Learning Outcomes

14.1 Discuss the pathology, treatment, and nursing care of pregnant women with diabetes mellitus.

14.2 Distinguish among the four major types of anemia associated with pregnancy with regard to signs, treatment, implications for pregnancy, and nursing care.

14.3 Summarize the effects of alcohol and illicit drugs on the childbearing woman and her fetus/newborn.

14.4 Explain the possible implications of maternal psychologic factors and disorders in caring for the childbearing family.

14.5 Discuss AIDS including care of the pregnant woman with HIV/AIDS, neonatal implications, ramifications for the childbearing family, and nursing care.

14.6 Describe the effects of various heart disorders on pregnancy, including their implications for nursing care.

14.7 Compare the effects of selected pregestational medical conditions on pregnancy.

Even though it is a normal process, for women with pre-existing (pregestational) conditions, pregnancy may become a life-threatening event. Effective prenatal care is directed toward identifying factors that increase a pregnant woman's risk and developing supportive therapies that will promote optimal health for the mother and her fetus.

This chapter focuses on women with pregestational medical disorders and the possible effects of these disorders on the pregnancy.

Healthy People 2020

(MICH-1.1) Reduce the rate of fetal deaths at 20 or more weeks of gestation

Care of the Woman With Diabetes Mellitus

Diabetes mellitus (DM), an endocrine disorder of carbohydrate metabolism, results from inadequate production or use of insulin. Insulin, produced by the β cells of the islets of Langerhans in the pancreas, lowers blood glucose levels by enabling glucose to move from the blood into muscle and adipose tissue cells.

Carbohydrate Metabolism in Normal Pregnancy

In early pregnancy the rise in serum levels of estrogen, progesterone, and other hormones stimulates increased insulin production by the maternal pancreas and increased tissue response to insulin. Thus an anabolic (building-up) state exists during the first half of pregnancy, with storage of glycogen in the liver and other tissues.

In the second half of pregnancy, placental secretion of human placental lactogen (hPL) and prolactin (from the decidua), as well as elevated cortisol and glycogen levels, cause increased resistance to insulin and decreased glucose tolerance. This decreased effectiveness of insulin results in a catabolic (destructive) state during fasting periods, such as during the night or after meal absorption. Because increasing amounts of circulating maternal glucose and amino acids are diverted to the fetus, maternal fat is metabolized much more readily during fasting periods than in a nonpregnant woman. As a result of this lipolysis (maternal metabolism of fat), ketones may be present in the urine.

The delicate system of checks and balances that exists between glucose production and glucose use is stressed by the growing fetus, who derives energy from glucose taken solely from maternal stores. This stress is known as the *diabetogenic effect of pregnancy*. Thus any pre-existing disruption in carbohydrate metabolism is augmented by pregnancy, and any diabetic potential may precipitate gestational diabetes mellitus.

Pathophysiology of Diabetes Mellitus

In diabetes mellitus, the pancreas fails to produce insulin or does not produce enough insulin to allow necessary carbohydrate metabolism. Without adequate insulin, glucose does not enter the cells and they become energy depleted. Blood glucose levels remain high (hyperglycemia), and the cells break down their stores of fats and protein for energy. Protein breakdown results in a negative nitrogen balance; fat metabolism causes ketosis.

These pathologic developments cause the four cardinal signs and symptoms of diabetes mellitus:

- *Polyuria* (frequent urination) results because water is not reabsorbed by the renal tubules due to the osmotic activity of glucose.
- *Polydipsia* (excessive thirst) is caused by dehydration from polyuria.
- *Polyphagia* (excessive hunger) is caused by tissue loss and a state of starvation, which results from the inability of the cells to use the blood glucose.
- *Weight loss* (seen with marked hyperglycemia) is because of the use of fat and muscle tissue for energy.

Diagnosis of diabetes is based on the presence of clinical symptoms and laboratory tests showing elevated glucose levels in the blood, glycosuria, and ketoacidosis.

Classification

The primary classification of diabetes is based on cause and includes four main categories American Diabetes Association [ADA], 2015):

- *Type 1 diabetes,* which develops because of β-cell destruction and generally results in an absolute insulin deficiency
- *Type 2 diabetes,* the most common form, which results from a combination of an insulin secretory defect and increased insulin resistance
- *Other specific types,* of which there are eight subcategories, including, for example, genetic defects, drug-induced diabetes, and endocrine disorders
- *Gestational diabetes mellitus (GDM)*

Gestational diabetes mellitus (GDM) is defined as any degree of glucose intolerance that has its onset or is first diagnosed during pregnancy. Diagnosis of GDM is important because even mild diabetes causes increased risk for perinatal morbidity and mortality. Furthermore, with time, many women with GDM progress to overt type 2 diabetes mellitus. *Note:* Gestational diabetes mellitus is not a pre-existing condition. It is included here, however, because many of the issues to consider in caring for a woman with GDM are similar to those involved in caring for a woman with pre-existing DM.

Influence of Pregnancy on Diabetes

Pregnancy can affect diabetes significantly because the physiologic changes of pregnancy can drastically alter insulin requirements. Pregnancy may also alter the progress of vascular disease secondary to DM. Pregnancy can affect diabetes in the following ways:

- DM may be difficult to control because insulin requirements are changeable.
- During the first trimester, the need for insulin frequently decreases. Levels of hPL, an insulin antagonist, are low, fetal needs are minimal, and the woman may consume less food because of nausea and vomiting.
- Nausea and vomiting may cause dietary fluctuations and increase the risk of hypoglycemia, formerly called insulin shock.
- Insulin requirements begin to rise late in the first trimester as glucose use and glucose storage by the woman and fetus increase. Insulin requirements may double or quadruple by the end of pregnancy as a result of placental maturation and hPL production.
- Increased energy needs during labor may require increased insulin to balance intravenous glucose.
- After delivery of the placenta, insulin requirements usually decrease abruptly as a result of the hPL in maternal circulation.
- A decreased renal threshold for glucose leads to a higher incidence of glycosuria.
- The risk of ketoacidosis, which may occur at lower serum glucose levels in a pregnant woman with DM than in a nonpregnant woman with diabetes, increases.
- The vascular disease that accompanies DM may progress during pregnancy.
- Hypertension may occur, contributing to vascular changes.

- Nephropathy may result from renal impairment and retinopathy may develop from occlusion of the microscopic blood vessels of the eye.

Influence of Diabetes on Pregnancy Outcome

The pregnancy of a woman who has diabetes carries a higher risk of complications, especially perinatal mortality and congenital anomalies. The risk can be reduced by tight metabolic control if these levels can be obtained without excessive hypoglycemia (fasting, pre-meal, and bedtime blood glucose levels of 60–99 mg/dL; peak postprandial blood glucose levels of 100–129 mg/dL; and HbA_{1c} less than 6%) (ADA, 2015).

MATERNAL RISKS

The prognosis for the pregnant woman with gestational, type 1, or type 2 diabetes without significant vascular damage is positive. However, diabetic pregnancy still carries a higher risk of complications than normal pregnancy. In addition, the risk of developing diabetes later in life is increased in women with GDM (American College of Obstetricians and Gynecologists [ACOG], 2013).

Hydramnios, an increase in the volume of amniotic fluid, occurs in 10% to 20% of pregnant women who have diabetes. It is thought to be a result of excessive fetal urination because of fetal hyperglycemia. Premature rupture of membranes and onset of labor may occasionally be a problem with hydramnios.

Preeclampsia–eclampsia occurs more often in diabetic pregnancies than in normal pregnancies, especially when vascular changes already exist.

Hyperglycemia, due to insufficient amounts of insulin, can lead to *ketoacidosis* as a result of the increase in ketone bodies (which are acidic) released in the blood from the metabolism of fatty acids. Decreased gastric motility and the contrainsulin effects of hPL also predispose the woman to ketoacidosis. Ketoacidosis usually develops slowly but, if untreated, can lead to coma and death for mother and fetus.

Another risk to the pregnant woman with diabetes is a difficult labor (*dystocia*), caused by fetopelvic disproportion if fetal macrosomia exists.

Pregnancy can also worsen *retinopathy* in women with diabetes. However, good control of blood glucose levels lessens the impact. Hence, women with pre-existing diabetes should be referred to an ophthalmologist for evaluation during pregnancy.

The pregnant woman with diabetes is also at increased risk for *monilial vaginitis* and *urinary tract infections* because of increased glycosuria, which contributes to a favorable environment for bacterial growth.

FETAL–NEONATAL RISKS

Many of the problems of the newborn result directly from high maternal plasma glucose levels. In the presence of untreated maternal ketoacidosis, the risk of fetal death increases dramatically.

The incidence of *congenital anomalies* in diabetic pregnancies is 6% to 12% and is the major cause of death among babies born to mothers with diabetes. Research suggests that this increased incidence is related to multiple factors including high glucose levels in early pregnancy (ACOG, 2012b). Most anomalies involve the heart, central nervous system, and skeletal system. One anomaly, *sacral agenesis*, appears almost exclusively in babies of mothers with diabetes. In sacral agenesis, the sacrum and lumbar spine fail to develop and the lower extremities develop incompletely. Preconception counseling and strict diabetes control before conception help reduce the incidence of congenital anomalies.

Characteristically, infants of diabetic mothers (IDMs) are *large for gestational age (LGA)* as a result of fetal insulin production stimulated by the high levels of glucose crossing the placenta from the mother. These elevated levels continually stimulate the fetal islets of Langerhans to produce insulin. This hyperinsulin state causes the fetus to use the available glucose, which leads to **macrosomia** (excessive growth) and fat deposits. If born vaginally, the macrosomic neonate is at increased risk for shoulder dystocia and traumatic birth injuries; thus cesarean birth may be considered if birth weight is expected to exceed 4500 g (ACOG, 2013). Macrosomia can be reduced significantly by strict maternal blood glucose control.

Once the umbilical cord is severed after birth, the generous maternal blood glucose supply stops. However, continued islet cell hyperactivity leads to high insulin levels and depleted blood glucose (hypoglycemia) in 2 to 4 hours. Newborns of mothers with advanced diabetes (vascular involvement) may demonstrate *intrauterine growth restriction (IUGR)*. This occurs because vascular changes in the woman with diabetes decrease the efficiency of placental perfusion and the fetus is not as well sustained in utero.

Respiratory distress syndrome (RDS) appears to result from inhibition, by high levels of fetal insulin, of some fetal enzymes necessary for surfactant production. *Polycythemia* (excessive number of red blood cells) in the newborn is due primarily to the diminished ability of glycosylated hemoglobin in the mother's blood to release oxygen. *Hyperbilirubinemia* is a direct result of the inability of immature liver enzymes to metabolize the increased bilirubin resulting from the polycythemia.

Clinical Therapy

DM occurs in about 6% to 7% of all pregnancies in the United States and of these cases, 90% are related to GDM (ACOG, 2013). Therefore, all pregnant women, regardless of risk factors, should have their risk for undiagnosed type 2 diabetes assessed at the first prenatal visit. Women at high risk (non-White, prior history of GDM or birth of an LGA baby, marked obesity, diagnosis of polycystic ovarian syndrome, hypertension, presence of glycosuria, or a strong family history of type 2 DM) should be screened for diabetes as soon as possible.

Various screening approaches may be used. HA1c equal to or greater than 6.5% would be considered diagnostic as would a fasting plasma glucose level equal to or greater than 126 mg/dL or a 2-hr plasma glucose equal to or greater than 200 mg/dL during an oral glucose tolerance test (OGTT) (see following discussion). Women who are determined to have diabetes at this visit should be diagnosed as having overt diabetes and not GDM (ADA, 2015).

Two approaches to prenatal screening are currently available and performed at 24 to 28 weeks' gestation for all pregnant women not previously diagnosed with overt DM (ADA, 2015). The two-step approach is the method most commonly used in the United States. A consensus panel has concluded that currently there is not enough evidence to recommend the use of the one-step approach universally as a screening tool (Johnson & Milio, 2015).

1. **Two-step approach** is recommended by a National Institutes of Health (NIH) Consensus Conference and ACOG (ACOG, 2013).

- **Step 1:** Women are given non-fasting, 50-g, 1-hour OGTT. The oral glucose load can be given at any time of the day with no requirement for fasting. One hour later plasma glucose is measured. If plasma glucose levels are elevated (equal to or greater than 140 mg/dL, depending on the laboratory used), a 100-g, 3-hour glucose test is done.

- **Step 2:** To do the 100 g, 3-hour OGTT, the woman eats an unrestricted diet, consuming at least 150 grams of carbohydrates per day for at least 3 days before her scheduled test. She then ingests 100-gram oral glucose solution in the morning after an overnight fast. Plasma glucose is measured fasting and at 1, 2, and 3 hours. Gestational diabetes is diagnosed if *two or more* of the following values are met or exceeded:

Fasting	95 mg/dL
1 hour	180 mg/dL
2 hours	155 mg/dL
3 hours	140 mg/dL

2. **One-step approach** is recommended by the International Association of Diabetes and Pregnancy Study Groups (IADPSG) (2010). ADA (2015) reports that either approach—one-step or two-step—can be used.

- In the morning, following an overnight fast, the woman ingests a 75-g oral glucose solution. Plasma glucose levels are determined fasting and at 1 and 2 hours. Gestational diabetes is diagnosed if any *one* of the following values are equaled or exceeded:

Fasting	92 mg/dL
1 hour	180 mg/dL
2 hours	153 mg/dL

LABORATORY ASSESSMENT OF LONG-TERM GLUCOSE CONTROL

Measurement of glycosylated hemoglobin levels provides information about the long-term (previous 4 to 8 weeks) control of hyperglycemia. It measures the percentage of glycohemoglobin in the blood. Glycohemoglobin, or HbA_{1c}, is the hemoglobin to which a glucose molecule is attached. Because glycosylation is a rather slow and essentially irreversible process, the test is not reliable for screening for gestational diabetes or for close daily control. However, in women with known pregestational DM, abnormal HbA_{1c} values correlate directly with the frequency of spontaneous abortion and fetal congenital anomalies. Consequently, women with pre-existing diabetes who plan to become pregnant should work to achieve HbA_{1c} levels at target levels (less than 7%) without significant hypoglycemia (ADA, 2015).

Antepartum Management of Diabetes Mellitus

To ensure an optimally healthy mother and newborn, good prenatal care using a team approach must be a top priority. The woman with gestational diabetes may find the diagnosis shocking and upsetting. She needs clear explanations about the actions she can take with regard to diet, weight gain, exercise, and the therapy that may be indicated to ensure a good outcome. The nurse-educator plays a major role in this counseling (Wong, Suwandarathne, & Russell, 2013).

The woman with pregestational diabetes needs to understand what changes she can expect during pregnancy; she should receive such teaching in preconception counseling. In addition, preconception care focuses on stringent blood glucose control before conception and during the first trimester. A pregnant woman with pre-existing diabetes may also require referral to specialists such as an ophthalmologist or nephrologist.

DIETARY REGULATION

The pregnant woman with diabetes needs to increase her caloric intake by about 300 kcal/day. During the first trimester the normal-weight woman generally requires about 30 kcal/kg of ideal body weight (IBW). During the second and third trimesters she needs about 35 kcal/kg IBW. Approximately 33% to 40% of the calories should come from complex carbohydrates, 20% from protein, and 40% from fats (ACOG, 2013). The food is divided among three meals and three snacks. The bedtime snack may be indicated to prevent nighttime hypoglycemia. A nutritionist should work out meal plans with the woman based on the woman's lifestyle, culture, and food preferences. The woman needs to be familiar with the use of food exchanges so she can plan her own meals.

It is possible to control GDM with diet alone. Daily food records, weekly weight checks, and regular ketone testing can assist in identifying an individual's energy requirements to help avoid the need for insulin therapy (Wong et al., 2013).

GLUCOSE MONITORING

Glucose monitoring is essential to determine the need for insulin and assess glucose control. Many physicians have the woman come in for weekly assessment of her fasting glucose levels and one or two postprandial levels. In addition, frequent self-monitoring of glucose levels is paramount in maintaining good glucose control. Self-monitoring is discussed shortly.

INSULIN ADMINISTRATION

Many women with gestational diabetes require insulin to maintain normal glucose levels. Individuals with pregestational diabetes typically have type 1 diabetes and are already on insulin. In either case, semisynthetic human insulin or an insulin analog such as lispro or aspart should be used. Insulin is given either in multiple injections or by continuous subcutaneous infusion. Multiple injections are more common and generally produce excellent results. Many women receive a combination of intermediate and regular insulin.

A three-dose approach is often used, with a combination of intermediate-acting insulin and short-acting insulin or an analog taken before breakfast, short-acting insulin or analog at dinner, and an intermediate-acting insulin at bedtime. Some women require a four-injection approach with a small dose of a short-acting insulin or analog before lunch (Landon, Catalano, & Gabbe, 2012).

Until recently oral hypoglycemics were not generally used during pregnancy because they cross the placenta and had not been well studied. Recent research suggests that glyburide, a second-generation sulfonylurea, and metformin, a biguanide, may be safe to use in women with gestational diabetes (ADA, 2015; Caritis & Hebert, 2013).

EVALUATION OF FETAL STATUS

Information about the well-being, size, and maturation of the fetus is important for planning the course of pregnancy and the timing of birth. See Table 14–1.

TABLE 14–1 Fetal Surveillance by Gestational Weeks

WEEKS GESTATION	FETAL SURVEILLANCE
8–10	Ultrasound crown–rump measurement for estimated date of birth (EDB)
16–18 or 20	Quadruple screen for neural tube defects (maternal serum alpha fetoprotein, hCG, unconjugated estriol, inhibin A)
18	Ultrasound confirms gestational age and diagnoses multiple pregnancy or congenital anomalies
20–22	Fetal echocardiogram
24	Begin ultrasounds for assessment of fetus and fetal growth.
28	Ultrasound for growth. Begin daily fetal movement counting. (See Chapter 13.)
	Start weekly non-stress testing (NST). If evidence of IUGR, preeclampsia, oligohydramnios, or poorly controlled blood glucose exists, testing may begin as early as 26 weeks and may be done more often.
32	Ultrasound for growth.
32	Increase to twice weekly non-stress test (NST) or weekly biophysical profile (BPP). If the NST is nonreactive, a fetal biophysical profile or contraction stress test is performed. If the woman requires hospitalization (e.g., to control glycemia or for complications), NSTs may be done daily.
36	Ultrasound for growth
37–39	Amniocentesis for women with poor glycemic control to document fetal pulmonary maturity prior to elective birth. Omit amniocentesis if maternal or fetal condition suggests jeopardy to either.
39–40	Birth without amniocentesis for women that have maintained good glycemic control and have excellent dating criteria

Note: Some physicians order fetal biophysical profiles (ultrasound evaluation of fetal well-being in which fetal breathing movements, fetal activity, reactivity, muscle tone, and amniotic fluid volume are assessed) as part of an ongoing evaluation of fetal status.

Intrapartum Management of Diabetes Mellitus

During the intrapartum period, medical therapy focuses on the following:

- **Timing of birth.** Most pregnant women with diabetes, regardless of the type, are allowed to go to full term, with spontaneous labor. Some clinicians opt to induce labor in a woman at full term to avoid problems related to decreased perfusion as the placenta ages. Cesarean birth may be indicated if evidence of nonreassuring fetal status exists. Birth before full term may be indicated for women with diabetes who are experiencing vascular changes and worsening hypertension or if evidence of IUGR exists. To determine fetal lung maturity, the following tests may be used (Cunningham et al., 2014):

Test	Lung Maturity Value
Lamellar body count	Greater than 50,000
Lecithin/sphingomyelin (L/S) ratio	2.0–3.5

- **Labor management.** Frequently maternal insulin requirements decrease dramatically during labor. Consequently maternal glucose levels are measured hourly to determine insulin need (Figure 14–1). The primary goal in controlling maternal glucose levels in the intrapartum period is to prevent neonatal hypoglycemia (American Academy of Pediatrics [AAP] & ACOG, 2012). Often two intravenous lines are used, one with a 5% dextrose solution and one with a saline solution. The saline solution is then available for piggybacking insulin or if a bolus is needed. Because insulin clings to plastic IV bags and tubing, the tubing should be flushed with insulin before the prescribed amount is added. During the second stage of labor and the immediate postpartum period, the woman may not need additional insulin. The intravenous insulin is discontinued with the completion of the third stage of labor.

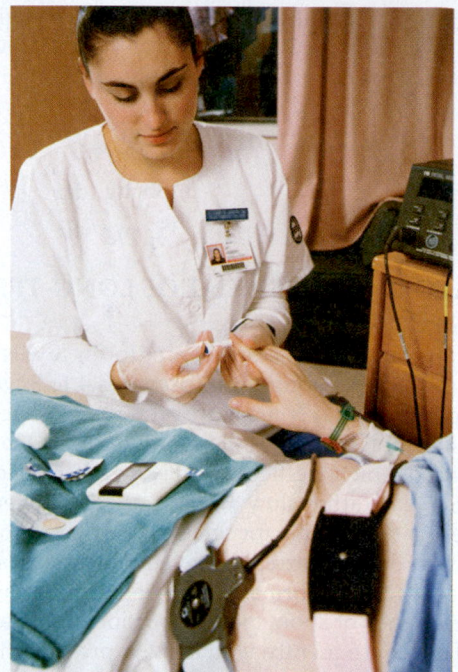

Figure 14–1 During labor the nurse closely monitors the blood glucose levels of the woman with diabetes mellitus.

Postpartum Management of Diabetes Mellitus

Generally, maternal insulin requirements fall significantly during the postpartum period because hormone levels fall after placental separation, and their anti-insulin effect ceases, resulting in decreased blood glucose levels. For the first 24 hours postpartum, a woman with pre-existing diabetes typically requires very little insulin and her insulin dosage is usually managed with a sliding scale. Afterward, a more regular insulin dosage pattern can be re-established based on blood glucose testing.

Women with GDM seldom need insulin during the postpartum period. Breastfeeding can be encouraged, but the nurse needs to remember that insulin requirements do decrease with breastfeeding, so a prenursing snack may be indicated (Hood, 2012). Maternal caloric needs increase during lactation to 500 to 800 kcal above prepregnant requirements, and insulin must be adjusted accordingly. Home blood glucose monitoring should continue for the woman with type 1 diabetes.

If elevated glucose levels develop, oral antihyperglycemic agents may be tried if the woman is not breastfeeding. Antihyperglycemics are contraindicated during breastfeeding. The woman should be reassessed 6 weeks postpartum to determine whether her glucose levels are normal. If the levels are normal, she should be reassessed at a minimum of 3-year intervals (ADA, 2015).

The establishment of parent–child relationships is a high priority during the postpartum period for all women with DM and their families. However, that may become more challenging if the newborn requires a special-care nursery. In such cases, the parents need ongoing information, support, and encouragement to visit and be involved in the newborn's care.

The woman and her partner, if he is involved, should also receive information on family planning. Barrier methods of contraception (diaphragm, cervical cap, condom) used with a spermicide are safe, effective, and economical and are the method of choice for women with insulin-dependent diabetes. The use of combined oral contraceptives (COCs) by women with diabetes is somewhat controversial. Many physicians who prescribe low-dose COCs to women with diabetes restrict them to women who have no vascular disease and do not smoke. The progesterone-only pill may also be used, as may Depo-Provera. Many couples who have completed their families choose elective sterilization.

Nursing Management

For the Woman With Diabetes Mellitus or Gestational Diabetes Mellitus

Nursing Assessment and Diagnosis

Whether diabetes has been diagnosed before pregnancy occurs or the diagnosis is made during pregnancy (GDM), careful assessment of the disease process and the woman's understanding of diabetes is important. A thorough physical examination—including assessment for vascular complications of the disease, any signs of infectious conditions, and urine and blood testing for glucose—is essential on the first prenatal visit. Follow-up visits are usually scheduled twice a month during the first two trimesters and once a week during the last trimester.

Assessment also yields vital information about the woman's ability to cope with the combined stress of pregnancy and diabetes and to follow a recommended regimen of care. It is necessary to determine the woman's knowledge about diabetes and self-care before formulating a teaching plan.

Nursing diagnoses that may apply to the pregnant woman with diabetes include the following (NANDA-I © 2014):

- *Overweight, Risk for,* related to imbalance between intake and available insulin

- *Injury, Risk for,* related to possible complications secondary to hypoglycemia or hyperglycemia

- *Family Processes, Interrupted,* related to the need for hospitalization secondary to diabetes mellitus

Nursing Plan and Implementation

For the woman with pre-existing diabetes, a nurse and a physician may provide prepregnancy counseling using a team approach. Ideally they see the couple before pregnancy so that the DM can be evaluated. The outlook for pregnancy is good if the diabetes is of recent onset without vascular complications, provided that glucose levels can be controlled.

For women with GDM, nursing care focuses heavily on client education about the condition, its implications, and its management. *Nursing Care Plan: For the Woman With Diabetes Mellitus* summarizes nursing management.

COMMUNITY-BASED NURSING CARE

In many cases, women with gestational diabetes mellitus are stabilized in the hospital and necessary teaching for self-care is begun. Women with pre-existing diabetes may also require hospitalization for stabilization of their diabetes. In either case, the majority of ongoing teaching and supervision of pregnant women with diabetes is then carried out by nurses in clinics, community agencies, and the women's homes.

Effective Insulin Use

Ensure that the woman and her partner understand the purpose of insulin, the types of insulin to be used, and the correct procedure for administering it. Instruct the woman's partner about insulin administration in case it becomes necessary for the partner to give it. For some highly motivated women whose glucose levels are not well controlled with multiple injections, the continuous infusion pump may improve glucose control.

Clinical Tip

Have a woman with GDM who is learning to test her blood glucose do a fingerstick while you watch. For many women actually sticking their finger can be a challenge to overcome. This also enables you to verify that correct technique is used.

Teach the woman how and when to monitor her blood glucose level, the desired range of blood glucose levels, and the importance of good control (Figure 14–2). Most women use a glucose meter to monitor blood sugar level because the meter provides a more accurate reading. Instruct the woman to follow the manufacturer's directions exactly; to wash her hands thoroughly before puncturing her finger; to touch the blood droplet,

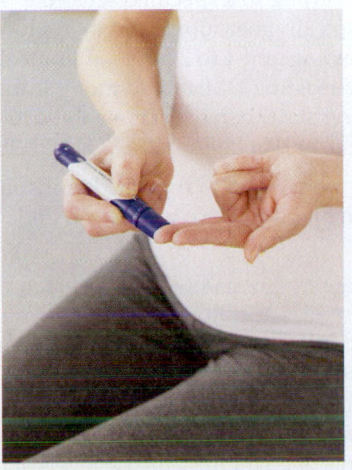

Figure 14–2 As she was taught, this pregnant woman regularly monitors her blood glucose at home.

not her finger, to the test pad on the strip; and to store the test strips as directed and discard them after the expiration date. Clients with diabetes need to keep a record of each blood sugar reading. Specific record sheets are available for this purpose.

Clinical Reasoning   Glucose Intolerance

Patti Chang, a 35-year-old G3P2, is a well-educated, active Chinese American woman with no history of glucose intolerance. Her two children were born healthy at 36 weeks' gestation. She receives the usual 50-g glucose tolerance test at 26 weeks' gestation, and her plasma level is 160 mg/dL. She seems irritated and frustrated when her obstetrician tells her that it would be best to perform a 3-hour fasting glucose tolerance test. After the physician leaves the room, Patti asks the nurse the following questions: "Will the glucose hurt my baby? What will the treatment be?"

How will you answer the questions? Why do you think Patti is so upset?

Planned Exercise Program

Regardless of the type of diabetes, unless otherwise medically contraindicated, encourage exercise for the woman's overall well-being. If she is used to a regular exercise program, encourage her to continue. In addition, advise the woman to exercise after meals when blood sugar levels are high, to wear diabetic identification, to carry a simple sugar such as hard candy (because of the possibility of exercise-induced hypoglycemia), to monitor her blood glucose levels regularly, and to avoid injecting insulin into an extremity that will soon be used during exercise.

If the woman has not been following a regular exercise plan, encourage her to begin gradually. Because of alterations in metabolism with exercise, the woman's blood glucose should be well controlled before she begins an exercise program.

Health Promotion   The Pregnant Woman and Diabetes
Glucose Monitoring

Home monitoring of blood glucose levels is the most accurate and convenient method to determine insulin dose and assess control.

- Teach the woman self-monitoring techniques that are done according to a specified schedule. Women with GDM typically measure their blood glucose 4 times a day (fasting and 1 to 2 hours after meals). Women with pre-existing DM should monitor their blood in the fasting state, before each meal, 1 to 2 hours after each meal, and at bedtime (ACOG, 2012b).

- Instruct the woman to regulate her insulin dosage based on blood glucose values and anticipated activity level.

- Encourage her to maintain blood glucose levels in normal ranges as follows: fasting (before eating or taking insulin), less than 95 mg/dL; 2 hours after each meal, less than 120 mg/dL (AAP/ACOG, 2012).

Review Symptoms of Hypoglycemia and Hyperglycemia

- Teach the pregnant woman with diabetes to recognize symptoms of changing glucose levels and to take

appropriate action by immediately checking her capillary blood glucose level.

- If blood glucose is less than 60 mg/dL, advise her to drink one 8-oz cup of skim milk or 1/2 cup of orange juice, apple juice, or regular soft drink; or eat four to six pieces of hard candy; or consume 1 tablespoon of honey, brown sugar, or corn syrup. Wait 15 minutes and recheck blood glucose (Cleveland Clinic, 2016). (*Note:* Many people overtreat their symptoms by continuing to eat, but doing so can cause rebound hyperglycemia.)

- Have the woman carry a snack at all times and have other fast sources of glucose (simple carbohydrates) at hand to treat an insulin reaction when milk or juice is not available.

- Ensure that family members learn how to inject glucagon in case food does not work or is not feasible (e.g., in the presence of severe morning sickness).

Smoking
- Ensure that the woman knows that smoking has harmful effects on both the maternal vascular system and the developing fetus and thus is contraindicated for both pregnancy and diabetes.

Travel
- Insulin can be kept at room temperature while traveling. Instruct woman to keep insulin supplies with her; they should not be packed in the baggage.

- On international flights most airlines can provide special meals if notified a few days before departure. If meals are not scheduled to be served, the woman should ensure that she has adequate food before boarding.

- Have her wear a diabetic identification bracelet or necklace and check with her physician for any instructions or advice before traveling.

Support Groups
- Many communities have diabetes support groups or education classes that are helpful to women with newly diagnosed diabetes. Refer her to them.

Cesarean Birth
- Chances for a cesarean birth increase if the pregnant woman is diabetic. Anticipate the possibility and suggest enrollment in cesarean birth preparation classes. The couple may prefer simply to discuss cesarean birth with the nurse and their obstetrician and read some books on the topic.

HOSPITAL-BASED NURSING CARE

Hospitalization may become necessary during the pregnancy to evaluate blood glucose levels and adjust insulin dosages. In such cases, monitor the woman's status and continue to provide teaching so that the woman is knowledgeable about her condition and its management.

During the intrapartum period, continue to monitor the woman's status, maintain her intravenous fluids, be alert for signs of hypoglycemia, and provide the care indicated for any woman in labor. If a cesarean birth becomes necessary, provide appropriate care, as described in Chapter 22.

Nursing Care Plan: For the Woman With Diabetes Mellitus

1. Nursing Diagnosis: *Nutrition, Imbalanced, Less than Body Requirements, related to poor carbohydrate metabolism (NANDA-I © 2014)*

GOAL: Client will maintain adequate nutrition throughout pregnancy.

INTERVENTION	RATIONALE
• Emphasize importance of regular prenatal visits for assessment of weight gain, controlled blood sugar, fetal heart tones, urine ketones, and fundal height measurement.	• Regular follow-up and assessment of weight, blood sugar levels, fetal heart tones, urine ketones, and fundal height will help promote a healthy pregnancy and outcome as well as allow for modifications in the treatment regimen if necessary.
• Coordinate care with a dietitian to assist client in meal planning and educate client on the daily caloric needs of pregnancy.	• A daily intake of high-quality foods promotes fetal growth and controls maternal glucose levels.
• Instruct client on signs and symptoms of hyperglycemia: polyphagia, nausea, hot flushes, polydipsia, polyuria, fruity breath, abdominal cramps, rapid deep breathing, headache, weakness, drowsiness, and general malaise. Instruct client on signs and symptoms of hypoglycemia: hunger, clammy skin, irritability, slurred speech, seizures, tachycardia, headache, pallor, sweating, disorientation, shakiness, blurred vision, and, if untreated, coma or convulsions.	• Maintaining a euglycemic state throughout pregnancy aids in preventing diabetic complications and promotes a positive pregnancy outcome.
• Instruct client on management of hyperglycemia and hypoglycemia.	
• Include family members in meal planning.	• Gives the family member a sense of involvement and an understanding of the importance of adequate nutrition in pregnancy.

EXPECTED OUTCOME: The client will maintain adequate nutrition as evidenced by adequate weight gain, normal blood sugar levels, normal fetal heart rate, verbalization of understanding of personal treatment regimen, and appropriate fetal growth and development during pregnancy.

2. Nursing Diagnosis: *Injury, Risk for,* to the fetus related to possible complications associated with altered tissue perfusion secondary to maternal diagnosis of diabetes mellitus (NANDA-I © 2014)

GOAL: Uncomplicated birth of a healthy newborn.

INTERVENTION	RATIONALE
• Assess fetal heart tones for reassuring variability and accelerations.	• Reassuring fetal heart rate variability and accelerations are interpreted as adequate placental oxygenation.
• Instruct mother on how to lie in a left recumbent position after eating and record how many fetal movements she feels in an hour.	• More than five fetal kicks in an hour are indicative of fetal well-being.
• **Collaborative:** Perform oxytocin challenge test (OCT), contraction stress test (CST), and non-stress tests as determined by physician.	• Fetal surveillance testing assesses fetal well-being and adequate placental perfusion.
• Prepare client for frequent ultrasound assessments.	• Ultrasonography is indicated in the first trimester to confirm gestational age and then repeated regularly to evaluate fetal well-being per physician's orders.
• Prepare client for possible amniocentesis procedure.	• A sample of amniotic fluid can be used to detect fetal lung maturity and enables medical personnel to prepare for a potential preterm birth.
• Assist physician with biophysical profile assessment.	• Helps ensure fetal well-being and a positive fetal outcome.

EXPECTED OUTCOME: The fetus will exhibit signs of adequate tissue perfusion as evidenced by positive fetal activity, reassuring fetal heart rate patterns, a biophysical profile score between 8 and 10, negative CST, L/S ratio indicating fetal lung maturity, and a reactive non-stress test.

(continued)

Nursing Care Plan: For the Woman With Diabetes Mellitus (*continued*)

3. Nursing Diagnosis: *Enhanced Knowledge, Readiness for,* about the effects of blood sugar on pregnancy related to an expressed desire to maintain stable blood glucose levels (NANDA-I © 2014)

GOAL: The client and her family will verbalize the importance of maintaining blood sugar within prescribed ranges during pregnancy.

INTERVENTION	RATIONALE
• Assess the woman's and family's cognitive level and develop a teaching strategy that will facilitate learning at that level.	• Behavior changes occur when teaching strategies are appropriate for the client's and family's cognitive level.
• Teach blood glucose monitoring, insulin administration, and predicted insulin needs throughout pregnancy, and then have client and family members repeat the discussion.	• Basic understanding of the relationship between blood sugar levels and how insulin needs change throughout pregnancy will foster compliance with prescribed regimen.
• Emphasize the importance of maintaining a healthy diet and exercise program during pregnancy. Encourage client and family to develop a sample diabetic diet and exercise regimen that is appropriate for pregnancy while present in the clinic or hospital and evaluate for appropriateness.	• Involves the client and her family members in the planning of her care, and the evaluation process promotes cooperation, positive reinforcement, and a time for modifications of regimen if necessary.
• Emphasize the importance of prenatal care for the purpose of maternal and fetal surveillance.	• Frequent prenatal visits allow for modifications in regimen and promote a healthy pregnancy outcome.

EXPECTED OUTCOME: The client and family members will verbalize understanding of the effects of blood sugar fluctuations on pregnancy as evidenced by asking questions and seeking health information when necessary. The client adheres to personal treatment regimen throughout pregnancy.

4. Nursing Diagnosis: *Infection, Risk for,* related to increased levels of glucose in urine (NANDA-I © 2014)

GOAL: The client will have no urinary tract infections (UTIs) during pregnancy.

INTERVENTION	RATIONALE
• Encourage client to utilize preventive measures to prevent UTIs: increasing intake of water and cranberry juice, wearing cotton underwear, wiping perineum from front to back, voiding frequently, and voiding before and immediately after sexual intercourse.	• Using preventive measures decreases the likelihood of client acquiring a UTI.
• Instruct client on the signs and symptoms of UTIs: urinary frequency, dysuria, cloudy urine, hematuria, lower back pain, and foul-smelling urine.	• Client will be aware of signs and symptoms of UTIs and report to physician for immediate intervention.
• **Collaborative:** Instruct client on how to obtain a clean-catch urine sample and send to laboratory for culture and sensitivity per physician's orders.	• A clean-catch urine sample will contain bacteria if a UTI is present.
• Administer prescribed antibiotic therapy and teach client about medication, adverse effects, and appropriate dosage.	• Antibiotic therapy is the appropriate treatment for a UTI. Compliance increases when a client fully understands medication regimen.
• Encourage client to drink 8–10 glasses of water each day.	• Increased fluid intake assists in flushing bacteria out of the urinary tract system.

EXPECTED OUTCOME: The client will remain free of UTIs during pregnancy as evidenced by verbalizing and complying with appropriate preventive measures, increasing fluid intake, and identifying negative urine samples during prenatal visits.

5. Nursing Diagnosis: *Anxiety* related to unfamiliarity with diagnosis (NANDA-I © 2014)

GOAL: The client expresses less anxiety.

INTERVENTION	RATIONALE
• Assess client's level of anxiety (mild—1, moderate—2, or severe—3) and have client verbalize causes of anxiety.	• Verbalization of anxiety provokers encourages expression of feelings and questions.
• Share information on diabetes care such as nutrition, exercise, and glucose control in a clear and concise manner.	• Accurate information gives the client a sense of control and comfort.
• Instruct client on anxiety-reducing techniques such as imagery, breathing exercises, and massage used in pregnancy.	• Gives client the tools necessary for decreasing anxiety.
• Refer client to a diabetes support group.	• A support group allows clients with similar problems to express concerns and share information with each other.

EXPECTED OUTCOME: The client will demonstrate appropriate coping strategies as evidenced by utilizing resources efficiently and verbalizing feelings of anxiety and the ways to deal with them.

SAFETY ALERT!

As a medication, insulin carries significant potential risks. Like all medications, nurses should use two client identifiers, administer it at the correct time, and monitor the client afterward. Nurses should have documented knowledge about its administration and demonstrate competency in administering, storing, and handling it and in the key assessments and findings indicated for maternity clients receiving insulin (Hurst, 2011).

Evaluation

Expected outcomes of nursing care include the following:

- The woman is able to discuss her condition and its possible impact on her pregnancy, labor and birth, and postpartum period.
- The woman participates in developing a healthcare regimen to meet her needs and follows it throughout her pregnancy.
- The woman avoids developing hypoglycemia or hyperglycemia.
- The woman gives birth to a healthy newborn.
- The woman is able to care for her newborn.

Care of the Woman With Anemia

Anemia indicates inadequate levels of hemoglobin (Hb) in the blood. During pregnancy, *anemia* is defined as hemoglobin less than 11 g/dL in the first and third trimesters and less than 10.5g/dL in the second trimester (King, Brucker, Kriebs, et al., 2015). The common anemias of pregnancy are caused by either insufficient hemoglobin production related to nutritional deficiency in iron or folic acid during pregnancy or by hemoglobin destruction in an inherited disorder such as sickle cell disease. Table 14–2 describes these common anemias.

KEY FACTS TO REMEMBER
Gestational Diabetes Mellitus (GDM)
and Diabetes Mellitus (DM)

- Gestational diabetes mellitus (GDM) refers to a carbohydrate intolerance that develops during pregnancy. If untreated, the risk of perinatal morbidity and mortality increases.
- All pregnant women should be screened for GDM.
- Women with GDM are often treated with diet therapy and regular exercise; in some cases insulin or an insulin analog is necessary.
- Women with pregestational DM require careful management. Their long-term glucose control is best assessed by determining the percentage of glycohemoglobin, or HbA1c, in the blood. The target level is less than 6%.
- To maintain normal glucose levels, women with pregestational DM typically receive doses of regular insulin or an insulin analog such as lispro before each meal and a dose of a longer-acting insulin or analog at bedtime.
- During labor, insulin requirements may decrease dramatically and require careful monitoring. The goal is to avoid neonatal hypoglycemia.

Healthy People 2020

(MICH-15) Reduce the proportion of women of childbearing potential who have low red blood cell folate concentrations

---

Care of the Woman With a Substance Abuse Problem

Substance abuse occurs when an individual experiences difficulties with work, family, social relations, and health as a result of alcohol or drug use. In general, the rate of illicit drug use among pregnant

TABLE 14–2 Anemia and Pregnancy

BRIEF DESCRIPTION	MATERNAL IMPLICATIONS	FETAL/NEONATAL IMPLICATIONS
IRON DEFICIENCY ANEMIA		
Most common medical complication of pregnancy. Condition caused by inadequate iron intake resulting in hemoglobin (Hb) levels below 11 g/dL. To prevent this, most women are advised to take supplemental iron during pregnancy and to eat an iron-rich diet.	A pregnant woman with this anemia tires easily, is more susceptible to infection, has an increased chance of preeclampsia–eclampsia and postpartum hemorrhage, and cannot tolerate even minimal blood loss during birth. Healing of episiotomy or incision may be delayed.	Risk of low birth weight, prematurity, stillbirth, and neonatal death increases in women with severe iron deficiency anemia (maternal Hb less than 6 g/dL). Fetus may be hypoxic during labor because of impaired uteroplacental oxygenation.
SICKLE CELL DISEASE (ALSO REFERRED TO AS SICKLE CELL ANEMIA)		
Recessive autosomal disease in which normal adult hemoglobin, hemoglobin A, is abnormally formed. It occurs primarily in people of African descent and occasionally in people of Southeast Asian or Mediterranean descent. The disease is characterized by sickling of the red blood cells (RBCs) in the presence of decreased oxygenation. Because the woman maintains her Hb levels by intense erythropoiesis, additional folic acid supplements (1–4 mg/day) are necessary (Resetkova & Szymanski, 2015). Condition may be marked by crisis with profound anemia, jaundice, high temperature, infarction, and acute pain. Crisis is treated by rehydration with intravenous fluids, administration of oxygen, antibiotics (if infection is present), and analgesics (Resetkova & Szymanski, 2015). The fetus is monitored throughout.	Pregnancy may aggravate sickle cell disease and bring on a vaso-occlusive crisis. Maternal mortality is rare but there is a significant risk of urinary tract infection, pneumonia, acute chest syndrome, and gestational hypertension (Cunningham, Leveno, Bloom, et al., 2014). Congestive heart failure or acute renal failure may also occur. The goal of treatment is to reduce anemia and maintain good health (Figure 14–3). Maternal infections are treated promptly because dehydration and fever can trigger sickling and crisis. Oxygen supplementation is used throughout labor and IV fluids are given to maintain hydration. Fetal heart rate is monitored closely. Antiembolism stockings are generally used postpartum.	The incidence of fetal death during and following an attack has greatly decreased in recent years. Prematurity and intrauterine growth restriction (IUGR) are associated with sickle cell disease. Fetal death is believed to be due to sickling attacks in the placenta (Andemariam & Browning, 2013).
FOLIC ACID DEFICIENCY ANEMIA		
Folic acid deficiency is the most common cause of megaloblastic anemia. In the absence of folic acid, immature RBCs fail to divide, become enlarged (megaloblastic), and are fewer in number. Increased folic acid metabolism during pregnancy and lactation can result in deficiency. All women who could become pregnant should take a multivitamin containing 400 mcg daily (generally found in prenatal vitamins) before conception and through at least the first trimester of pregnancy. The condition is treated with 1 mg folate daily (see Chapter 11 for more information about folic acid/folate).	Folate deficiency is the second most common cause of anemia in pregnancy. Severe deficiency increases the risk that the mother may need a blood transfusion following birth because of anemia. She also has an increased risk of hemorrhage caused by thrombocytopenia and is more susceptible to infection. Folic acid is readily available in foods such as fresh leafy green vegetables, red meat, fish, poultry, and legumes, but it is easily destroyed by overcooking or cooking with large quantities of water.	Maternal folic acid deficiency has been associated with an increased risk of neural tube defects (NTDs) such as spina bifida, meningomyelocele, and anencephaly in the newborn. Women who have already had one baby with a NTD are generally advised to take a larger dose of folic acid daily.

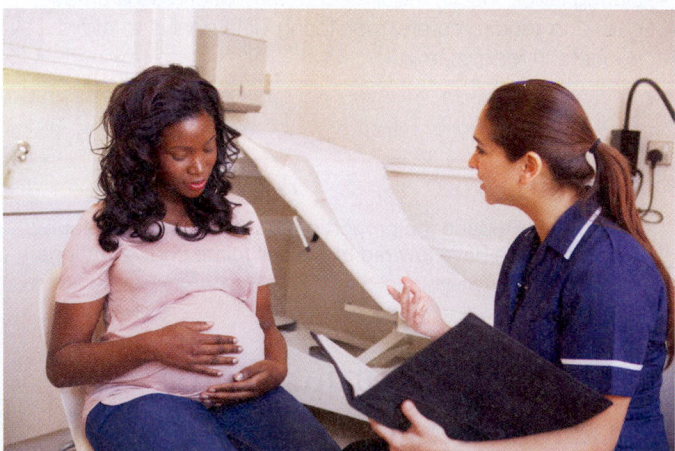

Figure 14–3 Health teaching is an important part of nursing care for the pregnant woman with sickle cell disease.

SOURCE: Monkey Business Images/Shutterstock.

women is less than half the rate among nonpregnant women. Specifically, approximately 5.4% of pregnant women ages 15 to 44 report having used an illicit drug in the past month as compared to 11.4% of nonpregnant women (Substance Abuse and Mental Health Services Administration [SAMHSA], 2014). However, illicit drug use varies significantly by age with the highest rate among the youngest pregnant women, specifically 14.6% among females ages 15 to 17; the rate was 8.6% among those ages 18 to 25, and 3.2% among prepregnant women ages 26 to 44 (SAMHSA, 2014).

Drugs that are commonly misused include tobacco, alcohol, cocaine, marijuana, amphetamines, barbiturates, hallucinogens, club drugs, heroin, and other narcotics. (Tobacco is discussed in Chapter 10 as a teratogenic substance.) *Polydrug use* involving multiple substances such as alcohol, tobacco, and illicit drugs is fairly common and contributes to the risks a pregnant woman faces. Table 14–3 identifies common addictive drugs and their effects on the fetus or newborn.

Drug use during pregnancy, particularly in the first trimester, may adversely affect the health of the woman and the growth and development of the fetus. Unfortunately, prenatal drug use may be the most frequently missed diagnosis in

TABLE 14–3 Possible Effects of Selected Drugs of Abuse/Addiction on Fetus and Newborn

MATERNAL DRUG	EFFECT ON FETUS/NEWBORN
DEPRESSANTS	
Alcohol	Intellectual disability, microcephaly, midfacial hypoplasia, cardiac anomalies, intrauterine growth restriction (IUGR), potential teratogenic effects, fetal alcohol syndrome (FAS), fetal alcohol spectrum disorder (FASD)
NARCOTICS	
Heroin	Withdrawal symptoms, known as neonatal abstinence syndrome (NAS), include tremors, irritability, sneezing, vomiting, fever, diarrhea, abnormal respiratory function, and possible seizures
Methadone	With abrupt maternal termination of the drug, severe withdrawal symptoms can include preterm labor, rapid labor, abruption, nonreassuring fetal status, and meconium aspiration. Neonates may present with NAS and be small for gestational age (SGA).
BARBITURATES	
Phenobarbital	Withdrawal symptoms Fetal growth restriction
TRANQUILIZERS	
Diazepam (Valium)	Withdrawal symptoms
ANTIANXIETY DRUGS	
Lithium	Congenital anomalies
STIMULANTS	
Amphetamine sulfate (Benzedrine)	Low birth weight; withdrawal symptoms
Cocaine	Cerebral infarctions, microcephaly, learning disabilities, poor state organization, decreased interactive behavior, CNS anomalies, cardiac anomalies, genitourinary anomalies, sudden infant death syndrome (SIDS)
Methamphetamine	Increased rates of preterm birth and abruptio placentae; impact on the SGA newborn; heart and brain abnormalities; decreased arousal, increased stress, and significant but subtle attention impairments (National Institute on Drug Abuse [NIDA], 2013b).
Nicotine (half to one pack cigarettes/day)	Increased rate of spontaneous abortion, increased incidence of placental abruption, SGA, small head circumference, decreased length, SIDS, attention-deficit/hyperactivity disorder (ADHD) in school-age children
PSYCHOTROPICS	
PCP (phencyclidine hydrochloride, "angel dust")	Withdrawal symptoms Newborn behavioral and developmental abnormalities
Marijuana	Possible impaired neurodevelopment in children exposed in utero; increased sensitivity to drugs of abuse; risks similar to those associated with smoking tobacco (ACOG, 2015b).

all of maternity care. Physicians and nurses may fail to ask women about drug and alcohol use because of their own lack of knowledge, discomfort, or biases. Often substance-abusing women wait until late in pregnancy to seek health care. Moreover, the substance-abusing woman who seeks early prenatal care may not voluntarily reveal her addiction, so caregivers should ask direct, nonjudgmental questions (see Chapter 9) and be alert for a history or physical signs that suggest substance abuse.

Providing effective prenatal care to chemically dependent women presents many challenges for clinicians. However, pregnancy represents a period in most women's lives when they recognize the need for and are receptive to caring interventions.

Healthy People 2020

(MICH 11) Increase abstinence from alcohol, cigarettes, and illicit drugs among pregnant women

Clinical Tip

Keep in mind that almost 1 out of 10 women in the United States, regardless of socioeconomic status or ethnic background, is currently abusing a substance. If you consider that possibility with every woman, you will ask the important questions about drug use and be alert for signs of substance abuse.

Substances Commonly Abused During Pregnancy

ALCOHOL

Alcohol is a central nervous system (CNS) depressant and a potent teratogen. An estimated 10.2% of pregnant women ages 15 to 44 use alcohol in a given month. This rate is significantly lower than the rate for nonpregnant women of that age (53.6%). The prevalence of binge drinking (four or more drinks on the same occasion) among pregnant women is 3.1% as compared to 18.2%

among those who are not pregnant (Tan, Denny, Cheal, et al., 2015). These figures are of concern because birth defects that are related to fetal alcohol exposure can occur in the first 3 to 8 weeks' gestation, often before the woman even knows she is pregnant. Alcohol use among pregnant women tends to decrease by trimester.

The effects of alcohol on the fetus may result in a group of signs known as *fetal alcohol spectrum disorder (FASD)*. FASD has characteristic physical and mental abnormalities that vary in severity and combination. (See discussion in Chapter 26.) There is no definitive answer to how much alcohol a woman can safely consume during pregnancy. Consequently, it is essential that nurses and other healthcare providers advise women about the dangers associated with drinking while pregnant (U.S. Department of Health and Human Services, 2012). Chronic abuse of alcohol can undermine maternal health by causing malnutrition (especially folic acid and thiamine deficiencies), bone marrow suppression, increased incidence of infections, and liver disease. As a result of alcohol dependence, a woman may have withdrawal seizures in the intrapartum period as early as 12 to 48 hours after she stops drinking. Delirium tremens (DTs) may occur in the postpartum period, and the newborn may suffer a withdrawal syndrome. The nursing staff in the maternal–newborn unit must be aware of the manifestations of alcohol abuse so they can prepare for the client's special needs. The care regimen includes sedation to decrease irritability and tremors, seizure precautions, intravenous fluid therapy for hydration, and preparation for an addicted newborn. Although high doses of sedatives and analgesics may be necessary for the woman, caution is advised because these medications can cause fetal depression.

Breastfeeding generally is not contraindicated, although alcohol is excreted in breast milk. Excessive alcohol consumption may intoxicate the baby and inhibit the maternal letdown reflex. Discharge planning for the alcohol-addicted mother and newborn needs to be coordinated with the social services department of the hospital.

COCAINE AND CRACK
Cocaine acts at the nerve terminals to prevent the reuptake of dopamine and norepinephrine, which in turn results in vasoconstriction, tachycardia, and hypertension. Placental vasoconstriction decreases blood flow to the fetus. The onset of cocaine effects occurs rapidly, but the euphoria lasts only about 30 minutes. Euphoria and excitement are usually followed by irritability, depression, pessimism, fatigue, and a strong desire for more cocaine. This pattern often leads the user to take repeated doses to sustain the effect. Cocaine metabolites may be present in the urine of a pregnant woman for as long as 4 to 7 days after use.

Cocaine can be taken by intravenous injection or by snorting the powdered form. Crack, a form of freebase cocaine that is made up of baking soda, water, and cocaine mixed into a paste and microwaved to form a rock, can be smoked. Smoking crack leads to a quicker, more intense high than cocaine because the drug is absorbed through the large surface area of the lungs.

The cocaine user is difficult to identify prenatally. Because cocaine is an illegal substance, many women are reluctant to volunteer information about their drug use. The nurse who is familiar with the woman may recognize subtle signs of cocaine use, including mood swings and appetite changes, and withdrawal symptoms such as depression, irritability, nausea, lack of motivation, and psychomotor changes.

Major adverse maternal effects of cocaine use include seizures and hallucinations, pulmonary edema, respiratory failure, and heart problems. Women who use cocaine have an increased incidence of spontaneous abortion, abruptio

placentae, preterm birth, and stillbirth (Cain et al., 2013). Fetal exposure to cocaine increases the risk of intrauterine growth restriction (IUGR), microcephaly, shorter body length, altered brain development, congenital anomalies, and neurobehavioral abnormalities (Niebyl & Simpson, 2012). Newborns exposed to cocaine in utero may have neurobehavioral disturbances, marked irritability, an exaggerated startle reflex, labile emotions, and an increased risk of sudden infant death syndrome (SIDS). (See Chapter 26 for further discussion.)

Cocaine crosses into breast milk and may cause symptoms in the breastfeeding baby, including extreme irritability, vomiting, diarrhea, dilated pupils, and apnea. Thus women who continue to use cocaine after childbirth should avoid nursing.

MARIJUANA
Marijuana is the most widely used illicit drug among women, both pregnant and nonpregnant. Evidence about the potential impact of marijuana use on the fetus is mixed. In reality, the impact of heavy marijuana use on pregnancy is difficult to evaluate because of the variety of social factors (e.g., polydrug use) that may influence the direct results of marijuana itself. Because of concerns about maternal and fetal exposure to smoking and the possibility of impaired neurodevelopment in the child, the American College of Obstetricians and Gynecologists (ACOG, 2015b) recommends that all pregnant women and women who are planning a pregnancy should be counseled about the potential negative effects of marijuana use and encouraged to discontinue marijuana use.

MDMA (ECSTASY)
MDMA (methylenedioxymethamphetamine), better known as *Ecstasy* or *Molly*, is the most commonly used of a group of drugs referred to as *club drugs*, so called because they have become popular among adolescents and young adults who frequent dance clubs and "raves." Other club drugs include flunitrazepam (Rohypnol), gamma hydroxybutyrate (GHB), and ketamine hydrochloride. Phencyclidine (PCP) and lysergic acid diethylamine (LSD) are sometimes classified as club drugs as well.

A stimulant, MDMA is taken by mouth, usually as a tablet. It produces euphoria and feelings of empathy for others. It has been widely perceived as a "safe" drug because of a relatively low incidence of adverse reactions. However, adverse responses are very unpredictable and their incidence is growing. MDMA can cause muscle tension, involuntary teeth clenching, nausea, confusion, sleep problems, drug cravings, memory deficits, and severe anxiety. In high doses it can lead to severe hypothermia by interfering with the body's temperature regulation. This can lead to organ failure and even death (National Institute on Drug Abuse, 2013a).

Data about the fetal and neonatal effects are sparse. Singer, Moore, Min, et al. (2012) followed a group of women who reported MDMA use during pregnancy and evaluated their infants at 1 year of age. They found that the amount of MDMA exposure during pregnancy predicted a dose-related delay on mental and motor development at 1 year of age. There appeared to be no effect on language, emotional regulation, or parenting stress.

HEROIN
Heroin is an illicit CNS depressant narcotic that alters perception and produces euphoria. It is an addictive drug that is generally administered intravenously (Figure 14–4). Pregnancy in women who use heroin is considered high risk because of the increased incidence in these women of poor nutrition, iron deficiency anemia, and preeclampsia. Women addicted to heroin

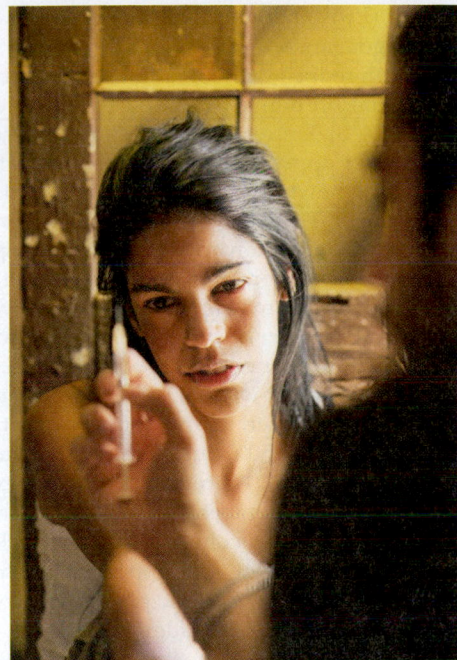

Figure 14–4 The use of illicit drugs puts the pregnant woman and her unborn child at increased risk for a variety of complications.

SOURCE: © Diego Cervo / Fotolia.

also have a higher incidence of sexually transmitted infections because many rely on prostitution to support their drug habit.

The fetus of a woman who is addicted to heroin is at increased risk for preterm birth, IUGR, meconium aspiration, and withdrawal symptoms after birth such as restlessness; shrill, high-pitched cry; irritability; fist sucking; vomiting; and seizures. Signs of withdrawal usually appear within 72 hours and may last for several days (Wang, 2014). These behaviors may interfere with successful maternal attachment and increase the risk for parenting problems or abuse in an already high-risk mother (Behnke & Smith, 2013). Buprenorphine, a partial opioid agonist, can decrease the severity of NAS in the newborn (National Institute on Drug Abuse, 2014).

Methadone is the most commonly used therapy for women who are dependent on opioids such as heroin. Methadone blocks withdrawal symptoms and reduces or eliminates the craving for narcotics. Dosage should be individualized at the lowest possible therapeutic level. Methadone does cross the placenta, and, consequently, newborns are at risk for NAS. However, various studies have demonstrated inconsistent long-term effects on the newborn (ACOG, 2012a).

Clinical Therapy

Antepartum care of the pregnant woman with substance abuse problems involves medical, socioeconomic, and legal considerations. A team approach allows for the comprehensive management necessary to provide safe labor and childbirth for the woman and her child.

The management of drug addiction may include hospitalization as necessary to initiate detoxification. "Cold turkey" withdrawal is not advisable during pregnancy because of potential risk to the fetus. Maintenance and support therapy are best individualized to the woman's history and condition. Urine screening is also done regularly throughout pregnancy if the woman has a known or suspected substance abuse problem

and should include maternal informed consent. This testing helps to identify the type and amount of drug being abused.

Nursing Management

For the Pregnant Woman With a Substance Abuse Problem

Nursing Assessment and Diagnosis

Because of the prevalence of substance abuse in society today, nurses and other care providers should screen all pregnant women for substance abuse during the health history. Several simple screening tools are available. In addition, be alert for clues in the history or appearance of the woman that suggest substance abuse (Table 14–4). If abuse is suspected, ask direct questions, beginning with less threatening questions about use of tobacco, caffeine, and over-the-counter medications. Then progress to questions about alcohol consumption and finally to questions focusing on past and current use of illicit drugs. A matter-of-fact, nonjudgmental approach is more likely to elicit honest responses.

When assessing a woman with a known substance abuse problem, focus on the woman's general health status, and pay specific attention to nutritional status, susceptibility to infections, and evaluation of all body systems. Also assess the woman's understanding of the impact of substance abuse on herself and on her pregnancy.

Nursing diagnoses that may apply to a woman at risk because of substance abuse include the following (NANDA-I © 2014):

- *Nutrition, Imbalanced: Less than Body Requirements,* related to inadequate food intake secondary to substance abuse

- *Infection, Risk for,* related to use of inadequately cleaned syringes and needles secondary to intravenous (IV) drug use

- *Health Maintenance, Ineffective,* related to a lack of information about the impact of substance abuse on the fetus

TABLE 14–4 Possible Signs of Substance Abuse

HISTORY

- History of vague or unusual medical complaints
- Family history of alcoholism or other addiction
- History of childhood physical, sexual, or emotional abuse
- History of cirrhosis, pancreatitis, hepatitis, gastritis, sexually transmitted infections, or unusual infections such as cellulitis or endocarditis
- History of high-risk sexual behavior
- Psychiatric history of treatment and/or hospitalization

PHYSICAL SIGNS

- Dilated or constricted pupils
- Inflamed nasal mucosa
- Evidence of needle "track marks" or abscesses
- Poor nutritional status
- Slurred speech or staggering gait
- Odor of alcohol on breath

BEHAVIORAL SIGNS

- Memory lapses, mood swings, hallucinations
- Pattern of frequently missed appointments
- Frequent accidents, falls
- Signs of depression, agitation, euphoria
- Suicidal gestures

Nursing Plan and Implementation

Prevention of substance abuse during pregnancy is the ideal nursing goal and is best accomplished through education. Unfortunately, many women who abuse substances do not receive regular health care and may not seek care until they are far along in pregnancy. Thus it is important to focus on ongoing assessment and client teaching.

Provide information about the relationship between substance abuse and existing health problems and the implications for the woman's unborn child. Establishing a relationship of trust and support helps ensure the woman's cooperation. If possible, discuss strategies to help the woman quit (addiction treatment programs, 12-step programs, individual counseling) and suggest a referral for more in-depth assessment by a specialist. Preparation for labor and birth should be part of prenatal planning. Fear, tension, or discomfort may be relieved through nonnarcotic psychologic support and careful explanation of the labor process. If pain medication is necessary, it should not be withheld; the notion that it will contribute to further addiction is mistaken. Preferred methods of pain relief include the use of psychoprophylaxis and regional blocks such as epidurals or local anesthetics such as pudendal block and local infiltration. Nitrous oxide is gaining increased popularity for its analgesic and antianxiety effects during labor and birth (Collins, 2015). It is an excellent alternative for women with substance abuse problems.

Immediate intensive care should be available for the newborn, who is often depressed, small for gestational age (SGA), and premature. (For care of the addicted newborn, see Chapter 26.)

Evaluation

Expected outcomes of nursing care include the following:

- The woman is able to describe the impact of her substance abuse on herself and her unborn child.

- The woman gives birth to a healthy newborn.

- The woman agrees to accept a referral to social services (or another appropriate community agency) for follow-up care after discharge.

Care of the Woman With a Psychologic Disorder

The prevalence of psychologic disorders among adults in the United States is 22.5% or almost one in four adults (Karg, Bose, Batts, et al., 2014). **Psychologic disorders** are characterized by alterations in thinking, mood, or behavior. Although many such disorders can affect labor and birth, only the most common are discussed here. Because an in-depth discussion of psychologic disorders is beyond the scope of this text, students are encouraged to consult a mental health nursing textbook for further reference. Postpartum psychologic disorders are discussed in Chapter 30.

Maternal Implications

Depression, a common disorder that affects many pregnant women, often goes undiagnosed or untreated. Estimates suggest that 9.4% to 12.7% of pregnant women will have a major depression (Shade, Miller, Borst, et al., 2011). Research findings are mixed, but women with depression may be more likely to have a preterm birth, intrauterine growth restriction (IUGR), a

low-birth-weight (LBW) newborn, or various birth complications (Staneva, Bogossian, & Wittkowski, 2015).

Depression can reduce the woman's ability to concentrate or process information being provided by healthcare team members (Figure 14–5). Untreated depression can lead to inadequate self-care, poor appetite, poor weight gain, self-medication, poor maternal–newborn/infant bonding, and maternal suicide (Daniels, 2013). The labor process may feel overwhelming to a woman with depression and she may feel hopelessness about the outcome of her labor. However, she may not be able to articulate these feelings and may appear irritable or withdrawn.

For women with *bipolar disorder (BD)*, pregnancy, birth, and the first postpartum year can be especially destabilizing. In particular, pregnant women with BD are susceptible to major depressive episodes; however, the rate of new-onset mania or psychosis may be as high as 50% during the postpartum (Battle, Weinstock, & Howard, 2014). A pregnant woman experiencing a manic episode may engage in behaviors that are dangerous to herself or her fetus including alcohol or drug use, reckless driving, driving without a seat belt, and unprotected sexual intercourse. If labor occurs during a manic phase, the woman may be hyperexcitable and exhibit poor judgment.

Anxiety disorders include a cluster of diagnoses such as panic disorder, obsessive-compulsive disorder (OCD), posttraumatic stress disorder (PTSD), general anxiety disorder, and other specific phobias. These disorders can cause a wide range of symptoms in pregnant women and laboring women. For example, women with OCD may need to repeat specific rituals as a means of coping, while women with PTSD may experience flashbacks and avoidance behaviors. Anxiety may cause the laboring woman to experience physical symptoms such as chest pain, shortness of breath, faintness, fear, or even terror. In general, laboring women with psychologic disorders tend to exhibit the behaviors characteristic of their disorder, but these behaviors may be somewhat exaggerated because of the intense emotions that are evoked in the woman's memory. Women with

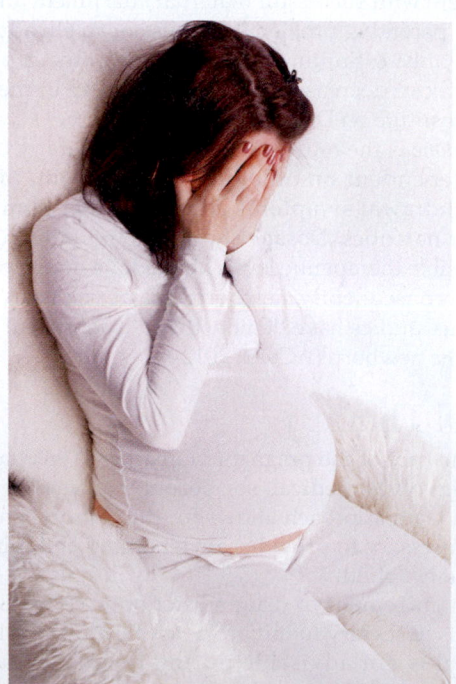

Figure 14–5 A depressed pregnant woman may be inarticulate and appear withdrawn.

SOURCE: Gladskikh Tatiana/Shutterstock.

a past history of abuse, including physical and sexual abuse, are often fearful of losing control.

Schizophrenia is the most disabling of the psychologic disorders. Women with uncontrolled schizophrenia may have difficulty managing emotions, interacting with the healthcare team, or thinking clearly. The woman's behavior may be dramatically inappropriate or she may simply be withdrawn. It is often difficult to treat schizophrenia in pregnant women because many of the medications are teratogenic and thus contraindicated. Specifically, antipsychotics can cause cardiovascular defects. These women have an increased incidence of preterm birth, low birth weight, small for gestational age newborns, placental abnormalities, and antenatal hemorrhage.

Clinical Therapy

ACOG (2015c) recommends that healthcare providers use a standardized tool to screen women for depression and anxiety at least once during pregnancy. Screening should be coupled with appropriate follow-up and treatment if indicated. The goal of clinical therapy is to provide strategies that will help decrease the woman's anxiety (as well as that of her partner), keep her oriented to reality, and promote optimal functioning during pregnancy and while in labor. Pharmacologic measures such as sedatives, analgesics, or antianxiety medications are determined on an individual basis following careful assessment.

Nursing Management

For the Pregnant Woman With a Psychologic Disorder

Use therapeutic communication and sharing of information to allay anxiety for both the woman and her support person during each prenatal visit and during labor and childbirth.

Nursing Assessment and Diagnosis

Because maternal mental illness can significantly impact pregnancy, maternal health, birth outcomes, and the child's subsequent development, healthcare providers are increasingly focused on screening for perinatal mental illness (Paschetta, Berrisford, Coccia, et al., 2014). At the first prenatal visit, begin the assessment by reviewing the woman's background. Factors such as age, marital and socioeconomic status, culture, methods of coping, support system, and understanding of the labor process contribute to the woman's psychologic response to pregnancy and birth. It is important to ask all women if they have ever been diagnosed with a psychologic disorder. If the woman has, ask her if she is currently receiving any treatment, including medications or psychotherapy. Also ask if she has ever had a psychiatric hospitalization or if she has ever had thoughts of hurting herself or others.

This same attention to detail is important when the woman goes into labor. The prenatal record should be reviewed for additional information regarding any psychiatric illnesses. During labor, assess the woman for objective cues indicating a psychologic disorder. Monotone replies and/or a flat affect may indicate depression. Women with schizophrenia may lack orientation to person, time, and place. Objective cues indicating acute anxiety or signs of a panic attack include tachycardia and hyperventilation.

As labor progresses, remain alert to the woman's verbal and nonverbal behavioral responses to the pain and anxiety. The woman who is too quiet and compliant, is disoriented, is agitated and seems uncooperative, or is experiencing acute anxiety symptoms may require further appraisal for psychologic disorders. These rare circumstances require one-on-one nursing care. A consult with a psychiatrist is often warranted.

Nursing diagnoses that may apply to the woman with a psychologic disorder include the following (NANDA-I © 2014):

- *Anxiety* related to stress of the labor process, unfamiliar environment, and unknown caregivers
- *Fear* related to unknown outcome of labor and invasive medical procedures
- *Pain, Acute,* related to increased anxiety and stress
- *Coping, Ineffective,* related to increased anxiety and stress

Nursing Plan and Implementation

The primary nursing interventions center on providing support to the pregnant woman and her partner or family. During labor, families that have had the opportunity to attend prenatal classes may benefit from encouragement as they employ some of the coping techniques they have learned (see Chapter 10). If the woman begins to lose her ability to cope or her orientation to reality, assist her in regaining control and orientation by explaining where she is, why she is there, and what is currently happening; providing reassurance; decreasing stimuli; and acknowledging her fears, concerns, and symptoms.

Your ability to help the woman and her partner cope with the stress of labor is directly related to the rapport you have established. By employing a calm, caring, confident, nonjudgmental approach, you may be able not only to acknowledge the anxiety or other emotions the woman is feeling but also to identify the source of the distress. Once the causative factors are known, implement appropriate interventions such as offering information, comfort measures, touch, or therapeutic communication. Some women with severe psychologic disorders may have excessive symptoms during their labor and birth. Although providing emotional support is imperative, care of these women should focus on maintaining a safe environment and ensuring maternal and fetal well-being. Pharmacologic interventions may be necessary for excessive symptoms. See Chapter 30 for a discussion of medications commonly used.

Evaluation

Anticipated outcomes of nursing care include the following:

- The woman experiences a decrease in physiologic and psychologic stress and an increase in physical and psychologic comfort.
- The woman remains oriented to person, time, and place.
- The woman uses effective coping mechanisms to manage her stress and anxiety in labor.
- The woman is able to verbalize feelings about her labor.
- The woman's and her family's fear is decreased.

Care of the Woman With HIV/AIDS

AIDS (acquired immunodeficiency syndrome), caused by the virus known as **HIV** (human immunodeficiency virus), is one of today's major health concerns. By the end of 2013, an estimated 1,218,400 persons ages 13 or older in the United States were living with HIV/AIDS, including 156,300 who did not know they were infected (Centers for Disease Control and Prevention [CDC], 2015a). Male adults and adolescents are the largest groups of infected individuals. Of these groups, new infections occurred as follows: male-to-male sexual contact (63%), IV drug use (8%), high-risk heterosexual contact (11%), and both male-to-male sexual contact and IV drug use (8%). Among females with HIV/AIDS, 84% were infected through high-risk heterosexual contact and 16% were infected because of IV drug use (CDC, 2015a).

Of the estimated 2,519 children under age 13 living with HIV/AIDS in the United States, 84% were exposed perinatally (CDC, 2015b). Fortunately, the incidence of new pediatric AIDS cases is declining rapidly.

Pathophysiology of HIV and AIDS

HIV-1, which causes AIDS, typically enters the body through blood, blood products, or other body fluids such as semen, vaginal fluid, and breast milk. HIV affects specific T cells, thereby decreasing the body's immune responses. This makes the affected person susceptible to opportunistic infections such as *Pneumocystis jiroveci*, which causes a severe pneumonia, candidiasis, cytomegalovirus infection, tuberculosis, and toxoplasmosis.

Once infected with the virus, the individual develops antibodies that can be detected with a reactive enzyme immunoassay (EIA) and confirmed with the Western blot test or immunofluorescence assay (IFA). A confirmed case is then categorized into one of four HIV infection stages for adults and adolescents over age 13. These stages are used for public health surveillance and not as a guide for diagnosis and therapy.

Developing Cultural Competence Variations in the Prevalence Rates of New HIV Infections

The prevalence rates per 100,000 of persons living with HIV/AIDS vary significantly among races and ethnic groups: at the end of 2012 the rates were 1,011 in the Black/African American population, 347.8 in the Hispanic/Latino population, 166.4 in the Native Hawaiian/Pacific Islander population, 124.1 in the American Indian/Alaska Native population, 149.2 in the White population, and 70.5 in the Asian population (CDC, 2015b).

The diagnosis of AIDS is made when an individual is HIV positive and is identified as having one of several specific opportunistic infections.

MATERNAL RISKS

Recent advances and the availability of antiretroviral therapy (ART) have led women who are HIV positive who adhere to their ART to consider pregnancy because of their increased life expectancy. If pregnancy is considered, priorities should focus on maintaining the health of the mother before, during, and after the pregnancy; preventing transmission to a potentially sero-negative father; and preventing mother-to-child transmission. Reproductive assisted technology is one possibility along with further interventions including cesarean birth to reduce risk of transmission to the fetus. More research is needed, however, to improve understanding of the health implications of pregnancy for women living with HIV (Loutfy, Sonnenberg-Schwan, Margolese, et al., 2013).

For women who have not had access to ART or who have not followed their plan of care, AIDS-defining symptoms that are more common in women than men include wasting syndrome, esophageal candidiasis, and herpes simplex virus disease. Kaposi sarcoma is rare in women. Non–AIDS-defining gynecologic conditions, such as vaginal *Candida* infections and cervical pathology, are prevalent among women at all stages of HIV infection.

FETAL/NEONATAL RISKS

HIV transmission can occur during pregnancy and through breast milk; however, it is believed that the majority of all infections occur during labor and birth. In the United States, the rate of transmission has dropped dramatically and is now less than 2% for pregnant women infected with HIV who receive prophylactic antiretroviral therapy, give birth by elective cesarean at 38 weeks before rupture of membranes, and avoid breastfeeding (Panel on Treatment of HIV-Infected Pregnant Women [Panel on Treatment], 2015). These decreases in transmission are dramatic and impressive.

Following birth, HIV infection in newborns should be diagnosed using HIV virologic assays as soon as possible, with initiation of antiretroviral prophylaxis immediately if the test is positive. For further discussion of the newborn who is HIV positive, see Chapter 26.

Clinical Therapy

The revised CDC HIV testing guidelines indicate that screening should be emphasized as a routine part of prenatal care while continuing to ensure that the testing of pregnant women is voluntary and informed (Panel on Treatment, 2015). Initial testing is done using enzyme-linked immunoabsorbent assay (ELISA). If the results are positive, the Western blot test is used to confirm the diagnosis. Women who test positive should be counseled about the implications of the diagnosis for themselves and their fetus to ensure an informed reproductive choice. All women who are infected with HIV and considering pregnancy should be receiving combination antiretroviral therapy (cART) and have a plasma viral load below the limit of detection. For pregnant women who have never received antiretroviral drugs, cART should be started as soon as HIV is diagnosed (Panel on Treatment, 2015).

Combination ART regimens should include a dual nucleoside reverse transcriptase inhibitor (NRTI) backbone that includes one or more NRTIs with high levels of transplacental passage such as tenofovir with lamivudine or emtricitabine. Zidovudine with lamivudine is also a preferred dual NRTI combination (Panel on Treatment, 2015).

Treatment recommendations have also been developed for the mother and newborn for the intrapartum and postpartum periods. Care of the baby is discussed in Chapter 26. The decision about which regimen is most appropriate should be determined following discussion with the woman about the risks and benefits based on her individual HIV status.

Women with HIV infection should be evaluated and treated for other sexually transmitted infections and for conditions occurring more commonly in women with HIV, such as tuberculosis, cytomegalovirus infection, toxoplasmosis, and cervical dysplasia. Women with HIV infection but no history of hepatitis B should receive the hepatitis vaccine, which is not contraindicated prenatally, as well as the pneumococcal vaccine and an annual flu shot. In addition to routine prenatal laboratory tests, a platelet count and a complete blood count with differential should be obtained at the first prenatal visit and repeated each trimester to identify anemia, thrombocytopenia, and leukopenia, which are associated both with HIV infection and with antiviral therapy.

The woman with HIV also should be assessed regularly for serologic changes that indicate the disease is progressing. This is determined by the absolute CD4+ T-lymphocyte count, which provides the number of helper T4 cells. When CD4+ counts fall to 200/mm^3 or lower, opportunistic infections such as *Pneumocystis jiroveci* pneumonia are more likely to develop, and prophylaxis may need to be instituted (Panel on Treatment, 2015).

At each prenatal visit, women with asymptomatic HIV infection are monitored for early signs of complications, such as weight loss in the second or third trimester or fever. The woman is asked about signs of vaginal infection. Her mouth is inspected for signs of infections such as thrush (candidiasis) or hairy leukoplakia; her lungs are auscultated for signs of pneumonia; and her lymph nodes, liver, and spleen are palpated for signs of enlargement. Each trimester the woman should have a visual examination and a funduscopic examination to detect such complications as toxoplasmosis retinitis. Further discussion of therapy for the pregnant woman who is HIV positive or who has AIDS may be found in journal articles and specialty texts.

A pregnancy complicated by HIV infection, even if asymptomatic, is considered high risk, and the fetus is monitored closely. Weekly non-stress testing (NST) is begun at 32 weeks' gestation, and serial ultrasounds are done to detect intrauterine growth restriction. Biophysical profiles are also indicated (see Chapter 13). Invasive procedures such as amniocentesis are avoided when possible to prevent the contamination of a noninfected fetus.

Scheduled cesarean birth at 38 weeks' gestation is indicated for women with HIV RNA levels greater than 1000 copies/ml and for women with unknown HIV RNA levels near the time of birth whether they are on antiretroviral therapy (ART) or not. If the indication for cesarean birth is prevention of perinatal transmission of HIV, the risks to a woman should be balanced with potential benefits expected for the neonate (Panel on Treatment of HIV-Infected Women, 2015).

Women who are HIV positive are at increased risk for complications such as intrapartum or postpartum hemorrhage, postpartum infection, poor wound healing, and infections of the genitourinary tract. Thus they need careful monitoring and appropriate therapy as indicated. To prevent exposure of an uninfected neonate to HIV during labor and birth, invasive procedures such as vaginal examinations following rupture of the membranes, fetal scalp electrode monitoring, fetal scalp sampling, and vacuum extraction should be done only after carefully evaluating the risks and benefits. Following childbirth, the woman who is HIV positive should be referred to a physician knowledgeable about treating individuals with HIV infection.

Nursing Management

For the Pregnant Woman Who Is HIV Positive

Nursing Assessment and Diagnosis

A woman who tests positive for HIV may be asymptomatic or may present with any of the following signs or symptoms: fatigue, anemia, malaise, progressive weight loss, lymphadenopathy, diarrhea, fever, neurologic dysfunction, cell-mediated immunodeficiency, or evidence of Kaposi sarcoma (purplish, reddish brown lesions either externally or internally).

If a woman tests positive for HIV or is involved in a relationship that places her at high risk, assess the woman's knowledge level about the disease, its implications for her and her fetus, and self-care measures the woman can take.

Examples of nursing diagnoses that might apply for a pregnant woman who tests positive for HIV include the following (NANDA-I © 2014):

- *Health Maintenance, Ineffective,* related to lack of information about HIV/AIDS and its long-term implications for the woman, her unborn child, and her family
- *Infection, Risk for,* related to altered immunity secondary to HIV infection
- *Family Processes, Interrupted,* related to the implications of a positive HIV test in one of the family members

Nursing Plan and Implementation

COMMUNITY-BASED NURSING CARE

Women need to understand that HIV/AIDS is a fatal disease. HIV infection can be avoided if women practice safe sex, including insisting that their partners wear a latex condom for each act of intercourse and avoid sharing IV drug needles. Women at high risk for HIV/AIDS should be offered premarital and prepregnancy screening for HIV antibodies.

In monitoring the asymptomatic pregnant woman who is HIV positive, be alert for nonspecific symptoms such as fever, weight loss, fatigue, persistent candidiasis, diarrhea, cough, skin lesions, and behavior changes. These may be signs of developing symptomatic HIV infection. Laboratory findings such as increased viral load, decreased hemoglobin, hematocrit, and CD4+ T lymphocytes; elevated erythrocyte sedimentation rate (ESR); and abnormal complete blood count, differential, and platelets may indicate complications such as infection or progression of the disease.

Education about optimal nutrition and maintenance of wellness is important, and the information should be reviewed frequently with the woman. *Nursing Care Plan: For the Pregnant Woman with HIV Infection* summarizes essential nursing management. Also see *Key Facts to Remember: Caring for a Pregnant Woman with HIV Infection.*

HOSPITAL-BASED NURSING CARE

Protocols have been established for postexposure treatment of a healthcare worker who experiences a needlestick or exposure to the body fluids of a person with positive or unknown HIV status. The effectiveness of the therapy, usually a combined drug approach, depends on starting rapidly. Thus such exposure should be reported immediately. See *Health Promotion: The Pregnant Woman With HIV Infection.*

SAFETY ALERT!

In 1987, the CDC stated that the increasing prevalence of HIV/AIDS and the risk of exposure faced by healthcare workers is significant enough that precautions should be taken with all clients (not only those with known HIV infection), especially in dealing with blood and body fluids. These precautions are called *standard precautions.*

Health Promotion
The Pregnant Woman With HIV Infection

The psychologic implications of HIV/AIDS for the child-bearing family are staggering.

- The woman is faced with the knowledge that she and her newborn, if infected, have a decreased life expectancy. If her baby is not infected, she must face the possibility that others will raise her child. She must also face the reality that she can hope only to lengthen her life by carefully following an expensive, exacting medical regimen.

- The couple must deal with the impact of the illness on the partner, who may or may not be infected, and on other children. The woman and her family may feel fearful, helpless, angry, and isolated.

- It is essential to provide complete, accurate information about the condition, transmission prevention, and ways of coping using language that is well understood by the woman and her partner.

- Ensure that the woman is referred to a comprehensive program that includes social services, psychologic support, and appropriate health care.

Evaluation

Expected outcomes of nursing care include the following:

- The woman discusses the implications of her HIV infection (or diagnosis of AIDS), its implications for her unborn child and for herself, the method of transmission, and the treatment options.

- The woman uses information about social services (or other agency referral) for follow-up assistance and counseling.

- The woman begins to verbalize her feelings about her condition and its implications for her and her family.

KEY FACTS TO REMEMBER
Caring for a Pregnant Woman With HIV Infection

- Following initial infection, antibodies usually become detectable within about 6 to 12 weeks, but it may take 6 months or longer. Despite this, the woman is infected, and infectious.

- HIV infection is spread primarily through sexual contact, through exposure to contaminated blood, and (perinatally) from infected mother to child.

- Many women who are HIV positive are asymptomatic and may be unaware they have the infection. Standard precautions are indicated in caring for all pregnant women.

- A pregnant woman found to be HIV positive should receive prenatal counseling about the possible implications of HIV for the fetus so that she can make an informed choice about continuing her pregnancy. Her choice should be supported.

- During pregnancy, caregivers should be alert to nonspecific symptoms such as weight loss and fatigue, which may indicate progression of HIV disease.

- The incidence of vertical transmission of HIV infection from mother to baby has decreased significantly because of the administration of cART to the mother prenatally and during labor and to the newborn for a specified period following birth.

- Invasive procedures during the intrapartum period increase the risk of exposure to HIV for the fetus (who may be uninfected) and should be undertaken only after carefully weighing the advantages and risks.

- The cardinal rule in caring for pregnant women, and indeed for any client, is: If it's wet and it's not yours, use protection when handling it.

Nursing Care Plan: For the Pregnant Woman With HIV Infection

1. Nursing Diagnosis: *Infection, Risk for,* related to inadequate defenses (leukopenia, suppressed inflammatory response) secondary to HIV-positive status (NANDA-I © 2014)

GOAL: Client will remain free of opportunistic infection during the course of pregnancy.

INTERVENTION	RATIONALE
• Obtain a complete health history and physical examination during first prenatal visit.	• A complete health history will help determine risk factors for the development of opportunistic infections, and a physical examination will assist in identifying any underlying problem symptoms or illnesses that may compromise the pregnancy or complicate the treatment of HIV.
• Educate the woman as to the signs and symptoms of infection.	• Early recognition of signs and symptoms of infection will allow for immediate treatment, which may decrease the severity of the infection. Signs and symptoms of infections include fever, weight loss, fatigue, persistent candidiasis, diarrhea, cough, and skin lesions (Kaposi sarcoma and hairy leukoplakia in the mouth).
• Obtain nutritional history and monitor weight gain at each prenatal visit.	• The HIV-infected woman needs to maintain optimal nutritional intake. A compromised nutritional status may affect maternal and fetal well-being. Depleted reserves of protein and iron may decrease the client's ability to fight infection, thereby making her more susceptible to opportunistic infections.

- **Collaborative:** Monitor the absolute CD4$^+$ T-lymphocyte count, erythrocyte sedimentation rate (ESR), complete blood count (CBC) with differential, and hemoglobin and hematocrit (H&H) at each prenatal visit.

- Laboratory results provide information about the woman's immune system and the potential for disease progression. Opportunistic infections are more likely to occur when the CD4$^+$ T-lymphocyte count drops below a level of 200/mm^3. ESR can rise above 20 mm/hr with anemia and with acute and chronic inflammation. CBC with differential and platelet count helps identify anemia, thrombocytopenia, and leukopenia. H&H can also identify anemia.

EXPECTED OUTCOME: Client will remain free of opportunistic infection as evidenced by CD4$^+$ T-lymphocyte count within normal limits; no complaints of chills, fever, or sore throat; normal weight gain throughout pregnancy.

---

2. **Nursing Diagnosis:** *Health Maintenance, Ineffective,* related to a lack of information about HIV/AIDS and its long-term implications for the woman, her unborn child, and her family (NANDA-I © 2014)

GOAL: The client and her family will verbalize the importance of following her medication regimen and of regular prenatal care.

INTERVENTION	RATIONALE
• Assess the client's and family's level of understanding of HIV infection, its modes of transmission, and the long-term implications.	• Knowledge of the woman's (and her family's) level of understanding about her HIV infection forms a starting point for further health teaching.
• Explain the risks of mother-to-child transmission of HIV infection.	• In untreated women the risk of transmission is 25%. That risk can be reduced to less than 2% with the availability of antiretroviral therapy, the use of cesarean birth when indicated, and formula-feeding rather than breastfeeding.
• Describe combination antiretroviral therapy (cART). Include the regimen prescribed, its purposes, and the procedures for taking it.	• Combination ART therapy approaches vary based on the health status of the individual woman and whether she is currently on cART therapy. Generally it includes oral Zidovudine (ZDV) daily, IV ZDV during labor and until birth, and ZDV therapy for the baby for 6 weeks following birth.
• Discuss signs the woman should be alert for, including fever, fatigue, weight loss, cough, skin lesions, and behavior changes.	• These symptoms may indicate that the woman is developing symptomatic loss, persistent candidiasis, diarrhea, HIV infection.

EXPECTED OUTCOME: Woman will actively seek information about her condition, her treatment regimen, and her pregnancy and will cooperate with her healthcare givers.

---

3. **Nursing Diagnosis:** *Family Processes, Dysfunctional,* related to the implications of positive maternal HIV status on fetal/neonatal well-being and long-term family functioning (NANDA-I © 2014)

GOAL: Family is able to manage stressors related to the maternal diagnosis.

INTERVENTION	RATIONALE
• Assess ability and readiness of family to learn about HIV and its long-term implications.	• Readiness is a key element in the teaching–learning process.
• Provide woman and her family with accurate, reliable information about her diagnosis, its prognosis for her and for her baby, and the immediate and long-term implications for her care.	• Fear and anxiety will lessen when the woman and her family understand her health status and the implications of the HIV diagnosis and can then plan for the future.
• Assess interactions between the woman and her family. Be alert for potentially destructive behaviors.	• If the HIV diagnosis was not expected, the couple may have to deal with issues of blame, concerns about mortality, and worries about the status of the baby. If the HIV diagnosis was known, concerns may focus on fetal/neonatal well-being. In either case, negative responses can lead to destructive behaviors.
• Assist family in realistically identifying the needs of the woman and the family unit.	• Once needs are identified realistically, it is possible to plan interventions to meet the needs.
• **Collaborative:** Explore available community resources and family support systems.	• Because HIV is a long-term condition, the family may require ongoing assistance.

EXPECTED OUTCOME: Family members actively participate in the treatment plan, are involved in planning for labor and birth in light of a positive HIV status, and are able to express unresolved feelings about the diagnosis.

Care of the Woman With Heart Disease

Pregnancy results in increased cardiac output, heart rate, and blood volume. The normal heart is able to adapt to these changes without undue difficulty. The woman with heart disease, however, has decreased cardiac reserve, making it more difficult for her heart to accommodate the higher workload of pregnancy.

Currently cardiac disease complicates about 1% of pregnancies (Cunningham et al., 2014). The pathology found in a pregnant woman with heart disease varies with the type of disorder. The more common conditions are discussed briefly here.

CONGENITAL HEART DEFECTS

Congenital heart defects have become more common in pregnant women as improved surgical techniques enable females born with heart defects to live to childbearing age. Congenital heart defects most commonly seen in pregnant women include atrial septal defect, ventricular septal defect, patent ductus arteriosus, coarctation of the aorta, and tetralogy of Fallot.

For women with congenital heart disease, the implications of pregnancy depend on the specific defect. If the heart defect has been surgically repaired and no evidence of organic heart disease remains, pregnancy may be undertaken with confidence. Women with chronic cyanosis are at increased risk for complications and so are their fetuses. A few conditions carry such great risk of complications and death that they can be considered absolute contraindications. These include, for example, Eisenmenger syndrome, pulmonary hypertension, uncorrected coarctation of the aorta, severe symptomatic aortic stenosis, and Marfan syndrome in certain instances (Harris, 2011).

RHEUMATIC HEART DISEASE

Rheumatic heart disease has declined rapidly in the past half century, primarily because of the availability of antibiotics for treatment. Rheumatic heart disease, which may develop in untreated group A β-hemolytic streptococcal infections, is an inflammatory connective tissue disease that can involve the heart, joints, central nervous system, skin, and subcutaneous tissue. When the heart is affected, mitral valve stenosis is the most common and serious lesion. Aortic valve involvement, manifested by aortic insufficiency, is the second most common problem. The tricuspid and pulmonic valves are rarely affected.

The increased blood volume of pregnancy, coupled with the pregnant woman's need for increased cardiac output, stresses the heart of a woman with mitral stenosis and increases her risk of developing congestive heart failure. Even the woman who has no symptoms at the onset of her pregnancy is at risk.

MITRAL VALVE PROLAPSE

Mitral valve prolapse (MVP) is a usually asymptomatic condition commonly found in women of childbearing age. The condition is more common in women than in men and seems to run in families. In MVP, the mitral valve leaflets tend to prolapse into the left atrium during ventricular systole because the chordae tendineae that support them are long, stretched, and thin. This produces a characteristic systolic click on auscultation. In more pronounced cases of MVP, mitral valve regurgitation occurs, producing a systolic murmur.

Women with MVP usually tolerate pregnancy well. Most women require assurance that they can continue with normal activities. A few women experience symptoms—primarily palpitations, chest pain, and dyspnea—which are often caused by arrhythmias. They are usually treated with propranolol hydrochloride (Inderal). Limiting caffeine intake also helps decrease palpitations.

PERIPARTUM CARDIOMYOPATHY

Peripartum cardiomyopathy is a relatively rare but serious dysfunction of the left ventricle that occurs in the last month of pregnancy or the first 5 months postpartum in a woman with no previous history of heart disease. The cause is unknown but mortality is increased with maternal age, in women who have had four or more live births, and in women of African descent (Elkayam, Jalnapurkar, & Barakat, 2012). The symptoms are similar to those of congestive heart failure: dyspnea, orthopnea, fatigue, cough, chest pain, palpitations, and edema. The condition usually presents with anemia and infection; consequently, treatment focuses on underlying abnormalities. Digitalis, diuretics, vasodilators, anticoagulants, sodium restriction, and strict bed rest are often part of the treatment. In over half of women, heart function returns to normal within 2 to 6 months with bed rest and careful monitoring (Elkayam et al., 2012). Subsequent pregnancy is strongly discouraged because the disease tends to recur during pregnancy.

Clinical Therapy

The primary goal of clinical therapy is early diagnosis and ongoing management of the woman with cardiac disease. Echocardiogram, chest X-ray, auscultation of heart sounds, and sometimes cardiac catheterization are essential for establishing the type and severity of the heart disease. The severity of the disease can also be determined by the individual's ability to perform ordinary physical activity. Table 14–5 outlines the functional capacity that has been standardized by the Criteria Committee of the New York Heart Association (1994).

TABLE 14–5 Severity of Heart Disease by Functional Capacity

CLASS	FUNCTIONAL CAPACITY
I	Asymptomatic. No limitation of physical activity.
II	Slight limitation of physical activity. Asymptomatic at rest; symptoms occur with ordinary physical activity.
III	Marked limitation of physical activity. Comfortable at rest but symptomatic during less-than-ordinary physical activity.
IV	Inability to carry on any physical activity without discomfort. Even at rest the person experiences symptoms of cardiac insufficiency or anginal pain; discomfort increases with any physical activity.

Women in classes I and II usually experience a normal pregnancy and have few complications, whereas those in classes III and IV are at risk for more severe complications. Because anemia increases the work of the heart, it should be diagnosed early and treated if present. Infections, even if minor, also increase cardiac workload and should be treated. As pregnancy progresses, the woman's activity should be limited to minimize cardiac workload. Similarly, weight gain and sodium intake may also be restricted.

DRUG THERAPY

Besides the iron and vitamin supplements prescribed during pregnancy, the pregnant woman with heart disease may need additional drug therapy to maintain health. Antibiotic prophylaxis is not indicated for uncomplicated vaginal or cesarean birth unless infection is suspected. If the woman develops coagulation problems, the anticoagulant heparin may be used. Heparin offers the greatest safety to the fetus because it does not cross the placenta (Fryearson & Adamson, 2014). The thiazide diuretics and furosemide (Lasix) may be used to treat congestive heart failure if it develops. Digitalis glycosides and common antiarrhythmic drugs may be used to treat cardiac failure and arrhythmias. These agents cross the placenta but have no reported teratogenic effect. However, they have not been adequately studied to establish their safety in pregnancy (Wilson, Shannon, & Shields, 2014).

LABOR AND BIRTH

Spontaneous natural labor with adequate pain relief is usually recommended for women in classes I and II. Special attention should be given to the prompt recognition and treatment of any signs of heart failure (Figure 14–6). Those in classes III and IV may have labor induced and may need to be hospitalized before

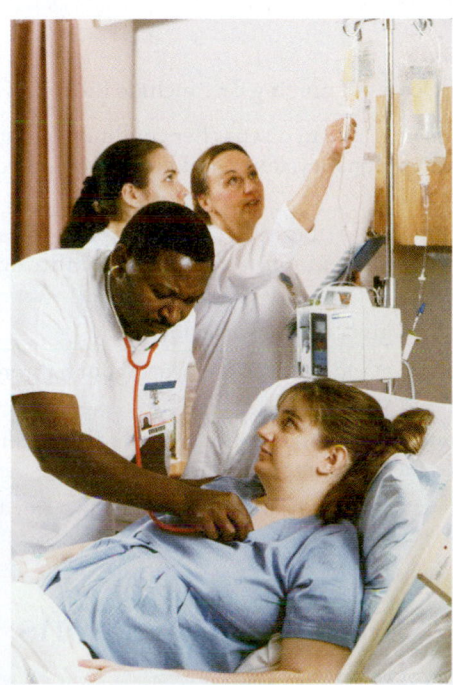

Figure 14–6 **When a woman with heart disease begins labor, the nursing students and instructor caring for her monitor her closely for signs of congestive heart failure.**

the onset of labor for cardiac stabilization. They also require invasive cardiac monitoring during labor.

Vaginal birth with low-dose regional analgesia (epidural) is recommended with the use of forceps or vacuum assistance if necessary to limit maternal pushing. The regional analgesia helps decrease maternal cardiac output and oxygen demand by reducing pain and related maternal anxiety. Cesarean birth is usually used only if fetal or maternal indications exist, not on the basis of heart disease alone.

Nursing Management

For the Pregnant Woman With Heart Disease

Nursing Assessment and Diagnosis

Assess the stress of pregnancy on the functional capacity of the heart during every antepartum visit. Note the category of functional capacity assigned to the woman; take the woman's pulse, respirations, and blood pressure; and compare the findings with the normal values expected during pregnancy. Then determine the woman's activity level, including rest, and any changes in the pulse and respirations that have occurred since previous visits. Also identify and evaluate other factors that would increase strain on the heart. These factors might include anemia, infection, anxiety, lack of a support system, and household and career demands.

The following signs and symptoms, if they are progressive, are indicative of congestive heart failure:

- Cough (frequent, with or without blood-stained sputum [hemoptysis])
- Dyspnea (progressive, on exertion)
- Edema (progressive, generalized, including extremities, face, eyelids)
- Heart murmurs (heard on auscultation)
- Palpitations
- Rales (auscultated in lung bases)
- Weight gain (related to fluid retention)

Progressiveness of the cycle is the critical factor because some of these same behaviors are seen to a minor degree in a pregnancy without cardiac problems.

Nursing diagnoses that might apply to the pregnant woman with heart disease include the following (NANDA-I © 2014):

- *Cardiac Output, Decreased,* resulting in easy fatigability
- *Gas Exchange, Impaired,* related to pulmonary edema secondary to cardiac decompensation
- *Fear* related to the effects of the maternal cardiac condition on fetal well-being

Nursing Plan and Implementation

Nursing care is directed toward maintaining a balance between cardiac reserve and cardiac workload.

ANTEPARTUM NURSING CARE

The priority of nursing action varies based on the severity of the disease process and the individual needs of the woman determined by the nursing assessment.

The woman and her family should thoroughly understand her condition and its management and should recognize signs of potential complications; this level of understanding will decrease anxiety. Giving thorough explanations using printed material and providing frequent opportunities to ask questions and discuss concerns lets the woman better meet her own healthcare needs and seek assistance appropriately.

As part of health teaching, explain the purposes of the dietary and activity changes that are required. A diet is instituted that is high in iron, protein, and essential nutrients but low in sodium, with adequate calories to ensure normal weight gain. Such a diet best meets the nutrition needs of the client with cardiac disease. To help preserve her cardiac reserves, the woman may need to restrict her activities. In addition, 8 to 10 hours of sleep, with frequent daily rest periods, are essential. Because upper respiratory infections may tax the heart and lead to decompensation, the woman must avoid contact with sources of infection.

During the first half of pregnancy, the woman is seen approximately every 2 weeks to assess cardiac status. During the second half of pregnancy, the woman is seen weekly. These assessments are especially important between weeks 28 and 30, when the blood volume reaches its maximum. If symptoms of cardiac decompensation occur, prompt medical intervention is indicated to correct the cardiac problem.

INTRAPARTUM PERIOD

Labor and birth exert tremendous stress on the woman and her fetus. This stress could be fatal to the fetus of a woman with cardiac disease because the fetus may be receiving a decreased oxygen and blood supply. Thus the intrapartum care of a woman with cardiac disease is aimed at reducing physical exertion and the accompanying fatigue.

Evaluate maternal vital signs frequently to determine the woman's response to labor. A pulse rate greater than 100 beats per minute or respirations greater than 24 per minute may indicate the onset of cardiac decompensation and require further evaluation. Auscultate the woman's lungs frequently for evidence of rales and carefully observe for other signs that she is developing congestive heart failure.

To ensure cardiac emptying and adequate oxygenation, encourage the laboring woman to assume either a semi-Fowler or side-lying position, with her head and shoulders elevated. Oxygen by mask, diuretics to reduce fluid retention, sedatives and analgesics, prophylactic antibiotics, and digitalis may also be used as indicated by the woman's status.

Remain with the woman to support her. It is essential to keep the woman and her family informed of labor progress and management plans, collaborating with them to fulfill their wishes for the birth experience as much as possible. Maintain an atmosphere of calm to lessen the anxiety of the woman and her family.

Continuous electronic fetal monitoring is used to provide ongoing assessment of the fetal response to labor. To prevent overexertion and the accompanying fatigue, encourage the woman to sleep and relax between contractions and provide her with emotional support and encouragement. Epidural anesthesia is often used to decrease exertion. During pushing, encourage the woman to use shorter, more moderate pushing, with complete relaxation between pushes (see Chapter 18). Forceps or vacuum extraction may be used if pushing is too difficult. Monitor vital signs closely during the second stage.

POSTPARTUM PERIOD

The postpartum period is a significant time for the woman with cardiac disease. As extravascular fluid returns to the bloodstream for excretion, cardiac output and blood volume increase. This physiologic adaptation places great strain on the heart and may lead to decompensation, especially in the first 48 hours after birth.

So that the health team can detect any possible problems, the woman may remain in the hospital longer postpartum than the low-risk woman. Her vital signs are monitored frequently, and she is assessed for signs of decompensation. She stays in the semi-Fowler or side-lying position, with her head and shoulders elevated, and begins a gradual, progressive activity program. Appropriate diet and stool softeners facilitate bowel movement without undue strain.

As the postpartum nurse, give the woman opportunities to discuss her birth experience and help her deal with any feelings or concerns that distress her. Also encourage maternal–newborn attachment by providing frequent opportunities for the mother to interact with her baby.

No evidence exists that breastfeeding compromises cardiac output. Thus the only concern about breastfeeding for women with cardiovascular disease is related to medications the mother may be taking. These should be evaluated for the likelihood of passing into the milk or affecting lactation. Assist the breastfeeding mother to a comfortable side-lying position, with her head moderately elevated, or to a semi-Fowler position. To conserve the mother's energy, position the newborn at the breast and be available to burp the baby and reposition him or her at the other breast. Encourage family members to assist the mother in this way.

In addition to providing the normal postpartum discharge teaching, ensure that the woman and her family understand the signs of possible problems from her heart disease or other postpartum complications. Plan an activity schedule with the woman and her family. Visiting nurse referrals may be necessary, depending on the woman's health status.

Evaluation

Expected outcomes of nursing care include the following:

- The woman is able to discuss her condition and its possible impact on pregnancy, labor and birth, and the postpartum period.
- The woman participates in developing an appropriate healthcare regimen and follows it throughout her pregnancy.
- The woman gives birth to a healthy baby.
- The woman avoids congestive heart failure, thromboembolism, and infection.
- The woman is able to identify signs and symptoms of possible postpartum complications.
- The woman is able to care effectively for her newborn.

Other Medical Conditions and Pregnancy

A woman with a pre-existing medical condition needs to be aware of the possible impact of pregnancy on her condition, as well as the impact of her condition on the successful outcome of her pregnancy. Table 14–6 discusses some of the less common medical conditions in relation to pregnancy.

TABLE 14–6 Less Common Medical Conditions and Pregnancy

BRIEF DESCRIPTION	MATERNAL IMPLICATIONS	FETAL/NEONATAL IMPLICATIONS
ASTHMA		
Asthma, an obstructive lung condition, is the most common respiratory disease found in pregnancy, complicating approximately 8% of all pregnancies (Cossette, Forget, & Beauchesne, 2013). Typical symptoms include wheezing, dyspnea, and episodic coughing. A severe asthmatic attack may require hospitalization. It is managed by long-term comprehensive drug therapy to prevent airway inflammation, combined with drug treatment to manage attacks or exacerbations. Client education focuses on triggers (such as cold air, dust, smoke, exercise, food additives), methods of prevention, and treatment options.	The severity of asthma may improve, worsen, or remain unchanged during pregnancy. The mechanisms associated with these variations remain undefined; however, poor asthma control is associated with increased maternal and neonatal complications, most likely from poor adherence to the treatment regime. Maternal complications include preeclampsia, growth restriction, and preterm birth. Asthma management during labor and birth focuses on maintenance of adequate hydration and analgesia as well as continuing asthma medications.	Prematurity and low birth weights are more common among the newborns of women who have asthma (Whitty & Dombrowski, 2012). The goal of therapy is to prevent maternal exacerbations because even a mild exacerbation can cause severe hypoxia-related complications in the fetus. If an exacerbation occurs, it should be managed in the same way as for a nonpregnant woman because the asthma drugs used are less of a threat to the fetus than a serious asthma attack (Martin & Graham, 2015).
EPILEPSY		
Chronic disorder characterized by seizures; may be idiopathic or secondary to other conditions, such as head injury, metabolic and nutritional disorders such as phenylketonuria (PKU) or vitamin B_6 deficiency, encephalitis, neoplasms, or circulatory interferences. Treated with anticonvulsants.	The vast majority of pregnancies in women with seizure disorders are uneventful and have an excellent outcome. Women with more frequent seizures before pregnancy may have exacerbations during pregnancy, but this may be related to lack of cooperation with drug regimen or sleep deprivation. During pregnancy the woman should continue to be treated with the medication that best controls her seizures. Folic acid therapy should be started prior to conception if possible. Folic acid and vitamin D are indicated throughout pregnancy (Kamyar & Varner, 2013).	Certain anticonvulsant medications are associated with increased incidence of congenital anomalies, especially cleft lip and heart defects, although the incidence has decreased in recent years. The lowest dose of a single effective medication is the goal of treatment to decrease the potential for fetal anomalies (Wheeler & Burd, 2015). Multiple medications and valproic acid should also be avoided for women planning pregnancy when possible.
HEPATITIS B		
Hepatitis B, caused by the hepatitis B virus (HBV), is a major, growing health problem. Groups at risk include those from areas with a high incidence (primarily developing countries), illegal IV drug users, prostitutes, homosexuals, those with multiple sex partners, or occupational exposure to blood, although many infected people have no identifiable source of infection. HBV transmission is bloodborne, primarily sexually and perinatally transmitted. Because of the dramatic increase and the difficulty of vaccinating high-risk individuals before they become infected, the CDC now recommends (1) testing all pregnant women for the presence of hepatitis B surface antigen (HBsAg) and prophylactic treatment for all babies born to women who are HBsAg positive or whose status is unknown; (2) routine newborn/infant vaccination; (3) vaccination of children and adolescents through age 18 years who have not been vaccinated; and (4) vaccination of unvaccinated adults who are at risk for hepatitis B (Schillie & Murphy, 2013).	In the United States estimates suggest 1% to 2% of the population has chronic hepatitis B (Apuzzio et al., 2012a). Hepatitis B does not usually affect the course of pregnancy. However, chronic HBV carriers have a great potential for infecting others when exposure to blood and body fluids occurs. It is now recommended that all pregnant women be screened for HBV at the first prenatal visit. A woman who is negative may be given the hepatitis vaccine. Women in labor whose HBV status is unknown and who are at increased risk for STIs should be rescreened (King, Brucker, Kriebs, et al., 2015).	Perinatal transmission most often occurs at or near the time of childbirth. Women who are positive for hepatitis B surface antigen (HBsAG) have almost a 100% chance of transmitting HBV to their newborn at birth (Apuzzio et al., 2012a). More important, the risk of becoming a chronic carrier of the HBV is inversely related to the age of the individual at the time of initial infection. Therefore neonates infected perinatally have the highest risk of becoming chronically infected if not treated. Routine vaccination of all neonates born to HBsAg-negative women is indicated. Babies born to HBsAg-positive mothers should receive hepatitis B immune globulin at birth or at least within the first 12 hours and should also receive the hepatitis B vaccine (Apuzzio et al., 2012b). Within 12 hours of birth, neonates born to HIV-positive women with HBV infection should be given hepatitis B immune globulin and the first dose of the HBV vaccine series. The second and third doses of vaccine should then be administered at ages 1 and 6 months, respectively (Panel on Treatment of HIV-Infected Pregnant Women, 2015).

(continued)

TABLE 14–6 Less Common Medical Conditions and Pregnancy (*continued*)

BRIEF DESCRIPTION	MATERNAL IMPLICATIONS	FETAL/NEONATAL IMPLICATIONS
HYPERTHYROIDISM (THYROTOXICOSIS)		
Hyperthyroidism is characterized by an enlarged, overactive thyroid gland, decreased TSH level, and increased free T_4 level (ACOG, 2015d). Symptoms include muscle weight loss, tremors, tachycardia, excessive sweating, insomnia, palpitations, hypertension, and exophthalmos. Treatment by antithyroid drug propylthiouracil (PTU) in the first trimester followed by a switch to methimazole in the second trimester while monitoring free T_4 levels because methimazole has been associated with some rare birth defects and propylthiouracil is toxic to the liver (ACOG, 2015d). Surgery used only if drug intolerance exists.	Mild hyperthyroidism is not dangerous. The incidence of severe preeclampsia and maternal heart failure increases if disease is not well controlled (ACOG, 2015d). Serious risk related to thyroid storm characterized by high fever, tachycardia, sweating, and congestive heart failure. Now occurs rarely. When diagnosed during pregnancy, may be transient or permanent.	Neonatal thyrotoxicosis is rare. Even low doses of antithyroid drug in mother may produce a mild fetal/neonatal hypothyroidism; higher dose may produce a goiter or mental deficiencies. Fetal loss not increased in euthyroid women. If untreated, rates of abortion, intrauterine death, and stillbirth increase. Breastfeeding contraindicated for women on antithyroid medication because it is excreted in the milk (may be tried by woman on low dose if neonatal T_4 levels are monitored).
HYPOTHYROIDISM		
Characterized by inadequate thyroid secretions, elevated TSH, decreased free T_4, lowered BMR, and enlarged thyroid gland (goiter). Other symptoms include fatigue, constipation, excessive weight gain, dry skin, hair loss, and cold intolerance. Iodine deficiency is the most common cause worldwide (Johnson & Milio, 2015). Hashimoto thyroiditis is the most common cause in the United States (King et al., 2015). Treated by thyroxine replacement therapy.	Long-term replacement therapy continues; often pregnant women need an increase in their thyroxine dose (Johnson & Milio, 2015). Serial ultrasounds are done to monitor fetal growth; non-stress tests are not necessary in well-controlled disease but are considered beginning at 32 to 34 weeks' gestation in cases of poorly controlled disease (Abel, 2011).	If mother is untreated, there is an increased risk of spontaneous abortion, preeclampsia, abruptio placentae, and fetal loss. Offspring are at increased risk of impaired neuropsychologic development although the incidence is low (ACOG, 2015d). Therefore newborns are screened for T_4 level. Mild TSH elevations present little risk because TSH does not cross the placenta.
MATERNAL PHENYLKETONURIA (PKU) (HYPERPHENYLALANINEMIA)		
Inherited recessive single gene anomaly causing a deficiency of the liver enzyme needed to convert the amino acid phenylalanine to tyrosine, resulting in high serum levels of phenylalanine. Brain damage and intellectual disability occur if not treated early. In the United States the incidence is approximately 1 in 15,000 births (ACOG, 2015a)	Lifelong diet therapy with a low phenylalanine diet improves the woman's quality of life and is essential for successful management. Women with PKU should achieve phenylalanine (Phe) levels less than 6 mg/dL for at least 3 months before conceiving and should maintain Phe levels at 2–6 mg/dL during pregnancy (ACOG, 2015a). The woman should be counseled that her children will either inherit the disease or be carriers, depending on the zygosity of the father for the disease. Treatment at a PKU center is recommended.	Risk to fetus if maternal treatment not begun preconception. In untreated women increased incidence of fetal intellectual disability, microcephaly, congenital heart defects, and growth retardation (ACOG, 2015a). Fetal phenylalanine levels are approximately 50% higher than maternal levels because Phe crosses the placenta by an active transport process. Breastfeeding is safe as long as the newborn does not have PKU. Neonates diagnosed with PKU should begin treatment within the first week of life (ACOG, 2015a).
MULTIPLE SCLEROSIS (MS)		
Neurologic disorder characterized by destruction of the myelin sheath of nerve fibers. The condition occurs primarily in young adults, more commonly in females, and is marked by periods of remission; progresses to marked physical disability in 10 to 20 years. Women who seek to become pregnant are generally advised to discontinue their disease-modifying medications for 1 to 3 months before conceiving, depending on the medication. Women are also advised not to take medication during pregnancy because of possible teratogenic effects (Coyle, 2014).	MS disease activity is reduced during the second and third trimester but increased during the 3 months following birth. Overall, disease progression is not increased by pregnancy (King et al., 2015). Rest is important; help with child care should be planned. Uterine contraction strength is not diminished, but because sensation is frequently lessened, labor may be almost painless.	MS itself should not influence method of birth. That is determined by the status of the mother and her fetus. Risk of genetic predisposition estimated at 2% to 2.5% (Coyle, 2014). Reproductive counseling is recommended for all couples when one partner has MS.

BRIEF DESCRIPTION	MATERNAL IMPLICATIONS	FETAL/NEONATAL IMPLICATIONS
RHEUMATOID ARTHRITIS		
Chronic inflammatory disease believed to be caused by a genetically influenced antigen–antibody reaction. Symptoms include fatigue, low-grade fever, pain and swelling of joints, morning stiffness, pain on movement. Treated with salicylates, physical therapy, and rest. Corticosteroids used cautiously if not responsive to above.	Usually there is remission of rheumatoid arthritis symptoms during pregnancy, often with a relapse postpartum. Anemia may be present due to blood loss from salicylate therapy. Mother needs extra rest, particularly to relieve weight-bearing joints, but needs to continue range-of-motion exercises. If in remission, may stop medication during pregnancy.	Babies of women taking prednisone or prednisolone during the first trimester have a slightly increased risk of cleft palate. Its use in the later part of pregnancy increases the risk of preterm premature rupture of the membranes and small-for-gestational age newborns (Bermas, 2014).
SYSTEMIC LUPUS ERYTHEMATOSUS (SLE)		
Chronic autoimmune collagen disease, characterized by exacerbations and remissions; symptoms range from characteristic rash to inflammation and pain in joints, fever, nephritis, depression, cranial nerve disorders, and peripheral neuropathies.	SLE during pregnancy needs to be actively managed with careful surveillance of blood pressure, proteinuria, and placental blood flow. SLE medications may be necessary to control exacerbations and lupus flare. Increased incidence of caesarean birth, postpartum hemorrhage, and blood transfusion (Latimer & Neale, 2015). Women with severe disease may be counseled to avoid pregnancy.	Women with SLE are more likely to give birth to premature babies, smaller babies, and babies with congenital heart block (Nili, McLeod, O'Connell, et al., 2013). Neonatal lupus is characterized by a photosensitive skin rash, thrombocytopenia, neutropenia, or anemia, all of which resolve by about 6 months of age. Complete congenital heart block is the most serious complication of SLE, typically diagnosed in utero. When diagnosed, the mother is given corticosteroids that cross the placenta and decrease fetal heart inflammation. The prognosis for these newborns varies based on the extent of the cardiac damage. Live-born neonates may require a pacemaker (Akin, Baykan, Sezer, et al., 2011).
TUBERCULOSIS (TB)		
Tuberculosis (TB) is a major health problem. Approximately one third of the world's population (about 1.75 billion people) carry the TB bacteria (Loto & Awowole, 2012). Worldwide, TB is one of the top killers of women (CDC, 2012). Infection is caused by *Mycobacterium tuberculosis*; an inflammatory process causes destruction of lung tissue, increased sputum, and coughing. Associated primarily with poverty and malnutrition, 80% of new cases are found in developing countries primarily in Asia and Africa. In the United States the majority of cases occur in foreign-born people. More than 75% of these individuals were born in just 15 countries (CDC, 2013). Treated with isoniazid and either ethambutol or rifampin, or both.	The incidence of pregnancy complications may be higher in women with TB. TB skin test screening is recommended for women in high-risk groups (healthcare workers; foreign-born women from countries with a high TB risk; women who have had known contact with an infectious person; those who are HIV infected, alcoholics, or illicit drug users; women living or working in homeless shelters; prisoners and detainees [Cunningham et al., 2014]). If TB is inactive due to prior treatment, isoniazid therapy is delayed until the postpartum period unless the woman is HIV positive, has close contact with a person with active TB, or has had a skin test convert to positive within the last 2 years. For those women, isoniazid is started during pregnancy (CDC, 2012). Women with active TB are treated with isoniazid, rifampin, and ethambutol during pregnancy (Cunningham et al., 2014). Extra rest and limited contact with others is required until disease becomes inactive.	Women with TB have a higher rate of spontaneous abortion, suboptimal weight gain, and preterm labor; there is also an increased incidence of neonatal mortality and low birth weight. Congenital TB is a rare complication of in utero infection but the risk of postnatal transmission to the newborn is higher (Loto & Awowole, 2012). If maternal TB is inactive, the mother may breastfeed and care for her baby. If TB is active, the newborn should not have direct contact with the mother until she is noninfectious. Isoniazid crosses the placenta, but most studies show no teratogenic effects. Rifampin crosses the placenta. Possibility of harmful effects is still being studied.

Focus Your Study

- Almost any health problem that a person can have when not pregnant can coexist with pregnancy as well. Some problems, such as anemias, may be exacerbated by pregnancy. Others, such as collagen disease, may go into temporary remission with pregnancy. Regardless of the health problem, careful health care is needed throughout pregnancy to improve the outcome for mother and fetus.

- The diagnosis of high-risk pregnancy can shock an expectant couple. Providing emotional support, teaching about the condition and prognosis, and educating for self-care are important nursing measures that help clients cope.

- The key point in the care of the pregnant woman with diabetes is scrupulous maternal plasma glucose control. This is best achieved by home blood glucose monitoring, multiple daily insulin injections, and a careful diet.

- To reduce the incidence of congenital anomalies and other problems in the newborn, the woman should maintain a normal blood glucose level before conception and throughout the pregnancy. Women with diabetes, even more than most other clients, need to be educated about their condition and involved with their own care.

- Anemia indicates inadequate levels of hemoglobin (Hb) in the blood. In pregnant women, anemia is defined as hemoglobin less than 11 g/dL in the first and third trimesters and less than 10.5 g/dL in the second trimester. Iron deficiency anemia is the most common form of anemia. Other anemias include folic acid deficiency, sickle cell disease, and thalassemia.

- Substance abuse (either drugs or alcohol) not only is detrimental to the mother's health but also may have profound, lasting effects on the fetus. Nurses need to be alert to signs of substance abuse and be nonjudgmental in their care of women with substance abuse problems.

- Psychologic disorders such as depression and acute anxiety may have a profound effect on labor, particularly when complications that might jeopardize the mother or fetus occur.

- HIV infection, which is transmitted via blood and body fluids, may also be transmitted vertically from the mother to the fetus. Currently there is no definitive treatment for HIV/AIDS.

- Vertical transmission of HIV infection has been reduced dramatically with the administration of ZDV to the mother prenatally and during labor and to the newborn.

- Nurses should employ blood and body fluid precautions (standard precautions) in caring for all women to avoid potential spread of infection.

- Cardiac disease during pregnancy requires careful assessment, limitation of activity, and knowing and reporting signs of impending cardiac decompensation by both client and nurse.

- Worldwide, more women die from TB than from any other infection. Most cases are concentrated in developing countries.

Clinical Reasoning in Action

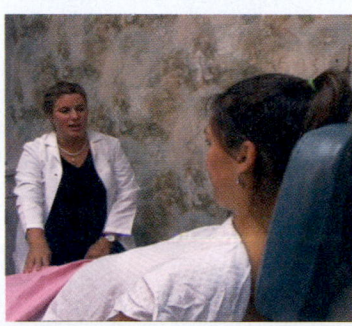

Jane Adams, a 23-year-old, G3P2, at 37 weeks' gestation, presents to you in the birthing unit complaining of "vaginal pressure" but no contractions. You assess her and find that her history includes being HIV positive for 2 years, second trimester cocaine and marijuana use, missed appointments, anemia (hematocrit 28%), and a positive syphilis serology. Jane tells you that she has other children and that they are being cared for by her mother, who has legal custody of them. You admit Jane and place her on the fetal monitor for evaluation of fetal well-being and contraction patterns. The monitor shows you that the fetal heart rate baseline is 120 to 130 with no decelerations; contractions are mild and irregular, lasting 20 to 30 seconds. You obtain vital signs of BP 130/88, temperature 97°F, P 88, R 14. A vaginal examination determines that Jane is 7 cm dilated at +1 station with intact membranes. She asks you if being HIV positive will affect her labor.

1. Discuss the prophylactic regimen for the prevention of HIV transmission to the fetus during labor.

2. Discuss the transmission of HIV to the fetus during pregnancy and birth.

3. Identify the emotional impact of HIV infection or other STIs on the woman.

4. On postpartum day 2 you inform Jane that her baby is HIV antibody positive. How would you clarify the results?

References

Abel, D. E. (2011). Thyroid disease during pregnancy: Part 1: Thyroid function testing and hypothyroidism. *The Female Patient, 36*(1), 16–22.

Akin, M. A., Baykan, A., Sezer, S., & Gunes, T. (2011). Review of literature for the striking clinic picture seen in two infants of mothers with systemic lupus erythematosus. *Journal of Maternal–Fetal and Neonatal Medicine, 24*(8), 1022–1026.

American Academy of Pediatrics (AAP) and American College of Obstetricians and Gynecologists (ACOG). (2012). *Guidelines for perinatal care* (7th ed.). Elk Grove Village, IL: American Academy of Pediatrics.

American College of Obstetricians and Gynecologists (ACOG). (2012a). *Opioid abuse, dependence, and addiction in pregnancy* (ACOG Committee Opinion No. 524). Washington, DC: Author.

American College of Obstetricians and Gynecologists (ACOG). (2012b). *Pregestational diabetes mellitus* (ACOG Practice Bulletin No. 60, issued 2005, reaffirmed 2012). Washington, DC: Author.

American College of Obstetricians and Gynecologists (ACOG). (2013). *Gestational diabetes mellitus*. (ACOG Practice Bulletin No. 137). Washington, DC: Author.

American College of Obstetricians and Gynecologists (ACOG). (2015a). *Management of women with phenylketonuria*. (Committee Opinion No. 636). Washington, DC: Author.

American College of Obstetricians and Gynecologists (ACOG). (2015b). *Marijuana use during pregnancy and lactation*. (Committee Opinion No. 637). Washington, DC: Author.

American College of Obstetricians and Gynecologists (ACOG). (2015c). *Screening for perinatal depression*. (Committee Opinion No. 630). Washington, DC: Author.

American College of Obstetricians and Gynecologists (ACOG). (2015d). *Thyroid disease in pregnancy*. (Practice Bulletin No. 148). Washington, DC: Author.

American Diabetes Association (ADA). (2015). Standards of medical care in diabetes—2015. *Diabetes Care, 38*(Suppl. 1), S1–S93.

Andemariam, B., & Browning, S. L. (2013). Current management of sickle cell disease in pregnancy. *Clinics in Laboratory Medicine, 33*(2), 293–310.

Apuzzo, J., Block, J. M., Cullison, S., Cohen, C., Leong, S. L., London, W. T., … McMahon, B. J. (2012a). Chronic hepatitis B in pregnancy: A workshop consensus statement on screening, evaluation, and management, Part 1. *The Female Patient, 37*(4), 22–27.

Apuzzo, J., Block, J. M., Cullison, S., Cohen, C., Leong, S. L., London, W. T., … McMahon, B. J. (2012b). Chronic hepatitis B in pregnancy: A workshop consensus statement on screening, evaluation, and management, Part 2. *The Female Patient, 37*(5), 30–34.

Battle, C. L., Weinstock, L. M., & Howard, M. (2014). Clinical correlates of perinatal bipolar disorder in an interdisciplinary obstetrical hospital setting. *Journal of Affective Disorders, 158*, 97–100.

Behnke, M., & Smith, V. C. (2013). Prenatal substance abuse: short- and long-term effects on the exposed fetus. *Pediatrics, 131*(3), e1009–24.

Bermas, B. (2014). Non-steroidal anti-inflammatory drugs, glucocorticoids and disease modifying antirheumatic drugs for the management of rheumatoid arthritis before and during pregnancy. *Current Opinion in Rheumatology, 26*(3), 334–340.

Cain, M. A., Bornick, P., & Whiteman, V. (2013). The maternal, fetal, and neonatal effects of cocaine exposure in pregnancy. *Clinical Obstetrics and Gynecology, 56*(1), 124–32.

Caritis, S. N., Hebert, M. F. (2013). A pharmacologic approach to the use of glyburide in pregnancy. *Obstetrics & Gynecology, 121*(6), 1309–12.

Centers for Disease Control and Prevention (CDC). (2012). *Global tuberculosis report 2012*. Retrieved from http://www.who.int/tb/publications/global_report/en/index.html

Centers for Disease Control (CDC). (2013). *Global tuberculosis 2013*. Retrieved from http://www.cdc.gov/tb/topic/globaltb/default.htm

Centers for Disease Control and Prevention (CDC). (2015a). *HIV in the United States: At a glance*. Retrieved from http://www.cdc.gov/hiv/statistics/basics/ataglance.html

Centers for Disease Control and Prevention (CDC). (2015b). Diagnosis of HIV infection in the United States and dependent areas, 2013. *HIV Surveillance Report, Vol. 25*. Retrieved from http://www.cdc.gov/hiv/pdf/statistics_2013_HIV_Surveillance_Report_vol_25.html

Cleveland Clinic. (2016). *Gestational diabetes*. Retrieved from http://my.clevelandclinic.org/disorders/Diabetes_Gestational/hic_Gestational_Diabetes.aspx

Collins, M. (2015). A case report on the anxiolytic properties of nitrous oxide during labor. *JOGNN: The Journal of Obstetric, Gynecologic & Neonatal Nursing, 44*(1), 87–92.

Cossette, B., Forget, A., Beauchesne, M. F., Rey, E., Lemière, C., Larivée, P., Battista, M. C., & Blais, L. (2013). Impact of maternal use of asthma-controller therapy on perinatal outcomes. *Thorax, 68*(8), 724–730.

Coyle, P. K. (2014). Multiple sclerosis in pregnancy. *Continuum: Lifelong Learning in Neurology, 20*(1), 42–59.

Criteria Committee of the New York Heart Association. (1994). *Nomenclature and criteria for diagnosis of diseases of the heart and great vessels* (9th ed.). Dallas, TX: American Heart Association.

Cunningham, F. G., Leveno, K. J., Bloom, S. L., Spong, C. Y., Dashe, J. S., Hoffman, B. L., … Sheffield, J. S. (2014). *Williams obstetrics* (24th ed.). New York, NY: McGraw-Hill.

Daniels, V. (2013). Antepartum depression—screening and treatment. *International Journal of Childbirth Education, 28*(3), 67–70.

Elkayam, U., Jalnapurkar, S., & Barakat, M. (2012). Peripartum cardiomyopathy. *Cardiology Clinics, 30*(3), 435–440.

Fryearson, J., & Adamson, D. L. (2014). Heart disease in pregnancy: Ischaemic heart disease. *Best Practice & Research, Clinical Obstetrics & Gynaecology, 28*(4), 551–562.

Harris, I. S. (2011). Management of pregnancy in patients with congenital heart disease. *Progress in Cardiovascular Diseases, 53*, 305–311.

Hood, D. G. (2012). Continuous subcutaneous insulin infusion for managing diabetes. *Nursing for Women's Health, 16*(4), 310–317.

Hurst, H. (2011). Insulin revisited: Safety in the maternity setting. *Nursing for Women's Health, 15*(3), 244–248.

International Association of Diabetes and Pregnancy Study Groups Consensus Panel (IADPSG). (2010). International Association of Diabetes and Pregnancy Study Groups recommendations on the diagnosis and classification of hyperglycemia in pregnancy. *Diabetes Care, 33*(3), 676–683.

Johnson, C. T., & Milio, L. A. (2015). Endocrine disorders of pregnancy. In C. T. Johnson, J. L. Hallock, J. L. Bienstock, H. E. Fox, and E. E. Wallach (Eds.), *The Johns Hopkins manual of gynecology and obstetrics* (5th ed.). Philadelphia, PA: Wolters Kluwer.

Kamyar, M., & Varner, M. (2013). Epilepsy in pregnancy. *Clinical Obstetrics and Gynecology, 56*(2), 330–341.

Karg, R. S., Bose, J., Batts, K. R., Forman-Hoffman, V. L., Liao, D., Hirsch, E., Pemberton, M. R., Colpe, L. J., & Hedden, S. L. (2014). Past year mental disorders among adults in the United States: Results from the 2008–2012 mental health surveillance study. Retrieved from http://www.samhsa.gov/data/sites/default/files/NSDUH-DR-N2MentalDis-2014-1/Web/NSDUH-DR-N2MentalDis-2014.htm

King, T. L., Brucker, M. C., Kriebs, J. M., Fahey, J. O., Gegor, C. L., & Varney, H. (2015). *Varney's midwifery* (5th ed.). Burlington, MA: Jones & Bartlett Learning.

Landon, M. B., Catalano, P. M., & Gabbe, S. G. (2012). Diabetes mellitus complicating pregnancy. In S. G. Gabbe, J. R. Niebyl, J. L. Simpson, M. B. Landon, H. L. Galan, E. R. M. Jauniaux, & D. A. Driscoll (Eds.), *Obstetrics: Normal and problem pregnancies* (6th ed.). Philadelphia, PA: Elsevier Saunders.

Latimer, K., & Neale, D. (2015). Autoimmune disease in pregnancy. In C. T. Johnson, J. L. Hallock, J. L. Bienstock, H. E. Fox, and E. E. Wallach (Eds.), *The Johns Hopkins manual of gynecology and obstetrics* (5th ed.). Philadelphia, PA: Wolters Kluwer.

Loto, O. M., & Awowole, I. (2012). Tuberculosis in pregnancy: A review. *Journal of Pregnancy*, Article ID 379271. Retrieved from http://www.hindawi.com/journals/jp/2012/379271

Loutfy, M. R., Sonnenberg-Schwan, U., Margolese, S., & Sherr, L. (2013). A review of reproductive health research, guidelines and related gaps for women living with HIV. *AIDS Care, 25*(6), 657–666.

Martin, S., & Graham, E. M. (2015). Cardiopulmonary disorders of pregnancy. In C. T. Johnson, J. L. Hallock, J. L. Bienstock, H. E. Fox, and E. E. Wallach (Eds.), *The Johns Hopkins manual of gynecology and obstetrics* (5th ed.). Philadelphia, PA: Wolters Kluwer.

National Institute on Drug Abuse. (2013a). *InfoFacts: MDMA (Ecstasy)*. Retrieved from http://www.drugabuse.gov/publications/drugfacts/mdma-ecstasy-or-molly

National Institute on Drug Abuse. (2013b). *Methamphetamine: What are the risks of methamphetamine abuse during pregnancy?* Retrieved from https://www.drugabuse.gov/publications/research-reports/methamphetamine/what-are-risks-methamphetamine-abuse-during-pregnancy

National Institute on Drug Abuse. (2014). *Drug Facts: Heroin*. Retrieved from http://www.drugabuse.gov/publications/drugfacts/heroin

Niebyl, J. R., & Simpson, J. L. (2012). Drugs and environmental agents in pregnancy and lactation: Embryology, teratology, epidemiology. In S. G. Gabbe, J. R. Niebyl, J. L. Simpson, M. B. Landon, H. L. Galan, E. R. M. Jauniaux, & D. A. Driscoll (Eds.), *Obstetrics: Normal and problem pregnancies* (6th ed.). Philadelphia, PA: Elsevier Saunders.

Nili, F., McLeod, L., O'Connell, C., Sutton, E., & McMillan, D. (2013). Maternal and neonatal outcomes in pregnancies complicated by systemic lupus erythematosus: A population-based study. *Journal of Obstetrics and Gynaecology Canada, 35*(4), 323–328.

Panel on Treatment of HIV-Infected Pregnant Women and Prevention of Perinatal Transmission. (2015, December 30). *Recommendations for use of antiretroviral drugs in pregnant HIV-1-infected women for maternal health and interventions to reduce perinatal HIV transmission in the United States*. Retrieved from https://aidsinfo.nih.gov/contentfiles/lvguidelines/perinatalgl.pdf

Paschetta, E., Berrisford, G, Coccia, F., Whitmore, J., Wood, A. G., Pretlove, S., & Ismail, K. M. K. (2014). Perinatal psychiatric disorders: An overview. *American Journal of Obstetrics and Gynecology, 210*(6), 501–509.

Resetkova, N., & Szymanski, L. M. (2015). Hematologic disorders of pregnancy. In C. T. Johnson, J. L. Hallock, J. L. Bienstock, H. E. Fox, and E. E. Wallach (Eds.), *The Johns Hopkins manual of gynecology and obstetrics* (5th ed.). Philadelphia, PA: Wolters Kluwer.

Schillie, S. F., & Murphy, T. V. (2013). Seroprotection after recombinant hepatitis B vaccination among newborn infants: A review. *Vaccine*, 31(21), 2506–2516. doi. 10.1016/j.vaccine.2012.12.012

Shade, M., Miller, L., Borst, J., English, B., Valliere, J., Downs, K., … Hare, I. (2011). Statewide innovations to improve services for women with perinatal depression. *Nursing for Women's Health, 15*(2), 127–136.

Singer, L. T., Moore, D. G., Min, M. O., Goodwin, J., Turner, J. J., Fulton, S., & Parrott, A. C. (2012). One-year outcomes of prenatal exposure to MDMA and other recreational drugs. *Pediatrics, 130*(3), 407–413.

Staneva, A. A., Bogossin, F., & Wittkowski, A. (2015). The experience of psychological distress, depression, and anxiety during pregnancy: A meta-synthesis of qualitative research. *Midwifery, 31*, 563–573.

Substance Abuse and Mental Health Services Administration (SAMHSA). (2014). *Results from the 2013 National Survey on Drug Use and Health: Summary of National Findings* (NSDUH Series H-48, DHHS Publication No. SMA 14-4863). Rockville, MD: Substance Abuse and Mental Health Services Administration.

Tan, C. H., Denny, C. H., Cheal, N. E., Sniezek, J. E., & Kanny, D. (2015). Alcohol use and binge drinking among women of childbearing age—United States, 2011–2013. *Morbidity and Mortality Weekly Reports (MMWR), 64*(37), 1042–1046.

U.S. Department of Health and Human Services. (2012). *Healthy people 2020: Maternal, infant, and child health.* Washington, DC: U.S. Department of Health and Human Services. Retrieved from http://www.healthypeople.gov/2020/topicsobjectives2020/objectiveslist.aspx?topicid=26

Wang, M. (2014). Perinatal drug abuse and neonatal withdrawal. *eMedicine.* Retrieved from http://emedicine.medscape.com/article/978492-overview

Wheeler, S. M., & Burd, I. (2015). Neurologic diseases in pregnancy. In C. T. Johnson, J. L. Hallock, J. L. Bienstock, H. E. Fox, and E. E. Wallach (Eds.), *The Johns Hopkins manual of gynecology and obstetrics* (5th ed.). Philadelphia, PA: Wolters Kluwer.

Whitty, J. E., & Dombrowski, M. P. (2012). Respiratory diseases in pregnancy. In S. G. Gabbe, J. R. Niebyl, J. L. Simpson, M. B. Landon, H. L. Galan, E. R. M. Jauniaux, & D. A. Driscoll (Eds.), *Obstetrics: Normal and problem pregnancies* (6th ed.). Philadelphia, PA: Elsevier Saunders.

Wilson, B. A., Shannon, M. T., & Shields, K. M. (2014). *Pearson Nurse's Drug Guide 2015.* Upper Saddle River, NJ: Pearson.

Wong, V. W., Suwandarathne, H., & Russell, H. (2013). Women with pre-existing diabetes under the care of diabetes specialist prior to pregnancy: Are their outcomes better? *Australian and New Zealand Journal of Obstetrics and Gynaecology, 53*, 207–210.

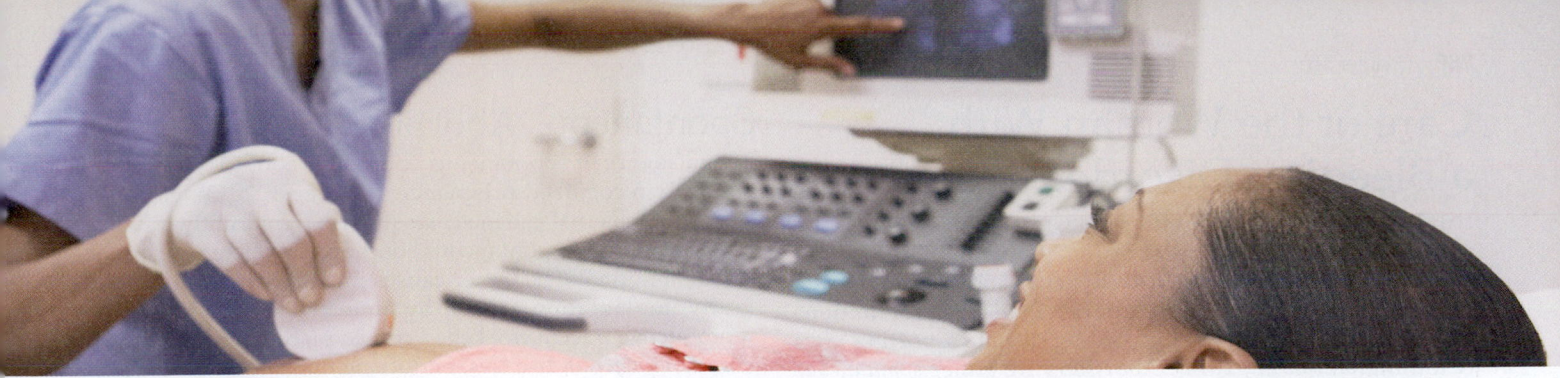

Chapter 15
Pregnancy at Risk: Gestational Onset

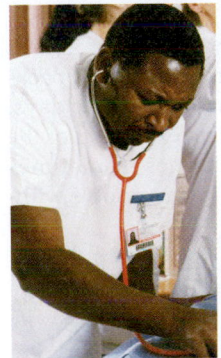

Working with women who are dealing with high-risk pregnancies has given me a much deeper appreciation of the stress a family faces when their unborn child is threatened or when the mother is ill. Some families seem so strong and resilient—they use me as a resource, and I am delighted to assist them in that way. Other families seem to crumble and have such needs. I do my best to help them gain the tools they need to cope. When I succeed, I am elated. When they can't seem to cope, no matter what any of us do, I feel such a sense of sadness for the family and their future.

—Maternity Nurse Working in a Large Medical Center

∨ Learning Outcomes

15.1 Contrast the etiology, medical therapy, and nursing interventions for the various bleeding problems associated with pregnancy.

15.2 Discuss the medical therapy and nursing care for a woman with hyperemesis gravidarum.

15.3 Describe the development and course of hypertensive disorders associated with pregnancy.

15.4 Describe the maternal and fetal/neonatal risks, clinical manifestations, and nursing care of the pregnant woman with a hypertensive disorder.

15.5 Summarize the risks and implications of surgical procedures performed during pregnancy.

15.6 Relate the impact of trauma caused by an automobile crash or a fall to the nursing care of the pregnant woman and her fetus.

15.7 Discuss the needs and care of the pregnant woman who experiences abuse.

15.8 Contrast the effects of various infections on the pregnant woman and her unborn child.

15.9 Explain the cause and prevention of hemolytic disease of the newborn secondary to Rh incompatibility.

15.10 Compare Rh incompatibility to ABO incompatibility with regard to occurrence, clinical treatment, and implications for the fetus or newborn.

P regnancy is usually an uncomplicated experience. In some pregnancies, however, problems arise that place the woman and her unborn child at risk. Regular prenatal care helps detect these complications quickly so that effective care can be provided. This chapter focuses on problems that primarily occur during pregnancy, those with a *gestational onset*. (*Note:* Conditions such as diabetes mellitus and anemia, which may occur prior to pregnancy or develop during pregnancy, are discussed in Chapter 14.)

Care of the Woman With a Bleeding Disorder

During the first and second trimesters of pregnancy, the major cause of bleeding is abortion. **Abortion** is the expulsion of the fetus before viability, which is considered to be 20 weeks' gestation or a fetal weight less than 500 g. Definitions of viability vary somewhat according to state reporting laws (Cunningham et al., 2014). Abortions are either *spontaneous* (occurring naturally) or *induced* (occurring as a result of medical or surgical means). **Miscarriage** is a lay term used for spontaneous abortion.

Other complications that can cause bleeding in the first half of pregnancy are ectopic pregnancy and gestational trophoblastic disease, discussed shortly. In the second half of pregnancy, particularly in the third trimester, the two major causes of bleeding are placenta previa and abruptio placentae. (These are discussed in detail in Chapter 20.)

General Principles of Nursing Intervention

Spotting is relatively common during pregnancy and usually occurs following sexual intercourse or exercise because of trauma to the highly vascular cervix. However, the woman is advised to report any spotting or bleeding that occurs during pregnancy so that it can be evaluated.

The nurse is often responsible for making the initial assessment of bleeding. In general, the following nursing measures are indicated:

- Monitor blood pressure and pulse frequently. The frequency is determined by the extent of the bleeding and the stability of the woman's condition.

- Observe the woman for behaviors indicative of shock, such as pallor, clammy skin, perspiration, dyspnea, or restlessness.

- Count and weigh pads to assess amount of bleeding over a given time period; save any tissue or clots expelled.

- If pregnancy is of 12 weeks' gestation or beyond, assess fetal heart tones with a Doppler.

- Prepare for intravenous (IV) therapy. There may be standing orders to begin IV therapy on clients who are bleeding.

- Prepare equipment for examination.

- Have oxygen available.

- Collect and organize all data, including antepartum history, onset of bleeding episode, and laboratory studies (hemoglobin, hematocrit, Rh status, hormonal assays) for analysis.

- Obtain an order to type and crossmatch for blood if evidence of significant blood loss exists.

- Assess coping mechanisms of the woman in crisis. Give emotional support to enhance her coping abilities by continuous, sustained presence; by clear explanation of procedures; and by communicating her status to her family. Prepare the woman for possible fetal loss. Assess her expressions of anger, denial, silence, guilt, depression, or self-blame.

- Assess the family's response to the situation.

Spontaneous Abortion (Miscarriage)

The incidence of spontaneous abortion is about 15% to 20% in clinically recognized pregnancies (Pflueger, 2013). However, advanced maternal age increases the risk significantly.

A majority of spontaneous abortions are related to chromosomal abnormalities. Other causes include teratogenic drugs, faulty implantation caused by abnormalities of the female reproductive tract, a weakened cervix, placental abnormalities, chronic maternal diseases, endocrine imbalances, and maternal infections. Women who use hot tubs or Jacuzzis may be at increased risk for miscarriage and neural tube defects because of the hyperthermia that results from increased core body temperature (Harms, 2012).

CLASSIFICATION

Spontaneous abortions are subdivided into the following categories:

- *Threatened abortion* (Figure 15–1A). The embryo or fetus is jeopardized by unexplained bleeding, cramping, and backache. The cervix is closed. Bleeding may persist for days. It may be followed by partial or complete expulsion of the embryo or fetus, placenta, and membranes (sometimes called the "products of conception") or it may resolve without threatening the fetus.

- *Imminent abortion* (Figure 15–1B). Bleeding and cramping increase. The internal cervical os dilates. Membranes may rupture. The term *inevitable abortion* also applies.

- *Complete abortion.* All the products of conception are expelled.

- *Incomplete abortion* (Figure 15–1C). Some of the products of conception are retained, most often the placenta. The internal cervical os is dilated slightly.

- *Missed abortion.* The fetus dies in utero but is not expelled. Uterine growth ceases, breast changes regress, and the woman may report a brownish vaginal discharge. The cervix is closed. If the fetus is retained beyond 6 weeks, the breakdown of fetal tissues results in the release of thromboplastin, and disseminated intravascular coagulation (DIC) may develop.

- *Recurrent pregnancy loss.* Abortion occurs consecutively in three or more pregnancies. Formerly called *habitual abortion*.

- *Septic abortion.* Presence of infection. May occur with prolonged, unrecognized rupture of the membranes; pregnancy with an intrauterine device (IUD) in utero; or attempts by unqualified individuals to terminate a pregnancy.

CLINICAL THERAPY

Pelvic cramping and backache are reliable indicators of potential spontaneous abortion. These symptoms are usually absent in bleeding caused by polyps, ruptured cervical blood vessels, or cervical erosion.

Speculum examination is done to determine the presence of cervical polyps or cervical erosion. Ultrasound scanning may detect the presence of cardiac activity and a gestational sac, or reveal a crown–rump length (CRL) that is small for gestational age. Laboratory determination of human chorionic gonadotropin (hCG) level can confirm a pregnancy, but because the hCG level falls slowly after fetal death, it cannot confirm a live embryo/fetus. Serial hCG levels may be indicated to confirm a diagnosis. Hemoglobin and hematocrit

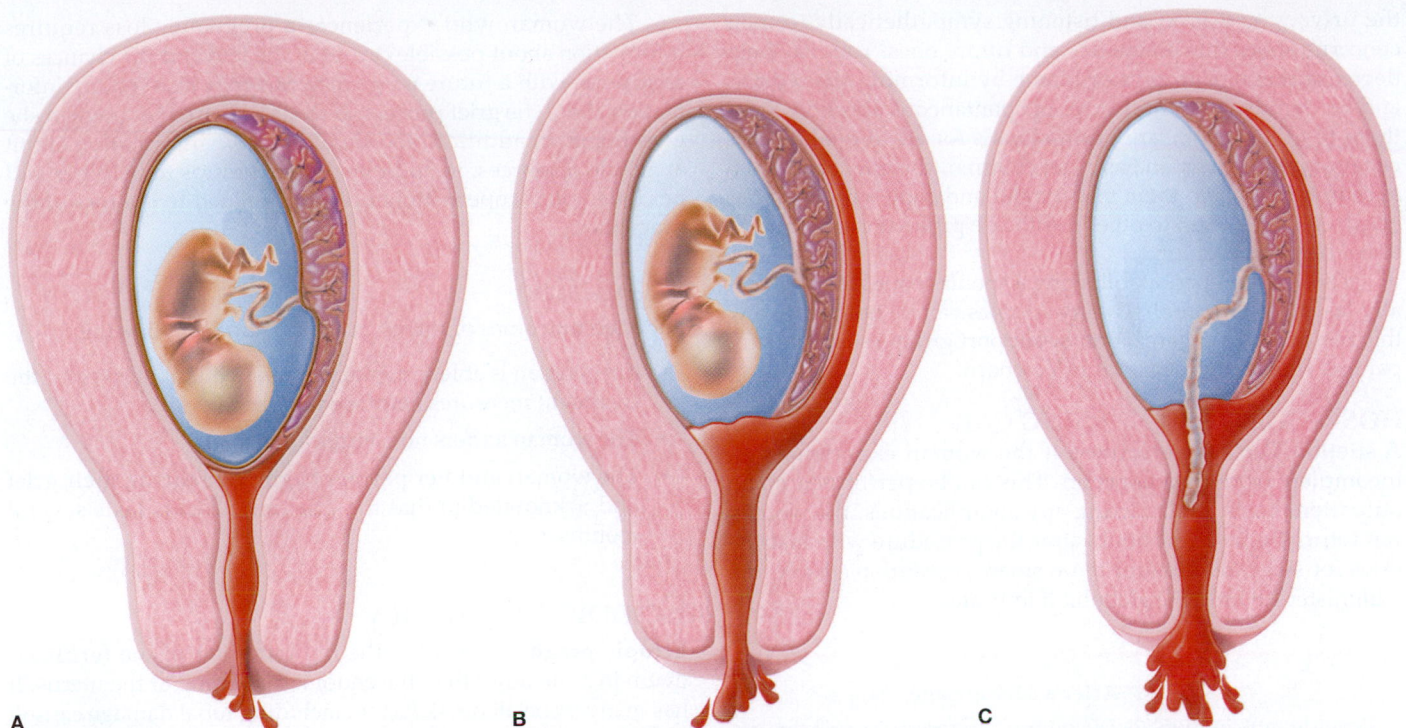

A   **B**   **C**

Figure 15–1 Types of spontaneous abortion. A. Threatened. The cervix is not dilated, and the placenta is still attached to the uterine wall, but some bleeding occurs. B. Imminent. The placenta has separated from the uterine wall, the cervix has dilated, and the amount of bleeding has increased. C. Incomplete. The embryo/fetus has passed out of the uterus; however, the placenta remains.

levels are obtained to assess blood loss. Blood is typed and crossmatched for possible replacement needs.

The therapy prescribed for the pregnant woman with bleeding is bedrest, abstinence from coitus, and emotional support. If bleeding persists and abortion is imminent or incomplete, the woman may be hospitalized, IV therapy or blood transfusions may be started to replace fluid, and dilatation and curettage (D&C) or suction evacuation is performed to remove the remainder of the products of conception. If the woman is Rh negative and not sensitized, Rh immune globulin (RhoGAM) is given within 72 hours (see discussion on Rh alloimmunization later in this chapter).

In missed abortions, the products of conception eventually are expelled spontaneously. If this does not occur within 4 to 6 weeks after embryo or fetal death, hospitalization is necessary. Dilatation and curettage or suction evacuation is done if the pregnancy is in the first trimester. In the second trimester, labor is induced or, alternatively, dilatation and evacuation (D&E) may be used.

Nursing Management

For the Woman Experiencing Spontaneous Abortion

Nursing Assessment and Diagnosis

Assess the woman's vital signs, amount and appearance of any bleeding, level of comfort, and general physical health. Identify the woman's blood type and antibody status to determine the need for Rh immune globulin. If the pregnancy is 10 to 12 weeks

or more, fetal heart rate should be assessed by Doppler. Also assess the responses of the woman and her family to this crisis and evaluate their coping mechanisms and ability to comfort each other.

Examples of nursing diagnoses that may apply include the following (NANDA-I © 2014):

- *Fluid Volume: Deficient,* related to excessive bleeding secondary to spontaneous abortion
- *Pain, Acute,* related to abdominal cramping secondary to threatened abortion
- *Grieving* related to expected loss of unborn child

Nursing Plan and Implementation

COMMUNITY-BASED NURSING CARE

If a woman in her first trimester of pregnancy begins cramping or spotting, she is often evaluated on an outpatient basis. Provide analgesics for pain relief if the woman's cramps are severe and explain what is occurring throughout the process.

Feelings of shock or disbelief are normal. Couples who approached the pregnancy with feelings of joy and excitement now feel grief, sadness, and possibly anger. Because many women, even with planned pregnancies, feel some ambivalence initially, guilt is also a common emotion. These feelings may be even stronger for women who were negative about their pregnancies. The women may even believe that the abortion may be a punishment for some wrongdoing.

Offer psychologic support to the woman and her family by encouraging them to talk about their feelings, allowing them the privacy to grieve, and listening sympathetically to their concerns about this pregnancy and future ones. You may help decrease feelings of guilt or blame by informing the woman and her family about the causes of spontaneous abortion. Refer them to other healthcare professionals for additional help as necessary. If the woman has older children, she may need guidance in how to help them understand and cope with what has occurred. Refer them to other healthcare professionals for additional help as necessary.

The grieving period following a spontaneous abortion usually lasts 6 to 24 months. Many couples can be helped during this period by an organization or support group established for parents who have lost a fetus or newborn.

HOSPITAL-BASED NURSING CARE

A suction D&C is performed if the woman experiences an incomplete or missed abortion. This can be performed on an outpatient basis, and, barring any complications, the woman can return home a few hours after the procedure with instructions for self-care. Monitor the woman's condition closely and administer Rh immune globulin if indicated.

Health Promotion   After a Miscarriage

Provide information about community resources to help the woman and her loved ones cope with the loss and advise her to:

- Report heavy or bright red vaginal bleeding, fever, chills, foul-smelling vaginal discharge, or abdominal tenderness

- Take the full course of antibiotics if any are prescribed

- If she has had a D&C, have someone remain with her for the first 12 to 24 hours.

- Delay pregnancy for at least 2 months to allow sufficient time for healing

---

Developing Cultural Competence   Response to Fetal Loss

Remember that individual responses to fetal loss following miscarriage may vary greatly and may be influenced by ethnic or cultural norms.

- Miscarriage may be viewed in many ways. For example, it may be seen as a punishment from God, as the result of the evil eye or of a hex or curse by an enemy, or as a natural part of life.

- When grieving over a pregnancy loss, women from some cultures and ethnic groups may show their emotions freely, crying and wailing, whereas other women may hide their feelings behind a mask of stoicism.

- In some cultures the woman's partner is her primary source of support and comfort. In others, the woman turns to her mother or close female relatives for comfort.

- Avoid falling into the trap of stereotyping women according to culture. Individual responses are influenced by many factors, including the degree of assimilation into the dominant culture.

The woman who experiences a pregnancy loss requires information about possible causes of the loss and the chances of recurrence with a future pregnancy. She may also require information about the grief process so she is prepared for it when she goes home. In addition, she should receive information about available resources, including support groups to help her and her loved ones cope with her feelings related to the loss of the pregnancy.

Evaluation

Expected outcomes of nursing care include the following:

- The woman is able to explain spontaneous abortion and the treatment measures employed in her care.

- The woman suffers no complications.

- The woman and her partner begin verbalizing their grief and acknowledge that the grieving process lasts several months.

Ectopic Pregnancy

Ectopic pregnancy (EP) is the implantation of the fertilized ovum in a site other than the endometrial lining of the uterus. It has many associated risk factors including tubal damage caused by pelvic inflammatory disease (PID), previous tubal surgery, congenital anomalies of the tube, endometriosis, previous ectopic pregnancy, presence of an IUD, and in utero exposure to diethylstilbestrol (DES).

Ectopic pregnancy occurs in about 2% of diagnosed pregnancies and accounts for about 6% of all pregnancy-related deaths (Mensah & Yates, 2015). Although the incidence of EP has increased, the mortality rate in the United States has decreased. This decrease can be credited to improved recognition of early signs and symptoms and better diagnostic methods, which allow detection before tubal rupture.

Ectopic pregnancy occurs when the fertilized ovum is prevented or slowed in its passage through the tube and thus implants before it reaches the uterus. The most common location for implantation is the ampulla of the fallopian tube. Figure 15–2 illustrates this and other implantation sites.

Initially the normal symptoms of pregnancy may be present—specifically, amenorrhea, breast tenderness, and nausea. The hormone hCG is present in the blood and urine. As the pregnancy progresses, the chorionic villi grow into the wall of the tube or site of implantation and a blood supply is established. The faulty implantation of the placenta causes fluctuation of hormone levels. Hormones first stimulate the endometrial lining of the uterus to grow, but fluctuation in levels cannot support the endometrium, and vaginal bleeding ensues. When the embryo outgrows this space, the tube ruptures and there is bleeding into the abdominal cavity. This bleeding irritates the peritoneum, causing the characteristic symptoms of sharp, one-sided pain, syncope, and referred right shoulder pain. The woman may also experience lower abdominal pain. Physical examination usually reveals adnexal tenderness. (The adnexae are the areas of the lower abdomen located over each ovary and fallopian tube.) An adnexal mass is palpable about half the time. Bleeding is slow and chronic, and the abdomen gradually becomes rigid and very tender. With extensive bleeding into the abdominal cavity, pelvic examination causes extreme pain, and a mass of blood may be palpated in the cul-de-sac of Douglas. Laboratory tests may reveal low hemoglobin and hematocrit levels and rising leukocyte levels. In a normal pregnancy β-hCG titers frequently double every 48 to 72 hours from 2 to 4 weeks' gestation. Ectopic

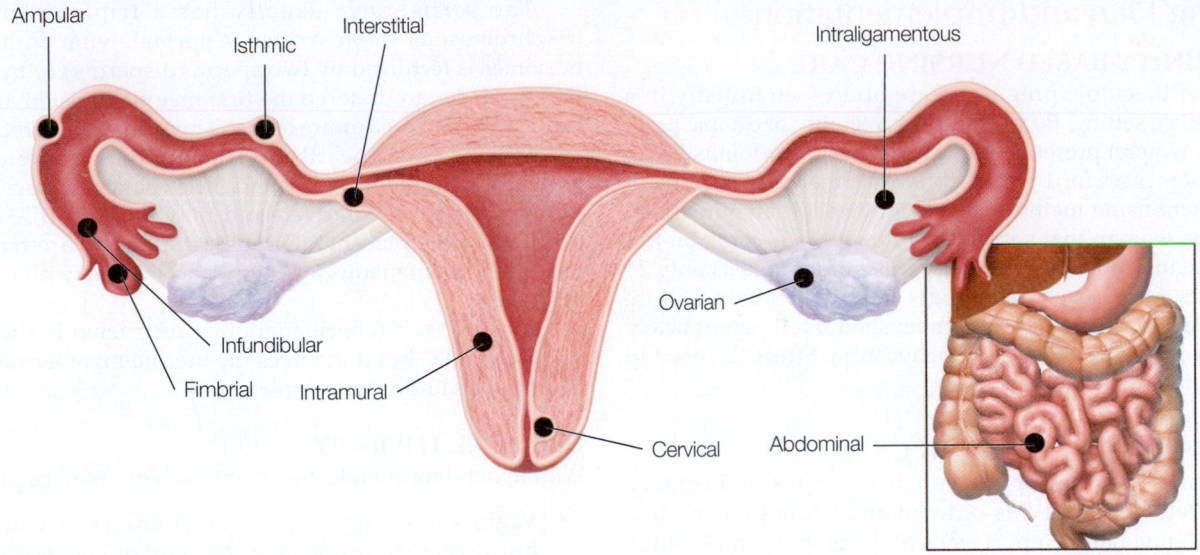

Figure 15–2 Various implantation sites in ectopic pregnancy. The most common site is within the fallopian tube, hence the name "tubal pregnancy."

pregnancies are associated with β-hCG titers that increase more slowly (Mensah & Yates, 2015).

CLINICAL THERAPY

The following measures are used to establish the diagnosis of ectopic pregnancy and assess the woman's status:

- A careful assessment of menstrual history, particularly the last menstrual period (LMP).
- Pelvic examination to identify any abnormal pelvic masses and tenderness.
- Laboratory testing completed as described previously.
- Transvaginal ultrasound, which is the test of choice to detect an intrauterine pregnancy or an adnexal mass (Mensah & Yates, 2015). Confirming an intrauterine pregnancy nearly eliminates the diagnosis of ectopic pregnancy.
- Serial measurements of serum hCG values, which should increase significantly every 2 days. Women with an ectopic pregnancy often have serial serum hCG values that increase more slowly than expected with a viable intrauterine pregnancy (Visconti & Zite, 2012).
- If the presence or absence of an ectopic pregnancy cannot be confirmed by other measures, laparoscopic intervention may be necessary for both diagnosis and treatment.

Treatment may be medical or surgical. Medical treatment using methotrexate is indicated for the woman who desires future pregnancy. The best success is obtained when the woman's ectopic pregnancy is unruptured and of 4 cm (1.6 in.) size or less, there is no fetal motion, and her condition is stable. In addition, woman must have no evidence of acute intra-abdominal bleeding, a blood disorder, or kidney or liver disease.

Methotrexate is a folic acid antagonist that interferes with the proliferation of trophoblastic cells. It is administered intramuscularly using either a single-dose, two-dose, or multiple-dose regimen. As an outpatient, the woman is monitored for increasing abdominal pain and β-hCG titers are determined. β-hCG titers are assessed on day 4 and day 7. If hCG levels do not decrease at least 15% from day 4 to day 7 after the initial injection, an additional dose of methotrexate is given on day 7 (Lipscomb, 2012). The multidose regimen includes methotrexate given IM and leucovorin administered orally on alternate days for up to 8 days (Visconti & Zite, 2012). This regimen is far more care intensive and is reserved for clients who present with high hCG levels.

If the woman is not clinically stable, surgical intervention may be required. When surgery is indicated and the woman desires future pregnancies, a laparoscopic linear salpingostomy will be performed to gently evacuate the ectopic pregnancy and preserve the tube. If the tube is ruptured or if future childbearing is not an issue, laparoscopic salpingectomy (removal of the tube) is performed, leaving the ovary in place unless it is damaged. If the woman is in shock and unstable, an abdominal incision will be made.

With both medical and surgical therapies for ectopic pregnancy, the Rh-negative nonsensitized woman is given Rh immune globulin to prevent sensitization.

Nursing Management

For the Woman With an Ectopic Pregnancy

Nursing Assessment and Diagnosis

When the woman with a suspected ectopic pregnancy is admitted to the hospital, assess the appearance and amount of vaginal bleeding and monitor vital signs for evidence of developing shock. Assess the woman's emotional state and coping abilities and determine the couple's informational needs. The woman may experience marked abdominal discomfort, so also determine the woman's level of pain. If surgery is necessary, perform the ongoing assessments that are appropriate postoperatively.

Nursing diagnoses that may apply for a woman with an ectopic pregnancy include the following (NANDA-I © 2014):

- *Pain, Acute,* related to abdominal bleeding secondary to tubal rupture
- *Fluid Volume: Deficient,* related to hypovolemia secondary to maternal blood loss
- *Grieving* related to loss of the pregnancy

Nursing Plan and Implementation

COMMUNITY-BASED NURSING CARE

Women with ectopic pregnancy are often seen initially in a clinic or office setting. Be alert to the possibility of ectopic pregnancy if a woman presents with complaints of abdominal pain and lack of menses for 1 to 2 months. A woman receiving medical treatment using methotrexate is followed as an outpatient. Advise the woman that some abdominal pain is common following the injection, but generally it is mild and lasts only 24 to 48 hours. More severe pain might indicate treatment failure and should be evaluated. The woman should also report heavy vaginal bleeding, dizziness, or tachycardia. Stress the need to return for follow-up β-hCG testing.

HOSPITAL-BASED NURSING CARE

Once a diagnosis of ectopic pregnancy is made and surgery is scheduled, start an IV as ordered and begin preoperative teaching. Immediately report signs of developing shock. If the woman is experiencing severe abdominal pain, administer analgesics and evaluate their effectiveness.

Regardless of the treatment used, the woman and her family will also need emotional support during this difficult time. Their feelings and responses to this crisis are generally similar to those that occur in cases of spontaneous abortion. As a result, similar nursing actions are required.

Evaluation

Expected outcomes of nursing care include the following:

- The woman is able to explain ectopic pregnancy, treatment alternatives, and implications for future childbearing.
- The woman and her caregivers detect possible complications early and manage them successfully.
- The woman and her partner are able to begin verbalizing their loss.

Gestational Trophoblastic Disease

Gestational trophoblastic disease (GTD) is the pathologic proliferation of trophoblastic cells (the trophoblast is the outermost layer of embryonic cells). In the United States the incidence is approximately 1 per 1000 to 1200 pregnancies (Cobb & Giuntoli II, 2015). GTD includes hydatidiform mole, invasive mole (chorioadenoma destruens), and choriocarcinoma, a form of cancer.

Hydatidiform mole (molar pregnancy) is a condition in which a proliferation of trophoblastic cells results in the formation of a placenta characterized by *hydropic* (fluid-filled) grapelike clusters. The disease results in the loss of the pregnancy and the possibility, though remote, of developing choriocarcinoma, a form of cancer, from the trophoblastic tissue.

Molar pregnancies are classified into two types, complete and partial, both of which meet the previously mentioned criteria. A *complete mole* develops from an ovum containing no maternal genetic material, an "empty egg," which is fertilized by a normal sperm. The embryo dies very early, no circulation is established, the hydropic vesicles are avascular, and no embryonic tissue or membranes are found. Choriocarcinoma seems to be associated exclusively with the complete mole (ACOG, 2012b). *Choriocarcinoma* is an invasive, malignant trophoblastic disease that is usually metastatic and can be fatal. It is discussed in more detail shortly.

The *partial mole* usually has a triploid karyotype (69 chromosomes). Most often, a normal ovum with 23 chromosomes is fertilized by two sperm (dispermy) or by a sperm that has failed to undergo the first meiotic division and therefore contains 46 chromosomes. There may be a fetal sac or even a fetus with a heartbeat. The fetus has multiple anomalies because of the triploidy and little chance for survival. The villi are often vascularized and may be fluid filled in only portions of the placenta. Often partial moles are recognized only after spontaneous abortion, and they may go unnoticed even then.

Invasive mole (chorioadenoma destruens) is similar to a complete mole, but it involves the uterine myometrium. Treatment is the same as for complete mole.

CLINICAL THERAPY

With hydatidiform mole, the following signs may be present:

- Vaginal bleeding occurs almost universally. It is often brownish (like prune juice) because of liquefaction of the uterine clot, but it may be bright red.
- Uterine enlargement greater than expected for gestational age is a classic sign of a complete mole, which is present in about half of cases. Enlargement is due to the proliferating trophoblastic tissue and to a large amount of clotted blood.
- Hydropic vesicles (grapelike clusters) may be passed; if so, they are diagnostic (Figure 15–3). With a partial mole the vesicles are often smaller and may not be noticed.
- Serum human chorionic gonadotropin (hCG) levels are markedly elevated because of continued secretion by the proliferating trophoblastic tissue.
- Hyperemesis gravidarum is present, probably because of the elevated hCG level.
- Very low levels of maternal serum α-fetoprotein (MSAFP) are found.

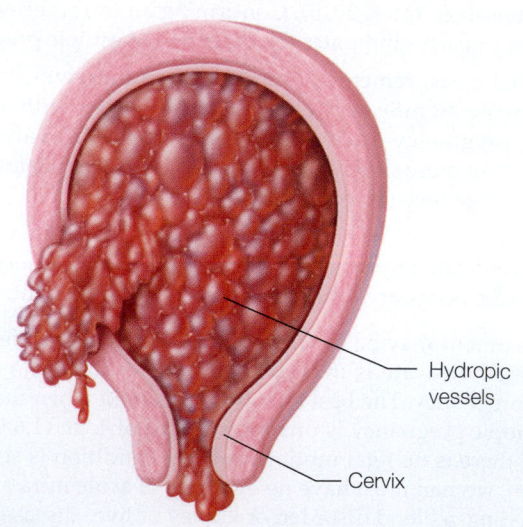

Hydropic vessels

Cervix

Figure 15–3 Hydatidiform mole. A common sign is vaginal bleeding, often brownish (the characteristic "prune juice" appearance) but sometimes bright red. In this figure, some of the hydropic vessels are being passed. This occurrence is diagnostic for hydatidiform mole.

- Anemia occurs frequently because of blood loss.
- Symptoms of preeclampsia are observed before 24 weeks' gestation.
- Fetal heart tones are absent despite other signs of pregnancy.

Transvaginal ultrasound is used for diagnosis. Therapy begins with suction evacuation of the mole and curettage of the uterus to remove all fragments of the placenta. Early evacuation decreases the possibility of other complications. Rh immune globulin is administered to women with an Rh-negative blood type. If the woman is older and has completed her childbearing, or if there is excessive bleeding, hysterectomy may be the treatment of choice to reduce the risk of choriocarcinoma.

Because of the risk of choriocarcinoma, the woman treated for hydatidiform mole should receive extensive follow-up therapy. Follow-up care includes a baseline chest x-ray to detect lung metastasis and a physical examination including a pelvic examination. Approaches to ongoing monitoring vary somewhat. Typically serum β-hCG levels are monitored weekly until negative results are obtained three consecutive times, then monthly for 6 to 12 months (Salani, Eisenhauer, & Copeland, 2012). The woman should avoid pregnancy during that time because the elevated hCG levels associated with pregnancy would cause confusion as to whether cancer had developed. If after a year of monitoring, the hCG serum titers are within normal limits, a couple may be assured that a normal pregnancy can be anticipated, with a low risk of recurring hydatidiform mole.

If hCG levels plateau for 3 consecutive weeks or rise, pregnancy must be ruled out and then the woman should be evaluated for metastatic disease and treated appropriately (Salani et al., 2012). Treatment at a center specializing in GTD is advised.

Nursing Management

For the Woman With Gestational Trophoblastic Disease

Nursing Assessment and Diagnosis

It is important for nurses involved in antepartum care to be aware of symptoms of hydatidiform mole and observe for them at each antepartum visit. The classic symptoms used to diagnose molar pregnancy are found more frequently with the complete than with the partial mole. Before evacuation, the partial mole may be difficult to distinguish from a missed abortion. If a molar pregnancy is diagnosed, assess the woman's (or the couple's) understanding of the condition and its implications.

Nursing diagnoses that may apply to a woman with a hydatidiform mole include the following (NANDA-I © 2014):

- *Fear* related to the possible development of choriocarcinoma
- *Grieving* related to the loss of the pregnancy secondary to GTD

Nursing Plan and Implementation

COMMUNITY-BASED NURSING CARE

When a molar pregnancy is suspected, the woman needs emotional support. Answer questions about the condition and explain what ultrasound and other diagnostic procedures will entail. If a molar pregnancy is diagnosed, support the parents as they deal with their grief about the lost pregnancy and their fear about the possibility of having a serious illness (DiGiulio, Wiedaseck, & Monchek, 2012). Healthcare counselors, a member of the clergy, or a professional counselor may also be of help.

HOSPITAL-BASED NURSING CARE

When the woman is hospitalized for evacuation of the mole, monitor vital signs and vaginal bleeding for evidence of hemorrhage. Determine whether abdominal pain is present and evaluate the woman's emotional state and coping ability. Typed and crossmatched blood must be available for surgery because of previous blood loss and the potential for hemorrhage. Administer oxytocin as ordered to keep the uterus contracted and to prevent hemorrhage. If the woman is Rh negative and not sensitized, give Rh immune globulin to prevent antibody formation.

Health Promotion   **Hydatidiform Mole**

- Stress the importance of follow-up visits.
- Advise the woman to delay another pregnancy until the follow-up program has been completed.

Evaluation

Expected outcomes of nursing care include the following:

- The woman has an uneventful recovery following successful evacuation of the mole.
- The woman is able to explain GTD and its treatment, follow-up, and long-term implications for pregnancy.
- The woman and her partner are able to begin verbalizing their grief at the loss of their anticipated child.
- The woman can discuss the importance of follow-up care and indicates her willingness to cooperate with the regimen.

Care of the Woman With Hyperemesis Gravidarum

Hyperemesis gravidarum, which is excessive vomiting during pregnancy, occurs in 0.3% to 2% of pregnancies (DeStephano & Aina-Mumuney, 2015). It may be mild at first, but true hyperemesis may progress to a point at which the woman not only vomits everything she swallows but also retches between meals.

Although the exact cause of hyperemesis is unclear, increased levels of human chorionic gonadotropin (hCG) may play a role. Higher levels of estradiol as well as lower levels of prolactin have been implicated as potential causes. Other mechanisms that may relate to hyperemesis are displacement of the gastrointestinal tract, hypofunction of the anterior pituitary gland and adrenal cortex, abnormalities of the corpus luteum, and psychologic factors.

In severe cases, hyperemesis causes dehydration, which leads to fluid–electrolyte imbalance and alkalosis from loss

EVIDENCE-BASED PRACTICE | Biologic Markers for Diagnosis of Hyperemesis Gravidarum

Clinical Question

Are there biologic markers for hyperemesis gravidarum that could help in the early detection, diagnosis, and treatment of this condition of pregnancy?

The Evidence

Nausea and vomiting are common symptoms in early pregnancy. More than half of all pregnant women will experience daily nausea in the first trimester. In up to 2% of women, though, nausea and vomiting may be so severe as to cause dehydration and weight loss that may require hospitalization. Diagnostic biomarkers could help in the early detection of hyperemesis gravidarum so that treatments can be initiated before adverse events occur. One group of clinicians conducted a systematic review of the literature to determine if there were biomarkers, and, if so, their relative usefulness in detecting either presence or severity of the condition. This type of unbiased approach to research review forms the strongest level of evidence for practice.

Historically, ketonuria has been hypothesized as a marker for the condition, but this review did not identify urinalysis for the condition as useful. Testing for human chorionic gonadotropin, thyroid hormones, estradiol, progesterone, and white blood count were inconsistently associated with the condition. Serology for *H. pylori* was predictive for hyperemesis gravidarum, and may be one marker that can identify the condition early in its onset (Niemeijer et al., 2014).

Best Practice

Early detection of hyperemesis gravidarum can enable interventions to decrease the prevalence of morbidity associated with the condition. The only test that has been shown to effectively predict the onset of the condition is serology for *H. pylori*. The test may be most useful if conducted when the first signs of protracted vomiting in pregnancy appear.

Clinical Reasoning

How would the nurse identify protracted vomiting in pregnancy, and how might it be distinguished from normal nausea and vomiting? Why might *H. pylori* be a causative agent for hyperemesis gravidarum?

---

of hydrochloric acid. Hypovolemia, hypotension, tachycardia, increased hematocrit and blood urea nitrogen (BUN), and decreased urine output can also occur. Dehydration may also lead to condensation of bile in the bile duct, resulting in less effective bile drainage with subsequent jaundice. If untreated, metabolic acidosis may develop. Severe potassium loss interferes with the ability of the kidneys to concentrate urine and may disrupt cardiac functioning. Starvation causes muscle wasting and severe protein and vitamin deficiencies. Fetal or embryonic death may result, and the woman may suffer irreversible metabolic changes or death.

The diagnostic criteria for hyperemesis include a history of intractable vomiting in the first half of pregnancy, dehydration, ketonuria, and a weight loss of 5% of prepregnancy weight.

Clinical Therapy

The goals of treatment include control of vomiting, correction of dehydration, restoration of electrolyte balance, and maintenance of adequate nutrition. If the woman does not respond to standard approaches to the control of nausea and vomiting in pregnancy, she may require intravenous (IV) fluids on an outpatient basis. If her symptoms do not improve, hospitalization may be indicated. Initially the woman is given nothing by mouth (NPO), and IV fluids are administered. Potassium chloride is typically added to the IV infusion to prevent hypokalemia.

Diclegis (a combination of doxylamine succinate and pyridoxine hydrochloride [vitamin B_6]) is the only FDA-approved treatment of nausea and vomiting during pregnancy. It is administered daily on an empty stomach (U.S. Food and Drug Administration (FDA), 2013). If this is not effective, other pharmacologic options include promethazine (Phenergan), metoclopramide (Reglan), and ondansetron (Zofran). Typically the woman remains NPO for 48 hours. If her condition does not improve, total parenteral nutrition may be needed. She then begins controlled oral feedings.

Nursing Management

For the Woman With Hyperemesis Gravidarum

Nursing Assessment and Diagnosis

When a woman is hospitalized for control of vomiting, assess the amount and character of any emesis, intake and output, fetal heart rate, signs of jaundice or bleeding, and the woman's emotional state.

Nursing diagnoses that may apply to a woman with hyperemesis gravidarum include the following (NANDA-I © 2014):

- *Nutrition, Imbalanced: Less than Body Requirements,* related to persistent vomiting secondary to hyperemesis
- *Fluid Volume: Deficient,* related to severe dehydration secondary to persistent vomiting
- *Fear* related to the effects of hyperemesis on fetal well-being

Nursing Plan and Implementation

COMMUNITY-BASED NURSING CARE

Parenteral nutrition therapy provided at home in collaboration with a physician and a registered dietitian is sometimes used to enable the woman to remain in her home. This therapy also gives an opportunity to observe family interactions and evaluate the home environment. This assessment is often useful in determining the pregnant woman's level of support, any significant stressors in her life, and her understanding of nutrition and self-care measures.

HOSPITAL-BASED NURSING CARE

Nursing care is supportive and directed at maintaining a relaxed, quiet environment away from food odors or offensive smells. Once oral feedings resume, food needs to be attractively served. Oral hygiene is important because the mouth is dry and may be irritated from vomitus. Monitor the woman's weight regularly. In some cases emotional factors have appeared to play a role in this condition, although that remains controversial. Nevertheless, psychotherapy may sometimes be recommended. With proper treatment, prognosis is favorable.

Evaluation

Expected outcomes of nursing care include the following:

- The woman is able to explain hyperemesis gravidarum, its therapy, and its possible effects on her pregnancy.
- The woman's condition is corrected and complications are avoided.

Care of the Woman With a Hypertensive Disorder

Hypertension, which affects 12% to 22% of pregnant women, is the most common medical complication in pregnancy. It is directly responsible for 17.6% of maternal deaths in the United States (ACOG, 2012a).

The classification of hypertension in pregnancy is as follows:

- Preeclampsia–eclampsia
- Chronic hypertension
- Chronic hypertension with superimposed preeclampsia
- Gestational hypertension

Healthy People 2020

(MICH-6) Reduce maternal illness and complications due to pregnancy (complications during hospitalized labor and delivery)

Preeclampsia and Eclampsia

Preeclampsia, the most common hypertensive disorder in pregnancy, is defined as an increase in blood pressure after 20 weeks' gestation accompanied by proteinuria in a previously normotensive woman. Previously edema was included in the definition but it was removed because it is such a common finding in pregnancy. However, sudden onset of severe edema warrants close evaluation to rule out preeclampsia or other pathologic processes such as renal disease.

Preeclampsia, typically categorized as mild or severe, is a progressive disorder. In its most severe form, eclampsia develops. **Eclampsia** is the occurrence of a seizure in a woman with preeclampsia who has no other cause for seizure. Eclamptic seizures may occur during the antepartum, intrapartum, or postpartum periods.

Most often preeclampsia is seen in the last 10 weeks of gestation, during labor, or in the first 48 hours after childbirth. Although birth of the fetus and removal of the placenta is the only known cure for preeclampsia, it can be controlled with early diagnosis and careful management.

PATHOPHYSIOLOGY OF PREECLAMPSIA

The exact cause of preeclampsia–eclampsia remains unknown, despite decades of research. Preeclampsia affects all the major systems of the body. The following pathophysiologic changes are associated with the disease:

- In normal pregnancy, the lowered peripheral vascular resistance and the increased maternal resistance to the pressor effects of angiotensin II result in lowered blood pressure. In preeclampsia, blood pressure begins to rise after 20 weeks' gestation, probably in response to a gradual loss of resistance to angiotensin II. This response has been linked to the ratio between the prostaglandins prostacyclin and thromboxane. Prostacyclin, a vasodilator produced by endothelial cells, decreases blood pressure, prevents platelet aggregation, and promotes uterine blood flow. Thromboxane, produced by platelets, causes vessels to constrict and platelets to clump together. Prostacyclin is decreased in preeclampsia, allowing the potent vasoconstrictor and platelet-aggregating effects of thromboxane to dominate. These hormones are produced partially by the placenta, which would help explain the reversal of the condition when the placenta is removed and why the incidence is increased when there is a larger-than-normal placental mass.

- Nitric oxide, a potent vasodilator and important regulator of maternal blood pressure, plays a role in the pregnant woman's resistance to vasopressors. Decreased nitric oxide production in women with preeclampsia may contribute to the development of hypertension.

- The loss of normal vasodilation of uterine arterioles and the concurrent maternal vasospasm result in decreased placental perfusion (see Figure 15–4). The effect on the fetus may be growth restriction, decrease in fetal movement, and chronic hypoxia or nonreassuring fetal status.

- In preeclampsia, normal renal perfusion is decreased. With a reduction of the glomerular filtration rate (GFR), serum levels of creatinine, blood urea nitrogen (BUN), and uric acid begin to rise from normal pregnant levels, whereas urine output decreases. Sodium is retained in increased amounts, which results in increased extracellular volume, increased sensitivity to angiotensin II, and edema. Stretching of the capillary walls of the glomerular endothelial cells allows the large protein molecules, primarily albumin, to escape in the urine, decreasing serum albumin levels. The decreased serum albumin concentration causes decreased plasma colloid osmotic pressure. This lowered pressure results in a further movement of fluid to the extracellular spaces, which also contributes to the development of edema.

- The decreased intravascular volume causes increased viscosity of the blood and a corresponding rise in hematocrit.

HELLP syndrome (**h**emolysis, **e**levated **l**iver enzymes, and **l**ow **p**latelet count) is sometimes associated with severe preeclampsia. Women who experience this multiple-organ-failure syndrome have high morbidity and mortality rates, as do their offspring.

The hemolysis that occurs is termed *microangiopathic hemolytic anemia*. It is thought that red blood cells are distorted or fragmented during passage through small, damaged blood vessels. Vascular damage is associated with vasospasm, and platelets aggregate at sites of damage, resulting in a low platelet count (less than 100,000/mm³). Elevated liver enzymes occur from blood flow that is obstructed by fibrin deposits. Hyperbilirubinemia and jaundice may also be seen. Liver distention causes epigastric pain and may ultimately result in liver rupture. Symptoms may include nausea, vomiting, flulike symptoms, or epigastric pain. HELLP syndrome is sometimes complicated by disseminated intravascular coagulation (DIC). See the discussion of DIC later in the chapter.

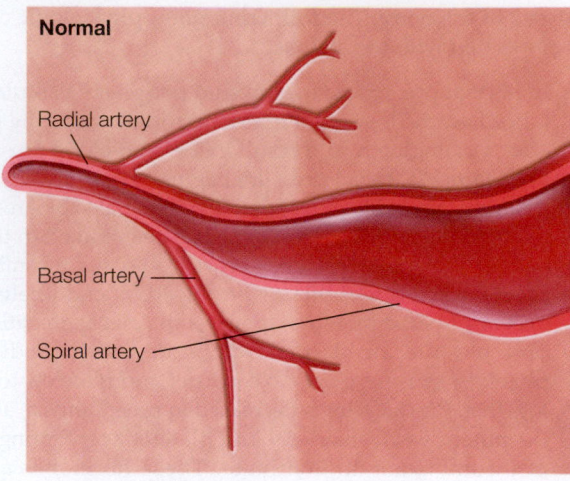

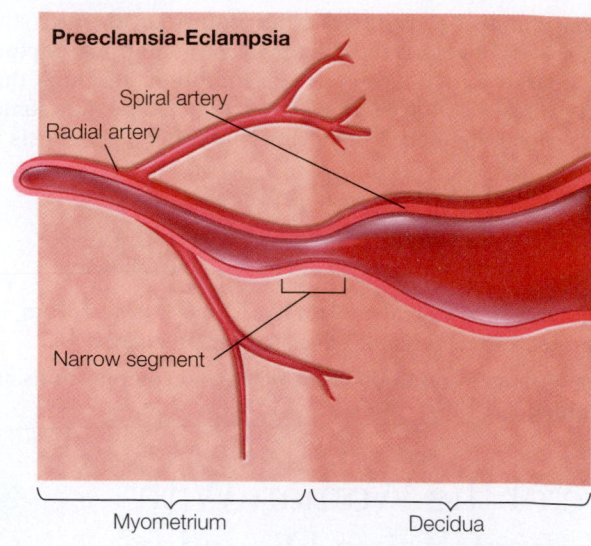

A   **B**

Figure 15–4 A. In a normal pregnancy, the passive quality of the spiral arteries permits increased blood flow to the placenta. B. In preeclampsia, vasoconstriction of the myometrial segment of the spiral arteries occurs.

Women with HELLP syndrome are best cared for in a tertiary care center. Initially the mother's condition should be assessed and stabilized, especially if her platelet counts are very low. The fetus is also assessed, using a non-stress test and biophysical profile. Regardless of gestational age, all women with true HELLP syndrome should give birth as expeditiously as possible.

Healthy People 2020

(MICH-5) Reduce the rate of maternal mortality

MATERNAL RISKS

Central nervous system changes associated with preeclampsia include hyperreflexia, headache, and seizures. Thrombocytopenia (platelet count less than 100,000/mm^3) is a frequent finding in preeclampsia. The exact mechanism is not fully understood, but platelet consumption is believed to be related to endothelial damage and activation of thrombin.

Women with severe preeclampsia or eclampsia are at increased risk for renal failure, abruptio placentae, DIC, ruptured liver, and pulmonary embolism.

FETAL/NEONATAL RISKS

Newborns of women with preeclampsia tend to be small for gestational age (SGA). The cause is related specifically to maternal vasospasm and hypovolemia, which result in fetal hypoxia and malnutrition. In addition, the newborn may be premature because of the necessity for early birth.

At birth, the newborn may be oversedated because of medications administered to the mother. The newborn may also have hypermagnesemia caused by treatment of the woman with large doses of magnesium sulfate.

CLINICAL MANIFESTATIONS AND DIAGNOSIS

Mild Preeclampsia.   Women with mild preeclampsia may exhibit few if any symptoms. The blood pressure is elevated to 140/90 mmHg or higher and the proteinuria is 1 g or less in 24 hours (2+ dipstick).

Although edema is no longer considered a diagnostic criterion, generalized edema, seen as puffy face or hands, and in dependent areas such as the ankles, may be present. Edema is identified by a weight gain of more than 1.5 kg (3.3 lb) per month

in the second trimester or more than 0.5 kg (1.1 lb) per week in the third trimester. Edema is assessed on a 1+ to 4+ scale.

Severe Preeclampsia.   Severe preeclampsia may develop suddenly. The following clinical signs are often present (ACOG, 2012a):

- Blood pressure of 160/110 mmHg or higher on two occasions at least 6 hours apart while the woman is on bedrest
- Proteinuria 5 g/L or higher in 24 hours or 3+ or greater on two random urine samples collected at least 4 hours apart
- Oliguria: urine output less than or equal to 500 mL in 24 hours
- Cerebral or visual disturbances
- Pulmonary edema or cyanosis
- Epigastric or right upper quadrant pain
- Impaired liver function (elevated hepatic enzymes–alanine aminotransferase (ALT) or aspartate aminotransferase (AST) to at least twice normal)
- Thrombocytopenia (less than 100,000 platelets per cubic millimeter)
- Fetal growth restriction

Other signs or symptoms that may be present include severe headache or one that persists despite analgesic therapy, blurred vision or scotomata (spots before the eyes), narrowed segments on the retinal arterioles when examined with an ophthalmoscope, retinal edema (retinas appear wet and glistening) on funduscopy, dyspnea due to pulmonary edema, moist breath sounds on auscultation, pitting edema of lower extremities while on bedrest, epigastric pain, hyperreflexia, nausea and vomiting, irritability, and emotional tension.

Eclampsia.   Eclampsia, characterized by a grand mal convulsion or coma, may occur before the onset of labor, during labor, or early in the postpartum period. Some women experience only one seizure; others have several.

CLINICAL THERAPY

The goals of medical management are prevention of cerebral hemorrhage, convulsion, hematologic complications, and renal and hepatic diseases, and birth of an uncompromised newborn as close to term as possible.

Antepartum Management. The clinical therapy for preeclampsia depends on the severity of the disease.

Home Care of Mild Preeclampsia. In general, women with preeclampsia are admitted to the hospital. However, for some women with mild preeclampsia, home care is now an option. The woman assesses her blood pressure, weight, and urine protein daily and does daily fetal movement monitoring. Weight gains of 1.4 kg (3 lb) in 24 hours or 1.8 kg (4 lb) in a 3-day period are generally cause for concern. Remote non-stress tests (NSTs) are performed twice per week or biophysical profiles are done weekly. Nursing contact varies from daily to weekly, depending on physician request. Laboratory testing regularly evaluates platelet counts, uric acid and BUN, liver enzymes, and 24-hour urine specimens for creatinine clearance and total protein. It is extremely important to advise the woman to report to the physician if she develops signs of worsening preeclampsia.

Health Promotion Preeclampsia

- The woman needs to know which symptoms are significant and should be reported at once.
- She is usually seen once or twice weekly. Explain that she may need to come in earlier than her next appointment if symptoms indicate that her condition is progressing.

Hospital Care of Mild Preeclampsia. The woman is placed on bedrest, primarily on her left side, to decrease pressure on the vena cava, thereby increasing venous return, circulatory volume, and placental and renal perfusion. She is weighed daily and evaluated for worsening edema, persistent headache, visual changes, or epigastric pain. Urine dipstick is done daily to assess for protein; blood pressure is checked at least four times per day. Diet should be well balanced and moderate to high in protein (80 to 100 g/day, or 1.5 g/kg/day) to replace protein lost in the urine. Sodium intake should be moderate, not to exceed 6 g/day. Excessively salty foods should be avoided, but sodium restriction and diuretics are no longer used in treating preeclampsia.

To achieve a safe outcome for the fetus, tests to evaluate fetal status are done more frequently as preeclampsia progresses. The following tests are used:

- Fetal movement record
- Non-stress test
- Ultrasonography at least every 3 or 4 weeks for serial determination of growth
- Biophysical profile
- Amniocentesis to determine fetal lung maturity
- Doppler velocimetry beginning at 30 to 32 weeks' gestation to screen for fetal compromise

Hospital Care of Severe Preeclampsia. If the uterine environment is considered detrimental to fetal well-being, birth may be the treatment of choice for both mother and fetus, even if the fetus is immature. Other medical therapies for severe preeclampsia include the following:

- *Bedrest.* Bedrest must be complete. Stimuli that may bring on a seizure should be reduced.
- *Diet.* A high-protein, moderate-sodium diet is given as long as the woman is alert and has no nausea or indication of impending seizure.

- *Anticonvulsants.* Magnesium sulfate is the treatment of choice for seizure prophylaxis and in the treatment of eclamptic convulsions because of its depressant action on the central nervous system (CNS).
- *Fluid and electrolyte replacement.* The goal of fluid intake is to achieve a balance between correcting hypovolemia and preventing circulatory overload. Fluid intake may be oral or supplemented with intravenous therapy. Intravenous fluids may be started "to keep lines open" in case they are needed for drug therapy even when oral intake is adequate. Electrolytes are replaced as indicated by daily serum electrolyte levels.
- *Corticosteroids.* Betamethasone or dexamethasone is often administered to the woman whose fetus has an immature lung profile. Corticosteroids may also have a beneficial effect in women with HELLP syndrome.
- *Antihypertensives.* Antihypertensive medications are the most commonly used methods of treatment. Antihypertensive therapy is generally given for sustained systolic blood pressure of at least 160 mmHg or diastolic blood pressures of 110 mmHg or higher (ACOG, 2013). Labetalol and hydralazine are first-line medications for the treatment of acute-onset, severe hypertension in pregnancy and are generally administered by IV boluses. Labetalol should be avoided in women with asthma, heart disease, or congestive heart failure (ACOG, 2015). Oral nifedipine acts rapidly and has favorable hemodynamic effects and fewer side effects than IV hydralazine. If these medications are not successful in controlling blood pressure, sodium nitroprusside may be indicated for extreme emergencies and used for the shortest amount of time possible (ACOG, 2015). Methyldopa is often used for long-term control of mild to moderate hypertension in pregnancy because it is effective and has a well-documented safety record.

Hospital Care of Eclampsia. An eclamptic seizure requires immediate, effective treatment. A bolus of 4 to 6 g magnesium sulfate is given intravenously in 100 mL IV fluid over 20 to 30 minutes followed by 2 g/hr IV infusion (Cunningham et al., 2014). Antihypertensive agents are used to keep the diastolic blood pressure between 90 and 100 mmHg, thus avoiding a potential reduction in uteroplacental blood flow or cerebral perfusion. A sedative such as diazepam or amobarbital is used only if the seizures are not controlled by magnesium sulfate. The lungs are auscultated for pulmonary edema. The woman is observed for circulatory and renal failure and signs of cerebral hemorrhage. Furosemide (Lasix) may be given for pulmonary edema; digitalis may be given for circulatory failure. An indwelling Foley catheter is often inserted and intake and output are monitored hourly.

The woman is assessed for signs of labor. She is also checked every 15 minutes for evidence of vaginal bleeding and abdominal rigidity, which might indicate abruptio placentae. While she is comatose, she is positioned on her side with the side rails up.

Because of the severity of her condition, the woman is often cared for in an intensive care unit. When the condition of the woman and the fetus have been stabilized, induction of labor is considered, because birth is the only known cure for preeclampsia. The woman and her partner should be given a careful explanation about her status and that of her unborn child and the treatment they are receiving. Plans for further treatment and for birth must be discussed with them.

Intrapartum Management. Labor may be induced by IV oxytocin when there is evidence of fetal maturity and cervical readiness. In severe cases, cesarean birth may be necessary even if the fetus is immature.

Assessment for signs of worsening preeclampsia continues. The woman may receive intravenous oxytocin and magnesium sulfate simultaneously. Infusion pumps should be used, and bags and tubing must be carefully labeled. Magnesium levels are assessed regularly.

Narcotics may be given intravenously for pain relief in labor. An epidural, spinal, or combined spinal-epidural can be safely administered to the woman with preeclampsia in the absence of thrombocytopenia. A preeclamptic woman is in total body fluid overload but has a depleted intravascular volume, making her prone to hypotension when the vascular bed dilates in response to spinal-epidural administration.

Electronic fetal monitoring is used to assess fetal status continuously. Birth in the Sims or semisitting position should be considered. If the lithotomy position is used, a wedge should be placed under the right buttock to displace the uterus. The wedge should also be used if birth is by cesarean. Oxygen is administered to the woman during labor if the need is indicated by fetal response to the contractions.

A pediatrician or neonatal nurse practitioner must be available to care for the newborn at birth. This caregiver must be informed of all amounts and times of medication the woman has received during labor.

Postpartum Management. The woman with preeclampsia usually improves rapidly after giving birth, although seizures can still occur during the first 48 hours postpartum. When the hypertension is severe, the woman may continue to receive hydralazine or magnesium sulfate postpartum.

Nursing Management

For the Woman With Preeclampsia

See *Nursing Care Plan: For the Woman With Preeclampsia* for additional information on nursing care.

Nursing Assessment and Diagnosis

Take and record the woman's blood pressure during each antepartum visit. If the blood pressure rises, or if the normal slight decrease in blood pressure expected between 8 and 28 weeks of pregnancy does not occur, the woman should be followed closely. Also check her urine for proteinuria at each visit.

If hospitalization becomes necessary, assess the following:

- **Blood pressure.** Assess every 1 to 4 hours, or more frequently if indicated by medication or other changes in the woman's status.

Clinical Tip

The following factors may lead to errors in measuring blood pressure (BP):

Incorrect cuff size—a cuff that is too small results in a falsely elevated blood pressure, whereas one that is too large falsely lowers blood pressure.

Elevating the arm above the level of the heart, such as occurs when a woman lying on her left side raises her right arm for a blood pressure measurement, will falsely lower the blood pressure 10 to 20 mmHg.

Korotkoff phase—when blood pressure is checked during pregnancy, the disappearance of the sound (phase V) is the preferred indicator rather than the muffling of the sound (phase IV).

Anxiety, exercise, and smoking can elevate blood pressure. Wait 10 minutes after the woman's arrival to check a resting blood pressure.

- **Temperature.** Take every 4 hours, or every 2 hours if elevated or if premature rupture of the membranes (PROM) has occurred.

- **Pulse and respirations.** Determine pulse rate and respirations along with blood pressure.

- **Fetal heart rate (FHR).** Check the FHR with the blood pressure or monitor continuously with the electronic fetal monitor if the situation indicates.

- **Urinary output.** Measure every voiding. The woman frequently has an indwelling catheter. In this case, urine output can be assessed hourly. Output should be 700 mL or greater in 24 hours, or at least 30 mL/hr.

- **Urinary protein.** Evaluate hourly if an indwelling catheter is in place or with each voiding. Readings of 3+ or 4+ indicate a loss of 5 g or more of protein in 24 hours.

- **Urine specific gravity.** Check hourly or with each voiding. Readings over 1.040 correlate with oliguria and proteinuria.

- **Edema.** Inspect and palpate the face (especially eyelids and cheekbone area), fingers, hands, arms (ulnar surface and wrist), legs (tibial surface), ankles, feet, and sacral area for edema. The degree of pitting is determined by pressing over bony areas.

- **Weight.** Weigh the woman daily at the same time, wearing the same robe or gown and slippers. Weighing may be omitted if the woman is to maintain strict bedrest.

- **Pulmonary edema.** Observe the woman for coughing, shortness of breath, or difficulty breathing. Auscultate the lungs for moist respirations.

- **Deep tendon reflexes.** Assess the woman for evidence of hyperreflexia in the brachial, wrist, patellar, or Achilles tendon. The patellar reflex is the easiest to assess (see *Clinical Skill: Assessing Deep Tendon Reflexes and Clonus*). Clonus should also be assessed by vigorously dorsiflexing the foot while the knee is held in a fixed position. Normally no clonus is present. If clonus is present, it is measured as beats and recorded as such.

- **Placental separation.** Assess the woman hourly for vaginal bleeding and/or uterine rigidity.

- **Headache.** Question the woman about the existence and location of any headache.

- **Visual disturbance.** Question the woman about any visual blurring or changes or scotomata. Record the results of the daily funduscopic examination in her medical record.

- **Epigastric pain.** Ask about any epigastric pain. It is important to differentiate it from simple heartburn, which tends to be familiar and less intense.

- **Laboratory blood tests.** Daily tests of hematocrit to measure hemoconcentration; blood urea nitrogen (BUN), creatinine, and uric acid levels to assess kidney function; clotting studies for any indication of thrombocytopenia or DIC; liver enzymes; and electrolyte levels for deficiencies are all indicated. Monitor magnesium levels regularly in women receiving magnesium sulfate.

- **Level of consciousness.** Observe for alertness, mood changes, and any signs of impending convulsion or coma.

- **Emotional response and level of understanding.** Assess the woman's emotional response so that support and teaching can be planned accordingly.

In addition, continue to assess the effects of any medications administered. Because the administration of prescribed medications is an important aspect of care, be familiar with the more commonly used medications and their purpose, implications, and associated untoward or toxic effects.

Clinical Skill 15–1
Assessing Deep Tendon Reflexes and Clonus

NURSING ACTION

Preparation

- Explain the procedure, indications for its use, and information that will be obtained.
- Check the patellar reflex and one other such as the biceps, triceps, or brachioradialis.

Rationale: Deep tendon reflexes (DTRs) are assessed to gain information about central nervous system (CNS) irritability secondary to preeclampsia and to assess the effects of magnesium sulfate if the woman is receiving it.

Equipment and Supplies

- Percussion hammer

Clinical Tip

If a percussion hammer is not available, you may use the side of your stethoscope or the side of your hand or the tips of the index and middle fingers to elicit DTRs.

Procedure

1. Elicit reflexes.
   - *Patellar reflex.* Position the woman with her legs hanging over the edge of the bed (feet should not be touching the floor). (See Figure 15–5.) Briskly strike the patellar tendon, which is located just below the patella. Normal response is extension or a thrusting forward of the foot.

Note: In an inpatient setting the patellar reflex is often assessed while the woman lies supine. Flex her knees slightly and support them.

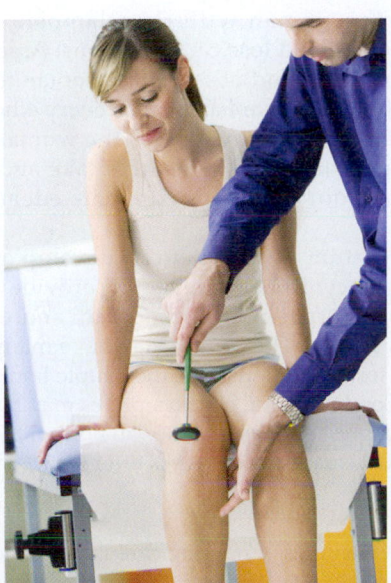

Figure 15–5 **Correct position for eliciting patellar reflex: sitting.**

SOURCE: © BSIP SA/Alamy.

Rationale: The correct position causes the muscle to be slightly stretched. Then when the tendon is stretched, with a tap the muscle should contract. Correct positioning and technique are essential to elicit the reflex.

- *Biceps reflex.* Flex the woman's arm 45 degrees at the elbow and place your thumb on the biceps tendon. Allow your fingers to hold the biceps muscle. Strike your thumb in a slightly downward motion and assess the response. Normal response is flexion of the arm.
- *Triceps reflex.* Flex the woman's arm up to 90 degrees and allow her hand to hang against the side of her body. Using the percussion hammer, strike the triceps tendon just above the elbow. Normal response is contraction of the muscle, which causes extension of the arm.
- *Brachioradialis reflex.* Flex the woman's arm slightly and lay it on your forearm with her hand slightly pronated. Using the percussion hammer, strike the brachioradialis tendon, which is found about 1 to 2 inches above the wrist. Normal response is pronation of the forearm and flexion of the elbow.

2. Grade reflexes. Reflexes are graded on a scale of 0 to 4+, as follows:

   4+ Hyperactive; very brisk, jerky, or clonic response; abnormal

   3+ Brisker than average; may not be abnormal

   2+ Average response; normal

   1+ Diminished response; low normal

   0 No response; abnormal

Rationale: Normally reflexes are 1+ or 2+. With CNS irritation, hyperreflexia may be present; with high magnesium levels, reflexes may be diminished or absent.

3. Assess for clonus. With the woman's knee flexed and the leg supported, vigorously dorsiflex the foot, maintain the dorsiflexion momentarily, and then release. With a normal response, the foot returns to its normal position of plantar flexion. Clonus is present if the foot "jerks" or taps against the examiner's hand. If so, record the number of taps or beats of clonus.

Rationale: Clonus occurs with more pronounced hyperreflexia and indicates CNS irritability.

4. Report and record findings. For example: DTRs 2+, no clonus; or DTRs 4+, 2 beats clonus.

Examples of nursing diagnoses that might apply to the woman with preeclampsia include the following (NANDA-I © 2014):

- ***Fluid Volume: Deficient,*** related to fluid shift from intravascular to extravascular space secondary to vasospasm
- ***Injury, Risk for,*** related to the possibility of seizure secondary to cerebral vasospasm or edema

Nursing Plan and Implementation

COMMUNITY-BASED NURSING CARE

A woman with preeclampsia has several major concerns. She may fear losing her fetus, she may worry about her personal relationship with her other children and her personal and sexual relationship with her partner, she may be concerned about finances, and she may also feel bored and a little resentful if she faces prolonged bedrest. If she has small children, she may have trouble providing for their care. Help the couple to identify and discuss these concerns. Offer information and explanations if certain aspects of therapy cause difficulty. Refer the woman and her family to community resources such as support groups or homemaker services as appropriate.

HOSPITAL-BASED NURSING CARE

The development of severe preeclampsia is a cause for increased concern for the woman and her family. The most immediate concerns usually are about the prognosis for the woman and her fetus. Explain medical therapy and its purpose and offer honest, hopeful information. Keep the couple informed of fetal status and discuss other concerns the couple may express. Provide as much information as possible and seek other sources of information or aid for the family as needed. Offer to contact a member of the clergy or hospital chaplain for additional support if the couple so chooses.

Maintain a quiet, low-stimulus environment for the woman. The woman is generally placed in a private room in a quiet location where she can be watched closely. Limit visitors to close family members or main support persons. The woman should maintain the left lateral recumbent position most of the time, with side rails up for her protection. Eliminate phone calls except for those that are planned because the phone ringing unexpectedly may be too jarring. To avoid a sense of isolation, however, some women find it preferable to limit calls to a certain time of day. Bright lights and sudden loud noises may precipitate seizures in the woman with severe preeclampsia.

SAFETY ALERT!

When caring for a woman with preeclampsia who is receiving IV magnesium sulfate, it is imperative to follow protocols for monitoring blood levels of magnesium. You are probably already aware of the common signs of increasing magnesium levels, such as diminished reflexes and decreased respiratory rate. However, you can also watch for some subtle clues that may suggest either the therapeutic or toxic range. When a woman's magnesium level is in the therapeutic range, she usually has some slurring of speech, awkwardness of movement, and decreased appetite. If the woman begins to have difficulty swallowing and begins to drool, she may be approaching the toxic range.

The occurrence of a convulsion is frightening to any family members who may be present, although the woman will not be able to recall it when she becomes conscious. Therefore, it is essential to offer explanations to the family members and the woman herself later.

A grand mal seizure has both a tonic phase, marked by pronounced muscular contraction and rigidity, and a clonic phase, marked by alternate contraction and relaxation of the muscles, which causes the woman to thrash about wildly. When the tonic phase of the contraction begins, turn the woman to her side (if she is not already in that position) to aid circulation to the placenta. Turn her head face down to allow saliva to drain from her mouth. Attempting to insert a padded tongue blade is no longer advocated in many facilities; in others, it is used if it can be inserted without force because it may prevent injury to the woman's mouth. The side rails should be padded or a pillow put between the woman and each side rail.

After 15 to 20 seconds the clonic phase starts. When the thrashing subsides, intensive monitoring and therapy begin. An oral airway is inserted, the woman's nasopharynx is suctioned, and oxygen is administered by nasal catheter. Fetal heart tones are monitored continuously. Maternal vital signs are monitored every 5 minutes until they are stable, then every 15 minutes.

NURSING MANAGEMENT DURING LABOR AND BIRTH

The laboring woman with preeclampsia must receive all the care and precautions necessary for normal labor, as well as those required for managing preeclampsia. Keep the woman positioned on her left side as much as possible. Monitor both the woman and the fetus carefully throughout labor. Note the progress of labor and be alert to signs of worsening preeclampsia or its complications.

During the second stage of labor, encourage the woman to push in the side-lying position if possible. If she is unable to do so comfortably or effectively, she can be helped to a semisitting position for pushing and she can then resume the lateral position between contractions. Birth is in the side-lying position or in the lithotomy position with a wedge placed under the woman's right hip.

Encourage a family member or other support person to stay with the woman as much as possible. Keep the woman in labor and the support person informed of the progress and plan of care. In addition, respect their wishes about the birth experience when possible.

NURSING MANAGEMENT DURING THE POSTPARTUM PERIOD

Because the woman with preeclampsia is hypovolemic, even normal blood loss can be serious. Assess the amount of vaginal bleeding and observe the woman for signs of shock. Monitor blood pressure and pulse every 4 hours for 48 hours. Check hematocrit daily. Assess the woman for any further signs of preeclampsia. Measure intake and output. Normal postpartum diuresis helps eliminate edema and is a favorable sign.

Postpartum depression can develop after such a difficult pregnancy. To help prevent it, provide opportunities for frequent maternal–newborn contact and encourage family members to visit. The couple may have many questions, so be available for discussion. Give the couple family-planning information. Combined oral contraceptives may be used if the woman's blood pressure has returned to normal by the time they are prescribed (usually 4 to 6 weeks after birth).

Evaluation

Expected outcomes of nursing care include the following:

- The woman is able to explain preeclampsia, its implications for her pregnancy, the treatment regimen, and possible complications.

KEY FACTS TO REMEMBER
Preeclampsia and Eclampsia

- Preeclampsia, which occurs after the 20th week of pregnancy, involves elevated BP and proteinuria. It may be mild or severe.

- A woman with preeclampsia who has a seizure is said to have eclampsia.

- The exact cause of preeclampsia is unknown.

- Vasospasm is responsible for most of the clinical manifestations, including the CNS signs of headache, hyperreflexia, and convulsion.

- Vasospasm also causes poor placental perfusion, which leads to IUGR.

- The only known cure for preeclampsia is birth of the baby, but symptoms may develop up to 48 hours postpartum.

- Management is supportive and includes anticonvulsant therapy, generally with magnesium sulfate; prevention of renal, hepatic, and hematologic complications; and careful assessment of fetal well-being.

- Nursing care focuses on implementing appropriate interventions based on the data gathered from regular assessment of vital signs, reflexes, degree of edema and proteinuria, response to therapy, fetal status, detection of developing complications, knowledge level, and psychologic state of the woman and her family.

- The woman suffers no eclamptic seizures.

- The woman and her caregivers detect early evidence of increasing severity of the preeclampsia or possible complications so that appropriate treatment measures can be instituted.

- The woman gives birth to a healthy newborn.

Chronic Hypertension in Pregnancy

Chronic hypertension in pregnancy is diagnosed when the blood pressure is 140/90 mmHg or higher before pregnancy or before the 20th week of gestation (ACOG, 2013). The cause of chronic hypertension has not been determined. In most women the condition is mild.

The woman is seen regularly for prenatal care (every 2 to 3 weeks during the first two trimesters and then weekly until birth). She is taught the importance of daily rest periods in the left lateral recumbent position and also learns to monitor her blood pressure at home. Sodium is limited to about 2.4 g/day. Antihypertensive medication is generally used for women with blood pressure over 150–160/100–110. Labetalol, nifedipine, and methyldopa are the antihypertensives recommended when medication is required (ACOG, 2013).

SAFETY ALERT!

Before administering labetalol be certain to check the woman's health history. Labetalol is contraindicated for people with bronchial asthma.

Nursing Care Plan: For the Woman With Preeclampsia

1. Nursing Diagnosis: *Fluid Volume: Deficient,* **related to fluid shift from intravascular to extravascular space secondary to vasospasm (NANDA-I © 2014)**

GOAL: Woman is restored to normal fluid volume levels.

INTERVENTION	RATIONALE
• Encourage woman to lie in the left lateral recumbent position.	• The left lateral recumbent position decreases pressure on the vena cava, thereby increasing venous return, circulatory volume, and placental and renal perfusion. Angiotensin II levels are decreased when renal blood flow is improved, which helps to promote diuresis and lower blood pressure.
• Assess blood pressure every 1 to 4 hours as necessary.	• Frequent monitoring will assess for progression of the disorder and allow for early intervention to ensure maternal and fetal health and well-being.
• Monitor urine for volume and proteinuria every shift or every hour per agency protocol.	• Monitoring provides information to assess renal perfusion. Proteinuria is the last cardinal sign of preeclampsia to appear. As the disorder worsens, the capillary walls of the glomerular endothelial cells stretch, allowing protein molecules to pass into the urine. Normally urine does not contain protein. Readings of 3+ and 4+ indicate loss of 5 g or more protein in 24 hours. Urinary output decreases when there is a reduction of the glomerular filtration rate. Urinary output that falls below 30 mL per hour or less than 700 mL in a 24-hour period should be reported.

(*continued*)

Nursing Care Plan: For the Woman With Preeclampsia (*continued*)

INTERVENTION	RATIONALE
• Assess deep tendon reflexes and clonus.	• Hyperreflexia may occur as preeclampsia worsens. Eliciting deep tendon reflexes provides information about central nervous system (CNS) status and is also used to assess for magnesium sulfate toxicity. Reflexes are graded on a scale of 0 to 4+ using the Deep Tendon Reflex Rating Scale. A rating of 4+ is abnormal and indicates hyperreflexia. A rating of 0 or no response is also abnormal and is seen with high maternal serum magnesium levels. Clonus, an abnormal finding, is present if the foot "jerks" or taps the examiner's hand, at which time the examiner counts the number of taps or beats. The presence of clonus indicates a more pronounced hyperreflexia and is indicative of CNS irritability.
• Assess for edema.	• Edema develops as fluid shifts from the intravascular to the extravascular spaces. Edema is assessed either by weight gain (more than 3.3 lb/month [1.5 kg] in the second trimester or more than 1.1 lb/week [0.5 kg] in the third trimester) or by assessing for pitting edema (assessed by using finger pressure to a swollen area, usually the lower extremities, and grading on a scale of 1+ to 4+).
• Administer magnesium sulfate per infusion pump as ordered.	• As preeclampsia worsens, the risk of an eclamptic seizure increases. Magnesium sulfate is the treatment of choice for seizures because of its CNS depressant action. As a secondary effect, magnesium sulfate relaxes smooth muscles and may therefore decrease the blood pressure. Magnesium sulfate is contraindicated in women with myasthenia gravis.
• Assess for magnesium sulfate toxicity.	• Side effects of magnesium sulfate are dose related. Therapeutic levels are in the range of 4.8 to 8.4 mg/dL. As maternal serum magnesium levels increase, toxicity may occur. Signs of toxicity include decreased or absent deep tendon reflexes (DTRs), urine output below 30 mL/hr, respirations below 12, and confusion.
• Provide a balanced diet that includes 80 to 100 g/day or 1.5 g/kg/day of protein.	• A diet rich in protein is necessary to replace protein that is excreted in the urine.

EXPECTED OUTCOME: The signs and symptoms of preeclampsia will diminish as evidenced by decreased blood pressure, urine protein levels of zero, and a return of the deep tendon reflexes to normal.

2. **Nursing Diagnosis:** *Injury, Risk for*, to the fetus related to uteroplacental insufficiency secondary to vasospasm (NANDA-I © 2014)

GOAL: The fetus will avoid complications related to uteroplacental insufficiency.

INTERVENTION	RATIONALE
• Instruct woman to count fetal movements three times a day for 20 to 30 minutes.	• Fetal activity provides reassurance of fetal well-being. Decrease in fetal movement or cessation of movement may indicate fetal compromise.
• Encourage woman to rest in the left lateral recumbent position.	• Lying in the left lateral recumbent position decreases pressure on the vena cava, which increases venous return, circulatory volume, and placental and renal perfusion. Blood flow to the fetus is increased, thereby reducing the risk of fetal hypoxia and malnutrition.
• **Collaborative:** Assist with serial ultrasounds.	• Maternal vasospasm and hypovolemia result from preeclampsia, which may lead to intrauterine growth restriction and oligohydramnios. Ultrasound provides assessment of fetal growth and fluid levels.

INTERVENTION	RATIONALE
• Perform non-stress test (NST) as ordered.	• NST is performed to assess the fetal heart rate in response to fetal movement. Accelerations of fetal heart rate with fetal movement may indicate the fetus has adequate oxygenation and an intact central nervous system. (Refer to Chapter 13 for interpretation of NST results.)
• Describe for the woman the purposes of a biophysical profile (BPP).	• Preeclampsia or eclampsia places the woman at risk for uteroplacental insufficiency due to the loss of normal vasodilation of uterine arterioles and maternal vasospasm. This results in decreased uteroplacental perfusion, which may lead to fetal hypoxia. A BPP is one assessment tool used to evaluate fetal well-being. Providing explanation of the diagnostic test helps relieve anxiety and ensures the woman understands what the test evaluates and what the results mean.
• Assist with amniocentesis to obtain lecithin/sphingomyelin (L/S) ratio.	• Women with preeclampsia may give birth before term. Amniotic fluid may be analyzed to determine the maturity of the fetal lungs. An L/S ratio of 2:1 or greater indicates fetal lung maturity and is usually achieved by 35 to 36 weeks' gestation.
• Explain the purpose of Doppler flow studies.	• Doppler flow studies (umbilical velocimetry) help to assess placental function and sufficiency. Uteroplacental insufficiency is a risk for a woman with preeclampsia. If fetal growth restriction is present, Doppler velocimetry of the umbilical artery is useful for fetal surveillance.

EXPECTED OUTCOME: The fetus will have an adequate supply of oxygen and nutrients as evidenced by absence of signs of nonreassuring fetal status and by fetal diagnostic test results within normal limits.

3. **Nursing Diagnosis:** *Health Maintenance, Ineffective,* **related to deficient knowledge about new diagnosis (preeclampsia) (NANDA-I © 2014)**

GOAL: The woman will describe the condition and treatment regimen.

INTERVENTION	RATIONALE
• Assess the woman and the family's understanding of preeclampsia and its implications for pregnancy.	• This assessment provides information about the woman's cognitive level and her understanding of her diagnosis. Behavior changes occur when teaching strategies are appropriate for the woman's and her family's cognitive level.
• Provide information about the disease process, impact on maternal well-being, risks of progression, implications for the fetus, and dangers of eclampsia.	• Basic understanding of the condition and its implications is necessary for the woman to understand the treatment plan. A woman who shows signs of early preeclampsia often feels well and may have difficulty accepting the need to rest.
• Emphasize the importance of self-monitoring for signs that her condition is worsening and the importance of regular prenatal care for the purpose of maternal and fetal surveillance.	• The woman should be able to identify signs of disease progression, including evidence of increasing edema, decreased urine output, signs of cerebral disturbance (frontal headache, blurred vision, scotomata), epigastric or right upper quadrant pain, nausea or vomiting, and increased irritability.

EXPECTED OUTCOME: The woman will demonstrate understanding of preeclampsia and its implications as evidenced by verbalization of basic condition, signs and symptoms of progression, importance of sufficient rest in side-lying position, and need to follow prescribed diet.

Twenty-four-hour urines, serum creatinine, uric acid, hematocrit, and ultrasound examinations are repeated at least once during the last two trimesters.

Nursing care is directed at providing sufficient information so that the woman can meet her healthcare needs. She is given information about her diet, the importance of regular rest, her medications, the need for blood pressure control, and any procedures used to monitor the well-being of her fetus.

Chronic Hypertension With Superimposed Preeclampsia

Preeclampsia may develop in women with chronic hypertension. After 20 weeks' gestation the onset of proteinuria and worsening hypertension are suggestive of superimposed preeclampsia. A rise in serum uric acid is helpful in identifying preeclampsia, which frequently occurs late in the second trimester or early in the third.

Gestational Hypertension

Gestational hypertension exists when transient elevation of blood pressure occurs for the first time after midpregnancy without proteinuria or other signs of preeclampsia. If preeclampsia does not develop and blood pressure returns to normal by 12 weeks postpartum, the diagnosis of gestational hypertension may be assigned. If the blood pressure elevation persists after 12 weeks postpartum, the woman is diagnosed with chronic hypertension.

Clinical Reasoning Pregnancy Complication

Jillian Rundus is a 31-year-old G1P0 who is 35 weeks pregnant. She presents for a routine office visit with complaints of nausea and abdominal pain rating 7/10. She has had a headache and general malaise for 2 days. She denies visual changes. Upon examination, you find her to be alert and oriented and her physical examination is unremarkable with the exception of abdominal tenderness and a blood pressure of 170/110. She has had no previous history of hypertension. Fetal heart rate ranges from 140 to 150 beats per minute.

What should the nurse do at this time?

Disseminated Intravascular Coagulation

Disseminated intravascular coagulation (DIC) occurs more often in pregnancies complicated by preeclampsia, abruptio placentae, intrauterine fetal demise, amniotic fluid embolism, maternal liver disease, and septic abortion. Although DIC is not considered a component of severe preeclampsia, eclampsia, or HELLP syndrome, it can occur as a complication when any of these conditions exist.

DIC occurs when there is an overactivation of the normal clotting process. In most instances, tissue factor entering the circulation is the primary trigger for DIC. When this occurs, there is an imbalance between the coagulation and the fibrinolytic systems. This mechanism leads to hemorrhage and shock. During these events, clots are being formed and fibrin deposited into the microcirculation, resulting in cell or tissue damage. This triggers further coagulation, which eventually depletes the plasma clotting factors. These fibrin clots can lead to intravascular obstruction and infarctions. In addition, the fibrinolytic system is activated, which results in the formation of fibrin–fibrinogen degradation products or fibrin split products. The release of these products decreases platelet functioning and further inhibits coagulation (Blackburn, 2013).

DIC is diagnosed when thrombocytopenia, low fibrinogen levels, and elevated fibrin split products are found in the laboratory findings. Serial platelet and serum fibrin degradation product counts are performed to monitor the mother's hematologic status. Supportive measures and reversing the causative factors are the primary interventions used to manage DIC.

Care of the Woman Requiring Surgery During Pregnancy

Although elective surgery should be delayed until the postpartum period, essential surgery can generally be undertaken during pregnancy. However, surgery poses some risks. The early second trimester is the best time to operate because there is less risk of spontaneous abortion or early labor, and the uterus is not so large as to impinge on the abdominal field.

Although general preoperative and postoperative care is similar for gravid and nongravid women, special considerations must be kept in mind when the surgical client is pregnant. If a chest x-ray is done, the fetus should be shielded from the radiation. To prevent uterine compression of major blood vessels while the woman is supine, a wedge must be placed under the woman's right hip to tilt the uterus during both surgery and recovery. The decreased intestinal motility and delayed gastric emptying that occur in pregnancy increase the risk of vomiting when anesthetics are given and during the postoperative period. Thus a nasogastric tube may be recommended before major surgery. An indwelling urinary catheter prevents bladder distention, decreases risk of injury to the bladder, and permits convenient monitoring of output. Fetal heart rate must be monitored electronically before, during, and after surgery.

Pregnancy causes increased secretions of the respiratory tract and engorgement of the nasal mucous membrane, often making breathing through the nose difficult. Consequently, pregnant women often need an endotracheal tube for respiratory support during surgery. Spinal or epidural anesthesia is preferred because local anesthetics are not associated with birth defects. Caution must be exercised because this type of anesthesia may produce hypotension and respiratory apnea in the pregnant woman.

Caregivers must guard against maternal hypoxia during surgery because uterine circulation will be decreased and fetal oxygenation can decline quickly. Blood loss is also closely monitored throughout the procedure and following it.

Postoperatively, the nurse encourages the woman to turn, breathe deeply, and cough regularly and to use any ventilation therapy, such as incentive spirometry, to avoid developing pneumonia. Sequential compression devices (SCDs) or support stockings during and after surgery help prevent venous stasis and the development of thrombophlebitis. The nurse encourages leg exercises while the woman is confined to bed and introduces ambulation as soon as possible.

Discharge teaching is especially important. The woman and her family should clearly understand what to expect regarding activity level, discomfort, diet, medications, and any special considerations. In addition, they should know the warning signs they need to report to the physician immediately.

Care of the Woman Suffering Major Trauma

Trauma complicates from 6% to 8% of pregnancies; trauma from motor vehicle crashes is the leading cause of fetal and maternal death (Mozurkewich & Pearlman, 2012). Falls and violence—including domestic violence—are the next most common causes of injury.

Late in pregnancy, when balance and coordination are adversely affected, the woman may fall. Her protruding abdomen is vulnerable to a variety of minor injuries. The fetus is usually well protected by the amniotic fluid, which distributes the force of a blow equally in all directions, and by the muscle layers of the uterus and abdominal wall. In early pregnancy, while the uterus is still in the pelvis, it is shielded from blows by the surrounding pelvic organs, muscles, and bones.

Trauma that causes concern includes blunt trauma (from an automobile crash, for example); penetrating abdominal injuries; and the complications of maternal shock, premature labor, and spontaneous abortion. Maternal mortality most often occurs from head trauma or hemorrhage. Uterine rupture is a rare but life-threatening complication of trauma. It may result from strong deceleration forces in an automobile crash, with or without seat belts. Traumatic separation of the placenta can occur, which causes a high rate of fetal mortality. Premature labor, often following rupture of membranes during a crash, is another serious hazard to the fetus. Premature labor can ensue even if the woman is not injured. To help prevent trauma from automobile crashes, all pregnant women should wear both lap seat belts and shoulder harnesses.

Penetrating trauma includes gunshot wounds and stab wounds. The mother generally fares better than the fetus if the penetrating trauma involves the abdomen because the enlarged uterus is likely to protect the mother's bowel from injury. Unfortunately, the fetal injury rate is high.

Treatment of major injuries during pregnancy focuses initially on life-saving measures for the woman. Such measures include establishing an airway, controlling external bleeding, and administering intravenous fluid to alleviate shock. The woman must be kept on her left side to prevent further hypotension. Oxygen is administered. Fetal heart rate and fetal movement are monitored. Exploratory surgery may be necessary following abdominal trauma to determine the extent of injuries. If the fetus is near term and the uterus has been damaged, cesarean birth is indicated. If the fetus is still immature, the uterus can often be repaired, and the pregnancy continues until term. In all cases, emotional support and information about the woman's condition and its implications for her and for her fetus are essential components of care.

In cases of trauma in which the mother's life is not directly threatened, fetal monitoring for 4 hours is suggested if there are no contractions, vaginal bleeding, uterine tenderness, or leaking amniotic fluid (American Academy of Pediatrics (AAP) & American College of Obstetricians and Gynecologists (ACOG), 2012). Abruptio placentae may occur following a blow to the abdomen. Increased uterine irritability in the first few hours after trauma helps identify women who may be at risk for this potentially catastrophic complication.

When cardiopulmonary resuscitation (CPR) is performed on the pregnant woman late in gestation, perimortem cesarean birth is advocated if CPR is unsuccessful in the first 4 minutes. Chest compressions are less effective in the third trimester because of compression of the inferior vena cava by the gravid uterus. Cesarean birth alleviates this compression and improves resuscitation efforts in both the fetus and the mother.

Care of the Pregnant Woman Who Has Experienced Intimate Partner Violence

Domestic abuse, also called *intimate partner violence (IPV)*, may be defined as the intentional injury of a woman by her partner. Domestic violence often begins or increases during pregnancy. Estimates suggest that approximately 25% of women in the United States have experienced physical and/or sexual violence by a current or former intimate partner (Devi, 2012). Physical abuse may result in loss of pregnancy, preterm labor, low-birth-weight newborns, and fetal death. Abused women have significantly higher rates of complications such as anemia, infection, low weight gain, pelvic fracture, and placental abruption.

Violence may escalate during pregnancy, and homicide by an intimate partner is a significant cause of maternal mortality (ACOG, 2012c).

The first step toward helping the battered woman is to identify her. Asking every woman about abuse at various times during pregnancy is crucial because a woman may not disclose abuse until she knows her caregivers better. Screening for abuse should be done at the first prenatal visit, at least once each trimester, and then again during the postpartum period (ACOG, 2012c).

Chronic psychosomatic symptoms can also be an indicator of abuse. The woman may have nonspecific or vague complaints. It is important to assess old scars around the head, chest, arms, abdomen, and genitalia and to evaluate any bruising or evidence of pain. The nurse should be especially alert for signs of bruising or injury to the woman's breasts, abdomen, or genitalia because these areas are common targets of violence during pregnancy. Other indicators include a decrease in eye contact; silence when the partner is in the room; and a history of nervousness, insomnia, drug overdose, or alcohol problems. Frequent visits to the emergency room and a history of accidents without understandable causes are possible indicators of abuse.

The goals of treatment are to identify the woman at risk, increase her decision-making abilities to decrease the potential for further abuse, and provide a safe environment for the pregnant woman and her unborn child. She needs to be aware of community resources available to her, such as emergency shelters; police, legal, and social services; and counseling. Ultimately, it is the woman's decision to either seek assistance or return to old patterns.

Because abuse often begins during pregnancy, it may be a new, unexpected experience for the woman, one she believes is an isolated incident. She needs to know that battering may continue after childbirth and may extend to the child as well. This is an important time for the nurse to provide information and establish a trusted link for the woman with a health professional. (For further discussion see Chapter 5.)

Care of the Woman With a Perinatal Infection Affecting the Fetus

Fetal infection may develop at any time during pregnancy. In general, perinatal infections are most likely to cause harm when the embryo is exposed during the first trimester when organ development is occurring. Infections that occur later in pregnancy create other concerns such as growth restriction, preterm birth, and neurologic changes. (The acronym TORCH—to identify **t**oxoplasmosis, **r**ubella, **c**ytomegalovirus, and **h**erpes—is occasionally used to identify the most common of these infections.) This section addresses several of the most commonly occurring viral and parasitic infections that may have an impact on the fetus if acquired during pregnancy.

Toxoplasmosis

Toxoplasmosis is caused by the protozoan *Toxoplasma gondii*. It is barely noticeable in adults, but, when contracted in pregnancy, it can profoundly affect the fetus and create long-term sequelae for affected children. The pregnant woman may contract the organism by eating raw or undercooked meat, by drinking unpasteurized goat's milk, or by contact with the feces of infected cats, either through the cat litter box or by gardening in areas frequented by cats.

FETAL/NEONATAL RISKS

The likelihood of fetal infection increases with each trimester of pregnancy, but the risk of serious impact on the fetus decreases. Thus maternal infection contracted during the first trimester is associated with the lowest incidence of fetal infection but the highest risk of severe fetal disease or death. The highest rate of fetal infection (70%) occurs when the mother contracts the infection in the third trimester (Martin & Satin, 2015). Most babies are born without clinical signs of infection. However, up to half of these babies will develop signs and symptoms if left untreated. In mild cases, retinochoroiditis (inflammation of the retina and choroid of the eye) may be the only recognizable damage, and it and other manifestations may not appear until adolescence or young adulthood. Severe neonatal disorders associated with congenital infection include convulsions, coma, microcephaly, and hydrocephalus. The newborn with a severe infection may die soon after birth. Survivors often are blind, are deaf, and have severe intellectual disabilities. Treatment of the mother can reduce the incidence of fetal infection and decrease the late sequelae of the infection (Duff, 2012).

CLINICAL THERAPY

Diagnosis can be made by serologic testing of antibody titers, specifically the IgG and IgM fluorescent antibody (IFA) tests. A positive IgG and negative IgM in the third trimester or any positive IgM result should be followed by confirmatory testing. Toxoplasmosis polymerase chain reaction (PCR) test of amniotic fluid is useful in diagnosing congenital toxoplasmosis. Ultrasound may be useful in detecting signs of fetal infection such as ascites, microcephaly, intracranial calcifications, and fetal growth restriction.

Pregnant women in whom maternal infection is established should receive spiramycin in the first and early second trimester and pyrimethamine/sulfadiazine and folinic acid (leucovorin) in the late second and third trimesters. Newborns with congenital infection are treated with pyrimethamine and leucovorin for one year (Centers for Disease Control and Prevention [CDC], 2015b).

Nursing Management

For the Pregnant Woman With Toxoplasmosis

Nursing Assessment and Diagnosis

The incubation period for the disease is 10 days. The woman with acute toxoplasmosis may be asymptomatic, or she may develop myalgia, malaise, rash, splenomegaly, and enlarged posterior cervical lymph nodes. Symptoms usually disappear in a few days or weeks.

Nursing diagnoses that might apply to the pregnant woman with toxoplasmosis include the following (NANDA-I © 2014):

- *Knowledge, Readiness for Enhanced,* related to a desire to understand the ways in which a pregnant woman can contract toxoplasmosis
- *Injury, Risk for,* related to toxoplasmosis infection

Nursing Plan and Implementation

Caring for women during the antepartum period provides the primary opportunity to discuss methods of preventing

toxoplasmosis. The woman must understand the importance of avoiding poorly cooked or raw meat, especially pork, beef, lamb, and, in the Arctic region, caribou. Fruits and vegetables should be washed. She should avoid contact with the cat litter box and have someone else clean it frequently, because it takes approximately 48 hours for a cat's feces to become infectious. Also discuss the importance of wearing gloves when gardening and of avoiding garden areas frequented by cats.

Evaluation

Expected outcomes of nursing care include the following:

- The woman is able to discuss toxoplasmosis, its methods of transmission, the implications for her fetus, and measures she can take to avoid contracting it.
- The woman implements health measures to avoid contracting toxoplasmosis.
- The woman gives birth to a healthy newborn.

Rubella

The effects of rubella (German measles) on the fetus and newborn are great because rubella causes a chronic infection that begins in the first trimester of pregnancy and may persist for months after birth. Fortunately, the success of the rubella vaccination program in the United States has led to a dramatic decrease in the incidence of rubella. Still, today there are pockets of unvaccinated people and cases continue to occur among babies born to women who emigrate from countries without rubella vaccination programs (AAP & ACOG, 2012).

FETAL/NEONATAL RISKS

The period of greatest risk for the teratogenic effects of rubella on the fetus is the first trimester. Defects are rare when infection develops after 20 weeks' gestation (AAP & ACOG, 2012). The most common clinical signs of congenital infection include congenital cataracts, sensorineural deafness, and congenital heart defects, particularly patent ductus arteriosus. Other abnormalities, such as intellectual disability or cerebral palsy, may become evident in infancy. Diagnosis in the newborn can be made in the presence of these conditions and with an elevated rubella IgM antibody titer at birth.

Neonates born with congenital rubella syndrome are infectious and should be isolated. These babies may continue to shed the virus for months.

CLINICAL THERAPY

The best therapy for rubella is prevention. Live attenuated vaccine is available and should be given to all children. Women of childbearing age should be tested for immunity and vaccinated if susceptible and if it is established that they are not pregnant. As part of the prenatal laboratory screen, the woman is evaluated for rubella using hemagglutination inhibition (HI), a serology test. The presence of an immunoglobulin G (IgG) titer of 1:10–1:20 or greater is evidence of immunity. A titer less than 1:8 indicates susceptibility to rubella. Because the vaccine is made with attenuated virus, pregnant women are not vaccinated. However, it is considered safe for newly vaccinated children to have contact with pregnant women.

If there is a question of an active rubella infection in a pregnant woman, serologic testing for IGM is done as early during the infection as possible and again 2 to 3 weeks later using an enzyme immunoassay test. If a woman who is pregnant becomes infected during the first trimester, therapeutic abortion may be an alternative.

Nursing Management

For the Woman Who Develops Rubella During Pregnancy

Nursing Assessment and Diagnosis

The woman may be asymptomatic or may show signs of a mild infection including a maculopapular rash, lymphadenopathy, muscular achiness, and joint pain. The presence of IgM antirubella antibody is diagnostic of a recent infection. These titers remain elevated for approximately 1 month after infection.

Nursing diagnoses that may apply to the woman who develops rubella early in her pregnancy include the following (NANDA-I © 2014):

- *Coping, Ineffective,* due to an inability to accept the possibility of fetal anomalies secondary to maternal rubella exposure
- *Health Maintenance, Ineffective,* related to lack of knowledge about the importance of rubella immunization before becoming pregnant

Nursing Plan and Implementation

Nursing support and understanding are vital for the couple contemplating abortion because of a diagnosis of rubella. Such a decision may initiate a crisis for the couple who has planned the pregnancy. The parents need objective data to understand the possible effects on their unborn fetus and the prognosis for the offspring.

Evaluation

Expected outcomes of nursing care include the following:

- The woman is able to describe the implications of rubella exposure during the first trimester of pregnancy.
- If exposure occurs in a woman who is not immune, she is able to identify her options and make a decision about continuing her pregnancy that is acceptable to her and her partner.
- The nonimmune woman receives the rubella vaccine during the early postpartum period.
- The woman gives birth to a healthy baby.

Cytomegalovirus

Cytomegalovirus (CMV) belongs to the herpes virus group and causes both congenital and acquired infections referred to as cytomegalic inclusion disease (CID). The significance of this virus in pregnancy is related to its ability to be transmitted by asymptomatic women across the placenta to the fetus or by the cervical route during birth.

The virus can be found in virtually all body fluids. It can be passed between humans by any close contact, such as kissing, breastfeeding, and sexual intercourse. Asymptomatic CMV infection is particularly common in children and pregnant women. It is a chronic, persistent infection in that the individual may shed the virus continually over many years. The cervix can harbor the virus, and an ascending infection can develop after birth. Although the virus is usually innocuous in adults and children, it may be fatal to the fetus.

Accurate diagnosis in the pregnant woman is best documented by seroconversion. Identification of the virus in amniotic fluid by polymerase chain reaction (PCR) or viral culture is the most specific way of diagnosing congenital infection (Bernstein, 2012). Ultrasound findings may include fetal hydrops, growth restriction, hydramnios, cardiomegaly, and fetal ascites. At present, no treatment exists for maternal CMV or for the congenital disease in the newborn.

CMV is the most frequent cause of viral infection in the human fetus. For the fetus/newborn, serious long-term complications most often follow a primary maternal infection in the first half of pregnancy (Bernstein, 2012). For the fetus, this infection can result in extensive intrauterine tissue damage that leads to fetal death; in survival with developmental delays, hearing loss, and visual and dental problems; or in survival with no damage at all (Martin & Satin, 2015). The infected newborn is often small for gestational age (SGA). The principal tissues and organs affected are the blood, brain, and liver; however, virtually all organs are potentially at risk.

At present, no treatment exists for maternal CMV. Thus, prevention is important. The pregnant woman should be advised to avoid areas with high concentrations of young children such as daycare centers, if possible, and to practice good handwashing techniques.

Herpes Simplex Virus

In the United States approximately 15.5% of people ages 14 to 49 are infected with genital herpes (CDC, 2015a). Herpes simplex virus (HSV-I or HSV-2) infection can cause painful lesions in the genital area. Lesions may also develop on the cervix. This condition and its implications for nonpregnant women are discussed in Chapter 6.

FETAL/NEONATAL RISKS

Primary infection poses the greatest risk to both the mother and her newborn. Primary infection has been associated with spontaneous abortion, low birth weight, and preterm birth. Transmission to the fetus almost always occurs after the membranes rupture and the virus ascends or during birth through an infected birth canal. Transplacental infection is rare. The risk to the fetus varies with the route of birth and whether the lesion that is present at the time of birth is primary or recurrent. If HSV-1 or HSV-2 is acquired close to the time of labor, the risk of transmission is 30% to 50% for a vaginal birth. Exposure of the newborn to a *recurrent* lesion drops the risk of transmission to less than 1% (CDC, 2015c).

The infected newborn is often asymptomatic at birth but develops symptoms of fever (or hypothermia), jaundice, seizures, and poor feeding any time after birth and up to 4 weeks of age. Approximately half of infected newborns develop the characteristic vesicular skin lesions. All newborns who have neonatal herpes should be evaluated promptly and treated with acyclovir (AAP & ACOG, 2012).

CLINICAL THERAPY

The vesicular lesions of herpes have a characteristic appearance, and they rupture easily. Definitive diagnosis is made by culturing active lesions.

Women with a primary HSV infection during pregnancy can be treated with oral acyclovir, valacyclovir, or famciclovir. Currently, there is no evidence that there are any adverse fetal effects related to exposure to any of these drugs during any trimester. For a woman with either a primary or a secondary outbreak of genital herpes during labor, or symptoms that may indicate an impending outbreak, the preferred method of childbirth is cesarean birth. Women who do not have any signs or symptoms of herpes or its prodromal symptoms at the onset of labor can give birth vaginally (CDC, 2015c).

Nursing Management

For the Pregnant Woman With Herpes Simplex Virus Infection

Nursing Assessment and Diagnosis

During the initial prenatal visit it is important to learn whether the woman or her partner has had previous herpes infections. Ongoing assessment is indicated as pregnancy progresses.

Nursing diagnoses that may apply to the pregnant woman with HSV infection include the following (NANDA-I © 2014):

- *Pain, Acute*, related to the presence of lesions secondary to herpes infection
- *Coping, Ineffective*, related to depression secondary to the risk to the fetus if herpes lesions are present at birth

Nursing Plan and Implementation

Client education about this fast-spreading disease is crucial. Inform women of the association of HSV infection with spontaneous abortion, newborn mortality and morbidity, and the possibility of cesarean birth. A woman needs to inform all healthcare providers of her infection. She should also know of the possible association of genital herpes with cervical cancer and the importance of a yearly Papanicolaou (Pap) smear.

The woman who acquired HSV infection as an adolescent may be devastated as a mature young adult who wants to have a family. Clients may be helped by counseling that allows them to express the anger, shame, and depression often experienced by those with herpes. Literature may be helpful and is available from many public health agencies.

Evaluation

Expected outcomes of nursing care include the following:

- The woman is able to describe her infection with regard to its method of spread, therapy and comfort measures, implications for her pregnancy, and long-term implications.
- The woman gives birth to a healthy newborn.

Group B Streptococcal Infection

Group B streptococcus (GBS) infection causes a bacterial infection found in the lower GI or urogenital tract. Women may transmit GBS infection to their fetus in utero or during childbirth. GBS is one of the major causes of early-onset neonatal infection. Newborns become infected in one of two ways: by vertical transmission from the mother during birth or by horizontal transmission from colonized nursing personnel or colonized babies.

GBS causes severe, invasive disease in newborns. The majority of cases occur within the first week of life and are designated as early-onset disease. Late-onset disease occurs 1 week or more after birth. Early-onset GBS is often characterized by signs of serious illness including pneumonia, apnea, and shock. Mortality is 11% to 50% (Martin & Satin, 2015). Babies with late-onset GBS often develop meningitis. Long-term neurologic complications are common in both types of

GBS. Fortunately, improved recognition and rapid treatment of infected newborns has reduced mortality and morbidity rates significantly.

Risk factors for GBS neonatal sepsis include young maternal age, African American or Hispanic race, preterm labor, maternal intrapartum fever, prolonged rupture of the membranes, previous birth of an infected baby, and GBS bacteriuria in the current pregnancy. Guidelines for the detection and preventive treatment of newborns at risk include the following (CDC, 2014):

- All pregnant women should be screened for both vaginal and rectal GBS colonization at 35 to 37 weeks' gestation. Treatment should be based on these results, even if cultures were done earlier in pregnancy.
- Women identified as GBS carriers should receive antibiotic prophylaxis at the onset of labor or the rupture of membranes.
- Women with GBS in their urine in any concentration should be treated according to guidelines for treating urinary tract infections (UTIs) during pregnancy and should receive antibiotic prophylaxis intrapartally. These women do not need vaginal and rectal cultures at 35 to 37 weeks' gestation because therapy is already indicated.
- Women who have already given birth to a newborn with invasive GBS disease should receive intrapartum antibiotic prophylaxis. Culture-based screening is not necessary for them.
- If the results of GBS screening are not known when labor begins, prophylaxis is indicated for women with any of the following risk factors: gestation less than 37 weeks, membranes ruptured 18 hours or longer, temperature equal to or greater than 38.0°C (100.4°F).

Intrapartum antibiotic therapy is recommended as follows: initial loading dose of penicillin G 5 million units intravenously (IV) followed by 2.5 million units IV every 4 hours until childbirth. Alternately, ampicillin may be used. In women at high risk for an anaphylactic reaction to penicillin because of marked allergy, testing is done to see if the organism is susceptible to clindamycin and erythromycin. If the organism is susceptible, clindamycin is used. If the organism is resistant or if susceptibility testing is not done, vancomycin is administered (Martin & Satin, 2015).

Intrapartum prophylaxis is *not* indicated for women with intact membranes who have a planned cesarean birth before labor begins, for women who had positive GBS screening culture in a previous pregnancy but have negative cultures in the current pregnancy, and women who have negative GBS cultures in late pregnancy regardless of risk factors (CDC, 2014).

Other Infections in Pregnancy

Table 15–1 summarizes other urinary tract, vaginal, and sexually transmitted infections that contribute to risk during pregnancy. (These are described in detail in Chapter 6.) Spontaneous abortion is frequently the result of a severe maternal infection. Some evidence links infection and prematurity. In addition, if the pregnancy is carried to term in the presence of infection, the risk of maternal and fetal morbidity and mortality increases. Thus it is essential to maternal and fetal health that infection be diagnosed and treated promptly.

TABLE 15–1 Infections That Put Pregnancy at Risk

CONDITION AND CAUSATIVE ORGANISM	SIGNS AND SYMPTOMS	TREATMENT	IMPLICATIONS FOR PREGNANCY
URINARY TRACT INFECTIONS (UTIS)			
Asymptomatic bacteriuria (ASB): *Escherichia, Klebsiella, Proteus* most common	Bacteria present in urine on culture with no accompanying symptoms.	Oral sulfonamides early in pregnancy, ampicillin and nitrofurantoin (Furadantin) in late pregnancy. Antibody sensitivity results will guide the selection of an appropriate antibiotic.	Women with ASB in early pregnancy may go on to develop cystitis or acute pyelonephritis by third trimester if not treated. They are also at risk for preterm labor. Oral sulfonamides taken in the last few weeks of pregnancy may lead to neonatal hyperbilirubinemia and kernicterus.
Cystitis (lower UTI): causative organisms same as for ASB	Dysuria, urgency, frequency; low-grade fever and hematuria may occur. Urine culture (clean catch) shows c leukocytes. Presence of 10^5 (100,000) or more colonies bacteria per milliliter of urine.	Same as for ASB	If not treated, infection may ascend and lead to acute pyelonephritis. Suppressive therapy is recommended for bacteriuria that persists after two or more courses of therapy during pregnancy.
Acute pyelonephritis: causative organisms same as for ASB	Sudden onset. Chills, high fever, flank pain. Nausea, vomiting, malaise. May have decreased urine output, severe colicky pain, dehydration. Increased diastolic blood pressure (BP), positive fluorescent antibody (FA) test, low creatinine clearance. Marked bacteremia in urine culture, pyuria, white blood cell (WBC) casts.	Hospitalization; IV antibiotic therapy. Other antibiotics safe during pregnancy include carbenicillin, methenamine, cephalosporins. Catheterization if there is no urine output. Supportive therapy for comfort. Follow-up urine cultures are necessary.	Increased risk of premature birth and intrauterine growth restriction (IUGR). These antibiotics interfere with urinary estriol levels and can cause false interpretations of estriol levels during pregnancy.
VAGINAL INFECTIONS			
Vulvovaginal candidiasis (yeast infection): *Candida albicans*	Often thick, white, curdy discharge; severe itching, dysuria, dyspareunia. Diagnosis based on presence of hyphae and spores in a wet-mount preparation of vaginal secretions.	Only topical agents are recommended. Intravaginal insertion of miconazole, butoconazole, or other topical azole preparation at bedtime for 7 days (CDC, 2015c).	If the infection is present at birth and the fetus is born vaginally, the fetus may contract thrush.
Bacterial vaginosis: *Gardnerella vaginalis*	Thin, watery, yellow-gray discharge with foul odor often described as "fishy." Wet-mount preparation reveals "clue cells." Application of potassium hydroxide (KOH) to a specimen of vaginal secretions produces a pronounced fishy odor.	Treatment recommended for symptomatic pregnant women. Metronidazole (Flagyl) 500 mg PO bid × 7 days or metronidazole gel 0.75%, one full applicator (5 g) intravaginally at bedtime × 7 days or clindamycin cream 2%, one full applicator (5 g) intravaginally at bedtime × 7 days (CDC, 2015c).	CDC (2015c) reports that multiple studies have failed to demonstrate a teratogenic effect from metronidazole.
Trichomoniasis: *Trichomonas vaginalis*	Occasionally asymptomatic. May have frothy greenish gray vaginal discharge, pruritus, urinary symptoms. Strawberry patches may be visible on vaginal walls or cervix. Wet-mount preparation of vaginal secretions shows motile flagellated trichomonas.	Single 2-g dose of metronidazole orally (CDC, 2015c). While tinidazole is an alternative treatment for nonpregnant women, it should be avoided during pregnancy.	Increased risk for premature rupture of membranes (PROM), preterm birth, and low birth weight.
SEXUALLY TRANSMITTED INFECTIONS			
Chlamydial infection: *Chlamydia trachomatis*	Women are often asymptomatic. Symptoms may include thin or purulent discharge, urinary burning and frequency, or lower abdominal pain. Lab test available to detect monoclonal antibodies specific for *Chlamydia*.	Doxycycline, ofloxacin, and levofloxacin are contraindicated during pregnancy. Thus, pregnant women are treated with azithromycin or amoxicillin followed by repeat culture in 3 weeks (CDC, 2015c).	Newborn of woman with untreated chlamydial infection may develop neonatal conjunctivitis, which can be treated with erythromycin eye ointment (but not silver nitrate). Newborn may also develop chlamydial pneumonia. May be responsible for premature labor and fetal death.

(continued)

TABLE 15–2 Infections That Put Pregnancy at Risk (continued)

CONDITION AND CAUSATIVE ORGANISM	SIGNS AND SYMPTOMS	TREATMENT	IMPLICATIONS FOR PREGNANCY
Syphilis: *Treponema pallidum*, a spirochete	Primary stage: chancre, slight fever, malaise. Chancre lasts about 4 weeks, then disappears. Secondary stage: occurs 6 weeks to 6 months after infection. Skin eruptions (condylomata lata) are also symptoms of acute arthritis, liver enlargement, iritis, chronic sore throat with hoarseness. Diagnosed by blood tests such as VDRL, RPR, FTA, ABS. Dark-field examination for spirochetes may also be done.	Treatment of pregnant woman follows the regimen recommended for the general population and is based on the stage of syphilis. For syphilis less than 1 year in duration: single dose of 2.4 million units benzathine penicillin G intramuscularly (IM). For syphilis of more than 1 year's duration or latent syphilis of unknown duration: 2.4 million units benzathine penicillin G once a week for 3 weeks. Sexual partners should also be screened and treated (CDC, 2015c).	Syphilis can be passed transplacentally to the fetus. If untreated, one of the following can occur: second trimester abortion, stillborn baby at term, congenitally infected newborn, uninfected live newborn.
Gonorrhea: *Neisseria gonorrhoeae*	Majority of women asymptomatic; disease often diagnosed during routine prenatal cervical culture. If symptoms are present they may include purulent vaginal discharge, dysuria, urinary frequency, inflammation, and swelling of the vulva. Cervix may appear eroded.	Quinolones (ofloxacin, levofloxacin) and tetracyclines are not used to treat pregnant women. Pregnant women are treated with ceftriaxone 250 mg. in a single IM dose and azithromycin 1 g. orally in a single dose (CDC, 2015c). All sexual partners are also treated.	Infection at time of birth may cause ophthalmia neonatorum in the newborn.
Condylomata acuminata (genital warts): caused by human papilloma virus (HPV)	Soft, grayish pink lesions on the vulva, vagina, cervix, or anus.	Podophyllin, podofilox, sinecatechins, and imiquimod are contraindicated during pregnancy. Some caregivers recommend removing warts by surgical methods or laser because the warts can proliferate and become friable (bleed easily) during pregnancy but the results may be poor or incomplete (CDC, 2015c).	Possible teratogenic effect of podophyllin. Large doses have been associated with fetal death. Cesarean birth is indicated only for women with warts that obstruct the pelvic outlet or if vaginal birth would result in significant bleeding (CDC, 2015c).

Clinical Reasoning Preventing Cystitis

Your friend Jena Yoo, G1P0, is 6 months pregnant and mentions to you that she is developing symptoms of a bladder infection. She has had several bladder infections over the past few years and feels she has warded off others by increasing her fluid intake and drinking acidic juices. Jena tells you that she plans to use the same approach this time because she just had her prenatal appointment last week. She assures you that if symptoms persist, she will discuss it with her caregiver at her next prenatal visit.

What advice would you give her?

Care of the Woman at Risk for Rh Alloimmunization

The Rh blood antigen, or Rh factor, is present on the surface of erythrocytes in a majority of the population. When it is present, a person is designated as Rh positive. Those without the factor are designated as Rh negative. If an Rh-negative individual is exposed to Rh-positive blood (antigen Rh[D]), an antigen–antibody response occurs, and the person forms anti-Rh agglutinin and is said to be *sensitized*. Subsequent exposure to Rh-positive blood can then cause a serious reaction that results in agglutination and hemolysis of red blood cells. In the United States about 15% of Whites and 8% of African Americans and Hispanic Americans are Rh-negative (Vander Tuig & Blakemore, 2015).

Rh *alloimmunization* (sensitization), also called *isoimmunization*, most often occurs when an Rh-negative woman carries an Rh-positive fetus, either to term or to termination by spontaneous or induced abortion. It can also occur if an Rh-negative nonpregnant woman receives an Rh-positive blood transfusion.

The red blood cells (RBCs) from the fetus invade the maternal circulation, thereby stimulating the production of Rh antibodies. Because this transfer of RBCs usually occurs at birth, the first child is not affected. In a subsequent pregnancy, however, Rh antibodies cross the placenta and enter the fetal circulation, causing severe hemolysis. The destruction of fetal RBCs causes anemia in the fetus (Figure 15–6).

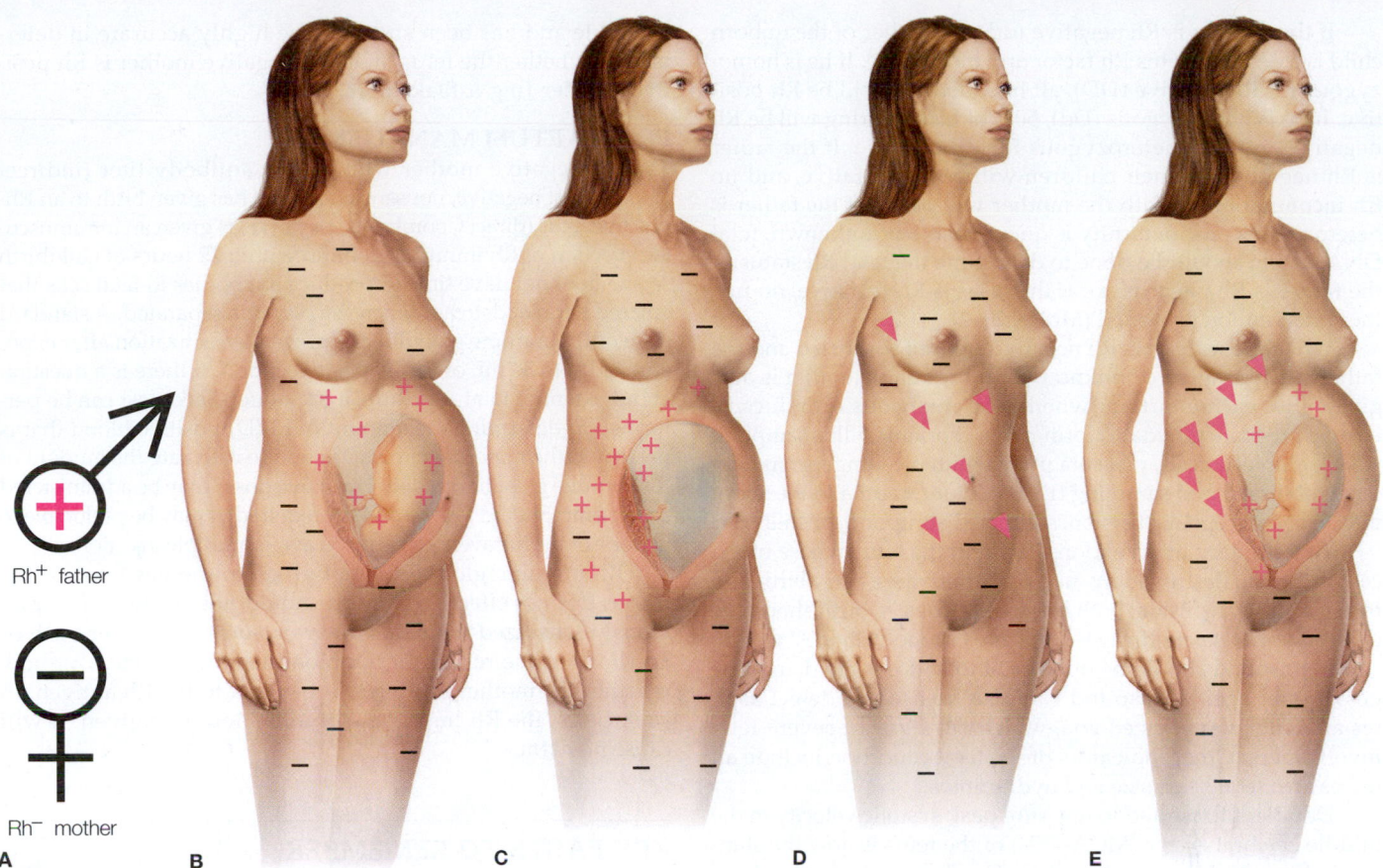

Figure 15–6 Rh alloimmunization sequence. A. Rh-positive father and Rh-negative mother. B. Pregnancy with Rh-positive fetus. Some Rh-positive blood enters the mother's blood. C. As the placenta separates, the mother is further exposed to the Rh-positive blood. D. The mother is sensitized to the Rh-positive blood; anti-Rh-positive antibodies (triangles) are formed. E. In subsequent pregnancies with an Rh-positive fetus, Rh-positive red blood cells are attacked by the anti-Rh-positive maternal antibodies, causing hemolysis of red blood cells in the fetus.

Healthy People 2020

(BDBS-18.4) Reduce the proportions of persons who develop adverse events due to alloimmunization among persons with hemoglobinopathies

---

Fetal/Neonatal Risks

If treatment with Rh immune globulin is not initiated, the hemolysis caused by the maternal IgG antibodies in the fetus will create fetal anemia. The anemia can cause marked fetal edema, called **hydrops fetalis**. Congestive heart failure may result; marked jaundice (called *icterus gravis*), which can lead to neurologic damage (*kernicterus*), is also possible. This severe hemolytic syndrome is known as **erythroblastosis fetalis**.

Screening for Rh Incompatibility and Alloimmunization

At the first prenatal visit, healthcare providers should do the following:

1. Take a history of past pregnancies, previous sensitization, abortions, blood transfusions, or children who developed jaundice or anemia during the newborn period.

2. Determine maternal blood type (ABO) and Rh factor and do a routine Rh antibody screen.

3. Identify other medical complications such as diabetes, infections, or hypertension.

An antibody screen (*indirect Coombs test*) is done to determine whether an Rh-negative woman is sensitized (has developed isoimmunity) to the Rh antigen. The test measures the number of antibodies in the maternal blood. If the pregnant woman is not sensitized, a second antibody screening test is done at 28 weeks' gestation. If the maternal antibody screen is positive, a maternal antibody titer is obtained. A woman with an elevated antibody titer should be considered sensitized and her pregnancy should be managed closely.

Clinical Therapy

ANTEPARTUM MANAGEMENT

If the antibody screen obtained at 28 weeks' gestation is negative, the woman is given 300 mcg of **Rh immune globulin (RhoGAM)** intramuscularly as a prophylactic (preventive) measure. Rh immune globulin provides passive antibody protection against Rh antigens. This "tricks" the body, which does not then produce antibodies of its own (active immunity).

Rh⁺ father

Rh⁻ mother

A   B   C   D   E

If the woman is Rh negative (dd), the father of the unborn child is assessed for his Rh factor and blood type. If he is homozygous for Rh positive (DD), all his offspring will be Rh positive. If he is heterozygous (Dd), 50% of his offspring will be Rh negative and 50% heterozygous for Rh positive. If the father is Rh negative, all their children will be Rh negative, and no Rh incompatibility with the mother will occur. If the father is heterozygous or if paternity is questionable or unknown, fetal DNA testing should be done to determine the fetal Rh status. If the father is Rh negative, or if the fetus is Rh negative, no further intervention is needed (Moise, 2012).

When the woman is Rh negative and not sensitized and the father is Rh positive or unknown, Rh immune globulin is also given after each abortion (whether spontaneous or induced), ectopic pregnancy, hydatidiform mole, chorionic villus sampling (CVS), amniocentesis, placenta previa with bleeding, percutaneous umbilical blood sampling (PUBS), blunt trauma to the abdomen, external cephalic version, suspected abruption, or stillbirth.

Two primary interventions can help the fetus whose blood cells are being destroyed by maternal antibodies: early birth and intrauterine transfusion; both carry risks. Ideally, birth should be delayed until fetal maturity is confirmed at about 36 to 37 weeks.

Ultrasound should be done at 14 to 16 weeks to determine gestational age. Ultrasound can also be used to detect ascites and subcutaneous edema, which are signs of severe fetal involvement. Other indicators of the fetal condition include an increase in fetal heart size and hydramnios.

Doppler ultrasound to measure peak systolic velocity in the middle cerebral artery (MCA-PSV) of the fetus is now the standard of care to detect fetal anemia. The decreasing fetal red cell mass and concurrent decrease in blood viscosity results in an increase in fetal cardiac output and an increase in the velocity of blood flow through the middle cerebral artery, which is demonstrated by an increase in the peak systolic velocities (Vander Tuig & Blakemore, 2015). MCA-PSV trends over time correlate well with increasing levels of bilirubin in the amniotic fluid and should be monitored regularly starting at 15 to 18 weeks. After 35 weeks' gestation, the reliability of MCA Doppler decreases.

Historically, management of Rh disease was done with ΔOD analysis (delta optical density), a test that determines the amount of bilirubin pigment found in the amniotic fluid. Normally the concentration of bilirubin pigments in the amniotic fluid declines during pregnancy. Elevated bilirubin levels are significant. Because the amount of bilirubin found in the amniotic fluid correlates roughly with the extent of the hemolysis, the ΔOD analysis serves as an indirect predictor of the severity of the fetal anemia. It should be used only if MCA screening is not available.

Negative antibody titers can consistently identify the fetus not at risk. However, the titers cannot reliably point out the fetus in danger, because titer level does not always correlate with the severity of the disease. Thus, if the maternal antibody titer is 1:16 or greater, further testing is indicated.

If MCA-PSV is elevated, indicating severe fetal anemia, or if fetal hydrops is present, percutaneous umbilical blood sampling (PUBS) (see Chapter 7) may be performed to determine fetal hematocrit. If the hematocrit is low (generally less than 30%), the fetus is given an intrauterine blood transfusion either intravascularly through PUBS or intraperitoneally. If the fetal hematocrit is greater than 30%, the PUBS is repeated in 1 to 2 weeks (Moise & Argoti, 2012). Severely sensitized fetuses may require birth at 32 to 34 weeks.

Fetal DNA can be found in the maternal circulation as early as day 38. Fetal genotyping from maternal blood is now available and has been shown to be highly accurate in determining whether the fetus of an Rh-negative mother is Rh positive (Vander Tuig & Blakemore, 2015).

POSTPARTUM MANAGEMENT

The Rh-negative mother who has no antibody titer (indirect Coombs test negative, nonsensitized) and has given birth to an Rh-positive fetus (direct Coombs test negative) is given an intramuscular injection of Rh immune globulin within 72 hours of childbirth so she does not have time to produce antibodies to fetal cells that entered her bloodstream when the placenta separated. A standard dose of Rh immune globulin can prevent sensitization after exposure of up to 30 mL of Rh(D) positive blood. If there is a question about extent of fetal exposure, a Kleihauer-Betke test can be performed to determine the amount of Rh(D)-positive blood that is present in the maternal circulation and to calculate the amount of Rh immune globulin needed. Up to five doses may be administered at one time. Should a large dose be required, it may be preferable to use one of the intravenous forms to avoid multiple injections.

Rh immune globulin is not given to the newborn or the father. It is not effective for, and should not be given to, a previously sensitized woman. However, sometimes after birth or an abortion the results of the blood test do not clearly show whether the mother is already sensitized to the Rh antigen. In such cases, the Rh immune globulin should be given; it will cause no harm.

KEY FACTS TO REMEMBER
Rh Sensitization

When trying to work through Rh problems, the nurse should remember the following:

- A potential problem exists when an Rh-negative mother and an Rh-positive father conceive a child who is Rh positive.
- In this situation, the mother may become sensitized or produce antibodies to her fetus's Rh-positive blood.

The following tests are used to detect sensitization:

- Indirect Coombs test—done on the mother's blood to measure the number of Rh-positive antibodies
- Direct Coombs test—done on the newborn's blood to detect antibody-coated Rh-positive red blood cells (RBCs)

Based on the results of these tests, the following may be done:

- If the mother's indirect Coombs test is negative and her newborn's direct Coombs test is negative (confirming that sensitization has not occurred), the mother is given Rh immune globulin within 72 hours of birth.
- If the mother's indirect Coombs test is positive and her Rh-positive newborn has a positive direct Coombs test, Rh immune globulin is *not* given; in this case, the baby is carefully monitored for hemolytic disease.
- It is recommended that Rh immune globulin be given antenatally at 28 weeks to decrease possible transplacental bleeding concerns.
- Rh immune globulin is also administered after each abortion (spontaneous or therapeutic), antepartum hemorrhage, mismatched blood transfusion, ectopic pregnancy, amniocentesis, chorionic villi sampling (CVS), percutaneous umbilical blood sampling (PUBS), fetal cephalic version, or maternal trauma.

Nursing Management

For the Pregnant Woman With Alloimmunization

Nursing Assessment and Diagnosis

As part of the initial prenatal history, ask the mother if she knows her blood type and Rh factor. Many women are aware that they are Rh negative and that this status has implications for pregnancy. If the woman knows she is Rh negative, assess the woman's knowledge of what that means. Ask the woman if she has ever received Rh immune globulin, if she has had any previous pregnancies and what their outcome was, and if she knows her partner's Rh factor. If the partner is Rh negative, there is no risk to the fetus, who will also be Rh negative.

If the woman does not know what Rh type she is, intervention cannot begin until the initial laboratory data have been obtained. Once that is done, plan care based on the findings.

If the woman becomes sensitized during her pregnancy, nursing assessment focuses on the knowledge and coping skills of the woman and her family. Provide ongoing assessment during procedures, such as ultrasound and amniocentesis, to evaluate fetal well-being.

After birth, review data about the Rh type of the fetus. If the newborn is Rh positive, the mother is Rh negative, and no sensitization has occurred, nursing assessment reveals the need to administer Rh immune globulin. If both the mother and her newborn are Rh negative, Rh immune globulin is not indicated.

Nursing diagnoses that might apply to the pregnant woman at risk for Rh sensitization include the following (NANDA-I © 2014):

- *Knowledge, Readiness for Enhanced*, related to an expressed desire to understand the treatment of Rh incompatibility and information about the purpose of RhIgG
- *Coping, Ineffective*, related to depression secondary to the development of indications of the need for fetal exchange transfusion

Nursing Plan and Implementation

During the antepartum period explain the mechanisms involved in alloimmunization and answer any questions the woman and her partner have. It is imperative that the woman understand the importance of receiving Rh immune globulin after every spontaneous or therapeutic abortion or ectopic pregnancy. Explain the purpose of the Rh immune globulin administered at 28 weeks' gestation if the woman is not sensitized.

If the woman is sensitized to the Rh factor, it poses a threat to any Rh-positive fetus she carries. Provide emotional support to the family to help the members deal with their grief and any feelings of guilt about the baby's condition. If an intrauterine transfusion becomes necessary, continue to provide emotional support while also assuming responsibility as part of the healthcare team.

During the labor of an Rh-negative woman who has not been sensitized, ensure that the woman's blood is assessed for any antibodies and also has been crossmatched for Rh immune globulin. On the postpartum unit, the nurse generally is responsible for administering the Rh immune globulin intramuscularly if the newborn is Rh positive (see *Clinical Skill: Intramuscular Administration of Rh Immune Globulin*).

Clinical Skill 15–2

Intramuscular Administration of Rh Immune Globulin (RhoGAM, HyperRHO, Rhophlac, WinRho-SDF)

NURSING ACTION

Preparation

- Confirm that Rh immune globulin is indicated by checking the woman's prenatal or intrapartum record to verify that she is Rh negative. Then confirm that sensitization has not occurred—maternal indirect Coombs negative. Postpartum, confirm that the baby is Rh positive but not sensitized (direct Coombs negative) and that the mother's indirect Coombs is negative. Rh immune globulin is *not* indicated if the newborn is Rh negative, too.

Rationale: Rh immune globulin is only indicated for Rh-negative, unsensitized women.

- Confirm that the woman does not have a history of allergies to immune globulin preparations by checking entries on medication allergies in her medical record and by asking her whether she has ever had any allergic reactions to medications, globulins, or blood products.

Rationale: Rh immune globulin is made from the plasma portion of blood. Allergic reactions are possible.

- Explain purpose and procedure. Have consent form signed if required by agency policy.

Rationale: Many agencies require separate consent for the administration of Rh immune globulin because it is a blood product. The woman should clearly understand the purpose of the Rh immune globulin, its rationale, the administration procedure, and any related risks. Generally the primary side effects are redness and tenderness at the injection site and allergic responses.

Equipment and Supplies

- Rh immune globulin, which is obtained from the blood bank or pharmacy according to agency protocol. Lot numbers for the drug and the crossmatch should be the same.
- Syringe and IM needle

Procedure

1. Confirm the woman's identity and administer one vial of 300 mcg Rh immune globulin IM in the deltoid muscle.

Rationale: The normal 300-mcg dose provides passive immunity following exposure to 15 mL of transfused RBCs or 30 mL of fetal blood.

(continued)

Clinical Skill 13–1 (*continued*)

2. An immune globulin microdose is used after miscarriage, elective abortion, ectopic pregnancy, or molar pregnancy occurring within the first 12 weeks' gestation. Antepartum, the Rh immune globulin is generally given within 3 hours of, but not longer than 72 hours after, the event.

3. If a larger bleed is suspected at birth (as in cases of severe abruptio placentae), additional doses may be administered at one time using multiple sites at regular intervals as long as all doses are given within 72 hours of childbirth.

4. Provide opportunities for the woman to ask questions and express concerns.

   Rationale: *Many women, especially primigravidas, are not aware of the risks for an Rh-positive fetus of a sensitized Rh-negative mother. They need to understand the importance of receiving Rh immune globulin for each pregnancy to ensure continued protection.*

5. Document according to agency policy. Most agencies document lot number, route, dose, and client education.

Clinical Tip

In most cases, Rh immune globulin is administered in the deltoid muscle. However, in an extremely thin woman, or in the cases of a larger-than-normal dose, consider administering the medication in the ventrogluteal or posterior gluteal site. You may also divide the dose into multiple injections. Both Rhophlac and WinRho-SDF may be administered intravenously.

Evaluation

Expected outcomes of nursing care include the following:

- The woman is able to explain the process of Rh sensitization and its implications for her unborn child and for subsequent pregnancies.

- If the woman has not been sensitized, she is able to discuss the importance of receiving Rh immune globulin when necessary and cooperates with the recommended dosage schedule.

- The woman gives birth to a healthy newborn.

- If complications develop for the fetus or newborn, they are detected quickly and therapy is instituted.

Care of the Woman at Risk Because of ABO Incompatibility

ABO incompatibility is somewhat common but rarely causes significant hemolysis. In most cases, ABO incompatibility is limited to type O mothers with a type A or B fetus. The group B fetus of a group A mother and the group A fetus of a group B mother are only occasionally affected. Group O fetuses, because they have no antigenic sites on the red blood cells (RBCs), are never affected regardless of the mother's blood type. The incompatibility occurs as a result of the maternal antibodies present in her serum and interaction between the antigen sites on the fetal RBCs.

Anti-A and anti-B antibodies are naturally occurring; that is, women are naturally exposed to the A and B antigens through the foods they eat and through exposure to infection by gram-negative bacteria. As a result, some women have high serum anti-A and anti-B titers before they become pregnant. Once they become pregnant, the maternal serum anti-A and anti-B antibodies cross the placenta and produce hemolysis of the fetal red blood cells. With ABO incompatibility, the first newborn is frequently involved, and no relationship exists between the appearance of the disease and repeated sensitization from one pregnancy to the next.

Unlike Rh incompatibility, antepartum treatment is not warranted because it does not cause severe anemia. As part of the initial assessment, however, the nurse should note whether the potential for an ABO incompatibility exists (type O mother and type A or B father). This alerts caregivers so that, following birth, the newborn can be assessed carefully for the development of hyperbilirubinemia (discussed in Chapter 27).

Focus Your Study

- Several health problems associated with bleeding arise from the pregnancy itself, such as spontaneous abortion, ectopic pregnancy, and gestational trophoblastic disease. The nurse needs to be alert to early signs of these situations, to guard the woman against heavy bleeding and shock, to facilitate the medical treatment, and to provide educational and emotional support.

- Hyperemesis gravidarum, excessive vomiting during pregnancy, may cause fluid and electrolyte imbalance, dehydration, and signs of starvation in the mother and, if severe enough, death of the fetus. Treatment is aimed at controlling the vomiting, correcting fluid and electrolyte imbalance, correcting dehydration, and improving nutritional status.

- Hypertension may exist before pregnancy or, more often, may develop during pregnancy. Preeclampsia can lead to growth retardation for the fetus and, if untreated, may lead to convulsions (eclampsia) and even death for the mother and the fetus.

A woman's understanding of the disease process helps motivate her to maintain the required rest periods in the left lateral position.

- The impact of surgery or trauma on the pregnant woman and her fetus is related to timing in the pregnancy, seriousness of the situation, and other factors influencing the situation.

- Physical violence often begins or continues during pregnancy. The nurse needs to be alert for signs of abuse, including bruising or injury to the breasts, abdomen, and genitals. The nurse should provide the woman information about violence and about community resources available to assist her.

- Therapy for severe preeclampsia usually includes bedrest, antihypertensives, anticonvulsive drugs, and careful monitoring of mother and fetus. Corticosteroids may also be indicated.

- Toxoplasmosis, rubella, cytomegalovirus, herpes, group B streptococcus (GBS) infection, and other perinatal infections all pose a grave threat to the fetus. Prevention is the best therapy. There is no known treatment for rubella, but antimicrobial drugs are available for toxoplasmosis, herpes, and GBS. A vaccine for CMV may be available in the near future.

- Universal screening for GBS is now recommended for all pregnant women at 35 to 37 weeks' gestation.

- Rh incompatibility can exist when an Rh-negative woman and an Rh-positive partner conceive a child who is Rh positive. The use of Rh immune globulin has greatly decreased the incidence of severe sequelae due to Rh incompatibility because the drug "tricks" the body into thinking antibodies have been produced in response to the Rh antigen.

Clinical Reasoning in Action

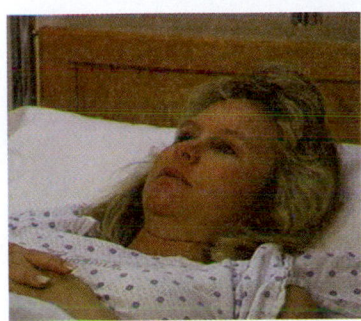

Carol Smith, a 40-year-old, single G2P0010, presents to you at 32 weeks' gestation while you are working in the birthing unit. Her chief complaint is severe headache, nausea, and trouble seeing. She describes "blackened areas" in her visual fields bilaterally. Her prenatal record reveals long-term substance abuse, depression, and hypertension currently treated with nifedipine 60 mg by mouth once in the morning. You note that she has had two prenatal visits with this pregnancy. You determine her blood pressure to be 170/110; deep tendon reflexes are 3+, clonus negative. She has general edema and 3+ proteinuria. You place Carol on the external fetal monitor to observe for fetal well-being and any contractions. You position her on her left side with her head elevated and use pillows for comfort. You observe that the fetal heart rate is 143–148 with decreased long-term variability. No fetal heart rate decelerations or accelerations are noted. The uterus is soft, and no contractions are palpated or noted on the fetal monitor.

Carol asks you why she should stay on her left side.

1. How would you explain the importance of the left side-lying position when on bedrest?

2. You administer nifedipine 10 mg sublingual and a loading dose of magnesium sulfate 4 gm IV piggyback to the main IV line of Ringer lactate. What findings would indicate that Carol has therapeutic levels of magnesium?

3. What signs of magnesium toxicity should you monitor Carol for?

4. Carol asks if magnesium sulfate will affect her baby. How would you answer her?

5. Identify the signs of premature labor that Carol should be alert for and report to you.

References

American Academy of Pediatrics (AAP) & American College of Obstetricians and Gynecologists (ACOG). (2012). *Guidelines for perinatal care.* Elk Grove Village, IL: Author.

American College of Obstetricians and Gynecologists (ACOG). (2012a). *Chronic hypertension in pregnancy* (Practice Bulletin No. 125). Washington, DC: Author.

American College of Obstetricians and Gynecologists (ACOG). (2012b). *Diagnosis and treatment of gestational trophoblastic disease* (ACOG Practice Bulletin No. 53). Washington, DC: Author.

American College of Obstetricians and Gynecologists (ACOG). (2012c). *Intimate partner violence* (Committee Opinion, No. 518). Washington, DC: Author.

American College of Obstetricians and Gynecologists (ACOG). (2013). *Hypertension in pregnancy.* Washington, DC: Author.

American College of Obstetricians and Gynecologists (ACOG). (2015). *Emergent therapy for acute-onset severe hypertension during pregnancy and the postpartum period* (Committee Opinion No. 623, Replaces No. 514). Washington, DC: Author.

Bernstein, H. B. (2012). Maternal and perinatal infection—Viral. In S. G. Gabbe, J. R. Niebyl, J. L. Simpson, M. B. Landon, H. L. Galan, E. R. M. Jauniaux, & D. A. Driscoll (Eds.), *Obstetrics: Normal and problem pregnancies* (6th ed.). Philadelphia, PA: Elsevier Saunders.

Blackburn, S. T. (2013). *Maternal, fetal, and neonatal physiology: A clinical perspective* (4th ed.). St. Louis, MO: Saunders.

Centers for Disease Control and Prevention (CDC). (2014). Prevention of perinatal group B streptococcal disease: Revised guidelines from CDC, 2010. *Morbidity and Mortality Weekly Report, 59*(RR10), 1–32.

Centers for Disease Control and Prevention (CDC). (2015a). Genital herpes—CDC fact sheet. Retrieved from http://www.cdc.gov/std/Herpes/STDFact-Herpes-detailed.htm

Centers for Disease Control and Prevention (CDC). (2015b). *Parasites—Toxoplasmosis (Toxoplasma infection).* Retrieved from http://www.cdc.gov/parasites/toxoplasmosis/health_professionals/index.html

Centers for Disease Control and Prevention (CDC). (2015c). Sexually transmitted diseases treatment guidelines, 2015. *Morbidity and Mortality Weekly Report (MMWR), 64*(RR3), 1–137.

Cobb, L., & Giuntoli II, R. L. (2015). Gestational Trophoblastic Disease. In C. T. Johnson, J. L. Hallock, J. L. Bienstock, H. E. Fox, and E. E. Wallach (Eds.), *The Johns Hopkins manual of gynecology and obstetrics* (5th ed.). Philadelphia, PA: Wolters Kluwer.

Cunningham, F. G., Leveno, K. J., Bloom, S. L., Spong, C. Y., Dashe, J. S., Hoffman, B. L., . . . , Sheffield, J. S. (2014). *Williams obstetrics* (24th ed.). New York, NY: McGraw-Hill.

DeStephano, C. C., & Aina-Mumuney, A. (2015). Gastrointestinal disease in pregnancy. In C. T. Johnson, J. L. Hallock, J. L. Bienstock, H. E. Fox, and E. E. Wallach (Eds.), *The Johns Hopkins manual of gynecology and obstetrics* (5th ed.). Philadelphia, PA: Wolters Kluwer.

Devi, S. (2012). U.S. guidelines for domestic violence screening spark debate. *The Lancet, 379,* 506.

DiGiulio, M., Wiedaseck, S., & Monchek, R. (2012). Understanding hydatidiform mole. *American Journal of Maternal–Child Nursing, 37*(1), 30–34.

Duff, P. (2012). Maternal and perinatal infection—bacterial. In S. G. Gabbe, J. R. Niebyl, J. L. Simpson, M. B. Landon, H. L. Galan, E. R. M. Jauniaux, & D. A. Driscoll (Eds.), *Obstetrics: Normal and problem pregnancies* (6th ed.). Philadelphia, PA: Elsevier Saunders.

Harms, R. W. (2012). *Is it safe to use a hot tub during pregnancy?* Retrieved from http://www.mayoclinic .org/healthy-living/pregnancy-week-by-week/ expert-answers/pregnancy-and-hot-tubs/ faq-20057844

Lipscomb, G. H. (2012). Medical management of ectopic pregnancy. *Clinical Obstetrics and Gynecology, 55*(2), 424–432.

Martin, S., & Satin, A. J. (2015). Perinatal infections. In C. T. Johnson, J. L. Hallock, J. L. Bienstock, H. E. Fox, and E. E. Wallach (Eds.), *The Johns Hopkins manual of gynecology and obstetrics* (5th ed.). Philadelphia, PA: Wolters Kluwer.

Mensah, V. & Yates, M. (2015). Ectopic pregnancy. In C. T. Johnson, J. L. Hallock, J. L. Bienstock, H. E. Fox, and E. E. Wallach (Eds.), *The Johns Hopkins manual of gynecology and obstetrics* (5th ed.). Philadelphia, PA: Wolters Kluwer.

Moise, K. J. (2012). Red cell alloimmunization. In S. G. Gabbe, J. R. Niebyl, J. L. Simpson, M. B. Landon, H. L. Galan, E. R. M. Jauniaux, & D. A. Driscoll (Eds.), *Obstetrics: Normal and problem pregnancies* (6th ed.). Philadelphia, PA: Elsevier Saunders.

Moise, K. J., & Argoti, P. S. (2012). Management and prevention of red cell alloimmunization in pregnancy: A systematic review. *Obstetrics & Gynecology, 5,* 1132–1139.

Mozurkewich, E. L., & Pearlman, M.D. (2012). Trauma and related surgery in pregnancy. In S. G. Gabbe, J. R. Niebyl, J. L. Simpson, M. B. Landon, H. L. Galan, E. R. M. Jauniaux, & D. A. Driscoll (Eds.), *Obstetrics: Normal and problem pregnancies* (6th ed.). Philadelphia, PA: Elsevier Saunders.

Niemeijer, M., Grooten, J., Vos, N., Bais, J., van der Post, J., Mol, B., … Painter, R. (2014). Diagnostic markers for hyperemesis gravidarum: A systematic review and meta-analysis. *American Journal of Obstetrics and Gynecology, 211(150),* e1–e15.

Pflueger, S. M.V. (2013). The cytogenics of SAB. In S. L. Gersen & M. B. Keagle (Eds.), *The principles of clinical cytogenetics* (3rd ed.). New York, NY: Springer.

Salani, R., Eisenhauer, E. L., & Copeland, L. J. (2012). Malignant diseases and pregnancy. In S. G. Gabbe, J. R. Niebyl, J. L. Simpson, M. B. Landon, H. L. Galan, E. R. M. Jauniaux, & D. A. Driscoll (Eds.), *Obstetrics: Normal and problem pregnancies* (6th ed.). Philadelphia, PA: Elsevier Saunders.

U.S. Food and Drug Administration (FDA). (2013). *FDA approves Diclegis for pregnant women experiencing nausea and vomiting.* Retrieved from http://www.fda. gov/newsevents/newsroom/pressannouncements/ ucm347087.htm?source=govdelivery

Vander Tuig, B. I. M., & Blakemore, K. J. (2015). Alloimmunization. In C. T. Johnson, J. L. Hallock, J. L. Bienstock, H. E. Fox, and E. E. Wallach (Eds.), *The Johns Hopkins manual of gynecology and obstetrics* (5th ed.). Philadelphia, PA: Wolters Kluwer.

Visconti, K., & Zite, N. (2012). hCG in ectopic pregnancy. *Clinical Obstetrics and Gynecology, 55*(2), 410–417.

Chapter 16

Processes and Stages of Labor and Birth

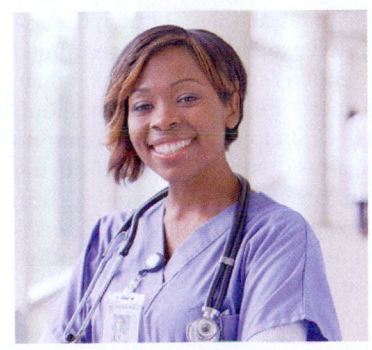

© Blend Images / Alamy

There is no doubt in my mind that I have the most wonderful job in nursing! What an enormous privilege to be allowed to share in the birth of a new life, in the birth of a new family. The sheer miracle of it never ceases to amaze and humble me. I only hope that I am able to demonstrate that sense of awe and respect even when things don't go as we would expect or like to see them.

—A Labor and Delivery Nurse

∨ Learning Outcomes

16.1 Compare methods of childbirth preparation.

16.2 Describe the five critical factors that influence labor in the assessment of an expectant woman's and fetus's progress in labor and birth.

16.3 Summarize the implications of abnormalities present in each of the five critical factors on the outcome of labor and the health of the expectant woman and the fetus.

16.4 Examine an expectant woman's and fetus's response to labor based on the physiologic processes that occur during labor.

16.5 Assess for the premonitory signs of labor when caring for an expectant woman.

16.6 Differentiate between false and true labor in an expectant woman.

16.7 Describe the physiologic changes occurring in an expectant woman during each stage of labor in the nursing care management of the expectant woman.

16.8 Predict an expectant mother's progression through the various stages of labor based on assessment data.

16.9 Explain the maternal systemic response to labor in the nursing care of an expectant woman.

16.10 Examine fetal responses to labor.

In the final weeks of pregnancy, both mother and baby begin to prepare for birth. The onset of labor begins a remarkable change in the relationship between the woman and her baby. In those hours and moments, the birth process may seem to carry all the power in the universe. The mother-to-be and her partner may feel stretched beyond their normal limits of concentration, purpose, endurance, and pain as they work to bring forth a precious new life.

This chapter focuses on the processes and stages of labor with a brief look at childbirth preparation methods. Subsequent chapters describe intrapartum assessment and nursing care.

Methods of Childbirth Preparation

Various types of childbirth preparation are taught in North America. Childbirth preparation classes are usually taught by certified childbirth educators. With both a theoretical and an educational component, childbirth education aims to reduce anxiety while providing physiologic- and psychosocial-based education along with labor-coping techniques, including relaxation tools, such as muscle relaxation and breathing exercises.

Childbirth preparation offers several advantages. It helps a pregnant woman and her support person understand the choices in the birth setting, promotes awareness of available options, and provides tools for them to use during labor and birth. Another advantage is the satisfaction of the parents, for whom childbirth becomes a shared and profound emotional experience. In addition, each method has been shown to shorten labor. All nurses should know how these techniques differ, so that they can support each birth experience effectively. A Cochrane review found that women who receive continuous support during labor require less analgesia, have fewer cesarean and instrument births, and experience a shorter period of labor (Hodnett, Gates, Hofmeyr, et al., 2011). This provides additional evidenced-based practice guidance regarding the need to provide ongoing support of the woman's partner during the labor and birth process.

Programs for Preparation

Some antepartum classes, specifically oriented to preparation for labor and birth, have a name associated with a theory of pain reduction in childbirth. The most common methods are described in Table 16–1.

SAFETY ALERT!

Explain to women who are using Internet childbirth education resources that some sites may not use health professionals or experts in the childbirth field and may be written by individuals who lack formal education and training. Advise women to look for resources that are supported by licensed professionals or well-known, credible organizations.

TABLE 16–1 Selected Childbirth Preparation Methods

- **Lamaze** (psychoprophylactic): Dissociative relaxation, controlled muscle relaxation, and specified breathing patterns are used to promote birth as a normal process.
- **Kitzinger** (sensory-memory): Women use chest breathing, abdominal breathing, and their sensory memory to help work through the birthing process.
- **Bradley** (partner-coached childbirth): Consists of a 12-week session in which the woman works on controlled breathing and deep abdominopelvic breathing with a focus on achieving natural childbirth.
- **HypnoBirthing**: Breathing and relaxation techniques help prepare the body to work in neuromuscular harmony to make the birth process easier, safer, and more comfortable.

One of the fundamental components of childbirth education is instilling confidence in the woman's ability to give birth, with contemporary models focusing on the interconnectedness of the body and the spirit (Hodnett et al., 2011). After that connection is established and understood by pregnant women, coping strategies, stress reduction, and relaxation techniques can be taught.

Another prominent organization that provides educational resources and certification for educators is the International Childbirth Education Association (ICEA) (2012), which stresses the importance of combining various techniques rather than adhering to one theoretical model. This approach provides each woman with the holistic framework to pick and choose from a variety of techniques that work best for her needs.

Body-Conditioning Exercises

Some body-conditioning exercises, such as the pelvic tilt, the pelvic rock, and Kegel exercises, are taught in childbirth preparation classes. Other exercises strengthen the abdominal muscles for the expulsive phase of labor. (See Chapter 10 for a description of some recommended exercises.) Exercises aimed at adducting the legs into an extended *McRoberts position*, which is performed by flexing the mother's thighs toward her shoulders while she is lying on her back, help enable the woman to stretch her hamstring muscles, a task usually required during the second stage of labor (King, Brucker, Kriebs, et al., 2015). Many childbirth methods utilize body-conditioning exercises and encourage the practice of daily exercise to help build endurance and strength for the labor and birth process.

Relaxation Exercises

Relaxation during labor allows the woman to conserve energy and the uterine muscles to work more efficiently. Most childbirth education methods use a form of relaxation exercise as part of their philosophical basis. Without practice, it is difficult to relax the whole body in the midst of intense uterine contractions. Progressive relaxation exercises such as those taught to induce sleep can be helpful during labor.

The *touch relaxation technique* is often used as a pain relief measure in which the partner's touch enhances the woman's ability to relax or release tense muscles. During labor, the partner's touch can include light touching, stroking, or massaging as a nonverbal cue to relax. The method often combines patterned abdominal breathing with focused touch relaxation. The laboring woman learns to release tension in the specific areas or in a generalized manner when her partner touches her. The partner observes and becomes attuned to the woman's tense, tightened muscles or to verbal cues that indicate discomfort. See *Teaching Highlights: Touch Relaxation Technique.*

An additional exercise is *disassociation relaxation*. The woman is taught to become familiar with the sensation of contracting and relaxing the voluntary muscle groups throughout her body. She then learns to contract a specific muscle group and relax the rest of her body. The exercise conditions the woman to relax uninvolved muscles while the uterus contracts, creating an active relaxation pattern.

See *Teaching Highlights: Visualization, Imagery, and Meditation* for other strategies to induce relaxation.

Breathing Techniques

Breathing techniques are a key element of most childbirth preparation programs. The Bradley method encourages abdominopelvic breathing, whereas the Kitzinger method utilizes chest

TEACHING HIGHLIGHTS | Touch Relaxation Technique

- The partner initially touches the woman's brow.

- The woman is encouraged to begin abdominal breathing, in which she breathes in through her nose, allowing her abdomen to rise as much as possible. The woman then breathes out through her mouth while simultaneously allowing her abdomen to fall. The partner reminds her to focus on muscle relaxation as the breath is released and to attempt to completely relax her body as she exhales.

- The partner continues gently touching the woman's brow while providing encouragement, telling her, "You are doing fine, you are releasing the tension in your forehead." After five or more breaths, the partner touches the woman's shoulders and the pattern described above is repeated.

- The partner then systematically focuses on the arms, chest, abdomen, thighs, and calves. The last instruction is for the woman to breathe in deeply and relax her entire body. The partner is advised to encourage this complete relaxation strategy at the end of each contraction to allow the woman to rest and reserve her energy between labor contractions.

- The couple should be encouraged to practice this technique prior to labor. Some couples may verbalize understanding of the technique, but actual practice should be encouraged prior to labor. This enables the woman to identify specific touch techniques that she personally finds helpful.

- Couples should be encouraged to practice the technique simulating a true labor pattern to become accustomed to the frequency needed to maintain the actual length of time and duration that will occur when the woman is in true labor. Women who regularly practice with their partners often become cued by touch alone and can begin the relaxation technique as soon as the partner touches her brow. Couples often individualize the technique to their own comfort levels and should be encouraged to make modifications that feel natural to them

Sources: Data from Perez, P., & Hutchins, C. (2014). *The nurturing touch at birth: A labor support handbook* (3rd ed.). Johson, VT: Cutting Edge Press; Simpkin, P., & Ancheta, R. (2011). *The labor progress handbook* (3rd ed.). New York, NY: Wiley-Blackwell.

TEACHING HIGHLIGHTS | Visualization, Imagery, and Meditation

Visualization and imagery	During pregnancy, visualization and imagery are used to induce a state of relaxation. The woman is advised to focus on a calming and relaxing image. Some women may envision a special peaceful place, while others may envision holding their baby or another pleasant event. Images can be suggested by the partner or healthcare practitioner or may be chosen by the woman herself. The partner or healthcare practitioner describes a tranquil image, such as a sparkling brook with sunshine peeking through the trees and birds singing gently in the background. During labor, this technique assists the woman with muscle relaxation and provides a positive distraction from uterine contractions, which helps conserve energy and fight fatigue.
Meditation	Meditation is a practice in which the woman remains upright in an alert position and focuses on stilling or emptying her mind. The woman focuses and repeats a particular word or sound, called a *mantra*, while attempting to reach a state of dissociation. In this state, she is detached from interacting with the environment and becomes an observer of her surroundings rather than an active participant. Mindfulness is a type of meditation that focuses on the present moment. The participant is aware of her environment and observes her thoughts and feelings without judgment. In mindfulness, the woman is encouraged to embrace the labor experience.

breathing in collaboration with abdominal relaxation. HypnoBirthing utilizes deep slow breathing as a center component of its philosophy. Breathing exercises help keep the mother and her unborn baby adequately oxygenated and help the mother relax and focus her attention appropriately. Breathing techniques are best taught during the final trimester of pregnancy. The nurse then supports the mother's use of breathing techniques during labor. See Chapter 18 for a discussion of breathing techniques.

Preparation for Childbirth That Supports Individuality

Childbirth educators stress the value of individuality when providing information to expectant parents. The goal is to encourage women to incorporate their own natural responses into

coping with the pain of labor and birth. Self-care activities that may be used include vocalization or "sounding" to relieve tension in pregnancy and labor, massage (light touch) to facilitate relaxation, use of warm water for showers or bathing during labor, visualization (imagery), relaxing music, subdued lighting, and the use of a birthing ball.

Additional ways in which the nurse can help the couple during labor and birth include the following:

- Identify the methods of childbirth preparation commonly used in your area and learn the basics of their approaches to relaxation and breathing; practice these methods so that you can support a laboring couple more effectively.

- Encourage expectant mothers and couples to make the birth a personal experience.

- Suggest the couple bring items from home that help create a more personal birthing space, such as warm socks, extra pillows or a favorite blanket, bath powder, lotion, or meaningful photos.
- Encourage the couple to listen to soothing music or watch favorite DVDs to increase personalization of the childbearing experience.

Critical Factors in Labor

Five factors are important in the process of labor and birth: the passage, the fetus, the relationship between the passage and the fetus, the physiologic forces of labor, and the psychosocial considerations. The progress of labor is critically dependent on the complementary relationship of these factors, which are summarized in *Key Facts to Remember: Critical Factors in Labor*. The first four factors are described in this chapter and psychosocial factors are discussed in detail in Chapter 17. Abnormalities affecting any one of these factors can alter the outcome of labor and jeopardize both the expectant woman and her baby. Complications of labor and birth are discussed in Chapter 21.

The Birth Passage

The true pelvis, which forms the bony canal through which the fetus must pass, is divided into three sections: the inlet, the pelvic cavity (midpelvis), and the outlet. (See Chapter 3 for a discussion of the pelvis and Chapter 9 for assessment techniques.)

The Caldwell-Moloy classification of pelvises is widely used to differentiate bony pelvis types. The four classic types of pelvis are *gynecoid*, *android*, *anthropoid*, and *platypelloid* (Figure 16–1).

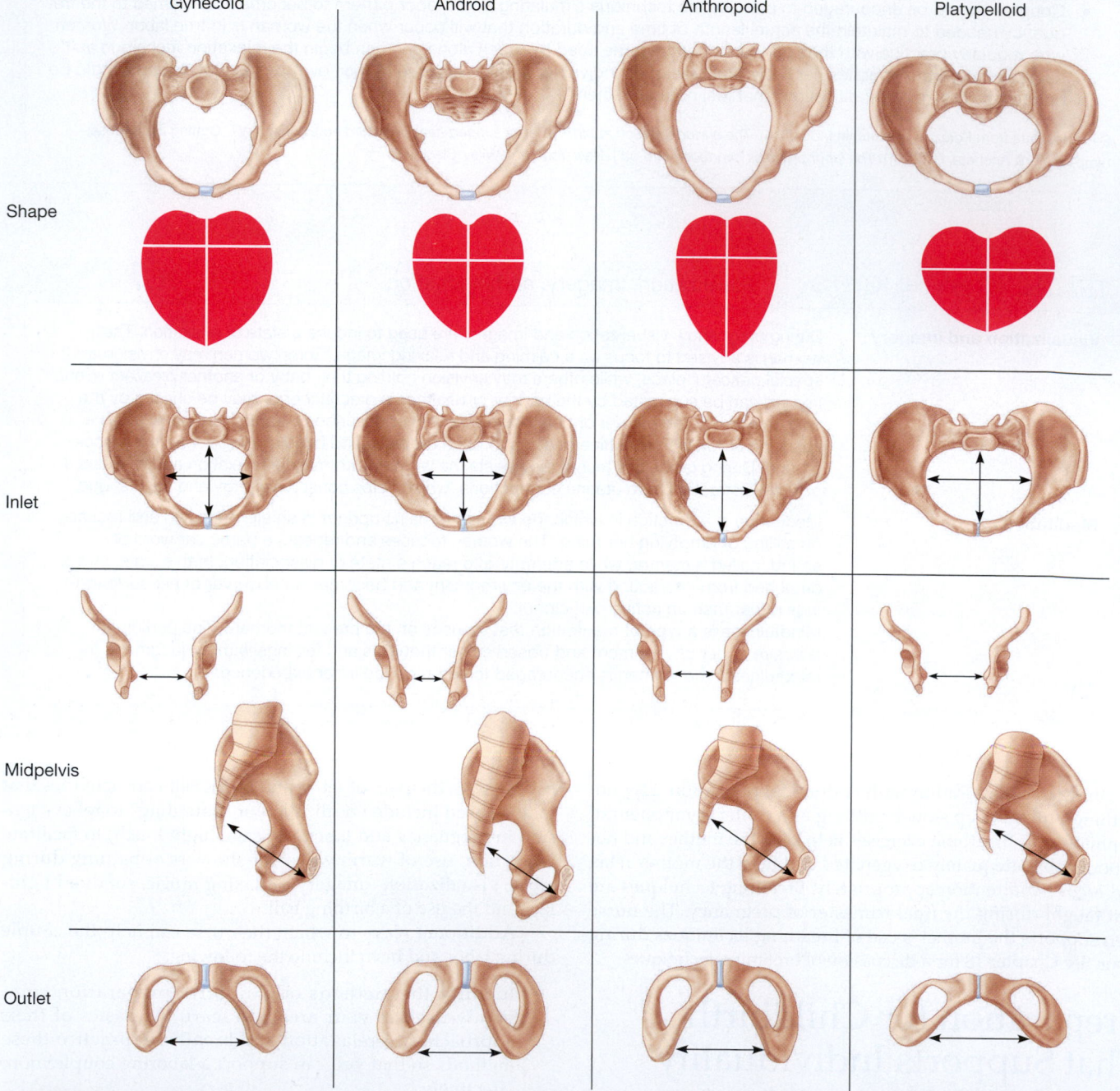

Figure 16–1 Comparison of Caldwell-Moloy pelvic types.

TABLE 16–2 Implications of Pelvic Type for Labor and Birth

PELVIC TYPE	PERTINENT CHARACTERISTICS	IMPLICATIONS FOR BIRTH
Gynecoid	Inlet rounded with all inlet diameters adequate Midpelvis diameters adequate with parallel side walls Outlet adequate	Favorable for vaginal birth
Android	Inlet heart shaped with short posterior sagittal diameter Midpelvis diameters reduced Outlet capacity reduced	Not favorable for vaginal birth Descent into pelvis is slow Fetal head enters pelvis in transverse or posterior position with arrest of labor frequent
Anthropoid	Inlet oval in shape, with long anteroposterior diameter Midpelvis diameters adequate Outlet adequate	Favorable for vaginal birth
Platypelloid	Inlet oval in shape, with long transverse diameters Midpelvis diameters reduced Outlet capacity inadequate	Not favorable for vaginal birth Fetal head engages in transverse position Difficult descent through midpelvis Frequent delay of progress at outlet of pelvis

Note: Description of pelvic shape is exaggerated for easier comprehension.

The gynecoid, or female, pelvis is most common, and all of its diameters are adequate for childbirth. Implications of each type of pelvis for childbirth are summarized in Table 16–2.

The Fetus

Several aspects of the fetal body and position are critical to the outcome of labor. Primary among these are the size and the orientation of the fetal head.

FETAL HEAD

The fetal head is the least compressible and largest part of the fetus. Once it has been born, the birth of the rest of the body is rarely delayed. The fetal skull (cranium) has three major parts: the face, the base of the skull, and the vault of the cranium (roof). The bones of the face and the cranial base are well fused and essentially fixed. The base of the cranium is composed of the two temporal bones, each with a sphenoid and an ethmoid bone. The bones composing the vault are the two frontal bones, the two parietal bones, and the occipital bone (Figure 16–2). These bones are not fused, allowing this portion of the head to adjust in shape as the presenting part passes through the narrow portions of the pelvis. The cranial bones overlap under pressure of the powers of labor and the demands of the unyielding pelvis. This overlapping is called **molding**.

The **sutures** of the fetal skull are membranous spaces between the cranial bones. The intersections of these sutures are called **fontanelles**. Cranial sutures allow for molding of the fetal head and help the clinician to identify the position of the fetal head during vaginal examination. The important sutures of the cranial vault are as follows (see Figure 16–2):

- *Frontal (metopic) suture.* Located between the two frontal bones, this becomes the anterior continuation of the sagittal suture.
- *Sagittal suture.* Located between the parietal bones, this divides the skull into left and right halves; it runs anteroposteriorly, connecting the two fontanelles.

- *Coronal suture.* Located between the frontal and parietal bones, this extends transversely left and right from the anterior fontanelle.
- *Lambdoidal suture.* Located between the two parietal bones and the occipital bone, this extends transversely left and right from the posterior fontanelle.

The anterior and posterior fontanelles are clinically useful (along with the sutures) in identifying the position of the fetal head in the pelvis and in assessing the status of the newborn after birth. The anterior fontanelle is diamond shaped and measures about 2 by 3 cm (0.8 to 1.2 in.). It permits growth of the

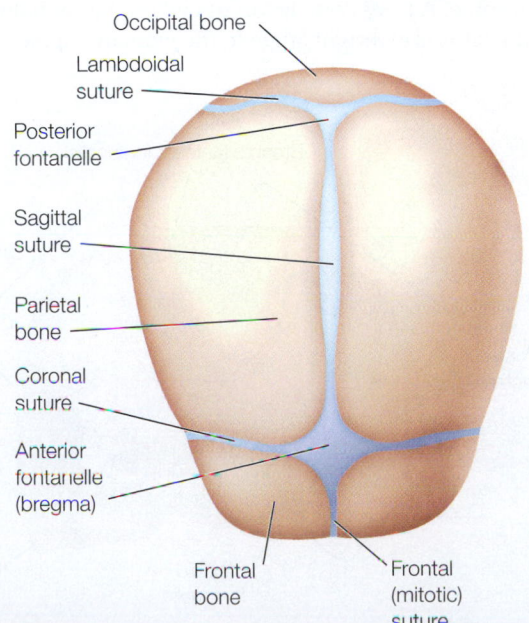

Figure 16–2 Superior view of the fetal skull.

brain by remaining unossified for as long as 18 months. The posterior fontanelle is much smaller and closes within 8 to 12 weeks after birth. It is shaped like a small triangle and marks the meeting point of the sagittal suture and the lambdoidal suture (Cunningham et al., 2014).

Following are several important landmarks of the fetal skull (Figure 16–3):

- *Mentum.* The fetal chin
- *Sinciput.* Anterior area known as the brow
- *Bregma.* Large diamond-shaped anterior fontanelle
- *Vertex.* The area between the anterior and posterior fontanelles
- *Posterior fontanelle.* The intersection between the posterior cranial sutures
- *Occiput.* The area of the fetal skull occupied by the occipital bone, beneath the posterior fontanelle.

The diameters of the fetal skull vary considerably within normal limits. Some diameters shorten and others lengthen as the head is molded during labor. Fetal head diameters are measured between the various landmarks on the skull. For example, the suboccipitobregmatic diameter is the distance from the undersurface of the occiput to the center of the bregma, or anterior fontanelle. Typical fetal skull measurements are given in Figure 16–4.

FETAL ATTITUDE

Fetal attitude refers to the relation of the fetal parts to one another. The normal attitude of the fetus is one of moderate flexion of the head, flexion of the arms onto the chest, and flexion of the legs onto the abdomen (Figure 16–5).

FETAL LIE

Fetal lie refers to the relationship of the cephalocaudal (spinal column) axis of the fetus to the cephalocaudal axis of the woman. The fetus may assume either a longitudinal (in an up-and-down position or vertical position) or a transverse lie (in a horizontal or side-to-side position). A longitudinal lie occurs when the cephalocaudal axis of the fetus is parallel to the woman's spine. A transverse lie occurs when the cephalocaudal axis of the fetus is at a right angle to the woman's spine.

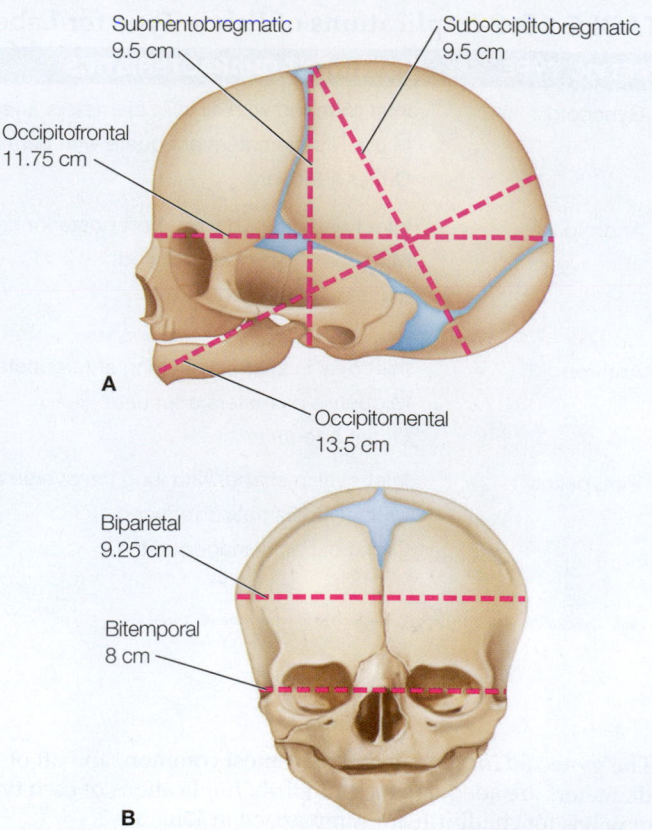

A

B

Figure 16–4 A. Anteroposterior diameters of the fetal skull. When the vertex of the fetus presents and the fetal head is flexed with the chin to the chest, the smallest anteroposterior diameter (suboccipitobregmatic) enters the birth canal. B. Transverse diameters of the fetal skull.

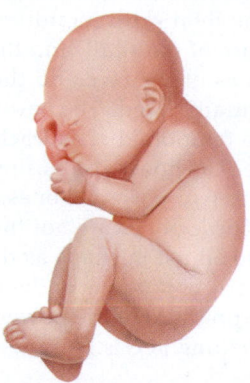

Figure 16–5 Fetal attitude. The attitude (or relationship of body parts) of this fetus is normal. The head is flexed forward with the chin almost resting on the chest. The arms and legs are flexed.

FETAL PRESENTATION

Fetal presentation is determined by fetal lie and by the body part of the fetus that enters the pelvic passage first. This portion of the fetus is referred to as the **presenting part**. Fetal presentation may be cephalic, breech, or shoulder. The most common presentation is cephalic. When this presentation occurs, labor and birth are likely to proceed normally. Breech and shoulder

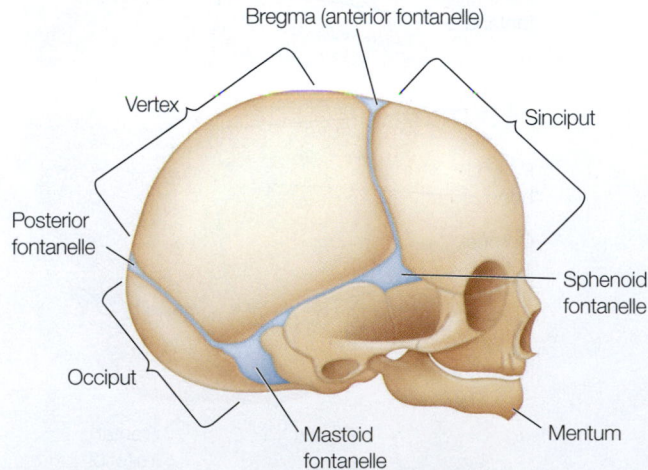

Figure 16–3 Lateral view of the fetal skull identifying the landmarks that have significance during birth.

presentations are associated with difficulties during labor, and labor does not proceed as expected; therefore, they are called **malpresentations** (see Chapter 21 for further discussion of malpresentations).

Cephalic Presentation. The fetal head presents itself to the passage in approximately 97% of term births. The cephalic presentation can be further classified (Figure 16–6) according to the degree of flexion or extension of the fetal head (attitude) as follows:

- *Vertex presentation.* The most common type of presentation; the fetal head is completely flexed onto the chest, and the smallest diameter of the fetal head (suboccipitobregmatic) presents to the maternal pelvis (Figure 16–6A); the occiput is the presenting part.
- *Sinciput presentation (also called military presentation).* The fetal head is neither flexed nor extended; the occipitofrontal diameter presents to the maternal pelvis (Figure 16–6B); the top of the head is the presenting part.
- *Brow presentation.* The fetal head is partially extended; the occipitomental diameter, the largest anteroposterior diameter, is presented to the maternal pelvis (Figure 16–6C); the sinciput is the presenting part (refer to Figure 16–3).
- *Face presentation.* The fetal head is hyperextended (complete extension); the submentobregmatic diameter presents to the maternal pelvis (Figure 16–6D); the face is the presenting part.

Breech Presentation. Breech presentations occur in 3% to 4% of all births (Cunningham et al., 2014). These presentations are classified according to the attitude of the fetus's hips and knees. In all the following variations of the breech presentation, the sacrum is the landmark to be noted:

- *Complete breech.* The fetal knees and hips are both flexed; the thighs are on the abdomen, and the calves are on the posterior aspect of the thighs; the buttocks and feet of the fetus present to the maternal pelvis (see Figure 21–7).
- *Frank breech.* The fetal hips are flexed, and the knees are extended; the buttocks of the fetus present to the maternal pelvis.
- *Footling breech.* The fetal hips and legs are extended, and the feet of the fetus present to the maternal pelvis. In a single footling, one foot presents; in a double footling, both feet present.

Shoulder Presentation. A shoulder presentation is also called a transverse lie. Most frequently, the shoulder is the presenting part and the acromion process of the scapula is the landmark to be noted. However, the fetal arm, back, abdomen, or side may present in a transverse lie. The incidence of shoulder presentation is 1% of all births (Cunningham et al., 2014). (See Chapter 21 for further discussion of transverse lie.)

Relationship of Maternal Pelvis and Presenting Part

We have discussed the birth passage and the fetus, but the third critical factor is the relationship between these two. When assessing the relationship of the maternal pelvis and the presenting part of the fetal body, the nurse considers engagement, station, and fetal position.

ENGAGEMENT

Engagement of the presenting part occurs when the largest diameter of the presenting part reaches or passes through the pelvic inlet (Figure 16–7). Whereas engagement confirms the adequacy of the pelvic inlet, it does not indicate whether the midpelvis and the outlet are also adequate.

Engagement can be determined by vaginal examinations and Leopold maneuvers. (See Chapter 17 for assessment techniques.) In primigravidas, engagement occurs approximately 2 weeks before term. Multiparas, however, may experience

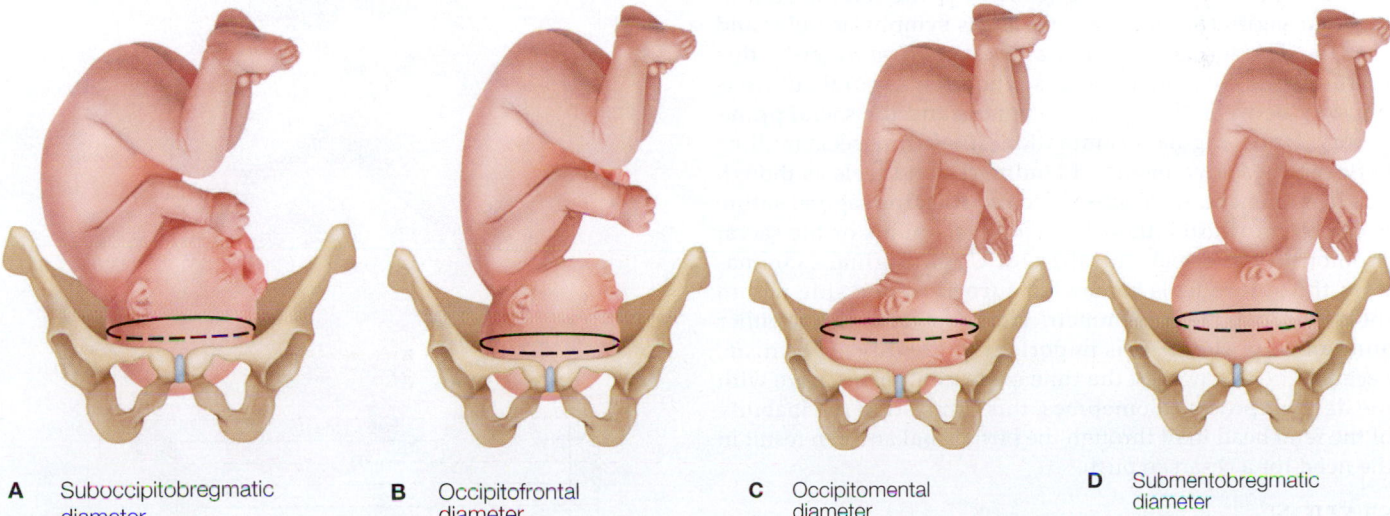

A Suboccipitobregmatic diameter   **B** Occipitofrontal diameter   **C** Occipitomental diameter   **D** Submentobregmatic diameter

Figure 16–6 Cephalic presentation. **A.** Vertex presentation. Complete flexion of the head allows the suboccipitobregmatic diameter to present to the pelvis. **B.** Sinciput (median vertex) presentation (also called military presentation) with no flexion or extension. The occipitofrontal diameter presents to the pelvis. **C.** Brow presentation. The fetal head is in partial (halfway) extension. The occipitomental diameter, which is the largest diameter of the fetal head, presents to the pelvis. **D.** Face presentation. The fetal head is in complete extension, and the submentobregmatic diameter presents to the pelvis.

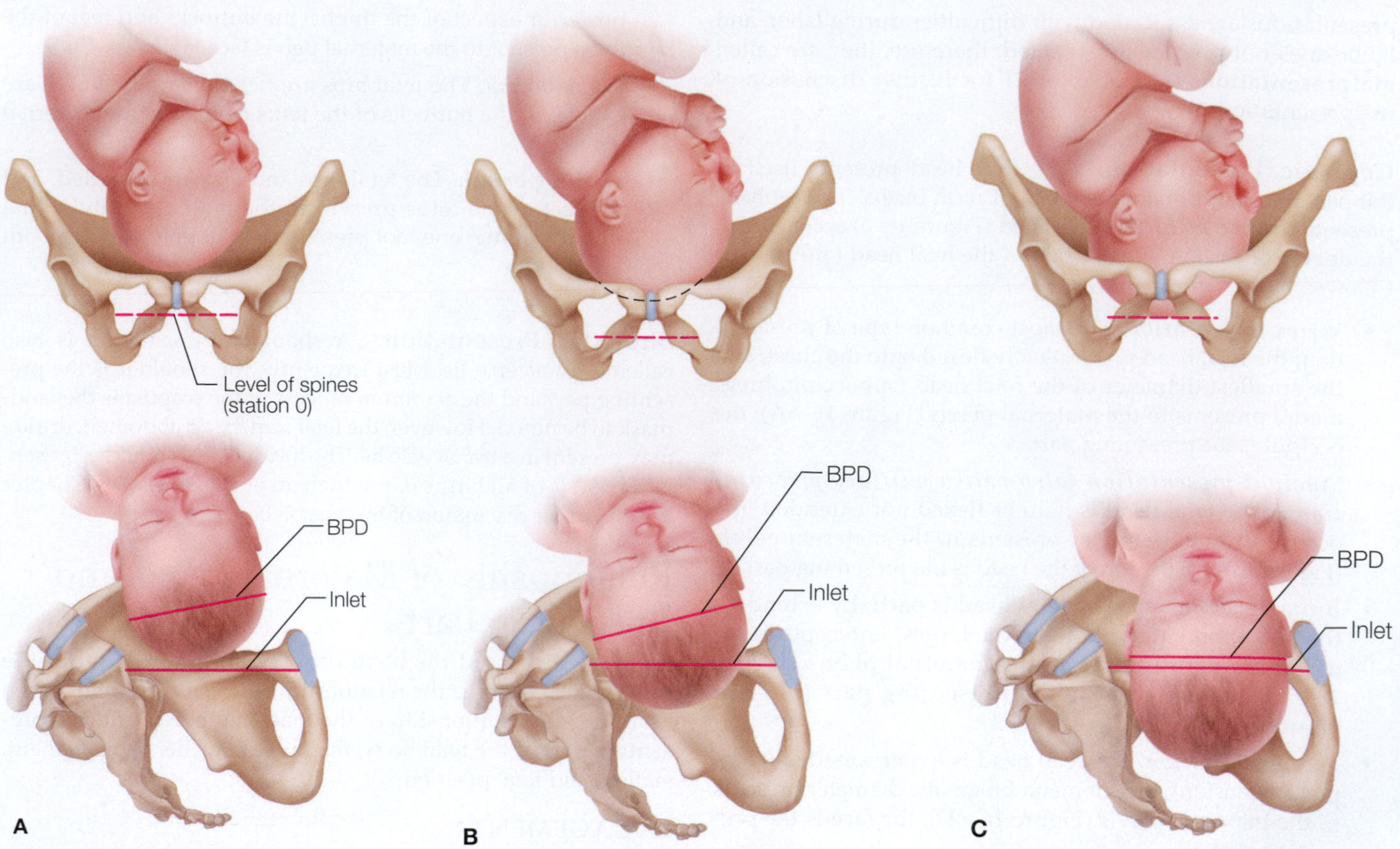

Level of spines
(station 0)

BPD

Inlet

BPD

Inlet

BPD

Inlet

A **B** **C**

Figure 16–7 Process of engagement in cephalic presentation. A. Floating. The fetal head is directed down toward the pelvis but can still easily move away from the inlet. B. Dipping. The fetal head dips into the inlet but can be moved away by exerting pressure on the fetus. C. Engaged. The biparietal diameter (BPD) of the fetal head is in the inlet of the pelvis. In most instances, the presenting part (occiput) will be at the level of the ischial spines (0 station).

engagement several weeks before the onset of labor or during the process of labor.

Another variable of engagement is the relationship of the fetal sagittal suture to the mother's symphysis pubis and sacrum. The terms *synclitism* and *asynclitism* describe this relationship. Synclitism occurs when the sagittal suture is midway between the symphysis pubis and the sacral promontory. Upon vaginal examination, the suture feels midline between these two maternal landmarks and feels as though it is in alignment. Asynclitism occurs when the sagittal suture is directed toward either the symphysis pubis or the sacral promontory and feels misaligned. Upon vaginal examination, the suture feels somewhat turned to one side within the pelvis, making it asymmetrical. Asynclitism can be either anterior or posterior. It is important to identify asynclitism, because it can lengthen the time of descent or interfere with the descent process. Sometimes, this can lead to the inability of the fetal head to fit through the birth canal and can result in the need for a cesarean birth.

STATION

Station refers to the relationship of the presenting part to an imaginary line drawn between the ischial spines of the maternal pelvis. In a normal pelvis, the ischial spines mark the narrowest diameter through which the fetus must pass. These spines are not sharp protrusions that harm the fetus, but blunted prominences at the midpelvis. As a landmark, the ischial spines have been designated as zero (0) station (Figure 16–8). If the

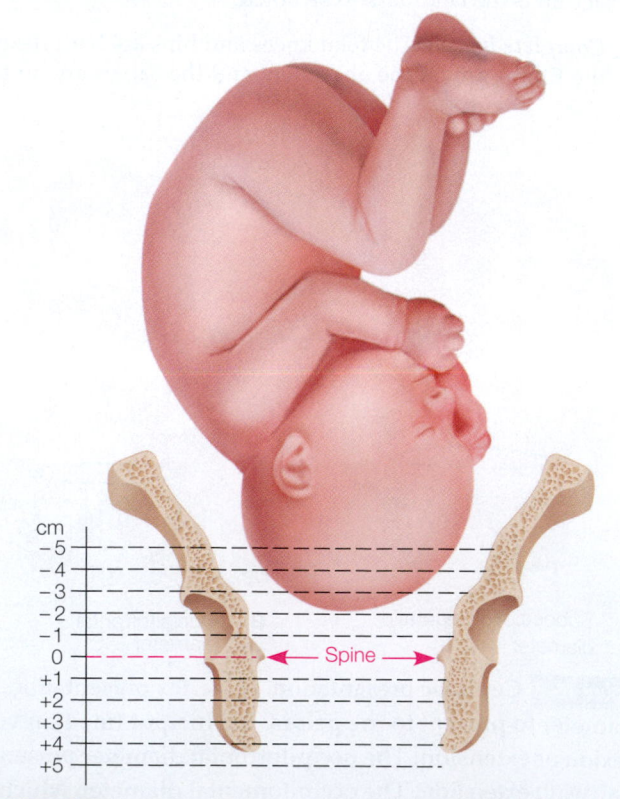

cm
−5
−4
−3
−2
−1
0 —— Spine ——
+1
+2
+3
+4
+5

Figure 16–8 Measuring the station of the fetal head while it is descending. In this view the station is −2.

presenting part is higher than the ischial spines, a negative number is assigned, noting centimeters above zero (0) station. Engagement is represented when the fetal head reaches the 0 station. Positive numbers indicate that the presenting part has passed the ischial spines. Station –5 is at the pelvic inlet, and station +5 is at the outlet.

During labor, the presenting part should move progressively from the negative stations to the midpelvis at zero (0) station and into the positive stations. If the presenting part can be seen at the woman's perineum, birth is imminent. Failure of the presenting part to descend in the presence of strong contractions may be caused by disproportion between the maternal pelvis and the fetal presenting part, malpresentation, asynclitism, or multiple fetuses. Station is determined by vaginal examination. (See Chapter 17 for assessment techniques.)

FETAL POSITION

Fetal position refers to the relationship between a designated landmark on the presenting fetal part and the front, sides, or back of the maternal pelvis. The chosen landmarks differ according to presentation:

- The landmark on the fetus for vertex presentations is the occiput.

- The landmark on the fetus for face presentations is the mentum.

- The landmark on the fetus for breech presentations is the sacrum.

- The landmark on the fetus for shoulder presentations is the acromion process on the scapula.

To determine position, the nurse notes which quadrant of the maternal pelvis the appropriate landmark is directed toward: the maternal left anterior, maternal right anterior, maternal left posterior, or maternal right posterior. If the landmark is directed toward the side of the maternal pelvis, fetal position is designated as *transverse*, rather than anterior or posterior. In documentation, the following abbreviations are used:

1. Right (R) or left (L) side of the maternal pelvis

2. The landmark of the fetal presenting part: occiput (O), mentum (M), sacrum (S), or acromion process (A)

3. Anterior (A), posterior (P), or transverse (T), depending on whether the landmark is in the front, back, or side of the pelvis.

These abbreviations help the healthcare team communicate the fetal position. Thus when the fetal occiput is directed toward the back and to the left of the birth passage, the abbreviation used is LOP (left-occiput-posterior). The term *dorsal* (D) is used when denoting the fetal position in a transverse lie; it refers to the fetal back. Thus RADA indicates that the acromion process of the scapula is directed toward the woman's right and the fetus's back is anterior.

The most common fetal position is occiput anterior. When this position occurs, labor and birth are likely to proceed normally. Positions other than occiput anterior, left occiput anterior, and right occiput anterior are more frequently associated with problems during labor; therefore they are called malpositions (see Chapter 21). The most commonly occurring positions and malpositions are illustrated in Figure 16–9.

Assessment techniques to determine fetal position include inspection and palpation of the maternal abdomen and vaginal examination. They are discussed in detail in Chapter 17.

Physiologic Forces of Labor

Primary and secondary forces work together to achieve birth of the fetus, the fetal membranes, and the placenta. The *primary force* is uterine muscular contractions, which cause the changes of the first stage of labor—complete effacement and dilatation of the cervix. The *secondary force* is the use of abdominal muscles to push during the second stage of labor. The pushing adds to the primary force after full dilatation.

CONTRACTIONS

In labor, uterine contractions are rhythmic but intermittent. Between contractions there is a period of relaxation. This allows uterine muscles to rest and provides respite for the laboring woman. It also restores uteroplacental circulation, which is important to fetal oxygenation and adequate circulation in the uterine blood vessels.

Each contraction has three phases. These are (1) *increment*, the building up of the contraction (the longest phase); (2) *acme*, or the peak of the contraction; and (3) *decrement*, or the letting up of the contraction.

When describing uterine contractions during labor, caregivers use the terms *frequency, duration,* and *intensity* (Figure 16–10):

- *Frequency.* The time between the beginning of one contraction and the beginning of the next contraction

- *Duration.* The time measured from the beginning of a contraction to the completion of that same contraction

- *Intensity.* The strength of the contraction during acme

In most instances intensity is estimated by palpating the uterine fundus during a contraction, but it may be measured directly with an intrauterine catheter. When estimating intensity by palpation, the nurse determines whether it is mild, moderate, or strong by judging how indentable the uterine wall is during the acme of a contraction. If the uterine wall can be indented easily, the contraction is considered mild. Strong intensity exists when the uterine wall cannot be indented. Moderate intensity falls between these two ranges. When intensity is measured with an intrauterine catheter, the normal resting pressure in the uterus (between contractions) averages 10 to 12 mmHg. During acme the intensity ranges from 25 to 40 mmHg in early labor, 50 to 70 mmHg in active labor, 70 to 90 mmHg during transition, and 70 to 100 mmHg while the woman is pushing in the second stage (Blackburn, 2013). (See Chapter 17 for further discussion of assessment techniques.)

At the beginning of labor, the contractions are usually mild. As labor progresses, the duration, intensity, and frequency of the contractions increase. Because the contractions are involuntary, the laboring woman cannot control their duration, intensity, or frequency.

BEARING DOWN

After the cervix is completely dilated, the maternal abdominal muscles contract as the woman pushes. This pushing action (called *bearing down*) aids in expulsion of the fetus and placenta. If the cervix is not completely dilated, however, bearing down can cause cervical edema (which retards dilatation), possible tearing and bruising of the cervix, and maternal exhaustion.

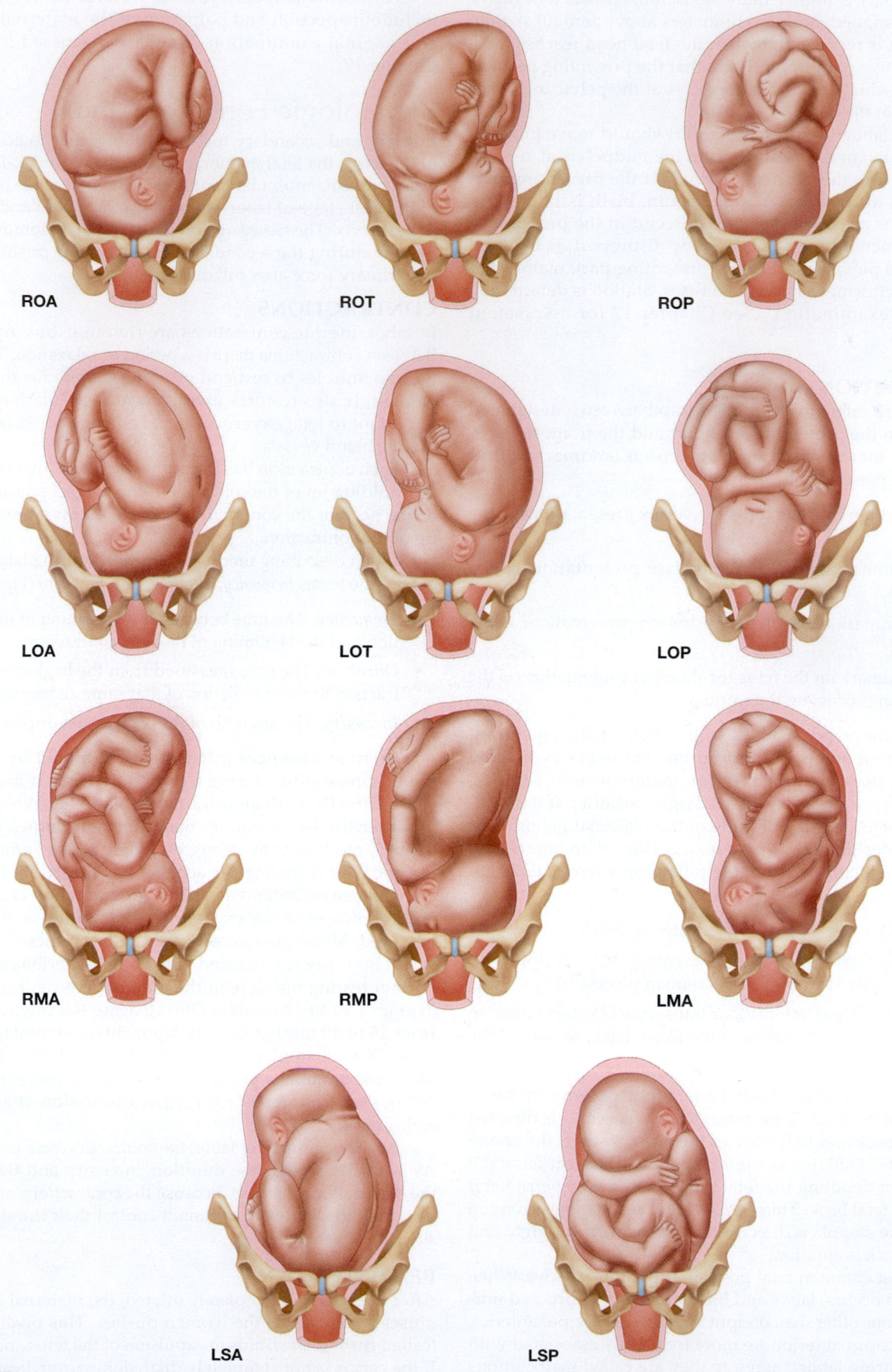

Figure 16–9 Categories of presentation.

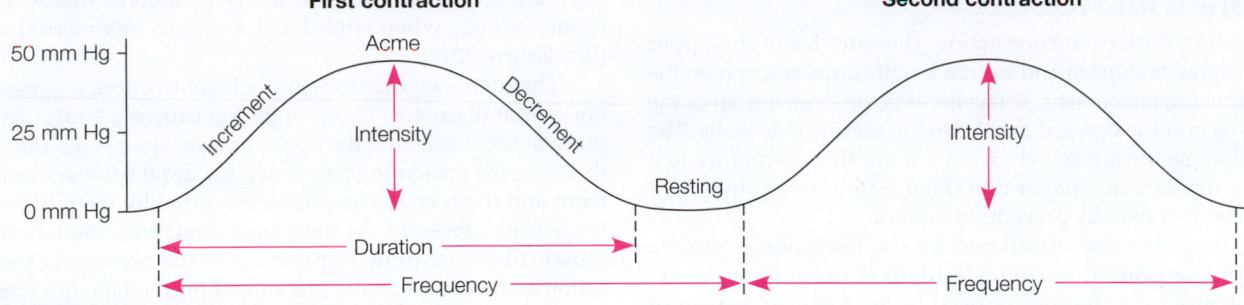

Figure 16–10 Characteristics of uterine contractions.

KEY FACTS TO REMEMBER
Critical Factors in Labor

1. Birth passage
   - Size of the maternal pelvis (diameters of the pelvic inlet, midpelvis, and outlet)
   - Type of maternal pelvis (gynecoid, android, anthropoid, platypelloid, or a combination)
   - Ability of the cervix to dilate and efface and ability of the vaginal canal and the external opening of the vagina (the introitus) to distend

2. Fetus
   - Fetal head (size and presence of molding)
   - Fetal attitude (flexion or extension of the fetal body and extremities)
   - Fetal lie
   - Fetal presentation (the body part of the fetus entering the pelvis in a single or multiple pregnancy)

3. The relationship between the passage and the fetus
   - Engagement of the fetal presenting part
   - Station (location of fetal presenting part in the maternal pelvis)
   - Fetal position (relationship of the presenting part to one of the four quadrants of the maternal pelvis)

4. Physiologic forces of labor
   - Frequency, duration, and intensity of uterine contractions as the fetus moves through the passage
   - Effectiveness of the maternal pushing effort

5. Psychosocial considerations
   - Mental and physical preparation for childbirth
   - Sociocultural values and beliefs
   - Previous childbirth experience
   - Support from significant others
   - Emotional status

The Physiology of Labor

In addition to considering the critical factors affecting the progress of labor and birth, it is essential to explore the physiology of the normal birth experience.

Possible Causes of Labor Onset

The process of labor usually begins between the 38th and the 42nd week of gestation, when the fetus is mature and ready for birth. Despite research, the exact cause of labor onset is not clearly understood. However, some important aspects have been identified: Progesterone relaxes smooth muscle tissue, estrogen stimulates uterine muscle contractions, and connective tissue loosens to permit the softening, thinning, and eventual opening of the cervix (Blackburn, 2013). Currently, researchers are focusing on the role of fetal membranes (chorion and amnion), the decidua, and the effect of progesterone withdrawal, of prostaglandin, and of corticotropin-releasing hormone in relation to labor onset (Blackburn, 2013).

PROGESTERONE WITHDRAWAL HYPOTHESIS

Progesterone, produced by the placenta, relaxes uterine smooth muscle by interfering with the conduction of impulses from one cell to the next. Therefore during pregnancy, progesterone exerts a quieting effect and the uterus generally is without coordinated contractions. Toward the end of gestation, biochemical changes decrease the availability of progesterone to myometrial cells and may be associated with an antiprogestin that inhibits the relaxant effect but allows other progesterone actions such as lactogenesis. With the decreased availability of progesterone, estrogen is better able to stimulate contractions (Tan, Yi, Rote, et al., 2012). Progesterone administration is now used as a mechanism to prevent preterm labor and childbirth (Tan et al., 2012).

PROSTAGLANDIN HYPOTHESIS

Although the exact relationship between prostaglandin and the onset of labor is not yet known, the effect is clinically demonstrated by the successful induction of labor after vaginal application of prostaglandin E. In addition, preterm labor may be stopped by using an inhibitor of prostaglandin synthesis (Tan et al., 2012).

The amnion and the decidua are the focus of research on the source of prostaglandins. Once prostaglandin is produced, stimuli for its synthesis may include rising levels of estrogen, decreased availability of progesterone, and increased levels of oxytocin, platelet-activating factor, and endothelin-1 (Tan et al., 2012).

CORTICOTROPIN-RELEASING HORMONE HYPOTHESIS

Corticotropin-releasing hormone (CRH) increases throughout pregnancy, with a sharp increase at term, and has a possible role in labor onset. There also is an increase in plasma CRH before preterm labor, and CRH levels are elevated in multiple gestation. CRH also is known to stimulate the synthesis of prostaglandin F and prostaglandin E by amnion cells (Ventolini, 2013).

Myometrial Activity

In true labor, with each contraction, the muscles of the upper uterine segment shorten and exert a longitudinal traction on the cervix, causing effacement. **Effacement** is the drawing up of the internal os and the cervical canal into the uterine side walls. The cervix changes progressively from a long, thick structure to a structure that is tissue-paper thin (Figure 16–11). In primigravidas, effacement usually precedes dilatation.

Contractions are stimulated by the hormone oxytocin. Oxytocin is a potent uterine stimulant (Cunningham et al., 2014). Oxytocin is frequently used as an agent to induce or augment labor in term fetuses or when delivery is necessitated. Uterine sensitivity to oxytocin is increased during pregnancy (Blackburn, 2013). Oxytocin is produced in the hypothalamus and secreted into the bloodstream but is also produced in uterine tissues during late gestation, with concentrations increasing at the onset of labor (Cunningham et al., 2014). The oxytocin receptors are most likely formed in the gestational tissues, which, when stimulated, produce myometrial activity (Blackburn, 2013).

The uterus elongates with each contraction, decreasing the horizontal diameter. This elongation causes a straightening of the fetal body, pressing the upper portion against the fundus and thrusting the presenting part down toward the lower uterine segment and the cervix. The pressure exerted by the fetus is called the *fetal axis pressure*. As the uterus elongates, the longitudinal muscle fibers are pulled upward over the presenting part. This action and the hydrostatic pressure of the fetal membranes cause cervical dilatation. The cervical os and cervical canal widen from less than 1 cm (0.4 in.) to approximately 10 cm (3.9 in.), allowing birth of the fetus. When the cervix is completely dilated and retracted up into the lower uterine segment, it can no longer be palpated. At the same time the round ligament pulls the fundus forward, aligning the fetus with the bony pelvis.

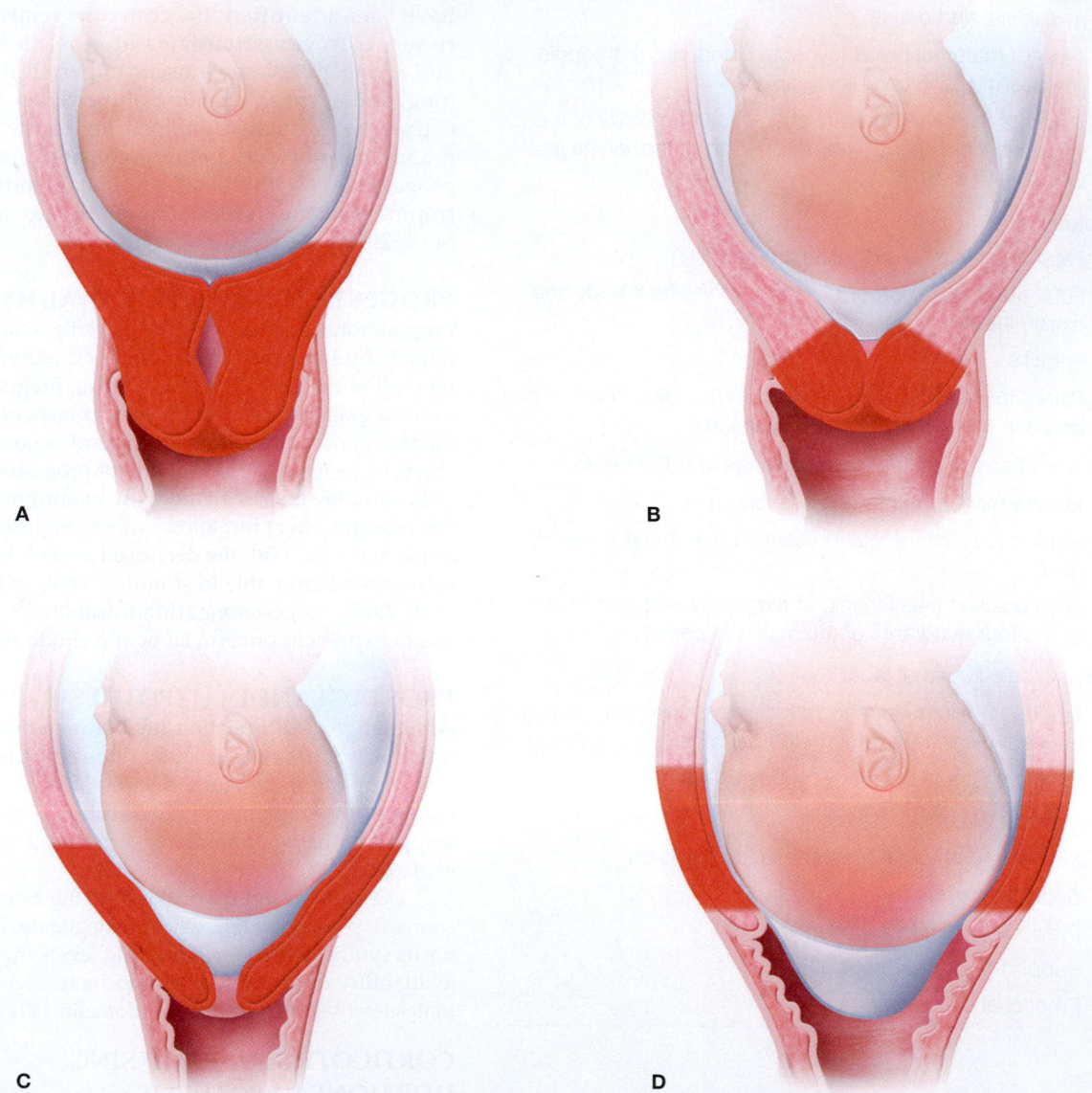

A

B

C

D

Figure 16–11 Effacement of the cervix in the primigravida. A. At the beginning of labor, there is no cervical effacement or dilatation. The fetal head is cushioned by amniotic fluid. B. Beginning cervical effacement. As the cervix begins to efface, more amniotic fluid collects below the fetal head. C. Cervix is about one-half (50%) effaced and slightly dilated. The increasing amount of amniotic fluid below the fetal head exerts hydrostatic pressure on the cervix. D. Complete effacement and dilatation.

Musculature Changes in the Pelvic Floor

The levator ani muscle and fascia of the pelvic floor draw the rectum and vagina upward and forward with each contraction, along the curve of the pelvic floor. As the fetal head descends to the pelvic floor, the pressure of the presenting part causes the perineal structure, which was once 5 cm (2 in.) in thickness, to change to a structure less than 1 cm (0.4 in.) thick. A normal physiologic anesthesia is produced as a result of the decreased blood supply to the area. The anus everts, exposing the interior rectal wall as the fetal head descends forward (Blackburn, 2013).

Premonitory Signs of Labor

Most primigravidas and many multiparas experience the following signs and symptoms of impending labor.

LIGHTENING

Lightening describes the effects that occur when the fetus begins to settle into the pelvic inlet (engagement). With fetal descent, the uterus moves downward, and the fundus no longer presses on the diaphragm, which eases breathing. However, with increased downward pressure of the presenting part, the woman may notice the following:

- Leg cramps or pains caused by pressure on the nerves that course through the obturator foramen in the pelvis
- Increased pelvic pressure
- Increased urinary frequency
- Increased venous stasis, leading to edema in the lower extremities
- Increased vaginal secretions resulting from congestion of the vaginal mucous membranes

BRAXTON HICKS CONTRACTIONS

Before the onset of labor, **Braxton Hicks contractions**, the irregular, intermittent contractions that have been occurring throughout the pregnancy, may become uncomfortable. The pain seems to be focused in the abdomen and groin but may feel like the "drawing" sensations experienced by some women with dysmenorrhea. When these contractions are strong enough for the woman to believe she is in labor, she is said to be in *false labor*. False labor is uncomfortable and may be exhausting. Because the contractions can be fairly regular, the woman has no way of knowing if they are the beginning of true labor. She may come to the hospital or birthing center for a vaginal examination to determine if cervical dilatation is occurring. Frequent episodes of false labor, as well as trips back and forth to the certified nurse-midwife (CNM), nurse practitioner, or physician's office or hospital, may frustrate or embarrass the woman who feels that she should know when she is really in labor. Reassurance by nursing staff can ease embarrassment. It is important to remember that women with contractions that occur on a regular basis before 38 weeks should be assessed to determine if they are experiencing preterm labor (PTL) (for a detailed discussion of PTL see Chapter 20).

CERVICAL CHANGES

Considerable change occurs in the cervix during the prenatal and intrapartum period. At the beginning of pregnancy, the cervix is rigid and firm, and it must soften so that it can stretch and dilate to allow the fetus passage. This softening of the cervix is called *ripening*.

As term approaches, collagen fibers in the cervix are broken down by the action of enzymes such as collagenase and elastase. As the collagen fibers change, their ability to bind together decreases because of increasing amounts of hyaluronic acid (which loosely binds collagen fibrils) and decreasing amounts of dermatan sulfate (which tightly binds collagen fibrils). The water content of the cervix also increases. All these changes result in a weakening and softening of the cervix.

BLOODY SHOW

During pregnancy, cervical secretions accumulate in the cervical canal to form a barrier called a *mucous plug*. With softening and effacement of the cervix, the mucous plug is often expelled, resulting in a small amount of blood loss from the exposed cervical capillaries. The resulting pink-tinged secretions are called **bloody show**. Bloody show is considered a sign that labor will begin within 24 to 48 hours. Vaginal examination that includes manipulation of the cervix may also result in a blood-tinged discharge, which is sometimes confused with bloody show.

RUPTURE OF MEMBRANES

Approximately 8% to 10% of women at term (37 through 41 weeks' gestation) experience **rupture of the amniotic membranes (ROM)** before the onset of labor (American College of Obstetricians & Gynecologists, 2016). **Spontaneous rupture of membranes (SROM)** and leakage of amniotic fluid before the onset of labor at any gestational age is known as **premature rupture of membranes (PROM)**. When the membranes rupture and leakage of amniotic fluid from the vagina occurs before 37 weeks of gestation, the term **preterm premature rupture of membranes (PPROM)** is used. After the membranes rupture, 50% of these women begin labor within 24 hours and 95% begin labor within 28 hours (American College of Obstetrics & Gynecology, 2016). When the membranes rupture, the amniotic fluid may be expelled in large amounts. If engagement has not occurred, there is danger of the umbilical cord washing out with the fluid (prolapsed cord). In addition, the open pathway into the uterus increases the risk of infection. Because of these threats, when the membranes rupture, the woman is advised to notify her healthcare provider and proceed to the hospital or birthing center. In some instances, the fluid is expelled in small amounts and may be confused with episodes of urinary incontinence associated with urinary urgency, coughing, or sneezing. The discharge should be checked to determine its source and the appropriate action. (See Chapter 17 for assessment techniques.)

The American College of Nurse Midwives (2012) recommends that women who present with ruptured membranes without contractions should be counseled on options for ongoing management. Some women may prefer *active management*, in which an oxytocin infusion or prostaglandin induction is immediately begun at the time of presentation to decrease the length of labor. While women in this group had a lower risk of maternal infection, they were 6.8 times more likely to undergo a cesarean birth (Pintucci, Meregalli, Colombo, et al., 2014).

Women who desire *expectant management* are those that prefer to wait until spontaneous labor begins and often prefer minimal interventions. Current research shows that these women do not increase their risk of newborn infection, cord prolapse, cesarean birth, or fetal death (Pintucci et al., 2014). Maternal infection rates in women who undergo expectant management are directly correlated with the number of vaginal examinations performed during labor; therefore, examinations should be kept to a minimum to avoid infection. Following these guidelines, women can wait 48 to 72 hours without showing signs of infection (Breakey, Reidner, & Dekker, 2013). If 48 hours elapse with no signs of labor, most practitioners opt to begin induction at that time (Breakey et al., 2013). The following parameters should be met before expectant management is pursued:

- Term singleton pregnancy
- No evidence of pregnancy complications
- Clear amniotic fluid
- Group beta strep negative
- Afebrile
- Normal fetal heart rate with negative non-stress test (NST)

Women with group B streptococcus (GBS) or those with no documented GBS culture have a higher incidence of neonatal infection; therefore antibiotic therapy should be started immediately (Breakey et al., 2013). Labor is induced if the pregnancy is beyond 34 weeks. Other risk factors that warrant induction of labor in women less than 34 weeks' gestation include chorioamnionitis, advanced labor, fetal distress, and placental abruption with nonreassuring fetal surveillance. If fetal lung maturity has been documented by amniocentesis or collection of vaginal fluid, birth should be facilitated regardless of gestational age. In a noncephalic fetus with advanced cervical dilatation (more than or equal to 3 cm) or if the risk of cord prolapse is present, labor induction is indicated.

Women between 34 and 37 weeks' gestation are administered GBS prophylactic antibiotics as needed and are able to progress to give birth. Women with preterm gestations of less than 34 weeks are managed conservatively provided both the mother and the fetus are stable (Jazayeri, 2014). Women with PPROM who are less than 34 weeks' gestation should be managed as follows (ACOG, 2016):

- Administration of a combination of erythromycin and ampicillin or amoxicillin to reduce maternal and neonatal infection at less than 34 0/7 weeks of gestation
- Intrapartum group B streptococcal (GBS) prophylaxis to prevent vertical transmission
- Single course corticosteroid administration
- Fetal neuroprotective treatment with intravenous magnesium sulfate
- Treatment for women with herpes simplex virus (HSV) infection
- Labor induction (if spontaneous labor does not occur at 37 0/7 weeks of gestation or more)
- Delivery (34 0/7 weeks of gestation or more)

The decision to induce, though, is based on maternal vital signs, stability, presence of maternal complications, status of fetal well-being, maternal preferences, and the healthcare provider's recommendations. Women should be counseled that expectant management does statistically result in higher rates of intrauterine infection, postpartum infection, and abruptio placentae (ACOG, 2016).

Clinical Tip

Nurses should avoid vaginal examinations whenever possible on women with PROM/PPROM. A good rule of thumb is to perform an examination only when the results would change the course of management. For example, examinations to assess cervical change should be performed only if a change of care will occur, such as the initiation of oxytocin or a decision to perform a cesarean section (C/S).

SUDDEN BURST OF ENERGY

Some women report a sudden burst of energy approximately 24 to 48 hours before labor. The cause of the energy spurt is unknown. In prenatal teaching the nurse should warn prospective mothers not to overexert themselves during this energy burst to avoid being overtired when labor begins.

Clinical Tip

Encourage mothers who experience a sudden burst of energy to eat small, frequent nutritious meals during this period, and to rest. Encourage the pregnant woman to have her partner or a friend do chores and activities that she feels are essential to complete before the baby arrives.

OTHER SIGNS

Additional premonitory signs include the following:

- Weight loss of 1 to 3 lb resulting from fluid loss and electrolyte shifts produced by changes in estrogen and progesterone levels.
- Diarrhea, indigestion, or nausea and vomiting just before onset of labor. The cause of these signs is unknown.

Differences Between True and False Labor

The contractions of true labor produce progressive dilatation and effacement of the cervix. They occur regularly and increase in frequency, duration, and intensity. The discomfort of true labor contractions usually starts in the back and radiates around to the abdomen. The pain is not relieved by ambulation (in fact, walking may intensify the pain).

The contractions of false labor do not produce progressive cervical effacement and dilatation. Classically, they are irregular and do not increase in frequency, duration, and intensity. The contractions may be perceived as a hardening or "balling up" without discomfort, or discomfort may occur mainly in the lower abdomen and groin. As with true labor contractions, the discomfort may be relieved by acupuncture, aromatherapy, freedom of movement, hydration, hydrotherapy, massage, therapeutic touch, music and song, and support. Additionally, a warm shower or tub bath are often helpful measures to promote relaxation and ease the discomfort associated with contractions of true or false labor (International Childbirth Education Association [ICEA], 2016).

The woman will find it helpful to know the characteristics of true labor contractions as well as the premonitory signs of ensuing labor. However, at times the only way to differentiate accurately between true and false labor is to assess dilatation. The woman must feel free to come in for accurate assessment of labor and should be counseled not to feel foolish if the labor is false. The nurse must reassure the woman that false labor is common and that it often cannot be distinguished from true labor except by vaginal examination.

Stages of Labor and Birth

To assist caregivers, common terms have been developed as benchmarks to subdivide the labor process into phases and stages of labor:

- *First stage.* Begins with the onset of true labor and ends when the cervix is completely dilated at 10 cm (3.9 in.).

- *Second stage.* Begins with complete dilatation and ends with the birth of the newborn.
- *Third stage.* Begins with the birth of the newborn and ends with the delivery of the placenta.
- *Fourth stage.* Begins with delivery of the placenta and lasts 1 to 4 hours, during which the uterus effectively contracts to control bleeding at the placental site.

It is important to note, however, that the stages of labor represent theoretical separations in the process. A laboring woman will not usually experience distinct differences from one stage to another.

KEY FACTS TO REMEMBER
Comparison of True and False Labor

True Labor	False Labor
Contractions are at regular intervals.	Contractions are irregular.
Intervals between contractions gradually shorten.	Usually no change.
Contractions increase in duration and intensity.	Usually no change.
Discomfort begins in back and radiates around to abdomen.	Discomfort is usually in abdomen.
Cervical dilatation and effacement are progressive.	No change.
Contractions do not decrease with rest or warm tub bath.	Rest and warm tub lessen contractions.

First Stage

The first stage of labor is divided into the latent, active, and transition phases. Each phase of labor is characterized by physical and psychologic changes and is summarized in Table 16–3.

LATENT PHASE

The *latent phase* starts with the beginning of regular contractions, which are usually mild. The woman feels able to cope with the discomfort. She may be relieved that labor has finally started and that the end of pregnancy has come. Although she may be anxious, she is able to recognize and express those feelings of anxiety. The woman is often smiling and eager to talk about herself and answer questions. Excitement is high, and her partner or other support person is often equally elated.

Uterine contractions become established during the latent phase and increase in frequency, duration, and intensity. They may start as mild contractions lasting 30 seconds with a frequency of 10 to 30 minutes and progress to moderate ones lasting 30 to 40 seconds with a frequency of 5 to 7 minutes. As the cervix begins to dilate, it also effaces, although little or no fetal descent is evident. For a woman in her first labor (nullipara), the latent (or early) phase of the first stage of labor averages 8.6 hours but should not exceed 20 hours. The latent phase in multiparas averages 5.3 hours but should not exceed 14 hours.

At the beginning of labor, the amniotic membranes bulge through the cervix in the shape of a cone. Spontaneous rupture of membranes (SROM) generally occurs at the height of an intense contraction with a gush of fluid out of the vagina. In many instances, the membranes are ruptured by the physician/CNM, using an instrument called an amnihook. This procedure is called *amniotomy*, or **artificial rupture of membranes (AROM)**, and is discussed in Chapter 22.

ACTIVE PHASE

When the woman enters the early *active phase*, her anxiety and her sense of the need for energy and focus tend to increase as she senses the intensification of contractions and pain. She may begin to fear a loss of control or may feel the need to "really work and focus" on the contractions. Women will use a variety of coping mechanisms. Some women exhibit a sense of purpose and the need for regrouping, whereas others may feel a decreased ability to cope and a sense of helplessness. Women who have support persons and family available often experience greater satisfaction and have less anxiety than those without support.

During this phase, the cervix dilates from about 4 to 7 cm (1.6 to 2.8 in.). Fetal descent is progressive. The cervical dilatation averages 1.2 cm/hr (0.5 in./hr) in nulliparas and 1.5 cm/hr (0.6 in./hr) in multiparas (Cheng, 2014). During the active and transition phases, contractions become more frequent and longer in duration, and they increase in intensity. By the end of the active phase, contractions have a frequency of 2 to 3 minutes, a duration of 60 seconds, and strong intensity.

TRANSITION PHASE

The *transition phase* is the last part of the first stage of labor. When the woman enters the transition phase, she may demonstrate an acute awareness of the need for her energy and attention to be completely focused on the task at hand. She may experience significant anxiety or feel out of control. She becomes

TABLE 16–3 Characteristics of Labor

| | FIRST STAGE | | | |
	LATENT PHASE	ACTIVE STAGE	TRANSITION PHASE	SECOND STAGE
Nullipara	8.6 hr	4.6 hr	3 hr	Up to 3 hr
Multipara	5.3 hr	2.4 hr	Less than 1 hr	Less than 1 hr, averages 15 min
Cervical dilatation	0 to 3 cm	4 to 7 cm	8 to 10 cm	
Contractions				
Frequency	Every 10 to 30 min	Every 2 to 5 min	Every 1½ to 2 min	Every 1½ to 2 min
Duration	30 sec	40 to 60 sec	60 to 90 sec	60 to 90 sec
Intensity	Begin as mild and progress to moderate; 25 to 40 mmHg by intrauterine pressure catheter (IUPC)	Begin as moderate and progress to strong; 50 to 70 mmHg by IUPC	Strong by palpation; 70 to 90 mmHg by IUPC	Strong by palpation; 70 to 100 mmHg by IUPC

acutely aware of the increasing force and intensity of the contractions. She may become restless, frequently changing position in an attempt to get comfortable. By the time the woman enters the transition phase, she is inner directed and often tired. She may not want to be left alone, while at the same time the support person may be feeling the need for a break. The nurse should reassure the woman that she will not be left alone. It is crucial for the nurse to be available as relief support at this time and to keep the woman informed about where her labor support people are if they have left the room. Some women have the intuition that the end of labor is occurring and know that birth is nearing, so an instinct to have support people remain with her often occurs.

During transition, contractions have a frequency of about every 1.5 to 2.0 minutes, a duration of 60 to 90 seconds, and strong intensity. Cervical dilatation slows as it progresses from 8 to 10 cm (3.1 to 3.9 in.) and the rate of fetal descent dramatically increases. The average rate of descent is 1.6 cm/hr (0.6 in./hr) and at least 1 cm/hr (0.4 in./hr) in nulliparas. In addition, the average rate of descent is 5.4 cm/hr (2.1 in./hr) and at least 2.1 cm/hr (0.8 in./hr) in multiparas. The transition phase does not usually last longer than 3 hours for nulliparas or longer than 1 hour for multiparas. The total duration of the first stage can be increased by approximately 1 hour if epidural anesthesia is used.

As dilatation approaches 10 cm (3.9 in.), there may be increased rectal pressure and an uncontrollable desire to bear down, increased amount of bloody show, and rupture of membranes (if it has not already occurred). With the peak of a contraction, the woman may experience a sensation of pressure so great that she may fear that she will be "torn open" or "split apart." She may also fear that the sensations indicate that something is wrong. Thus, the nurse should inform the woman that what she is feeling is normal in this stage of labor. Even with assurance, the woman may increasingly doubt her ability to cope with labor and may become apprehensive, irritable, and withdrawn. She may be terrified of being left alone, though she does not want anyone to talk to or touch her. However, with the next contraction she may ask for verbal and physical support.

Other characteristics of this phase may include the following:

- Increasing bloody show
- Hyperventilation, as the woman increases her breathing rate
- Generalized discomfort, including low backache, shaking and cramping in legs, and increased sensitivity to touch
- Increased need for partner's and/or nurse's presence and support
- Restlessness
- Increased apprehension and irritability
- An inner focusing on her contractions
- A sense of bewilderment, frustration, and anger at the contractions
- Requests for medication
- Hiccupping, belching, nausea, or vomiting
- Beads of perspiration on the upper lip or brow
- Increasing rectal pressure and feeling the urge to bear down

The woman in this phase is anxious to "get it over with." She may be amnesic and sleep between her now-frequent contractions. Her support persons may start to feel fatigue and may feel helpless. They may turn to the nurse for increased participation as their efforts to alleviate her discomfort seem less effective.

Second Stage

The second stage of labor begins with complete cervical dilatation and ends with birth of the baby. For primigravidas, the second stage is typically completed within 2 hours if the woman has no epidural anesthesia and 3 hours if she has an epidural after the cervix becomes fully dilated; the stage averages 15 minutes for multiparas (Cheng, 2014). Refer to Table 16–3. Contractions continue with a frequency of about every 1.5 to 2.0 minutes, a duration of 60 to 90 seconds, and strong intensity. Descent of the fetal presenting part continues until it reaches the perineal floor.

Some practitioners have further subdivided the second stage into two phases including the latent/passive fetal descent stage in which the woman may initially experience the urge to push. During this time, passive fetal descent occurs in response to the uterine contractions. Nursing tasks during this phase include (Association of Women's Health, Obstetric and Neonatal Nurses [AWHONN], 2013):

- Assessing the woman's perception of the need or urge to push
- Evaluating the maternal–fetal oxygenation status to ensure adequate uteroplacental perfusion is occurring
- Assessing fetal status through recommended monitoring protocols

Developing Cultural Competence   Presence of the Father

The presence of the father during labor and at birth, although common in countries such as the United States, Canada, and Australia, is not a universal norm. Rather it is strongly influenced by cultural practices. The father is not present at the birth in many countries, including Algeria, Brazil, China, Ethiopia, and Korea. Similarly, Orthodox Judaism does not allow men to attend the labor and birth (McFarland & Wehbe-Alamah, 2014).

The second phase (within the second stage of labor) is known as the active pushing phase and occurs once the urge to push has been established and the woman begins to actively push with her contractions. Nursing tasks during this phase include (AWHONN, 2013):

- Assessing the effectiveness of the maternal pushing efforts
- Providing encouragement and direction to obtain a more adequate pushing effort
- Assessing fetal response that occurs as maternal pushing is performed including continued fetal assessment measures

While some women may be encouraged to begin pushing immediately after the identification of complete dilatation, others may be encouraged to delay pushing and allow for passive fetal descent, an act known as "laboring down." A recent systematic review comparing both methods of pushing did not identify any differences in maternal or fetal outcomes; however, women in the passive descent or laboring down group experienced a longer second stage of labor that resulted in a reduction of active pushing efforts (King et al., 2015). Laboring down does aid the woman who is extremely fatigued and does prevent extensive pushing efforts that may occur before the urge to push is experienced by the woman.

As the fetal head descends, the woman usually has the urge to push because of pressure of the fetal head on the sacral and obturator nerves. As she pushes, intra-abdominal pressure is exerted from contraction of the maternal abdominal muscles. As the fetal head continues its descent, the perineum begins to bulge, flatten, and move anteriorly. Most women feel acute, increasingly severe pain and a burning sensation as the perineum distends. The amount of bloody show may increase. The labia begin to part with each contraction. Between contractions the fetal head appears to recede. With succeeding contractions and maternal pushing effort, the fetal head descends farther. **Crowning** occurs when the fetal head is encircled by the external opening of the vagina (introitus), and it means birth is imminent.

The woman may feel some relief that the transition phase is over, the birth is near, and she can push. Some women feel a sense of purpose now that they can be actively involved. The woman may be focused and should be encouraged to center all her energy into pushing. Resting between contractions should be encouraged. There are often many opportunities for the support person to assist the woman by providing support to the legs, offering ice chips, fanning the woman, who is often overheated and fatigued, and giving verbal encouragement. For women without childbirth preparation, this stage can become frightening; the woman should be encouraged to work with her contractions and not fight them. A support person who has never seen a labor may become disconcerted during this time. The nurse can assist the support person in performing activities and offering encouragement that assists the woman during the birth process. The woman may feel she has lost her ability to cope and become embarrassed, or she may demonstrate extreme irritability toward the staff or her supporters as she attempts to regain control over her body. Some women feel a great sense of purpose and are unrelenting in their efforts to work with each and every contraction. Some women will be very forceful and directive with staff and support persons. Again, all of these reactions and emotions are common and should be supported as the woman works toward the birth.

SPONTANEOUS BIRTH (VERTEX PRESENTATION)

As the fetal head distends the vulva with each contraction, the perineum becomes extremely thin and the anus stretches and protrudes. With time, the head extends under the symphysis pubis and is born. When the anterior shoulder meets the underside of the symphysis pubis, a gentle push by the mother aids in the birth of the shoulders. The body then follows (Figure 16–12). (Birth of a fetus in other than a vertex presentation [fetal malposition] is discussed in Chapter 21.)

POSITIONAL CHANGES OF THE FETUS

For the fetus to pass through the birth canal, the fetal head and body must adjust to the passage by certain positional changes. These changes, called **cardinal movements** or *mechanisms of labor*, are described in the order in which they occur (Figure 16–13).

Descent. *Descent* occurs because of four forces: (1) pressure of the amniotic fluid, (2) direct pressure of the uterine fundus on the breech, (3) contraction of the abdominal muscles, and (4) extension and straightening of the fetal body. The head enters

the inlet in the occiput transverse or oblique position because the pelvic inlet is widest from side to side. The sagittal suture is an equal distance from the maternal symphysis pubis and the sacral promontory.

Flexion. *Flexion* occurs as the fetal head descends and meets resistance from the soft tissues of the pelvis, the muscles of the pelvic floor, and the cervix. As a result of the resistance, the fetal chin flexes downward onto the chest.

Internal Rotation. The fetal head must rotate to fit the diameter of the pelvic cavity, which is widest in the anteroposterior diameter. As the occiput of the fetal head meets resistance from the levator ani muscles and their fascia, the occiput rotates—usually from left to right—and the sagittal suture aligns in the anteroposterior pelvic diameter.

Extension. The resistance of the pelvic floor and the mechanical movement of the vulva opening anteriorly and forward assist with extension of the fetal head as it passes under the symphysis pubis. With this positional change, the occiput, then brow and face, emerge from the vagina.

Restitution. The shoulders of the fetus enter the pelvis inlet obliquely and remain oblique when the head rotates to the anteroposterior diameter through internal rotation. Because of this rotation, the neck becomes twisted. Once the head is born and is free of pelvic resistance, the neck untwists, turning the head to one side (restitution), and aligns with the position of the back in the birth canal.

External Rotation. As the shoulders rotate to the anteroposterior position in the pelvis, the head turns farther to one side (external rotation).

Expulsion. After the external rotation, and through the pushing efforts of the laboring woman, the anterior shoulder meets the undersurface of the symphysis pubis and slips under it. As lateral flexion of the shoulder and head occurs, the anterior shoulder is born before the posterior shoulder. The body follows quickly.

Third Stage

The third stage of labor is defined as the period of time from the birth of the neonate until the completed delivery of the placenta. The third stage should be completed within 30 minutes of the birth of the baby. If the time of placenta delivery is delayed, the cervix begins to close as the uterus contracts and the risk of hemorrhage and placenta retention (retained placenta) occurs.

PLACENTAL SEPARATION

After the baby is born, the uterus contracts firmly, diminishing its capacity and the surface area of placental attachment. The placenta begins to separate because of this decrease in surface area. As this separation occurs, bleeding results in the formation of a hematoma between the placental tissue and the remaining decidua. This hematoma accelerates the separation process. The membranes are the last to separate. They are peeled off the uterine wall as the placenta descends into the vagina.

Signs of placental separation usually appear about 5 minutes after the birth of the newborn. These signs are (1) a globular shaped uterus, (2) a rise of the fundus in the abdomen, (3) a sudden gush or trickle of blood, and (4) further protrusion of the umbilical cord out of the vagina.

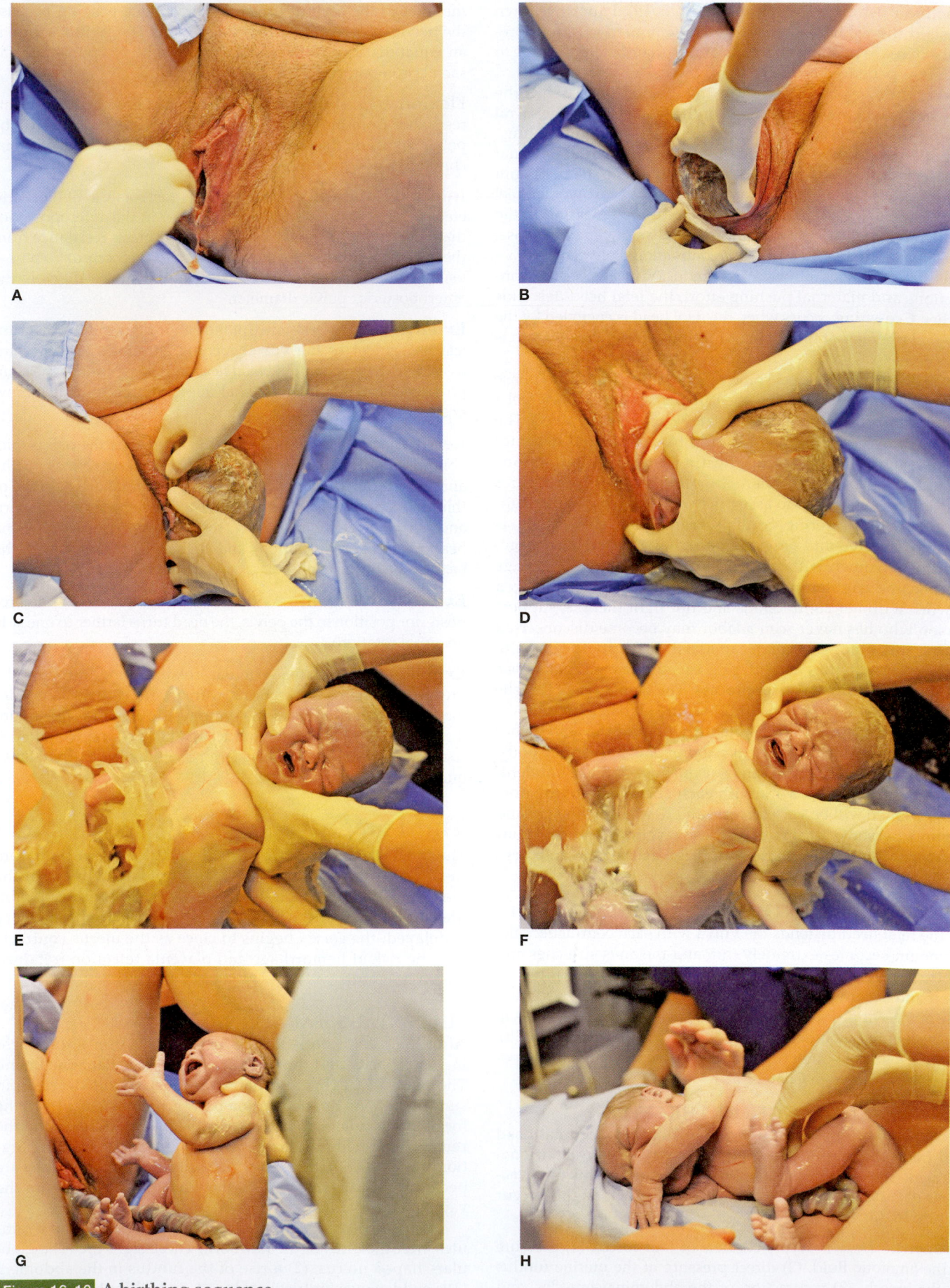

Figure 16–12 A birthing sequence.

SOURCE: Michele Davidson.

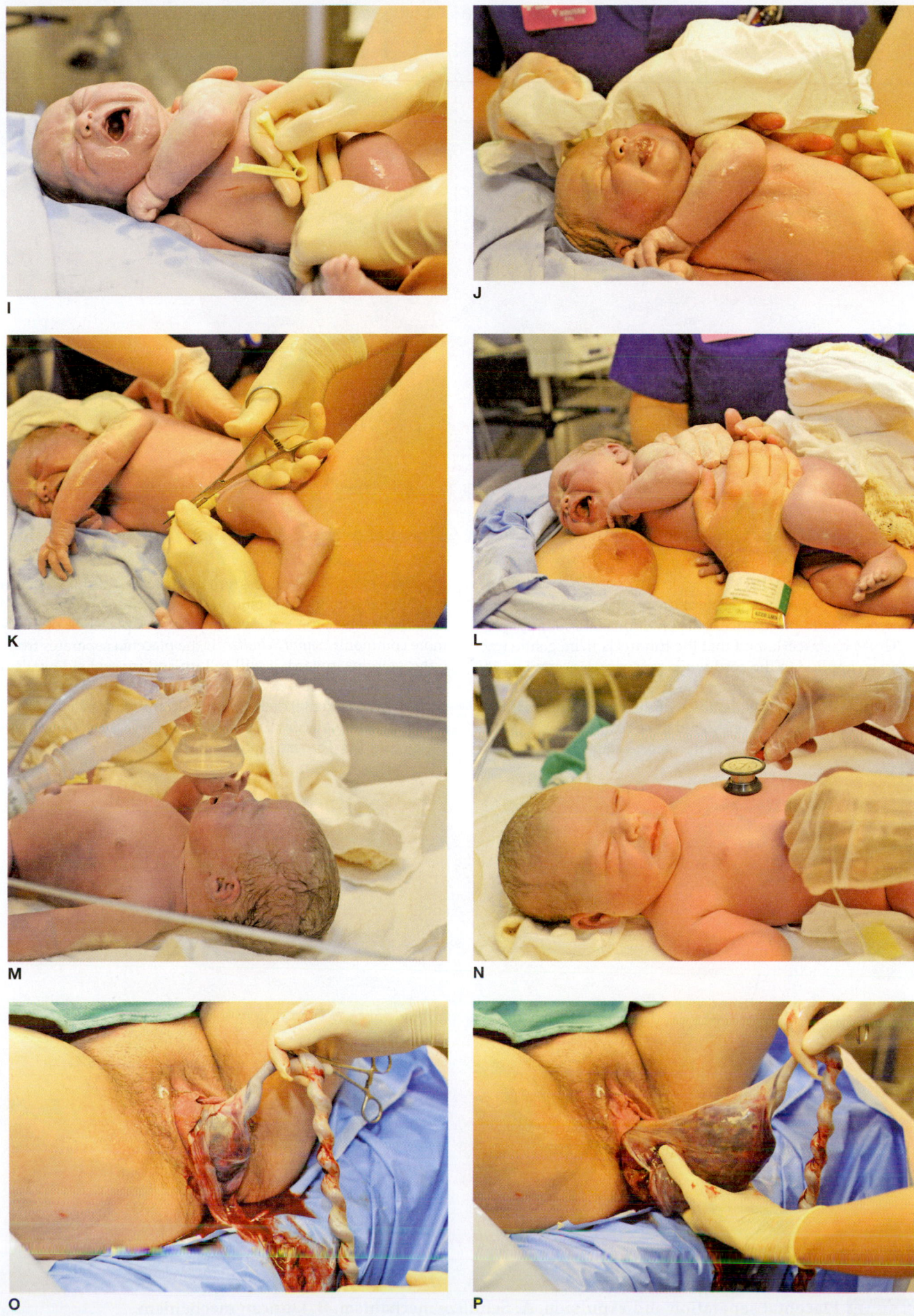

I

J

K

L

M

N

O

P

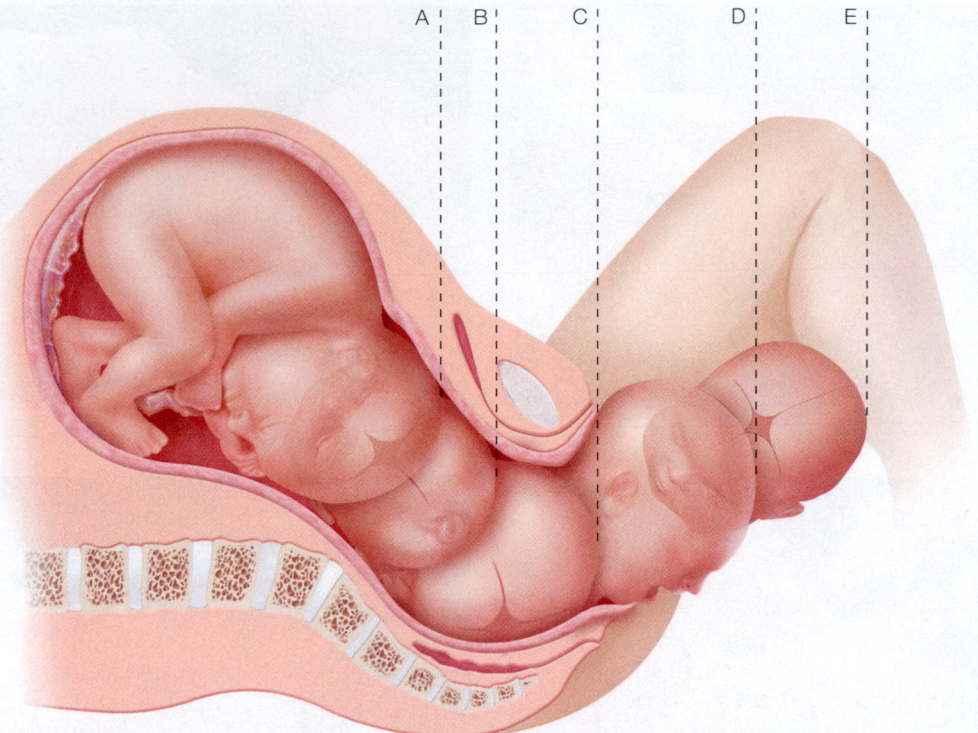

Figure 16–13 Mechanisms of labor. A. Descent. B. Flexion. C. Internal rotation. D. External rotation. E. Extension.

PLACENTAL DELIVERY

When the signs of placental separation appear, the woman may bear down to aid in placental expulsion. If this fails and the physician/CNM has ascertained that the fundus is firm, gentle traction may be applied to the cord while pressure is exerted on the fundus. The weight of the placenta as it is guided into the placental collection pan aids in the removal of the membranes from the uterine wall. A placenta is considered to be retained if 30 minutes have elapsed from completion of the second stage of labor.

If the placenta separates from the inside to the outer margins, it is delivered with the fetal (shiny) side presenting (Figure 16–14A). This is known as the *Schultze mechanism* of placental delivery or, more commonly, *Shiny Schultze*. If the placenta separates from the outer margins inward, it will roll up and present sideways with the maternal surface delivering first. This is known as the *Duncan mechanism* of placental delivery and is commonly called *Dirty Duncan* because the placental surface is rough (Figure 16–14B). Also see Figures 4–8 (Duncan) and 4–9 (Schultze).

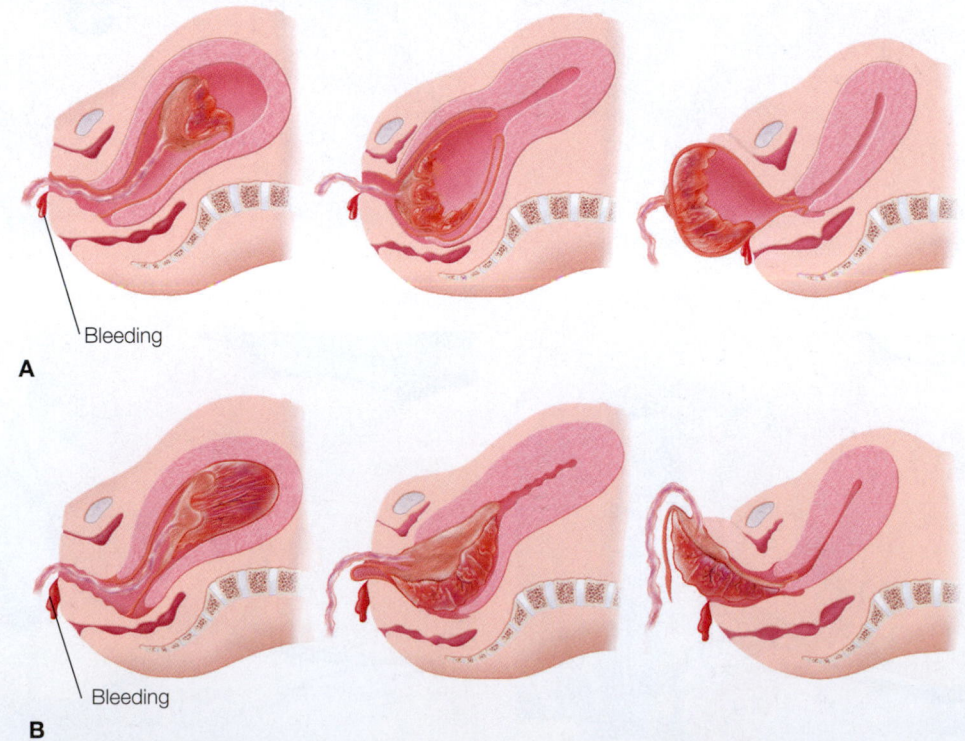

Figure 16–14 Placental separation and expulsion. A. Schultze mechanism. B. Duncan mechanism.

Fourth Stage

The fourth stage of labor is the time, from 1 to 4 hours after birth, during which physiologic readjustment of the mother's body begins. With the birth, hemodynamic changes occur. Blood loss ranges from 250 to 500 mL. With this blood loss and removal of the weight of the pregnant uterus from the surrounding vessels, blood is redistributed into venous beds. This results in a moderate drop in both systolic and diastolic blood pressure, increased pulse pressure, and moderate tachycardia (Cunningham et al., 2014).

The uterus remains contracted in the midline of the abdomen. The fundus is usually midway between the symphysis pubis and the umbilicus. Its contracted state constricts the vessels at the site of placental implantation. Immediately after birth of the placenta, the cervix is widely spread and thick.

Nausea and vomiting usually cease. The woman may be thirsty and hungry. She may experience a shaking chill, which is thought to be associated with the ending of the physical exertion of labor. The bladder is often hypotonic because of trauma during the second stage and/or the administration of anesthetics that decrease sensations. Hypotonic bladder can lead to urinary retention.

Maternal Systemic Response to Labor

The labor and birth process affects nearly all of the maternal physiologic systems.

Cardiovascular System

The woman's cardiovascular system is stressed both by the uterine contractions and by the pain, anxiety, and apprehension she experiences. During pregnancy, there is a 50% increase in circulating blood volume. The increase in cardiac output peaks between the second and third trimester although during labor there is a significant increase in cardiac output. With each contraction, 300 to 500 mL of blood volume is forced back into the maternal circulation, which results in an increase in cardiac output of as much as 10% to 15% over the typical third-trimester levels (Blackburn, 2013). Further increases in cardiac output occur as the laboring woman experiences pain with uterine contractions and her anxiety and apprehension increase.

Maternal position also affects cardiac output. In the supine position, cardiac output lowers as a result of the gravid uterus, heart rate increases, and stroke volume decreases. When the woman turns to a lateral (side-lying) position, cardiac output increases (Blackburn, 2013). Women with pre-existing heart disease have higher rates of arrhythmias in labor (Naderi & Raymond, 2015).

BLOOD PRESSURE

As a result of increased cardiac output, blood pressure (both systolic and diastolic) rises during uterine contractions. The nurse should ensure that blood pressure measurements are not obtained during uterine contractions because this can result in an inaccurate reading. In the first stage, systolic pressure increases by 35 mmHg and diastolic pressure increases by about 25 mmHg. There may be further increases in the second stage during pushing (Blackburn, 2013).

Respiratory System

Oxygen demand and consumption increase at the onset of labor because of the presence of uterine contractions. As anxiety and pain from contractions increase, hyperventilation frequently occurs. With hyperventilation there is a fall in $PaCO_2$, and respiratory alkalosis results.

By the end of the first stage, most women have developed a mild metabolic acidosis compensated by respiratory alkalosis. As they push in the second stage of labor, the women's $PaCO_2$ levels may rise along with blood lactate levels (because of muscular activity), leading to mild respiratory acidosis. By the time the baby is born (end of second stage), there is metabolic acidosis uncompensated for by respiratory alkalosis (Blackburn, 2013).

The changes in acid–base status that occur in labor are quickly reversed in the fourth stage because of changes in women's respiratory rates. Acid–base levels return to pregnancy levels by 24 hours after birth, and nonpregnant values are attained a few weeks after birth (Blackburn, 2013).

Renal System

During labor there is an increase in maternal renin, plasma renin activity, and angiotensinogen. This elevation is thought to be important in the control of uteroplacental blood flow during birth and the early postpartum period (Blackburn, 2013).

Structurally, the base of the bladder is pushed forward and upward when engagement occurs. The pressure from the presenting part may impair blood and lymph drainage from the base of the bladder, leading to edema.

Gastrointestinal System

During labor, gastric motility and absorption of solid food are reduced. Gastric emptying time is prolonged, and gastric volume (amount of contents that remain in the stomach) remains increased, regardless of the time the last meal was taken (Blackburn, 2013). Some narcotics also delay gastric emptying time and add to the risk of aspiration if general anesthesia is used.

Immune System and Other Blood Values

The white blood cell (WBC) count increases to 25,000 to 30,000/mm³ during labor and the early postpartum period. The change in WBCs is mostly because of increased neutrophils resulting from a physiologic response to stress. The increased WBC count makes it difficult to identify the presence of an infection.

Maternal blood glucose levels decrease because glucose is used as an energy source during uterine contractions. The decreased blood glucose levels lead to a decrease in insulin requirements (Blackburn, 2013).

Pain

Pain during labor comes from a complexity of physical causes. Each woman will experience and cope with pain differently. Multiple factors affect a woman's reaction to labor pain.

CAUSES OF PAIN DURING LABOR

The pain associated with the first stage of labor is unique in that it accompanies a normal physiologic process. Even though perception of the pain of childbirth varies among women, there is a physiologic basis for discomfort during labor. Pain during the first stage of labor arises from (1) dilatation of the cervix, which is the primary source of pain; (2) stretching of the lower uterine segment; (3) pressure on adjacent structures; and (4) hypoxia of the uterine muscle cells during contraction (Blackburn, 2013). The areas of pain include the lower abdominal wall and the areas over the lower lumbar region and the upper sacrum (Figure 16–15).

During the second stage of labor, pain is caused by (1) hypoxia of the contracting uterine muscle cells, (2) distention of the vagina and perineum, and (3) pressure on adjacent structures. The area of pain increases as shown in Figures 16–16 and 16–17.

Pain during the third stage results from uterine contractions and cervical dilatation as the placenta is expelled. This

stage of labor is short, and after it anesthesia is needed primarily for episiotomy repair.

FACTORS AFFECTING RESPONSE TO PAIN

Many factors affect the individual's perception and response to pain. For example, childbirth preparation classes may reduce the need for analgesia during labor. Preparing for labor and birth through reading, talking with others, or attending a childbirth preparation class frequently has positive effects for the laboring woman and her partner. The woman who knows what to expect and what techniques she may use to increase comfort

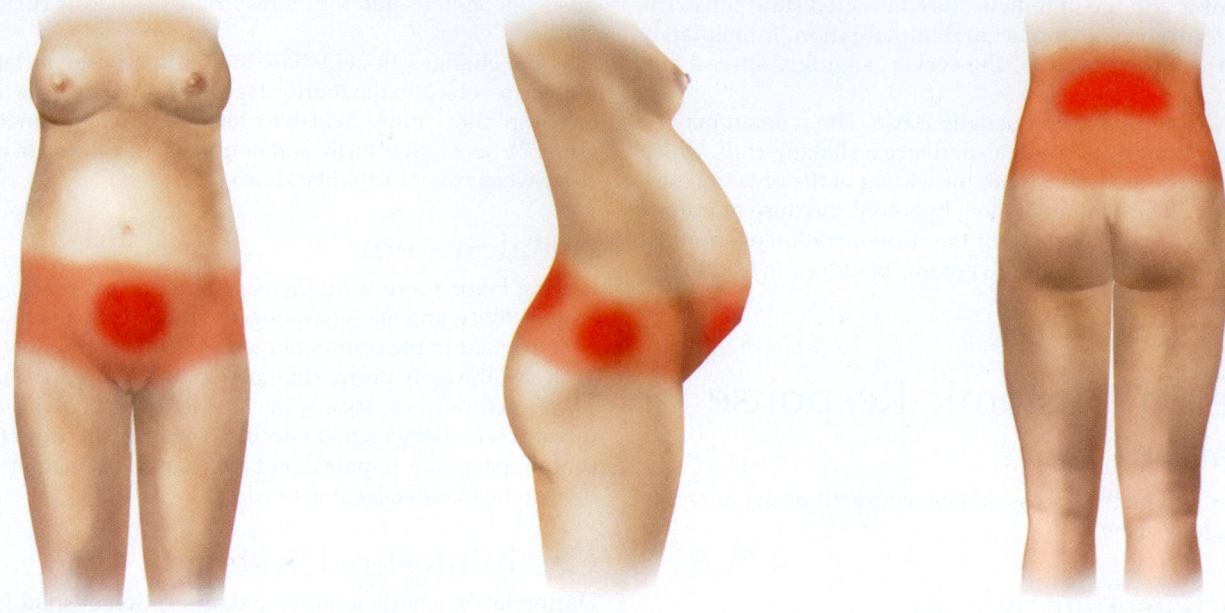

Figure 16–15 Area of reference of labor pain during the first stage. Pain is most intense in the darkened areas.

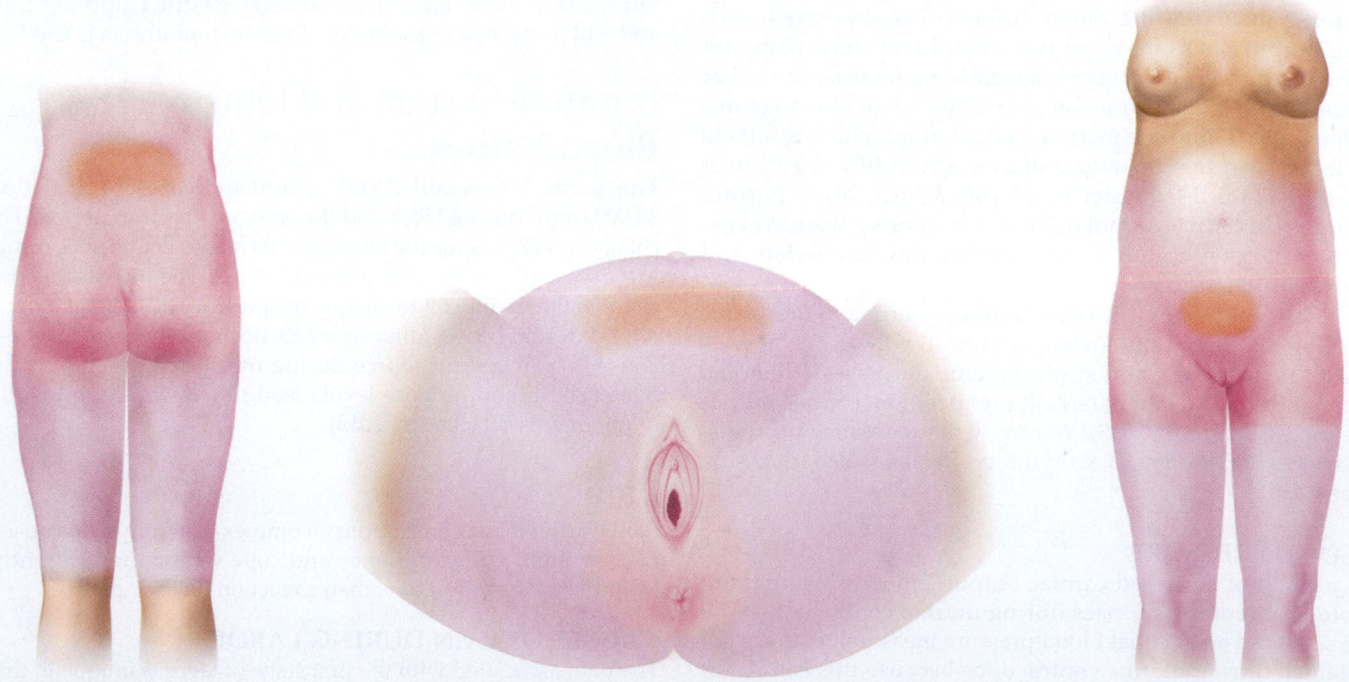

Figure 16–16 Distribution of labor pain during the later phase of the first stage and early phase of the second stage. The darkest colored areas indicate the location of the most intense pain; moderate color, moderate pain; and light color, mild pain. The uterine contractions, which at this stage are very strong, produce intense pain.

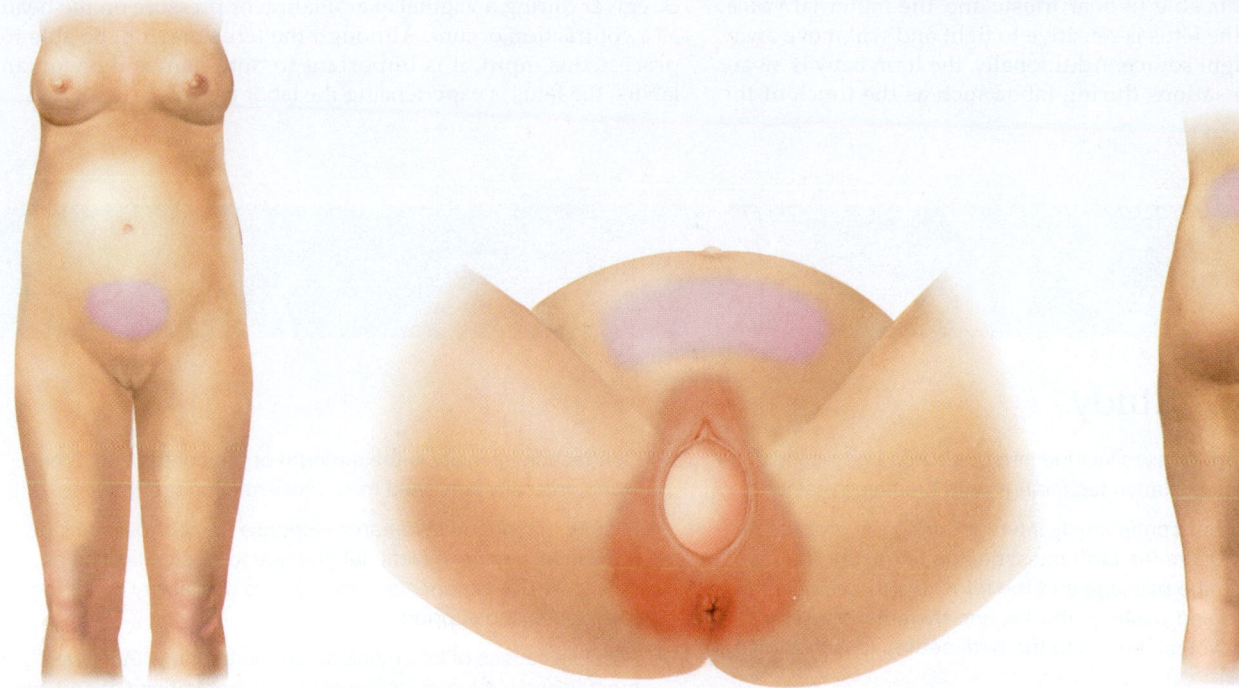

Figure 16–17 Distribution of labor pain during the later phase of the second stage and actual birth. The perineal component is the primary cause of discomfort. Uterine contractions contribute much less to the level of pain.

tends to be less anxious during the labor. A tour of the birthing center and an opportunity to see and feel the environment also help reduce anxiety because during admission (especially with the first child) many new things are happening and they seem to occur all at once.

In addition, individuals tend to respond to painful stimuli in the way that is acceptable in their culture. In some cultures, it is natural to communicate pain, no matter how mild, whereas members of other cultures stoically accept pain out of fear or because it is expected. Nurses need to be aware of cultural norms and demonstrate culturally sensitive care to women and their families in the intrapartum setting (Galanti, 2014).

Response to pain may also be influenced by fatigue and sleep deprivation. The fatigued woman has less energy and ability to use such strategies as distraction or imagination to deal with pain. As a result, she may lose her ability to cope with labor and choose analgesics or other medications to relieve the discomfort.

The woman's previous experience with pain and her anxiety level also affect her ability to manage current and future pain. Those who have had experience with pain seem more sensitive to painful stimuli than those who have not. Unfamiliar surroundings and events can increase anxiety, as does separation from family and loved ones. Anticipation of discomfort and questions about whether she can cope with the contractions may also increase anxiety.

Both attention and distraction influence the perception of pain. When pain sensation is the focus of attention, the perceived intensity is greater. A sensory stimulus such as a back rub can be a distraction that focuses the woman's attention on the stimulus rather than the pain.

Fetal Response to Labor

When the fetus is healthy, the mechanical and hemodynamic changes of normal labor have no adverse effects.

Heart Rate Changes

Early fetal heart rate decelerations can occur with intracranial pressures of 40 to 55 mmHg, as the head pushes against the cervix. The currently accepted explanation of this early deceleration is hypoxic depression of the central nervous system, which is under vagal control. The absence of these head-compression decelerations in some fetuses during labor is explained by the existence of a threshold that is reached more gradually in the presence of intact membranes and lack of maternal resistance. These early decelerations are harmless in a normal fetus.

Acid–Base Status in Labor

Blood flow is decreased to the fetus at the peak of each contraction, which leads to a slow decrease in pH status. During the second stage of labor, as uterine contractions become longer and stronger and the woman often holds her breath to push, the fetal pH decreases more rapidly. Although women are encouraged to maintain slow paced breathing, holding of the breath does often occur. As the base deficit increases, fetal oxygen saturation drops approximately 10% (Blackburn, 2013).

Hemodynamic Changes

The adequate exchange of nutrients and gases in the fetal capillaries and intervillous spaces depends in part on the fetal blood pressure. Fetal blood pressure is a protective mechanism for the normal fetus during the anoxic periods caused by the contracting uterus during labor. The fetal and placental reserve is usually enough to see the fetus through these anoxic periods unharmed (Blackburn, 2013).

Fetal Sensation

Beginning at about 38 weeks' gestation (full term), the fetus is able to experience sensations of light, sound, and touch. The full-term fetus is able to hear music and the maternal voice. Even in utero, the fetus is sensitive to light and will move away from a bright light source. Additionally, the term baby is aware of pressure sensations during labor such as the touch of the caregiver during a vaginal examination or pressure on the head as a contraction occurs. Although the fetus may not be able to process this input, it is important to note that as the woman labors, the fetus is experiencing the labor as well.

Focus Your Study

- Most childbirth classes include information on body-conditioning exercises, relaxation techniques, and breathing methods.

- Five factors that continuously interact during the process of labor and birth are the birth passage, the fetus, the relationship between the passage and the fetus, the forces of labor (contractions and pushing efforts), and the emotional components the woman brings to the birth setting (psychosocial status).

- Important parts of the maternal pelvis include the pelvic inlet, pelvic cavity, and pelvic outlet.

- The fetal head contains bones that are not fused. This allows for some overlapping and for a change in the shape of the head, called molding, to facilitate birth.

- Fetal attitude refers to the relation of the fetal parts to one another. The head is usually moderately flexed at midline, and the extremities are flexed close to the body.

- Fetal lie refers to the relationship of the cephalocaudal axis of the fetus to the maternal spine. The fetal lie is either longitudinal or transverse.

- Fetal presentation is determined by the body part lying closest to the maternal pelvis. Fetal presentation can be cephalic (head down), breech (buttocks or one or both feet), or shoulder.

- Fetal position is the relationship of the landmark on the presenting fetal part to the front, sides, or back of the maternal pelvis.

- Engagement of the presenting part takes place when the largest diameter of the presenting part reaches or passes through the pelvic inlet.

- Station refers to the relationship of the presenting part to an imaginary line drawn between the ischial spines of the maternal pelvis. Negative numbers (–5 through –1) are above the ischial spines, and the fetus is not engaged. Zero (0) station is at the pelvic inlet, and descent below the ischial spines is indicated by positive numbers (+1 through +4).

- Each uterine contraction has an increment, acme, and decrement. Contraction frequency is the time from the beginning of one contraction to the beginning of the next contraction.

- Contraction duration is the time from the beginning to the end of one contraction.

- Contraction intensity is the strength of the contraction during acme. Intensity is termed mild, moderate, or strong.

- Factors that affect a woman's response to labor pain include education, cultural beliefs, fatigue, personal significance of pain, previous experience, anxiety, and availability of coping techniques and support.

- Possible causes of labor include progesterone withdrawal, prostaglandin release, or increased concentrations of corticotropin-releasing hormone (CRH).

- Premonitory signs of labor include lightening, Braxton Hicks contractions, cervical softening and effacement, bloody show, sudden burst of energy, weight loss, and sometimes rupture of membranes.

- True labor contractions occur regularly, with an increase in frequency, duration, and intensity over time. The contractions usually start in the back and radiate around the abdomen. The discomfort is not relieved by ambulation or rest. False labor contractions do not produce progressive cervical effacement and dilatation. They are usually irregular and do not increase in intensity. The discomfort may be relieved by changes in activity.

- There are four stages of labor and birth: The first stage is from the beginning of true labor to complete dilatation of the cervix, the second stage is from complete dilatation of the cervix to birth, the third stage is from birth to expulsion of the placenta, and the fourth stage is from expulsion of the placenta to a period of 1 to 4 hours afterwards.

- The fetus accommodates itself to the maternal pelvis in a series of movements called the cardinal movements of labor, which include descent, flexion, internal rotation, extension, restitution, external rotation, and expulsion.

- Placental separation is indicated by lengthening of the umbilical cord, a small spurt of blood, change in uterine shape, and a rise of the fundus in the abdomen.

- The placenta is delivered by the Schultze or the Duncan mechanism, which is determined by the way it separates from the uterine wall.

- Maternal systemic responses to labor involve the cardiovascular, respiratory, renal, gastrointestinal, and immune systems.

- The fetus is usually able to tolerate the labor process with no untoward changes.

Clinical Reasoning in Action

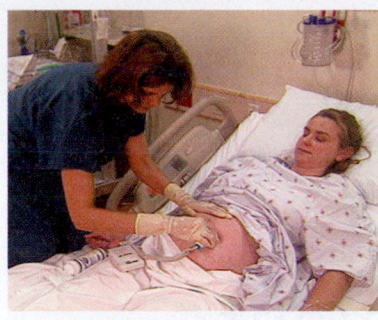

Ann Nelson, a 28-year-old, G2P0010 at 41 weeks' gestation, is admitted to the birthing unit where you are working. She is here for cervical ripening and induction of labor due to postdate pregnancy and decreased amniotic fluid volume. A review of her prenatal medical record reveals a pertinent history of infertility (Clomid-included pregnancy) and asthma (treated with inhalers on a PRN basis). The Doppler picks up a fetal heart rate of 120 beats/min. You place Ann on the electronic fetal monitor and obtain the following data: BP 126/76, T 98°F, P 82, R 16; vaginal examination reveals a 20% effaced cervix, 1 cm dilatation in the posterior position, and vertex at −2 station. The fetal monitor shows a fetal heart rate baseline of 120 to 128 with occasional variable decelerations, accelerations to 140 with fetal activity. No contractions are noted on the monitor or palpated. Ann asks you what to expect with "cervical ripening" using prostaglandin gel.

1. Discuss the action of prostaglandin gel.
2. Ann asks you why cervical ripening and induction of labor are recommended for her and her baby. How would you best respond to her?
3. Ann asks how she will know if she is getting contractions. How would you answer her?
4. Discuss the difference between mild, moderate, and strong contractions.
5. Describe the latent phase of labor.

References

American College of Nurse Midwives (ACNM). (2012). Premature rupture of membranes at term. Position statement. Silver Spring, MD: ACNM.

American College of Obstetricians & Gynecologists (ACOG). (2016). *Premature rupture of membranes* (Practice Bulletin No. 160). Washington, DC: Author.

Association of Women's Health, Obstetric and Neonatal Nurses (AWHONN). (2013). *Evidence-based clinical practice guideline: Nursing care and management of the second stage of labor* (3rd ed.). Washington, DC: Author.

Blackburn, S. T. (2013). *Maternal, fetal, and neonatal physiology: A clinical perspective* (4th ed.). Philadelphia, PA: Saunders.

Breakey, A. A., Reidner, A., & Dekker, R. (2013). *What is the evidence for inducing labor if your water breaks at term?* Retrieved from http://evidencebasedbirth.com/evidence-inducing-labor-water-breaks-term/

Cheng, Y. (2014). Normal labor and delivery. *Medscape.* Retrieved from http://emedicine.medscape.com/article/260036-overview

Cunningham, F. G., Leveno, K. J., Bloom, S. L., Spong, C. Y., Dashe, J. S., Hoffman, B. L., . . . Sheffield, J. S.

(2014). *Williams obstetrics* (24th ed.). New York, NY: McGraw-Hill.

Galanti, G. A. (2014). *Caring for patients from different cultures* (5th ed.). Philadelphia, PA: University of Pennsylvania Press.

Hodnett, E. D., Gates, S., Hofmeyr, G. J., Sakala, C., & Weston, J. (2011). Continuous support for women during childbirth. *Cochrane Database of Systematic Reviews,* Issue 2. Art. No.: CD003766. doi:10.1002/14651858.CD003766.pub3

International Childbirth Education Association (ICEA). (2012). *ICEA philosophy statement.* Retrieved from http://www.icea.org/content/mission

International Childbirth Education Association. (ICEA). (2016). *ICEA position paper: Comfort measures.* Retrieved from http://icea.org/wp-content/uploads/2016/01/Comfort_Measues_PP.pdf

Jazayeri, A. (2014). Premature rupture of membranes. *Medscape.* Retrieved from http://emedicine.medscape.com/article/261137-overview#aw2aab6b3

King, T. K., Brucker, M. C., Kriebs, J. M., & Fahey, J. (2015). *Varney's midwifery* (5th ed.). New York, NY: Jones Bartlett Learning.

McFarland, M. R., & Wehbe-Alamah, H. B. (2014). *Leininger's culture care diversity and universality: A worldwide nursing theory* (3rd ed.). New York, NY: Jones & Bartlett.

Naderi, S., & Raymond, R. (2015). Pregnancy and heart disease. *Cleveland Clinic Continuing Education.* Retrieved from http://www.clevelandclinicmeded.com/medicalpubs/diseasemanagement/cardiology/pregnancy-and-heart-disease/Default.htm#factors

Pintucci, A., Meregalli, V., Colombo, P., & Fiorilli, A. (2014). Premature rupture of membranes at term in low risk women: How long should we wait in the "latent phase"? *Journal of Perinatal Medicine, 42*(2), 189–196.

Tan, H., Yi, L., Rote, N. S., Hurd, W. W., Mesiano, S. (2012). Progesterone receptor-A and -B have opposite effects on proinflammatory gene expression in human myometrial cells: Implications for progesterone actions in human pregnancy and parturition. *Journal of Clinical Endocrinology Metabolism, 97*(5), E719–E730. doi:http://dx.doi.org/10.1210/jc.2011–3251

Ventolini, G. (2013). Activation of simultaneous pathways in the initiation of parturition in humans. *OA Medical Hypothesis, Aug. 01,1*(2),11.

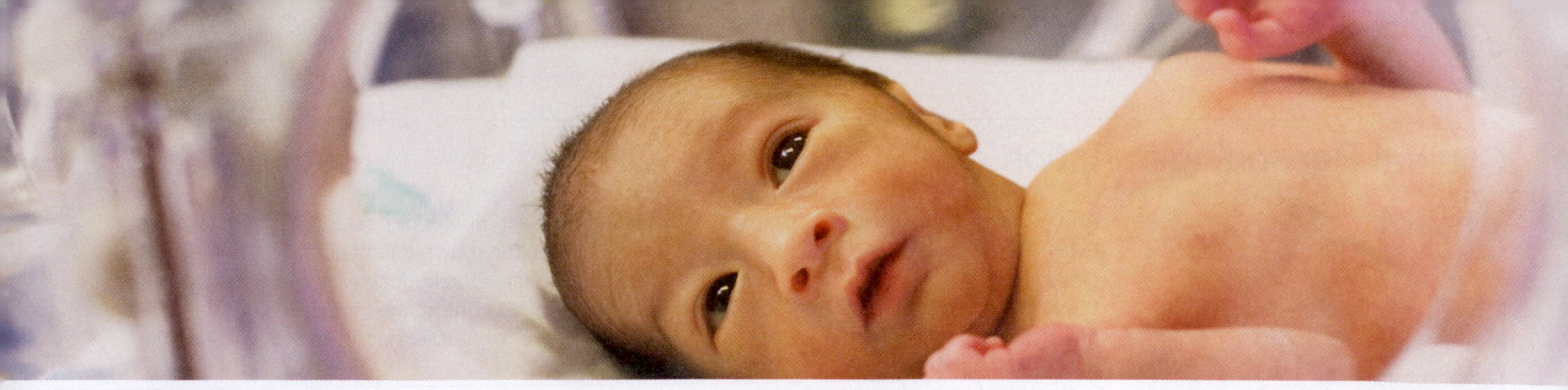

Chapter 17
Intrapartum Nursing Assessment

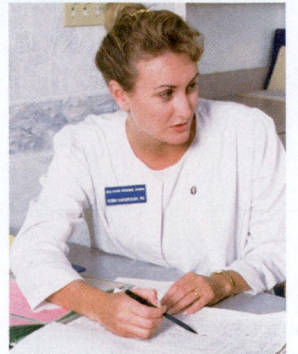

As charge nurse on a busy birthing unit, sometimes I feel like I'm meeting myself coming and going. At any one time I may be called upon to do a great number of things, seemingly all at once: maintain a safe and adequate staffing level, be the extra pair of hands at a high-risk delivery, consult with members of the hospital's support services team, arrange for the smooth transfer of a laboring woman to the operating room for a cesarean, help a mom who is having difficulty breastfeeding, or simply cuddle a newborn whose parents (and nurse) need a few minutes of rest. Would I trade this bustle for anything else? Not on your life!

—Birth Center Charge Nurse

∨ Learning Outcomes

17.1 Describe a maternal assessment of the laboring woman that includes the client history, high-risk screening, and physical and psychosociocultural factors.

17.2 Evaluate the progress of labor by assessing the laboring woman's contractions, cervical dilatation, and effacement.

17.3 Describe an intrapartum fetal assessment to determine fetal position and presentation, fetal heart rate, and fetal status.

17.4 Describe the steps and frequency for performing auscultation of fetal heart rate.

17.5 Delineate the procedure for performing Leopold maneuvers and the information that can be obtained.

17.6 Describe the indications, methods, and steps for performing and recording electronic fetal monitoring.

17.7 Distinguish between baseline and periodic changes in fetal heart rate monitoring, and the appearance and significance of each.

17.8 Evaluate fetal heart rate tracings using a systematic approach.

17.9 Compare nonreassuring fetal heart rate patterns to appropriate nursing responses.

17.10 Explain the family's responses to electronic fetal monitoring in nursing management.

The physiologic and psychologic events that occur during labor call for continual and rapid adaptations by the mother and the fetus. Frequent and accurate assessments are crucial to the progress of these adaptations. In current nursing practice, the traditional assessment techniques of observation, palpation, and auscultation are augmented by the judicious use of technology such as ultrasound and electronic monitoring. These tools may provide more detailed information for assessment; however, it is important for the nurse to remember that the technology only provides data. It is the nurse who monitors the mother and her baby.

Maternal Assessment

Assessment of the mother begins with a client history and screening for intrapartum risk factors.

History

The nurse obtains a brief oral history when the woman is admitted to the birthing area. Typically the maternal and fetal vital signs are immediately assessed. If the vital signs are within normal limits, the interview continues. If there is an identified problem, nursing care is then prioritized.

It is common for the provider to send the prenatal records to the labor and birthing unit before the woman's due date. The information should be reviewed in a nonjudgmental manner to ensure changes have not occurred since the information was documented. During the initial interview, the nurse is building a trusting relationship. It is often helpful if the nurse sits down and appears unrushed, makes direct eye contact (if culturally appropriate), and begins the interview with a statement such as "I am going to be asking you some very personal and specific questions so that we can provide the best care for both you and your baby." This conveys a nonjudgmental approach, shows respect, and makes the woman feel more at ease. Each agency has its own admission forms, but they usually include the following information:

- Woman's name and age
- Last menstrual period (LMP) and estimated date of birth (EDB)
- Attending physician or certified nurse-midwife (CNM)
- Personal data: blood type; Rh factor; results of serology testing; group B streptococcus status; prepregnant and present weight; allergies to medications, foods, or other substances; prescribed and over-the-counter medications taken during pregnancy; and history of drug and alcohol use and smoking during the pregnancy
- History of previous illness, such as tuberculosis, heart disease, diabetes, convulsive disorders, and thyroid disorders; asthma; sickle cell/Tay–Sachs and other inherited disorders; pregnancy-related complications (such as preterm labor, gestational diabetes, preeclampsia, low platelets)
- Problems in the prenatal period, such as elevated blood pressure, bleeding problems, recurrent urinary tract infections, other infections, abnormal laboratory findings (such as abnormal glucose screen indicating gestational diabetes or low hemoglobin or hematocrit indicating anemia), mental health issues, or sexually transmitted infections
- Pregnancy data: gravida, para, preterm births, term births, abortions, living children, and neonatal deaths
- The method chosen for newborn/infant feeding
- Type of childbirth education or newborn/infant care classes
- Previous newborn/infant care experience
- Woman's preferences regarding labor and birth, such as mobility preferences, no analgesics or anesthetics, or the presence of the father, partner, or others at the birth
- Pediatrician, family practice physician, or nurse practitioner
- Additional data: history of special tests such as non-stress test (NST), biophysical profile (BPP), or ultrasound; history of any preterm labor; onset of labor; amniotic fluid membrane status; and brief description of any previous labor and birth
- Onset of labor, status of amniotic membranes (intact, ruptured, time of rupture, color, and odor)

PSYCHOSOCIAL CONSIDERATIONS

Assessment of psychosocial history is a critical component of intrapartum nursing assessment. The parents' psychosocial readiness, including their fears, anxieties, birth fantasies, excitement level, feelings of joy and anticipation, and level of social support can be critical factors in a successful birth experience. Both the mother and the father are making a transition into a new role, and both have expectations of themselves during the labor and birth experience, and as caregivers for their child and their new family. Psychosocial factors affecting labor and birth include the couple's accomplishment of the tasks of pregnancy, usual coping mechanisms in response to stressful life events, support system, preparation for childbirth, and cultural influences. Even mothers and fathers who attend childbirth preparation classes and have a solid support system can be concerned about what labor will be like, whether they will be able to perform the way they expect, whether the pain will be more than the mother expects or can cope with, and whether the father can provide helpful support. The physical and emotional stress of birth can impact a couple's responses to the labor itself.

Some women may fear the pain of contractions, whereas others welcome the opportunity to feel the birth process. Some women view the pain as threatening and associate it with a loss of control over their bodies and emotions. Other women see pain as a rite of passage into motherhood and a necessary means to an end. It is helpful for women to realize that the pain of labor is natural. Assurances that labor is progressing normally can go a long way toward reducing anxiety and thereby reducing pain, and providing positive reinforcement that the mother is doing "a good job." Empowerment and having control over one's body play key roles in determining whether the woman views her labor and birth positively (Empowered Birth Summit, 2015). Women who viewed their births as a positive experience were also more likely to have a sense of well-being about themselves after the experience (Empowered Birth Summit, 2015). A wide variety of coping techniques to assist both the laboring woman and her partner are discussed in Chapter 18 and Chapter 19.

How the woman views the birth experience in hindsight may affect her mothering behaviors. It appears that any activities by the expectant woman or by healthcare providers that enhance the birth experience will be beneficial to the mother–baby connection. Some studies have shown that when women are disappointed with their birth experience or are disappointed with their attempts at breastfeeding, they may be more prone to postpartum mood disorders (Coates, Ayers, & de Visser, 2014). Psychosocial factors associated with a positive birth experience are summarized in Table 17–1.

The laboring woman's support system also influences the course of labor and birth. Some women prefer not to have a support person or family member with them. They may feel that the birth process is a private moment that they wish to reserve for themselves. However, most women choose to have significant persons (father or partner, family members, friends) with them during labor and birth. Social support tends to have a positive effect. For some families, the birth event is a celebration, and they want to create a joyful, festive atmosphere with many loved ones present. For many women, a partner's presence at the bedside provides a means to enhance communication and to demonstrate feelings of love.

TABLE 17–1 Psychosocial Factors Associated with a Positive Birth Experience

- Motivation for the pregnancy
- Attendance at childbirth education classes
- A sense of competence or mastery
- Self-confidence and self-esteem
- Feelings of empowerment
- Positive relationship with mate
- Maintaining control during labor
- Support from mate or other person during labor
- Not being left alone in labor
- Trust in the medical/nursing staff
- Personal control of breathing patterns and comfort measures
- A physician/CNM who has a similar philosophy of care
- Clear information from healthcare providers regarding necessary procedures
- Perceived positive birth experience
- Early success with breastfeeding

Clinical Tip

Many nurses have difficulty asking questions about domestic violence, sexual abuse, and drug or alcohol use during pregnancy. However, this information is necessary to provide the best nursing care possible. To create a relationship of trust in which the woman feels safe answering uncomfortable questions, the following tips may be helpful:

- Explore your own beliefs and values.
- Use open-ended questions.
- Be receptive of the answers.
- Be accepting of others' life experiences.

Clinical Reasoning   Identifying Domestic Violence

You are the birthing center nurse and you have reason to suspect that Lynn Ling, who has just been admitted in labor, may be in an abusive relationship.

How could you set up an interview so that the partner would leave the room (and take any accompanying children) without feeling that you are possibly increasing the risk to the woman? What communication techniques would you use to encourage Lynn to reveal if her partner is abusive?

Psychosocial Risk Factors. It is estimated that 20% of women are diagnosed with an anxiety or mood disorder during pregnancy or in the postpartum period (Massachusetts General Hospital Center for Women's Mental Health, 2015). It is estimated that up to 25% of pregnant women may experience depression during pregnancy and in the postpartum period. One study found that 13% of women were prescribed an antidepressant during pregnancy. Although concerns have been raised about possible adverse effects of psychotropic use in pregnancy, untreated depression can also have potentially lethal adverse effects. In a study that examined pregnant women in France with a history of antenatal depression, 15% of unmedicated depressed pregnant women attempted suicide during pregnancy. Suicide accounted for 20% of all postpartum maternal deaths. Women who did not take antidepressants during pregnancy had a 5 times higher rate of relapse of depressive symptoms in the postpartum period (Friedmann & Hall, 2013).

Other mental illnesses that may occur in pregnancy include bipolar disorder, anxiety disorders, and schizophrenia. It is also not uncommon for women to be diagnosed with eating disorders, autism, learning disabilities, and attention deficit or attention-deficit/hyperactivity disorder. All of these diagnoses can play a role in how the woman copes with the labor and birth experience and should be assessed by the admitting nurse. Women with identified disorders will need ongoing assessment during the labor and birth. In addition, they are at greater risk for postpartum mood disorders and posttraumatic stress disorders and warrant additional evaluation in the immediate, intermediate, and extended postpartum periods.

Women who have been sexually assaulted in the past or those with a history of sexual abuse in childhood are at greater risk and experience significant vulnerability in the obstetric setting. They may become anxious in the intrapartum setting, especially when vaginal examinations need to be performed. Women should be questioned on admission about intimate partner violence, past sexual abuse, and sexual assault. These questions should be asked in a private, secure area without the partner or family members present.

Intrapartum High-Risk Screening

Screening for intrapartum high-risk factors is an integral part of assessing the normal laboring woman. As the history is obtained, the nurse notes the presence of any potential risk factors that may be considered high-risk conditions. For example, the woman who reports a physical symptom such as intermittent bleeding needs further assessment to rule out abruptio placentae or placenta previa before the admission process continues. It is important to determine the difference between vaginal bleeding and bloody show. Bloody show is usually brown to reddish brown in color with a tinged vaginal discharge that has a consistency similar to mucus, whereas vaginal bleeding is bright red in color and is more like the type of bleeding encountered from a cut or laceration. In addition to identifying the presence of a high-risk condition, the nurse must recognize the implications of the condition for the laboring woman and her fetus. For example, if there is an abnormal fetal presentation, the nurse understands that the labor may be prolonged, prolapse of the umbilical cord is more likely, and the possibility of a cesarean birth is increased.

Although physical conditions are frequently listed as the major factors that increase risk in the intrapartum period, psychosocial, socioeconomic, and cultural variables such as poverty, poor nutrition, the amount of prenatal care, crowded living conditions, cultural beliefs regarding pregnancy, and communication patterns may also precipitate a high-risk situation. Mental illness is also a risk factor because it can result in episodic prenatal care or the need to take psychotropic medications during the pregnancy (Davidson, 2012). In addition, recent research indicates that women who suffer from posttraumatic stress disorder (PTSD) may be at increased risk for stress during pregnancy, engagement in high-risk behaviors during pregnancy, low birth weight neonate, preterm birth, and postpartum mood disorders and postpartum PTSD (Yonkers, Smith, & Forray, 2014). The nurse can quickly review the prenatal record for number of prenatal visits; weight gain during pregnancy;

progression of fundal height; exposure to environmental agents; and history of traumatic life events, including abuse.

The nurse can begin gathering data about sociocultural factors as the woman enters the birthing area. The nurse observes the communication pattern between the woman and her support person(s) and their responses to admission questions and initial teaching. If the woman and her support person(s) do not speak English and translators are not available among the birthing unit staff, the course of labor and the nurse's ability to interact and provide support and education are affected. The couple must receive information in their primary language to make informed decisions. Communication may also be affected by cultural practices such as beliefs about when to speak, who should ask questions, or whether it is acceptable to let others know about discomfort. People from certain cultures may want to experience birth naturally and may decline pain medications. In some cultures, the father is not expected to be present in the birthing area. Nurses need to be culturally sensitive so that this is not interpreted as being disinterested in the birth, the mother, or the newborn (Burnard & Gill, 2015).

A partial list of intrapartum risk factors appears in Table 17–2. The factors precede the *Assessment Guide: Intrapartum—First Stage of* Labor at the end of this chapter because they must be kept in mind during the assessment.

TABLE 17–2 Intrapartum High-Risk Factors

FACTOR	MATERNAL IMPLICATION	FETAL/NEONATAL IMPLICATION
Abnormal presentation	↑ Incidence of cesarean birth ↑ Incidence of prolonged labor	↑ Incidence of placenta previa Prematurity ↑ Risk of congenital abnormality Neonatal physical trauma ↑ Risk of intrauterine growth restriction (IUGR)
Multiple gestation	↑ Uterine distention → ↑ risk of postpartum hemorrhage ↑ Risk of cesarean birth ↑ Risk of preterm labor	Low birth weight Prematurity ↑ Risk of congenital anomalies Twin-to-twin transfusion
Hydramnios/polyhydramnios	↑ Discomfort ↑ Dyspnea ↑ Risk of preterm labor Edema of lower extremities Increased risk of cord prolapse with artificial rupture of membranes/spontaneous rupture of membranes (AROM/SROM)	↑ Risk of esophageal or other high alimentary tract atresias ↑ Risk of CNS anomalies (myelocele)
Oligohydramnios	Maternal fear	↑ Incidence of congenital anomalies ↑ Incidence of renal lesions ↑ Risk of IUGR ↑ Risk of fetal acidosis ↑ Risk of cord compression Postmaturity
Meconium staining of amniotic fluid	Psychologic stress due to fear for baby	↑ Risk of fetal asphyxia ↑ Risk of meconium aspiration ↑ Risk of pneumonia due to aspiration of meconium
Premature rupture of membranes	↑ Risk of infection (chorioamnionitis) ↑ Risk of preterm labor ↑ Anxiety Fear for the baby Prolonged hospitalization ↑ Incidence of tocolytic therapy	↑ Perinatal morbidity Prematurity ↑ Birth weight ↑ Risk of respiratory distress syndrome Prolonged hospitalization
Induction of labor	↑ Risk of hypercontractility of uterus ↑ Risk of uterine rupture Length of labor if cervix not ready ↑ Anxiety	Prematurity if gestational age not assessed correctly Hypoxia if hyperstimulation occurs Nonreassuring fetal status can occur
Abruptio placentae	Hemorrhage Uterine atony ↑ Incidence of C/S Severe maternal abdominal pain	Fetal hypoxia/acidosis Fetal exsanguination ↑ Perinatal mortality

(continued)

TABLE 17–2 Intrapartum High-Risk Factors (*continued*)

FACTOR	MATERNAL IMPLICATION	FETAL/NEONATAL IMPLICATION
Placenta previa	Hemorrhage Uterine atony Increased incidence of cesarean birth Painless vaginal bleeding	Fetal hypoxia/acidosis Fetal exsanguination Increased perinatal mortality
Failure to progress in labor	Maternal exhaustion ↑ Incidence of augmentation of labor ↑ Incidence of cesarean birth	Fetal hypoxia/acidosis Intracranial birth injury
Precipitous labor (less than 3 hr)	Perineal, vaginal, cervical lacerations ↑ Risk of postpartum hemorrhage Maternal hematomas	Tentorial tears
Prolapse of umbilical cord	↑ Fear for baby Cesarean birth	Acute fetal hypoxia/acidosis
Fetal heart abnormalities	↑ Fear for baby ↑ Risk of cesarean, forceps-assisted, or vacuum extraction birth Continuous electronic monitoring and intervention in labor	Tachycardia, chronic asphyxic insult, bradycardia, acute asphyxic insult Chronic hypoxia Congenital heart block
Uterine rupture	Maternal hemorrhage Cesarean birth for hysterectomy ↑ Risk of death	Fetal anoxia Fetal hemorrhage Neonatal morbidity and mortality Fetal neurologic sequelae
Postdates (greater than 42 weeks)	↑ Anxiety ↑ Incidence of induction of labor ↑ Incidence of cesarean birth ↑ Use of technology to monitor fetus ↑ Risk of shoulder dystocia Placental calcifications/advanced placental grading	Postmaturity syndrome ↑ Risk of fetal/neonatal mortality and morbidity ↑ Risk of antepartum fetal death ↑ Incidence or risk of large baby ↑ Risk of intrauterine growth restriction Fetal hypoxia Increased nonreassuring fetal status
Diabetes (gestational and preexisting)	↑ Risk of hydramnios ↑ Risk of hypoglycemia or hyperglycemia ↑ Risk of preeclampsia/eclampsia	↑ Risk of malpresentation ↑ Risk of macrosomia ↑ Risk of IUGR ↑ Risk of respiratory distress syndrome ↑ Risk of congenital anomalies ↑ Risk of fetal death Neonatal hypoglycemia
Preeclampsia/eclampsia	↑ Risk of seizures ↑ Risk of stroke ↑ Risk of HELLP (**h**emolysis, **e**levated **l**iver enzymes, and **l**ow **p**latelet count) syndrome and DIC (disseminated intravascular coagulation)	↑ Risk of small-for-gestational-age baby ↑ Risk of preterm birth ↑ Risk of mortality
HIV/sexually transmitted infection (STI)	↑ Risk of additional infections	↑ Risk of transplacental transmission ↑ Risk of infection during birth process or with invasive medical procedures

Intrapartum Physical and Psychosociocultural Assessment

A physical examination is part of the admission procedure and part of the ongoing care of the woman. Although the intrapartum physical assessment is not as complete and thorough as the initial prenatal physical examination (see Chapter 9), it does involve assessment of some body systems and the actual labor process. See *Assessment Guide: Intrapartum—First Stage of Labor* later in the chapter for a framework the maternity nurse can use when examining the laboring woman.

The physical assessment portion includes assessments performed immediately on admission as well as ongoing assessments. Nurses should conduct ongoing assessments in all clinical situations. For example, when the woman is changing into her gown, the nurse can assess the skin for bruises, needle marks,

While performing the intrapartum assessment, it is imperative for the nurse to follow Centers for Disease Control and Prevention (CDC) guidelines to prevent exposure to body substances. Gloves should be worn at all times when performing vaginal assessments or providing pericare. A waterproof apron and mask or eye protection should be worn if fluid exposure is likely.

burns, or other abnormalities. The possibility that the woman may be in an abusive relationship must be considered by the nurse in the presence of bruises. The nurse can also determine if the woman appears under- or overnourished. When labor is progressing rapidly, the nurse may not have time for a complete assessment. In that case, the critical physical assessments include maternal vital signs, labor status, fetal status, and laboratory findings.

The cultural assessment portion provides a starting point for this important aspect of assessment. Individualized nursing care can best be planned and implemented when the values and beliefs of the laboring woman are known and honored (Burnard & Gill, 2015). To avoid stereotyping clients, the nurse always asks the woman and her family about individual beliefs and preferences. Nurses who feel uncertain about what to ask or consider need to explore the varying cultural values and beliefs of the people residing in their community. Some communities have a prominent culture that may follow certain rituals but it is still important for the nurse to ask each woman about her own beliefs and preferences.

The final section of the assessment guide addresses psychosocial factors, including ideas, knowledge, fantasies, and fears about childbearing. In addition, women with a previous history of psychologic disorders, such as anxiety or depression, may have unique needs during labor. The nurse should specifically ask the woman if she has any special needs, but must recognize that some women may not know what needs will arise. This makes ongoing assessments imperative. It is important for the nurse to pay specific attention to body language, eye contact, and other nonverbal cues that may indicate that the woman is experiencing anxiety or other feelings. By assessing her psychosocial status, the nurse can meet the woman's needs for information and support. The nurse can then assist the woman and her partner; in the absence of a partner, the nurse may become the support person.

Methods of Evaluating Labor Progress

The nurse assesses the woman's contractions and cervical dilatation and effacement to evaluate labor progress.

CONTRACTION ASSESSMENT

Uterine contractions may be assessed by palpation or continuous electronic monitoring.

Palpation. The nurse assesses contractions for frequency, duration, and intensity by placing one hand on the uterine fundus. The hand is kept relatively still because excessive movement may stimulate contractions or cause discomfort. The nurse determines the frequency of the contractions by noting the time from the beginning of one contraction to the beginning of the next. If contractions begin at 7:00, 7:04, and 7:08, for example, their frequency is every 4 minutes. To determine contraction duration, the nurse notes the time when tensing of the fundus is first felt (beginning of contraction) and again as relaxation occurs (end of contraction). During the peak or acme of the contraction, intensity can be evaluated by estimating the indentability of the fundus. The nurse should assess at least three successive contractions to provide enough data to determine the contraction pattern.

KEY FACTS TO REMEMBER
Contraction and Labor Progress Characteristics

Contraction Characteristics	
Latent phase	Every 10 to 30 min × 30 sec; mild, progressing to every 5 to 7 min × 30 to 40 sec; moderate
Active phase	Every 2 to 5 min × 40 to 60 sec; moderate to strong
Transition phase	Every 1.5 to 2.0 min × 60 to 90 sec; strong
Labor Progress Characteristics	
Primipara	At least 1.2 cm/hr dilatation
	At least 1 cm/hr descent
	Less than 2 hr in second stage
Contraction Characteristics	
Multipara	At least 1.5 cm/hr dilatation
	At least 2.1 cm/hr descent
	Less than 1 hr in second stage

Clinical Tip

Many experienced nurses note that mild contractions are similar in consistency to the tip of the nose, moderate contractions feel more like the chin, and with strong contractions, there is little indentability, much like the forehead. When palpating the fundus of a woman's uterus during a contraction, compare the consistency to your nose, chin, and forehead to determine the intensity.

This is also a good time to assess the laboring woman's perception of pain. How does she describe the pain? What is her affect? Is this contraction more uncomfortable than the last one? Is the nurse's palpation of intensity congruent with the woman's perception? (For instance, the nurse might evaluate a contraction as mild in intensity whereas the laboring woman evaluates it as very strong.) A nurse's assessment is not complete unless the laboring woman's affect and response to the contractions are also noted and documented in the medical record.

Electronic Monitoring of Contractions. Electronic monitoring of uterine contractions provides continuous data. In many birth settings electronic monitoring is routine for high-risk women and those who are having oxytocin-induced labor; other facilities monitor all laboring women. Although electronic monitoring offers many advantages, it is useless unless it is coupled with careful nursing assessment.

Electronic monitoring may be done externally, with a device that is placed against the maternal abdomen, or internally, with an **intrauterine pressure catheter (IUPC)**. When monitoring by external means, the portion of the monitoring equipment called a *tocodynamometer*, or "toco," is positioned against the fundus of the uterus and held in place with an elastic belt (Figure 17–1). The toco contains a flexible disk that responds to pressure. When the uterus contracts, the fundus tightens and the change in pressure against the toco is amplified and transmitted to the electronic fetal monitor. The monitor displays the uterine contraction as a pattern on graph paper.

External monitoring offers several advantages including providing a continuous recording of the frequency and duration of uterine contractions and it is noninvasive. However, it does not accurately record the intensity of the uterine contraction, and it is difficult to obtain an accurate fetal heart rate (FHR) in some women, such as those who are very obese, those who have hydramnios (an

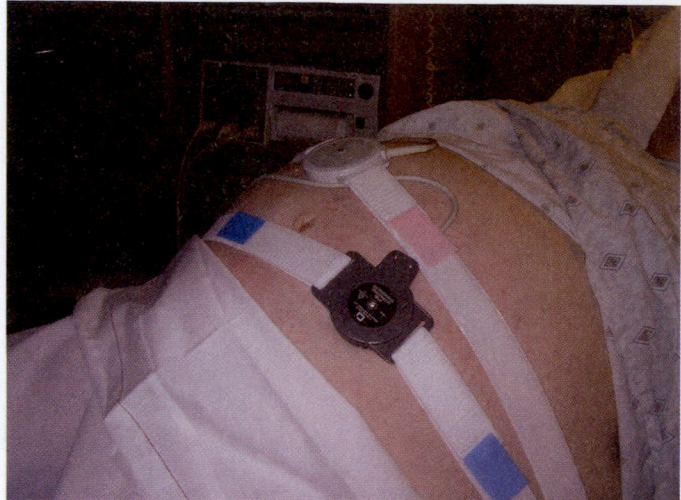

Figure 17–1 Woman in labor with external monitor applied. The tocodynamometer placed on the uterine fundus is recording uterine contractions. The lower belt holds the ultrasonic device that monitors the fetal heart rate. The belts can be adjusted for comfort.

SOURCE: Wilson Garcia.

abnormally large amount of amniotic fluid), or those whose fetus is very active. In addition, the woman may be bothered by the belt if it requires frequent readjustment when she changes position.

External monitoring allows the nurse to continually monitor the fetus if there are concerns about the FHR. Continuous monitoring also enables the nurse and physician/CNM to observe the pattern of the FHR over a period of time, enabling them to examine the electronic fetal monitoring strip. Electronic monitoring of the fetal heart rate is discussed in detail in the Fetal Assessment section of this chapter.

Internal intrauterine monitoring provides the same data and also provides accurate measurement of uterine contraction intensity (the strength of the contraction and the actual pressure within

the uterus). After membranes have ruptured, the physician/CNM (or the nurse in some facilities) inserts the IUPC into the uterine cavity and connects it by a cable to the electronic fetal monitor. It is important to first assess the fetal position and to review a past ultrasound to determine placenta placement. The internal monitor should be placed away from the placenta. If an ultrasound has not been previously obtained, the physician/CNM may wish to do one on the unit or have the radiologist perform an exam.

The pressure within the uterus in the resting state and during each contraction is measured by a small micropressure device located in the tip of the catheter. Internal electronic monitoring is used when it is imperative to have accurate intrauterine pressure readings to evaluate the stress on the uterus or to determine the adequacy of contractions. The advantage of the intrauterine pressure monitor is that it can directly measure the intensity of the contraction. It can be used in cases where the external monitor may not be accurately assessing the contraction strength, such as in cases of maternal obesity. It can also be used when oxytocin is being administered to ensure that uterine contractions are adequate.

The nurse should also evaluate the woman's labor status by palpating the intensity and resting tone of the uterine fundus during contractions. Technology is a useful tool if used as an adjunct to good assessment skills.

Internal monitoring has both risks and benefits. It provides a more accurate fetal tracing and is more effective in monitoring the fetal status. Placement of an intrauterine pressure catheter can cause vaginal bleeding. In rare cases, the scalp electrode can be placed on the fetal fontanelle or on an eye if the fetus is in a face presentation, thus causing fetal injury. Women with certain medical conditions, such as a positive HIV status, should not be monitored with internal monitoring because it can increase the risk of viral transmission.

Cervical Assessment. Cervical dilatation and effacement are evaluated directly by vaginal examination (see *Clinical Skill: Performing an Intrapartum Vaginal Examination*). The vaginal examination can provide information about the adequacy of the maternal pelvis, membrane status, characteristics of amniotic fluid, and fetal position and station.

Clinical Skill 17–1

Performing an Intrapartum Vaginal Examination

NURSING ACTION

Preparation

- Explain the procedure, the indications for the exam, what the exam may feel like, and that it may cause discomfort.

- Assess for latex allergies.

- Position the woman with her thighs flexed and abducted. Instruct her to put the heels of her feet together. Drape the woman with a sheet, leaving a flap to access the perineum.

Rationale: This position provides access to the woman's perineum. The drape ensures privacy.

- Encourage the woman to relax her muscles and legs.

Rationale: Relaxation decreases muscle tension and increases comfort.

- Inform the woman before touching her. Be gentle.

Equipment and Supplies

- Clean disposable gloves if membranes not ruptured
- Sterile gloves if membranes ruptured
- Lubricant
- Nitrazine test tape
- Slide
- Sterile cotton-tipped swab (Q-tip)

Before the Procedure: Test for Fluid Leakage

If fluid leakage has been reported or noted, use Nitrazine test tape and Q-tip with slide for fern test before performing the exam.

Procedure: Clean Gloves (Sterile if Membranes Ruptured)

1. Pull glove onto dominant hand.

Rationale: A single glove is worn when membranes are intact. If a sterile exam is needed, both hands will be gloved with sterile gloves.

2. Using your gloved hand, position the hand with the wrist straight and the elbow tilted downward. Insert your well-lubricated second and index fingers of the gloved hand

gently into the vagina until they touch the cervix. Use care when positioning your hand.

Rationale: This position allows the fingertips to point toward the umbilicus and find the cervix.

3. If the woman verbalizes discomfort, acknowledge it and apologize. Pause for a moment and allow her to relax before progressing.

Rationale: This validates the woman's discomfort and helps her feel more in control.

4. To determine the status of labor progress, perform the vaginal examination during and between contractions.

Rationale: Cervical effacement, dilatation, and fetal station are affected by the presence of a contraction.

5. Palpate for the opening, or a depression, in the cervix and cervical length. Estimate the diameter of the depression to identify the amount of dilatation and the length to identify the degree of effacement (Figure 17–2).

Rationale: Allows determination of effacement and dilatation.

6. Determine the status of the fetal membranes by observing for leakage of amniotic fluid. If fluid is expressed, test for amniotic fluid.

Rationale: The status of the amniotic membranes influences management decisions. Women with ruptured membranes are at a greater risk for infection.

7. Palpate the presenting part (Figure 17–3).

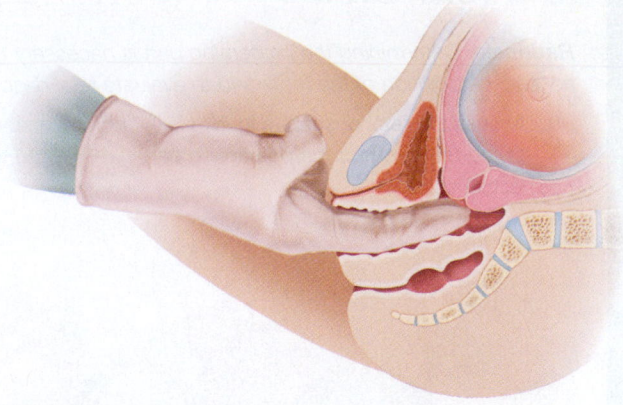

Figure 17–2 To gauge cervical dilatation, the nurse places the index and middle fingers against the cervix and determines the size of the opening. Before labor begins, the cervix is long (approximately 2.5 cm [1 in.]), the sides feel thick, and the cervical canal is closed, so an examining finger cannot be inserted. During labor, the cervix begins to dilate, and the size of the opening progresses from 1 to 10 cm (0.4 to 3.9 in) in diameter.

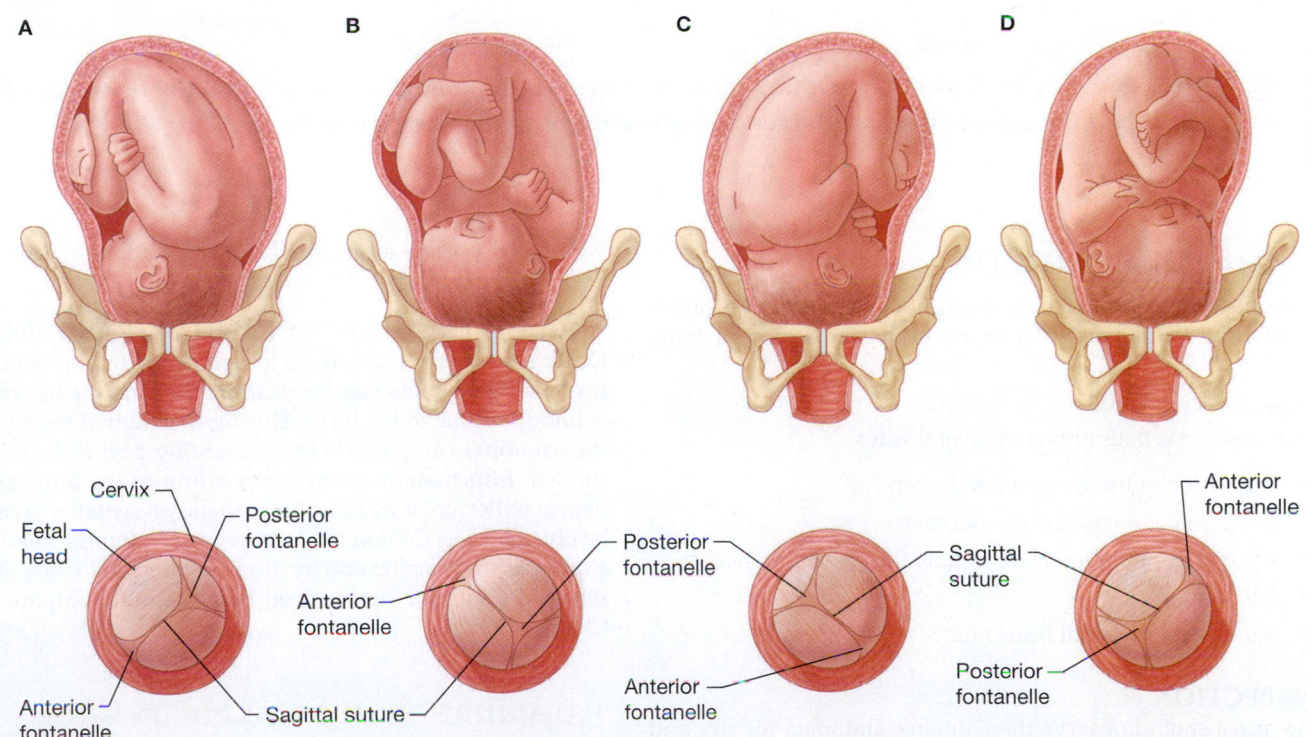

Figure 17–3 Palpating of the presenting part (the portion of the fetus that enters the pelvis first). A. Left occiput anterior (LOA). The occiput (area over the occipital bone on the posterior part of the fetal head) is in the left anterior quadrant of the woman's pelvis. When the fetus is in LOA, the posterior fontanelle (located just above the occipital bone and triangular in shape) is in the upper left quadrant of the maternal pelvis. B. Left occiput posterior (LOP). The posterior fontanelle is in the lower left quadrant of the maternal pelvis. C. Right occiput anterior (ROA). The posterior fontanelle is in the upper right quadrant of the maternal pelvis. D. Right occiput posterior (ROP). The posterior fontanelle is in the lower right quadrant of the maternal pelvis.

Clinical Skill 17–1 (*continued*)

Rationale: Determining the presenting part is necessary to assess the position of the fetus and to evaluate fetal descent.

8. Assess the fetal descent (Figure 17–4) and station by identifying the depth of the presenting part in relation to the ischial spines.

9. Record findings on woman's electronic medical record (EMR).

Note: The anterior fontanelle is diamond shaped. Because of the roundness of the fetal head, only a portion of the anterior fontanelle can be seen in each of the views, so it appears to be triangular in shape.

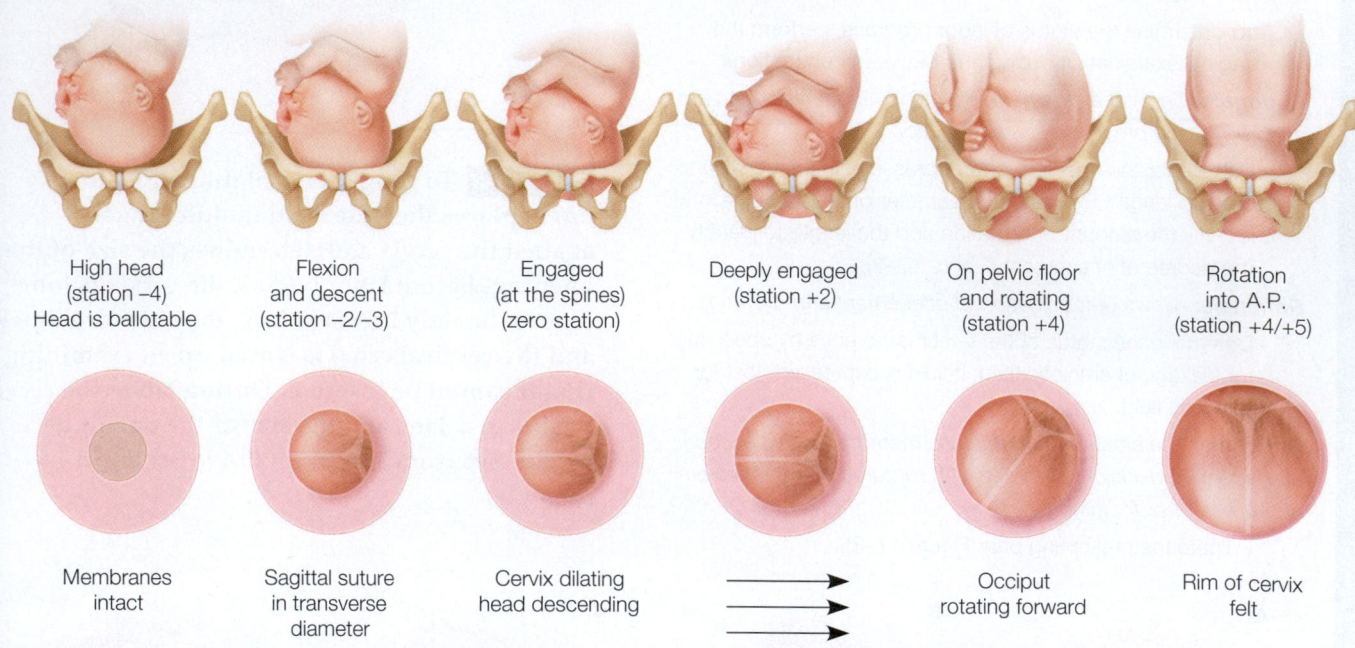

| High head (station −4) Head is ballotable | Flexion and descent (station −2/−3) | Engaged (at the spines) (zero station) | Deeply engaged (station +2) | On pelvic floor and rotating (station +4) | Rotation into A.P. (station +4/+5) |

| Membranes intact | Sagittal suture in transverse diameter | Cervix dilating head descending | | Occiput rotating forward | Rim of cervix felt |

Figure 17–4 **Top: The fetal head progressing through the pelvis. Bottom: The changes that the nurse will detect on palpation of the occiput through the cervix while doing a vaginal examination.**

Fetal Assessment

A complete intrapartum fetal assessment requires determination of the fetal position and presentation, and evaluation of the fetal status.

Fetal Position

Fetal position is determined in several ways:

- Inspection of the woman's abdomen
- Palpation of the woman's abdomen
- Vaginal examination to determine the presenting part
- Ultrasound
- Auscultation of fetal heart rate

INSPECTION

The nurse should observe the woman's abdomen for size and shape. The lie of the fetus should be assessed by noting whether the uterus projects up and down (longitudinal lie) or left to right (transverse lie).

PALPATION: LEOPOLD MANEUVERS

Leopold maneuvers are a systematic way to evaluate the maternal abdomen. Frequent practice increases the examiner's skill in determining fetal position by palpation. Leopold maneuvers may be difficult to perform on an obese woman or on a woman who has excessive amniotic fluid (hydramnios). See *Clinical Skill: Performing Leopold Maneuvers*.

VAGINAL EXAMINATION AND ULTRASOUND

Other assessment techniques to determine fetal position and presentation include vaginal examination and the use of ultrasound to visualize the fetus. During the vaginal examination, the examiner can palpate the presenting part if the cervix is dilated. Information about the position of the fetus and the degree of flexion of its head (in cephalic presentations) can also be obtained (see *Clinical Skill: Performing an Intrapartum Vaginal Examination*). Visualization by ultrasound is used when the fetal position cannot be determined by abdominal palpation (see Chapter 15).

Auscultation of Fetal Heart Rate

The handheld Doppler ultrasound device or the electronic fetal monitor transducer is used to auscultate the fetal heart rate (FHR) between, during, and immediately after uterine contractions. A fetoscope can also be used. Instead of listening haphazardly over the woman's abdomen for the FHR, the nurse may choose to perform Leopold maneuvers first. Leopold maneuvers not only indicate the probable location of the FHR but also help determine the presence of multiple fetuses, fetal lie, and fetal presentation.

Clinical Skill 17–2

Performing Leopold Maneuvers

NURSING ACTION

Preparation

- Have the woman empty her bladder.

Rationale: Palpating the abdomen may be uncomfortable if the woman's bladder is full. A full bladder may also make it difficult to complete the third and fourth maneuvers. See later discussion.

- Ask the woman to lie on her back with her feet on the bed and her knees bent.

Rationale: This position provides good access to the woman's abdomen. Flexing the knees helps relax the abdominal muscles.

- Perform the procedure between contractions.

Rationale: It is difficult to identify fetal parts when the abdominal muscles are contracted.

Procedure

1. First maneuver: Facing the woman, palpate the fundus of the uterus with both hands. Note the shape, consistency, and mobility of the palpated part (see Figure 17–5A).

Rationale: The fetal head is firm, hard, and round and moves independently of the trunk. The breech (fetal buttocks) feels softer and symmetric and has small bony prominences; it moves with the trunk.

2. Second maneuver: After determining whether the head or the buttocks occupy the fundus, try to determine the location of the fetal back. Still facing the woman, palpate the abdomen with gentle but deep pressure, using the palms. Hold the right hand steady while the left hand

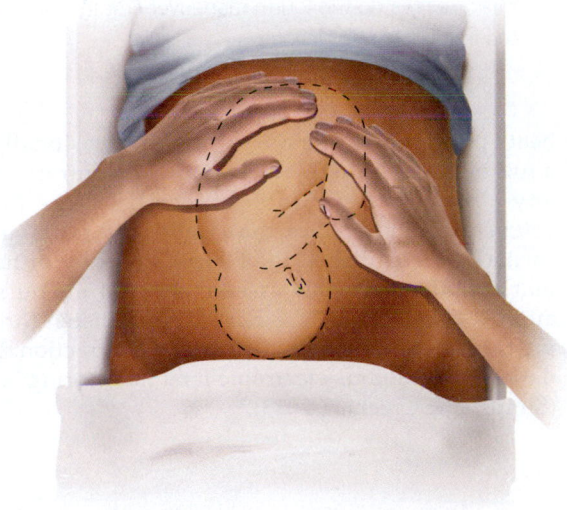

A. First maneuver

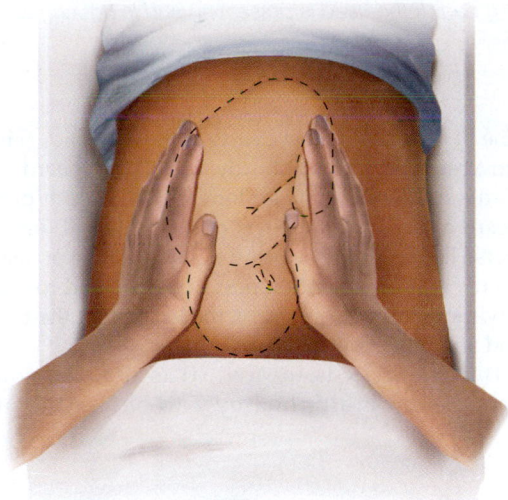

B. Second maneuver

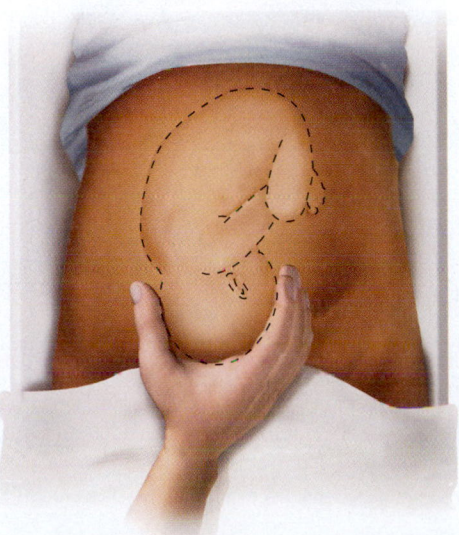

C. Third maneuver

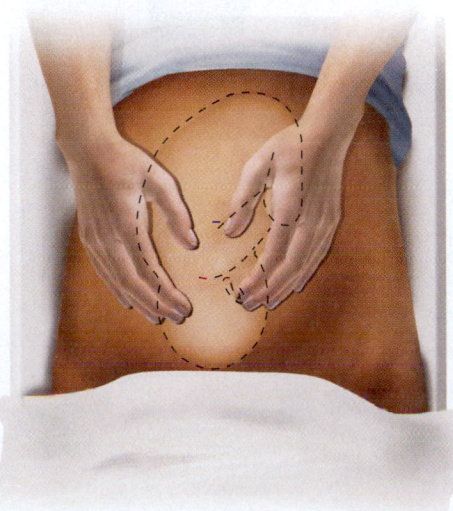

D. Fourth maneuver

Figure 17–5 Leopold maneuvers for determining fetal position, presentation, and lie.

Clinical Skill 17–2 (*continued*)

explores the right side of the uterus. Then repeat the maneuver, holding the left hand steady while exploring the left side of the woman's abdomen with your right hand (see Figure 17–5B).

Rationale: The fetal back, on one side of the abdomen, feels firm and smooth and should connect what was found in the fundus with a mass in the outlet. The fetal extremities, which feel small and knobby, should be found on the other side.

3. Third maneuver: Determine what fetal part is lying just above the pelvic outlet. To do this, gently grasp the abdomen with the thumb and fingers just above the symphysis pubis. Note whether the presenting part feels like the fetal head or the buttocks and whether it is engaged (see Figure 17–5C).

Rationale: This maneuver yields the opposite information from that gained with the first maneuver and validates the presenting part. If the head is presenting and is not engaged, it may be gently pushed back and forth.

4. Fourth maneuver: Facing the woman's feet, place both hands on the lower abdomen and move the hands gently down the sides of the uterus toward the pubis. Attempt to locate the cephalic prominence or brow (see Figure 17–5D).

Rationale: The brow is located on the side where there is the greatest resistance to the descent of the fingers toward the pubis. It is located on the side opposite the fetal back if the head is well flexed. However, when the fetal head is extended, the occiput is the first cephalic prominence felt, and it is located on the same side as the fetal back. Thus when completing the fourth maneuver, if the first cephalic prominence palpated is on the same side as the back, the head is not flexed. If the cephalic prominence is found opposite the back, the head is well flexed.

Note: Some practitioners may perform the sequence differently. Many nurses do the fourth maneuver first to identify the part of the fetus in the pelvic inlet.

The FHR is heard most clearly at the fetal back (Figure 17–6). Thus in a cephalic presentation, the FHR is best heard in the lower quadrants of the maternal abdomen. In a breech presentation, it is heard at or above the level of the maternal umbilicus. In a transverse lie, FHR may be heard best just above or just below the umbilicus. As the presenting part descends and rotates through the pelvic structure during labor, the location of the FHR tends to descend and move toward the midline.

After the FHR is located, it is usually counted for 30 seconds and multiplied by 2 to obtain the number of beats per minute. The nurse should occasionally listen for a full minute, through and just after a contraction, to detect any abnormal heart rate, especially if the FHR is over 160 beats/min (tachycardia), under 110 beats/min (bradycardia), or irregular. If the FHR is irregular or has changed markedly from the last assessment or if the nurse hears an audible deceleration, the nurse should listen for a full minute through and immediately after a contraction. In these situations, continuous electronic fetal monitoring is warranted (Simpson & Creehan, 2013).

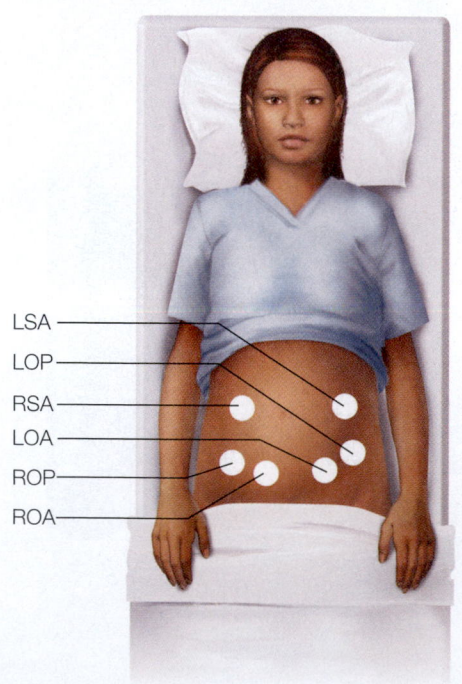

LSA
LOP
RSA
LOA
ROP
ROA

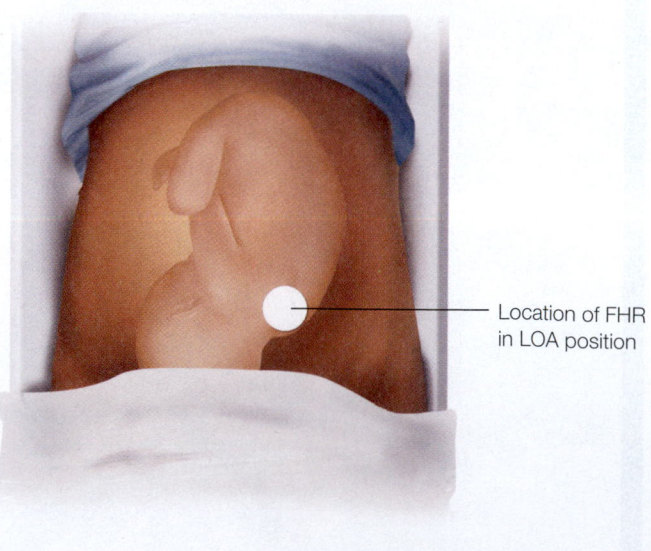

Location of FHR in LOA position

Figure 17–6 Location of the fetal heart rate (FHR) in relation to the more commonly seen fetal positions. The FHR is heard more clearly over the fetal back.

| EVIDENCE-BASED PRACTICE | Best Practices for Fetal Heart Rate Assessment |

Clinical Question

What is the most effective way to monitor fetal status in laboring women who are low risk?

The Evidence

Monitoring of the fetal heart rate is one way of assessing the well-being of the fetus during labor. The primary interest is fetal oxygenation; threats to fetal oxygenation are never higher than during labor. Electronic fetal heart rate monitoring has become widespread, even though there is little evidence that it reduces risks for low-risk mothers. Currently, nearly 97% of births in U.S. hospitals are accompanied by electronic fetal monitoring. A military nurse-researcher undertook a systematic review of the evidence to determine best practices for fetal monitoring in low-risk labor and delivery. Included in the review were the best practice bulletins of the American College of Obstetricians and Gynecologists (ACOG) and the Association for Women's Health, Obstetric and Neonatal Nurses (AWOHNN). This type of review of practice guidelines is considered the strongest level of evidence for practice.

The recommended means of fetal monitoring in low-risk mothers is intermittent auscultation (Riffle, 2014). Using this low-technology monitoring method saves costs and results in lower rates of unnecessary assisted and surgical births. In addition, intermittent auscultation is noninvasive and requires no special equipment. Laboring mothers are free to walk, which generally enhances labor progress, and to change positions as frequently as needed to manage pain. Overall, both physiologic and psychologic outcomes were superior with intermittent auscultation.

Best Practice

Intermittent auscultation of fetal heart rate is superior to electronic fetal monitoring for low-risk mothers. This method of assuring fetal well-being is low cost, involves no special technology, and enables full mobility of the mother.

Clinical Reasoning

How can the nurse help implement this important change in practice when current practices are ingrained? What is appropriate childbirth education to empower parents to choose a low-technology option?

It is important to note that intermittent auscultation has been found to be as effective as the electronic method for fetal surveillance. A growing number of healthcare professionals, doctors and nurses alike, are beginning to question the widespread usage of this technology. Although fetuses who are monitored continuously have a reduced risk of seizures, there is no reduction in cerebral palsy, neonatal mortality, or adverse neonatal outcomes. Women who receive continuous fetal monitoring are more likely to undergo a cesarean birth or an instrument-assisted birth and do not have better outcomes than low-risk women who undergo intermittent fetal auscultation (Simpson & Creehan, 2013). Figure 17–7 shows the use of a Doppler to auscultate the FHR. *Clinical Skill: Auscultation of Fetal Heart Rate* describes the procedure. For guidelines about how often to auscultate the FHR, see *Key Facts to Remember: Frequency of Auscultation: Assessment and Documentation*.

Electronic Monitoring of Fetal Heart Rate

Electronic fetal monitoring (EFM) produces a continuous tracing of the FHR, which allows visual assessment of many characteristics of the FHR (see *Clinical Skill: Electronic Fetal Monitoring*).

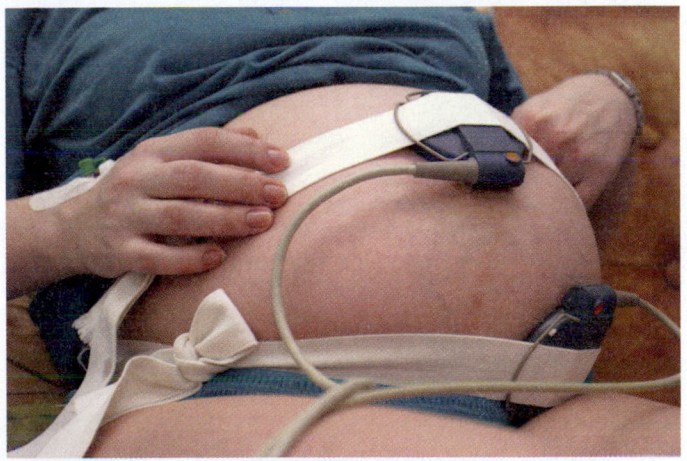

Figure 17–7 The nurse uses a Doppler to assess the fetal heart rate. Doppler monitors can be used for intermittent labor monitoring or in the outpatient or community setting.

SOURCE: © Artur Steinhagen/Fotolia

Clinical Skill 17–3

Auscultation of Fetal Heart Rate

NURSING ACTION

Preparation

- Explain the procedure, the indications for it, and the information that will be obtained.
- Uncover the woman's abdomen.

Equipment and Supplies

- Doppler device
- Ultrasonic gel

Procedure

1. To use the Doppler:
   - Place ultrasonic gel on the diaphragm of the Doppler. Gel is used to maintain contact with the maternal abdomen and enhances conduction of sound.

(continued)

Clinical Skill 17–3 (*continued*)

- The diaphragm should be warmed prior to using the Doppler.

- Place the Doppler diaphragm on the woman's abdomen halfway between the umbilicus and the symphysis and in the midline. You are most likely to hear the FHR in this area. Listen carefully for the sound of the fetal heartbeat.

2. Check the woman's pulse against the fetal sounds you hear. If the rates are the same, reposition the Doppler and try again.

Rationale: If the rates are the same, you are probably hearing the maternal pulse and not the FHR.

3. If the rates are not similar, count the FHR for 1 full minute. Note that the FHR has a double rhythm and only one sound is counted.

4. If you do not locate the FHR, move the Doppler laterally.

5. Auscultate the FHR between, during, and for 30 seconds following a uterine contraction (UC).

6. Frequency recommendations:
   - Low-risk women: Every 30 minutes during the first stage, and every 15 minutes in the second stage.
   - High-risk women: Every 15 minutes during the first stage, and every 5 minutes in the second stage.

Rationale: This evaluation provides the opportunity to assess the fetal status and response to labor.

Auscultation with the Fetoscope

The fetoscope is an older assessment tool; however, some clinicians prefer it because it is "natural" and does not rely on ultrasound. Some women seeking prenatal care outside of a traditional care environment may request the use of a fetoscope.

KEY FACTS TO REMEMBER
Frequency of Auscultation: Assessment and Documentation

Low-Risk Laboring Women	High-Risk Laboring Women
First stage of labor: q30 min	First stage of labor: q15 min
Second stage of labor: q15 min	Second stage of labor: q5 min

Note: When oxytocin is used, frequency should be every 15 minutes during active labor (Simpkin & Creehan: Association of Women's Health, Obstetric and Neonatal Nurses [AWHONN], 2013).

Labor Events

Assess FHR before:

Initiation of labor-enhancing procedures (e.g., artificial rupture of membranes)

Periods of ambulation

Administration of medications

Administration or initiation of analgesia/anesthesia

Assess FHR following:

Rupture of membranes

Recognition of abnormal uterine activity patterns, such as increased base tone or tachysystole

Evaluation of oxytocin (maintenance, increase, or decrease of dosage)

Administration of medications (at time of peak action)

Expulsion of enema

Voiding, bowel movement, or urinary catheterization

Vaginal examination

Periods of ambulation

Evaluation of analgesia and/or anesthesia (maintenance, increase, or decrease of dosage)

Source: Adapted from American College of Obstetricians & Gynecologists. (2009). *Intrapartum fetal heart rate monitoring* (Practice Bulletin No. 106). Washington, DC: Author.

INDICATIONS FOR ELECTRONIC MONITORING

If one or more of the following factors are present, the fetal heart rate and contractions are monitored by EFM:

1. Previous history of a stillbirth at 38 or more weeks' gestation

2. Presence of a complication of pregnancy (e.g., preeclampsia, placenta previa, abruptio placentae, multiple gestation, prolonged or premature rupture of membranes)

3. Induction of labor (labor that is begun as a result of some type of intervention such as an intravenous infusion of Pitocin)

4. Preterm labor

5. Decreased fetal movement

6. Nonreassuring fetal status

7. Meconium staining of amniotic fluid (Meconium has been released into the amniotic fluid by the fetus, which may indicate a problem.)

8. Trial of labor after cesarean birth (TOLAC)

9. Maternal fever

10. Placental problems

11. Category II or III tracings

METHODS OF ELECTRONIC MONITORING OF FHR

External monitoring of the fetus is usually accomplished by ultrasound. A transducer, which emits continuous sound waves, is placed on the maternal abdomen. When placed correctly, the sound waves bounce off the fetal heart and are picked up by the electronic monitor. The actual moment-by-moment FHR is displayed graphically on a screen (Figure 17–8). In some instances, the monitor may track the maternal heart rate instead of the fetal heart rate. However, the nurse can avoid this error by comparing the maternal pulse to the FHR. In cases of fetal demise, only the maternal heart rate is detected.

Recent advances in technology have led to the development of new ambulatory methods of external monitoring. Using

Clinical Skill 17–4
Electronic Fetal Monitoring

NURSING ACTION

Preparation

- Explain the procedure, the indications for it, and the information that will be obtained.

Equipment and Supplies

- Monitor
- Two elastic monitor belts
- Tocodynamometer ("toco")
- Ultrasound transducer
- Ultrasound gel

Procedure

1. Turn on the monitor.
2. Place the two elastic belts around the woman's abdomen.
3. Place the "toco" over the uterine fundus off the midline on the area palpated to be most firm during contractions. Secure it with one of the elastic belts.

Rationale: The uterine fundus is the area of greatest contractility.

4. Note the UC tracing. The resting tone tracing (that is, without a UC) should be recording on the 10 or 15 mm Hg pressure line. Adjust the line to reflect that reading.

Rationale: If the resting tone is set on the zero line, the toco should be reset to baseline resting tone when the uterus is relaxed.

5. Apply the ultrasonic gel to the diaphragm of the ultrasound transducer.

Rationale: Ultrasonic gel is used to maintain contact with the maternal abdomen. The ultrasonic beam is directed toward the fetal heart.

6. Place the diaphragm on the maternal abdomen in the midline between the umbilicus and the symphysis pubis.
7. Listen for the FHR, which will have a whiplike sound. Move the diaphragm laterally if necessary to obtain a stronger sound.
8. When the FHR is located, attach the second elastic belt snugly to the transducer.

Rationale: Firm contact is necessary to maintain a steady tracing.

9. Place the following information on the beginning of the fetal monitor paper: date, time, woman's name, gravida, para, membrane status, and name of physician or certified nurse-midwife.
10. Ongoing documentation should provide information about FHR including baseline rate in beats per minute (beats/min), variability, response to uterine contractions (accelerations or decelerations), procedures performed, changes in position, and the like, as well as any therapy initiated. The maternal pulse should be assessed and documented to ensure the tracing is not detecting the maternal heartbeat. Tracing should be categorized using the three-tier system (see later discussion).

Note: Each birthing unit may have specific guidelines about additional information to include. A full description of fetal monitoring analysis is beyond the scope of this text.

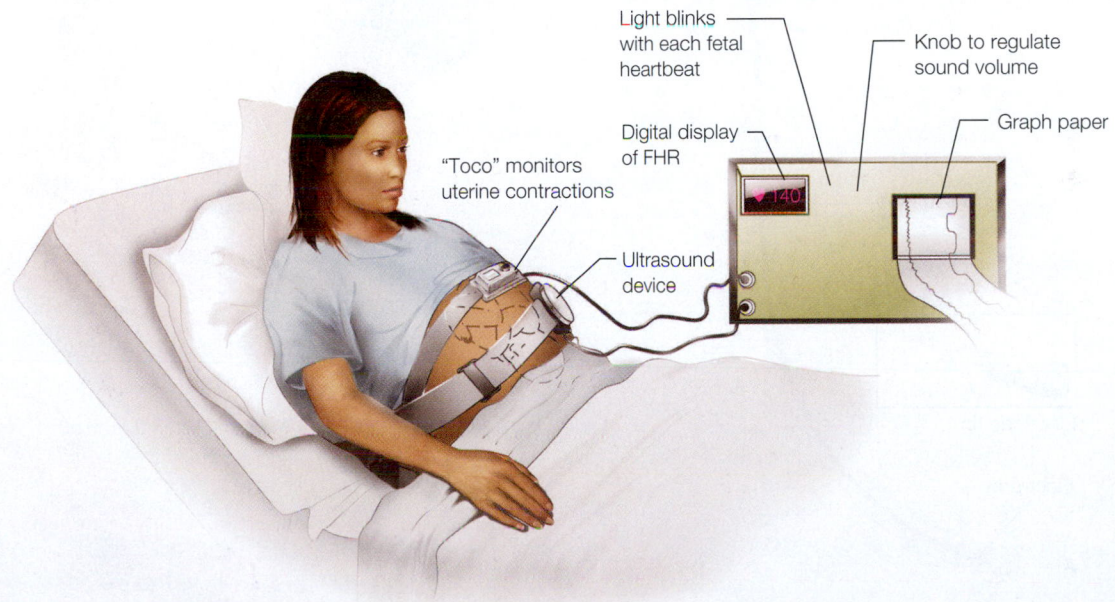

Light blinks with each fetal heartbeat

Knob to regulate sound volume

Digital display of FHR

Graph paper

"Toco" monitors uterine contractions

Ultrasound device

Figure 17–8 Electronic fetal monitoring by external technique. The tocodynamometer ("toco") is placed over the uterine fundus. The toco provides information that can be used to monitor uterine contractions. The ultrasound device is placed over the area of the fetal back. This device transmits information about the FHR. Information from both the toco and the ultrasound device is transmitted to the electronic fetal monitor. The FHR is displayed in a digital display (as a blinking light), on the special monitor paper, and audibly (by adjusting a button on the monitor). The uterine contractions are displayed on the special monitor paper as well.

a telemetry system, a small, battery-operated transducer transmits signals to a receiver connected to the monitor. This system, which is held in place with a shoulder strap, allows the woman to ambulate, helping her to feel more comfortable and less confined during labor. Many of the newer models can also be worn in the tub and can be completely submerged in water, making a more natural birthing experience possible even for women who require continuous monitoring for medical indications. In contrast, the system depicted in Figure 17–8 requires the woman to remain close to the electrical power source for the monitor.

Internal monitoring requires an internal spiral electrode. Women who require internal monitoring are typically confined to bed and cannot ambulate. To place the spiral electrode on the fetal occiput, the amniotic membranes must be ruptured, the cervix must be dilated at least 2 cm, the presenting part must be down against the cervix, and the presenting part must be known (i.e., the nurse must be able to detect the actual part of the fetus that is down against the cervix). In cases of a breech presentation, the electrode can be placed on the fetal buttocks. The exact position should be identified because the electrode should not be placed on the external genitalia. If all these factors are present, the labor and birth nurse (if specialty training has been completed) or the physician/CNM inserts a sterile internal spiral electrode into the vagina and places it against the fetal presenting part. The spiral electrode is rotated clockwise until it is attached to the presenting part. It is essential that the electrode not be placed over the eye or a fontanelle, so the fetal position

should be determined before a scalp electrode is applied. Wires that extend from the spiral electrode are attached to a leg plate (which is placed on the woman's thigh) and then attached to the electronic fetal monitor. This method of monitoring the FHR provides more accurate continuous data than external monitoring, because the signal is clearer and movement of the fetus or the woman does not interrupt it (Figure 17–9).

Change affecting the baseline is called **variability**, which is a change in FHR over a few seconds to a few minutes. The FHR tracing at the top of Figure 17–10 was obtained by internal monitoring with a spiral electrode; the uterine contraction tracing at the bottom of the figure was obtained by external monitoring with a toco. Note that the FHR is variable (the tracing moves up and down instead of in a straight line). In this figure each dark vertical line represents 1 minute; therefore, contractions are occurring about every 2 to 3 minutes. The FHR is evaluated by assessing an electronic monitor tracing for baseline rate, baseline variability, and periodic changes.

BASELINE FETAL HEART RATE

The **baseline rate** refers to the average FHR rounded to increments of 5 beats/min observed during a 10-minute period of monitoring. This excludes periodic or episodic changes, periods of marked variability, and segments of the baseline that differ by more than 25 beats/min. The duration should be at least 2 minutes. Normal FHR (baseline rate) ranges from 110 to 160 beats/min. There are two abnormal variations of the baseline

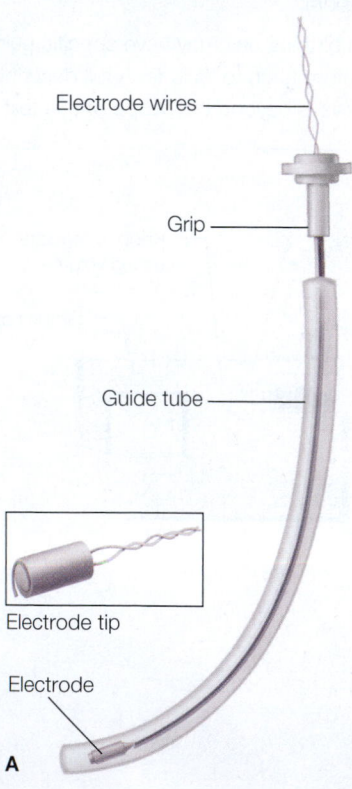

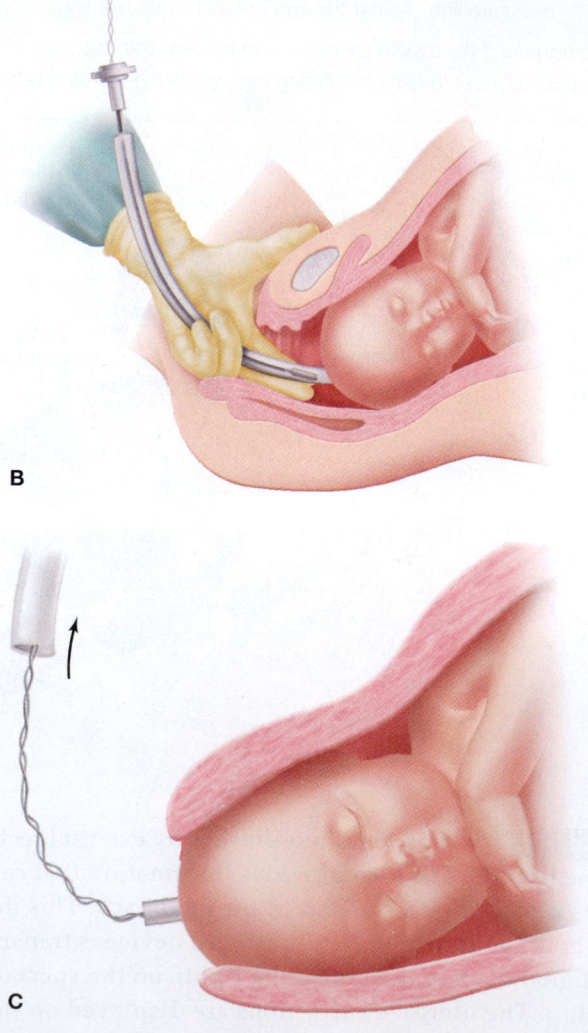

Figure 17–9 Technique for internal, direct fetal monitoring. A. Spiral electrode. B. Attaching the spiral electrode to the scalp. C. Attached spiral electrode with the guide tube removed.

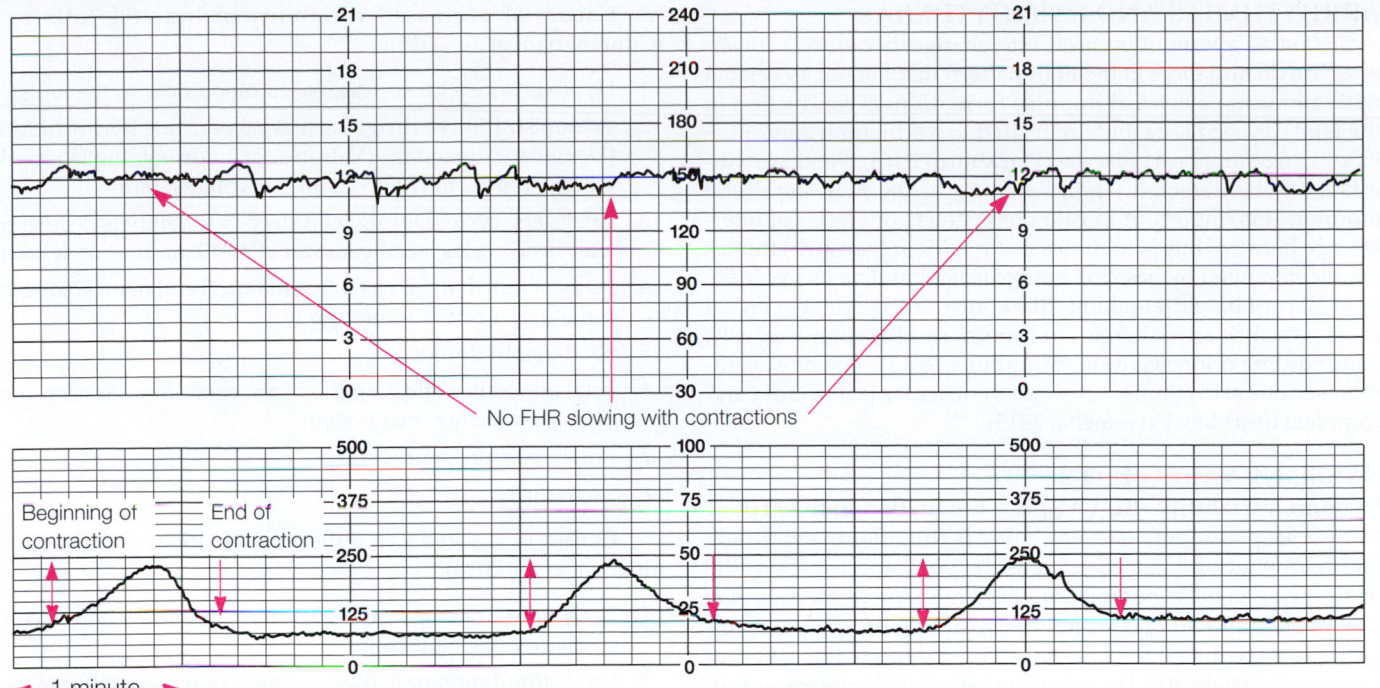

No FHR slowing with contractions

Beginning of contraction — End of contraction

←—1 minute—→

Figure 17–10 Top: A fetal heart rate (FHR) tracing obtained by internal monitoring. Normal FHR range is from 110 to 160 beats/min. This tracing indicates an FHR range of 140 to 155 beats/min. Bottom: A uterine contraction tracing obtained by external monitoring. Each dark vertical line marks 1 minute, and each small rectangle represents 10 seconds. The contraction frequency is about every 3 minutes, and the duration of the contractions is 50 to 60 seconds.

rate: those above 160 beats/min (tachycardia) and those below 110 beats/min (bradycardia).

A **wandering baseline** fluctuates between 120 and 160 beats/min in an unsteady wandering pattern and can be associated with neurologic impairment of the fetus or a preterminal event (Cunningham et al., 2014).

Fetal tachycardia is a sustained rate of 161 beats/min or above. *Marked tachycardia* is 180 beats/min or above. Causes of tachycardia include the following (Cunningham et al., 2014):

1. Early fetal hypoxia, which leads to stimulation of the sympathetic system as the fetus compensates for reduced blood flow

2. Maternal fever, which accelerates the metabolism of the fetus

3. Maternal dehydration

4. Beta-sympathomimetic drugs such as terbutaline, atropine, and isoxsuprine, which have a cardiac stimulant effect

5. Amnionitis (Fetal tachycardia may be the first sign of developing intrauterine infection.)

6. Maternal hyperthyroidism (Thyroid-stimulating hormones may cross the placenta and stimulate fetal heart rate.)

7. Fetal anemia (The heart rate is increased as a compensatory mechanism to improve tissue perfusion.)

8. Tachydysrhythmias (Fetal dysrhythmias occur in less than 1% of all pregnancies.)

Tachycardia is considered an ominous sign if it is accompanied by late decelerations, severe variable decelerations, or decreased variability. If tachycardia is associated with maternal fever, treatment may consist of antipyretics and/or antibiotics.

Fetal bradycardia is a rate less than 110 beats/min during a 10-minute period or longer. Causes of fetal bradycardia include the following (Cunningham et al., 2014):

1. Late (profound) fetal hypoxia (depression of myocardial activity)

2. Maternal hypotension, which results in decreased blood flow to the fetus

3. Prolonged umbilical cord compression (Fetal baroreceptors are activated by cord compression and this produces vagal stimulation, which results in decreased FHR.)

4. Fetal arrhythmia, which is associated with complete heart block in the fetus

5. Uterine hyperstimulation

6. Abruptio placentae

7. Uterine rupture

8. Vagal stimulation in the second stage (Because this does not involve hypoxia, the fetus can recover.)

9. Congenital heart block

10. Maternal hypothermia

Bradycardia may be a benign or an ominous (preterminal) sign. If there is variability, the bradycardia may be considered benign, although the degree of the rate change and length of time it occurs are significant factors. Bradycardia accompanied by decreased variability and late decelerations is considered ominous and a sign of nonreassuring fetal status (Cunningham et al., 2014).

ARRHYTHMIAS AND DYSRHYTHMIAS

Arrhythmias, a term often used interchangeably with *dysrhythmias*, are disturbances in the FHR pattern that are not associated with abnormal electrical impulse formation or conduction in the fetal cardiac tissue, but are related to a structural abnormality or congenital heart disease (Blackburn, 2013). Fetal arrhythmias may be detected when listening to the FHR on a fetal monitor. It is important to rule out artifacts or electrical interference because this sometimes occurs. Most true arrhythmias are accompanied by baseline bradycardia, baseline tachycardia, or an abrupt baseline spiking (Blackburn, 2013). Ninety percent of fetal cardiac arrhythmias are benign, resolve spontaneously, and require no intervention (Blackburn, 2013). The most common serious arrhythmias are supraventricular tachycardia and complete heart block (Gomella, 2013).

BASELINE VARIABILITY

Baseline variability (BL VAR) is a fluctuation in the FHR of two cycles per minute or greater that is irregular in amplitude and frequency and is measured as the peak and trough of the fetal tracing in beats per minute. It is a measure of the interplay (the push–pull effect) between the sympathetic and parasympathetic nervous systems. Figure 17–11 depicts the different ranges of variability. The amplitudes of peak and trough in beats per minute are defined as follows (King, Brucker, Kriebs, et al., 2015):

- *Marked:* amplitude greater than 25 beats/min
- *Moderate (normal):* amplitude 6 to 25 beats/min
- *Minimal:* amplitude detectable but 5 beats/min or less
- *Absent:* amplitude undetectable

Reduced variability is the best single predictor for determining fetal compromise. Fetal acidosis and subsequent hypoxia are highest in fetuses that have absent or minimal variability (Cunningham et al., 2014).

Causes of decreased variability include the following (Cunningham et al., 2014):

1. Hypoxia and acidosis (decreased blood flow to the fetus)
2. Administration of drugs such as meperidine hydrochloride (Demerol), diazepam (Valium), or hydroxyzine (Vistaril), which depress the fetal central nervous system
3. Fetal sleep cycle (During fetal sleep, variability is decreased; fetal sleep cycles usually last for 20 to 40 minutes each hour.)
4. Fetus of less than 32 weeks' gestation (Fetal neurologic control of heart rate is immature.)
5. Fetal dysrhythmias
6. Fetal anomalies affecting the heart, central nervous system, or autonomic nervous system
7. Previous neurologic insult
8. Tachycardia

Causes of marked variability include the following (Cunningham et al., 2014):

1. Early mild hypoxia (Variability increases as a result of compensatory mechanism.)
2. Fetal stimulation or activity (stimulation of autonomic nervous system because of abdominal palpation, maternal vaginal examination, application of spiral electrode on fetal head, or acoustic stimulation)
3. Fetal breathing movements
4. Advancing gestational age (greater than 30 gestational weeks)

Absent variability that does not appear to be associated with a fetal sleep cycle or the administration of drugs is a warning sign of nonreassuring fetal status. It is especially ominous if absent or minimal variability is accompanied by late decelerations (explained shortly). If decreased variability is noted on

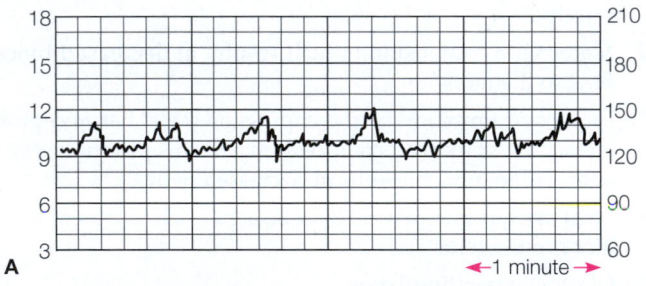

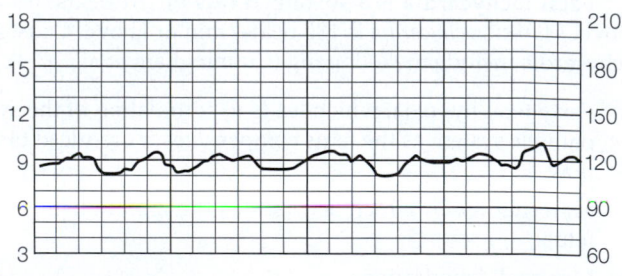

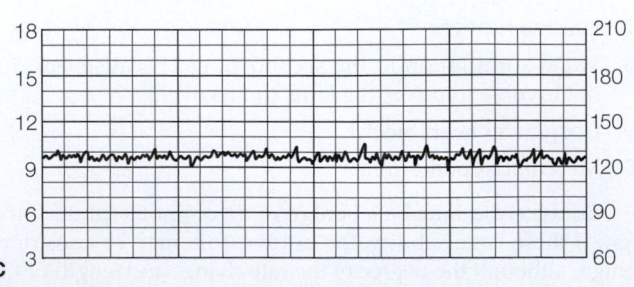

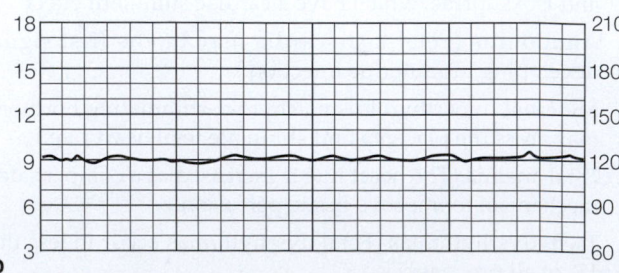

Figure 17–11 Variability. A. Marked variability. B. Moderate variability. C. Minimal variability. D. Absent variability.

monitoring, application of a spiral electrode should be considered to obtain more accurate information.

ACCELERATIONS

Accelerations are transient increases in the FHR normally caused by fetal movement. When the fetus moves, its heart rate increases, just as the heart rates of adults increase during exercise. Often accelerations accompany uterine contractions, usually because the fetus moves in response to the pressure of the contractions or as a result of sympathetic stimulation in response to chemoreceptor signals when a reduction in oxygen supply occurs as a result of the contraction. Accelerations of this type are thought to be a sign of fetal well-being and adequate oxygen reserve. They indicate a mature autonomic nervous system and the absence of acidosis (Blackburn, 2013; Cunningham et al., 2014). The accelerations with fetal movement are the basis for non-stress tests (see Chapter 15).

DECELERATIONS

Decelerations are periodic decreases in FHR from the normal baseline. They are categorized as early, late, and variable according to the time of their occurrence in the contraction cycle and their waveform (Figure 17–12). An **early deceleration** occurs when the fetal head is compressed; cerebral blood flow is decreased, which leads to central vagal stimulation and results in a reduction in the fetal heart rate. The onset of early deceleration is associated with the onset of the uterine contraction. This type of deceleration is usually of uniform shape, is usually considered benign, and does not require intervention.

Clinical Tip

The presence of repetitive early decelerations may be a sign of advanced dilatation or the beginning of the second stage of labor. If the monitoring strip shows reoccurring early decelerations, ask the laboring woman if she is experiencing any pressure. Pressure that occurs only with the contractions typically indicates advanced dilatation. Intense pressure that does not change or ease up when the contractions cease may indicate the beginning of the second stage. A vaginal examination may be performed to establish the dilatation.

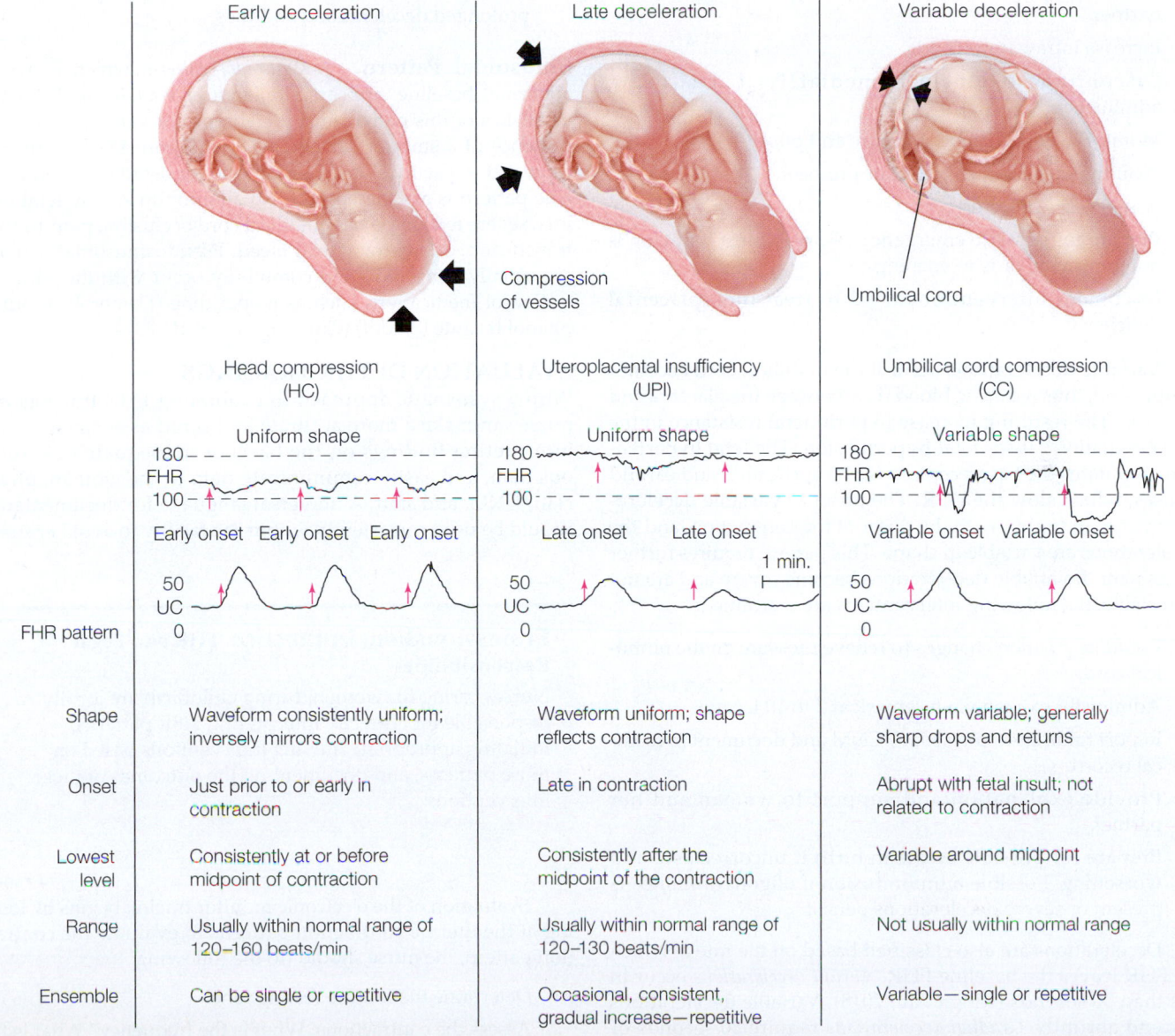

FHR pattern	Early deceleration	Late deceleration	Variable deceleration
	Head compression (HC)	Uteroplacental insufficiency (UPI)	Umbilical cord compression (CC)
Shape	Waveform consistently uniform; inversely mirrors contraction	Waveform uniform; shape reflects contraction	Waveform variable; generally sharp drops and returns
Onset	Just prior to or early in contraction	Late in contraction	Abrupt with fetal insult; not related to contraction
Lowest level	Consistently at or before midpoint of contraction	Consistently after the midpoint of the contraction	Variable around midpoint
Range	Usually within normal range of 120–160 beats/min	Usually within normal range of 120–130 beats/min	Not usually within normal range
Ensemble	Can be single or repetitive	Occasional, consistent, gradual increase—repetitive	Variable—single or repetitive

Figure 17–12 Types and characteristics of early, late, and variable decelerations.

A **late deceleration** is caused by uteroplacental insufficiency resulting from decreased blood flow and oxygen transfer to the fetus through the intervillous spaces during uterine contractions. The most common causes of late decelerations are maternal hypotension resulting from the administration of epidural anesthesia and uterine tachysystole associated with oxytocin infusion (King et al., 2015). Maternal hypertension, diabetes, collagen-vascular disorders, placental abruption, or placental dysfunction are also causative factors (Cunningham et al., 2014). The onset of the deceleration occurs after the onset of a uterine contraction and is of a uniform shape that tends to reflect associated uterine contractions. The late deceleration pattern is considered a nonreassuring sign and requires continuous assessment and immediate intervention to correct or improve uteroplacental blood flow. If late decelerations continue, and the time until birth is not imminent, a cesarean birth may be indicated. Nursing interventions required include the following:

- Facilitate a left lateral position with changes in position as warranted until FHR improves or stabilizes.
- Administer oxygen via facemask at 7 to 10 L/min.
- Alert physician/CNM of status immediately.
- Provide explanation and support to woman and her partner.
- Increase intravenous fluids.
- Discontinue oxytocin immediately if it is being administered.
- Monitor maternal blood pressure and pulse.
- Treat hypotension per orders or protocol.
- Assess cervical status.
- Prepare for possible emergency cesarean birth if tracing is not improving or is worsening.
- Document interventions used to treat uteroplacental deficiency.

Variable decelerations occur if the umbilical cord becomes compressed, thus reducing blood flow between the placenta and the fetus. The resulting increase in peripheral resistance in the fetal circulation causes fetal hypertension. The fetal hypertension stimulates the baroreceptors in the aortic arch and carotid sinuses, which slow the FHR. The onset of variable decelerations varies in timing with the onset of the contraction, and the decelerations are variable in shape. This pattern requires further assessment. If variable decelerations become severe and are not correctable, the following interventions are warranted:

- Facilitate position changes to relieve pressure on the umbilical cord.
- Administer oxygen via facemask at 7 to 10 L/min.
- Report findings to physician/CNM and document in medical record.
- Provide explanation and support to woman and her partner.
- Prepare for possible cesarean birth if uncorrectable and worsening. Possible amnioinfusion if oligohydramnios is present or severe decelerations persist.

Decelerations are also classified based on the rate at which the FHR leaves the baseline FHR. *Abrupt decelerations* occur in less than 30 seconds (King et al., 2015). Variable decelerations descend abruptly. *Gradual decelerations* require 30 seconds or more to descend. Both early and late decelerations descend

gradually. Decelerations can also be episodic or periodic. *Episodic decelerations* occur independently of the uterine contractions and are frequently the result of external stimulations, such as vaginal exams. *Periodic decelerations* refer to decelerations that occur with the contractions and are considered repetitive if they occur with 50% of the contractions (King et al., 2015).

Decelerations that leave the baseline for more than 2 minutes but less than 10 minutes are known as *prolonged decelerations*. Nursing interventions for prolonged decelerations include the following:

- Perform a vaginal examination to rule out a prolapsed umbilical cord.
- Change maternal position.
- Discontinue oxytocin if being administered.
- Notify physician/CNM of findings and responses to interventions.
- Provide explanation and support to woman and her partner.
- Increase intravenous fluid administration rate.
- Administer tocolytic if tachysystole is occurring.
- Anticipate physician/CNM intervention upon arrival if prolonged deceleration continues.

Sinusoidal Pattern. A *sinusoidal pattern*, which is a very abnormal baseline, appears similar to a waveform. The characteristics of this pattern include absence of variability and the presence of a smooth wavelike shape (Figure 17–13). This can represent a pseudosinusoidal or true sinusoidal pattern. The true pattern is associated with Rh alloimmunization, fetal anemia, severe fetal hypoxia, umbilical cord occlusion, twin-to-twin transfusion, or a chronic fetal bleed. Pseudosinusoidal patterns are usually temporary and commonly occur with the administration of medications such as meperidine (Demerol) or butorphanol tartrate (Stadol) (Cunningham et al., 2014).

EVALUATION OF FHR TRACINGS

With a systematic approach to evaluating FHR tracings, the nurse can make a more accurate and rapid assessment, avoid interpreting findings on the basis of inadequate or erroneous data, and easily communicate data to the woman, physician/CNM, and staff. A universal language for documentation should be used consistently within the facility to avoid errors.

Professionalism in Practice FHR and Legal Responsibilities

Nurses caring for women during childbirth are legally responsible for correctly interpreting FHR patterns, initiating appropriate nursing interventions based on those patterns, and documenting the outcomes of those interventions.

Evaluation of the electronic monitor tracing begins by looking at the uterine contraction pattern. To evaluate the contraction pattern, the nurse should do the following:

1. Determine the uterine resting tone.
2. Assess the contractions: What is the frequency? What is the duration? What is the intensity?

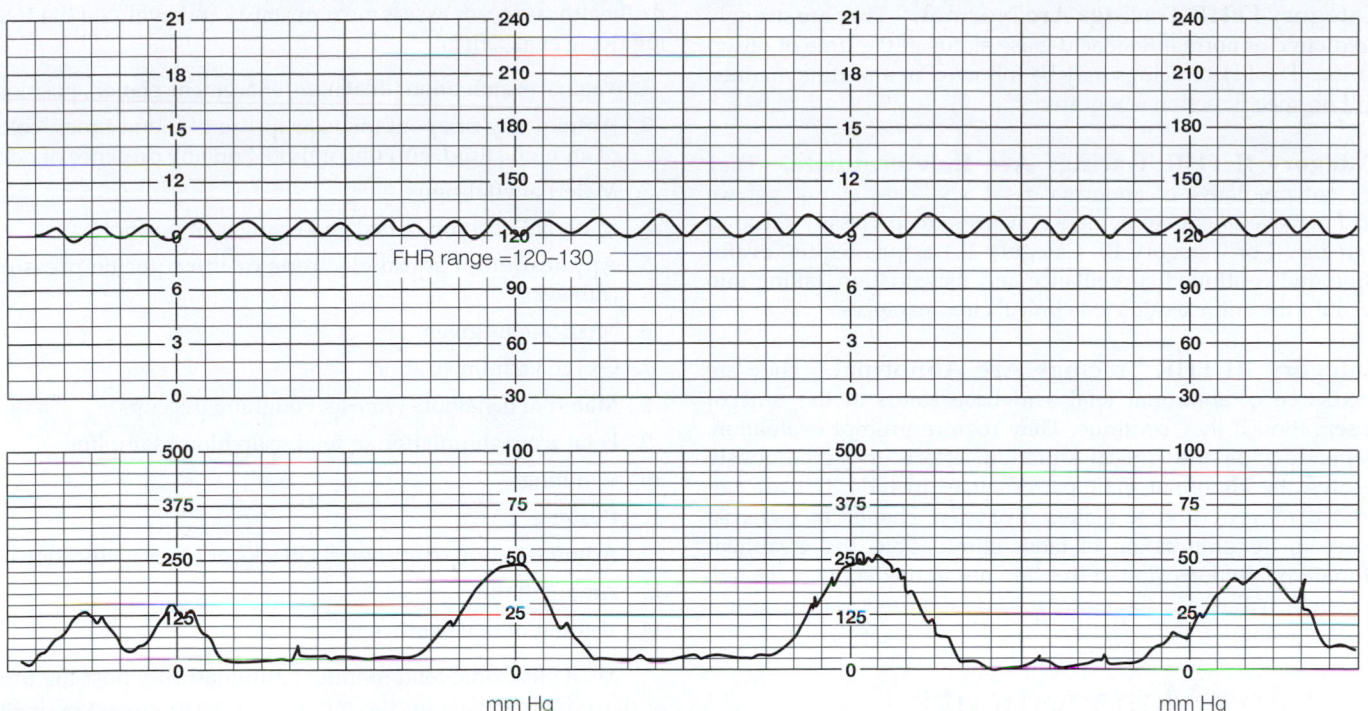

Figure 17–13 Sinusoidal pattern. Note the undulating waveform evenly distributed between the 120 and 130 beats/min baseline. There is minimal variability.

After evaluating the FHR tracing for the contraction pattern, the nurse may categorize the tracing according to the Three-Tier FHR Interpretation System (Table 17–3). The three-tier system for the categorization of FHR patterns is recommended by ACOG, AWHONN, and the National Institute of Child Health and Human Development (Cunningham et al., 2014). Categorization of the FHR tracing evaluates the fetus at that point in time; tracing patterns can and will change. A FHR tracing may move back and forth between categories depending on the clinical situation and management strategies employed.

TABLE 17–3 Three-Tier Fetal Heart Rate Interpretation System

CATEGORY I	CATEGORY II	CATEGORY III
REASSURING FETAL HEART RATE TRACINGS	**PATTERNS WARRANTING CONTINUAL ASSESSMENT**	**PATTERNS OF NONREASSURING FETAL STATUS THAT WARRANT IMMEDIATE INTERVENTION**
<ul><li>Normal range FHR 110–160 beats/min</li><li>Normal FHR variability in the moderate range</li><li>Absence of variable or late decelerations</li><li>Accelerations may be present or may be absent</li><li>Early decelerations may be present or may be absent; they do not represent a nonreassuring status</li></ul>	<ul><li>Baselines that include bradycardia with continued variability, or tachycardia</li><li>Baseline changes in variability that include minimal variability, absent variability without decelerations, or marked baseline variability</li><li>Lack of accelerations with scalp stimulation</li><li>Episodic decelerations that include recurrent variable decelerations with minimal or moderate variability, prolonged decelerations lasting > 2 minutes but < 10 minutes in duration, or recurrent late decelerations that maintain moderate variability</li><li>Variable deceleration patterns that include overshoots, shoulders, or slow return to baseline status</li></ul>	<ul><li>Absent variability in baseline FHR with recurrent late decelerations, recurrent variable decelerations, and/or bradycardia</li><li>Sinusoidal FHR patterns</li></ul>

Source: Data from American College of Obstetricians & Gynecologists (ACOG). (2009, reaffirmed 2013). Intrapartum fetal heart rate monitoring: Nomenclature, interpretation, and general management principles. ACOG Practice Bulletin No. 106. Washington, DC: ACOG.

Category I FHR Tracings Are Normal. They are strongly predictive of normal fetal acid–base status at the time of observation. The FHR tracings may be followed in a routine manner, and no specific action is required.

Category II FHR Tracings Are Indeterminate. They are not predictive of abnormal fetal acid–base status, yet we do not have adequate evidence at present to classify these as Category I or Category III. Category II tracings require evaluation and continued surveillance and reevaluation, taking into account the entire associated clinical circumstances.

Category III FHR Tracings Are Abnormal. They are predictive of abnormal fetal acid–base status at the time of observation if they continue. They require prompt evaluation. Depending on the clinical situation, efforts to expeditiously resolve the abnormal FHR pattern may include, but are not limited to, provision of maternal oxygen, change in maternal position, discontinuation of labor stimulation, and treatment of maternal hypotension. If they are not immediately corrected, acidemia will occur; therefore, birth is required via the fastest route possible.

Nursing Management

Technology has been advancing at a rapid rate in the labor and birthing arena, and each new development challenges nurses to understand, include, and balance technology with holistic nursing practice. A key strength of technology is its potential to explain and predict health patterns or problems with precision. It can also save time and reduce the risk of more invasive procedures. However, technology also has the potential to dehumanize the nurse–client relationship. This can happen when nurses focus on a device instead of the client; or in other words, on data that are objectively measurable, tangible, and visible rather than cues that may arise from intuition or from observations of or interactions with the client and family. In addition, the technical language of EFM and other procedures may act as a barrier, isolating the client and deemphasizing her experience.

For these reasons, it is important to recognize that every encounter with the childbearing family offers you an opportunity to provide education and empowerment. These encounters include times when technology is utilized. By helping to provide information when needed, answering questions, and encouraging the family to make decisions, a trusting relationship can be established. Within this bond of trust resides an awareness of the client's whole being and the healing power of each moment.

Before using the electronic fetal monitor, fully explain to the woman the reason for its use and the information that it can provide. After the monitor is applied, basic information can be recorded on the monitor strip. These data should include the date, client's name, physician's or CNM's name, hospital identification number, age, gravida, para, estimated date of birth (EDB), membrane status, and maternal vital signs.

It is important for the laboring woman to feel that what is happening to her is the central focus. Acknowledge this need by always speaking to and looking at the woman when entering the room, before looking at the monitor.

As the monitor strip runs and care is provided, the following occurrences should be recorded not only in the medical record but also on the monitoring strip. This information helps the healthcare team assess current status and evaluate the tracing (King et al., 2015).

1. Vaginal examination (dilatation, effacement, station, position)
2. Amniotomy or spontaneous rupture of membranes, color of amniotic fluid, amount of fluid, and any presence of odor
3. Maternal vital signs
4. Maternal position in bed and changes of position
5. Application of spiral electrode or intrauterine pressure catheter
6. Medications given
7. Oxygen administration
8. Maternal behaviors (emesis, coughing, hiccups)
9. Fetal scalp stimulation or fetal scalp blood sampling
10. Vomiting
11. Pushing
12. Administration of anesthesia blocks or other medications
13. Ambulation
14. Voiding or bowel movements

Most electronic fetal monitors automatically post the time at periodic intervals on the monitoring strip; however, if the monitor does not automatically add the time, the time should be included when recording any information. When adding information to the monitoring strip, it is essential to initial each note. The tracing is considered a legal part of the woman's medical record and is submissible as evidence in court.

Fetal Scalp Stimulation Test

When there is a question regarding fetal status, a scalp stimulation test can be used before the more invasive **fetal blood sampling (FBS)**. In this test, the examiner applies pressure to the fetal scalp while doing a vaginal examination. The fetus with a category II or III tracing who is not in any stress and responds with an acceleration of the FHR is unlikely to have acidemia and labor can likely continue (Cunningham et al., 2014).

Cord Blood Analysis at Birth

In cases where significant abnormal FHR patterns have been noted, meconium-stained amniotic fluid is present, or the neonate is depressed at birth, umbilical cord blood may be analyzed immediately following the birth to determine if acidosis is present. Blood gases should be performed in cases where the Apgar score is below 7 at 5 minutes of age (a normal Apgar score is 7 to 10). Other indications include fetal compromise, severe growth restriction, abnormal fetal heart rate tracing, maternal thyroid disease, intrapartum fever, or multifetal gestation (Ramin, 2015).

The cord is clamped before the neonate takes the first breath. Using a third hemostat, the practitioner clamps an 8- to 10-inch portion of the umbilical cord. A small amount of blood (1.0 ml is required for a full panel) is aspirated with a syringe from one of the umbilical arteries. An artery is selected because it gives a more reliable blood gas reading and fetal tissue pH level. If the cord blood will not be analyzed immediately, a heparinized syringe should be used. Normal fetal blood pH should be above 7.25 (Ramin, 2015). Lower levels indicate acidosis and hypoxia. Many practitioners obtain a cord blood analysis to minimize medicolegal exposure.

See *Assessment Guide: Intrapartum—First Stage of Labor.*

ASSESSMENT GUIDE | Intrapartum—First Stage of Labor

Physical Assessment/Normal Findings	Alterations and Possible Causes*	Nursing Responses to Data†
Vital Signs		
Blood pressure (BP): Less than or equal to 120 systolic and 80 diastolic in adult 18 years of age or older or no more than 15 to 20 mmHg rise in systolic pressure over baseline BP during early pregnancy	High blood pressure (essential hypertension, preeclampsia, renal disease, apprehension, anxiety, or pain)	Evaluate history of preexisting disorders and check for presence of other signs of preeclampsia.
	Low blood pressure (supine hypotension, epidural administration) Hemorrhage/hypovolemia	Do not assess during contractions; implement measures to decrease anxiety and reassess.
	Shock	Turn woman on her side and recheck BP.
	Drugs	Provide quiet environment.
Pulse: 60 to 100 beats/min	Increased pulse rate (excitement or anxiety, cardiac disorders, early shock, drug use, pain)	Have O_2 available. Evaluate cause, reassess to see if rate continues; report to physician/CNM.
Respirations: 12 to 20/min (or pulse rate divided by 4)	Marked tachypnea (respiratory disease), hyperventilation in transition phase	Assess between contractions; if marked tachypnea continues, assess for signs of respiratory disease or respiratory distress.
Pulse oximetry 95% or greater	Decreased respirations (narcotics)	
	Hyperventilation (anxiety/pain)	Encourage slow breaths if woman is hyperventilating.
	Less than 90%: hypoxia, hypotension, hemorrhage	Apply O_2; notify physician/CNM.
Temperature: 36.2° to 37.6°C (97° to 99.6°F)	Elevated temperature (infection, dehydration, prolonged rupture of membranes, epidural regional block)	Assess for other signs of infection or dehydration.
Weight		
25 to 35 lb (for average body mass index [BMI]) greater than pre-pregnant weight	Weight gain greater than 35 lb (fluid retention, obesity, large baby, diabetes mellitus, preeclampsia), weight gain less than 15 lb for average BMI (small for gestational age [SGA], substance abuse, psychosocial problems)	Assess for signs of edema.
Lungs		
Normal breath sounds, clear and equal	Rales, rhonchi, friction rub (infection), pulmonary edema, asthma	Reassess; refer to physician/CNM.
Fundus		
At 40 weeks' gestation located just below xiphoid process	Uterine size not compatible with estimated date of birth (SGA, large for gestational age [LGA], hydramnios, oligohydramnios, multiple pregnancy, placental/fetal anomalies, malpresentation)	Reevaluate history regarding pregnancy dating. Refer to physician/CNM for additional assessment.
Edema		
Slight amount of dependent edema	Excessive edema of face, hands; pitting edema in legs; edema in abdomen, sacral area, and labia (preeclampsia)	Check deep tendon reflexes for hyperactivity; check for clonus; refer to physician/CNM.
Hydration		
Normal skin turgor, elastic	Poor skin turgor (dehydration)	Assess skin turgor; refer to physician for deviations. Provide fluids per physician/CNM orders.
Perineum		
Tissues smooth, pink color (see Assessment Guide: Initial Prenatal Assessment in Chapter 9)	Varicose veins of vulva, herpes lesions/genital warts	Note on client record need for follow-up in postpartum period; reassess after birth, refer to physician/CNM.
Clear mucus; may be blood tinged with earthy or human odor	Profuse, purulent, foul-smelling drainage	Suspected gonorrhea or chorioamnionitis; report to physician/CNM; initiate care to newborn's eyes; notify neonatal nursing staff and pediatrician.
Presence of small amount of bloody show that gradually increases with further cervical dilatation	Hemorrhage	Assess BP and pulse, pallor, diaphoresis; report any marked changes. Standard precautions.

(continued)

ASSESSMENT GUIDE | Intrapartum—First Stage of Labor (*continued*)

Physical Assessment/Normal Findings	Alterations and Possible Causes*	Nursing Responses to Data†
Labor Status		
Uterine contractions: Regular pattern	Failure to establish a regular pattern, prolonged latent phase Tachysystole Hypotonicity Dehydration	Evaluate whether woman is in true labor. Ambulate if in early labor. Evaluate client status and contractile pattern. Obtain a 20-minute electronic fetal monitoring (EFM) strip. Notify physician/CNM. Provide hydration.
Cervical dilatation: Progressive cervical dilatation from size of fingertip to 10 cm (see *Clinical Skill: Performing an Intrapartum Vaginal Examination*)	Rigidity of cervix (frequent cervical infections, scar tissue, failure of presenting part to descend)	Evaluate contractions, fetal engagement, position, and cervical dilatation. Inform woman of progress.
Cervical effacement: Progressive thinning of cervix (see *Clinical Skill: Performing an Intrapartum Vaginal Examination*)	Failure to efface (rigidity of cervix, failure of presenting part to engage); cervical edema (pushing effort by woman before cervix is fully dilated and effaced; trapped cervix)	Evaluate contractions, fetal engagement, and position. Notify physician/CNM if cervix is becoming edematous; work with woman to prevent pushing until cervix is completely dilated. Keep vaginal exams to a minimum.
Fetal descent: Progressive descent of fetal presenting part from station −2 to +4 (see Figure 17–4)	Failure of descent (abnormal fetal position or presentation, macrosomic fetus, inadequate pelvic measurements)	Evaluate fetal position, presentation, and size.
Membranes: May rupture before or during labor	Rupture of membranes more than 12 to 24 hours before onset of labor	Assess for ruptured membranes using Nitrazine test tape before doing vaginal exam. Follow standard precautions. Instruct woman with ruptured membranes to remain on bed rest if presenting part is not engaged and firmly down against the cervix. Keep vaginal exams to a minimum to prevent infection. When membranes rupture in the birth setting immediately assess FHR to detect changes associated with prolapse of umbilical cord (fetal heart rate [FHR] slows).
Findings on Nitrazine test tape: Membranes probably intact: Yellow pH 5.0 Olive pH 5.5 Olive green pH 6.0 Membranes probably ruptured: Blue-green pH 6.5 Blue-gray pH 7.0 Deep blue pH 7.5	False-positive results may be obtained if large amount of bloody show is present, previous vaginal examination has been done using lubricant, or tape is touched by nurse's fingers	Assess fluid for consistency, amount, odor; assess FHR frequently. Assess fluid at regular intervals for presence of meconium staining. Follow standard precautions while assessing amniotic fluid. Teach woman that amniotic fluid is continually produced (to allay fear of "dry birth"). Teach woman that she may feel amniotic fluid trickle or gush with contractions. Change chux pads often.
Amniotic fluid clear, with earthy or human odor, no foul-smelling odor	Greenish amniotic fluid (fetal stress, postterm pregnancy, breech presentation) Bloody fluid (vasoprevia, abruptio placentae, placenta previa) Strong or foul odor (amnionitis)	Assess FHR; do vaginal exam to evaluate for prolapsed cord; apply fetal monitor for continuous data; report to physician/CNM. Take woman's temperature and report to physician/CNM.
Fetal Status		
FHR: 110 to 160 beats/min	Less than 110 or greater than 160 beats/min (nonreassuring fetal status); abnormal patterns on fetal monitor: decreased variability, late decelerations, variable decelerations, absence of accelerations with fetal movement	Initiate interventions based on particular FHR pattern.
Presentation: Cephalic, 97% Breech, 3%	Face, brow, breech, or shoulder presentation	Report to physician/CNM; after presentation is confirmed as face, brow, breech, or shoulder, woman may be prepared for cesarean birth.

Physical Assessment/Normal Findings	Alterations and Possible Causes*	Nursing Responses to Data†
Position: Left-occiput-anterior (LOA) most common	Persistent occipital-posterior (OP) position; transverse arrest	Carefully monitor maternal and fetal status. Reposition mother side-lying or hands/knee to promote rotation of fetal head.
Activity: Fetal movement	Hyperactivity (may precede fetal hypoxia)	Carefully evaluate FHR; apply fetal monitor.
	Complete lack of movement (nonreassuring fetal status or fetal demise)	Carefully evaluate FHR; apply fetal monitor. Report to physician/CNM.
Laboratory Evaluation		
Hematologic tests **Hemoglobin:** 12 to 16 g/dL	Less than 11 g/dL (anemia, hemorrhage, sickle cell disorders, pernicious anemia)	Evaluate woman for problems associated with decreased oxygen-carrying capacity caused by lowered hemoglobin.
CBC **Hematocrit:** 38% to 47% **RBC:** 4.2 to 5.4 million/mm³ **WBC:** 4500 to 11,000/mm³, although leukocytosis to 20,000/mm³ is not unusual **Platelets:** 150,000 to 400,000/mm³	Presence of infection or blood dyscrasias, loss of blood (hemorrhage, disseminated intravascular coagulation [DIC])	Evaluate for other signs of infections, petechiae, bruising, or unusual bleeding.
Serologic testing STS or VDRL test: nonreactive Rh	Positive reaction (see Assessment Guide: Initial Prenatal Assessment in Chapter 9)	For reactive test notify newborn nursery and pediatrician.
	Rh-positive fetus in Rh-negative woman	Assess prenatal record for titer levels during pregnancy. Obtain cord blood for direct Coombs test at birth.
Urinalysis **Glucose:** negative	Glycosuria (low renal threshold for glucose, diabetes mellitus)	Assess blood glucose; test urine for ketones; ketonuria and glycosuria require further assessment of blood sugars.
Ketones: negative	Ketonuria (starvation ketosis)	
Proteins: negative	Proteinuria (urine specimen contaminated with vaginal secretions, fever, kidney disease); proteinuria of 2+ or greater found in uncontaminated urine may be a sign of ensuing preeclampsia	Instruct woman in collection technique; incidence of contamination from vaginal discharge is common. Report any increase in proteinuria to physician/CNM.
Red blood cells: negative	Blood in urine (calculi, cystitis, glomerulonephritis, neoplasm)	Assess collection technique (may be bloody show).
White blood cells: negative	Presence of white blood cells (infection in genitourinary tract)	Assess for signs of urinary tract infections.
Casts: none	Presence of casts (nephrotic syndrome)	
Cultural Assessment§	**Variations to Consider**	**Nursing Responses to Data†**
Cultural influences determine customs and practices regarding intrapartum care.	Individual preferences may vary.	
Ask the following questions: Who would you like to remain with you during your labor and birth?	She may prefer only her partner/significant other to remain or may also want family and/or friends. Some cultures prefer only female relatives or friends.	Provide support for her wishes by encouraging desired people to stay. Provide information to others (with the woman's permission) who are not in the room.
What would you like to wear during labor?	She may be more comfortable in her own clothes.	Offer supportive materials such as chux pads if needed to protect her own clothing. Avoid subtle signals to the woman that she should not have chosen to remain in her own clothes. Have other clothing available if the woman desires. If her clothing becomes contaminated, it will be simple to place it in a plastic bag.

(continued)

Cultural Assessment§	Variations to Consider	Nursing Responses to Data†
What activity would you like during labor?	She may want to ambulate most of the time, stand in the shower, sit in a whirlpool bath, sit on a chair/stool/birthing ball, remain on the bed, and so forth.	Support the woman's wishes; provide encouragement and complete assessments in a manner so her activity and positional wishes are disturbed as little as possible.
What position would you like for the birth?	She may feel more comfortable in lithotomy with stirrups and her upper body elevated, or side-lying or sitting in a birthing bed, or standing, or squatting, or on hands and knees.	Collect any supplies and equipment needed to support her in her chosen birthing position. Provide information to the coach regarding any changes that may be needed based on the chosen position.
Is there anything special you would like?	She may want the room darkened or to have curtains and windows open, music playing, a Leboyer birth, her coach to cut the umbilical cord, to save a portion of the umbilical cord, to save the placenta, to videotape the birth, and so forth.	Support requests, and communicate requests to any other nursing or medical personnel (so requests can continue to be supported and not questioned). If another nurse or physician does not honor the request, act as advocate for the woman by continuing to support her unless her desire is truly unsafe.
Ask the woman if she would like fluids, and ask what temperature she prefers.	She may prefer clear fluids other than water (tea, clear juice). She may prefer iced, room-temperature, or warmed fluids.	Provide fluids as desired.
Observe the woman's response when privacy is difficult to maintain and her body is exposed.	Some women do not seem to mind being exposed during an exam or procedure; others feel acute discomfort.	Maintain privacy and respect the woman's sense of privacy. If the woman is unable to provide specific information, the nurse may draw from general information regarding cultural variation.
If the woman is to breastfeed, ask if she would like to feed her baby immediately after birth.	She may want to feed her baby right away or may want to wait a little while.	

Psychosocial Assessment	Variations to Consider	Nursing Responses to Data†
Preparation for Childbirth		
Woman has some information regarding process of normal labor and birth.	Some women do not have any information regarding childbirth.	Add to present information base.
Woman has breathing and/or relaxation techniques to use during labor.	Some women do not have any method of relaxation or breathing to use, and some do not desire them.	Support the breathing and relaxation techniques that the woman is using; provide information if needed.
Woman and support person have done extensive preparation for childbirth (Bradley classes, Lamaze).	Some women have strong opinions regarding labor and birth preparation.	Support woman's wishes to participate in her birth experience; support birth plan.
Response to Labor		
Latent phase: Relaxed, excited, anxious for labor to be well established	May feel unable to cope with contractions because of fear, anxiety, or lack of information	Provide support and encouragement, establish trusting relationship.
Active phase: Becomes more focused on coping as contractions become more intense, begins to tire	May remain quiet and without any sign of discomfort or anxiety; may insist that she is unable to continue with the birthing process	Provide support and coaching if needed.
Transitional phase: Feels tired, may feel unable to cope, needs frequent coaching to maintain breathing patterns		
Coping mechanisms: Ability to cope with labor through use of support system, breathing, relaxation techniques, and comfort measures including frequent position changes in labor, warm water immersion, and massage	May feel marked anxiety and apprehension, may not have coping mechanisms that can be brought into this experience, or may be unable to use them at this time. Many women are unable to maintain a lying position and may need to sit up or change position frequently.	Support coping mechanisms if they are working for the woman; provide information and support if she exhibits anxiety or needs alternative to present coping methods.

Psychosocial Assessment	Variations to Consider	Nursing Responses to Data†
	Women may fear needles and intravenous fluids. Some women may not feel comfortable with male care providers.	Encourage participation of coach/significant other if a supportive relationship seems apparent. Establish rapport and a trusting relationship. Provide information that is true and offer your presence.
	Survivors of sexual abuse may demonstrate fear of IVs or needles, may recoil when touched, may insist on a female caregiver, may be very sensitive to body fluids and cleanliness, and may be unable to labor lying down.	
Anxiety		
Showing some anxiety and apprehension is within normal limits	May show anxiety through rapid breathing, nervous tremors, frowning, grimacing, clenching of teeth, thrashing movements, crying, increased pulse and blood pressure.	Provide support, encouragement, and information. Teach relaxation technique. The nurse needs to determine if the etiology is an anxious response or related to pain.
		Support controlled breathing efforts. May need to provide a paper bag to breathe into if woman says her lips are tingling. Note FHR.
Sounds During Labor		
	Some women are very quiet; others moan or make a variety of noises.	Provide a supportive environment. Encourage woman to do what feels right for her.
Support System		
Physical intimacy between mother and father (or mother and support person/doula); caretaking activities such as soothing conversation, touching	Some women would prefer no contact; others may show clinging behaviors.	Encourage caretaking activities that appear to comfort the woman; encourage support for the woman; if support is limited, the nurse may take a more active role.
Support person stays in proximity	Limited interaction may come from a desire for quiet.	Encourage support person to stay close (if this seems appropriate).
Relationship between mother and father/partner or support person: involved interaction	The support person may seem to be detached and maintain little support, attention, or conversation.	Support interactions; if interaction is limited, the nurse may provide more information and support.
		Ensure that partner/significant other has short breaks, especially before transition.

*Possible causes of alterations are identified in parentheses.

†This column provides guidelines for further assessment and initial nursing intervention.

§These are only a few suggestions. We do not mean to imply that this is a comprehensive cultural assessment; rather, it is a tool to encourage cultural sensitivity.

Focus Your Study

- Intrapartum assessment includes attention to both the physical and the psychosociocultural parameters of the laboring woman, assessment of the fetus, and ongoing assessment for conditions that place the woman and her fetus at increased risk.

- A vaginal examination determines the status of fetal membranes; cervical dilatation and effacement; and fetal presentation, position, and station.

- Uterine contractions may be assessed by palpation or by an electronic monitor.

- Leopold maneuvers provide a systematic evaluation of fetal presentation and position.

- Fetal presentation and position may also be assessed by vaginal examination or ultrasound.

- The fetal heart rate may be assessed by auscultation (with a fetoscope or Doppler) or by electronic monitoring.

- Electronic fetal monitoring is accomplished by indirect ultrasound or by direct methods that require the placement of a spiral electrode on the fetal presenting part.

- Indications for electronic monitoring include fetal, maternal, and uterine factors; presence of pregnancy complications; regional anesthesia; and elective monitoring.

- Variability is the single most important indicator of fetal compromise.

- Baseline FHR refers to the range of FHR observed between contractions, during a 10-minute period of monitoring.

- The normal range of FHR is 110 to 160 beats/min.

- Baseline changes of the FHR include tachycardia, bradycardia, and variability.

- Fetal tachycardia is defined as a rate of more than 160 beats/min for a 10-minute period.

- Fetal bradycardia is defined as a rate of less than 110 beats/min for a 10-minute period.

- Baseline variability is an important parameter of fetal well-being.

- Periodic changes are transient decelerations or accelerations of the FHR from the baseline. Accelerations are normally caused by fetal movement; decelerations may be termed early, late, variable, or sinusoidal.

- Early decelerations are caused by compression of the fetal head during contractions and are considered reassuring.

- Late decelerations are associated with uteroplacental insufficiency and are considered ominous.

- Variable decelerations are associated with compression of the umbilical cord and require further assessment.

- Sinusoidal patterns are characterized by an undulant sine wave.

- Psychologic reactions to monitoring vary between feelings of relief and feelings of being tied down.

- Birthing room nurses have responsibilities in recognizing and interpreting fetal monitoring patterns, notifying the physician/CNM of problems, and initiating corrective and supportive measures when needed.

- Fetal scalp stimulation can be used when fetal status is in question.

- Cord blood analysis can be obtained from the umbilical artery immediately after birth to determine the acid–base status.

Clinical Reasoning in Action

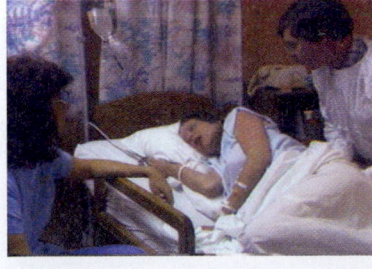

Cindy Bell, a 20-year-old gravida 2, para 1 at 40 weeks' gestation, presents to you in the birthing unit with contractions every 5 to 7 minutes. She is accompanied by her husband. Spontaneous rupture of membranes occurred 2 hours prior to admission. Cindy tells you that the fluid was colorless and clear. You orient Cindy and her family to the birthing room and perform a physical assessment, documenting that vital signs are normal. A vaginal examination demonstrates the cervix is 75% effaced, 4 cm dilated with a vertex at −1 station in the LOP position. You place Cindy on an external fetal monitor. The fetal heart rate baseline is 140 to 147 with accelerations to 156; no decelerations are noted. Contractions are 5 to 6 minutes apart, moderate intensity and lasting 40 to 50 seconds. Cindy states she would like to stay out of bed as long as possible because lying down seems to make the contractions more painful, especially in her back.

1. Discuss the benefits of ambulation in labor.

2. Cindy would like her 5-year-old daughter to be present for the baby's birth. What would you discuss with her about the impact of having a young sibling present during labor and birth?

3. What fetal heart rate assessment will best ensure fetal well-being during the period Cindy is ambulating?

4. When a nonreassuring fetal heart pattern is detected, what remedial nursing intervention is carried out?

5. What are indications for continuous fetal monitoring in labor?

References

Blackburn, S. (2013). *Maternal, fetal, & neonatal physiology: A clinical perspective* (4th ed.). St. Louis, MO: Saunders.

Burnard, P., & Gill, P. (2015). *Culture, communication, and nursing.* London, UK: Routledge.

Coates, R., Ayers, S., & de Visser, R. (2014). Women's experiences of postnatal distress: a qualitative study. *BMC Pregnancy & Childbirth, 14*(359) doi:10.1186/1471-2393-14-359

Cunningham, F. G., Leveno, K. J., Bloom, S. L., Spong, C. Y., Dashe, J. S., Hoffman, B. L., . . . Sheffield, J. S. (2014). *Williams obstetrics* (24th ed.). New York, NY: McGraw-Hill.

Davidson, M.R. (2012). *A nurse's guide to women's mental health.* New York, NY: Springer.

Empowered Birth Summit. (2015). *The mother's guide to a happy, healthy, holistic birth experience.* Retrieved from http://shebirths.com/empowered-birth-online-summit

Friedman, S. H., & Hall, R. C. (2013). Antidepressant use during pregnancy: How to avoid clinical and legal pitfalls. *Clinical Psychiatry, 12*(2), 134–136.

Gomella, T. (2013). *Neonatology* (7th ed.). St. Louis, MO: McGraw-Hill.

King, T. K., Brucker, M. C., Kriebs, J. M., & Fahey, J. (2015). *Varney's midwifery.* (5th ed.). New York, NY: Jones Bartlett Learning.

Massachusetts General Hospital Center for Women's Mental Health. (2015). *Psychiatric disorders during pregnancy.* Retrieved from http://womensmentalhealth.org/specialty-clinics/psychiatric-disorders-during-pregnancy/

Ramin, S.M. (2015). Umbilical cord blood acid-base analysis at delivery. Up-to-date. Retrieved from http://www.uptodate.com/contents/umbilical-cord-blood-acid-base-analysis-at-delivery

Riffle, E. (2014). Fetal heart rate assessment best practice. *International Journal of Childbirth Education, 29*(4), 55–58.

Simpson, K. R., & Creehan, P. A. (2013). AWHONN's perinatal nursing (4th ed.). Washington, DC: AWHONN.

Yonkers, K. A., Smith, M. V., & Forray, A. (2014). Pregnant women with posttraumatic stress disorder and risk of preterm birth. *JAMA Psychiatry, 71*(8), 897–904. doi: 10.1001/jamapsychiatry.2014.558

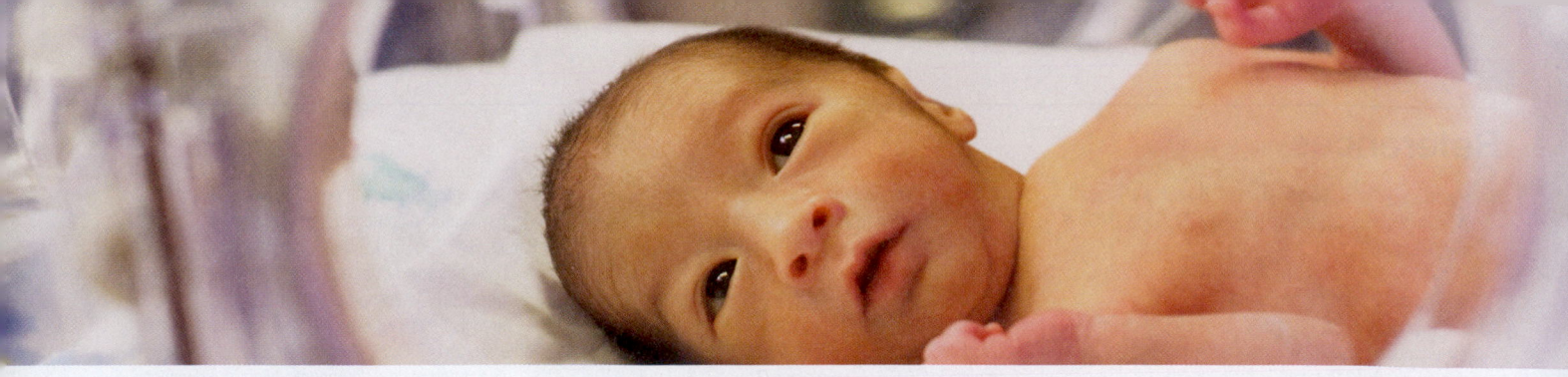

Chapter 18

The Family in Childbirth: Needs and Care

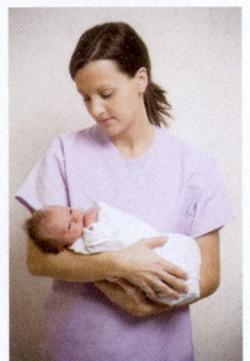

For as long as I can remember I have been fascinated with birth. I began as a hospital volunteer, then taught childbirth preparation, and then became a labor nurse before going back to school to become a certified nurse-midwife. It has been a challenge, and sometimes I wondered if I would make it. But here I am, practicing in the same hospital that I used to volunteer in. I'm still fascinated with birth.

—A Certified Nurse-Midwife

Source: © RubberBall / SuperStock

⌄ Learning Outcomes

18.1 Identify admission data for a woman admitted to the birthing area.

18.2 Describe the nursing care of a woman and her partner/family upon admission to the birthing area.

18.3 Use assessment data to determine the nursing interventions to meet the psychologic, social, physiologic, and spiritual needs of the woman and her partner/family during each stage of labor.

18.4 Compare methods of promoting comfort during the first and second stages of labor.

18.5 Explain the immediate needs and physical assessment of the newborn following birth in the provision of nursing care.

18.6 Examine the unique needs of the adolescent during birth in the provision of nursing care.

18.7 Describe the role and responsibility of the nurse in management of a precipitous labor and birth.

It is time for a child to be born. The waiting is over; labor has begun. The dreams and wishes of the past months fade as the mother-to-be or the expectant parents face the reality of the childbearing and childrearing tasks that lie ahead.

The parents are about to undergo one of the most meaningful and stressful events of their lives. The adequacy of their preparation for childbirth, including the coping mechanisms, communication, and support systems that they have established, will be put to the test. In particular, the childbearing woman may feel that her psychologic and physical limits are about to be challenged. Social and peer relationships may dramatically change after the birth of a child. These events may be even more challenging for a single woman or an adolescent, especially if she lacks a strong support system.

Family-centered care is a model of care based on the philosophy that physical, sociocultural, spiritual, and economic needs of the family are combined and considered collectively when planning care for the childbearing family (Institute for Patient and Family-Centered Care, 2015). To reflect the consumer demand for family-centered care, most birthing centers now have **birthing rooms**, single rooms where the woman and her partner or other family members or support persons will stay for the labor, birth, recovery, and possibly the postpartum period. These rooms may be called *labor, delivery, recovery, and postpartum (LDRP) rooms* or *single-room maternity care (SRMC)*.

The atmosphere of a birthing room is more relaxed than that of a traditional hospital room and families seem to feel more comfortable in them. Another benefit to a birthing room is that the woman does not have to be transferred from one area to another for the actual birth. A birthing room setting helps the laboring woman create her own space to labor in and enhances the family's comfort and involvement. Birthing rooms usually have beds that can be adapted for birth by removing a small section near the foot. The decor is designed to produce a home-like atmosphere in which families can feel both safe and at ease.

Maternal–newborn nursing has kept pace with the changing philosophy of childbirth. Nurses who choose positions in birthing areas are presented with opportunities to interact with clients in a wide variety of situations, from a family that wants maximum interaction to one that wants to be left alone as much as possible. In addition, the nurse must always be ready to meet the needs and concerns of the single woman who is laboring alone. In every case, nurses strive to provide high-quality, individualized care.

The previous two chapters provided a database about physiologic and psychologic changes during labor and birth and needed nursing assessments. This chapter presents nursing care during labor and birth.

Nursing Diagnoses During Labor and Birth

When a plan of care is devised for the intrapartum period, the nurse can develop a general plan that encompasses the total process, from the beginning of labor through the fourth stage, or a plan can be developed for each stage of labor and birth. A general plan presents an overview of the whole process, whereas a plan of care that identifies nursing diagnoses for each stage provides an opportunity to identify more specific nursing care.

In the first stage, examples of appropriate nursing diagnoses may include the following (NANDA-I © 2014):

- *Fear* related to discomfort of labor and unknown labor outcome
- *Pain, Acute,* related to uterine contractions, cervical dilatation, and fetal descent

- *Knowledge, Readiness for Enhanced,* related to the normal labor process and comfort measures
- *Family Processes, Readiness for Enhanced,* related to the opportunity to incorporate newborn into the family

Examples of nursing diagnoses for the second and third stages may include the following (NANDA-I © 2014):

- *Pain, Acute,* related to uterine contractions, the birth process, and/or perineal trauma from birth
- *Knowledge, Readiness for Enhanced,* related to pushing methods to assist in the birth
- *Anxiety* related to the outcome of the birth process

In the fourth stage, possible nursing diagnoses include the following (NANDA-I © 2014):

- *Pain, Acute,* related to perineal trauma
- *Knowledge, Readiness for Enhanced,* related to the involution process and self-care needs
- *Family Processes, Readiness for Enhanced,* related to incorporation of the newborn into the family

Nursing Care During Admission

Nursing Management

During prenatal visits, instruct the woman to come to the birthing unit if any of the following occurs:

- Rupture of membranes (ROM)
- Regular, frequent uterine contractions (nulliparas, 5 minutes apart for 1 hour; multiparas, 6 to 8 minutes apart for 1 hour)
- Vaginal bleeding
- Decreased fetal movement

The woman in labor and her partner or support person(s) tend to be concerned about arriving at the birth center in time for the birth. Sometimes the labor is advanced and birth is imminent, but usually the woman is in early labor at admission. If time permits and the family is not familiar with what will occur during labor, provide necessary information. (See *Teaching Highlights: What to Expect During Labor.*)

The way you greet the woman and her partner influences the course of the woman's hospital stay. The sudden environmental change and the sometimes impersonal and technical aspects of admission can produce significant stress. If women and their families are greeted in a brusque, harried manner, they are less likely to look to the nurse for support. A calm, pleasant manner indicates to the woman that she is important. It helps to instill a sense of confidence in the staff's ability to provide quality care during this critical time.

Following the initial greeting, escort the woman to the birthing room and provide a quick yet thorough orientation to the facility, including the location of the restrooms, public phones, and nurse-call or emergency-call system. These simple steps can go a long way toward helping the woman and her partner feel more at ease. Explain the monitoring equipment or

| TEACHING HIGHLIGHTS | What to Expect During Labor |

- Describe aspects of the admission process:
  - Abbreviated history
  - Physical assessment (maternal vital signs, fetal heart rate, contraction status, status of membranes)
  - Assessment of uterine contractions (frequency, duration, intensity)
  - Orientation to surroundings
  - Introductions to other staff
  - Determination of the woman's and support person's expectations of the nurse
- Present aspects of ongoing physical care, such as when to expect assessment of maternal vital signs, fetal heart rate, and contractions.
- If an electronic fetal monitor is used, describe how it works and the information it provides. Orient the woman to sights and sounds of the monitor.
- Explain what "normal" data look like and what characteristics are being watched for.
- Be sure to note that assessments will increase as the labor progresses, especially during the transition phase, to help keep the mother and baby safe by noting any changes from the normal course.
- Explain the vaginal examination and the information it can provide.
- Review comfort techniques that may be used in labor and ascertain what the woman thinks will promote comfort.
- Review breathing techniques the woman has learned so that you can support her technique.
- Review comfort and support measures such as positioning, back rub, effleurage, touch, distraction techniques, and ambulation.
- If the woman is in early labor, offer her a tour of the birthing area.
- Have printed materials available for reference, especially for the partner or support person.
- If time permits, a brief video describing procedures may be helpful.

other unfamiliar technology and make every effort to make the environment less frightening for the laboring woman and her support person(s).

Some women prefer that their partner remain with them during the admission process, and others prefer to have the partner wait outside. While helping the woman undress and get into a hospital gown, begin to develop rapport and establish a nursing database. The experienced labor and birth nurse can obtain essential information about the woman and her pregnancy within a few minutes after admission, initiate any immediate interventions needed, and establish individualized priorities.

The woman may be facing a number of unfamiliar procedures that seem routine for healthcare providers. Remember that all women have the right to determine what happens to their bodies. The woman's informed consent should be obtained prior to any procedure that involves touching her.

If indicated, assist the woman into bed. A side-lying or semi-Fowler position rather than a supine position is most comfortable and avoids supine hypotensive syndrome (vena caval syndrome). After obtaining the essential information from the woman and her records, begin the intrapartum assessment (see Chapter 17). Once the assessment is complete, it is possible to make effective nursing decisions about care, such as the following:

- Should ambulation, bedrest, or a combination of both be encouraged?
- Is more frequent or continuous electronic fetal monitoring needed?
- What does the woman want during her labor and birth?

- Is a support person available?
- What special needs do this woman and her partner have?

Auscultate the fetal heart rate (FHR). Determine the woman's blood pressure, pulse, respirations, and oral temperature and assess contraction frequency, duration, and intensity (possibly while gathering other data). Before the vaginal examination, inform the woman about the procedure and its purpose; afterward, report the findings. If signs of advanced labor exist (frequent contractions, an urge to bear down, and so on), a vaginal examination must be done immediately. If there are signs of excessive bleeding or if the woman reports episodes of painless bleeding in the last trimester, suspect placenta previa. Do not do a vaginal examination, and notify the physician/CNM immediately.

Results of FHR assessment, uterine contraction evaluation, and the vaginal examination help determine whether the rest of the admission process can proceed at a leisurely pace or whether additional interventions are required. For example, an FHR of less than 110 beats per minute (beats/min) on auscultation indicates that a fetal monitor should be applied immediately to obtain additional data. The woman's vital signs can be assessed once the monitor is in place.

After obtaining admission data, collect a clean voided midstream urine specimen. The woman with intact membranes may collect her specimen in the bathroom. If the membranes are ruptured and the presenting part is not engaged, the woman generally remains in bed to avoid prolapse of the umbilical cord. Views vary about the wisdom of ambulation once the membranes are ruptured. The decision is generally based on history and physical findings (e.g., history of precipitous labors, indications for continuous fetal monitoring, presence of meconium), clinician orders, the woman's desires, agency policy, and safety concerns.

Use a dipstick to test the woman's urine for the presence of protein, ketones, and glucose before sending the sample to the laboratory. This procedure is especially important if edema or elevated blood pressure is noted on admission. Proteinuria of 1+ or more may be a sign of impending preeclampsia. Glycosuria (sugar in the urine) is found frequently in pregnant women because of the increased glomerular filtration rate in the proximal tubules and the inability of these tubules to increase reabsorption of glucose. However, it may also be associated with gestational diabetes, so do not discount it. Ketones can be associated with inadequate calorie intake, dehydration, vomiting, skipping meals, insulin resistance, or gestational diabetes. While the woman is collecting the urine specimen, gather the equipment needed for any procedures ordered by the physician/CNM.

Laboratory tests are done during early admission. Hemoglobin and hematocrit values help determine the oxygen-carrying capacity of the circulatory system and the woman's ability to withstand blood loss at birth. Elevation of the hematocrit may reveal hemoconcentration of blood, which occurs with edema or dehydration. A low hemoglobin, in the absence of other evidence of bleeding, suggests anemia. Blood may be typed and cross-matched if the woman is in a high-risk category. Platelets are also evaluated because low platelets can lead to bleeding problems. Additional serologic testing may be performed as indicated. HIV testing should be offered to all women who have not been previously screened (Centers for Disease Control & Prevention [CDC], 2015).

Depending on how rapidly labor is progressing, notify the physician/CNM before or after completing the admission procedures. The report should include the following information: parity, cervical dilatation and effacement, station, presenting part, status of the membranes, contraction pattern, FHR, vital signs that are not in the normal range, any significant prenatal history, the woman's birth preferences, and her reaction to labor.

Enter a nursing admission note into the medical record system. The admission note should include the reason for admission, the date and time of the woman's arrival and notification of the physician/CNM, the condition of the woman and her baby, and labor and membrane status.

Nursing Care During the First Stage of Labor

After completing the nursing assessment and diagnosis steps, the nurse creates a plan of care to achieve identified nursing goals. For instance, if the woman and her support person did not have the opportunity to attend childbirth education classes, the nursing goal is to provide desired information. To accomplish this goal, the nurse assesses the current level of the couple's understanding and then plans to provide brief explanations as labor progresses.

Integration of Family Expectations

Laboring families have specific expectations of the labor and birth experience, of themselves, of the nurse, and of the physician/CNM. Sometimes families have unrealistic expectations, which can increase anxiety, create stress, and end in

disappointment if expectations are not met. All families should be encouraged to discuss their preferences and special requests with the nurse. Some families may present to the birthing center with a birth plan. Reviewing the plan provides the nurse with the opportunity to explore the family's wishes. If a request cannot be met, the reason why should be explained thoroughly. All members of the healthcare team should be informed of the family's requests.

Some families may want the nurse present at all times, whereas others will desire privacy and want to spend time alone. Couples may want a great deal of support if they have not attended childbirth education classes or if they are anxious. Others may want to enjoy the experience as a couple, with as few outside interruptions as possible. In this case, the nurse informs the couple of her or his availability and of the need to make intermittent assessments.

Integration of Cultural Beliefs

Knowledge of values, customs, and practices of different cultures is as important during labor as it is in the prenatal period. Without this knowledge, a nurse is less likely to understand a family's behavior and may attempt to impose personal values and beliefs on the family. As cultural sensitivity increases, so does the likelihood of providing high-quality care (Burnard & Gill, 2015).

The following sections briefly present a few possible responses to labor. General examples about any culture or belief system need to be viewed as background information only. The nurse must always remain aware that an individual example of a birthing practice will never be pertinent to all women in a given group. Within every culture, each person develops his or her own beliefs, values, and behaviors.

Clinical Tip

When providing care for a culturally diverse woman and her family, ask yourself what your assumptions are regarding their expectations. Ask the woman direct questions to ensure that you are not making false assumptions based on her cultural identity alone. Consider how these factors will affect her behavior during the labor and birth and incorporate these into your plan of care.

MODESTY

Modesty is an important consideration for most women regardless of culture. Many women are uncomfortable with the degree of exposure needed for certain procedures during labor and the birth. Some women may be particularly uncomfortable when men are present and feel more comfortable with women; in particular, some Middle Eastern women are not accustomed to male physicians and attendants. Others may be uncomfortable with exposure regardless of the gender of the healthcare givers. The nurse needs to be alert to the woman's responses to examinations and procedures and provide appropriate draping and privacy. It is more prudent to assume that embarrassment will occur with exposure and take measures to provide privacy than to assume that it will not matter to the woman if she is exposed.

Orthodox Jewish women may follow several Jewish laws during the childbearing period. The law of *Tznius* requires the woman to maintain modesty in order to preserve dignity. The woman may prefer a gown that covers her elbows and knees. She may also wish to wear a hair covering such as a wig or scarf. The men typically do not observe the woman while she is changing and should be given the opportunity to leave the room to maintain the woman's dignity (Andrews, 2014).

Clinical Reasoning Gender-Specific Care Preference

Fatima Al Ahala is a 22-year-old, G1 who presents in labor. Fatima and her husband Samir are from Pakistan. The couple has stated that they can accept care only from female providers. The couple is being attended to by a female nurse-midwife and the backup physician is also a female. When her labor intensifies, Fatima requests an epidural. The only anesthesiologist available is a male physician.

What actions can you take to help this family meet their cultural preferences?

EXPRESSION AND MEANING OF PAIN

The manner in which a woman chooses to deal with the discomfort of labor varies widely. Some women seem to turn inward and remain very quiet during the whole process. They speak only to ask others to leave the room or cease conversation. Others may be very vocal, with behaviors such as counting out loud, moaning, crying, or shouting. They may also turn from side to side or change positions frequently, often appearing restless.

In many Asian cultures, it is important for individuals to act in a way that will not bring shame on the family. Therefore, the Korean woman may not express pain outwardly for fear of shaming herself or her family, and a Filipina woman may say it is best to lie quietly. Silence is valued in Chinese society, so a Chinese woman may be quiet and stoic to avoid dishonoring herself or her family. Japanese women often prefer natural childbirth and prefer to eat during labor. The male partner is often present for the birth. Mexican women often chant the phrase "Aye yie yie" while in labor, which is actually a form of "folk Lamaze." Repeating the phrase in succession several times necessitates taking long, slow, deep breaths. Thus, it is a cultural method for alleviating pain (Burnard & Gill, 2014). Many Mexican women will want their partners and female relatives present during the birthing process. European Americans demonstrate a wide variety of behaviors in response to pain, from silence to shouting. The nurse supports a woman's individual expression, as long as it is not harmful, in order to enhance the birthing experience for mother, baby, and family.

Different cultures also have differing beliefs about the meaning and value of labor pain. Because childbearing is considered a woman's "career" by ancient Chinese custom, elders advise the pregnant woman not to fear childbirth. South or Central American women may view pain during labor as a symbol of love toward the baby—the more intense the pain, the more intense the love. Native American women typically view labor pain as natural, and may use meditation, self-control, or indigenous plants or herbs, such as black cohosh, throughout their labor as well as to aid them during birth (Burnard & Gill, 2014). European American women may value pain as aiding in the birth of their baby and signaling that all is well, or they may find themselves feeling angry about the intensity of the pain and fearful of losing control.

EXAMPLES OF CULTURAL BELIEFS

Although it is important to avoid stereotyping, descriptions of a few women's responses to labor may be helpful. The following are "snapshots" from Hmong, Vietnamese, Hispanic, Muslim, and Orthodox Judaism cultures.

Hmong women from Laos report that squatting during childbirth is common in their culture. During labor they may want to be active and move about. The husband is frequently present and actively involved in providing comfort. Traditionally, the woman prefers that the amniotic membranes not be ruptured until just before birth. It is thought that the escape of fluid at this time makes the birth easier. During labor the woman usually prefers only "hot" foods and warm water to drink (Burnard & Gill, 2014). As soon as the baby is born, the family may request that the mother be given a soft-boiled egg to restore her energy.

Vietnamese women usually maintain self-control and may even smile throughout labor. They may prefer to walk about during labor and to give birth in a squatting position. In labor, the mother often prefers cold beverages because pregnancy is viewed as a "hot" condition. However, during the postpartum period, which is viewed as a "cold" condition, she will prefer warm liquids (Burnard & Gill, 2014). The newborn is protected from praise and the "evil eye" to prevent jealousy (Burnard & Gill, 2014).

Latina women have identified expectations of their partners during labor and birth such as wanting their partners to stay with them and to reassure them that everything will be all right. As they labor, the women want their partners to show their love and to speak using affectionate words. Latina women also typically want their mothers present during the birth process.

Muslim women may have their husband or a female friend or relative with them during childbirth. However, the father may take a very passive, hands-off approach, speaking up only as an advocate as needed. Family support may be particularly important but does not preclude the importance of the nurse's presence. The woman may want to retain her head covering (*khimar*), and the nurse can offer two long-sleeved gowns. It is important for a female nurse or physician/CNM to perform examinations when possible. If a male physician or nurse is involved, the woman may want her husband to remain in the room. After the birth Muslim fathers may call praise to Allah (*adhan*) in the newborn's right ear and clean the newborn.

Orthodox Jews observe the law of *niddah*, which begins with the onset of regular uterine contractions or the appearance of bloody show or membrane rupture. Once this occurs, the *niddah* law mandates a physical separation of husband and wife. Usually, husbands will not touch their wives during this time, but may remain in the room, or just outside the curtain. The nurse can encourage the father to offer verbal support, prayer, and eye contact if the couple feels comfortable with these interventions. Once the father stops providing physical care, the nurse will need to assist the woman and serve as the primary caretaker and coach. Sometimes, the laboring woman's mother or another female friend or relative may be present. It is common for the father to read prayers during this time. It is also usual practice for the husband not to observe the birth and he reenters the room only after the woman is draped (Andrews, 2014).

Maternity nurses can provide culturally sensitive care by first becoming acquainted with the beliefs and practices of the various cultures in their communities. In the birthing situation, the truly effective nurse supports the family's cultural practices as long as it is safe to do so. Nurses should not assume that because a woman is from a certain ethnic group, her preferences will always follow cultural norms. Instead, the nurse should assess her individualized preferences and wishes.

Nursing Management

For the Woman in the First Stage of Labor

Latent Phase

As discussed in Chapter 17, it is important to evaluate the physical parameters of the woman and her fetus. Monitor maternal temperature every 4 hours unless the temperature is over 37.5°C (99.6°F); in such cases it is taken every hour. When the amniotic membranes have ruptured, assess maternal temperature every 1 to 2 hours depending on the policy of the institution.

Monitor blood pressure, pulse, respirations, and response to pain every hour. If the woman's blood pressure is over 120/80 mmHg or her pulse is more than 100, notify the physician/CNM and reevaluate the blood pressure and pulse more frequently. Monitor the woman's pain level continually because this can elevate the blood pressure and pulse, especially during contractions.

Palpate uterine contractions for frequency, intensity, and duration every 30 minutes. Auscultate the fetal heart rate (FHR) every 30 minutes for low-risk women and every 15 minutes for high-risk women as long as it remains between 110 and 160 beats per minute (beats/min) and is reassuring (King, Brucker, Kriebs, et al., 2015). Auscultate the FHR throughout one contraction and for about 15 seconds after the contraction to ensure that there are no decelerations. If the FHR baseline is not in the 110 to 160 range or decelerations are heard, continuous electronic monitoring is recommended. See Table 18–1 for nursing assessments during the four stages of labor.

Offer the woman fluids in the form of clear liquids or ice chips at frequent intervals, unless complications exist that may necessitate general anesthesia. Some certified childbirth educators advise the woman to bring lollipops to help combat the dryness that occurs with some of the labor breathing patterns. Avoiding both liquids and solids during labor, which was once standard practice, is no longer so because evidence-based practice research and new guidelines indicate that clear fluids can be consumed throughout labor and up to 1 to 2 hours before an elective cesarean birth (Ghorashi, Ashori, Aninzadeh, et al., 2014).

TABLE 18–1 Nursing Assessments During the Stages of Labor

STAGE	MATERNAL ASSESSMENTS	FETAL ASSESSMENTS
FIRST STAGE *Latent phase*	Blood pressure (BP), respirations each hour if in normal range. Temperature every 4 hr unless over 37.5°C (99.6°F) or membranes ruptured, then every 2 hr. Uterine contractions every 30 min.	Fetal heart rate (FHR) every 30 min for low-risk women and every 15 min for high-risk women if normal characteristics present (average variability, baseline in the 110–160 beats/min range, without late or variable decelerations). Note fetal activity. If electronic fetal monitor is in place, assess for reactive non-stress test (NST).
Active phase	BP, pulse, respirations every hour if in normal range. Uterine contractions palpated every 15–30 min.	FHR every 30 min for low-risk women and every 15 min for high-risk women if normal characteristics are present.
Transition phase	BP, pulse, respirations every 30 min. Contractions palpated at least every 15 min.	FHR every 30 min for low-risk women and every 15 min for high-risk women if normal characteristics are present.
SECOND STAGE	BP, pulse, and respirations every 5–15 minutes. Temperature every 2 hr. Uterine contractions palpated continuously.	FHR every 15 min for low-risk women and every 5 min for high-risk women.
THIRD STAGE	BP, pulse, and respirations every 5 min. Palpate uterine contractions intermittently to assess for signs of placenta separation.	Newborn assessment at time of birth, gestational age assessment, and neurologic assessment within first hour of birth. Apgars at 1 and 5 min. Assess initial BP, apical pulse, respirations, and temperature. Assess umbilical cord for the presence of three vessels.
FOURTH STAGE	Assess maternal vital signs including temperature, BP, pulse, and respirations every 5–15 min for first hour. Assess fundus, lochia, perineum, laceration/episiotomy site, bladder distention, and rectum every 15 min.	Perform complete examination to include vital signs, gestational age assessment, physical examination, and neurologic reflexes once between 1 and 4 hr postbirth. After initial 8 hr, assess vitals and perform assessment every 8 hr. Skin color should be assessed every 4 hr.

Research shows that the volume of liquid consumed is less important than the presence of particulate matter ingested because this increases the risk of aspiration. Certain women with specific risk factors for aspiration should be evaluated on a case-by-case basis to assess their specific risk factors and determine the most appropriate recommendation. Current guidelines suggest avoiding solids for 6 to 8 hours before an elective cesarean birth, although evidence supporting this guideline is not based on research outcomes but is a standard of practice. It should be noted that women who have not been fasting prior to emergency cesarean birth also have demonstrated a low incidence of pulmonary aspiration (Santos, 2014). Women with certain risk factors, including diabetes, obesity, and increased risk of cesarean birth should be evaluated on a case-by-case basis to determine the best practice for intake of solids during labor.

Eating during labor has not been associated with an increase in aspiration and is therefore no longer contraindicated. Previously, it was believed that drinking fluids should be avoided because doing so could lead to vomiting caused by the decreased gastric emptying time. Although vomiting is common during the first stage of labor, many women have more energy and tolerate labor better with oral intake and have higher satisfaction with their labor and birth experience (Santos, 2014). If vomiting does occur, the nurse provides reassurance and oral care.

Active Phase

During the active phase, contractions have a frequency of 2 to 5 minutes, a duration of 40 to 60 seconds, and an intensity from moderate to strong. Palpate contractions every 15 to 30 minutes. As the contractions become more frequent and intense, vaginal examinations assess cervical dilatation and effacement and fetal station and position. During the active phase, the cervix dilates from 4 to 7 cm, and vaginal discharge and bloody show increase. Monitor maternal blood pressure, pulse, and respirations every hour for low-risk women (unless elevated, as previously noted) and every 30 minutes for high-risk women. Auscultate the FHR every 30 minutes for low-risk women and every 15 minutes for high-risk women (Narendra, Shah, Pratap, et al., 2014).

A woman who has been ambulatory up to this point may wish to sit in a chair or on a bed. If the woman wants to lie on the bed, encourage her to assume a side-lying position, help her into a comfortable position, and place pillows to support her body. To increase comfort, offer a back rub or effleurage or place a cool cloth on the woman's forehead or across her neck. Because vaginal discharge increases, change the chux pad frequently. Washing the perineum with warm soapy water removes secretions and increases comfort. During such procedures it is essential to wear disposable gloves to avoid exposure to vaginal discharge.

If the amniotic membranes have not ruptured previously, they may do so during this phase. When the membranes rupture, immediately note the FHR on the monitor if one is being used (if the woman is not on a monitor, auscultate FHR) and then note the color, odor, and consistency of the amniotic fluid and the time of rupture. The fluid should be clear, with no odor. The presence of any frank bright red vaginal bleeding should be noted because it is not considered a normal finding. Fetal stress leads to intestinal and anal sphincter relaxation, and meconium may be released into the amniotic fluid, which turns the fluid greenish brown. Whenever meconium-stained fluid is present, apply an electronic monitor to assess the FHR continuously. Note the time of rupture because infection increases as the duration of ruptured membranes is prolonged.

Prolapse of the umbilical cord is a possible risk when membranes rupture and the fetus is not engaged, because the amniotic fluid coming through the cervix might wash the umbilical cord out through the cervix. With each contraction the cord would then become trapped between the presenting part and the maternal pelvis. The FHR is auscultated because a drop in the rate might indicate an undetected prolapsed cord. Immediate intervention is necessary to remove pressure on a prolapsed umbilical cord (see Chapter 20). (See Table 18–2 for additional deviations from the normal labor process.)

Transition

During transition the contraction frequency is every 1.5 to 2.0 minutes, duration is 60 to 90 seconds, and intensity is strong. Cervical dilatation increases from 8 to 10 cm, effacement is complete (100%), and there is usually a heavy amount of bloody show. Palpate contractions at least every 15 minutes. Sterile vaginal examinations may be done more frequently because this stage of labor usually is accompanied by rapid change. Take the maternal blood pressure, pulse, and respirations at least every 30 minutes, and auscultate FHR every 15 to 30 minutes.

Comfort measures are important in this phase of labor, but continual assessment is required to intervene appropriately. The woman may rapidly change from wanting a back rub and other hands-on care to wanting to be left completely alone. You and the support person need to follow her cues and change interventions as needed. Because the woman is breathing more rapidly, increase her comfort by offering small spoonfuls of ice chips to moisten her mouth or offer an emollient for her dry lips. Encourage the woman to rest between contractions. If analgesics have been administered, a quiet environment enhances the quality of rest between contractions. Awaken the woman just before a contraction begins so that she can begin patterned breathing.

Some women have difficulty coping during this time and need help with their breathing. Either you or the support person can breathe along with the woman during each contraction to help her maintain her pattern. It is helpful to encourage the woman and to assure her that she is doing a good job. The woman will begin to feel increased rectal pressure as the fetal presenting part moves down the birth canal. To help prevent cervical edema, encourage the woman to refrain from pushing until the cervix is completely dilated.

The end of transition and the beginning of the second stage may be indicated by a change in the woman's voice or the sounds she is making. As the fetus moves down and she feels increased pressure and a bearing-down sensation, her voice tends to deepen. A moan during a contraction takes on a more guttural quality.

Promotion of Comfort in the First Stage

The nurse's first step in planning care is to talk with the woman and her partner or support person to identify their goals. Usually the woman or the couple is concerned with discomfort, so it is helpful to identify factors that may contribute to discomfort. These factors include uncomfortable positions or infrequent position changes, diaphoresis, continual leaking of amniotic fluid, a full bladder, a dry mouth, anxiety, and fear. Nursing interventions can minimize the effects of these factors. These interventions are described later in this section.

There are many types of responses to pain. As the intensity of the contractions increases with the progress of labor, the woman becomes less aware of the environment and may have difficulty hearing and understanding verbal instructions. Some women may become irritable during this time. The pattern of

TABLE 18–2 Deviations from Normal Labor Process Requiring Immediate Intervention

PROBLEM	IMMEDIATE ACTION
Woman admitted with vaginal bleeding or history of painless vaginal bleeding	Do not perform vaginal examination. Assess fetal heart rate (FHR). Evaluate amount of blood loss and initiate a pad count. Evaluate labor pattern. Notify physician/CNM immediately.
Presence of greenish or brownish amniotic fluid	Continuously monitor FHR. Evaluate dilatation of cervix and determine if umbilical cord is prolapsed. Evaluate presentation (vertex or breech). Maintain woman on complete bed rest on left side. Notify physician/CNM immediately.
Absence of FHR and fetal movement	Notify physician/CNM. Provide truthful information and emotional support to laboring couple. Remain with the couple.
Prolapse of umbilical cord	Relieve pressure on cord manually. Continuously monitor FHR; watch for changes in FHR pattern. Notify physician/CNM. Assist woman into knee–chest position or place in Trendelenburg position. Administer oxygen. Prepare for possible cesarean birth.
Woman admitted in advanced labor; birth imminent	Prepare for immediate birth. Obtain critical information: Estimated date of birth (EDB), history of bleeding problems, history of medical or obstetric problems Past and/or present use/abuse of prescription/over-the-counter/illicit drugs Problems with this pregnancy. FHR and maternal vital signs. Whether membranes are ruptured and how long since rupture. Blood type and Rh. Direct another person to contact physician/CNM. Do not leave woman alone. Provide support to couple. Put on gloves.

coping with labor contractions varies from the use of highly structured breathing techniques to turning inward. Low moaning that begins deep in the throat, rocking or swaying, counting, facial grimacing, and using loud vocalizations are all effective means of dealing with the discomfort of labor and birth. Some women feel that making sounds helps them cope and do the work of labor, whereas others make loud sounds only as they lose their perception of control.

The most frequent physiologic manifestations of pain are increased pulse and respiratory rates, dilated pupils, increased blood pressure, and muscle tension. In labor, these reactions are transitory because the pain is intermittent. Increased muscle tension is most significant because it may impede the labor process. Women in labor frequently tighten skeletal muscles voluntarily during a contraction and remain motionless. This method of dealing with the contractions may actually increase her discomfort, but the woman may believe it is the only acceptable way to cope with the pain.

A woman generally wants touching, massage, effleurage, and other forms of physical contact during the first part of labor, but when she moves into the transition phase, she may pull away. Alternatively, the woman may beseech her partner or nurse to hold her hand or rub her back, or may even reach out and grasp the support person. Some women are uncomfortable with being touched at all, regardless of the phase of labor, whereas others do not welcome touch from a nonfamily member. It is important to validate the unique strengths and coping techniques of the individual and to meet each family on its own terms, always keeping in mind that this is *their* experience. Cultural influences can also affect how a woman will react to support and touch in labor. The nurse should take cues from the woman and make adjustments in her care to meet her specific needs.

Clinical Tip

The following nonpharmacologic pain relief techniques can be introduced and facilitated during labor to encourage maternal comfort and facilitate coping: massage, effleurage, hydrotherapy, position changes, hypnosis, aromatherapy, sitting in a rocking chair or glider or on a birthing ball, walking, leaning against the bed or her partner, using a transcutaneous electrical nerve stimulation (TENS) unit, visualization, relaxation techniques, prayer or meditation, and breathing techniques.

Most nurses like to incorporate comfort measures into their nursing care, and they readily respond to the woman's needs. As the nurse and woman or couple work together to increase comfort during contractions, a ritual of supportive measures begins to develop. The nurse watches for cues and nonverbal behaviors and asks for feedback from the woman. As labor progresses, the nurse and couple will use their prior experience and growing rapport to change comfort measures as needed.

A decrease in the intensity of discomfort is one of the goals of nursing support during labor. Nursing measures used to decrease pain include the following:

- Ensuring general comfort
- Providing information to decrease anxiety
- Using specific supportive relaxation techniques
- Encouraging controlled breathing
- Administering pharmacologic agents as ordered by the physician/CNM (see Chapter 19)

Clinical Tip

Acupressure is an ancient Chinese medical treatment that involves using the fingers to press key pressure points on the surface of the skin. This pressure ultimately stimulates the immune system to promote healing by triggering the release of endorphins, reducing stress through muscle relaxation, and promoting circulation. The use of acupressure in labor has been associated with shorter labors and lower subjective and objective pain scores. Women who receive acupressure typically use less pain medication than those who do not receive acupressure (Simpkin & Creehan, 2013).

GENERAL COMFORT

General comfort measures are of great importance during labor. By relieving minor discomforts, the nurse helps the woman optimize her coping abilities to deal with pain.

The woman is encouraged to ambulate as long as there are no contraindications, such as vaginal bleeding or rupture of membranes (ROM) before the fetus is engaged in the pelvis. Ambulation can increase comfort and aid in fetal descent (Figure 18–1).

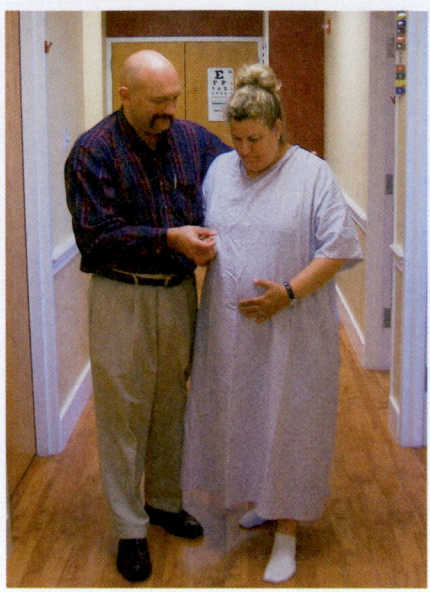

Figure 18–1 Increasing comfort and aiding in fetal descent, this woman and her partner are walking in the hospital during labor.

SOURCE: Michele Davidson.

EVIDENCE-BASED PRACTICE | Movement During Labor

Clinical Question
How does walking, moving around, and changing positions during labor affect the birth process?

The Evidence
Birth in the United States has become a high-technology venture and one of the consequences is limitation on the mother's mobility and positions. Many women remain recumbent after fetal monitoring has been initiated, if an intravenous line is inserted, or, subsequently, after administration of an epidural anesthetic. *The Journal of Perinatal Education* published a review of consensus statements of the American College of Nurse-Midwives, the Midwife Alliance of North America, and the National Association of Certified Professional Midwives regarding maternal position and movement during labor. This type of aggregation of practice guidelines forms the strongest evidence for practice.

The guidelines recommend supportive care practices that use relatively little technology and that support the normal physiologic processes of labor. Women who moved, walked, and changed position during labor reported less pain and more satisfaction with the childbirth process than women who

remained in the recumbent position in bed (Ondeck, 2014). Movement during labor actually resulted in a shorter labor, by more than an hour on average. These women also have fewer interventions during labor. Best practice means supporting the woman's natural physiologic processes without restricting movement through initiation of unnecessary intravenous lines and the use of intermittent versus continuous fetal monitoring for low-risk mothers. Despite these widely replicated findings, more than half of all laboring women remain in bed or in a recumbent position.

Best Practice
Supportive practices during labor include minimizing the use of technology so that mothers can move around, walk, and change position during labor. These women will have shorter, less painful labor and will be more satisfied with the process.

Clinical Reasoning
How can the nurse help implement this important change in practice when current practices are ingrained? What is appropriate childbirth education to empower parents to choose a low-technology option?

Even if the woman prefers not to walk around, upright positions such as sitting in a rocker or leaning against a wall or bed can enhance comfort. A woman can also utilize a birthing ball for comfort during labor. If she stays in bed, the nurse can encourage the woman to assume positions that she finds comfortable (Figure 18–2).

A side-lying position is generally the most advantageous for the laboring woman, although frequent position changes seem to achieve more efficient contractions. In one facility where evidence-based practice was embraced, changes were implemented to benefit the care of laboring women. Care should be taken to support all body parts, with the joints kept slightly flexed. For instance, when the woman is in a side-lying position, pillows may be placed against her chest and under the uppermost arm. The nurse should place a pillow or folded bath towel between her knees to support the uppermost leg and relieve tension or muscle strain. Placing a pillow at the woman's midback and placing one to support the uterus also help provide support.

If the woman is more comfortable on her back, the head of the bed should be elevated to relieve the pressure of the uterus on the vena cava. Pillows may be placed under each arm and under the knees to provide support. Because a pregnant woman is at increased risk for thrombophlebitis, excessive pressure behind the knee and calf should be avoided. The nurse needs to assess pressure points frequently. Frequent changes of position contribute to comfort and relaxation.

The lithotomic position was once the position of choice but has recently been associated with adverse outcomes compared to other positions. One study compared lithotomy and squatting positions and found a higher incidence of extensions of episiotomy, third- and fourth-degree laceration, forceps assisted birth, persistent occiput posterior position, retained placenta, and postpartum hemorrhage in the women who maintained a lithotomy position (Zaibunnisa, Firdos, Bilqees, et al., 2015).

Women may find it comfortable to utilize water or water therapy as a means to increase their comfort level.

Some facilities offer whirlpool tubs while others may have bathtubs or showers that can be utilized during labor. The woman needs to be monitored per protocol during water therapy. Some facilities have handheld Doppler devices that can be submerged in water while others may offer the option of continuous monitoring during water therapy. The nurse should provide supervision while the woman is entering and exiting the tub and check on her frequently when water therapy is in use.

Wearing socks or slippers may alleviate cold feet and adjusting the room's thermostat can offset excessive warmth. Attention to such details allows the woman to focus on the more important issues of giving birth. The woman may be offered a warmed or cooled facial cloth, which is placed on her forehead or across or behind her neck. Providing a toothbrush and toothpaste for oral care can also increase comfort.

Diaphoresis and the constant leaking of amniotic fluid can dampen the woman's gown and bed linen. Offering fresh, smooth, dry bed linen promotes comfort. To avoid having to change the bottom sheet following rupture of the membranes, the nurse may replace absorbent underpads at frequent intervals (following standard precautions). The perineal area should be kept as clean and dry as possible to promote comfort and to prevent infection. A full bladder adds to discomfort during a contraction and may prolong labor by interfering with the descent of the fetus. The bladder should be kept as empty as possible. Even if the woman is voiding, urine may be retained because of the pressure of the fetal presenting part. The nurse can detect a full bladder by palpating directly over the symphysis pubis. Some of the regional procedures for analgesia and anesthesia during labor contribute to the inability to void, and catheterization may be necessary. The woman should be encouraged to empty her bladder every 1 to 2 hours.

Family members also need to be encouraged to maintain their own comfort. Because their attention is directed toward the laboring woman, they may forget their own needs.

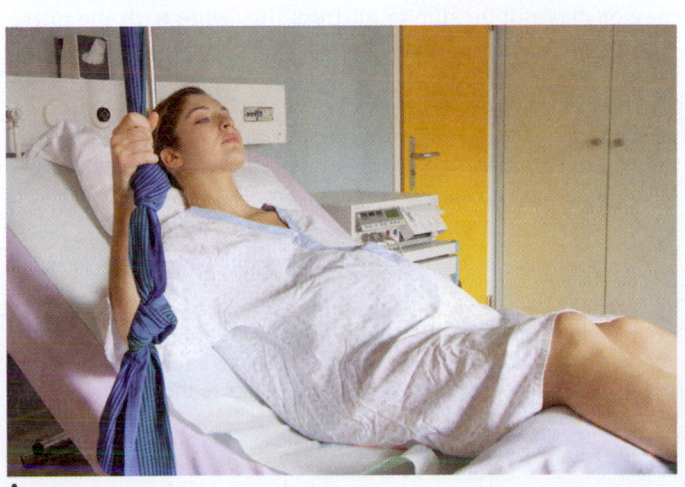
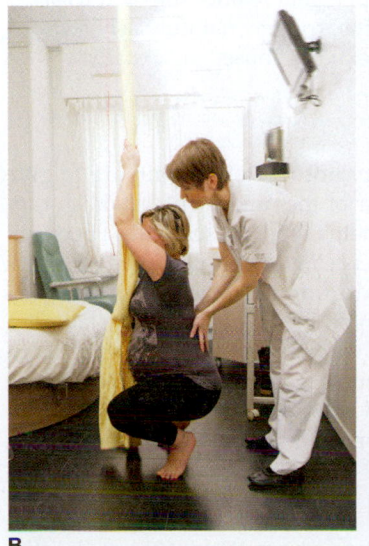
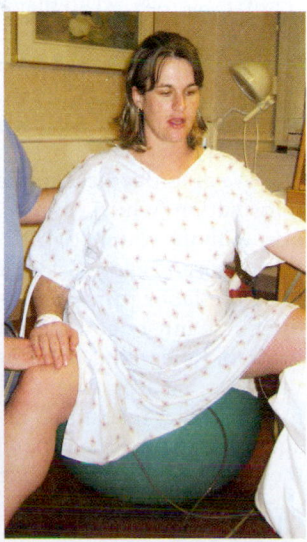

A   B   C

Figure 18–2 The laboring woman is encouraged to choose a position of comfort. A, B. The nurse modifies assessments and interventions as necessary. C. While often promoting maternal comfort during labor, the birthing ball also facilitates fetal descent and rotation and helps increase the diameter of the pelvis.

SOURCE: A: © olly/Fotolia; B: © BSIP SA / Alamy.

The nurse may have to encourage them to take breaks, to maintain food and fluid intake, and to rest.

Clinical Tip

Clinical Tip

Many support persons and family members are reluctant to leave the woman unattended while they meet their own personal needs. Offer to stay with the woman during their absence. This provides reassurance to the support person or family member that the woman will be well cared for in his or her absence.

HANDLING ANXIETY

The anxiety experienced by women beginning labor is related to a combination of factors inherent to the process. A moderate amount of anxiety about pain enhances the woman's ability to deal with it. In contrast, an excessive degree of anxiety decreases her ability to cope with the pain. Women in the latent phase of labor who are experiencing increased levels of anxiety about their ability to cope and their own personal safety are much more likely to describe their pain as unbearable. Women at risk for greater anxiety during labor include women who are young, poor, minority, and unmarried. Women with preexisting mental illness, such as depression and anxiety, are at a greater risk for developing posttraumatic stress disorder (PTSD) related to their labor and birth experience. Women who have unplanned cesarean births, have limited coping skills, and perceive the pain as intense also are at greater risk of PTSD (Davidson, 2012). Women with mental illness issues may need additional support to assist them with identifying effective coping mechanisms during the labor and birth.

Women With Special Needs Mental Health Disabilities

Women with mental health disabilities, such as posttraumatic stress disorder (PTSD), may experience flashbacks and excessive fear during labor. Supportive care with one nurse is preferred so that a personal relationship and trust can be established. Labor often triggers painful flashbacks in women who have been sexually abused or sexually assaulted.

Ways to decrease anxiety not related to pain are to give information (which eases fear of the unknown), establish rapport with the couple (which helps them preserve their personal integrity), and express confidence in the couple's ability to work with the labor process. In addition to being a good listener, the nurse must demonstrate genuine concern for the laboring woman. Remaining with the woman as much as possible conveys a caring attitude and dispels fears of abandonment. Praise for breathing, relaxation, and pushing efforts not only encourages repetition of the behavior but also decreases anxiety about the ability to cope with labor.

CLIENT TEACHING

Providing truthful information about the nature of the discomfort that will occur during labor is important. Stressing the intermittent nature and maximum duration of the contractions can be helpful. The woman can cope with pain better when she knows that a period of relief will follow. Describing the type of discomfort and specific sensations that will occur as labor progresses helps the woman recognize these sensations as normal and expected when she does experience them.

Clinical Tip

Advise women that the strength and intensity of contractions are different for each person, but they may feel like a tightening sensation or a menstrual cramp initially. Over time as the labor progresses, the contractions become more intense and more uncomfortable with the uterus tightening and becoming very hard, with the pain radiating from the back around to the front. For some women, the pain takes their breath away or they may feel anxiety and fear. As the contractions become more painful, they also occur closer together. The sensation of having to push occurs as the head progresses into the pelvis and feels like the woman has to have a bowel movement. Once the contraction goes away, this intense feeling of having to have a bowel movement usually lets up to some degree.

Descriptions of sensations are best accompanied by information on specific comfort measures. As previously noted, some women experience the urge to push during transition, when the cervix is not fully dilated and effaced. This sensation can be controlled by pant-blow breathing (it is difficult to pant or blow and bear down at the same time); the nurse should provide instructions about this technique before it is required (see next sections).

Labor and childbirth may be a critical time for the woman with a history of childhood sexual abuse or rape. It is estimated that of the approximately 899,000 children abused in some way annually, 9.3% have experienced sexual abuse (American Humane Association, 2015). Each year, there are approximately 270,000 victims of sexual assault (Bureau of Justice Statistics, 2013). Women with a history of sexual abuse experiencing current life stressors, such as pregnancy, are more apt to have medical complications than those with no history of abuse.

To develop a competent plan of care, all women entering the healthcare arena should be evaluated for a history of sexual abuse, rape, or intimate partner violence. Culturally diverse women may need specific examples of abuse to determine if they have had these types of experiences because some behaviors that are considered abusive in our society may be considered normal patterns of behavior in other cultures. Women may or may not be able to address this issue with the nurse, because sharing such personal information is difficult and may stir up painful memories. It is therefore especially important for the nurse to be alert for nonverbal cues, such as excessive unexplained anxiety, unrelenting pain, and/or intense fear during vaginal examinations, and to be prepared to offer additional teaching to help offset the woman's anxiety.

Clinical Tip

If a woman is experiencing severe fear or anxiety about a vaginal examination, advise her to slowly count to 10 during the examination while continually wiggling her toes. This source of distraction may lessen her fear and anxiety. It also enables the woman to have a sense of control.

SUPPORTIVE RELAXATION TECHNIQUES

Tense muscles increase resistance to the descent of the fetus and contribute to maternal fatigue. This fatigue increases pain perception and decreases the woman's ability to cope with the pain. Comfort measures, massage, techniques for decreasing anxiety, and client teaching can contribute to relaxation. Adequate sleep and rest are also important. The laboring woman needs to be encouraged to use the period between contractions for rest and relaxation. A prolonged prodromal phase of labor may interfere with sleep. An aura of excitement naturally accompanies the onset of labor, making it difficult for the woman to sleep even though the contractions are mild and infrequent. The nurse may have to act as an advocate for the woman to limit the number of her visitors, interruptions, and phone calls.

Distraction is another method of increasing relaxation and coping with discomfort. During early labor, conversation or activities such as watching television, light reading, or playing cards or other games can serve as distractions. One technique that is effective for relieving moderate pain is to have the woman concentrate on a pleasant experience she has had in the past. Other techniques include the use of a specific visual or mental focal point (such as a picture of a loved one), breathing techniques, counting or humming, or visualization.

Touch is another type of distraction (Figure 18–3). Although some women regard touching as an invasion of privacy or threat to their independence, many want to touch and be touched during a painful experience. To determine whether the woman desires touch, the nurse can place a hand on the side of the bed within the woman's reach. The woman who needs touch will reach out for contact, and the nurse can follow through with this behavioral cue.

Some nurses utilize *intuitive touch*, the use of physical contact with the laboring woman with the intent of helping her to slow down and regulate her breathing pattern and encouraging a reduction of anxiety and decrease of stress levels. Evidence suggests that touch induces the relaxation response, which is mediated through the neuroendocrine and sympathetic nervous systems (Konda, Vikas, Yarlagadda, 2014).

A variety of techniques can be used. These include hand holding; stroking or patting of a woman's arm, face, or legs; placing one hand on her shoulder; putting an arm around her shoulders; and hugging. To implement intuitive touch, the nurse uses long, slow, up-and-down strokes on the woman's limbs. Special training is not needed to use this intervention; all that is needed is the intention to help regulate the breathing pattern and the willingness to use a little time to achieve this goal (Konda et al., 2014).

Mild to moderate abdominal discomfort during contractions may be relieved or lessened by effleurage. Firm pressure on the lower back or sacral area may relieve back pain associated with labor. To apply firm pressure, the nurse can place a hand or a rolled, warmed towel or blanket in the small of the woman's back. In addition to the measures just described, the woman's relaxation can be enhanced by providing encouragement and support for her controlled breathing techniques.

In some instances, analgesics or regional anesthetic blocks may be used to enhance comfort and relaxation during labor. (See Chapter 19 for in-depth information.)

BREATHING TECHNIQUES

Breathing techniques may help the laboring woman. Used correctly, they increase the woman's pain threshold, permit relaxation, enhance the woman's ability to cope with contractions, provide a sense of control, and allow the uterus to function more efficiently. Many women learn patterned-paced breathing during prenatal education classes (Table 18–3).

Hyperventilation is the result of an imbalance of oxygen and carbon dioxide (i.e., too much carbon dioxide is exhaled, and too much oxygen remains in the body). Hyperventilation may occur when a woman breathes very rapidly over a prolonged period. The signs and symptoms of hyperventilation are tingling or numbness in the tip of the nose, lips, fingers, or toes; dizziness; spots before the eyes; or spasms of the hands or feet (carpal–pedal spasms). If hyperventilation occurs, the woman should be encouraged to slow her breathing rate and take shallow breaths. With instruction and encouragement, many women are able to change their breathing to correct the problem. Encouraging the woman to relax and counting out loud for her so she can pace her breathing during contractions are also helpful actions. If the signs and symptoms continue or become more severe (they progress from numbness to spasms), the woman can breathe into a paper surgical mask or a paper bag (causes rebreathing of carbon dioxide) until symptoms abate. The nurse should remain with the woman to reassure her because a great deal of anxiety often occurs.

ROLE OF THE DOULA

Throughout the first stage of labor, the nurse assesses and supports the interaction between the woman and her partner. In the absence of a partner, or when the partner desires a less active role, it is becoming more common for women to employ a paid caregiver who has experience in caring for laboring women. The caregiver, often called a **doula**, has typically received special training and may even be certified. The doula's role is to enhance the laboring woman's comfort and decrease her anxiety. A doula can be a valuable advocate for the laboring woman and her family, as well as an asset to the labor nurse. For example, the doula might support the woman by helping to identify the beginning of each contraction and encouraging her as she breathes through it. A constant presence offering continued encouragement and support with each contraction throughout labor has immeasurable benefits.

Table 18–4 summarizes labor progress, possible responses of the laboring woman, and support measures.

Nursing Care During the Second Stage of Labor

The second stage is reached when the cervix is completely dilated (10 cm [3.9 in.]). The uterine contractions continue as in the transition phase. Maternal pulse is assessed at the onset of the second stage. The blood pressure is assessed every 5 to 15 minutes, but may be done more frequently if fetal decelerations or bradycardia occur. The fetal heart rate (FHR) is assessed every 15 minutes in low-risk women and every 5 minutes in women with high-risk complications (ACOG, 2015). Once the second stage has been reached, the nurse remains with the woman continually and does not generally leave the room.

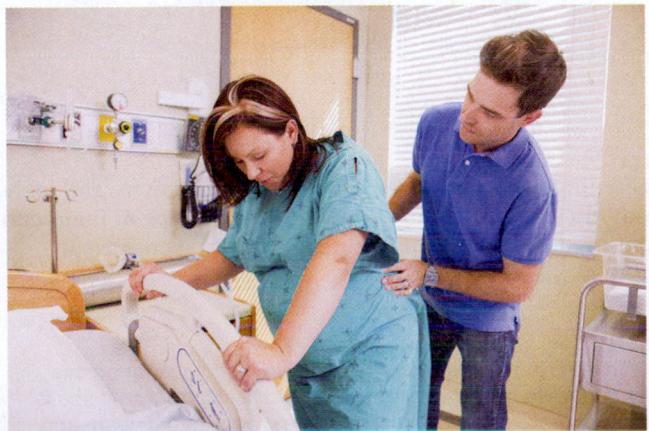

Figure 18–3 The woman's partner provides support and encouragement during labor.

SOURCE: Tyler Olson/Shutterstock.

TABLE 18–3 Nursing Support of Patterned-Paced Breathing

Determine which breathing method the woman has learned. Provide encouragement as needed in maintaining breathing pattern. Provide support to the labor coach and assist as needed.

LAMAZE BREATHING PATTERN

First Level (Slow Paced)

Pattern begins and ends with a cleansing breath (in through the nose and out through pursed lips as if cooling a spoonful of hot food). While inhaling through the nose and exhaling through pursed lips, slow breaths are taken, moving only the chest. The rate should be approximately 6–9/minute or 2 breaths/15 seconds. The coach or nurse may assist by reminding the woman to take a cleansing breath, and then the breaths could be counted out if needed to maintain pacing. The woman inhales as someone counts "one one thousand, two one thousand, three one thousand, four one thousand." Exhalation begins and continues through the same count.

First level for use during uterine contractions (the level begins and ends with a cleansing breath [CB]).

First Level (Slow Paced)

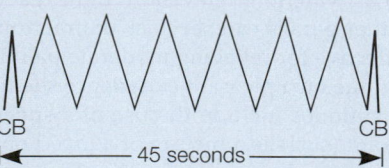

Second Level (Modified Paced)

Pattern begins and ends with a cleansing breath. Breaths are then taken in and out silently through the mouth at approximately 4 breaths/5 seconds. The jaw and entire body need to be relaxed. The rate can be accelerated to 2 to 2½ breaths/second. The rhythm for the breaths can be counted out as "one and two and one and two and . . ." with the woman exhaling on the numbers and inhaling on "and."

Second level

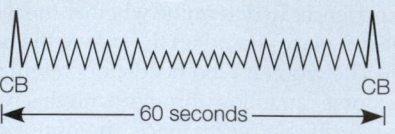

Third Level (Pattern Paced)

Pattern begins and ends with a cleansing breath. All breaths are rhythmical, in and out through the mouth. Exhalations are accompanied by a "hee" or "hoo" sound in a varying pattern, 2:1, which begins as 3:1 (hee hee hee hoo) and can change to 2:1 (hee hee hoo) or 1:1 (hee hoo) as the intensity of the contraction changes. The rate should not be more rapid than 2 to 2½ breaths/second. The rhythm of the breaths would match a "one and two and" count.

Third level (Darkened spike represents "hoo.")

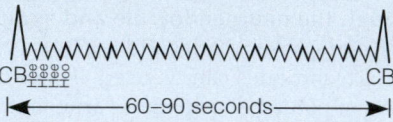

ABDOMINAL BREATHING PATTERN CUES

The abdomen moves outward during inhalation and inward during exhalation. The rate remains slow with approximately 6 to 9 breaths/minute.

Breathing sequence for abdominal breathing

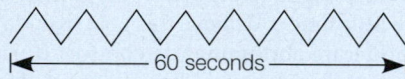

QUICK METHOD

When the woman has not learned a particular method and is in the active phase of labor, the nurse may teach her a combination of two patterns. Abdominal breathing may be used until labor is more advanced. Then a more rapid pattern consisting of two short blows from the mouth followed by a longer blow can be used. (This pattern is called "pant-pant-blow" even though all exhalations are a blowing motion.)

Pant-pant-blow breathing pattern

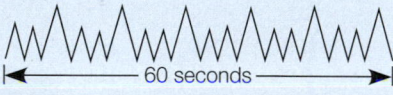

As the woman pushes during the second stage, she may make a variety of sounds. A low-pitched, grunting sound ("uhhh") usually indicates that the woman is working with the pushing. The nurse who feels comfortable with maternal sounds and stays sensitive to changes in the sounds may be able to detect if the woman is losing her ability to cope. For instance, if the woman feels afraid of the sensations produced by her pushing effort, her sound may change to a high-pitched cry or whimper.

It is not uncommon for the woman to be afraid to push. In these situations, the woman may talk or cry out during the contraction instead of actively pushing. During this time, the nurse should provide support, reassurance, and clear directions for the woman to follow. Often it is helpful to direct the woman to

concentrate on a single voice, listen for suggestions, and let her body do the work. Many women find this type of interaction comforting because it allows them to focus on one person.

Clinical Tip

When teaching the woman the effective technique for pushing, instruct her to bear down and push into her bottom as if she is having a bowel movement. Watch the woman's perineum and rectum while she is pushing and give verbal praise and encouragement when change in the perineum or rectum is seen, indicating she is successfully pushing.

TABLE 18–4 Normal Progress, Psychologic Characteristics, and Nursing Support During the First and Second Stages of Labor

PHASE	CERVICAL DILATATION	UTERINE CONTRACTIONS	WOMAN'S RESPONSE	SUPPORT MEASURES
Stage 1 *Latent phase*	1–3 cm	Every 10–20 min, 15–20 sec duration Mild intensity progressing to every 5–7 min, 30–40 sec duration Moderate intensity	Usually happy, talkative, and eager to be in labor. Exhibits need for independence by taking care of own bodily needs and seeking information.	Establish rapport on admission and continue to build during care. Assess information base and learning needs. Be available to consult regarding breathing technique if needed; teach breathing technique if needed and in early labor. Orient family to room, equipment, monitors, and procedures. Encourage woman and partner to participate in care as desired. Provide needed information. Assist woman into position of comfort; encourage frequent change of position; encourage ambulation during early labor. Offer fluids or ice chips. Keep couple informed of progress. Encourage woman to void every 1–2 hr. Assess need for an interest in using visualization to enhance relaxation, and teach if appropriate.
Active phase	4–7 cm	Every 2–3 min, 50–60 sec duration Moderate to strong intensity	May experience feelings of helplessness. Exhibits increased fatigue and may begin to feel restless and anxious as contractions become stronger. Expresses fear of abandonment. Becomes more dependent because she is less able to meet her needs.	Encourage woman to maintain breathing patterns. Provide quiet environment to reduce external stimuli. Provide reassurance, encouragement, support; keep couple informed of progress. Promote comfort by giving back rubs, sacral pressure, cool cloth on forehead, assistance with position changes, support with pillows, effleurage. Provide ice chips, ointment for dry mouth and lips. Encourage to void every 1–2 hr. Offer shower, whirlpool, or warm bath if available.
Transition phase	8–10 cm	Every 1.5–2.0 min, 60–90 sec duration Strong intensity	Tires and may exhibit increased restlessness and irritability. May feel she cannot keep up with labor process and is out of control. Exhibits physical discomforts. Fears being left alone. May fear tearing open or splitting apart with contractions.	Encourage woman to rest between contractions. If she sleeps between contractions, wake her at beginning of contraction so she can begin breathing pattern (increases feeling of control). Provide support, encouragement, and praise for efforts. Keep couple informed of progress; encourage continued participation of support persons. Promote comfort as listed earlier but recognize that many women do not want to be touched when in transition. Provide privacy. Provide ice chips, ointment for lips. Encourage to void every 1–2 hr.
Stage 2	Complete	Every 1.5–2.0 min	May feel out of control, helpless, panicky	Assist woman in pushing efforts. Encourage woman to assume position of comfort. Provide encouragement and praise her efforts. Keep couple informed of progress. Provide ice chips. Maintain privacy as woman desires.

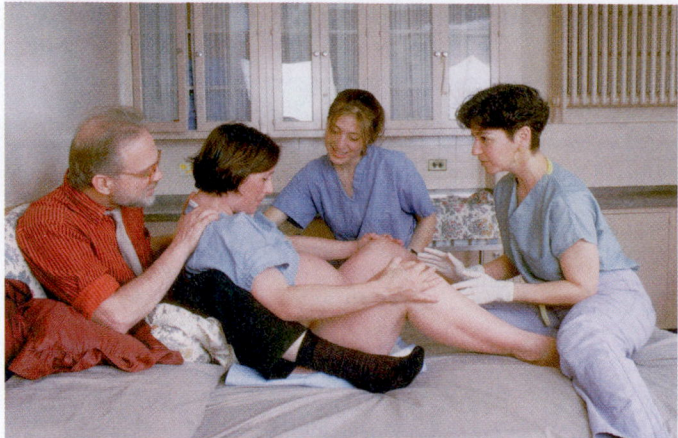

Figure 18–4 The nurse provides encouragement and support during pushing efforts.

SOURCE: Margaret Miller/Science Source.

During the second stage, the woman may feel intense rectal pressure. The instinctive response is to resist and to tighten muscles rather than bear down (push). A sensation of splitting apart or burning also occurs in the latter part of the second stage when the woman is pushing. The woman who expects these sensations and understands that bearing down contributes to progress at this stage is more likely to do so. When the urge to bear down becomes uncontrollable and pushing begins, the nurse can help by encouraging her and by supporting her efforts (Figure 18–4).

Most women push spontaneously and effectively in response to messages from their body. While the more natural approach, which lets the mother wait to bear down until she feels an urge to push, may not shorten the pushing phase, it does reduce the incidence of physiologic stress in the mother and acidosis in the newborn (King et al., 2015). In some settings, however, sustained, forceful pushing is still advocated. In that case, when the contraction begins, the nurse tells the woman to take a cleansing breath or two, then to take a third large breath and hold it while pushing down with her abdominal muscles (called the *Valsalva maneuver*).

A nullipara is usually prepared for birth when perineal bulging is noted. A multipara usually progresses much more quickly, so she may be prepared for birth when the cervix is dilated 7 to 8 cm. As the birth approaches, the woman's partner or support person also prepares for the birth.

KEY FACTS TO REMEMBER
Indications of Imminent Birth

Birth is imminent if the woman shows the following changes:

- Bulging of the perineum
- Uncontrollable urge to bear down
- Increased bloody show

The woman's blood pressure and the FHR are monitored between contractions, and the contractions are palpated at least every 5 minutes until the birth. The nurse continually assesses the woman's level of pain or her ability to cope with the discomfort of labor. The nurse continues to assist the woman in her pushing efforts, to keep both the woman and the coach informed of procedures and progress, and to support them both throughout the birth.

Promotion of Comfort in the Second Stage

Most of the comfort measures that have been used during the first stage remain appropriate at this time. Applying cool cloths to the face and forehead may help cool the woman involved in the intense physical exertion of pushing. The woman may feel hot and want to remove some of her clothing or bed linens. Care still needs to be taken to provide privacy even though covers are removed. The woman can be encouraged to rest and relax all muscles during the periods between contractions. The nurse and support person(s) can assist the woman into a pushing position with each contraction to further conserve energy. Between contractions, the woman should be assisted into a comfortable position. Sips of fluids or ice chips may be used to provide moisture and relieve dryness of the mouth. Positive reinforcement and encouragement should be continually provided.

Assisting During Birth

In addition to assisting the woman and her partner, the nurse also assists the physician/CNM in preparing for the birth. The physician/CNM dons a sterile gown and gloves and may place sterile drapes over the woman's abdomen and legs. An episiotomy may be performed just before the actual birth. (See the discussion of episiotomy in Chapter 22.)

Shortly before the birth, the birthing room or delivery room is prepared with the equipment and materials that may be needed. These materials typically come in a prepackaged kit and contain the instruments and disposable drapes, gowns, and containers that will be used during the birth. The nurse ensures that all supplies and a pair of sterile gloves are placed on the instrument table. This table can be prepared before the birth and covered with a sterile drape. Family members do not need to change into other clothing if the birth occurs in a birthing room; they don a disposable scrub suit or scrubs provided by the facility if the birth is to occur in a delivery room or surgery suite. Thorough hand washing is required of the nurses and physician/CNM. Nurses who will be in direct contact with the mother at the time of birth need to wear protective clothing such as an apron or gown with a splash apron, disposable gloves, and eye covering. The physician/CNM also needs to wear a plastic apron or a gown with a splash apron, eye covering, and sterile gloves.

Clinical Tip

Some physicians/CNMs may routinely use other equipment or supplies during the birth. Examples of equipment include mineral oil, warm water, and clean washcloths for perineal massage. Gathering these supplies early can save time and enable you to stay with the woman during pushing.

If the laboring woman is to give birth in a location other than the birthing room (such as in the case of a cesarean birth), she is moved on her bed or a cart shortly before birth. It is important for the woman to move from one bed to another *between contractions*. During the contraction, the woman feels increased discomfort and may be involved in pushing efforts. Perineal bulging may be occurring, which adds to the discomfort and difficulty in moving. Care should be taken to preserve her privacy during the transfer, and safety must be provided by raising the side rails. The bed itself should be placed in a locked position. The labor bed or transfer cart must be carefully braced against the delivery table to ensure the woman's safety during the transfer.

Even in the delivery room setting, the family can still be together during the birth. It is important to provide encouragement for family members to participate, because the delivery room environment may be unfamiliar and seem intimidating. The family member may hesitate to continue providing support because of fear of interfering or being in the way. The nurse provides clear, simple directions that help the support person participate throughout the birth process. The nurse can ensure the support person is sitting as close as possible to the woman. The nurse can also encourage hand holding and touching or stroking of the woman's face.

MATERNAL BIRTHING POSITIONS

The upright posture for birth was considered normal in most societies until modern times. Women variously selected squatting, kneeling, standing, and sitting positions for birth. During the mid-20th century, the recumbent position (lithotomy) became common in North American hospitals because of the convenience it offered in applying new technology. In recent years, however, consumers and healthcare professionals have begun searching for alternative positions, refocusing on the comfort of the laboring woman rather than on the convenience of the physician/CNM (Figure 18–5). Evidence-based practice research has shown that the squatting position results in fewer instrumental deliveries, fewer episiotomy extensions, fewer perineal tears, and a reduction in persistent occiput-posterior fetal position than are associated with lithotomic positions (Ara, Ara, Kaker, et al., 2015). An upright position, which has been found to be the most effective birthing position, is possible even for women who have epidural anesthesia (Ara et al., 2015). See Table 18–5 for a comparison of birthing positions.

The woman may be positioned for birth on a bed with use of leg supports, in a squatting position, or perhaps on her hands and knees. If a birthing bed is used, the back is elevated 30 to 60 degrees to help the woman bear down. Stirrups, if needed and used, are padded to alleviate pressure. If assisting the woman to place her legs in the stirrups, both legs should be lifted simultaneously to avoid strain on abdominal, back, and perineal muscles. Stirrups are sometimes needed if the woman is unable to control her legs following epidural anesthesia, if forceps or a

vacuum extractor is being used, or if a difficult birth is anticipated. The stirrups should be adjusted to fit the woman's legs. The feet are supported in the stirrup holders. The height and angle of the stirrups are adjusted so there is no pressure on the back of the knees or the calves, which might cause discomfort and postpartum vascular problems. Some practitioners may opt to leave the bed assembled and instead lower the foot of the bed into a lower position. Many times, women are more comfortable with this position. When stirrups are not used for the birth, the woman's legs may be placed in stirrups after the birth if a repair of the perineum is needed.

CLEANSING THE PERINEUM

After the woman has been positioned for the birth, her vulvar and perineal area are cleansed to increase her comfort, to remove the bloody discharge that is present before the actual birth, and to prevent infection. Perineal cleansing methods range from use of warm soapy water to aseptic technique depending on the agency protocol or on physician/CNM orders. Once the cleansing has been completed, the woman returns to the desired birthing position.

CONTINUED LABOR SUPPORT

Both the woman's partner and the nurse who has been with the woman during the labor continue to provide support during contractions. The woman is encouraged to push with each contraction and, as the fetal head emerges, is asked to take shallow breaths or to pant to prevent pushing. The physician/CNM may instruct her to "push and breathe, push and breathe" in an effort to ease the fetal head out to prevent perineal trauma and tearing. While supporting the head, the physician/CNM assesses whether the umbilical cord is around the fetal neck and removes it if it is, then suctions the mouth and nose with a bulb syringe. The mouth is suctioned first to prevent reflex inhalation of mucus when the sensitive nares are touched with the bulb syringe tip. The woman is encouraged to push again as the rest of the newborn's body is born. Figure 16–12 depicts an entire birthing experience.

Nursing Care During the Third and Fourth Stages of Labor

Nursing care during the third and fourth stages focuses on initial care of the newborn, assisting with placenta delivery, enhancing attachment, and providing care for the mother.

Initial Care of the Newborn

The physician/CNM places the newborn on the mother's abdomen or under the radiant-heated unit. Placing the newborn on the maternal abdomen promotes attachment and bonding and gives the mother the opportunity to immediately interact with her baby. Placing the baby on the mother's chest also promotes early breastfeeding opportunities. Even though the baby may not breastfeed immediately, placement on the mother's chest enables the baby to smell, touch, and lick the mother's nipples. The newborn is maintained in a modified Trendelenburg position, which aids drainage of mucus from the nasopharynx and trachea by gravity. Newborns should be dried immediately and kept warm by covering them with warmed blankets or by placing them in skin-to-skin contact with their mothers. If newborns are in a radiant-heated unit, they should be dried, placed on a dry blanket, and left uncovered. Because radiant heat warms the outer surface of objects, newborns wrapped in blankets will receive no benefit from the unit.

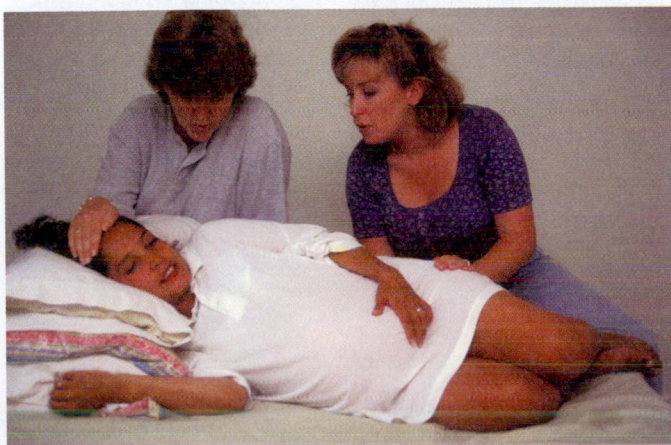

Figure18–5 Side-lying laboring or birthing position.

SOURCE: © Angela Hampton Picture Library/Alamy.

TABLE 18–5 Comparison of Birthing Positions

POSITION	ADVANTAGES	DISADVANTAGES	NURSING ACTIONS
Recumbent	Enhances ability to maintain sterile field. May be easier to monitor FHR. Easier to perform episiotomy or laceration repair.	May decrease blood pressure. It is difficult for the woman to breathe because of pressure on the diaphragm. There is an increased risk of aspiration. May increase perineal pressure, making laceration more likely. May interfere with uterine contractions. May increase lacerations, episiotomies, instrument-assisted births, and unfavorable fetal positions.	Ensure that stirrups do not cause excess pressure on the legs. Assess legs for adequate circulation and support.
Left lateral Sims or side-lying	Does not compromise venous return from lower extremities. Increases perineal relaxation and decreases need for episiotomy; assists in preserving perineal integrity. Appears to prevent rapid descent.	It is difficult for the woman to see the birth.	Adjust position so that the upper leg lies on the bed (scissor fashion) or is supported by the partner or on pillows.
Squatting	Size of pelvic outlet is increased. Gravity aids descent and expulsion of newborn. Second stage may be shortened. Decreases lacerations, episiotomy performance, instrument-assisted birth.	It may be difficult to maintain balance while squatting. Can result in perineal edema. Can cause maternal fatigue.	Help woman maintain balance. Use a birthing bar if available. Help woman sit back and rest between contractions.
Semi-Fowler	Does not compromise venous return from lower extremities. Woman can view birth process.	If legs are positioned wide apart, relaxation of perineal tissues is decreased.	Assess that upper torso is evenly supported. Increase support of body by changing position of bed or using pillows as props.
Sitting in birthing bed	Gravity aids descent and expulsion of the fetus. Does not compromise venous return from lower extremities. Woman can view the birth process. Leg position may be changed at will.		Ensure that legs and feet have adequate support.
Sitting on birthing stool	Gravity aids descent and expulsion of neonate. Does not compromise venous return from lower extremities. Woman can view birth process.	It is difficult to provide support for the woman's back.	Encourage woman to sit in a position that increases her comfort.
Hands and knees	Increases perineal relaxation and decreases need for episiotomy. Increases placental and umbilical blood flow and decreases fetal distress. Improves fetal rotation. Better able to assess perineum. Better access to fetal nose and mouth for suctioning at birth. Facilitates birth of neonate with shoulder dystocia.	Woman cannot view birth. There is decreased contact with birth attendant. Healthcare givers cannot use instruments. There may be increased maternal fatigue. Some women may feel uncomfortable delivering in nontraditional position.	Adjust birthing bed by dropping the foot down. Supply extra pillows for increased support. Provide verbal updates on how pushing is progressing. Offer woman mirror if she desires to see perineum and pushing efforts.

The newborn's nose and mouth are suctioned with a bulb syringe as needed. Most immediate care of the newborn can be accomplished while the newborn is in the parent's arms or under the radiant-heated unit. Many women request that their newborns be left on their abdomen or chest while initial care is given. Unless a medical complication exists, the nurse should complete assessments in this position because it promotes maternal attachment. See Figure 16–12H–N.

APGAR SCORING SYSTEM

The Apgar scoring system (Table 18–6) is used to evaluate the physical condition of the newborn at birth. The newborn is rated 1 minute after birth and again at 5 minutes and receives a total score (**Apgar score**) ranging from 0 to 10 based on the following assessments. If the Apgar score is less than 7 at 5 minutes, the scoring should be repeated every 5 minutes up to 20 minutes (Lanting & van Woewe, 2015).

1. Heart rate is auscultated or palpated at the junction of the umbilical cord and skin. This is the most important assessment. A newborn heart rate of less than 100 beats per minute indicates the need for immediate resuscitation.

2. Respiratory effort is the second most important Apgar assessment. Complete absence of respirations is termed apnea. A vigorous cry indicates adequate respirations.

3. Muscle tone is determined by evaluating the degree of flexion and resistance to straightening of the extremities. A normal newborn's elbows and hips are flexed, with the knees positioned up toward the abdomen.

4. Reflex irritability is evaluated by stroking the baby's back along the spine or by flicking the soles of the feet. A cry merits a full score of 2. A grimace is 1 point, and no response is 0.

5. Skin color is inspected for cyanosis and pallor. Generally, newborns have blue extremities, with a pink body, which merits a score of 1. This condition is termed *acrocyanosis* and is present in 85% of normal newborns at 1 minute after birth. A completely pink newborn scores a 2, and a totally cyanotic, pale newborn scores 0. Newborns with darker skin pigmentation will not be pink in color. Their skin color is assessed for pallor and acrocyanosis, and a score is selected based on the assessment.

A score of 7 to 10 indicates a newborn in good condition who requires only nasopharyngeal suctioning and perhaps some oxygen near the face (called "blow-by" oxygen). An Apgar score between 4 and 7 indicates the need for stimulation; resuscitative measures may need to be instituted if the score is less than 4. Apgar scores of less than 3 at 5 minutes postbirth may correlate with neonatal mortality (Lanting & van Wouwe, 2015).

ASSISTING WITH CLAMPING THE CORD

If the physician/CNM has not placed some type of cord clamp on the newborn's umbilical cord, the nurse must do so. Before applying the cord clamp, the nurse examines the cut end of the cord for the presence of two arteries and one vein. The umbilical vein is the largest vessel, and the arteries are seen as smaller vessels. The number of vessels is recorded on the birth and newborn records. The cord is clamped approximately 0.5 to 1.0 in. from the abdomen to allow room between the abdomen and the clamp as the cord dries. Abdominal skin must not be clamped because this will cause necrosis of the tissue. The cord clamp is removed in the newborn nursery approximately 24 hours after the cord has dried. The most common type of cord clamp is the plastic Hollister cord clamp (Figure 18–6).

In recent years, the timing of umbilical cord clamping has been the focus of discussion and research. In one study of preterm newborns (less than 37 gestational weeks), babies in the group with delayed cord clamping had fewer intraventricular hemorrhages and less late-onset sepsis. Newborns that are preterm and term benefit from an increase in red blood cells which can reduce anemia in the first 12 months of life and reduce the need for blood transfusions in the early neonatal period. Evidence-based practice therefore suggests that delayed clamping in premature neonates may yield more benefits than immediate cord clamping because the increased blood volume can potentially supply immunoglobulins and stem cells, which provide the potential for improved organ repair and rebuilding after injury from disorders caused by preterm birth although immunologic status remains unchanged (ACOG, 2012a). In full-term newborns, delayed cord clamping can result in polycythemia; however, this appears to be benign. Newborns with polycythemia may have to undergo phototherapy for jaundice. These babies were more likely to have improved hematocrit, ferritin, and iron levels resulting in a reduction in anemia (ACOG, 2012a). Based on these findings, delayed cord clamping is now the preferred approach (ACOG, 2012a).

Delayed cord clamping should not be performed if there are maternal or neonatal complications that require prompt interventions, such as postpartum hemorrhage, and bleeding complications from placenta previa or placentae abruption. Neonates that require immediate resuscitation should have their umbilical cord promptly cut so that neonatology intervention is not delayed.

CORD BLOOD COLLECTION FOR BANKING

A growing number of parents are arranging for cord blood banking. Cord blood banking involves collecting the newborn's umbilical cord blood immediately following birth. Since cord blood, like

TABLE 18–6 The Apgar Scoring System

SIGN	SCORE		
	0	1	2
Heart rate	Absent	Slow; less than 100 beats/min	Greater than 100 beats/min
Respiration	Absent	Slow; irregular	Good breathing with crying
Muscle tone	Flaccid	Some flexion of extremities	Active movement of extremities
Reflex response	Absent	Grimace; noticeable facial movement	Vigorous cry; coughs; sneezes; pulls away when touched
Skin color	Pale or blue	Pink body, blue extremities	Pink body and extremities

Source: Data from Apgar, V. (1966). *The newborn (Apgar) scoring system, reflections and advice.* http://profiles.nlm.nih.gov/ps/access/CPBBJY.pdf

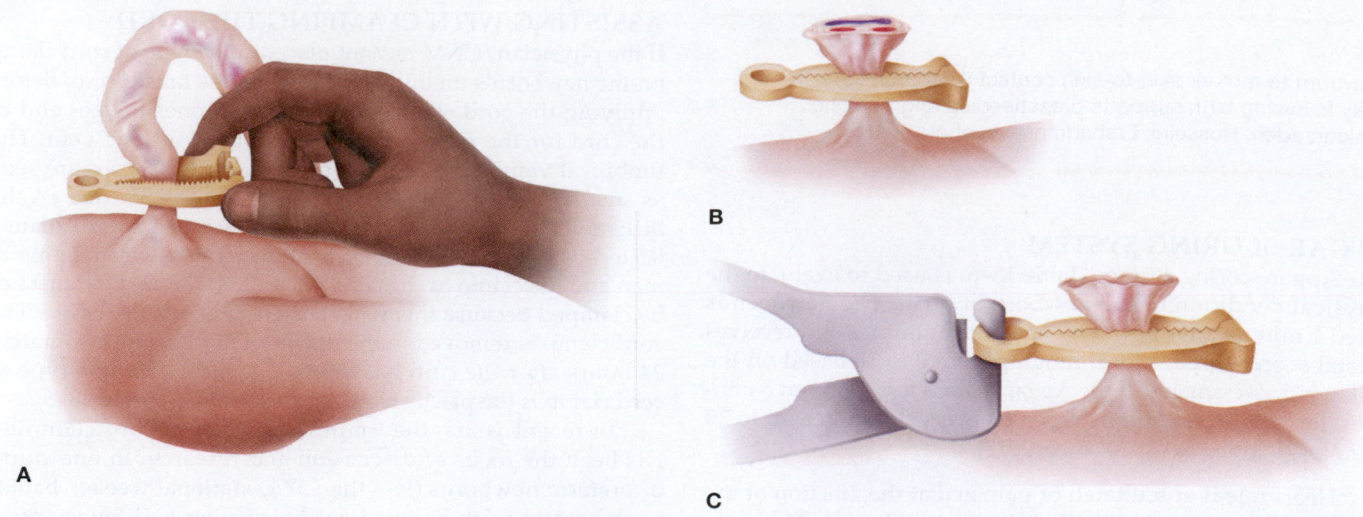

Figure 18–6 Hollister cord clamp. A. Clamp is positioned 0.5 to 1.0 inch from the abdomen and then secured. B. Cut cord. The one vein and two arteries can be seen. C. Plastic device for removing clamp after the cord has dried. After the cord has dried, the nurse grasps the Hollister clamp on either side of the cut area and gently separates it.

bone marrow, contains hematopoietic stem cells, it can be used to treat numerous cancers, genetic and blood disorders, cerebral palsy, and immune disorders. Cord blood has advantages over bone marrow. It is a no-risk procedure and causes no discomfort to the newborn or the mother and is less likely to trigger a potentially fatal rejection response. Cord blood can also work with a less than perfect match and is more readily available than bone marrow. Although cord blood banks have been established in the United States, universal cord blood collection does not exist. While some facilities collect volunteer donations, the majority of hospitals do not. Most of the banking performed in the United States is done by for-profit agencies where the parents pay a set fee to collect the blood and have it processed and then pay an annual storage fee. The main drawback of cord blood banking is the high cost.

Cord blood transplants can be utilized to treat a growing number of disorders. It is estimated that more than 30,000 transplants have been performed globally (Ballen, Gluckman, & Boxmeyer, 2013). Both ACOG (2012b) and the American Academy of Pediatrics have issued position statements on the importance of cord blood banking and the need to discuss the advantages and disadvantages with parents. While universal cord blood banking is not routinely recommended, parents who have an older child affected by a condition that may benefit from a cord blood transfusion should consider cord blood banking.

Once collected, the blood is tested for infectious and genetic disorders before it is frozen. Abnormal blood results are communicated to the parents. Written consent is required for both collection and storage of cord blood, preferably upon admission or prior to the onset of labor.

Immediately after the newborn's umbilical cord is clamped and cut, the physician/CNM withdraws blood from the remaining umbilical cord by inserting a large-gauge needle into the umbilical vein. The needle allows the blood to be collected into a special container that parents receive from the Cord Blood Registry and bring with them for the birth. The nurse labels the specimen immediately and follows the directions required for storage and pickup.

PHYSICAL ASSESSMENT OF THE NEWBORN

The nurse performs an abbreviated systematic physical assessment in the birthing area to detect any abnormalities (Table 18–7).

First, the size of the newborn and the contour and size of the head in relationship to the rest of the body are noted. The newborn's posture and movements indicate tone and neurologic functioning.

TABLE 18–7 Initial Newborn Evaluation

ASSESS	NORMAL FINDINGS
Respirations	Rate 30 to 60, irregular; no retractions, no grunting
Apical pulse	Rate 120 to 160 and somewhat irregular
Temperature	Skin temp above 36.5°C (97.8°F)
Skin color	Body pink with bluish extremities
Umbilical cord	Two arteries and one vein
Gestational age	Should be 37 to 42 weeks to remain with parents for extended time
Sole creases	Sole creases that involve the heel

In general, expect scant amount of vernix on upper back, axilla, groin; lanugo only on upper back; ears with incurving of upper two thirds of pinnae and thin cartilage that springs back from folding; male genitals—testes palpated in upper or lower scrotum; female genitals—labia majora larger; clitoris nearly covered.

In the following situations, newborns should generally be stabilized rather than remain with parents in the birth area for an extended period of time:

- Apgar less than 8 at 1 minute and less than 9 at 5 minutes or baby requires resuscitation measures (other than whiffs of oxygen)
- Respirations below 30 or above 60, with retractions and/or grunting
- Apical pulse below 120 or above 160 with marked irregularities
- Skin temperature below 36.5°C (97.8°F)
- Skin color pale blue or circumoral pallor
- Baby less than 37 weeks' or more than 42 weeks' gestation
- Baby very small or very large for gestational age
- Congenital anomalies involving open areas in the skin (meningomyelocele)

The skin should be inspected for discoloration, presence of vernix caseosa and lanugo, and evidence of trauma and desquamation (peeling of skin). Vernix caseosa is a white, cheesy substance found normally on newborns. It is absorbed within 24 hours after birth. Vernix is abundant on preterm newborns and absent on postterm newborns. A large quantity of fine hair (lanugo) is often seen on preterm newborns, especially on the shoulders, foreheads, backs, and cheeks. Desquamation of the skin is seen in postterm newborns.

The nurse observes the nares for flaring and, as the newborn cries, inspects the palate for cleft palate. The nurse looks for mucus in the nose and mouth and removes it with a bulb syringe as needed. The nurse inspects the chest for respiratory rate and the presence of retractions. If retractions are present, the nurse assesses the newborn for grunting or stridor. A normal respiratory rate is 30 to 80 per minute. The nurse auscultates the lungs bilaterally for breath sounds. Absence of breath sounds on one side could indicate a pneumothorax. Crackles may be heard immediately after birth because a small amount of fluid may remain in the lungs; this fluid will be absorbed.

Rhonchi indicate aspiration of oral secretions. If there is excessive mucus or respiratory distress, the nurse suctions the newborn with a mucus trap. (See *Clinical Skill: Performing Nasal Pharyngeal Suctioning.*) The nurse notes and records elimination of urine or meconium on the newborn record.

NEWBORN IDENTIFICATION AND SECURITY MEASURES

Identification bands typically come in a set, all preprinted with identical numbers. The nurse places two bands on the newborn—one on the wrist and one on the ankle. The newborn bands must fit snugly to prevent their loss. The nurse then gives the mother and the partner each a band. The band number is recorded in both the maternal and the newborn medical records. The bands allow access to the neonatal care areas and must not be removed until the baby is discharged. In most facilities, as a security measure, only individuals with a band are given unlimited access to the newborn.

Although some institutions rely on an umbilical band system to ensure the safety of newborns, others attach an alarm to the

---

Clinical Skill 18–1
Performing Nasal Pharyngeal Suctioning

NURSING ACTION

Preparation

- Suction equipment is always available in the birthing area to clear secretions from the newborn's nose or oropharynx if respirations are depressed or if amniotic fluid was meconium stained.

- Tighten the lid on the DeLee mucus trap or other suction device collection bottle.

Rationale: This avoids spillage of secretions and prevents air from leaking out of the lid.

- Connect one end of the DeLee tubing to low suction.

Equipment and Supplies

- DeLee mucus trap or other suction device

Procedure: Clean Gloves

1. Don gloves.

2. Without applying suction, insert the free end of the DeLee tubing 3 to 5 inches into the newborn's nose or mouth (Figure 18–7).

Rationale: Applying suction while passing the tube would interfere with smooth passage of the tube.

3. Place your thumb over the suction control and begin to apply suction. Continue to suction as you slowly remove the tube, rotating it slightly.

Rationale: Suctioning during withdrawal removes fluid and avoids redepositing secretions in the newborn's nasopharynx.

4. Continue to reinsert the tube and provide suction for as long as fluid is aspirated.

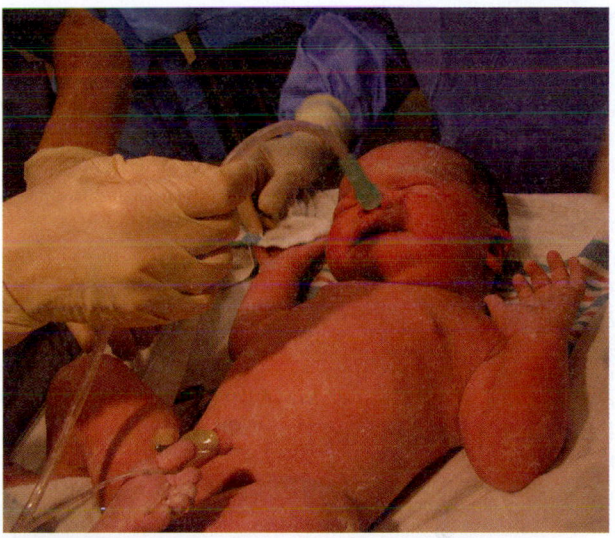

Figure18–7 DeLee mucus trap being used to suction a newborn's mouth to remove excess secretions.
SOURCE: Wilson Garcia.

Note: Excessive suctioning can cause vagal stimulation, which decreases the heart rate.

5. If it is necessary to pass the tube into the newborn's stomach to remove meconium secretions that the newborn swallowed before birth, insert the tube through the newborn's mouth into the stomach. Apply suction and continue to suction as you withdraw the tube.

Rationale: Because the newborn's nares are small and delicate, it is easier and faster to pass the suction tube through the mouth.

6. Document the completion of the procedure and the amount and type of secretions.

Rationale: This documentation provides a record of the intervention and the status of the newborn at birth.

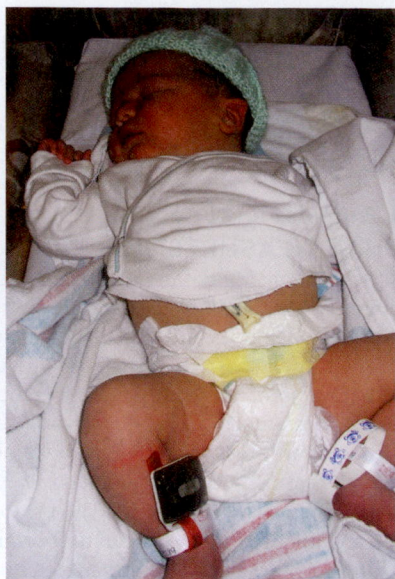

Figure 18–8 **A newborn with a security device in place on one ankle.**

SOURCE: Anne Garcia.

ankle band (Figure 18–8). The alarm is triggered if the device is tampered with or if the baby is removed from the parameters of the security field.

Additional hospital security measures are now commonplace in maternity settings. This includes mandating that all staff wear appropriate identification at all times. Parents are instructed that individuals without appropriate identification should not be allowed to remove their baby under any circumstances. The nurse also advises the parents to place the newborn on the side of the room away from the door opening, and to have the baby returned to the nursery whenever the mother naps or showers and no other family member is present.

Although hospital abductions are rare, they are catastrophic in nature to the family, hospital, and community. Many abductors pose as medical personnel to gain access to the mother and baby. Women should be advised to ask all hospital personnel for proper identification. If the mother or family members feel unsure of the individual, they should immediately call on the call bell to alert the nurse and ask for other verification. If a woman is reluctant to allow a student nurse to transport her baby, the staff nurse should be asked to assist the student.

Delivery of the Placenta

After birth, the physician/CNM prepares for the delivery of the placenta (see Placental Delivery in Chapter 16; see Figure 16–12O–P). The following signs suggest placental separation:

1. The uterus rises upward in the abdomen.
2. As the placenta moves downward, the umbilical cord lengthens.
3. A sudden trickle or spurt of blood appears.
4. The shape of the uterus changes from a disk to a globe.

While waiting for these signs, the nurse palpates the uterus to check for bogginess and fullness caused by uterine relaxation and subsequent bleeding into the uterine cavity. After the placenta has separated, the woman may be asked to bear down to aid delivery of the placenta.

Oxytocics are frequently given at the time of the delivery of the placenta, so that the uterus will contract and bleeding will be minimized. Oxytocin (Pitocin), 10 to 20 units, may be added to an intravenous (IV) infusion or 10 units may be given intramuscularly. In the presence of hemorrhage caused by uterine atony, some physicians/CNMs may order up to 40 units to a liter of intravenous fluid, methylergonovine maleate (Methergine), 0.2 mg, administered intramuscularly, or carboprost tromethamine (Hemabate), 250 mcg/mL, administered intramuscularly. Cytotec has been commonly used when other pharmacologic interventions have failed; however, current studies show it is not any more effective than Pitocin. It has been shown to decrease the risk of postpartum hemorrhage by 50% in women at risk for postpartum hemorrhage. Cytotec is administered rectally in dosages of 25 mcg (a 100 mcg tablet scored with ¼ tablet administered vaginally (ACOG, 2014). Cytotec can be administered every 3 to 6 hours. If Pitocin is to be administered, it should be held until a 4-hour time period has elapsed from the last dose of Cytotec. In addition to administering the ordered medications, the nurse assesses and records maternal blood pressure before and after administration of oxytocics and assesses the amount of bleeding. The nurse documents on the birth record the time of delivery of the placenta.

After delivery of the placenta, the physician/CNM inspects the placental membranes to make sure they are intact and that all cotyledons are present. If there is a defect or a part missing from the placenta, a manual uterine examination or *uterine exploration* is done.

Enhancing Attachment

Dramatic evidence indicates that the first few hours and even minutes after birth are an important period for the attachment of mother and newborn.

If contact can occur during the first hour after birth, the newborn will be in the quiet state and able to interact with parents by looking at them. Newborns also turn their heads in response to a spoken voice. (See Chapter 23 for further discussion of newborn states.) If possible and desired by the mother, the baby should be placed on the woman's chest so she can directly see her baby. This early interaction promotes attachment, early breastfeeding, and family interaction.

The first parent–newborn contact may be brief (a few minutes), and may be followed by a more extended contact after the mother completes other uncomfortable procedures (delivery of the placenta and suturing of the episiotomy or laceration). When the newborn is returned to the mother, the nurse can assist her to begin breastfeeding if she so desires. The baby may seek out the mother's breast, and early contact between the two can greatly affect breastfeeding success. Even if the newborn does not actively nurse, the baby can lick, taste, and smell the mother's skin. This activity by the newborn stimulates the maternal release of prolactin, which promotes the onset of lactation. These early interactions are associated with greater breastfeeding success.

Darkening the birthing room by turning out most of the lights causes newborns to open their eyes and gaze around. This in turn enhances eye-to-eye contact with the parents. (Note: If the physician/CNM needs a light source, the spotlight can be left on.)

Treatment of the newborn's eyes with antibiotic eye ointment may also be delayed up to an hour after birth. Many parents who establish eye contact with the newborn are content to quietly gaze at their baby. Others may show more active involvement by touching or inspecting the newborn. Some mothers talk to their babies in a high-pitched voice, which seems to be soothing to newborns. Some couples verbally express amazement and pride when they see they have produced a beautiful, healthy baby. Their verbalization enhances feelings of accomplishment and happiness.

Both parents need to be encouraged to do whatever they feel most comfortable doing. Some parents prefer only limited contact with the newborn immediately after birth and instead desire private time together in a quiet environment. In spite of the current zeal for providing immediate attachment opportunities, nursing personnel need to be aware of parents' wishes. The desire to delay interaction with the newborn does not necessarily imply a decreased ability of the parents to bond with their newborn.

Provision of Care in the Fourth Stage

The physician/CNM inspects the vagina, cervix, and perineum for lacerations and makes any necessary repairs. The episiotomy may be repaired now if it has not been done previously.

The nurse assesses the uterus for firmness by palpating the fundus. The normal position is at the midline and below the umbilicus. A displaced fundus may be caused by a full bladder or blood collected in the uterus. The clots or blood accumulation in the uterus may be expelled by grasping it with one hand anteriorly and posteriorly and squeezing. The nurse continues to palpate the uterine fundus at frequent intervals for at least 4 hours to ensure that it remains firmly contracted (Figure 18–9). It is palpated but not massaged unless it is soft (boggy). If it becomes boggy or appears to rise in the abdomen, the fundus is massaged until firm; then the nurse exerts firm pressure on the fundus in an attempt to express retained clots. During all aspects of fundal massage, the nurse uses one hand to provide support for the lower portion of the uterus and prevent damage to the round ligaments. The uterus is very tender at this time; all palpation and massage should be done as gently as possible. See *Clinical Skill: Assessing the Status of the Uterine Fundus After Vaginal or Cesarean Birth* in Chapter 28.

The nurse washes the woman's perineum with gauze squares and warmed solution and dries the area well with a towel before placing the sanitary pad. Many times, an ice pack is also placed against the perineum to promote comfort and decrease swelling. If stirrups have been used, the woman's legs are removed from the stirrups at the same time to avoid muscle strain. The woman is encouraged to move her legs gently up and down in a bicycle motion. The woman remains in the same bed or is transferred to a recovery room bed, and the nurse helps her don a clean gown. Soiled linens are removed and the woman is typically offered something to drink.

During the recovery period (1 to 4 hours) the woman is monitored closely. Frequent checking for deviations from normal in vital signs is required. The maternal blood pressure is monitored at 5- to 15-minute intervals to detect any changes. Blood pressure should return to the prelabor level because an increased volume of blood is returning to the maternal circulation from the uteroplacental shunt. Pulse rate should be slightly lower than it was during labor. Baroreceptors cause a vagal response, which slows the pulse. A rise in blood pressure may be a response to oxytocic drugs or may be caused by preeclampsia. Blood loss may be reflected by a lowered blood pressure and a rising pulse rate. See Table 18–8 for maternal adaptations after giving birth.

The nurse also monitors the woman's temperature. Frequently women have tremors or uncontrollable shaking in the

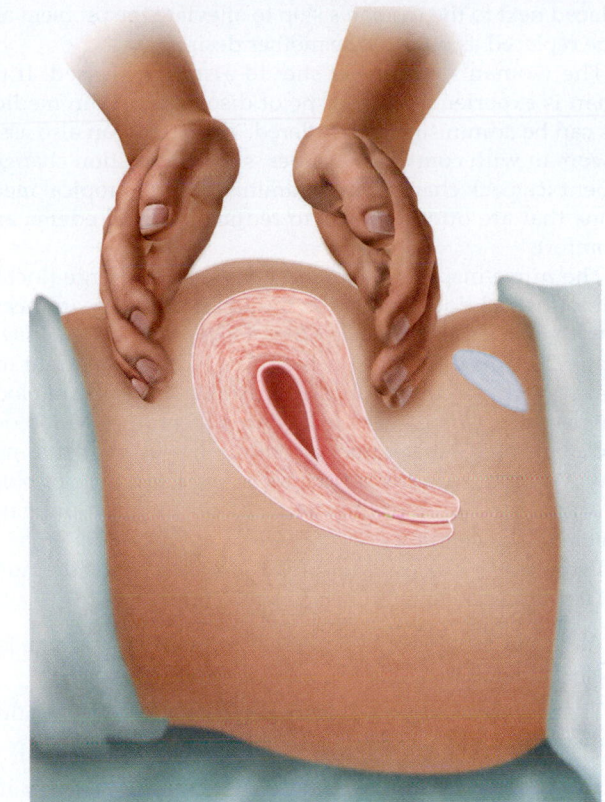

Figure 18–9 Suggested method of palpating the fundus of the uterus during the fourth stage. The left hand is placed just above the symphysis pubis, and gentle downward pressure is exerted. The right hand is cupped around the uterine fundus.

TABLE 18–8 Maternal Adaptations Following Birth

CHARACTERISTIC	NORMAL FINDING
Blood pressure	Returns to prelabor level
Pulse	Slightly lower than in labor
Uterine fundus	In the midline at the umbilicus or 1 to 2 fingerbreadths below the umbilicus
Lochia	Red (rubra), small to moderate amount (from spotting on pads to one quarter to one half of pad covered in 15 minutes); doesn't exceed saturation of one pad in first hour
Bladder	Nonpalpable
Perineum	Smooth, pink, without bruising or edema
Emotional state	Wide variation, including excited, exhilarated, smiling, crying, fatigued, verbal, quiet, pensive, and sleepy

immediate postpartum period that may be caused by a difference in internal and external body temperatures (higher temperature inside the body than outside). Another theory is that the woman is reacting to the fetal cells that have entered the maternal circulation at the placental site. A heated blanket may be placed next to the woman's skin to alleviate the problem and can be replaced as often as the mother desires.

The woman's pain level should also be assessed. If the woman is experiencing any type of discomfort, pain medications can be administered as ordered. The nurse can also assist the woman with comfort measures, such as position changes, frequent ice pack changes, and administration of topical medications that are often ordered to reduce perineal edema and discomfort.

The nurse inspects the bloody vaginal discharge (lochia) for amount and documents it as minimal, moderate, or heavy and with or without clots. See *Clinical Skill: Evaluating Lochia* in Chapter 28. This discharge, lochia rubra, should be bright red. A soaked perineal pad contains approximately 100 mL of blood. If the perineal pad becomes soaked in a 15-minute period or if blood pools under the buttocks, continuous observation is necessary. When the fundus is firm, a continuous trickle of blood may signal laceration of the vagina or cervix or an unligated vessel in the episiotomy.

If the fundus rises and displaces to the right, the nurse must be concerned about two factors:

1. As the uterus rises, the uterine contractions become less effective and increased bleeding may occur.

2. The most common cause of uterine displacement is bladder distention.

The nurse palpates the bladder to determine whether it is distended. The bladder fills rapidly with the extra fluid volume returned from the uteroplacental circulation (and with any fluid received intravenously during labor and birth). The postpartum woman may not realize that her bladder is full because trauma to the bladder and urethra during childbirth and the use of regional anesthesia decrease bladder tone and the urge to void.

All measures should be taken to enable the mother to void. The nurse may place a warm towel across the lower abdomen or pour warm water over the perineum to relax the urinary sphincter and facilitate voiding. The woman may also try running warm water over her hand. If the woman is unable to void, catheterization is necessary. The perineum is inspected for edema and hematoma formation.

The couple may be tired, hungry, and thirsty. Some agencies serve the couple a meal. Most women are very hungry after birth. The tired mother will probably drift off into a welcome sleep. The partner can also be encouraged to rest, because his supporting role is physically and mentally tiring. If the mother is not in a birthing room, she is usually transferred from the birthing unit to the postpartum or mother–baby area after 2 hours or more, depending on agency policy and whether the following criteria are met:

- Stable vital signs
- Stable bleeding
- Undistended bladder
- Firm fundus
- Sensations fully recovered from any anesthetic agent received during birth

For some women, the childbirth experience has been extremely painful, filled with hours of feeling powerless or out of control. In this circumstance, the woman is at higher risk for developing posttraumatic stress disorder (PTSD).

KEY FACTS TO REMEMBER
Immediate Postbirth Danger Signs

In the immediate postbirth recovery period, the following conditions should be reported to the physician/CNM:

- Hypotension
- Tachycardia
- Uterine atony
- Excessive bleeding
- Hematoma

Support of the Adolescent During Birth

As with all women, each adolescent in labor is different. The nurse must assess what each teen brings to the experience by asking the following questions:

- Has the adolescent received prenatal care?
- What are her attitudes and feelings about the pregnancy?
- Who will attend the birth and what is the person's relationship to her?
- What preparation has she had for the experience?
- What are her expectations and fears regarding labor and birth?
- How has her culture influenced her?
- What are her usual coping mechanisms?
- Does she plan to keep the newborn?

Any adolescent female who has not had prenatal care requires close observation during labor. Fetal well-being is established by fetal monitoring. Adolescents are at risk for pregnancy and labor complications and must be assessed carefully. The nurse should be especially alert for any physiologic complications of labor. The adolescent's prenatal record is carefully reviewed for risks, and she is screened for preeclampsia, cephalopelvic disproportion (CPD), anemia, cigarette smoking, alcohol and drugs ingested during pregnancy, sexually transmitted infections, and size–date discrepancies.

The support role of the nurse depends on the young woman's support system during labor. The adolescent may not be accompanied by someone who will stay with her during childbirth, or she may have her mother, the father of the baby, or a close friend as her labor partner. Regardless of whether the teen has a support person, it is important for the nurse to establish a trusting relationship with her. In this way, the nurse can help her understand what is happening to her. Establishing a nurturing rapport is essential. Some nurses may view adolescent pregnancy as a negative event; however, it is important to treat the young woman with respect. The adolescent who is given positive reinforcement for "work well done" will leave the experience with increased self-esteem, despite the emotional problems that may accompany her situation.

If a support person accompanies the adolescent, that person also needs the nurse's encouragement and support. The nurse must explain changes in the young woman's behavior and substantiate her wishes. The nursing staff should reinforce the adolescent's feelings that she is wanted and important.

The adolescent female who has taken childbirth education classes is generally better prepared for labor than one who has not. However, the nurse must keep in mind that the younger the adolescent, the less she may be able to participate actively in the process, even if she has taken prenatal classes. The adolescent's response to labor and birth often depends on the age of the mother-to-be, as follows:

- *Young adolescent.* A girl age 14 and under typically has fewer coping mechanisms and less experience to draw on than her older counterparts. Because her cognitive development is incomplete, the younger adolescent may have fewer problem-solving capabilities. Her ego integrity may be more threatened by the experience, and she may be more vulnerable to stress and discomfort. Thus, she needs someone to rely on at all times during labor. She may be more childlike and dependent than older teens. The nurse must be sure that instructions and explanations are simple and concrete. During the transition phase, she may become withdrawn and unable to express her need to be nurtured. Touch, soothing encouragement, and measures to provide comfort help her maintain control and meet her needs for dependence. During the second stage of labor, the young adolescent may feel as if she is losing control and may reach out to those around her. By remaining calm and giving directions, the nurse helps her cope with feelings of helplessness.

- *Middle adolescent.* The young woman age 15 to 17 years often attempts to remain calm and unflinching during labor. The experienced nurse realizes that a caring attitude will still help the young woman. Many older adolescents believe that they "know it all," but they may be no more prepared for childbirth than their younger counterparts. The nurse's reinforcement and nonjudgmental manner will help them save face. If the adolescent has not taken childbirth preparation classes, she may require preparation and explanations.

- *Older teenager.* The 18- to 19-year-old young woman's response to the stresses of labor may be similar to that of an older adult woman.

Adolescents, regardless of their age, need ongoing education throughout labor and in the early postpartum period (Figure 18–10). Clear explanations should be provided. They should be encouraged to ask questions and seek out information.

Even if the adolescent is planning to relinquish her newborn, she should be given the option of seeing and holding the baby. She may be reluctant to do this at first, but the grieving process is facilitated if the mother sees the baby. However, seeing or holding the newborn should be the adolescent's choice. (See Chapter 29 for further discussion of the relinquishing mother and the adolescent parent.)

Adolescents need individualized care for the issues that they face in the postpartum period. They may experience psychosocial issues unique to their age group and their developmental level. Adolescents are also at an increased risk for unintended subsequent pregnancies and abortions. Proper discharge teaching should include contraceptive options.

Nursing Care During Precipitous Labor and Birth

Occasionally labor progresses so rapidly that the nurse is faced with the task of managing the actual birth of the baby.

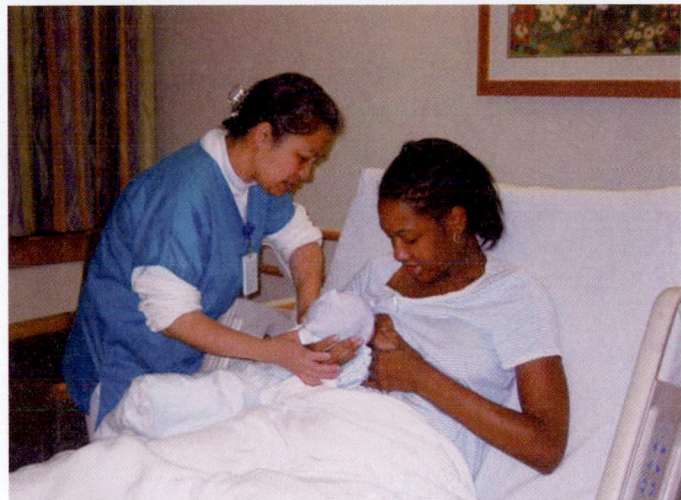

Figure 18–10 An adolescent mother receives breastfeeding assistance in the immediate postpartum period.

SOURCE: Michele Davidson.

Precipitous labor and **precipitous birth** occur when the labor and birth occur in 3 hours or less. Contributing factors include multiparity, large pelvis, previous precipitous birth, and small fetus in a favorable position. One of these contributing factors in addition to strong labor contractions and rapid descent in the birth canal can result in a precipitous birth. The incidence of precipitous birth is approximately 2% (Cunningham et al., 2014). A careful assessment in the antepartum period can identify many women at risk for precipitous birth. Cervical examinations starting at 38 weeks can be performed to assess for advanced dilatation. If advanced dilatation occurs, an elective induction can be scheduled to reduce the risk of precipitous birth or an unattended labor and birth.

During precipitous labor and birth, the attending nurse has the primary responsibility for providing a physically and psychologically safe experience for the woman and her baby. A woman whose physician/CNM is not present may feel disappointed, frightened, abandoned, angry, and cheated. She may fear what is going to happen and feel that everything is out of her control. In working with the woman, the nurse provides support by keeping her informed about the labor progress and assuring her that the nurse will stay with her. If birth is imminent, the nurse must not leave the mother alone. Auxiliary personnel can be directed to contact the physician/CNM and retrieve the emergency birth pack ("precip pack"), which should be readily accessible to birthing rooms. A typical pack contains the following items:

1. Small drape that can be placed under the woman's buttocks to provide a sterile field
2. Bulb syringe to clear mucus from the newborn's mouth
3. Two sterile clamps (Kelly or Rochester) to clamp the umbilical cord before applying a cord clamp
4. Sterile scissors to cut the umbilical cord
5. Sterile umbilical cord clamp, either Heseltine or Hollister
6. Baby blanket to wrap the newborn in after birth
7. Package of sterile gloves

At all times during the birth, the nurse remains calm; the woman is reassured by the composure of the nurse and feels that the nurse is competent.

Risks of Precipitous Labor and Precipitous Birth

The risks associated with precipitous labor and precipitous birth include:

- Loss of coping skills
- Lacerations of the cervix, vagina, and perineum caused by rapid descent of the fetal head
- Postpartum hemorrhage
- Nonreassuring fetal status
- Hypoxia
- Brachial plexus injury

Precipitous Birth

The nurse attends the precipitous birth by first encouraging the woman to assume a comfortable position. Women who give birth in the lateral positions are less prone to perineal lacerations (King et al., 2015). If time permits, the nurse scrubs his or her hands with soap and water and puts on sterile gloves. Sterile drapes may be placed under the woman's buttocks if time allows. The bed should be left in an intact position without the use of the stirrups. The nurse may place an index finger inside the lower portion of the vagina and the thumb on the outer portion of the perineum and gently massage the area to help stretch perineal tissues and prevent perineal lacerations. Warm compresses also protect against lacerations, although there may not be time to implement them (King et al., 2015).

Clinical Tip

When birth is imminent and a physician/CNM is not present, do not take the bed apart (or "break the bed") because this increases the risk that the newborn could be dropped at the time of birth. Lower the foot of the bed slightly to create space beneath the buttocks so you are able to adequately deliver the head without the risk of a newborn fall.

As the neonate's head crowns, the nurse should support the perineum with her thumb on one side and four fingers on the other side providing manual support while instructing the woman to pant, which decreases her urge to push. The nurse checks whether the amniotic sac is intact. If it is, the nurse tears the sac, usually with a Kelly clamp, so the newborn will not breathe in amniotic fluid with the first breath.

With one hand, the nurse applies gentle pressure in a downward motion against the fetal head to prevent it from popping out rapidly. The nurse does not hold the head back forcibly. Rapid birth of the head may result in tears in the woman's perineal tissues. In the fetus, the rapid change in pressure within the fetal head may cause subdural or dural tears. The nurse supports the perineum with the other hand and allows the head to be born between contractions.

As the woman continues to pant, the nurse inserts one or two fingers along the back of the fetal head to check for the umbilical cord. If there is a nuchal cord (umbilical cord around the neck), the nurse's fingers should be bent like a fish hook in order to grasp the cord and pull it over the baby's head. It is important to check that the cord is not wrapped around the neck more than one time. If the cord is tightly looped and cannot be slipped over the baby's head, two clamps are placed on the cord, the cord is cut between the clamps, and the cord is unwound.

Immediately after birth of the head, the nurse suctions the baby's mouth and nasal passages. The head will then rotate to one side or the other. The head will move in one direction; the nurse does not attempt to rotate the head to one side or another. The nurse then places one hand on each side of the head, over the fetal ears. Care should be taken to ensure that the hands are not exerting pressure on the fetal neck. The nurse then exerts gentle downward traction until the anterior shoulder passes under the symphysis pubis. After the anterior shoulder is seen, gentle upward traction is used to aid the birth of the posterior shoulder. The nurse then instructs the woman to push gently so that the rest of the body can be born quickly. As the newborn emerges, support should be provided.

The newborn is held at the level of the uterus to facilitate blood flow through the umbilical cord. The combination of amniotic fluid and vernix makes the newborn very slippery, so the nurse must be careful to avoid dropping the baby. Leaving the birthing bed in an intact position provides the nurse with an area to place the newborn immediately after the birth. The nose and mouth of the newborn are suctioned again, using a bulb syringe. The nurse then dries the newborn and removes the wet blankets to prevent heat loss.

The umbilical cord may now be cut. The nurse places two sterile Kelly clamps approximately 0.5 to 1.0 in. from the newborn's abdomen. The cord is cut between the Kelly clamps with sterile scissors. The nurse places a sterile umbilical cord clamp adjacent to the Kelly clamp on the newborn's cord, between the clamp and the newborn's abdomen. The clamp must not be placed snugly against the abdomen, because the cord will dry and shrink. As soon as the nurse determines that the newborn's respirations are adequate, the baby can be placed on the mother's abdomen. The newborn's head should be slightly lower than the body to aid drainage of fluid and mucus. The weight of the newborn on the mother's abdomen stimulates uterine contractions, which aid in placental separation. The umbilical cord should not be pulled.

The nurse is alert for signs of placental separation (slight gush of dark blood from the vagina, lengthening of the cord, or a change in uterine shape from discoid to globular). The nurse can also place a hand in the vagina to see if the placenta is present. When these signs are present, the mother is instructed to push so that the placenta can be delivered. The nurse inspects the placenta to determine whether it is intact. Cord blood can be obtained from the placenta after delivery.

The nurse checks the firmness of the uterus. The fundus may be gently massaged to stimulate contractions and decrease bleeding. Putting the newborn to breast also stimulates uterine contractions through release of oxytocin from the pituitary gland.

The nurse cleanses the area under the mother's buttocks and inspects her perineum for lacerations. Bleeding from lacerations may be controlled by pressing sterile gauze or a clean perineal pad against the perineum and instructing the woman to keep her thighs together.

If the physician/CNM's arrival is delayed or if the newborn is having respiratory distress, the newborn should be transported immediately to the nursery. Newborns must be properly identified before they leave the birth area. The nurse notes and places on a birth record the following information:

- Position of fetus at birth
- Presence of cord around neck or shoulder (nuchal cord)
- Time of birth
- Apgar scores at 1 and 5 minutes after birth
- Gender of newborn
- Time of expulsion of placenta
- Method of placental expulsion
- Appearance and intactness of placenta
- Mother's condition
- Any medications that were given to mother or newborn (per agency protocol)

Evaluation

Evaluation provides an opportunity to determine the effectiveness of nursing care. As a result of comprehensive nursing care during the intrapartum period, the following outcomes may be anticipated:

- The mother's physical and psychologic well-being has been maintained and supported.
- The baby's physical and psychologic well-being has been protected and supported.
- The woman and her family members have had input into the birth process and have participated as much as they desired.
- The mother and her baby have had a safe birth.

Focus Your Study

- Nursing diagnoses in the intrapartum period typically include a general plan that includes the beginning of labor through the fourth stage.

- During labor, before procedures are begun, it is important to explain what will be done, the reasons, potential benefits and risks, and possible alternatives. These explanations help the woman determine what happens to her body.

- Behavioral responses to labor vary with the phase of labor, the preparation the woman has had, and her previous experience, cultural beliefs, and developmental level.

- The childbearing family may have a variety of expectations of the nurse during labor and birth. Some families want to make all decisions themselves with limited nursing contact, whereas others want a moderate amount of contact and see the relationship as a cooperative venture. Still other families want a lot of involvement and look to the nurse to instill confidence in them that everything will be all right.

- Each woman's cultural beliefs affect her need for privacy, expression of discomfort, and expectations for the birth and the role she wishes the father to play in the birth event.

- The phases of the first stage of labor include the latent phase (dilatation up to 3 cm [1.2 in.]), the active phase (dilatation from 4 to 7 cm [1.6 to 2.8 in.]), and the transition phase (dilatation from 8 to 10 cm [3.1 to 3.9 in.]).

- The laboring woman's comfort may be increased by general comfort measures, methods of handling anxiety, client teaching, supportive relaxation techniques, controlled breathing, and support by a caring person.

- During the second stage of labor, the nurse assists the woman with establishing an effective pattern for pushing, finding a comfortable pushing position, and providing continuous encouragement for her efforts.

- Maternal birthing positions include a wide variety of possibilities, from side-lying (lateral) to sitting, squatting, and semi-Fowler.

- Immediate assessments of the newborn include evaluation of the Apgar score and an abbreviated physical assessment. These early assessments help determine the need for resuscitation and whether the newborn's adaptation to extrauterine life is progressing normally. The newborn who is not experiencing problems may remain with the parents for an extended period after birth.

- Immediate care of the newborn includes maintenance of respirations, promotion of warmth, prevention of infection, and accurate identification.

- The placenta separates from the uterine wall and is expelled with either the maternal or the fetal side emerging from the vagina. The maternal side contains the cotyledons, appears rough in texture, and may be associated with retention of placental fragments.

- The fourth stage includes the first 1 to 4 hours following birth. Many physiologic and psychologic changes occur during this period.

- The adolescent mother has special needs in the birth setting. Her developmental needs require specialized nursing care.

- At times a baby is born rapidly, in less than 3 hours, without the physician/CNM present. This event is referred to as a precipitous birth. The nurse in the birthing area remains with the woman and attends to her needs during the birth until the physician/CNM arrives.

- Precipitous labor is extremely rapid labor and birth that lasts less than 3 hours. It is associated with an increased risk to the mother and the newborn.

Clinical Reasoning in Action

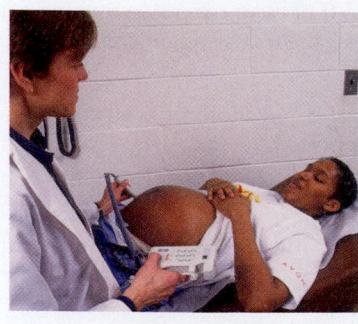

Anita Grey, a 22-year-old primigravida at 40 weeks' gestation, is admitted by you to the birthing center in labor. Anita was sent from her physician's office after being evaluated at her prenatal visit. While in the office, she was assessed to be 4 cm dilated, 100% effaced, vertex at 0 station with bulging membranes. She tells you that her husband is on his way to the birthing center and that she is anxious for him to arrive. A review of her prenatal record shows no complications affecting this pregnancy. Anita's vital signs are within normal limits. You assess the fetal heart rate and contraction pattern with the fetal monitor and observe a fetal heart rate of 140 to 150 bpm with accelerations to 160s. Contractions are every 3 to 4 minutes × 30 seconds of moderate intensity by palpation. Anita seems to be tolerating the contractions well, but still seems anxious about her husband's arrival.

1. What steps can you take to reduce the stress and anxiety of the laboring woman and her family?
2. When you notify the physician/CNM, what pertinent information should the report contain?
3. What support measures can you give in the active phase of labor?
4. What measures can be used to decrease discomfort/pain as labor progresses?
5. What observations reflect the physiologic manifestations of pain?

References

American College of Obstetricians and Gynecologists (ACOG). (2012a). *Timing of umbilical cord clamping after birth* (ACOG Practice Bulletin No. 543). Washington, DC: Author.

American College of Obstetricians and Gynecologists (ACOG). (2012b). *Umbilical cord blood banking* (Committee Opinion No. 399). Washington, DC: Author.

American College of Obstetricians and Gynecologists (ACOG). (2014). *Induction of labor.* (ACOG Practice Bulletin No. 107). Washington, DC: Author.

American College of Obstetricians and Gynecologists (ACOG). (2015). *Management of intrapartum fetal heart rate tracings* (Practice Bulletin No. 116). Washington, DC: Author.

American Humane Association. (2015). Child abuse and neglect statistics. Retrieved from http://www.americanhumane.org/children/stop-child-abuse/fact-sheets/child-abuse-and-neglect-statistics.html

Andrews, C. S. (2014). Developing a measure of cultural-, maturity-, or esteem-driven modesty among Jewish women. *Research and Theory for Nursing Practice, 28*(1), 9–37.

Ara, F., Ara, B., Kaker, P., & Aslam, M. (2015). Childbirth: Comparison of complications between lithotomy and squatting positions during labor. *Professional Medical Journal, 22*(4), 390–394.

Ballen, K. K., Gluckman, E., & Boxmeyer, H. E. (2013). Umbilical cord blood transplantation: The first 25 years and beyond. *Blood, 122*(4), 401–420. doi: http://dx.doi.org/10.1182/blood-2013-02-453175

Bureau of Justice Statistics. (2013). Over 60 percent decline in sexual violence against females from 1995 to 2010. Retrieved from http://www.bjs.gov/content/pub/press/fvsv9410pr.cfm

Burnard, P., & Gill, P. (2015). *Culture, communication, and nursing.* London, UK: Routledge.

Centers for Disease Control and Prevention. (2015). *Opt out HIV testing: HIV screening for prenatal care.* Retrieved from http://www.cdc.gov/Features/1Test2Lives

Cunningham, F. G., Leveno, K. J., Bloom, S. L., Spong, C. Y., Dashe, J. S., Hoffman, B. L., . . . Sheffield, J. S. (2014). *Williams obstetrics* (24th ed.). New York, NY: McGraw-Hill.

Davidson, M. R. (2012). *A nurse's guide to women's mental health.* New York, NY: Springer.

Ghorashi, Z., Ashori, V., Aminzadeh, F., & Mokhtari, M. (2014). The effects of oral fluid intake an hour before cesarean section on regurgitation incidence. *Iranian Journal of Nursing & Midwifery Research, 19*(4): 439–442.

Heidarzadeh, M., Hosseini, M., Ershadmanesh, M., & Tabari, M. G. (2013). The effect of kangaroo mother care (KMC) on breast feeding at the time of NICU discharge. *Iranian Red Crescent Medical Journal, 15*(4), 302–306. doi:10.5812/ircmj.2160

Institute for Patient and Family-Centered Care. (2015). *Family-centered care.* Retrieved from http://www.ipfcc.org/faq.html

King, T. L., Brucker, M. C., Kriebs, J. M., & Fahey, J. O. (2015). *Varney's midwifery* (5th ed.). New York, NY: Jones & Bartlett Learning.

Konda, A., Vikas, R., & Yarlagadda, P. (2014). An intuitive multi-touch surface and gesture based interaction for video surveillance systems. *International Journal of Future Computer and Communication, 3*(3), 197–201.

Lanting, C. I., & van Wouwe, J. P. (2015). Apgar score and risk of cause-specific infant mortality. *The Lancet, 385*(9967), 504–505. doi: http://dx.doi.org/10.1016/S0140-6736(15)60194-5

Narendra, M., Shah, P. K., Pratap, K., & Prashap, A. (2014). *Ultrasound in obstetrics & gynecology.* (4th ed.). Pradesh, India: Jaypee Brothers Medical.

Ondeck, M. (2014). Healthy birth practice #2: Walk, move around, and change positions throughout labor. *The Journal of Perinatal Education, 23*(4), 188–193.

Santos, A. (2014). *Obstetric anesthesia.* St. Louis, MO: McGraw-Hill.

Simpkin, P., & Creehan, M. (2013). Nonpharmacologic approaches to relieve labor pain: Acupuncture and acupressure (shiatsu). *Medscape.* Retrieved from http://www.medscape.com/viewarticle/494120_8

Zaibunnisa, A., Firdos, A., Bilqees, K., & Palwasha, A. M. (2015). Childbirth: Comparison of complications between lithotomy position and squatting position. *Professional Medical Journal, 22*(4), 390–394.

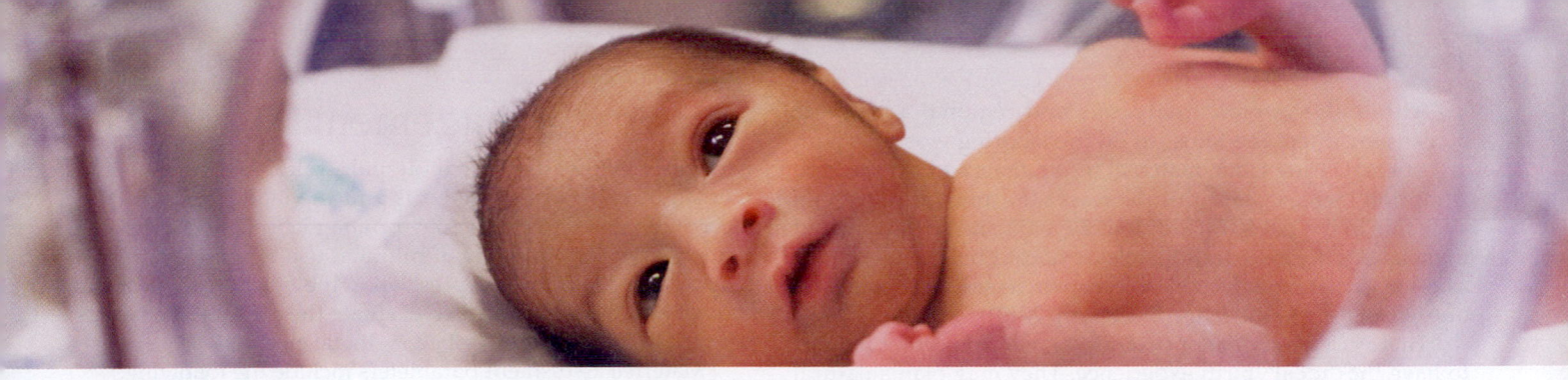

Chapter 19
Pharmacologic Pain Management

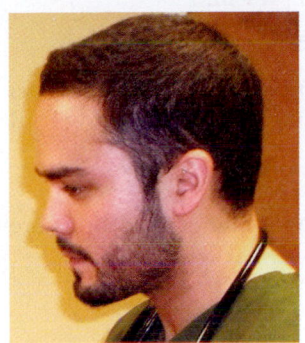

I had the unique opportunity to join the staff of a brand-new women's hospital as it was opening. The team I work with is very tight knit, and we really support each other. Our schedule rotates so that I cover the regular (daytime) surgical cases for 2 days a week and then I have a 24-hour call shift on the birthing unit. I may do 10 to 12 epidurals during that call period, so I really have to be efficient. Still, it is important to me (and the others on my team) to spend as much time as that laboring woman needs, to explain things, and help her feel comfortable with her choice of pain relief.

—Certified Registered Nurse Anesthetist

Learning Outcomes

19.1 Describe the use, administration, dose, onset of action, and adverse effects of systemic drugs to promote pain relief during the nursing management of the woman in labor and her fetus.

19.2 Compare the major types of regional analgesia and anesthesia, including area affected, advantages, disadvantages, techniques, and nursing management of the laboring woman and her fetus.

19.3 Explain the possible complications of regional anesthesia in nursing management of the laboring woman and her fetus.

19.4 Discuss the increasing use of nitrous oxide in the United States and the benefits of its use in contemporary obstetric practice.

19.5 Describe the nursing management for the laboring woman and her fetus related to general anesthesia.

19.6 Describe the major complications of general anesthesia during labor in nursing management of the woman in labor and her fetus.

Childbearing women experience varying levels of pain and other demanding sensations during labor and birth. As discussed in Chapter 18, nursing interventions directed toward pain relief begin with psychologic measures such as providing information, support, and encouragement. Measures to promote physical comfort include back rubs, showers, whirlpool baths, and the application of cool cloths. Some laboring women need no further interventions.

For other women, the progression of labor brings increasing pain that interferes with their ability to cope. These women may elect to use pharmacologic agents such as systemic medications, regional nerve blocks (epidural, spinal, or combined epidural–spinal), nitrous oxide, and local anesthetic blocks (pudendal and perineal) to decrease discomfort, increase relaxation, and reestablish their ability to participate more effectively in the labor and birth experience. The methods are not all mutually exclusive, and any of them may be used in combination with nonpharmacologic comfort measures. The use of general anesthesia has very limited use in modern obstetrics. It is occasionally used during emergency cesarean births, although this trend continues to decrease because of the associated adverse maternal and fetal effects.

Although systemic analgesics and regional anesthetic blocks may affect the fetus, so do the laboring woman's pain and stress. During labor, maternal respirations and oxygen consumption increase, and this decreases the amount of oxygen available to the fetus. In addition, the pain and stress can lead to metabolic acidosis and the release of catecholamines, which cause maternal blood vessels to constrict, lessening oxygen and nutrient supply to the fetus (Blackburn, 2013).

There is a good deal of peer pressure on expectant parents to have the "ideal" birth experience. They may plan a natural childbirth, in which case the need for analgesia may make them feel inadequate and guilty. Reassurance that accepting analgesia for discomfort is not a failure can help maintain the woman's self-esteem. The emphasis should be on achieving a healthy, satisfying outcome for the family. Evidence has shown that women who have continuous one-to-one support during labor are more likely to have a spontaneous vaginal birth, less likely to require analgesia, and less likely to report dissatisfaction with their childbirth experience (Anderson & Stone, 2013). Also, the American College of Obstetricians and Gynecologists has concluded that a woman's request is sufficient justification for pain relief during labor (Anderson & Stone, 2013).

Systemic Medications

Note that this discussion of obstetric analgesia and anesthesia applies only to a healthy woman and fetus. Pain relief during labor and birth for women with high-risk conditions, such as preterm labor, preeclampsia, blood disorders, asthma, obstructive sleep apnea, substance abuse issues, or diabetes mellitus, requires skilled decision making, close observation, and awareness of all the potential threats to both the woman and her baby (Wong, 2014). Few conditions warrant a contraindication to systemic medications. However, women with myasthenia gravis should not be given systemic medications and instead are better candidates for epidural anesthesia (Wong, 2014). The goal of pharmacologic analgesia during labor is to provide maximum pain relief at minimum risk for the mother and the fetus. To reach this goal, clinicians must consider a number of factors, including the following:

- All systemic medications used for pain relief during labor cross the placental barrier by simple diffusion, but some medications cross more readily than others.
- Medication action in the body depends on the rate at which the substance is metabolized by liver enzymes and excreted by the kidneys.
- High medication doses may remain in the fetus for long periods because fetal liver enzymes and kidney excretion are inadequate for metabolizing analgesic agents.

Clinical Reasoning **Anesthesia During Labor**

Luisa Silva, a 33-year-old G1P0, is 32 weeks pregnant. She is trying to decide whether she should accept any analgesia during her labor. She has finished childbirth education classes and wants an unmedicated labor and birth. She says, "I want to do this on my own, but I'm afraid it may be too much. Will it be OK if I need to take something?"

What will you tell her?

Nursing Management

Analgesic medications provide pain relief for the laboring woman but also affect the fetus and the labor process. Pain medication given too early may prolong labor and depress the fetus; if given too late it is of minimal use to the woman and may lead to respiratory depression in the newborn. Assess the mother and the fetus and also evaluate the contraction pattern before administering prescribed systemic medications.

Maternal assessment parameters include the following:

- Desire to receive medication after being advised about the risks and benefits of medication
- Stable vital signs
- Contraindications (such as specific medication allergy, respiratory compromise, myasthenia gravis, or current medication dependence) are not present.

Fetal assessment parameters include:

- Fetal heart rate (FHR) baseline is between 110 and 160 beats per minute and no late decelerations or nonreassuring FHR patterns are present
- Variability is present
- Fetus exhibits normal movement and accelerations are present with fetal movement
- Fetus is term

Assessment of labor includes:

- Documentation of the contraction pattern
- Cervical status, including cervical position, consistency, effacement, dilatation, and station

Before administering the medication, once again ascertain whether the woman has a history of any medication reactions or allergies and provide information about the medication. (See *Teaching Highlights: What Women Need to Know About Pain-Relief Medications.*) Maternal vital signs, FHR, contraction pattern, and pain level should be assessed and documented before administering any pain medication. After giving the medication, record the medication name, dose, route, and site, as well as the woman's blood pressure (BP) and pulse, within the medical record. If the woman is alone, side rails should be raised to provide safety. Assess the FHR for possible adverse effects of the medication. After the medication has been administered, document the woman's pain level, the effectiveness of the medication, and any adverse effects if they occurred.

When an analgesic medication is administered by intramuscular or subcutaneous route, it takes a few minutes for the effect to be felt. Continue with other supportive measures to enhance comfort until the pharmacologic agent is effective. Provide continued reassurance and verbal praise. When the medication begins to take effect, the woman may sleep between contractions. This short period of rest helps her relax and can restore her energy. When the physician/certified nurse-midwife (CNM) orders an intravenous route, the effect of the medication will be felt within a few minutes, so if any change of position is necessary or if the woman needs to void, suggest that the woman complete these activities before receiving the medication. Some women may be so uncomfortable that they do not want anything except the medication. In this case, administering the medication first would be more helpful for the women.

Before receiving medications, the woman should understand the following:

- Type of medication administered
- Route of administration
- Expected effects of medication
- Implications for fetus or newborn
- Safety measures needed (e.g., remain in bed with side rails up)

Developing Cultural Competence   Cultural Influence on Responses to Pain

A woman's cultural background may influence her responses to pain. Following are generalizations of how some cultures perceive pain and pain responses:

- Mexican American women may moan rhythmically and massage their thighs and abdomen when in pain.
- Haitian women may prefer massage, movement, and position changes to increase comfort.
- Filipino women may lie quietly because they believe that noise and activity increase labor pain.
- Black, Puerto Rican, and Middle Eastern women are often verbally expressive of pain.
- Native American women may be viewed as stoic, using meditation, self-control, and traditional herbs.
- Thai women's silent but restless behavior can reflect high levels of pain.
- Japanese, Chinese, Vietnamese, Laotian, and other women of Asian descent may feel that crying out during labor is shameful.
- Samoan women may believe no verbal response is allowed.

Opioid Analgesics

Opioid analgesic agents that are injected into the circulation have their primary action at sites in the brain, activating the neurons that descend to the spinal cord. The opioid analgesics used in early labor are given in either intermittent doses or, less commonly, by patient-controlled administration. It is unclear if these medications work by providing an analgesic effect or by inducing sedation; however, the medications do have a quieting effect that reduces pain for the laboring woman (Anderson & Stone, 2013). See Table 19–1 for information about analgesics used in labor. Opiod analgesics should be used with caution with women with a history of substance abuse (Wong, 2014).

BUTORPHANOL TARTRATE (STADOL) AND NALBUPHINE HYDROCHLORIDE (NUBAIN)

Butorphanol tartrate (Stadol) is a synthetic agonist–antagonist opioid analgesic agent used to reduce pain intensity in labor. Respiratory depression of both the mother and the fetus or newborn can occur if given late in the first stage of labor but can be reversed with naloxone (Narcan).

The most common side effects include:

- Drowsiness
- Dizziness
- Fainting
- Hypotension
- Urinary retention.

Clinical Tip

Butorphanol needs to be protected from light and stored at room temperature (Wilson, Shannon, & Shields, 2015).

SAFETY ALERT!

Because the most common side effect of butorphanol tartrate (Stadol) is drowsiness, the mother should be advised to remain in bed with side rails up to prevent falls or injuries after administration of the medication.

Like butorphanol, nalbuphine hydrochloride (Nubain) is a synthetic agonist–antagonist opioid analgesic. Both nalbuphine and butorphanol can have a ceiling effect where the pain reduction qualities do not increase, but the side effects increase. Nalbuphine is often the medication of choice because it is associated with less nausea and vomiting and a lower incidence of respiratory depression. Nalbuphine is also associated with increased maternal sedation, which allows the mother an opportunity to rest between contractions.

FENTANYL (SUBLIMAZE)

Fentanyl is a short-acting opiate that has been used during labor to relieve pain and induce sedation. Fentanyl is 50 to 100 times more potent than morphine. Fentanyl has less neonatal neurobehavioral depression than meperidine hydrochloride (Demerol) because it does not cross the placenta. However, neonatal depression can still occur, although at much lower rates when compared with meperidine. Fentanyl results in less sedation, nausea, vomiting, and pruritus compared with meperidine. See Table 19–1.

SAFETY ALERT!

Fentanyl has a variety of drug interactions that should be evaluated prior to administration, including CNS depressants; antipsychotics; anxiolytics; certain antihistamines such as diphenhydramine (Benadryl) and hydroxyzine (Vistaril); barbiturates; tricyclic antidepressants; high levels of alcohol; and skeletal muscle relaxants, such as cyclobenzaprine (Flexeril) and baclofen (Lioresal). Cimetidine (Tagamet) has been associated with confusion, disorientation and seizures when given concurrently with fentanyl (Chestnut, Wong, Tsen, et al., 2014).

TABLE 19–1 Analgesics Used in Labor

DRUG/CLASS	DOSAGE, ROUTE, FREQUENCY	COMMON SIDE EFFECTS	LIFE-THREATENING REACTIONS	CONTRAINDICATIONS
Stadol (butorphanol tartrate): CNS agent, analgesic, narcotic agonist/antagonist	IM 1–2 mg every 4 hr IV 0.5–2 mg every 4 hr; rapid onset; peak: 30–60 min; duration 3–4 hr Intranasal: 1 mg (1 puff) may repeat in 90 sec (max dose every 3–4 hr)	Sedation; sweaty, clammy skin; nausea and vomiting	Respiratory depression	Narcotic dependency, breastfeeding, women with chronic hypertension or preeclampsia, monoamine oxidase inhibitors (MAOIs) for depression
Nubain (nalbuphine hydrochloride): CNS agent analgesic, narcotic agonist	10–20 mg every 3–6 hr PRN subcutaneous IM/IV IV infusion should be administered over 3 to 5 minutes	Sedation, dizziness, fainting, hypotension, hypertension	Nonreassuring fetal heart rate, respiratory depression	Hypersensitivity to the drug, withdrawal symptoms in opioid-dependent women
Demerol (meperidine hydrochloride): CNS agent, analgesic, narcotic agonist	IV 2.5–15 mg every 4 hr	Pruritus, dizziness, sedation, nausea, constipation	Respiratory depression, convulsions, cardiovascular collapse, cardiac arrest, respiratory depression in newborn, bronchoconstriction, neonatal neurotoxicity	Hypersensitivity to the drug, convulsive disorders, breastfeeding, undiagnosed acute abdominal pain
Fentanyl (Sublimaze): Short-acting opiate agonist, analgesic	50–100 mcg every 2 hr IV/IM IV give over 1–2 min; immediate onset; peak 30–60 min, duration limited to 30–60 min IM onset 7–15 min	Bradycardia, hypotension, nausea, vomiting, and respiratory depression	Muscle rigidity, especially in the respiratory muscles	Women with opioid dependency

Additive Medications

The use of additive medications can decrease anxiety and increase the effectiveness of analgesics when given simultaneously. These medications, which are classified as tranquilizers, have no specific properties that decrease pain; however, they do work well to provide relief without increasing unwanted side effects and allow a smaller dose of the opioid to be administered. These medications can also be used to manage the unpleasant side effects, such as nausea or vomiting, associated with the administration of opioid analgesics.

Commonly used additive medications include promethazine (Phenergan), hydroxyzine (Vistaril), propiomazine (Largon), and promazine (Sparine). The main side effect is sedation, which may be helpful in promoting rest in women who have had a prolonged labor or who have had little sleep; however, the effect may be undesirable to other women.

Opiate Antagonist: Naloxone (Narcan)

Because naloxone is an antagonist with little or no agonistic effect, it exhibits little pharmacologic activity in the absence of opioids. Naloxone can be used to reverse the mild respiratory depression that follows administration of opiates. Naloxone is the medication of choice when the depressant is unknown because it will cause no further depression (Wilson et al., 2015). An initial dose of 0.4 to 2.0 mg may be administered intravenously to the laboring woman. If the woman is nonresponsive, the medication can be readministered every 2 to 3 minutes. The nurse should be prepared to provide basic airway management, including the chin-lift/jaw-thrust maneuver, and initiation of respirations through a bag-valve-mask device when the woman is not immediately responsive and respiratory depression is occurring. It is typically administered to mothers who have received opioids within 4 hours of the birth (Wilson et al., 2015).

When naloxone is given, other resuscitative measures may be indicated, and trained personnel should be readily available. The duration of the medication's effect is shorter than that of the analgesic medication for which it is acting as an antagonist, so the nurse must be alert to the return of respiratory depression and the need for repeated doses. Naloxone should not be given to women with known or suspected opiate dependency because it may precipitate severe withdrawal (Wilson et al., 2015). Naloxone may be given to the newborn if needed after birth. The newborn dose is 0.1 mg/kg and may need to be repeated if respiratory effort remains abnormal.

Regional Anesthesia and Analgesia

Regional anesthesia is the temporary loss of sensation produced by injecting an anesthetic agent (called a *local*) into direct contact with nervous tissue. Loss of sensation happens because the local agents stabilize the cell membrane, which prevents initiation and transmission of nerve impulses. The regional anesthetic blocks most commonly used in childbirth include the epidural, the spinal, and combined epidural-spinal blocks, which can be used for both vaginal and cesarean births.

An epidural relieves pain associated with the first stage of labor by blocking the sensory nerves supplying the uterus. Pain associated with the second stage of labor and with birth can be

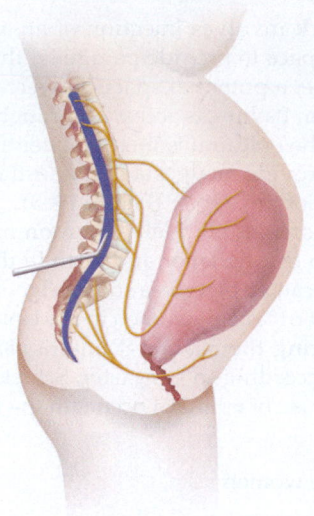
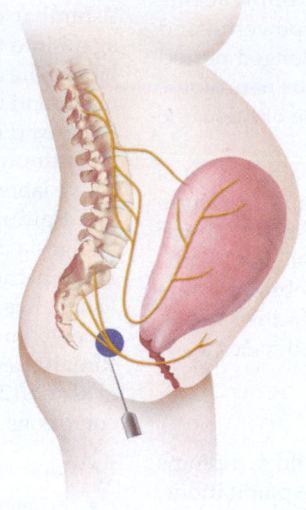
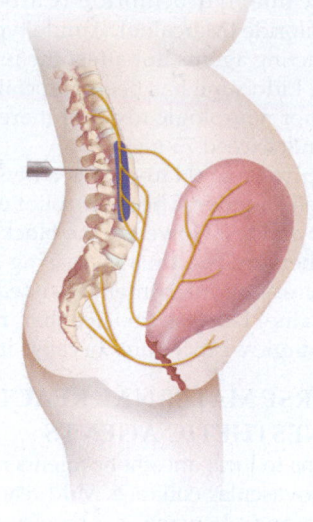

A   **B**   **C**

Figure 19–1 Schematic diagram showing pain pathways and sites of interruption. A. Lumbar sympathetic (spinal) block: relief of uterine pain only. B. Pudendal block: relief of perineal pain. C. Lumbar epidural block: dark area demonstrates peridural (epidural) space and nerves affected, and the gray tube represents a continuous plastic catheter.

alleviated with epidural, combined epidural-spinal, and pudendal blocks (see Figure 19–1).

Until recently, the same anesthetic agents used for regional epidurals were also used to produce **regional analgesia** (pain relief to a body region) during labor. The use of these agents produced undesirable side effects such as voiding difficulty, hypotension, reduced sensation in lower extremities, slowed fetal descent, and an increased risk of severe perineal lacerations. These effects occur in primigravida women more commonly when epidural anesthesia is used (Loewenberg-Weisband, Grisaru-Granovsky, Ioscovich, et al., 2014). In current practice, regional analgesia is now obtained by injecting an opioid such as fentanyl along with only a small amount of anesthetic agent. New medication combinations relieve the woman's pain while minimizing the side effects discussed above (Anderson & Stone, 2013).

The intrathecal injection of opioids results in another type of regional analgesia. In this case, the opioid is injected into the subarachnoid space. It is important for the anesthesia provider to provide a test dose before giving the entire dose to determine that the catheter is correctly placed. Fentanyl citrate and preservative-free morphine are the most commonly used medications. This typically results in more effective pain relief over the subsequent 24 hours after birth, although the incidence of nausea, pruritus, and urticaria may be increased in some women (Chestnut et al., 2014).

Nursing care during administration of regional analgesia is directed toward helping the woman void before administration, assisting her with positioning during and after the procedure, monitoring and assessing vital signs and respiratory status, monitoring analgesic effect, monitoring the fetus, and providing thorough explanations and reassurance to help decrease anxiety and fear. Additional measures may be needed to address pruritus, nausea and vomiting, and urinary retention.

As with other procedures, the woman needs to know how the block is given, the expected effect on her and the fetus, advantages and disadvantages, and possible complications.

Anesthetic Agents for Regional Blocks

Local anesthetic agents block the conduction of nerve impulses from the periphery to the central nervous system by preventing the propagation of an action potential from the source of pain (Chestnut et al., 2014). The types of nerve fibers are differentially sensitive to the various anesthetic agents. In general, the smaller the fiber, the more sensitive it is to local agents.

Absorption of local anesthetics depends primarily on the vascularity of the area of injection. The agents themselves contribute to increased blood flow by causing vasodilation. High concentrations of medications cause greater vasodilation. Good maternal physical condition or a high metabolic rate aids absorption. Malnutrition, dehydration, electrolyte imbalance, and cardiovascular and pulmonary problems increase the potential for toxic effects. The pH of tissues affects the rate of absorption, which has implications for fetal complications such as acidosis. The addition of vasoconstrictors such as epinephrine delays absorption and prolongs the anesthetic effect because vasoconstrictors decrease uteroplacental blood flow. The breakdown of local anesthetics in the body is accomplished by the liver and plasma esterase, and the resulting substance is eliminated by the kidneys. It is important to use the weakest concentration and the smallest amount necessary to produce the desired results.

Types of Local Anesthetic Agents

Two types of local anesthetic agents are currently available: esters and amides. The ester type includes procaine hydrochloride (Novocain), chloroprocaine hydrochloride (Nesacaine), and tetracaine hydrochloride (Pontocaine). Esters are rapidly metabolized; therefore, toxic maternal levels are not as likely to be reached, and placental transfer to the fetus is prevented. Ester-linked agents have a higher incidence of allergic reactions when compared with amides. However, they do not appear to have a higher incidence of fetal effects (Chestnut et al., 2014).

Amide types include lidocaine hydrochloride (Xylocaine), mepivacaine hydrochloride (Carbocaine), and bupivacaine hydrochloride (Marcaine). Amide types are more powerful and longer acting agents but affect the fetus for a prolonged period of time. Lidocaine has been associated with major neurologic and minor neurologic toxicity; therefore, the dose of lidocaine should not exceed 75 mg.

Ropivacaine (Naropin) is a new-generation amide that is also used in labor. The pain relief effects are similar to those of other amides. However, the blockade effect is slightly lower than other amides, thus increasing the rates of vaginal births and decreasing instrument-assisted births. Levobupivacaine (Chirocaine) has less toxicity than ropivacaine and is safer in longer surgical procedures because it has decreased toxicity.

ADVERSE MATERNAL REACTIONS TO ANESTHETIC AGENTS

Reactions to local anesthetic agents range from mild symptoms to cardiovascular collapse. Mild reactions include palpitations, tinnitus, apprehension, confusion, and a metallic taste in the mouth. Moderate reactions include more severe degrees of mild symptoms plus nausea and vomiting, hypotension, and muscle twitching, which may progress to convulsions. Severe reactions are sudden loss of consciousness, coma, severe hypotension, bradycardia, respiratory depression, and cardiac arrest. Anesthetic agents should not be used unless an intravenous line is in place.

The preferred treatment for a mild toxic reaction is administration of oxygen and IV injection of a short-acting barbiturate to diminish anxiety.

NEONATAL NEUROBEHAVIORAL EFFECTS OF ANESTHESIA AND ANALGESIA

Many studies have focused on the neurobehavioral effects on the newborn of pharmacologic agents used during labor and birth. Although analgesic and anesthetic agents may alter the behavioral and adaptive function of the newborn, physiologic factors such as hunger, degree of hydration, and time within the sleep–wake cycle may also exert an influence. Note that more neurologic impairment occurs in the newborn resulting from the normal birth process than from epidural complications.

Box 19–1 Acupressure and Manual and Electrical Stimulation as a Means to Reduce Epidural Use for Labor Pain

Acupressure with the addition of manual or electrical stimulation can reduce the risk of receiving epidural anesthesia in labor (Vixner, Schytt, Stener-Victorin, et al., 2014). The acupressure point for labor and birth is found in the webbing between the thumb and the index finger. This point should never be stimulated during pregnancy because it stimulates uterine contractions. The mother places her right thumb on the back of her left hand and her right index finger on the front of the left hand at the acupressure point. She can rub the point to stimulate labor and squeeze the point to decrease labor pain. Another acupressure point is found between the inner ankle bone and the Achilles tendon. Squeezing for 1 minute on each ankle reduces labor pain. Electrical stimulation of these sites can also be used. While these methods did not show a reduction in labor pain itself, it did reduce epidural use.

Epidural Block

A lumbar **epidural block** involves injection of an anesthetic agent into the epidural space to provide pain relief throughout labor. The epidural space, a potential space between the dura mater and the ligamentum flavum, is accessed through the lumbar area (Figure 19–2). The epidural is most frequently used as a continuous block to provide analgesia and anesthesia from active labor through episiotomy repair (Figure 19–3).

Epidurals have become a relatively common method of analgesia and anesthesia during labor and birth in the United States because epidurals can be placed as soon as labor is established. It is estimated that 61% of all women in the United States receive an epidural during their labor (Rimaitis, Klimenko, Rimaitis, et al., 2015). According to Lancaster, Schick, Osman, et al., (2012), the highest use of epidural occurs in the following conditions:

- Non-Hispanic White women
- Foreign-born Asian women
- Induced labors
- Maternal smoking

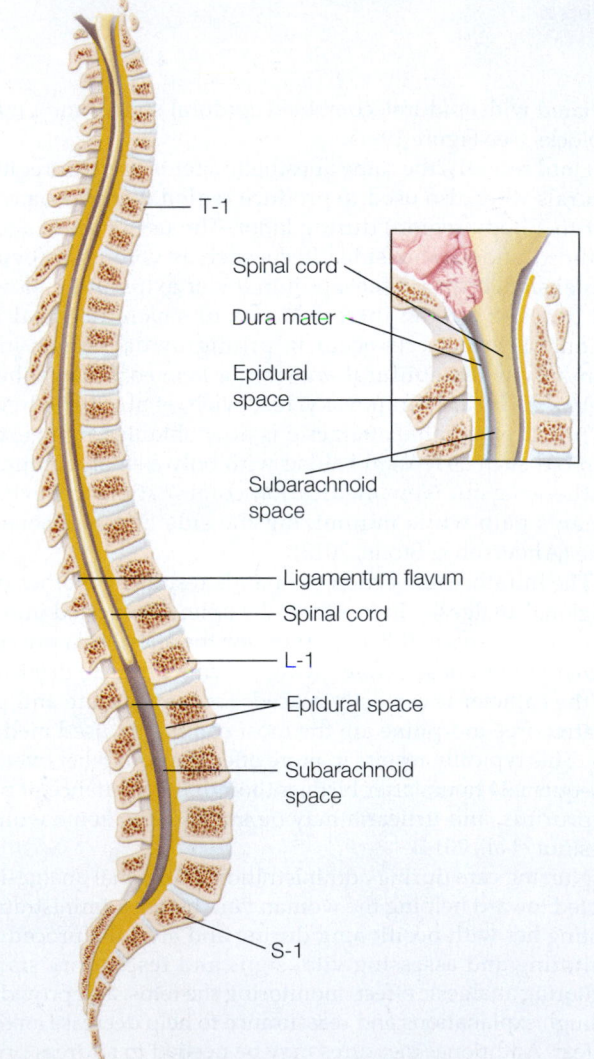

Figure 19–2 The epidural space lies between the dura mater and the ligamentum flavum, extending from the base of the skull to the end of the sacral canal.

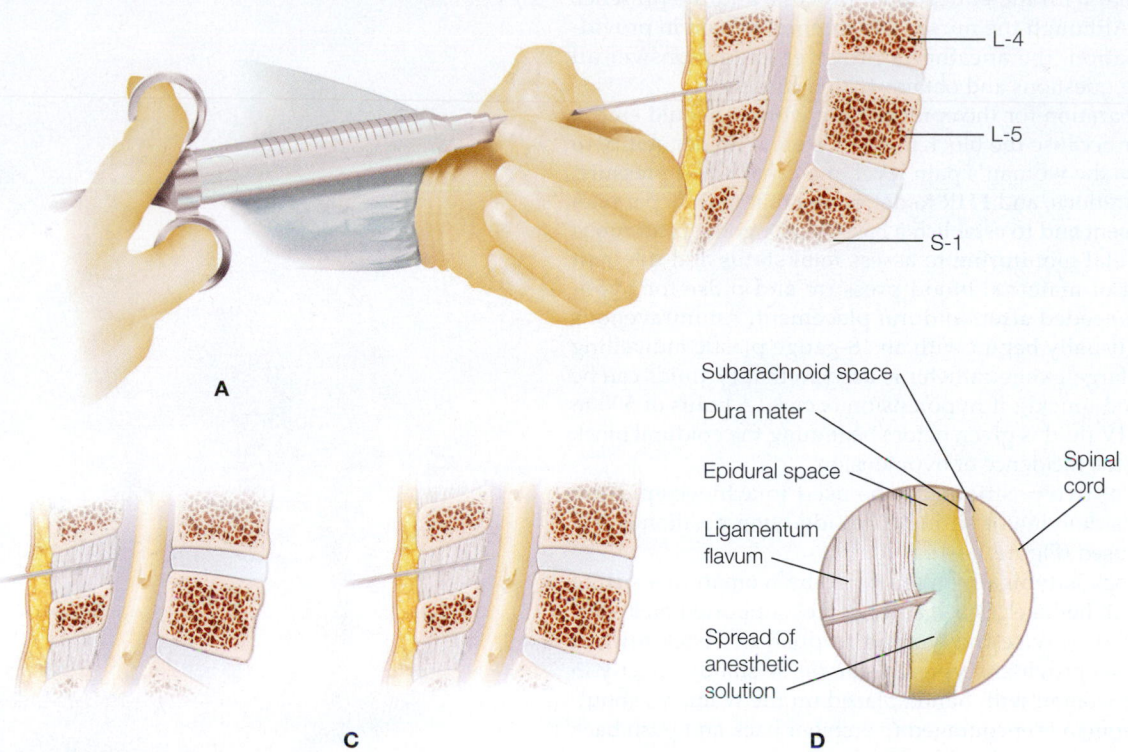

Figure 19–3 Technique for lumbar epidural block. A. Proper position for insertion. B. Needle in the ligamentum flavum. C. Tip of needle in epidural space. D. Force of injection pushing dura away from tip of needle.

- Higher educational achievement
- Giving birth in secondary or tertiary perinatal units, urban hospitals, or for-profit hospitals

As the childbearing population is becoming older, many pregnant women have various high-risk medical conditions. Some of these conditions create additional risk factors for the woman undergoing epidural anesthesia. Risk factors that warrant increased observation include maternal obesity, asthma, obstructive sleep apnea, cardiac disease, coagulopathy, spinal cord injuries, substance abuse, and women with a history of liver disease (Wong, 2014).

ADVANTAGES

The epidural block relieves discomfort during labor and birth, and the woman is fully awake and a part of the birth process. Epidural anesthesia results in fewer adverse fetal effects when compared with intravenous analgesia or general anesthesia. It can also allow the woman to rest and regain strength before she needs to push during the second stage. The continuous epidural allows different blocking for each stage of labor, so that the fetus is able to descend and rotate in the maternal pelvis; many times the woman's urge to bear down is preserved. Epidurals that combine anesthesia and an opioid agent are often effective in providing postoperative pain relief for longer periods of time.

Opioids are used with epidural blocks for labor. Some of the agents used include morphine and fentanyl (Chestnut et al., 2014). When only opioids are used epidurally, rather than in combination with another type of agent, the amount of pain relief is not as effective, especially toward the end of labor; therefore, a combination of opioids and a low dose of local anesthesia is given (Chestnut et al., 2014).

DISADVANTAGES

The most common complication of an epidural block is maternal hypotension, which is generally prevented by administering intravenous fluid before epidural placement, left uterine displacement, and maternal positioning on her side. In some instances, labor progress and fetal descent may be slowed, and pushing efforts in the second stage may be less effective because of a decrease in sensation. There appears to be an increase in forceps or vacuum use related to epidural anesthesia (King, Brucker, & Krebs, 2015). Delay in return of bladder sensation may result in urinary retention and the need for catheterization during labor and in the fourth stage (King et al., 2015). Low back pain can also occur after an epidural and is usually more common in women who have undergone vaginal deliveries. Women with a history of prepregnancy back pain or back surgery tend to have less relief with an epidural (Wong, 2014). Typically, epidurals do not cause chronic low back pain, although the woman can have soreness at the insertion site for a few days.

CONTRAINDICATIONS

The absolute contraindications for epidural block are client refusal, infection at the site of the needle puncture, maternal problems with blood coagulation (coagulopathies), raised intracranial pressure, specific medication allergy to the agent being used, and hypovolemic shock (King et al., 2015).

Nursing Management

Education and assessment of the woman's understanding of epidural block is essential. Before providing information, determine the woman's current knowledge and evaluate factors related to learning, such as the mother's education level, primary language spoken, the presence of any disabilities that may interfere with the educational process, and the presence of anxiety. Although the nurse is an integral person in providing information, the anesthesia provider should answer all outstanding questions and obtain written consent.

In preparation for the epidural, the woman should empty her bladder because the block may interfere with her ability to void. Assess the woman's pain level, maternal blood pressure, pulse, respirations, and FHR to determine that normal parameters are present and to establish a baseline. Ongoing continuous electronic fetal monitoring to assess fetal status and frequent monitoring of maternal blood pressure and pulse for hypotension are needed after epidural placement. An intravenous infusion is usually begun with an 18-gauge plastic indwelling catheter. A large-gauge catheter is used so that IV fluids can be administered quickly if hypotension occurs. A bolus of 500 to 1000 mL of IV fluid is given before beginning the epidural block to decrease the incidence of hypotension.

Either of two positions can be used to achieve epidural placement: side-lying or sitting. The side-lying position is less commonly used (Figure 19–4).

The block is typically given with the woman in a sitting position, with her back flexed and her feet supported on a stool (Figure 19–5). Advise the woman to push her back toward the anesthesia provider. Typically, the nurse stands directly in front of the woman with hands placed on the woman's shoulders. The woman is encouraged to arch her back and push back toward the analgesia provider. After positioning, continue to provide support and try to ensure that the woman does not move during the procedure. After the needle and catheter are placed, assist the woman into a reclining position.

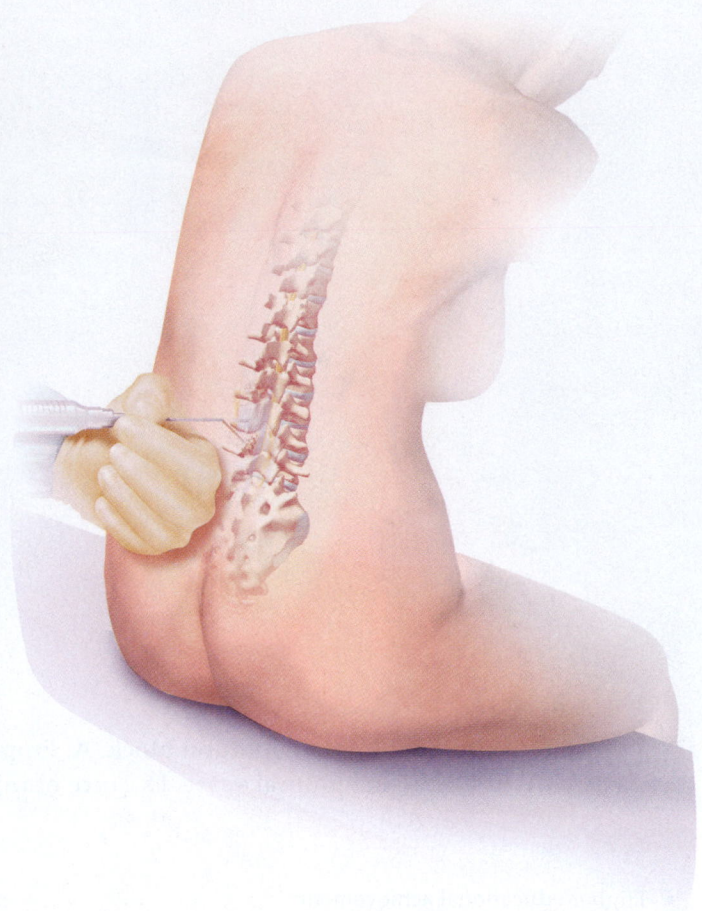

Figure 19–5 Correct sitting position for woman having an epidural anesthesia block: shoulders rolled forward and back exposed for needle insertion.

Clinical Tip

Advise the woman to identify when uterine contractions are occurring. Tell her that you will monitor contractions and will notify the anesthesia provider when a contraction is starting. Reassure her that the anesthesiologist will administer the injection between contractions when she is comfortable. Provide encouragement and reposition the woman as needed after a contraction occurs, since it is common for the woman to slouch during intense uterine contractions.

Clinical Tip

Frequent position changes from one side to the other facilitate proper rotation and assist with fetal descent.

Assess maternal vital signs frequently per protocol until the block wears off. Blood pressure can be monitored by a mechanical blood pressure device or directly by the nurse. Record vital signs in the medical record. Encourage the woman to maintain a side-lying position to maximize uteroplacental blood flow and to change her position (from side to side) frequently to increase

circulation, promote comfort, and avoid a one-sided block. Assess the woman's ability to lift her legs and her level of sensation every 30 minutes to monitor the effects of the nerve block.

Palpate the woman's bladder for distention at frequent intervals because the epidural block decreases the urge to urinate. During the second stage of labor, the woman with an epidural block may need assistance with pushing. This is best achieved when the bladder is emptied since a full bladder can interfere with fetal descent. Utilize a catheter if needed to empty the woman's bladder prior to pushing. You may need to tell the woman when contractions begin and give extra assistance by holding her legs during pushing efforts. The woman's legs need to be protected from pressure applied to them while sensation is diminished. If the woman has little or no control of her legs, her legs need bilateral support and should be placed on the bed between contractions. Some providers may use stirrups to avoid injury.

The most common side effect of epidural regional block is hypotension. See *Nursing Care Plan: For Epidural Anesthesia.*

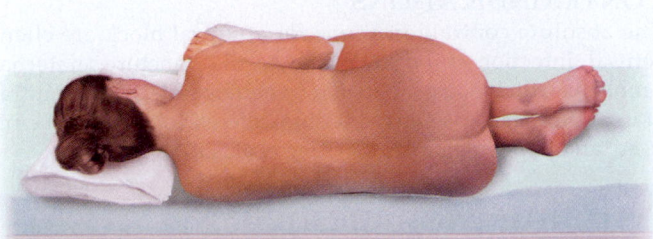

Figure 19–4 Correct maternal side-lying position for epidural anesthesia block placement. The back is straight and vertical, the shoulders are square, and the upper leg is prevented from rolling forward.

Nursing Care Plan: For Epidural Anesthesia

1. Nursing Diagnosis: *Injury, Risk for,* related to maternal hypotension associated with epidural anesthesia secondary to vasodilation and venous pooling (NANDA I © 2014)

GOAL: Maternal and fetal effects associated with hypotension will be minimized.

INTERVENTION	RATIONALE
• Obtain baseline maternal vital signs and fetal heart rate.	• Normal ranges include temperature 98 to 99.6°F/36.6 to 37.5°C, pulse 60 to 90, respirations 14 to 22/min, blood pressure 90–140/60–90, fetal heart rate 110 to 160 beats/min.
• Insert IV with large-gauge catheter.	• Allows for IV fluid to be administered quickly if hypotension occurs.
• Provide hydration with 500 to 1000 mL of intravenous solution (e.g., lactated Ringer solution) 15 to 30 min before procedure. Dextrose-free solution is recommended.	• Increases intravascular volume and maintains cardiac output by preloading the patient before epidural anesthesia. Rapid infusion of dextrose solution can cause fetal hyperglycemia and rebound neonatal hypoglycemia.
• Educate the patient about treatment measures to expect if unwanted side effects from the epidural occur.	• Advance preparation will decrease anxiety and the patient will be more compliant. Treatment measures include oxygen administration, increase of IV fluids, possible administration of a vasopressor such as ephedrine, and repositioning the patient.
• Assist the patient into position for the procedure.	• Place patient in a supine position for 5 to 10 min following administration of block to allow medication to diffuse bilaterally. After 5 to 10 min, position patient on side.
• Monitor blood pressure every 1 to 2 min for the first 10 min, then every 5 to 15 min until the block wears off.	• Hypotension is the most common side effect of epidural anesthesia. Close monitoring will allow for quick assessment and treatment of any changes from baseline blood pressure before the procedure.

EXPECTED OUTCOMES: Decrease in blood pressure is identified and treated successfully.

• Observe, record, and report symptoms of hypotension, including systolic pressure <100 mmHg or a 20% to 30% fall in systolic pressure, apprehension, restlessness, dizziness, tinnitus, and headache.	• These signs are related to hypotension and must be treated immediately to avoid health risk to mother and fetus.

EXPECTED OUTCOMES: Hypotension is identified and treatment measures started.

• Initiate treatment measures to reverse hypotension.	• Treatment measures include placing patient in left lateral position as directed, increase IV rate, administer oxygen by face mask at 7 to 10 L/min as needed, administer vasopressors as ordered (usually ephedrine 5 to 10 mg IV), manually displace uterus laterally to left using a wedge or pillow. Notify analgesia provider or certified nurse anesthetist immediately.

EXPECTED OUTCOMES: Hypotension is treated successfully, and blood pressure returns to normal limits.

• Observe, record, and report fetal bradycardia (FHR less than 110 beats/min) and loss of beat-to-beat variability.	• Maternal hypotension results in decreased blood flow to the fetus.
	• Normal fetal heart rate ranges between 110 and 160 beats/min. (Fetal bradycardia occurs when the fetal heart rate falls below 110 beats/min during a 10-min period of continuous monitoring. When fetal bradycardia is accompanied by decreased variability, it is considered ominous and could be a sign of fetal compromise.)

EXPECTED OUTCOMES: Treatment of maternal hypotension increases blood flow to the fetus, reversing fetal bradycardia. Fetal heart rate stays within normal limits with variability.

The epidural may cause elevation of maternal temperature (pyrexia). Pyrexia may be confused with maternal infection and frequently results in additional testing of the newborn to rule out infection (Gabbe et al., 2012).

Headache (which may occur with spinal blocks) is not a side effect of epidural anesthesia because the dura mater of the spinal canal has not been penetrated and there is no leakage of spinal fluid. Motor control of the legs is weak but not totally absent after birth. Return of complete sensation and the ability to control the legs are essential before ambulation is attempted. Recovery may take several hours, depending on the anesthetic agent and the dose given.

To assess sensation, touch various parts of the woman's legs and abdomen bilaterally to determine if the touch can be felt. Evaluate motor control by asking the woman to raise her knees, to lift her feet (one at a time) off the bed, or to dorsiflex her foot. Even though assessments may indicate that sensation and motor control have returned, be ready to support the woman's weight as she stands and quickly return her to bed if motor control is inadequate. In addition, blood pressure assessments will help to determine the safety of ambulation. Assess blood pressure while the woman is lying down, then sitting in the bed. As long as blood pressure values remain stable (no evidence of orthostatic hypotension), a standing blood pressure is assessed. To maintain safety, it is advisable to have additional assistance when the woman stands for the first time.

Women With Special Needs Spinal Cord Injury

Women with a spinal cord injury may be prone to autonomic dysreflexia, which is the most significant medical complication, especially when their injury is above T5 through T6 level. This condition is attributed to a loss of hypothalamic control of sympathetic spinal reflexes and occurs in clients with viable spinal cord segments distal to the level of injury. Epidural anesthesia is recommended as a means to decrease autonomic dysreflexia and should be introduced early in labor to reduce the incidence of this complication.

Continuous Epidural Infusion

Epidural anesthesia may be given with a continuous infusion pump. Some of the benefits include good to excellent analgesia, infrequent nausea, minimal sedation, decreased anxiety, earlier mobilization, retained cough reflex, decreased risk of deep vein thrombosis, decreased myocardial oxygen demand, and ease of administration. A continuous infusion reduces the use of bolus dosages, which may provide intermittent pain control.

SAFETY ALERT!

Ease of epidural administration should not imply lack of need for close observation. Malfunctioning equipment with subsequent overdose is always a possibility. Infusion pumps designed specifically for use in epidural anesthesia have safety factors incorporated into them. Continuous epidural infusions should be administered with the same precautions used for intermittent injections.

Some of the potential problems of epidural infusions include breakthrough pain, sedation, nausea and vomiting, pruritus, and hypotension. When complications or adverse effects

occur, the analgesia care provider should be notified. Some side effects may be treated with standing orders; however, the provider should still be notified. Breakthrough pain may occur at any time but usually occurs when the infusion rate is below the recommended therapeutic dose. It may also occur when there is a pump or epidural line malfunction. When breakthrough pain occurs, the nurse checks the integrity of the epidural infusion line, checks the pump settings, and notifies the analgesia provider. There may be standing orders for a bolus dose of medication. In rare circumstances, the epidural itself may need to be replaced.

Some women may experience *hot spots*, or areas of incomplete anesthesia coverage. Nursing interventions include position changes. If the hot spot becomes too uncomfortable, an anesthesia provider can administer additional medication. In some cases, the epidural will need to be replaced.

General sedation and resulting respiratory depression may occur from the systemic effect of the epidural agents as they are absorbed into the circulation. The respiratory rate, along with the quality of respirations, should be assessed no less frequently than every 15 to 30 minutes. The nurse should notify the anesthetist of any significant decreases in respiratory rate or respiratory pattern change. If the respiratory rate decreases below 12 respirations per minute, naloxone may be given to counteract the effect of the anesthetic agent; typically respirations then return to a normal rate.

Nausea and vomiting can occur at any time and can be treated with an antiemetic. Nausea and vomiting can make the woman very uncomfortable, and the infusion rate of the epidural may need to be decreased or terminated to alleviate this discomfort. Nausea and vomiting can sometimes occur as a result of transition rather than as a direct side effect of the epidural infusion.

Pruritus (itching and rash) may occur at any time during the epidural infusion. It usually appears first on the face, neck, or torso and is usually the result of the agent in the epidural infusion. Treatment generally involves administration of diphenhydramine hydrochloride (Benadryl). The epidural infusion may need to be decreased or terminated.

Hypotension may occur from hypovolemia or from the effect of the epidural. Treatment involves administering oxygen by mask, administering a bolus of crystalloid fluid, and notifying the anesthetist. Usually standing orders for treatment of hypotension are graded in terms of the degree of hypotension. The epidural infusion may have to be terminated and the woman placed in the Trendelenburg position.

Epidural Opioid Analgesia After Birth

To provide analgesia for approximately 24 hours after the birth, the analgesia provider may inject an opioid, such as morphine sulfate (Duramorph) or fentanyl (Sublimaze), into the epidural space immediately after the birth. The analgesic effect begins approximately 30 to 60 minutes after the injection. The side effects include pruritus, nausea and vomiting, and urinary retention (Wilson et al., 2015). The onset seems to occur early, and it resolves within 14 to 16 hours after the birth.

Spinal Block

In a **spinal block**, a local anesthetic agent is injected directly into the spinal fluid in the spinal canal to provide anesthesia for cesarean birth and occasionally for vaginal birth. This technique involves passing through the epidural space and dura mater and injecting the medication directly into the cerebral spinal

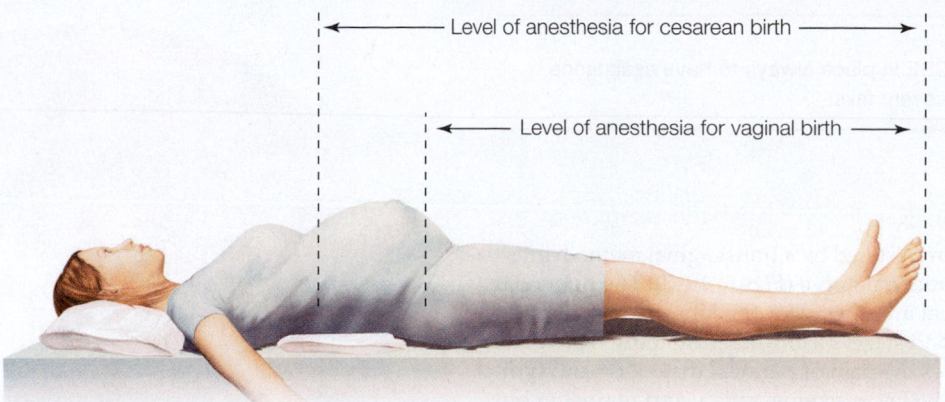

← Level of anesthesia for cesarean birth →

← Level of anesthesia for vaginal birth →

Figure 19–6 Levels of spinal anesthesia for vaginal and cesarean births.

fluid. The technique of administration varies depending on whether the spinal block is being given for a cesarean or vaginal birth (Figure 19–6).

ADVANTAGES

The advantages of spinal block are immediate onset of anesthesia, relative ease of administration, a need for smaller medication volume, and maternal compartmentalization of the medication. This approach is favored when an emergency cesarean birth is rapidly needed and anesthesia is immediately warranted.

DISADVANTAGES

The primary disadvantage of spinal block is blockade of sympathetic nerve fibers, resulting in a high incidence of hypotension, which can alter the fetal heart rate and result in fetal hypoxia. In addition, uterine tone is maintained, which makes intrauterine manipulation difficult.

CONTRAINDICATIONS

Contraindications for spinal block include severe hypovolemia, infection over the puncture site, sepsis, coagulation problems, and client refusal (Suresh, Segal, Preston, et al., 2013).

Nursing Management

If an intravenous infusion is not already in place, it is started with a 16- to 18-gauge plastic catheter. A bolus of 500 to 1000 mL is infused rapidly. Assess maternal vital signs, pain level, and the FHR to establish a baseline and then position the woman in a sitting (or a side-lying) position. The woman sits on the side of the bed or operating room table and places her feet on a stool. She places her arms between her knees or up around your shoulders, places her head to her chest, and arches her back to widen the intervertebral spaces. Support the woman in this position and palpate the uterus to identify the beginning of uterine contractions (if labor is present). The analgesia provider injects the anesthetic agent between contractions. If the anesthetic agent is injected during a contraction, the level of anesthesia obtained is higher and may compromise respirations.

The woman remains in a sitting position for 30 seconds and then returns to a lying position, with a rolled towel or blanket under her right hip to displace the uterus from the vena cava. Monitor maternal blood pressure and pulse frequently per protocol or physician's order. The blood pressure is also reassessed when the woman is moved after birth because movement may lower blood pressure.

If the spinal block is being used during vaginal birth, monitor uterine contractions and instruct the woman to bear down during a contraction. The block may reduce the woman's ability to push, although the new combinations of medications tend to decrease this side effect. Sometimes, the birth may be assisted with forceps or vacuum extractor (see Chapter 22).

After birth, the temporary motor paralysis of the woman's legs continues. Exercise caution when moving the woman from the birthing bed (or operating room table) to protect her from injury. The woman remains in bed for 6 to 12 hours following the block; she may not regain sensation and control of her bladder for 8 to 12 hours and may need to be catheterized. An indwelling bladder catheter is usually inserted before surgery for women undergoing cesarean birth.

The epidural or spinal catheter is removed by either you or an analgesia provider. Remove the tape used to secure the block. Then grasp the catheter between your fingers and slowly remove with gentle traction. Inspect the catheter to ensure the tip did not break off. Place a bandage or gauze and tape over the site. It is not unusual for a small amount of bleeding to occur initially upon removal. Continuous bleeding warrants a call to the anesthesia provider. Document removal of the catheter and any adverse effects in the medical record.

Combined Spinal–Epidural Block

Spinal anesthesia may be combined with an epidural block. The combined spinal–epidural (CSE) block can be used for labor analgesia and for cesarean birth. The anesthetic and analgesic agents used differ according to the purpose of the CSE block. A CSE is accomplished by inserting an epidural needle into the epidural space. A narrow-gauge atraumatic (24- to 27-gauge pencil point) needle is inserted through the epidural needle, through the dura, and into the cerebral spinal fluid. A small amount of local anesthetic agent, opioid, or both is injected, and the atraumatic needle is withdrawn. An epidural catheter is then threaded through the epidural needle and into the epidural space. The epidural needle is removed, and the epidural catheter is secured.

An advantage of CSE block is that the spinal (intrathecal) anesthetic and/or analgesic agent has a faster onset than medications that are injected into the epidural space. Most medications are used in low dose, so spinal analgesia may be given in early labor to assist in alleviating labor pain. The epidural is activated when active labor begins. Another advantage of a CSE block is that laboring women can ambulate after the CSE is placed.

Pudendal Block

A **pudendal block**, administered by a transvaginal method, intercepts signals to the pudendal nerve (Figure 19–7). The pudendal block provides perineal anesthesia for the latter part of the first stage of labor, the second stage, birth, and episiotomy repair. The pudendal block relieves the pain of perineal distention and typically relieves pain in the lower vagina, vulva, and perineum but not the discomfort of uterine contractions (King et al., 2015).

Advantages of the pudendal block are ease of administration and absence of maternal hypotension. It also may be used to decrease the discomfort of low forceps or vacuum-assisted birth. Because a pudendal block does not alter maternal vital signs or FHR, additional assessments are not necessary. The nurse explains the procedure and answers any questions.

The disadvantages of the pudendal block include possible broad ligament hematoma, perforation of the rectum, and trauma to the sciatic nerve. A moderate dose of anesthetic agent has minimal ill effects on the course of labor, but the urge to push may decrease.

Local Infiltration Anesthesia

Local infiltration anesthesia is accomplished by injecting an anesthetic agent into the intracutaneous, subcutaneous, and intramuscular areas of the perineum (Figure 19–8). It is generally used at the time of birth, in preparation for an episiotomy

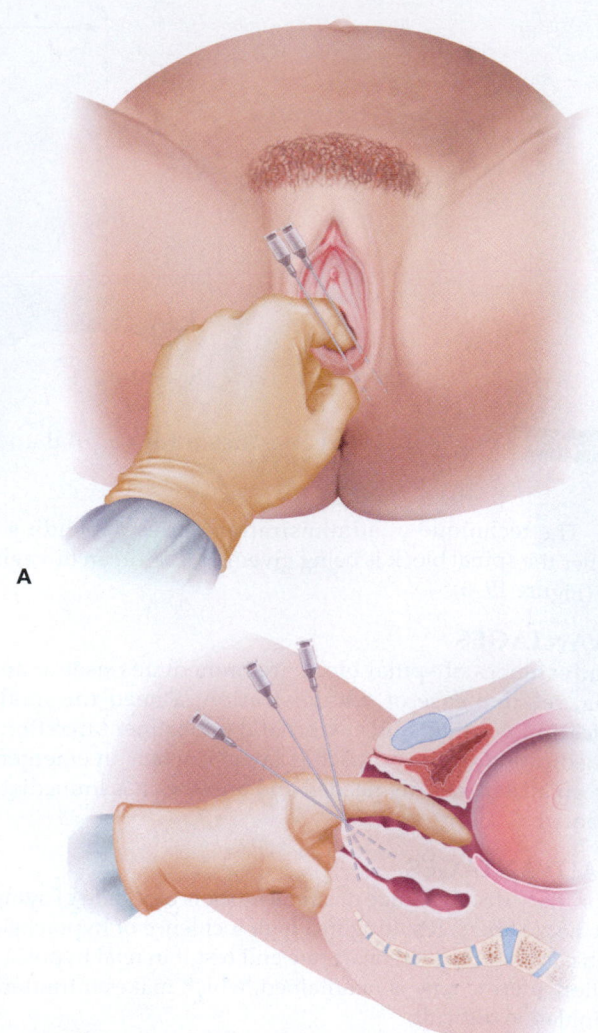

B

Figure 19–8 Local infiltration anesthesia. A. Technique of local infiltration for episiotomy and repair. B. Technique of local infiltration showing fan pattern for the fascial planes.

and for the repair of lacerations or an episiotomy. Women who have followed some type of prepared childbirth method and want minimal analgesia and anesthesia usually do not object to local anesthesia for the episiotomy or laceration repair. The administration procedure is technically uncomplicated and is practically free from complications.

A disadvantage of local infiltration is that large amounts of local anesthetic must be used to infuse the tissues. Although any local anesthetic may be used, chloroprocaine hydrochloride (Nesacaine), lidocaine hydrochloride (Xylocaine), tetracaine hydrochloride (Pontocaine), and mepivacaine hydrochloride (Carbocaine) are the agents of choice because of their capacity for diffusion. Because local anesthetic agents have no effect on maternal vital signs or FHR, additional assessments are unnecessary.

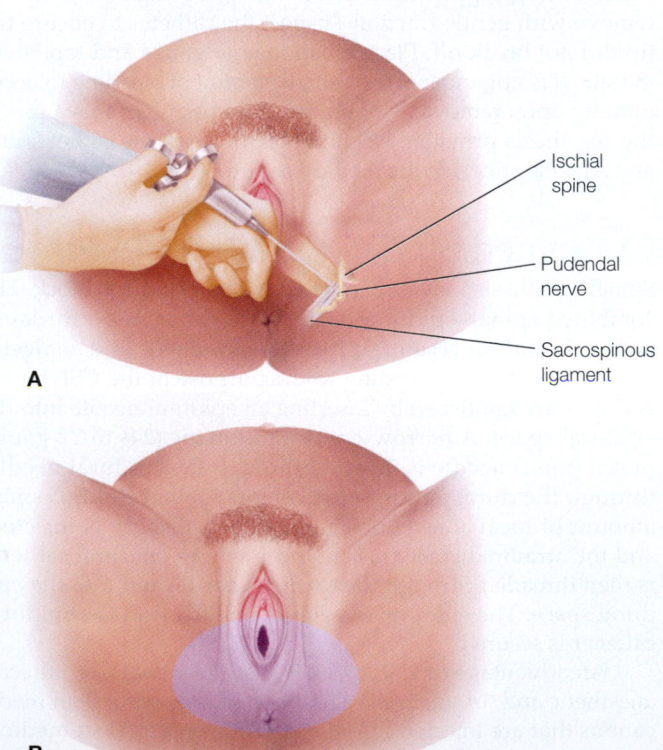

Ischial spine

Pudendal nerve

Sacrospinous ligament

A

B

Figure 19–7 Pudendal block. A. Pudendal block by the transvaginal approach. B. Area of perineum affected by pudendal block.

Inhalation Nitrous Oxide

While inhalation nitrous oxide is widely used in other Western countries, its use remains limited in the United States. The nitrous oxide used in labor is 50% nitrous oxide and

50% oxygen. At this titration, it is considered an analgesic and not an anesthetic agent. Nitrous oxide gas is self-administered by the laboring woman. When she begins to feel a contraction, the gas is inhaled through a face mask. Effects are usually felt within 30 seconds and the mask is then removed upon completion of the contraction.

Nitrous oxide offers several advantages over other forms of analgesia and anesthesia. The gas is quick to provide relief and dissipates quickly when the facial mask is removed. It gives the woman complete control in deciding to use the agent. Some women may use it with every contraction while others may use it periodically as a coping tool. Epidural and systematic medications can take hours to wear off, whereas nitrous oxide dissipates with several deep breaths of room air. The gas is also easier to administer and does not require the skilled training required of an anesthesiologist but instead can be administered by nurses or midwives. Like systemic agents, nitrous oxide gas does not provide complete pain relief, but it does take the edge off pain. For women who desire complete pain relief, the epidural will likely remain the gold standard. Nitrous oxide can be provided at a fraction of the cost of epidural anesthesia and narcotic agents.

Side effects from nitrous oxide are rare but may include drowsiness, dizziness, or nausea. Because the medication is filtered through the lungs, rather than the liver, it is safer for the fetus and does not appear to affect fetal heart rate or the mother's blood pressure.

Nursing Management

Advise the woman of the possible side effects and potential benefits of using nitrous oxide as a means of pain relief. Explain that if the gas is not effective, or if stronger medication is desired, an epidural can be placed. Instruct the woman on proper use of the mask, including when to apply it and when to remove it. Advise her to report any side effects, to avoid ambulation, and to call the nurse for assistance if she wishes to get out of bed. Continue to monitor maternal vital signs and fetal heart rate throughout labor to assess maternal and fetal well-being.

While nitrous oxide used intermittently will have no effect on a woman's respiratory or cardiovascular systems, pulse oximetry is recommended with continuous use or when nitrous oxide is used in conjunction with narcotic agents (Collins, Starr, Bishop, et al., 2012).

General Anesthesia

Rarely, **general anesthesia** (induced unconsciousness) is used for emergency cesarean birth or if epidural anesthesia is contraindicated for a cesarean birth. The method used to achieve general anesthesia is usually a combination of intravenous injection and inhalation of anesthetic agents. Maternal complications include difficulty in maternal intubation resulting in vomiting and aspiration, increased blood loss due to uterine relaxation, and possible memory loss in the early postpartum period (Gabbe, Niebyl, Galan, et al., 2012).

A common fetal complication is fetal depression, which is directly proportional to the depth and duration of the anesthesia. Babies born to mothers who have received general anesthesia have lower 1-minute Apgar scores and a higher incidence of metabolic acidosis than those who are given regional anesthesia for an emergency cesarean birth (King et al., 2015). General anesthesia is not advocated when the fetus is considered to be at high risk, particularly in preterm birth.

Nursing Management

Because pregnancy results in decreased gastric motility, and the onset of labor halts the process almost entirely, food eaten hours earlier may remain undigested in the stomach. It is important to find out when the laboring woman last ate and record this information in the medical record. Even when food and fluids have been withheld, the gastric juice produced during fasting is highly acidic and can cause chemical pneumonitis if aspirated. Prophylactic antacid therapy to reduce the acidic content of the stomach before general anesthesia is common practice. A nonparticulate antacid (such as sodium citrate/citric acid), H2-receptor antagonists (such as cimetidine [Tagamet] or famotidine [Pepsid]), or the use of prokinetic medications (such as metoclopramide), may also help empty gastric contents.

Before induction of anesthesia, the following interventions should be performed:

- Placement of a wedge under the woman's right hip
- Administration of 100% oxygen for 3 to 5 minutes
- Immediate administration of intravenous fluids
- Provision of client education and reassurance.

During the process of rapid induction of anesthesia, apply cricoid pressure to occlude the esophagus and prevent possible aspiration; the esophagus is occluded by applying 1 to 2 kg before the loss of consciousness and increasing that to 2 to 4 kg after the induction of anesthesia. The amount of pressure applied is critical because too much pressure can result in difficulty in performing a successful intubation. Too little pressure can result in aspiration. Cricoid pressure is maintained until the anesthesia provider has placed the endotracheal tube and indicates that the pressure can be released. Figure 19–9 shows the appropriate technique.

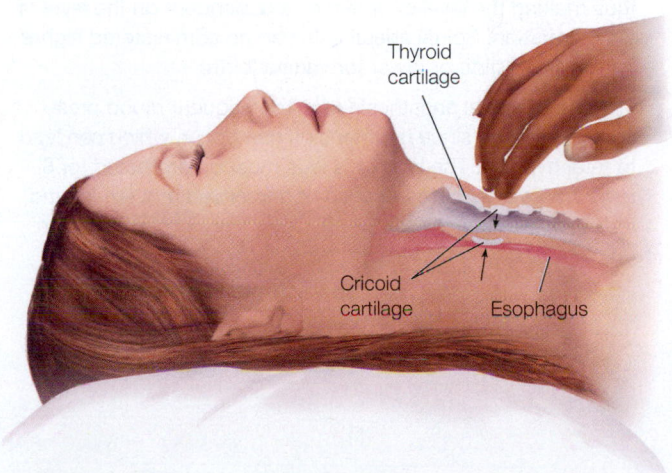

Thyroid cartilage

Cricoid cartilage

Esophagus

Figure 19–9 Cricoid pressure technique. Proper position for fingers in applying cricoid pressure until a cuffed endotracheal tube is placed by the analgesia provider or certified nurse-anesthetist. The cricoid cartilage is depressed 2 to 3 cm posteriorly so that the esophagus is occluded.

Focus Your Study

- The goal of systemic analgesia is to provide maximum pain relief with minimum risk to the mother and the fetus after cervical dilatation has occurred and maternal and fetal vital signs are stable.

- Systemic drug administration may cause fetal respiratory depression at birth if given too late in labor. Naloxone (Narcan) should be available at birth to treat respiratory depression in the newborn.

- Epidural anesthesia is an injectable anesthetic agent whose administration requires a preload intravenous bolus with a crystalloid solution that then results in little to no sensation below the uterus.

- Because of the numbness caused by epidural anesthesia, reduced pushing during the second stage and inability to urinate may occur. Urinary catheterization may be needed to facilitate bladder emptying as a result of a reduction in sensation.

- Women receiving epidural anesthesia require frequent blood pressure monitoring along with monitoring when a position change occurs to detect hypotension, a side effect that can lead to fetal hypoxia. Evaluation of motor and sensory sensation is also required.

- Continuous epidural anesthesia provides effective pain relief and is usually associated with less nausea and a greater ability to cough, although it is sometimes associated with breakthrough pain, sedation, itching, hypotension, and respiratory depression.

- Spinal blocks utilize a local anesthetic agent that is injected directly into the spinal column resulting in immediate onset, thus making the level of anesthesia dependent on the level of administration. Spinal anesthesia can be administered higher for cesarean birth or lower for vaginal birth.

- The use of spinal anesthesia requires frequent blood pressure monitoring since hypotension can occur, which can lead to fetal hypoxia. The woman's legs must be protected for 8 to 12 hours after birth because of decreased movement and reduced sensation.

- Women receiving spinal anesthesia typically have an indwelling urinary catheter due to decreased bladder sensation and tone.

- A pudendal block uses a local anesthesia at the end of labor that is directly injected into the pudendal nerve to produce anesthesia to the lower vagina, vulva, and perineum without having any effect on the labor or the fetus.

- Pudendal blocks can be associated with several complications including hematoma, perforation of the rectum, and trauma to the sciatic nerve.

- Local infiltration anesthesia is typically injected in laboring women prior to birth if an episiotomy is anticipated or for the repair of a laceration or episiotomy after birth.

- Local infiltration requires large amounts of anesthetic and provides pain relief only at the site of insertion and has no maternal or fetal side effects.

- Regional anesthesia, either spinal or epidural, is associated with maternal hypotension, bladder distention, less ability to effectively push in second stage, higher perineal laceration rates, and possible neurologic damage.

- While spinal anesthesia can result in a severe headache, epidural anesthesia can result in an elevated maternal temperature.

- Nitrous oxide is used to provide pain relief without compromising maternal or fetal well-being. The use of nitrous oxide is slowly increasing in the United States but it is used often in other countries with positive maternal satisfaction.

- General anesthesia for obstetric use is rare; however, its use necessitates a variety of interventions including obtaining a history of last oral consumption; administering prescribed medications, such as antacids; placing a wedge under the mother's right hip; providing oxygen prior to the start of surgery; ensuring patent intravenous access; and possible assistance to the anesthesia provider in applying cricoid pressure during endotracheal tube placement.

- General anesthesia can result in fetal depression, uterine relaxation, vomiting, and aspiration.

Clinical Reasoning in Action

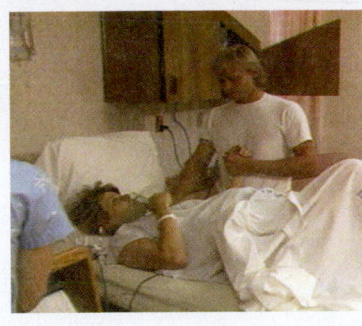

Sandra, a 26-year-old G1P0, is in active labor when she presents to you at the birthing center. She has been in labor for 5 hours and is clearly tired and seems to be having difficulty coping with the pain. Her contractions are occurring every 2 to 4 minutes lasting 50 to 60 seconds, and are moderate to strong in intensity. You assess the fetal heart rate of 120 to 130 beats/min with early decelerations; moderate variability is present. Sandra's vital signs are stable and her laboratory results are within normal limits. She is requesting an epidural analgesia for pain control. A vaginal examination demonstrates the cervix is 100% effaced, 6 cm dilated with the vertex at 0 station in the left occiput transverse (LOT) position. You notify the physician of Sandra's wish for pain relief and labor progress. You review the client's record for written consent for regional analgesia and assist the anesthesia provider with the procedure.

1. Discuss the advantages of regional analgesia.
2. Describe the nursing responsibility during the administration of regional analgesia.
3. Discuss the side effects of regional analgesia.
4. What are the absolute contraindications for an epidural block?
5. How do you assist Sandra with the second stage of labor when she cannot feel her contractions?

References

Anderson, B. A., & Stone, S. E. (2013). *Best practices in midwifery: Using the evidence to implement care.* New York, NY: Springer Publishing Company.

Blackburn, S. T. (2013). *Maternal, fetal, & neonatal physiology.* (4th ed.). Maryland Heights, MO: Elsevier.

Chestnut, D. H., Wong, C. A., Tsen, L. C., Kee, W. D. N., Beilin, Y., & Mhyre, J. (2014). *Chestnut's obstetric anesthesia: Principles & practice: Expert consult.* Philadelphia, PA: Saunders.

Collins, M. R., Starr, S. A., Bishop, J. T., & Baysinger, J. T. (2012). Nitrous oxide for labor analgesia: Expanding analgesic options for women in the United States. *Reviews in Obstetrics & Gynecology, 5*(3–4): e126–e131.

Gabbe, S. G., Niebyl, J. R., Galan, H., Jauniaux, E. R. M., Landon, M., Simpson, J. L., & Driscoll, D. (2012).

Obstetrics: Normal & problem pregnancies (6th ed.). Philadelphia, PA: Saunders.

King, T., Brucker, M., & Krebs, J. (2015). *Varney's midwifery* (5th ed.). Boston, MA: Jones & Bartlett.

Lancaster, S. M., Schick, U. M., Osman, M. M., & Equnobahrie, D. A. (2012). Risk factors associated with epidural use. *Journal of Clinical Medicine Research, 4*(2), 119–126. doi:10.4021/jocmr810w

Loewenberg-Weisband, Y., Grisaru-Granovsky, S., Ioscovich, A., Samueloff, A., & Calderon-Margalit, R. (2014). Epidural analgesia and severe perineal tears: A literature review and large cohort study. *Journal of Maternal-Fetal and Neonatal Medicine, 27*(17). doi: 10.3109/14767058.2014.889113.

Rimaitis, K., Klimenko, O., Rimaitis, M., Morkunaite, A., & Macas, A. (2015). Labor epidural analgesia and the incidence of instrumental assisted

delivery. *Medicina, 51*(2), 76–80. doi:10.1016/j.medici.2015.02.002

Suresh, M. S., Segal, B. S., Preston, R. L., Fernando, C., & Mason, L. (2013). *Shnider & Levinson's anesthesia for obstetrics* (5th ed.). Philadelphia, PA: Lippincott, Williams, & Wilkins.

Vixner, L., Schytt, E., Stener-Victorin, E., Waldenstrom, U., Pettersson, H., & Martensson, L.B. (2014). Acupuncture with manual and electrical stimulation for labour pain: A longitudinal randomised controlled trial. *BMC Complementary and Alternative Medicine, 14,* 187. doi:10.1186/1472-6882-14-187

Wilson, B. A., Shannon, M. T., & Shields, K. L. (Eds.). (2015). *Pearson's nurse's drug guide: 2016.* Upper Saddle River, NJ: Prentice Hall.

Wong, C. (2014). Anesthesia in high-risk obstetrics. *Global Library of Women's Medicine.* doi 10.3843/glowm.10217

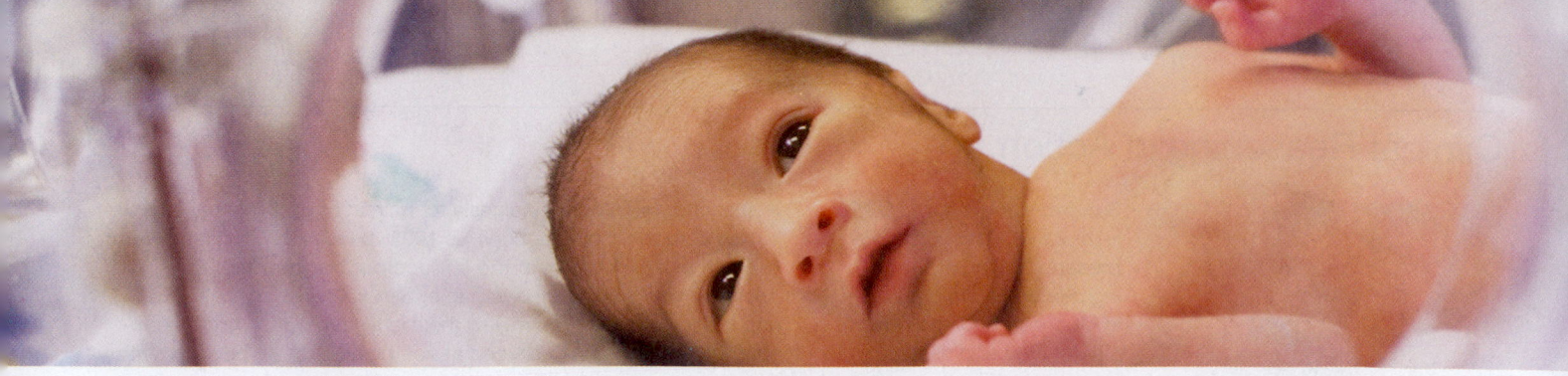

Chapter 20
Childbirth at Risk: Prelabor and Intrapartum Complications

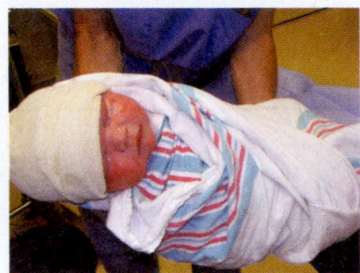

As a nurse-midwife who has worked with high-risk pregnant women for over a decade, I have gained some insight into the challenges high-risk women face in trying to follow medical advice and in dealing with the realities of that advice. It was not until I spent nearly 6 months on bedrest with my fourth child, however, that I truly understood the hardships and difficulties they endure. As I found myself unable to care for my other children or to work as a nurse-midwife, as I faced a variety of physical, emotional, and financial strains, I gained a new appreciation for all that a high-risk mother sacrifices for the well-being of her unborn child. These women need a great deal of support, education, and reassurance to deal with the daily struggles of a high-risk pregnancy.

—A Certified Nurse-Midwife and Former High-Risk Maternity Client

⌄ Learning Outcomes

20.1 Explain the possible causes, risk factors, and clinical therapy for premature rupture of the membranes or preterm labor in determining the hospital-based and community-based nursing management of the woman and her fetus/newborn.

20.2 Compare placenta previa and abruptio placentae, including implications for the mother and the fetus, as well as nursing care.

20.3 Describe the clinical therapies and appropriate nursing interventions for the mother with cervical insufficiency and her fetus.

20.4 Explain the maternal and fetal/neonatal implications and the clinical therapy in determining the community-based and hospital-based nursing care management of the woman with multiple gestation.

20.5 Compare the identification, maternal and fetal/neonatal implications, clinical therapy, and nursing care management of women with hydramnios and oligohydramnios.

After the first trimester, the majority of pregnancies progress smoothly to term. In some cases, however, complications can occur before the onset of labor that significantly impact the outcome of pregnancy. This chapter presents content related to the most common of these conditions. Labor-related complications are discussed in Chapter 21.

Care of the Woman with Premature Rupture of Membranes

Premature rupture of membranes (PROM) is spontaneous rupture of the membranes before the onset of labor. PROM affects up to 10% of all pregnancies. *Preterm PROM (PPROM)*, which affects approximately 3% of all pregnancies, is the rupture of membranes occurring before 37 weeks' gestation (Jazayeri, 2014). PROM and PPROM are associated with the following (Jazayeri, 2014):

- Abruptio placentae
- Amniocentesis
- Bleeding during pregnancy
- Cervical insufficiency
- History of laser conization or loop electrosurgical excision procedure (LEEP)
- Hydramnios
- Infection
- Low body mass index
- Low socioeconomic status
- Maternal genital tract anomalies
- Multiple pregnancy
- Placenta previa
- Previous history of PPROM
- Tobacco use
- Trauma
- Urinary tract infection (UTI)

Maternal risk of PROM/PPROM is related to infection, specifically *chorioamnionitis* and *endometritis* (postpartum infection of the endometrium). In addition, abruptio placentae occurs more frequently in women with PROM/PPROM. Other rare complications include retained placenta and hemorrhage, maternal sepsis, and maternal death.

Fetal/newborn complications may include the following (Guillet, Wilson-Smith, & Caughey, 2015):

- Compression of the umbilical cord
- Fetal sepsis
- Increased perinatal morbidity and mortality
- Malpresentation
- Nonreassuring fetal heart rate tracings
- Premature birth
- Prolapse of the umbilical cord
- Respiratory distress syndrome (with PPROM)

PROM that occurs at term is associated with favorable outcomes. Gestations from 32 to 37 weeks generally have favorable outcomes although there may be some complications. In general, babies born before 30 weeks have an increased risk of more serious complications, including respiratory distress syndrome (RDS), necrotizing enterocolitis (NEC), intraventricular hemorrhage (IVH), retinopathy of prematurity (ROP), sepsis, and fetal/neonatal death (Guillet et al., 2015). The earlier the gestational age, the greater the likelihood of newborn complications (Guillet et al., 2015).

Clinical Therapy

A sterile speculum examination is done to detect the presence of amniotic fluid in the vagina. If fluid is not obviously pooling, the diagnosis can be supported with Nitrazine paper (which turns deep blue). Because certain bacterial pathogens can also result in a positive Nitrazine test, a microscopic examination (ferning test) should be used as a confirmation of rupture because it is considered a definitive test. Digital examination increases the risk and is not recommended.

Management of PPROM in the absence of infection and gestation of less than 37 weeks is usually conservative. On admission, complete blood cell count (CBC), C-reactive protein, and urinalysis are obtained. Cultures, including chlamydia, gonorrhea, and group B streptococcus, should be obtained. An ultrasound is obtained to determine gestational age, amniotic fluid level, and fetal well-being. Regular non-stress tests (NSTs) or biophysical profiles are used to monitor fetal well-being. (These tests are discussed in Chapter 13.) Maternal blood pressure, pulse, temperature, and fetal heart rate (FHR) are assessed every 4 hours. Guidelines vary slightly for earlier gestational ages. The use of antibiotics is typically given in PPROM.

Women with PROM and PPROM should also receive intrapartum group B streptococci (GBS) prophylaxis when intrapartum indications exist, regardless of any past treatment (ACOG, 2013). Women with ruptured membranes >12 hours who receive intravenous antibiotics have lower rates of endometritis and chorioamnioitis than women who are left untreated (Saccone & Berghella, 2015). Women with PPROM have an increased risk of neonatal complications, so when possible, a consultation with a pediatrician or neonatologist provides an opportunity for the parents to ask questions and for the woman to understand potential risks and treatments that may be warranted after birth. Women with earlier gestational ages may benefit from corticosteroid and magnesium sulfate administration (discussed in the next section). Upon admission to the nursery, the newborn is assessed for sepsis and placed on antibiotics. (See Chapter 27 for information about the newborn with sepsis.) See *Key Facts to Remember: Management of Premature Rupture of Membranes Based on Gestational Age.*

KEY FACTS TO REMEMBER
Management of Premature Rupture of Membranes Based on Gestational Age

Gestational Age	Use of Antibiotic Therapy	Interventions Needed Prior to Birth	Recommendation for Birth
>34 weeks	Intrapartum group B streptococci (GBS) prophylaxis	Continuous electronic fetal monitoring (EFM)	If spontaneous labor does not begin, induction.
<34 weeks	7-day course of therapy with a combination of erythromycin and ampicillin or amoxicillin Intrapartum group B streptococci (GBS) prophylaxis	Continuous EFM Single course of corticosteroids Neonatology consult	Expectant management
24–32 weeks	7-day course of therapy with a combination of erythromycin and ampicillin or amoxicillin Intrapartum group B streptococci (GBS) prophylaxis	Continuous EFM Single course of corticosteroids Neonatology consult If birth anticipated, magnesium sulfate is indicated for neuroprotection	Expectant management

| EVIDENCE-BASED PRACTICE | Antibiotics for Premature Rupture of Membranes |

Clinical Question

Should antibiotics be used to prevent infection after premature rupture of membranes?

The Evidence

Premature rupture of membranes is linked to a higher risk of infection for the mother and potential morbidity for the baby. However, antibiotics carry the risks of potential maternal anaphylaxis and bacterial resistance and should not be used unless evidence supports clear benefit for both mother and neonate. Two Cochrane Reviews were conducted on the use of antibiotics for PROM; one review focused on pregnancies that were near term (37+ weeks) and the other focused on those that were preterm (less than 37 weeks). Cochrane Reviews are systematic reviews of randomized trials that are highly structured and peer reviewed. These reviews form the strongest level of evidence for practice.

No clear benefit was determined for mothers or babies for the administration of antibiotics when the pregnancy was near term (Wojcieszek, Stock, & Flenady, 2014). These studies encompassed nearly 3000 women and demonstrated that there was a higher surgical birth rate in those women who were administered antibiotics without clear demonstrated benefit for mother or child.

The reverse was true for PROM in pregnancies of less than 37 weeks' duration. These mothers had a lower rate of infection, a longer pregnancy, and better neonatal outcomes (Kenyon, Boulvain, & Neilson, 2013). The risk of perinatal death was not affected by the administration of antibiotics in either group. No clear direction was given for the specific antibiotic that was best, although one—co-amoxiclav—should be avoided because it was associated with subsequent necrotizing enterocolitis in neonates.

Best Practice

The use of antibiotics for treatment of PROM depends on the term of the pregnancy. They are not helpful for those women whose pregnancy has passed 37 weeks and no clear benefit emerges. For women with pregnancies of less than 37 weeks' duration, both maternal and neonatal outcomes are improved when antibiotics are administered.

Clinical Reasoning

What education can be provided to the parents to support using a full round of antibiotics for early PROMs? What side effects should the nurse observe for when administering antibiotics to these women?

Maternal corticosteroid administration promotes fetal lung maturity and helps to prevent respiratory distress syndrome, intraventricular hemorrhage, necrotizing enterocolitis, perinatal death, and long-term neurologic morbidity. Currently a single course of corticosteroids is recommended.

Healthy People 2020

(MICH-1.5) Reduce the rate of postneonatal deaths (between 28 days and 1 year)

(MICH-8.1) Reduce low birth weight (LBW)

(MICH-8.2) Reduce very low birth weight (VLBW)

Nursing Management

For the Woman with Premature Rupture of Membranes

Nursing Assessment and Diagnosis

Determining the duration of the rupture of the membranes is a significant component of the intrapartum assessment. Ask the woman when her membranes ruptured and when labor began. Gestational age is determined to prepare for the possibility of a preterm birth. Observe the mother for signs and symptoms of infection, especially by reviewing her white blood cell (WBC) count, temperature, pulse rate, and the character of her amniotic fluid. When a preterm or cesarean birth is anticipated, evaluate the childbirth preparation and coping abilities of the woman and her partner.

Nursing diagnoses that may apply to a woman with PROM include the following (NANDA-I © 2014):

- *Infection, Risk for,* related to premature rupture of membranes
- *Gas Exchange, Impaired,* of the fetus related to compression of the umbilical cord secondary to prolapse of the cord
- *Coping, Ineffective,* related to unknown outcome of the pregnancy

Nursing Plan and Implementation

Uterine activity and fetal response to the labor are evaluated, but vaginal examinations are not done unless absolutely necessary because this increases the risk of infection. Encourage the woman to rest on her left side to promote optimal uteroplacental perfusion. Comfort measures may help promote rest and relaxation. Ensure that hydration is maintained, particularly if the woman's temperature is elevated.

Education is another important aspect of nursing care. The woman and her partner, if he or she is involved, need to understand the implications of PROM and all treatment methods. It is important to address side effects and alternative treatments. The couple needs to know that although the membranes are ruptured, amniotic fluid continues to be produced.

| TEACHING HIGHLIGHTS | Explaining Amniotic Membranes |

To help a laboring woman and her family understand how the amniotic membranes provide protection, use a color chart that shows a side view of the fetus in the uterus with the membranes intact. Ask them to visualize what happens if the membranes rupture. They will be able to see that pathogens have direct access to the uterus, increasing the risk of infection. They will also see that when the membranes rupture and the fluid escapes, the cord could "wash out" with the fluid and become trapped between the pelvis and the fetal head, causing cord compression.

Providing psychologic support for the couple is critical. The nurse may reduce anxiety by listening empathetically, relaying accurate information, and providing explanations of procedures. Preparing the couple for a cesarean birth, a preterm newborn, and the possibility of fetal or newborn demise may be necessary. Consultation with the neonatologist or pediatric healthcare provider can give the woman and her partner an opportunity to ask questions if a preterm birth is anticipated.

Evaluation

Expected outcomes of nursing care include the following:

- The woman's risk of infection and of cord prolapse decrease.
- The couple is able to discuss the implications of PROM and all treatments and alternative treatments.
- The couple verbalizes understanding that they did not cause the event.
- The pregnancy is maintained without trauma to the mother or the fetus.

Care of the Woman at Risk Because of Preterm Labor

Labor that occurs between 20 and 36 completed weeks of pregnancy is called **preterm labor (PTL)**. Prematurity continues to be the number one perinatal and neonatal problem in the United States, with 10% of all live births occurring prematurely (Centers for Disease Control & Prevention [CDC], 2014). (Complications that may ensue with preterm newborns and their management are discussed in Chapter 26.) Often PTL is related to multiple risk factors; only rarely is there a single cause. Table 20–1 presents a list of risk factors for spontaneous preterm labor.

Maternal implications of PTL include psychologic stress related to the baby's condition and physiologic stress related to medical treatment for preterm labor.

Fetal/neonatal implications include increased morbidity and mortality, especially caused by respiratory distress syndrome (RDS), increased risk of trauma during birth, neurological injuries, and maturational deficiencies (fat storage, heat regulation, immaturity of organ systems).

Clinical Therapy

Women who are at risk for PTL are taught to recognize the symptoms associated with preterm labor and, if any symptoms are present, to notify their physician/CNM immediately. Prompt diagnosis is necessary to stop preterm labor before it progresses to the point at which intervention will be ineffective.

TABLE 20–1 Risk Factors for Spontaneous Preterm Labor

Abdominal surgery during second or third trimester	Interval of less than 6 to 9 months between pregnancies
Abdominal trauma	Known cervical insufficiency
Age (less than 17 or over 35 years)	Lack of social support
Anemia	Long work hours with prolonged standing or lifting
Bacterial vaginosis, *Escherichia coli* (ascending intrauterine infection)	Low maternal weight, poor weight gain
Bleeding after 12 weeks	Low socioeconomic status; low educational level
Cervical cerclage in situ	More than two first-trimester abortions
Cervical shortening (<25 mm diagnosed between 16–22 weeks)	Multiple gestation
Cervix dilated (1 cm at 32 weeks)	Non-White race
Clotting disorders	Pollutants
Diabetes	Poor social support
Domestic violence	Previous preterm birth, family history of preterm birth
Febrile illness	Previous preterm labor with term birth
Fetal abnormality	Second-trimester abortion
Foreign body (e.g., intrauterine device [IUD])	Sexually transmitted infection (STI) (e.g., trichomoniasis, chlamydial infection)
History of cervical surgery (cone biopsy, LEEP procedure)	Stress
History of pyelonephritis or other maternal infection	Substance abuse (cigarettes/alcohol/drug use)
Hypertension (preeclampsia, gestational hypertension, chronic hypertension)	Thrombophilias
In vitro fertilization (singleton or multiple gestation)	Uterine anomaly, uterine irritability
Inadequate or no prenatal care	Uteroplacental ischemia
	Weight variations (underweight, overweight, obesity, inadequate maternal weight gain)

Prompt diagnosis of PTL is often difficult because many of the symptoms are common in normal pregnancy. Research suggests that the strongest predictors of preterm birth include the following: multiple gestation, bleeding during pregnancy, cervicovaginal fibronectin, abnormal cervical length on ultrasound, history of previous preterm birth, abnormal vaginal flora, and the presence of infection (discussed later in this chapter) (Ross, 2015). Recently there has been an association between paternal smoking, exposure to second-hand smoke by family members, and environmental smoke exposure and preterm birth (Ko, Tsai, Chu, et al., 2014).

Fetal fibronectin (fFN) is a protein normally found in the fetal membranes and decidua. It is in the cervicovaginal fluid in early pregnancy but is not usually present in significant quantities between 22 and 37 weeks' gestation (Kuhrt, Hezelgrave, Foster, et al., 2015). A positive fFN test (fFN found in the cervicovaginal fluid) during this time puts the woman at increased risk for preterm birth. Conversely, a negative fFN in a woman with preterm contractions is associated with a very low risk of birth within 7 to 14 days (Kuhrt et al., 2015). The test is over 99% accurate for predicting no preterm birth within 7 days. The procedure for collecting a sample is similar to that of the Pap smear; results can be available within 1 hour. New research has shown promising results that other cervicovaginal fluid (CVF) biomarkers may be used in the future to predict women who are likely to give birth prematurely (Liong, Di Quinzio, Fleming, et al., 2015).

The length of the cervix can be measured fairly reliably after 16 weeks' gestation using an ultrasound probe inserted into the vagina. A cervix that is shorter than expected may be useful in assisting a physician to identify the need for a cerclage to prevent preterm birth because of cervical insufficiency. In general, cervical length less than 25 mm before term is abnormal (Suhag, Reina, Sanapo, et al., 2015). Cervical insufficiency is discussed in detail later in this chapter.

Diagnosis of preterm labor is confirmed if the pregnancy is between 20 and 36 completed weeks, there are documented uterine contractions (four in 20 minutes or eight in 1 hour), and there is documented cervical change or cervical dilatation of greater than 1 cm (0.4 in.) or cervical effacement of 80% or more. Electronic fetal monitoring is commonly used to evaluate the frequency and duration of contractions as well the use of a nonstress test (NST) to determine fetal well-being.

Labor is not interrupted if one or more of the following conditions are present: severe preeclampsia or eclampsia, chorioamnionitis, hemorrhage, maternal cardiac disease, poorly controlled diabetes mellitus or thyrotoxicosis, severe abruptio placentae, fetal anomalies incompatible with life, fetal death, nonreassuring fetal status, or fetal maturity.

The goal of clinical therapy is to prevent preterm labor from advancing to the point that it no longer responds to medical treatment. The initial management of preterm labor is directed toward maintaining good uterine blood flow, detecting uterine contractions, and ensuring that the fetus is stable. The mother is asked to lie on her side to increase placental profusion, an IV infusion is started to promote maternal hydration, and maternal laboratory studies including CBC, C-reactive protein, vaginal cultures, fetal fibronectin (fFN), and urine culture are completed. An ultrasound may be obtained to determine cervical shortening or funneling and to assess fetal well-being.

Tocolysis is the use of medications in an attempt to stop labor so that preventative medications to promote fetal lung maturity and provide fetal neuroprotection can be administered. Drugs currently used as tocolytics include the β-adrenergic agonists (also called β-mimetics) and calcium channel blockers.

Although tocolytic drugs suppress uterine contractions and allow pregnancy to continue, they may cause maternal side effects; the most serious are maternal pulmonary edema, maternal myocardial ischemia, maternal hyperglycemia, maternal hypokalemia, and fetal cardiac side effects (Padovani, Guyatt, & Lopes, 2015). The use of injectable terbutaline (Brethine) and calcium channel blockers should be used to facilitate the administration of corticosteroids and magnesium sulfate and to allow ample time for transport to a medical facility that is capable of handling preterm neonatal needs (Theplib & Phupong, 2015).

Recent research has indicated that nifedipine (Procardia) has significantly few maternal side effects and is considered a first-line treatment in managing preterm labor. It is easily administered orally or sublingually and has few serious maternal side effects. It decreases smooth muscle contractions by blocking the slow calcium channels at the cell surface. The most common side effects are related to arterial vasodilation and include hypotension, tachycardia, facial flushing, and headache. Nifedipine may be coadministered with the β-mimetics. However, it should *not* be used with magnesium sulfate (which is often administered for its neuroprotective benefits) because both drugs block calcium and simultaneous administration has been implicated in serious maternal side effects related to low calcium levels.

ACOG (2014a) recommends that corticosteroids (typically betamethasone or dexamethasone) be administered antenatally to women at risk for preterm birth because of their beneficial effect on the prevention of neonatal respiratory distress syndrome (RDS), IVH, NEC, and neonatal mortality (ACOG, 2014a). Women who are candidates for short-term tocolysis are candidates for antenatal corticosteroids, regardless of fetal gender, race, or availability of surfactant therapy for the newborn, especially between 24 and 34 weeks' gestation. Betamethasone is primarily used and should be administered in two intramuscular doses. When dexamethasone is used, four doses are given.

Magnesium sulfate administration in preterm gestations has been associated with a reduction in cerebral palsy (ACOG, 2015). It is administered for neuroprotection in preterm fetuses when birth is imminent or preterm delivery is likely to occur. Ideally, the infusion should be administered for at least 4 hours prior to birth and should be discontinued at 24 hours if birth has not occurred. The loading dose is 4 g administered over 30 minutes followed by 1g/hr until birth or 24 hours is reached. Magnesium sulfate needs to be administered via an infusion pump. Maternal side effects may include flushing, sweating, feeling of warmth, sharply lowered blood pressure, slurred speech, blurred vision, hypothermia, nausea, vomiting, headache, and stupor. Signs of toxicity include a reduction or lack of reflexes, oliguria, confusion, respiratory depression, circulatory collapse, and respiratory paralysis (Wilson, Shannon, & Shields, 2016).

Progesterone therapy has been shown to be effective in reducing the incidence of preterm birth, at least in certain high-risk populations including women with a previous preterm birth. Progesterone therapy may also be considered for women with a shortened cervix (Conde-Agudelo & Romero, 2015).

Healthy People 2020

(MICH-9.1) Reduce total preterm births

(MICH-9.2) Reduce late preterm or live births at 34 to 36 weeks of gestation

(MICH-9.3) Reduce live births at 32 to 33 weeks of gestation

(MICH-9.4) Reduce very preterm or live births at less than 32 weeks of gestation

Nursing Management

For the Woman at Risk for Preterm Labor

Nursing Assessment and Diagnosis

During the antepartum period, identify the woman at risk for preterm labor by noting the presence of risk factors. During the intrapartum period, assess the progress of labor and the physiologic impact of labor on the mother and the fetus.

Nursing diagnoses that may apply to the woman with preterm labor include the following (NANDA-I © 2014):

- *Fear* related to risk of early labor and birth
- *Coping, Ineffective,* related to need for constant attention to pregnancy
- *Acute Pain* related to uterine contractions

Nursing Plan and Implementation

COMMUNITY-BASED NURSING CARE

All pregnant women in the third trimester should be taught about the importance of recognizing the onset of labor (see *Teaching Highlights: Preterm Labor*). This teaching is often provided by clinic or office nurses.

Increasing the woman's awareness of the signs and symptoms of preterm labor will be one of your most important teaching objectives. Some clinics or offices may utilize calls to the woman between appointments to assess the woman's condition. Increasingly, insurance companies are offering programs to high-risk women that include monitoring calls to assess for symptoms. These symptoms include the following:

- Uterine contractions that occur every 10 minutes or less, with or without pain
- Mild menstrual-like cramps felt low in the abdomen
- Constant or intermittent feelings of pelvic pressure that feel like the baby pressing down
- Rupture of membranes
- Constant or intermittent low, dull backache
- A change in the vaginal discharge (an increase in amount, a change to more clear and watery, or a pinkish tinge)
- Abdominal cramping with or without diarrhea

Teach the woman to evaluate contraction activity once or twice a day. She does so by lying down tilted to one side with a pillow behind her back for support. The woman places her fingertips on the fundus of the uterus, which is above the umbilicus (navel). She checks for contractions (hardening or tightening in the uterus) for about 1 hour. It is important for the pregnant woman to know that uterine contractions occur occasionally throughout the pregnancy. If they occur every 10 minutes for 1 hour, however, the cervix could begin to dilate, and labor could ensue.

Ensure that the woman knows when to report signs and symptoms. If contractions occur every 10 minutes (or more frequently) for 1 hour, if any of the other signs and symptoms are present for 1 hour, or if clear fluid begins leaking from the vagina, the woman should telephone her physician/CNM or clinic and make arrangements for a complete assessment. Caregivers need to be aware that the woman's call must be taken seriously. When a woman is at risk for preterm labor, she may have many episodes of contractions and other signs or symptoms. If she is treated positively, she will feel freer to report problems as they arise.

Preventive self-care measures are also important. You have a vital role in communicating the self-care measures described in Table 20–2.

HOSPITAL-BASED NURSING CARE

Supportive nursing care is important to the woman in preterm labor during hospitalization. This care consists of promoting bedrest, monitoring vital signs (especially blood pressure and respirations), measuring intake and output, and continuous monitoring of fetal heart rate (FHR) and uterine contractions.

TABLE 20–2 Self-Care Measures to Prevent Preterm Labor

- Rest two or three times a day lying on your left side.
- Drink 2 to 3 quarts of water or fluid each day. Avoid caffeine drinks. Filling a quart container and drinking from it will eliminate the need to keep track of numerous glasses of fluid.
- Empty your bladder at least every 2 hours during waking hours.
- Avoid lifting heavy objects. If small children are in the home, work out alternatives for picking them up, such as sitting on a chair and having them climb on your lap.
- Avoid prenatal breast preparation such as nipple rolling or rubbing nipples with a towel. This is meant not to discourage breastfeeding but to avoid the potential increase in uterine irritability.
- Pace necessary activities to avoid overexertion.
- Curtail or eliminate sexual activity, if necessary.
- Find pleasurable ways to help compensate for limitations of activities and boost the spirits.
- Try to focus on 1 day or 1 week at a time rather than on longer periods of time.
- If on bedrest, get dressed each day and rest on a couch rather than becoming isolated in the bedroom.

Source: Prepared in consultation with the Prematurity Prevention Program at the University of Washington Medical Center.

TEACHING HIGHLIGHTS Preterm Labor

- Describe the dangers of preterm labor, especially the risk of prematurity in the newborn and the potential long-term effects.
- Explain that many of the early symptoms of labor, such as backache and increased bloody show, may be subtle initially.
- Summarize self-care measures (see Table 20–2) that the woman can take to prevent preterm labor.
- Teach the woman how to palpate for uterine contractions. Demonstrate and ask for a return demonstration.

Placing the woman on her left side facilitates maternal–fetal circulation. Vaginal examinations are kept to a minimum. If medications are being used, administer them and closely monitor the mother and the fetus for any adverse effects.

Whether preterm labor is arrested or proceeds, the woman and her partner, if involved, experience intense psychologic stress. Decreasing the anxiety associated with the risk of a preterm newborn by providing emotional support is a primary aim of the nurse. Recognize the stress of bedrest and of lack of sexual contact and help the couple find satisfactory ways of dealing with those stresses. With empathetic communication, you can assist the couple to express their feelings, which commonly include guilt and anxiety, thereby helping the couple identify and implement coping mechanisms. Keep the couple informed about the labor progress, the treatment regimen, and the status of the fetus. In the event of imminent vaginal or cesarean birth, the couple should be offered brief but ongoing explanations to prepare them for the actual birth process and the events following the birth. Arrange for consultations for the neonatologist or pediatrician to assist the couple in anticipating potential neonatal complications and risks for the newborn.

Evaluation

Expected outcomes of nursing care include the following:

- The woman is able to discuss the possible cause, identification, and treatment of preterm labor.

- The woman states that she feels comfortable in her ability to cope with her situation and has resources available to her.

- The woman can describe appropriate self-care measures and can identify characteristics that need to be reported to her caregiver.

- The woman receives pharmacological interventions to increase neonatal outcomes prior to birth when possible.

- The woman facing imminent birth verbalizes understanding of the process and feels comfortable asking for clarification or communicating her needs to her healthcare providers.

Care of the Woman at Risk Because of Bleeding During Pregnancy

Bleeding during pregnancy always requires assessment. The most common causes of bleeding during the first and second trimesters, namely, spontaneous abortion, ectopic pregnancy, and gestational trophoblastic disease, are addressed in Chapter 15. Cervical insufficiency and the two most clinically significant causes of bleeding in the second half of pregnancy, placenta previa and abruptio placentae, are discussed in this chapter. Placental problems that are labor related are addressed in Chapter 21.

Placenta Previa

In **placenta previa**, the placenta is implanted in the lower uterine segment rather than the upper portion of the uterus. This implantation may be on a portion of the lower segment or over the internal cervical os. As the lower uterine segment contracts and dilates in the later weeks of pregnancy, the placental villi are torn from the uterine wall, thus exposing the uterine sinuses at the placental site. Bleeding begins, but because the amount

depends on the number of sinuses exposed, initially it may be either scanty or profuse.

Placenta previa has been classified in several ways since it was first categorized in 1709 (Silver, 2015). Some clinicians continue to use terms to describe the relationship between the placenta edge and the cervical os. This terminology-based system has been modified and changed over the years. A *complete previa* is defined as complete coverage of the cervical os by the placenta. If the leading edge of the placenta is less than 2 cm from the internal os, but not fully covering it, it is considered a *marginal previa* (Joy, 2015). In response to the use of subjective terminology, the American College of Radiology (ACR) (2015) created the American College of Radiology Appropriateness Criteria, which recommends a grading system that includes four grades that provide a quantifiable description of the relationship between the cervical os and the placenta, as shown in Table 20–3.

The cause of placenta previa is unknown. Statistically it occurs in about 3.5 to 4.6 per 1000 births (Silver, 2015). As the cesarean section rate has risen dramatically in recent years, the incidence of placenta previa has also increased. The risk factors for placenta previa include a previous uterine surgery, maternal age greater than 35 years, prior cesarean birth, multiple spontaneous or elective abortions, grandmultiparity, and a prior history of placenta previa (Kollmann, Gaulhofer, Lang, et al., 2014). Additional risk factors include multiparity, non-White race, cigarette smoking, cocaine use, and a large placenta (multiple gestation, erythroblastosis) (Räisänen, Kancherla, Kramer, et al., 2014).

FETAL/NEONATAL IMPLICATIONS

The prognosis for the fetus depends on the extent of placenta previa. In cases of a Grade 1 or 2 placenta previa, the woman may be allowed to labor. Changes in the fetal heart rate (FHR) and meconium staining of the amniotic fluid may be apparent. In a profuse bleeding episode, the fetus is compromised and suffers some hypoxia. FHR monitoring is imperative when the woman is admitted, particularly if a vaginal birth is anticipated, because the presenting part of the fetus may obstruct the flow of blood from the placenta or umbilical cord. If nonreassuring fetal status occurs, cesarean birth is indicated. Women who are diagnosed with a Grade 3 or 4 placenta previa will need to undergo a cesarean birth because the risk of intrapartum hemorrhage is high. After birth, blood sampling should be done to determine whether the intrauterine bleeding episodes of the woman have caused anemia in the newborn.

CLINICAL THERAPY

The goal of medical care is to identify the cause of bleeding and to provide treatment that will ensure birth of a mature newborn. Indirect diagnosis is made by localizing the placenta through tests that require no vaginal examination, such as a transabdominal

TABLE 20–3 Grades of Placenta Previa

GRADE	DESCRIPTION
Grade 1	Placenta lies in lower uterine segment but its lower edge does not abut the internal cervical os (i.e., lower edge 0.5–5.0 cm from internal os) (Figure 20–1A)
Grade 2	Placental tissue reaches the margin of the internal cervical os, but does not cover it
Grade 3	Placenta partially covers the internal cervical os (Figure 20-1B)
Grade 4	Placenta completely covers the internal cervical os (Figure 20–1C)

Source: Data from Posner, G., & Black, A. (2013). Oxorne & Foote human labor and birth. (6th ed.). Philadelphia, PA: McGraw-Hill

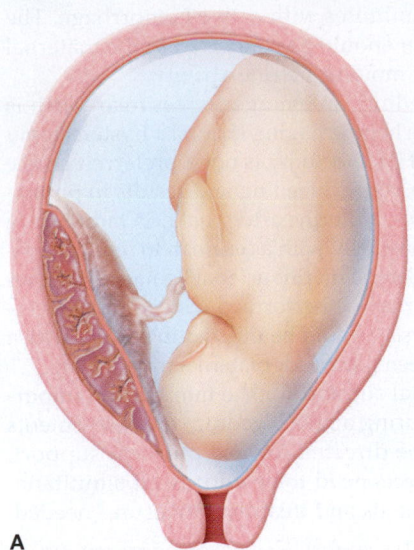 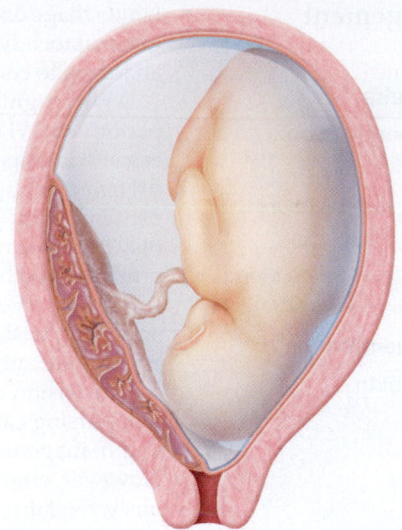 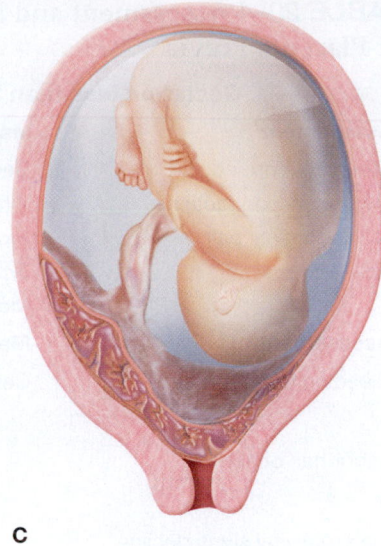

A   B   C

Figure 20–1 Grades of placenta previa. A. Grade 1, low-lying placental implantation. B. Grade 3, partial placenta previa. C. Grade 4, complete placenta previa.

ultrasound scan. Until placenta previa is ruled out, vaginal examinations should never be performed on a woman with bleeding because the examiner's fingers could perforate the placenta if cervical dilatation has occurred. Once placenta previa has been ruled out, a vaginal examination can be performed with a speculum to determine the cause of bleeding (such as cervical lesions).

The differential diagnosis of placental or cervical bleeding takes careful consideration. Partial separation of the placenta may also present with painless bleeding, and true placenta previa may not demonstrate overt bleeding until labor begins, thus confusing the diagnosis.

Care of the woman with painless late-gestational bleeding depends on (1) the week of gestation during which the first bleeding episode occurs and (2) the amount of bleeding. If the pregnancy is less than 37 weeks' gestation, expectant management is employed to delay birth until about 37 weeks' gestation to allow the fetus to mature. Women who have had two episodes of bleeding once viability has been reached are best managed in an acute care setting (Joy, 2015). Expectant management involves stringent regulation as follows:

1. Provide bedrest with bathroom privileges as long as the woman is not bleeding.

2. Perform no vaginal examinations.

3. Monitor blood loss, pain, and uterine contractility.

4. Evaluate FHR with an external fetal monitor.

5. Monitor maternal vital signs.

6. Perform a complete laboratory evaluation: hemoglobin, hematocrit, Rh factor, and urinalysis. DIC studies should be obtained, which include clotting studies (e.g., prothrombin time/activated partial thromboplastin time [PT/aPTT], fibrinogen, and fibrin split products).

7. Provide intravenous fluid (lactated Ringer solution).

8. Have two units of crossmatched blood available for transfusion.

9. If the fetus is less than 34 weeks' gestation, tocolytics can be used for 48 hours in order to provide ample time to administer corticosteroids. If the fetus is 24 to 32 weeks' gestation, magnesium sulfate for neuroprotection should be administered.

If frequent, recurrent, or profuse bleeding persists, or if fetal well-being appears threatened, a cesarean birth may be required. See Table 20–4 for assessment and management of placenta previa.

Clinical Tip

Women on bedrest may suffer from orthostatic hypotension upon rising and should be cautioned to sit at the edge of the bed with legs dangling prior to arising to prevent falls and other injuries.

Nursing Management

For the Woman with Placenta Previa

Nursing Assessment and Diagnosis

Assessment of the woman with placenta previa must be ongoing to prevent or treat complications that are potentially lethal to the mother and the fetus. Painless, bright-red vaginal bleeding is the most accurate diagnostic sign of placenta previa. If this sign develops during the last 3 months of pregnancy, placenta previa should always be considered until ruled out by ultrasound examination. The first bleeding episode is generally scanty. If no vaginal examinations are performed, it often subsides spontaneously. However, each subsequent hemorrhage is more profuse.

The uterus remains soft; if labor begins, it relaxes fully between contractions. The FHR usually remains stable unless profuse hemorrhage and maternal shock occur. As a result of the placement of the placenta, the fetal presenting part is often unengaged, and transverse lie is common.

Assess blood loss, pain, and uterine contractility both subjectively and objectively. Maternal vital signs and the results of blood and urine tests provide additional data about the woman's condition. Evaluate the FHR with continuous external fetal monitoring. Another pressing nursing responsibility is to observe and verify the family's ability to cope with the anxiety associated with an unknown outcome.

TABLE 20–4 Assessment and Management of Placenta Previa

Gestation less than 37 weeks

Assessment	Management/Action
Bleeding stopped	Bed rest
No uterine contractions	Vital signs every 4 hours
No abdominal pain	Provide IV fluids
NST reactive	Type and crossmatch blood
	Monitor client closely

Assessment	Management/Action
Bleeding begins again	Cesarean birth
or	
Labor has begun	
or	
Maternal vital signs decline	
or	
Fetal status is nonreassuring	

Assessment	Management/Action
Complete previa	Cesarean birth

Note: Gestation more than 34 but less than 37 weeks—administer corticosteroids.

Gestation 24 to 34 weeks—administer corticosteroids and magnesium sulfate.

Gestation more than 37 weeks

Assessment	Management/Action
Bleeding minimal or stopped Reassuring fetal status	Induction of labor possible if:
	Grade 1 or 2
	Cervix is ripe
	Cephalic presentation
	Fetal head down in pelvis

Assessment	Management/Action
Bleeding continues	Cesarean birth
or	
Complete previa	

Source: Data from Silver, R. (2015). Abnormal placentation: Placenta previa, vasa previa, and placenta accreta. *Obstetrics & Gynecology, 126*(3), 654–668; Joy, S. (2015). Placenta previa. *Medscape.* Retrieved from http://emedicine.medscape.com/article/262063-overview#a0156

Nursing diagnoses that may apply include the following (NANDA-I © 2014):

- *Fluid Volume: Deficient,* related to hypovolemia secondary to excessive blood loss
- *Gas Exchange, Impaired,* of the fetus related to decreased blood volume and maternal hypotension
- *Anxiety* related to concern for own personal status and the baby's safety

Nursing Plan and Implementation

Monitor the woman and her fetus to determine the status of the bleeding and the responses of the mother and the baby. Vital signs, intake and output, and other pertinent assessments must be made frequently. Use electronic monitor tracing to evaluate fetal status. A whole-blood setup should be ready for intravenous infusion and a patent intravenous line established before caregivers undertake any invasive procedures. Maternal vital signs should be monitored every 15 minutes in the absence of hemorrhage and every 5 minutes with active hemorrhage. The external tocodynamometer should be connected to the maternal abdomen to continuously monitor uterine activity.

With significant bleeding, an emergency cesarean birth is performed. When massive hemorrhaging occurs, a hysterectomy is sometimes performed. Hysterectomy is not a preferred choice for treatment because it increases bleeding and results in permanent infertility. In rare cases, a uterine artery balloon tamponade may be performed simultaneously with a cesarean to reduce hemorrhaging and bleeding. Bilateral uterine arterial ligation is another surgical intervention that may be performed instead of a hysterectomy. Intensive care nurses should be utilized in cases where a Swan-Ganz catheter has been placed for maternal monitoring.

Provision of emotional support for the family is an important nursing care goal. During active bleeding, the assessments and management must be directed toward physical support. However, emotional aspects need to be addressed simultaneously. Explain the assessments and treatment measures needed.

Clinical Tip

When emergent actions are necessary for severe hemorrhage, reassure the woman that she should follow your instructions, but as soon as time allows, you will provide a more complete explanation of the circumstances. Explain that you are doing everything possible for her and her newborn's care.

Time can be provided for questions, and you can act as an advocate in obtaining information for the family. Offer emotional support by staying with the family and using touch.

Promotion of neonatal physiologic adaptation is another important nursing responsibility. The newborn's hemoglobin, cell volume, and erythrocyte count should be checked immediately and then monitored closely. The newborn may require oxygen, administration of blood, and admission into a special-care nursery.

Evaluation

Anticipated outcomes of nursing care include the following:

- The cause of hemorrhage is recognized promptly and corrective measures are taken.
- The woman's vital signs remain in the normal range.
- Any other complications are recognized and treated early.
- The family understands what has happened and the implications and associated problems of placenta previa.
- The woman and her baby have a safe labor and birth.

Abruptio Placentae (Placental Abruption)

Abruptio placentae (placental abruption) is the premature separation of a normally implanted placenta from the uterine wall. Premature separation, the leading cause of perinatal mortality, is considered a catastrophic event because of the severity of the resulting hemorrhage. The incidence of abruptio placentae is 1.0% of all pregnancies but it accounts for 12% of all perinatal deaths (Ananath & Kinzler, 2015). The incidence of placental abruption appears to be increasing in frequency (Deering, 2015).

The cause of abruptio placentae is largely unknown, although there are a large number of potential risk factors associated with it, including increased maternal age, maternal age less than 20 years, increased parity, previous cesarean birth, cocaine use, blunt force trauma, falls, motor vehicle accidents, intimate partner violence, preeclampsia, maternal hypertension, bleeding in the second or third trimester, prolonged rupture of membranes, chorioamnionitis, rapid uterine decompression associated with hydramnios or multiple gestation, preterm premature rupture of membranes (PPROM), previous placental abruption, uterine malformations, placental anomalies, placenta previa, amniocentesis, retroplacental fibromyoma, shortened umbilical cord, male sex, low socioeconomic status, subchorionic hematoma, and elevated alpha fetoprotein in the second trimester. Black women have a higher incidence of abruption but it is unclear if this is a direct result of socioeconomic or of genetic variations (Deering, 2015).

Cigarette smoking has long been identified as a risk factor for abruptio placentae. Tikkanen (2014) examined 46,742 pregnancies, identified 198 that resulted in a placental abruption, and compared the pregnancies with those of a control group of 396 women. Women with a history of smoking had an increased risk of abruption, as did women with partners who smoked. Smoking by both partners further elevated this risk. Other studies have shown that the risk of abruption increased by 40% for each year of smoking prior to pregnancy (Deering, 2015).

Abruptio placentae is classified based on the extent of separation (i.e., partial or complete) and location of separation (i.e., marginal or central) and subdivided into four types (Figure 20–2):

- **Marginal.** The placenta separates at its edges, the blood passes between the fetal membranes and the uterine wall, and the blood escapes vaginally (also called *marginal sinus rupture*).

- **Central.** The placenta separates centrally, and the blood is trapped between the placenta and the uterine wall. Entrapment of the blood results in concealed bleeding.

- **Partial.** Separation occurs but is not complete. May be minimal or moderate. Partial separation can progress to complete separation.

- **Complete.** Massive vaginal bleeding is seen in the presence of total separation.

Abruptio placentae may also be graded according to the severity of clinical and laboratory findings as follows (Deering, 2015):

- **Grade 1 (Mild).** Mild separation with slight vaginal bleeding. FHR pattern and maternal blood pressure unaffected. Accounts for 48% of abruptions.

- **Grade 2 (Moderate).** Partial abruption with moderate bleeding. Significant uterine irritability is present. Maternal pulse may be elevated although blood pressure is stable. Signs of fetal compromise evident in FHR. Accounts for 27% of abruptions.

- **Grade 3 (Severe).** Large or complete separation with moderate to severe bleeding. Maternal shock and painful uterine contractions present. Fetal death common. Accounts for about 24% of abruptions.

In severe cases of central abruptio placentae, the blood invades the myometrial tissues between the muscle fibers. This occurrence accounts for the uterine irritability that is a significant sign of abruptio placentae. If hemorrhage continues, eventually the uterus turns entirely blue because the muscle fibers are filled with blood. After birth the uterus contracts poorly. This condition is known as a *Couvelaire uterus* and frequently necessitates hysterectomy.

A comparison of the signs and symptoms of placenta previa and abruptio placentae are shown in Table 20–5.

MATERNAL IMPLICATIONS

As a result of the damage to the uterine wall and the retroplacental clotting with central abruption, large amounts of thromboplastin are released into the maternal blood supply. This thromboplastin in turn triggers the development of disseminated intravascular coagulation (DIC) and resultant hypofibrinogenemia. Fibrinogen levels, which are ordinarily elevated in pregnancy, may drop in minutes to the point at which blood will no longer coagulate. See Chapter 15 for discussion of disseminated intravascular coagulation.

Perinatal mortality occurs in 119 of 1000 women and accounts for 6% of maternal deaths. Death rates are higher in women who smoke. Postpartum problems depend in large part on the severity of the intrapartum bleeding, coagulation defects such as DIC, hypofibrinogenemia, and time between separation and birth. Moderate to severe hemorrhage results in hemorrhagic shock, which may prove fatal to the mother if it is not rapidly reversed. In the postpartum period, women with this disorder are at risk for hemorrhage and renal failure caused by shock, vascular spasm, intravascular clotting, or a combination of these factors.

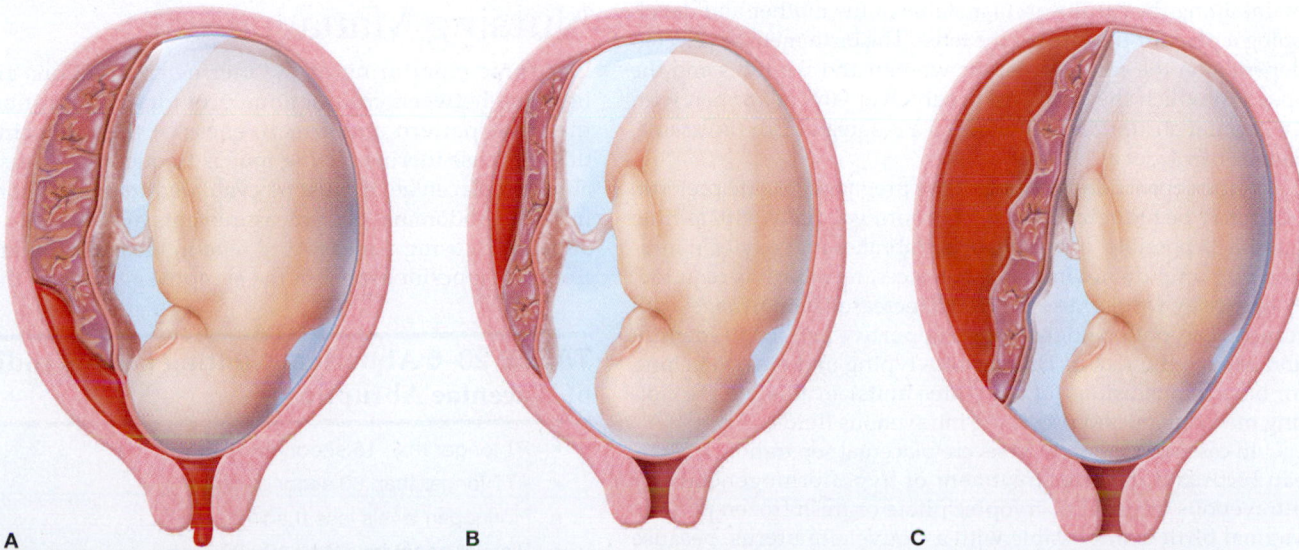

A   **B**   **C**

Figure 20–2 Abruptio placentae. A. Marginal abruption with external hemorrhage. B. Central abruption with concealed hemorrhage. C. Complete separation.

TABLE 20–5 Differential Signs and Symptoms of Placenta Previa and Abruptio Placentae

	PLACENTA PREVIA	ABRUPTIO PLACENTAE
Onset	Quiet and sneaky	Sudden and stormy
Bleeding	External	External or concealed
Color of blood	Bright red	Dark venous
Anemia	Equal to blood loss	Greater than apparent blood loss
Shock	Equal to blood loss	Greater than apparent blood loss
Preeclampsia/eclampsia	Absent	May be present
Pain	Only labor	Usually severe and steady
Uterine tenderness	Absent	Present
Uterine tone	Soft and relaxed	Firm to stony hard
Uterine contour	Normal	May enlarge and change shape
Fetal heart tones	Usually present	Present or absent
Engagement	Absent	May be present
Presentation	May be abnormal	No relationship

Source: Data from Posner, G., & Black, A. (2013). *Oxorn & Foote human labor and birth* (6th ed.). Philadelphia, PA: McGraw-Hill.

FETAL/NEONATAL IMPLICATIONS

Perinatal morbidity associated with abruptio placentae is about 12% (Ananath & Kinzler, 2015). Fetal death occurs as a result of the abruption or can occur due to prematurity. Fetal death typically occurs with complete placental separation. In less severe separation, fetal outcome depends on the level of maturity and the length of time to birth. The most serious complications in the newborn arise from preterm labor, anemia, and hypoxia. Fetal death and adverse outcomes also occur when prompt access to medical care is not available.

CLINICAL THERAPY

Because of the risk of DIC, evaluating the results of coagulation tests is imperative. In DIC, fibrinogen levels and platelet counts usually decrease; prothrombin times and partial thromboplastin times are normal to prolonged. If the values are not markedly abnormal, serial testing may be helpful in establishing an abnormal trend indicative of coagulopathy. Another test determines levels of fibrin-degradation products; these values rise with DIC. See Table 20–6.

After establishing the diagnosis, immediate priorities are maintaining the cardiovascular status of the mother and developing a plan for the birth of the fetus. The birth method selected depends on the condition of the woman and the fetus and the speed in which the birth will occur. Over 90% of women with a placental abruption will undergo a cesarean birth (Boisramé, Sananès, Fritz, et al., 2014).

If the separation is mild and the pregnancy is late preterm, labor may be induced and the fetus born vaginally with as little trauma as possible. If rupture of membranes and oxytocin infusion by pump do not initiate labor, a cesarean birth is required. A long delay would raise the risk of increased hemorrhage, with resulting hypofibrinogenemia. Supportive actions to identify and reduce the risk of DIC include typing and crossmatching for blood transfusions (at least three units), evaluating the clotting mechanism, and providing intravenous fluids.

In cases of moderate to severe placental separation, a cesarean birth is done after treatment of hypofibrinogenemia by intravenous infusion of cryoprecipitate or fresh frozen plasma. Vaginal birth is impossible with a Couvelaire uterus, because the uterus would not contract properly in labor, and a hysterectomy is often needed.

The hypovolemia that accompanies severe abruptio placentae is life threatening and must be combated with whole blood. If the fetus is alive but experiencing stress, emergency cesarean birth is the method of choice. With a stillborn fetus, vaginal birth is preferable if bleeding has stabilized, unless maternal shock from hemorrhage is uncontrollable. Intravenous fluids are administered. Central venous pressure (CVP) monitoring may be needed to evaluate intravenous fluid replacement. An absolute level is not as important as the response to fluid replacement. CVP is evaluated hourly, and the results are communicated to the physician. Elevations of CVP may indicate fluid overload and pulmonary edema. Laboratory testing is ordered to provide ongoing data regarding hemoglobin, hematocrit, and coagulation status. The hematocrit is maintained at 30% through the administration of packed red blood cells or whole blood (Cunningham et al., 2014). Measures are taken to stimulate labor to effect a vaginal birth, if possible. An amniotomy may be performed, and oxytocin is given. Progressive dilatation and effacement usually occur.

Nursing Management

Electronic monitoring of the uterine contractions and resting tone between contractions provides information about the labor pattern and effectiveness of the oxytocin induction. Because uterine resting tone is frequently increased with abruptio placentae, it must be evaluated frequently for further increase. Abdominal girth measurements may be ordered every 30 minutes using a measuring tape to measure fundal height from the superior aspect of the symphysis pubis to the top of

TABLE 20–6 Abnormal Clotting Factors Indicative of Placentae Abruptio

- PT longer than 15 seconds
- PTT longer than 60 seconds
- Fibrinogen levels less than 150 mg/dL
- Platelet count less than 100,000/mm³
- Fibrinogen degradation products greater than 100 mg/mL

the uterine fundus. Another method of evaluating uterine size, which increases as more bleeding occurs at the site of abruption, involves placing a mark at the top of the uterine fundus; the distance from the symphysis pubis to the mark may be measured hourly. Overdistention of the uterus can lead to a ruptured uterus, another life-threatening complication. See *Nursing Care Plan: For the Woman with Hemorrhage in the Third Trimester.*

Nursing Care Plan: For the Woman with Hemorrhage in the Third Trimester

1. Nursing Diagnosis: *Fluid Volume: Deficient, Risk for,* **related to excessive vascular loss during pregnancy (NANDA-I © 2014)**

GOAL: Woman will not experience significant fluid volume deficit during the third trimester of pregnancy.

INTERVENTION	RATIONALE
• Monitor vital signs: i.e., temperature—normal range is 96.8°–100.4°F (36°–38°C), pulse—normal is 60–90, respirations—normal is 12–22, blood pressure (BP)—normal range is 110/70 to 135/85, central venous pressure—normal range is 5–10 mmHg. Compare present BP with woman's baseline BP. Note pulse pressure.	• Any deviations in a woman's baseline vital signs could indicate intravascular fluctuations.
• Weigh pads and chux. If the woman has bathroom privileges, instruct her on initiating pad counts. Teach the woman how to weigh pads and chux, with each gram equal to approximately 1 mL of blood loss.	• The combination of weighing and counting pads and chux assists medical personnel in determining the woman's blood loss.
• Report amount of blood loss within a specific period (e.g., 50 mL of bright-red blood on pad in 20 min).	
• Monitor urinary output hourly and measure urine specific gravity (normal: 1.010–1.025).	• A decrease in urinary output (less than 30 mL/hr) and an increase in specific gravity suggest dehydration and a need for an increase in fluid intake.
• Palpate bilateral peripheral pulses (normal: equal and strong) and note capillary refill (normal: less than 3 sec). Also, assess skin color and temperature (normal: pink, warm, dry, and intact).	• Helps determine signs of circulatory loss or hypovolemic shock, which include weak pulses, capillary refill greater than 3 sec, skin color that is cyanotic or pallor, and skin temperature that is cool and clammy.
• Assess mental status at frequent intervals.	• Excessive blood loss can lead to changes in mentation.
• Assess the woman for signs and symptoms of disseminated intravascular coagulation.	• Provides vital information on maternal status.
• Instruct the woman on the importance of strict bedrest and avoidance of any sexual activity that involves nipple stimulation or that might lead to orgasm.	• Bleeding may cease with limited activity. Pressure on the abdomen and orgasms can stimulate uterine activity, thereby causing bleeding. Nipple stimulation may result in uterine contractions, as can orgasm.
• Monitor fetal status and uterine activity by continuous fetal monitoring.	• May determine the origin of bleeding and fetal well-being.

Collaborative:

INTERVENTION	RATIONALE
• Collect and review blood work: complete blood count (CBC), type and crossmatch, Rh titer, fibrinogen levels, platelet count, activated partial thromboplastin time (APTT), and prothrombin time (PT).	• Determines blood loss and need for intervention if blood work is abnormal.
• Administer appropriate isotonic IV solutions and blood products (e.g., plasma expanders, whole blood, serum albumin, or packed red blood cells) as ordered by the physician.	• Reverses shock symptoms by increasing blood volume.
• Insert Foley catheter.	• Close monitoring of urinary output will aid in determining adequate renal perfusion.

EXPECTED OUTCOME: The woman will show signs of adequate fluid volume during pregnancy as evidenced by vital signs within normal limits, capillary refill in less than 3 sec, adequate sensorium, and urine output greater than 30 mL/hr.

(*continued*)

Nursing Care Plan: For the Woman with Hemorrhage in the Third Trimester (*continued*)

2. Nursing Diagnosis: *Tissue Perfusion: Peripheral, Ineffective,* (uteroplacental) related to hypovolemia secondary to excessive maternal blood loss (NANDA-I © 2014)

GOAL: The fetus will have no evidence of hypoxia during pregnancy.

INTERVENTION	RATIONALE
• Assess maternal vital signs.	• Closely monitoring maternal physiologic status and circulatory status will assist in determining if an episode of bleeding has occurred and allow for interventions to protect maternal and fetal well-being.
• Monitor fetal heart tones continuously, assessing for variability, accelerations, and decelerations, and record.	• Continuous electronic fetal monitoring will aid in detecting signs of fetal hypoxia and allow time for appropriate intervention.
• Assess fundal height.	• Determines an approximate gestational age.
	• Determining fundal height and monitoring for increased size can reflect active bleeding.
• Assess labor progression by determining cervical dilatation and effacement if contractions are present.	• This provides information on maternal labor status.

Collaborative:

• Perform scalp stimulation to assess fetal accelerations.	• FHR acceleration is considered 15 beats above the baseline lasting for 15 sec and is indicative of fetal well-being.
• Assess amniotic fluid for meconium.	• Impaired gas exchange relaxes fetal intestinal motility, causing expulsion of meconium into amniotic fluid.
• Assist the physician during ultrasonography and amniocentesis for lecithin/sphingomyelin (L/S) ratio sample.	• Determines viability and alerts appropriate medical personnel of fetal age if birth is imminent.

EXPECTED OUTCOME: Fetus will demonstrate adequate tissue perfusion as evidenced by fetal heart tones that remain within 110–160 beats/min, long-term variability and short-term variability present, positive periodic changes (no variable or late decelerations), and fetal scalp blood pH greater than 7.25.

3. Nursing Diagnosis: *Fear/Anxiety* related to personal and fetal well-being secondary to third-trimester hemorrhage (NANDA-I © 2014)

GOAL: The woman will verbalize a decrease in fear and anxiety.

INTERVENTION	RATIONALE
• Maintain frequent contact with the woman and family members.	• Establishes trust with the woman and her family members, so they will not feel alone or abandoned.
• Provide the woman with accurate, reliable information concerning diagnosis and prognosis.	• Fear and anxiety will lessen when the woman is informed of health status and is allowed to make decisions based on present situation.

EXPECTED OUTCOME: The woman will actively seek information about diagnosis and prognosis.

• Allow the woman and family members to verbalize the origin of fears.	• Recognizing the origin of fear gives the woman and her family the appropriate tool to begin the process of developing coping strategies for dealing with the fears.
• Explain all procedures in an easy-to-understand, nonthreatening manner, and allow the woman and family members to ask questions.	• Accurate information prepares the woman and family members for the impending procedures, thereby reducing fear of the unknown.

EXPECTED OUTCOME: The woman and her family members develop appropriate coping strategies that decrease fear and anxiety.

Care of the Woman With Cervical Insufficiency

Cervical insufficiency is "a presumed physical weakness of the cervical tissue that causes or contributes to the early delivery of an otherwise healthy pregnancy" (Berghella, 2015, para 10). It is identified by painless dilatation of the cervix without contractions, which the pregnant woman is typically unaware of. The incidence of cervical insufficiency is 1% or less of all pregnancies (Sandberg, Einarsson, & McElrath, 2015). Cervical effacement occurs from the internal os out and can be seen on an ultrasound as "funneling." Alteration is apparent in a transvaginal scan when fundal pressure is applied or the woman assumes a standing position.

Clinical Tip

Women should be advised that cervical insufficiency can be asymptomatic or may present with mild symptoms, such as pelvic pressure, premenstrual-like cramping or backache, and/or a change in vaginal discharge. These symptoms often begin between 14 and 20 weeks and may be present for several days or weeks before diagnosis is made.

Cervical insufficiency often is due to congenital or acquired cervical abnormalities. Congenital abnormalities include genetic disorders affecting collagen (e.g., Ehlers-Danlos syndrome), uterine anomalies, and biologic variations such as a shortened cervical length (less than 25 mm as revealed on transvaginal ultrasound [TVU] examination) or other cervical changes (Berghella, 2015). Acquired risk factors are more common and include cervical trauma that occurred during previous labor or delivery (spontaneous, forceps-assisted, or vacuum-assisted cesarean birth), rapid mechanical cervical dilation before a gynecologic procedure, or treatment of cervical intraepithelial neoplasia (Berghella, 2015).

A comprehensive obstetrical history can identify women with historical risk factors who warrant prophylactic placement of a cerclage at 12 to 14 weeks' gestation. Historical risk factors include the following (Berghella, 2015):

- Two prior consecutive second-trimester pregnancy losses associated with relatively painless early cervical dilatation

- Three early (<34 weeks) preterm births, not including those that are directly related to other causes such as infection, placental bleeding, multiple gestation, and preterm labor.

Diagnosis of cervical insufficiency is made utilizing the woman's obstetrical history, TVU, and physical examination.

Clinical Management

The management and interventions for cervical insufficiency are complex and are dependent on the gestational age, history, TVU results, and physical examination. Fetal fibronectin screening has limited use in women between 22 to 34 weeks. While this test is predictive of preterm birth, typically the results cannot be used for clinical decision making (Norwitz, 2015). See Table 20–7.

TABLE 20–7 Clinical Management of Cervical Insufficiency

PREVIOUS OBSTETRICAL HISTORY/RISK FACTORS	PROGESTERONE SUPPLEMENTATION RECOMMENDATIONS	TRANSVAGINAL ULTRASOUND (TVU) MONITORING FREQUENCY	CERCLAGE RECOMMENDATIONS
Two consecutive second-trimester pregnancy losses associated with relatively painless early cervical dilatation **or** three early (<34 weeks) preterm births in which other causes of pregnancy loss or preterm birth have been ruled out.	Begin hydroxyprogesterone caproate weekly from 16 to 36 weeks' gestation.	Begin TVU monitoring after cerclage placement every 2 weeks or more frequently if bleeding or possible cervical change suspected.	Prophylactic cerclage placement at 12–14 gestational weeks in singleton pregnancy based on mother's history.
Uterine and collagen disorders, identified biological variation.	Begin hydroxyprogesterone caproate weekly from 16 to 36 weeks' gestation.	Begin TVU monitoring at 14 weeks; continue every 2 weeks if cervical length >30 mm. If cervical change occurs, increase screening to every week if cervical length >25 mm but <30 mm.	If cervical length is <25 mm, cerclage placement is indicated.
Prior preterm birth between 28 and 36 weeks' gestation	Begin hydroxyprogesterone caproate weekly from 16 to 36 weeks' gestation	Begin TVU screening at 16 weeks, then every 2 weeks if cervical length >30 mm. If cervical change occurs, increase screening to every week if cervical length >25 mm but <30 mm.	Cerclage placement if cervical length <25 mm.
Physical examination with cervical change and ultrasound showing cervical length <25 mm.	Begin hydroxyprogesterone caproate weekly from 16 to 36 weeks of gestation.	TVU every 2 weeks if cervical length is 25 mm to 30 mm. Cervical length <25 mm requires weekly or more frequent monitoring.	If <24 gestational weeks, cerclage placement is indicated.

(continued)

TABLE 20–7 **Clinical Management of Cervical Insufficiency (*continued*)**

PREVIOUS OBSTETRICAL HISTORY/RISK FACTORS	PROGESTERONE SUPPLEMENTATION RECOMMENDATIONS	TRANSVAGINAL ULTRASOUND (TVU) MONITORING FREQUENCY	CERCLAGE RECOMMENDATIONS
Previous cerclage placed for shortened cervix, with full-term pregnancy.	Not indicated unless documented shortened cervix or if cerclage is placed.	TVU monitoring at 16–24 weeks.	Cerclage placed only if shortened cervical length.
Previous cerclage placed for shortened cervix with subsequent preterm birth or perinatal loss in second semester.	Begin hydroxyprogesterone caproate weekly at time of cerclage placement.	TVU every 2 weeks if stable; if shortening continues, weekly or PRN.	Transabdominal cerclage indicated.

Source: Data from Berghella, V. (2015). *Cervical insufficiency*. Retrieved from http://www.uptodate.com/contents/cervical-insufficiency; Posner, G., Black, A., Jones, G., & Dy, J. (2014). *Oxorn & Foote's human labor and birth* (6th ed.). Philadelphia, PA: McGraw-Hill.

Additional risk factors include multiple gestations, progressively earlier births with each subsequent pregnancy, and precipitous labors and births. Women with multiple gestations are at higher risk for preterm labor and birth, but are generally excluded from cervical cerclage placement (Norwitz, 2015). In the past, clinical recommendations included bedrest and discontinuing work and home activities. Research has not shown that prohibiting these activities has led to improved clinical outcomes; thus, it is not routinely recommended. Studies have shown that women with cervical insufficiency should refrain from intercourse until after 34 weeks' gestation (Berghella, 2015).

Cerclage Procedures

A **cerclage** is a surgical procedure in which a stitch is placed in the cervix to prevent a spontaneous abortion or premature birth. See Figure 20–3. Most cerclages are placed through the vagina; however, some medical indications warrant an abdominal placement. These include failed vaginally placed cerclage, congenitally short or amputated cervix, cervical defects, a cervix previously scarred, unhealed lacerations, and subacute cervicitis. In the past, placement typically involved undergoing a laparotomy; however, it is now preferred that placement be done via a laparoscopic procedure (Hill & Burgis, 2015).

A prophylactic, history-based cervical cerclage placed at 12 to 14 weeks has an 89% success rate in preventing fetal loss and premature labor and birth (Adeniran, Aboyeji, Okpara, et al., 2014). History-based cerclages are typically done as an outpatient procedure and do not require antibiotic therapy. Emergent or rescue cerclages may warrant inpatient observation. Prolonged antibotics have not been shown to improve outcomes, but many women will receive a single dose during the surgical procedure.

Emergency or rescue cerclage placement, when dilatation and effacement have already occurred, has been shown to increase the chance of women maintaining the pregnancy until the age of viability, but the majority of these pregnancies result in preterm birth, 10% occurring between 24 and 28 weeks' gestation with risk for adverse neonatal outcomes (Hill & Burgis, 2015).

After 37 completed weeks' gestation, the cerclage suture may be cut and vaginal birth permitted, or the suture may be left in place and a cesarean birth performed to avoid repeating the procedure in subsequent pregnancies.

Care of the Woman with Multiple Gestation

In part because of advances in infertility treatments, the incidence of twins in the United States has increased from 1980 by 65%, with an incidence of 33.7 per 1000 births in 2013 (CDC, 2015).

The incidence of triplet and higher-order multiples has decreased since ACOG (2014b) and the American Society for Reproductive Medicine (ASRM) (2013) issued policy statements that the continued use of artificial reproductive technology should aim to reduce the number of multiples due to adverse fetal outcomes primarily related to prematurity. The incidence of spontaneous twins varies but is highest among Black women, women of greater age and parity, women with a family history of fraternal twins, women undergoing infertility treatment, and women who are tall and overweight. The incidence is low in the Asian and Hispanic populations (CDC, 2015). The physiology of multiple gestation is discussed in Chapter 4.

Twins that occur from two separate ova are called dizygotic (two zygotes) or fraternal twins. The fetuses may be the same sex or different sexes and are no more closely related genetically than any other siblings. In contrast, 33% of twins are monozygotic or identical twins; they develop from one fertilized ovum. They are genetically identical and always the same sex (CDC, 2015).

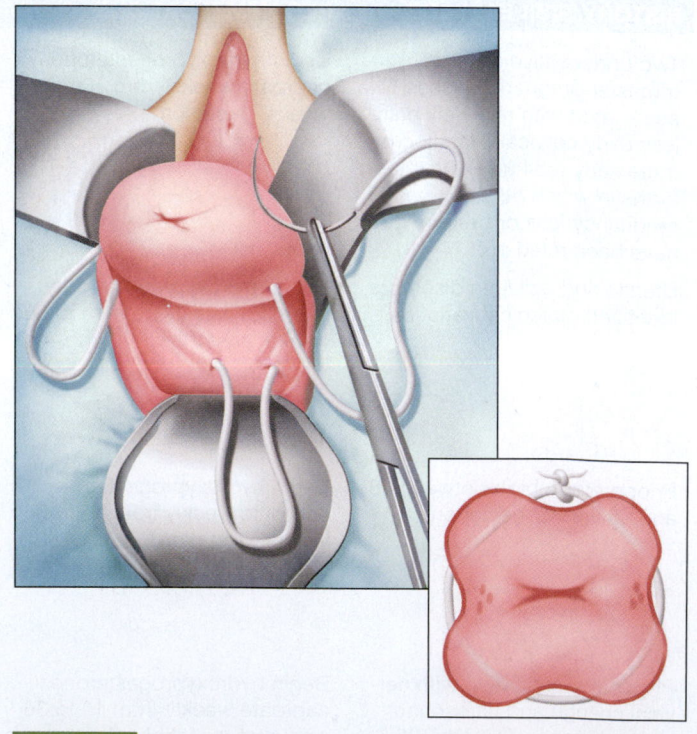

Figure 20–3 A cerclage, or purse-string suture, is inserted in the cervix to prevent preterm cervical dilatation and pregnancy loss. After placement, the string is tightened and secured anteriorly.

During the prenatal period, visualization of two gestational sacs at 5 to 6 weeks, fundal height greater than expected for the length of gestation, and auscultation of heart rates that differ by at least 10 beats per minute are the most likely clues to multiple-gestation pregnancies. In addition, the alpha-fetoprotein level on the quadruple screen is usually elevated and many women experience severe nausea and vomiting (caused by elevated levels of the human chorionic gonadotropin [hCG] hormone) (ASRM, 2013).

Maternal Implications

During her pregnancy, the woman may experience physical discomfort such as shortness of breath, dyspnea on exertion, backaches and musculoskeletal disorders, and pedal edema. Other associated problems include hyperemesis; iron deficiency anemia; urinary tract infections; threatened abortion; anemia; gestational hypertension; preeclampsia; gestational diabetes; preterm labor and birth; premature rupture of membranes; thromboembolism; placenta previa, abruptio placentae, and other types of placental disorders; cesarean section birth; and postpartum depression (ASRM, 2013). Complications during labor include abnormal fetal presentations, uterine dysfunction, prolapsed cord, and hemorrhage at or shortly after birth.

Fetal/Neonatal Implications

The perinatal mortality rate is approximately three times greater for twins than for a single fetus, and the mortality rate for triplets and higher-order multiple births is six times higher (ACOG, 2014b). It is estimated that 20% of triplet births result in one or more babies having a severe disability (ASRM, 2013). The perinatal mortality rate is substantially higher for mono-amniotic siblings. Fetal problems include decreased intrauterine growth rate for each fetus, increased incidence of fetal anomalies, increased risk of prematurity and its associated problems, abnormal presentations, and increased cord accidents. Neonatal risks include respiratory distress syndrome, intellectual disability, low birth weight, birth defects, high-grade intraventricular hemorrhage, periventricular leukomalacia, and an increase in cerebral palsy (ACOG, 2014b). Twins are more likely to have long-term disabilities when compared with children who were singleton births. Primiparous women have higher rates of complications than multiparous women. Multifetal pregnancies that are conceived spontaneously have better outcomes than those achieved with assisted reproductive technology (ASRM, 2013).

Clinical Therapy

Once the presence of twins has been detected, preventing and treating problems that infringe on the development and birth of normal fetuses are the most significant clinical goals. Prenatal visits are more frequent for women with twins than for those with one fetus. Women with multiple-gestation pregnancies need to understand the nutritional implications of multiple fetuses, the assessment of fetal activity, the signs of preterm labor, and the danger signs of pregnancy.

Women should begin serial ultrasound surveillance beginning in the second trimester (at 18 to 22 weeks' gestation). Women with monochorionic twins should undergo an ultrasound every 2 to 3 weeks to look for evidence of twin-to-twin transfusion syndrome. In dichorionic twins, surveillance can be done every 4 to 6 weeks (ACOG, 2014b). ACOG does not recommend specific antenatal testing for multiple gestations that lack additional risk factors and recommends that practitioners use the same guidelines that apply to singleton risk factors. Because multiple gestations have a higher incidence of stillbirth and complications, many practitioners continue to perform antepartum testing at 32 weeks' gestation despite the newer ACOG (2014b) guidelines.

Intrapartum management requires careful attention to maternal and fetal status. The mother should have an IV with a large-bore needle in place. Anesthesia and crossmatched blood should be readily available. The twins are monitored by continuous dual electronic fetal monitoring.

The decision about method of birth, which depends on a variety of factors, may not be made until labor occurs. The presence of maternal complications such as placenta previa, abruptio placentae, or severe preeclampsia usually indicates the need for cesarean birth. Fetal factors such as severe intrauterine growth restriction (IUGR), preterm birth, fetal anomalies, nonreassuring fetal status, and unfavorable fetal position or presentation also require cesarean birth.

Any combination of presentations and positions can occur with multiple births. Figure 20–4 shows some possible presentations of twins. When the presenting fetus is in a nonvertex position, cesarean birth is indicated.

Nursing Management

For the Woman With Multiple Gestation

COMMUNITY-BASED NURSING CARE

During pregnancy the woman may need counseling about diet and daily activities. Nutritional requirements vary based on the mother's prepregnancy body mass index (BMI). Women with BMIs of 18.5 to 24.9 are advised to gain 37 to 54 lb; women considered overweight (BMIs of 25 to 29.9) are advised to gain 31 to 50 lb; and women considered obese (BMIs above 30) are advised to gain 25 to 42 lb (Heard, 2015).

A prenatal vitamin and 1 mg of folic acid should also be taken daily. Additional iron and calcium are recommended.

Counseling about daily activities may include encouraging rest periods during the day, adjusting exercise to an appropriate level (walking), promoting sleep, and reducing stress. Rest periods in a side-lying position (which increases uteroplacental blood flow) with elevation of lower legs and feet help reduce edema. Back discomfort may be relieved by pelvic rocking, maintaining good posture, consistent use of a pregnancy belt to support the abdomen and lower back, and using good body mechanics when lifting objects and moving about.

HOSPITAL-BASED NURSING CARE

During labor, the fetal heart rates (FHRs) of the fetuses are monitored continuously by an electronic fetal monitor (EFM). All fetuses are monitored throughout labor until birth occurs: women undergoing a cesarean should continue to have EFM until the incision is completed. Most multiple gestations are now delivered via cesarean birth.

After the birth, prepare to receive two or more newborns instead of one. This means duplicating everything, including resuscitation equipment, radiant warmers, and newborn identification papers and bracelets. Additional staff members should be available for newborn resuscitation, monitoring, and newborn care. Special precautions should be taken to ensure correct identification of the newborns. The first born is usually tagged Baby A; the second, Baby B; and so on.

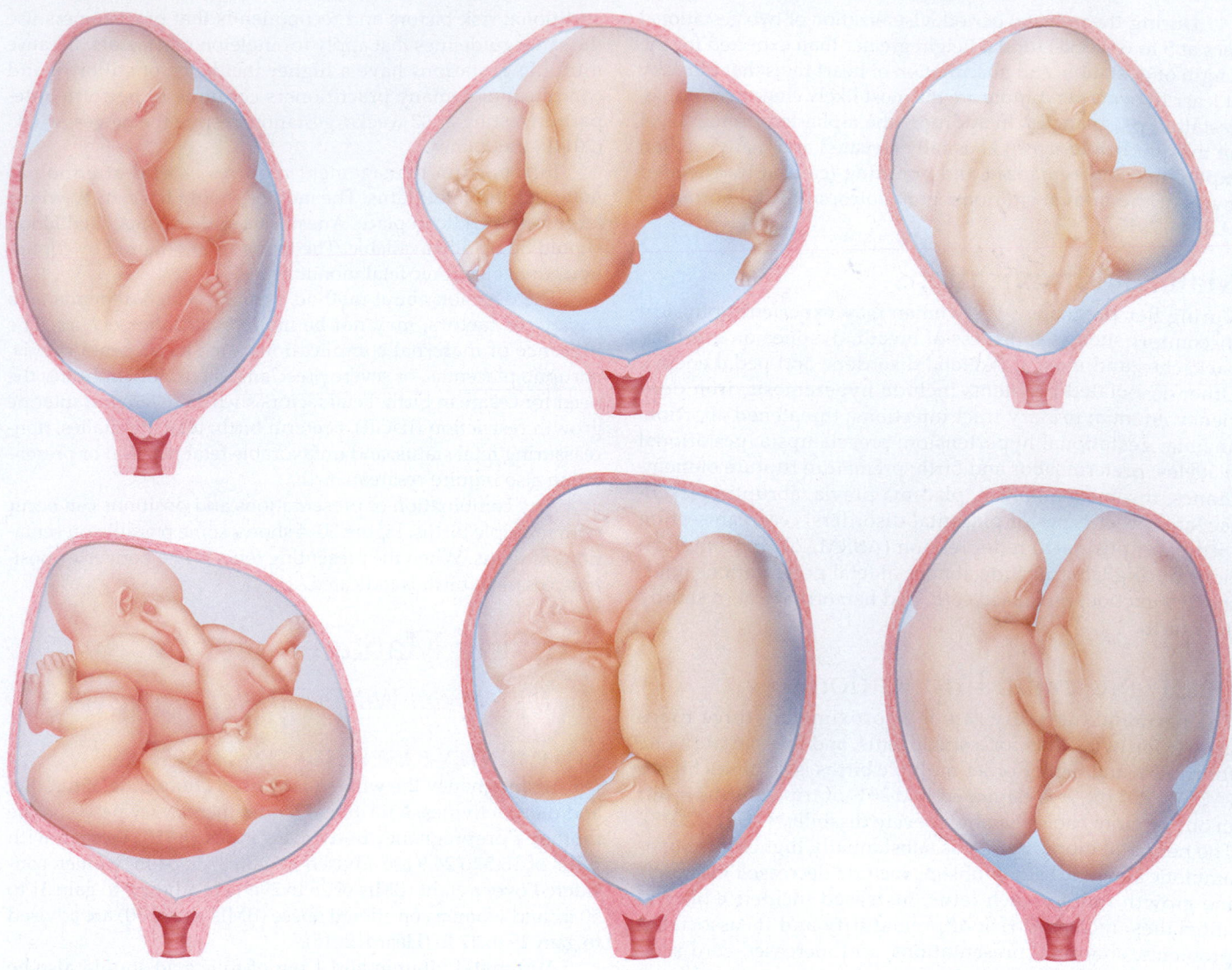

Figure 20–4 Twins may be in any of these presentations while in utero.

Care of the Woman with Abnormal Amniotic Fluid Volume

Amniotic fluid serves many important functions during pregnancy. Some pregnancies are complicated by either an excessive amount of amniotic fluid (hydramnios) or a reduced amount of fluid (oligohydramnios).

Hydramnios

Hydramnios (also called *polyhydramnios*), a situation in which there is more than 2000 mL of amniotic fluid (approximately 500 mL is considered normal), occurs in about 1% of all pregnancies (Cunningham et al., 2014). The exact cause of hydramnios is unknown; however, it often occurs in cases of major congenital anomalies.

During the second half of a normal pregnancy, the fetus begins to swallow and inspire amniotic fluid and to urinate, which contributes to the amount of amniotic fluid present. In cases of hydramnios, no pathology has been found in the amniotic epithelium. However, hydramnios is associated with fetal malformations that affect the fetal swallowing mechanism and neurologic disorders in which the fetal meninges are exposed in the amniotic cavity. This condition is also found in cases of anencephaly, in which the fetus is thought to urinate excessively because of overstimulation of the cerebrospinal centers. When monozygotic twins manifest hydramnios, it is because the twin with the increased blood volume urinates excessively. Because the weight of the placenta has been found to be increased in some cases of hydramnios, increased functioning of the placental tissue may be a factor.

There are two types of hydramnios: chronic and acute. In the chronic type, the fluid volume gradually increases and becomes a problem during the third trimester. Most cases are of this variety. In acute cases, the volume increases rapidly over a period of a few days. The acute type is usually diagnosed between 20 and 24 weeks' gestation.

MATERNAL IMPLICATIONS

When the amount of amniotic fluid is over 3000 mL, the woman experiences shortness of breath and edema in the lower extremities from compression of the vena cava. Milder forms of hydramnios occur more frequently and are associated with minimal symptoms. Hydramnios is associated with maternal disorders such as diabetes and Rh sensitization and with multiple-gestation pregnancies. It can also occur as a result of infections such as syphilis, toxoplasmosis, cytomegalovirus, herpes, and rubella.

If the amniotic fluid is removed rapidly before birth, abruptio placentae can result from too sudden a change in the size of the uterus. Because of overdistention of uterine muscles, uterine dysfunction can occur in the intrapartum period, and the incidence of postpartum hemorrhage increases.

FETAL/NEONATAL IMPLICATIONS

Fetal malformations and preterm birth are common with hydramnios; thus the perinatal mortality rate is fairly high. A prolapsed cord can result when the membranes rupture, creating a further complication for the fetus. The incidence of malpresentations also increases. In addition, the incidence of preterm labor and cesarean birth is significantly increased in pregnancies complicated by hydramnios.

CLINICAL THERAPY

Hydramnios is managed with supportive treatment unless the intensity of the woman's distress and symptoms dictates otherwise. If the accumulation of amniotic fluid is severe enough to cause maternal dyspnea and pain, hospitalization and removal of the excessive fluid are required. Fluid can be removed vaginally or by amniocentesis. The dangers of performing the technique vaginally are a prolapsed cord and the inability to remove the fluid slowly. If amniocentesis is performed, it should be done with the aid of sonography to prevent inadvertent damage to the fetus and the placenta. In addition, the fluid should be removed slowly to prevent abruption.

Nursing Management

Hydramnios should be suspected when the fundal height increases out of proportion to the gestational age. As the amount of fluid increases, you may have difficulty palpating the fetus and auscultating the fetal heart rate (FHR). In more severe cases, the maternal abdomen appears extremely tense and tight on inspection. On sonography, large spaces of fluid pockets can be identified between the fetus and the uterine wall.

When amniocentesis is performed, it is vital to maintain sterile technique to prevent infection. Offer support to the couple by explaining the procedure to them.

If the fetus has been diagnosed with a congenital defect in utero or is born with a defect, the family needs psychologic support. You may need to collaborate with social services to offer the family this additional help.

Oligohydramnios

Oligohydramnios is defined as a less-than-normal (<500 mL) amount of amniotic fluid. This condition affects 1% to 3% of all pregnancies (Cunningham et al., 2014). Oligohydramnios is diagnosed when the largest vertical pocket of amniotic fluid visible on ultrasound examination is 5 cm (2 in.) or less (Cunningham et al., 2014).

The exact cause of this condition is unknown. It is found in cases of postmaturity; with maternal hypertensive disorders; with intrauterine growth restriction (IUGR) secondary to placental insufficiency; and in fetal conditions associated with major renal malformations, including renal aplasia with dysplastic kidneys and obstructive lesions of the lower urinary tract. If oligohydramnios occurs in the first part of pregnancy,

there is a danger of fetal adhesions (one part of the fetus may adhere to another part).

MATERNAL IMPLICATIONS

When oligohydramnios exists, labor can be dysfunctional, and progress is slow. The woman should be monitored for hypertensive disorders.

> ### Health Promotion Oligohydramnios
>
> Because oligohydramnios is often associated with hypertensive complications and hyperglycemia, women should be carefully assessed for these risk factors at the initial prenatal visit. Obese women have a higher incidence of these risk factors and should strive to maintain a healthy weight gain during pregnancy. Healthy dietary practices, regular exercise, monitoring for blood pressure and glucose level abnormalities are all practices that can help reduce risk factors for oligohydramnios.

FETAL/NEONATAL IMPLICATIONS

During the gestational period, fetal skin and skeletal abnormalities may occur because fetal movement is impaired as a result of reduced amniotic fluid volume. Because there is less fluid available for the fetus to use during fetal breathing movements, pulmonary hypoplasia may develop. During the labor and birth, oligohydramnios reduces the cushioning effect for the umbilical cord, and cord compression is more likely to occur. Decreased amniotic fluid also contributes to fetal head compression.

CLINICAL THERAPY

During the antepartum period oligohydramnios may be suspected when the uterus does not increase in size according to the dates, the fetus is easily palpated and outlined by the examiner, and the fetus is not ballottable. The fetus can be assessed by biophysical profiles (BPPs), non-stress tests (NSTs), and serial ultrasounds. As soon as the fetus is term, induction is typically scheduled because the fetus is at an increased risk for intrauterine fetal demise. During labor, the fetus is monitored by continuous electronic fetal monitoring (EFM) to detect cord compression, which is indicated by variable decelerations. *Amnioinfusion* (a transcervical instillation of 250 mL of warmed sterile saline, followed by a continuous infusion rate of 100 to 200 mL/hr) after membranes have ruptured in the presence of nonreassuring fetal status may be utilized to decrease fetal heart decelerations; however, routine use is generally not recommended (Roque, Gillen-Goldstein, & Funai, 2015).

Nursing Management

Continuous electronic fetal monitoring is an important part of the assessment during labor and birth. Evaluate the EFM tracing for the presence of variable decelerations or other nonreassuring signs (such as increasing or decreasing baseline, decreased variability, presence of late decelerations). If variable decelerations are noted, change the woman's position (to relieve pressure on the umbilical cord), and notify the physician/CNM. If the tracing is not reassuring, a cesarean birth is performed. After the birth, the newborn is evaluated for signs of congenital anomalies, pulmonary hypoplasia, and postmaturity. The newborn affected by oligohydramnios should have a renal ultrasound to rule out renal agenesis, renal dysplasia, or obstructive uropathy (Carter, 2015).

Focus Your Study

- Both premature rupture of the membranes (PROM) and preterm labor (PTL) place the fetus at risk. Women with preterm PROM and no signs of infection are managed conservatively with bedrest and careful monitoring of fetal well-being. If preterm labor develops, tocolytics are often effective in delaying labor, but they have associated side effects.

- Placenta previa occurs when the placenta implants low in the uterus near or over the cervix. Placenta previa is classified into 4 grades. Grade 1, low-lying placenta, is the mildest form. Grade 2 is also known as a marginal previa; the placenta lies near the cervix. Grade 3 is considered a partial placenta previa; part of the placenta lies over the cervix. Grade 4 represents a complete placenta previa; the cervix is completely covered.

- Abruptio placentae is the separation of the placenta from the side of the uterus before the birth of the baby. Abruptio placentae may be central, marginal, or complete. Further classification by grades (0–3) provides quantitative terminology to explain the amount of bleeding. Grade 0 represents an undiagnosed bleed that is identified only through placental examination after birth. Grade 1 represents mild bleeding and uterine tenderness with no maternal or fetal compromise.

- Grade 2 occurs when bleeding is noted and maternal compromise occurs warranting continuous EFM. Grade 3 is the most severe and is diagnosed when severe maternal bleeding is present that results in maternal shock and/or fetal death.

- Cervical insufficiency refers to premature dilatation of the cervix with no uterine contractions. It is the most common cause of second-trimester abortion. It is treated surgically with a cerclage, which involves placing a suture in the cervix to keep it from opening.

- Hydramnios, also known as polyhydramnios, occurs when more than 2000 mL of amniotic fluid is contained within the amniotic membranes. Hydramnios is associated with fetal malformations that affect fetal swallowing, maternal diabetes mellitus, Rh sensitization, infection, and multiple-gestation pregnancies.

- Oligohydramnios occurs when there is a severely reduced volume of amniotic fluid (less than 500 mL). Oligohydramnios is associated with intrauterine growth restriction (IUGR), postmaturity, and fetal renal or urinary malformations. The fetus is more likely to experience variable decelerations because the amniotic fluid is insufficient to keep pressure off the umbilical cord.

Clinical Reasoning in Action

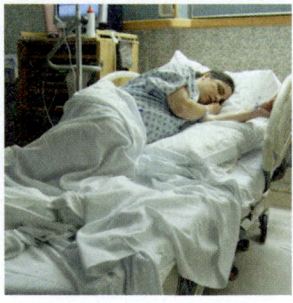

Monique Waleski, a 34-year-old G1P0 at 32 weeks' gestation, contacts her physician's office because she has been experiencing labor contractions that have gradually increased in frequency. She reports that she has been having about 8 contractions an hour for the past two hours. She is instructed to meet her doctor at the birthing unit for further evaluation.

At the birthing unit a vaginal examination reveals that Monique's cervix is dilated 3 cm and 80% effaced. Contractions continue to occur every 7 to 8 minutes. Her fFN test is positive. She is diagnosed with preterm labor. She is given two doses of terbutaline (Brethine) 0.25 mg subcutaneous injection, which decreases her contractions. Her physician orders magnesium sulfate for neuroprotection because she is 32 gestational weeks and prescribes 2 doses of betamethasone. You position her on her left side and start an IV infusion.

You explain to Monique and her partner that you will be giving her the magnesium sulfate by infusion pump and the betamethasone by IM injection once a day today and tomorrow. She asks you about the two medications, including their specific purposes.

1. Explain the concept of neuroprotection and the purpose of magnesium sulfate.

2. Describe the concept of a loading dose and a maintenance dose.

3. How will you know if Monique is developing toxic levels of magnesium?

4. Describe the role of corticosteroids used during preterm labor.

References

Adeniran, A. S., Aboyeji, A. P., Okpara, E. U., Fawole, A. A., & Adesina, K. T. (2014). Pregnancy outcome in cervical incompetence: Comparison of outcome before and after intervention. *Tropical Journal of Obstetrics and Gynaecology, 31*(1), 23–29.

American College of Obstetricians and Gynecologists (ACOG). (2013). *Premature rupture of membranes.*

(ACOG Practice Bulletin No. 139). Washington, DC: Author.

American College of Obstetricians and Gynecologists (ACOG). (2014a). *ACOG Practice Advisory on use of antenatal corticosteroids.* Washington, DC: Author.

American College of Obstetricians and Gynecologists (ACOG). (2014b). *Multifetal gestations: Twin, triplet,*

and higher-order multifetal pregnancies. (ACOG Practice Bulletin No. 114.) Washington, DC: ACOG.

American College of Obstetricians and Gynecologists (ACOG). (2010, reaffirmed 2015). *Magnesium sulfate before anticipated preterm birth for neuroprotection.* (ACOG Committee Opinion No. 455.) Washington, DC: ACOG.

American College of Radiology (ACR). (2015). American College of Radiology appropriateness criteria. Retrieved from https://acsearch.acr.org/list

American Society for Reproductive Medicine (ASRM). (2013). *Multiple pregnancy and birth: Twins, triplets, and high-order multiples.* Retrieved from https://www.asrm.org/BOOKLET_Multiple_Pregnancy_and_Birth/

Ananath, C. V., & Kinzler, W. L. (2015). Placental abruption: Clinical features and diagnosis. Retrieved from http://www.uptodate.com/contents/placental-abruption-clinical-features-and-diagnosis

Berghella, V. (2015). Cervical insufficiency. Retrieved from http://www.uptodate.com/contents/cervical-insufficiency

Boisramé, T., Sananès, N., Fritz, G., Boudier, E., Aissi, G., Favre, R., & Langer. B. (2014). Placental abruption: Risk factors, management and maternal–fetal prognosis: Cohort study over 10 years. *European Journal of Obstetrics & Gynecology and Reproductive Biology, 179,* 100–104. doi:10.1016/j.ejogrb.2014.05.026

Carter, B. S. (2015). Polyhydramnios and oligohydramnios follow up. Retrieved from http://reference.medscape.com/article/975821-followup#e6

Centers for Disease Control & Prevention (CDC). (2014). Preterm birth. Retrieved from http://www.cdc.gov/reproductivehealth/maternalinfanthealth/pretermbirth.htm

Centers for Disease Control & Prevention (CDC). (2015). Multiple births. Retrieved from http://www.cdc.gov/nchs/fastats/multiple.htm

Conde-Agudelo, A., & Romero, R. (2015). Vaginal progesterone to prevent preterm birth in pregnant women with a sonographic short cervix: Clinical and public health implications. *American Journal of Obstetrics and Gynecology.* Retrieved from http://www.sciencedirect.com/science/article/pii/S0002937815012168

Cunningham, F. G., Leveno, K. J., Bloom, S. L., Spong, C. Y., Dashe, J. S., Hoffman, B. L., . . . Sheffield, J. S. (2014). *Williams obstetrics* (24th ed.). New York, NY: McGraw-Hill.

Deering, S. H. (2015). Abruptio placentae. *eMedicine.* Retrieved from http://emedicine.medscape.com/article/252810-overview#a0101

Guillet, A., Wilson-Smith, M. R., & Caughey, A. B. (2015). Outcomes of neonates from pregnancies with preterm premature rupture of membranes [313].

Obstetrics & Gynecology, 125, 100S. doi:10.1097/01.AOG.0000463564.91457.b4

Heard, A.J. (2015). Multifetal pregnancy treatment and management. Retrieved from http://emedicine.medscape.com/article/1618038-treatment#d12

Hill, M. G., & Burgis, J. T. (2015). Success of rescue cervical cerclage at a single institution. *American Journal of Clinical Experts in Obstetrics & Gynecology, 2*(1), 34–38.

Jazayeri, A. (2014). Premature rupture of membranes. *Medscape.* Retrieved from http://emedicine.medscape.com/article/261137-overview

Joy, S. (2015). Placenta previa. *Medscape.* Retrieved from http://emedicine.medscape.com/article/262063-overview#a0156

Kenyon, S., Boulvain, M., & Neilson, J. (2013). Antibiotics for preterm rupture of membranes. *Cochrane Database of Systematic Reviews.* Issue 12, Art. No.: CD001058.

Ko, T. J., Tsai, L. Y., Chu, L. C., Yeh, S. J., Leung, C., Chen, C. Y., Chou, H. C., Tsao, P. N., Chen, P. C., & Hsieh, W. S. (2014). Parental smoking during pregnancy and its association with low birth weight, small for gestational age, and preterm birth offspring: A birth cohort study. *Pediatric Neonatology, 55*(1), 20–7. doi:10.1016/j.pedneo.2013.05.005

Kollmann, M., Gaulhofer, J., Lang, U., & Klaritsch, P. (2014). Placenta previa: Incidence, risk factors and outcome. *Ultrasound in Obstetrics & Gynecology, 44,* 332–333. doi:10.1002/uog.14485

Kuhrt, K., Hezelgrave, N., Foster, C., Seed, P. T., & Shennan, A. H. (2015). Development and validation of a predictive tool for spontaneous preterm birth, incorporating quantitative fetal fibronectin, in symptomatic women. *Ultrasound in Obstetrics & Gynecology, 47*(2), 129–264. doi:10.1002/uog.14894

Liong, S., Di Quinzio, M. K. W., Fleming, G., Permezel, M., Rice, G. E., & Georgiou, H. M. (2015). New biomarkers for the prediction of spontaneous preterm labour in symptomatic pregnant women: A comparison with fetal fibronectin. *BJOG: An International Journal of Obstetrics & Gynaecology, 122*(3), 370–379. doi:10.1111/1471-0528.12993

Norwitz, E. R. (2015). Cervical insufficiency treatment and management. Retrieved from http://emedicine.medscape.com/article/1979914-treatment

Padovani, T. R., Guyatt, G., & Lopes, L. C. (2015). Nifedipine versus terbutaline, Tocolytic effectiveness

and maternal and neonatal adverse effects: A randomized, controlled pilot trial. *Basic & Clinical Pharmacology & Toxicology, 116*(3), 244–250. doi:10.1111/bcpt.12306

Räisänen, S., Kancherla, V., Kramer, M. R., Gissler, M., & Heinonen, S. (2014). Placenta previa and the risk of delivering a small-for-gestational-age newborn. *Obstetrics & Gynecology, 124*(2, PART 1), 285–291. doi:10.1097/AOG.0000000000000368

Roque, H., Gillen-Goldstein, J., & Funai, E. F. (2015). Amnioinfusion technique. Retrieved from http://www.uptodate.com/contents/amnioinfusion-technique

Ross, M. G. (2015). Preterm birth. Retrieved from http://emedicine.medscape.com/article/260998-overview

Saccone, G., & Berghella, V. (2015). Antibiotic prophylaxis for term or near-term premature rupture of membranes: Meta-analysis of randomized trials. *American Journal of Obstetrics & Gynecology, 212,* 627, e1–9.

Sandberg, E. M., Einarsson, J. I., & McElrath, T. F. (2015). Laparascopic cerclage. In O. Istre (Ed.), *Minimally invasive gynecological surgery* (pp. 139–147). New York, NY: Springer Publishing Company.

Silver, R. (2015). Abnormal placentation: Placenta previa, vasa previa, and placenta accreta. *Obstetrics & Gynecology, 126*(3), 654–668. doi:10.1097/AOG.0000000000001005

Suhag, A., Reina, J., Sanapo, L., Martinelli, P., Saccone, G., Simonazzi, G., . . . & Berghella, V. (2015). Prior ultrasound-indicated cerclage: Comparison of cervical length screening or history-indicated cerclage in the next pregnancy. *Obstetrics & Gynecology, 126*(5), 962–968. doi:10.1097/AOG.0000000000001086

Theplib, A., & Phupong, V. (2015). Success rate of terbutaline in inhibiting preterm labor for 48 h. *The Journal of Maternal-Fetal & Neonatal Medicine,* (0), 1–4. doi:10.3109/14767058.2015.1021671

Tikkanen, M. (2014). Placental abruption: Epidemiology, risk factors and consequences. *Acta Obstetricia et Gynecologica Scandinavica, 90,*140–149. doi:10.1111/j.1600-0412.2010.01030x

Wilson, B. A., Shannon, M. T., & Shields, K. M. (2015). *Pearson nurse's drug guide 2016.* Upper Saddle River, NJ: Pearson.

Wojcieszek, A., Stock, O., & Flenady, V. (2014). Antibiotics for pre-labour rupture of membranes at or near term. *Cochrane Database of Systematic Reviews.* Issue 10. Art. No.: CD001807.

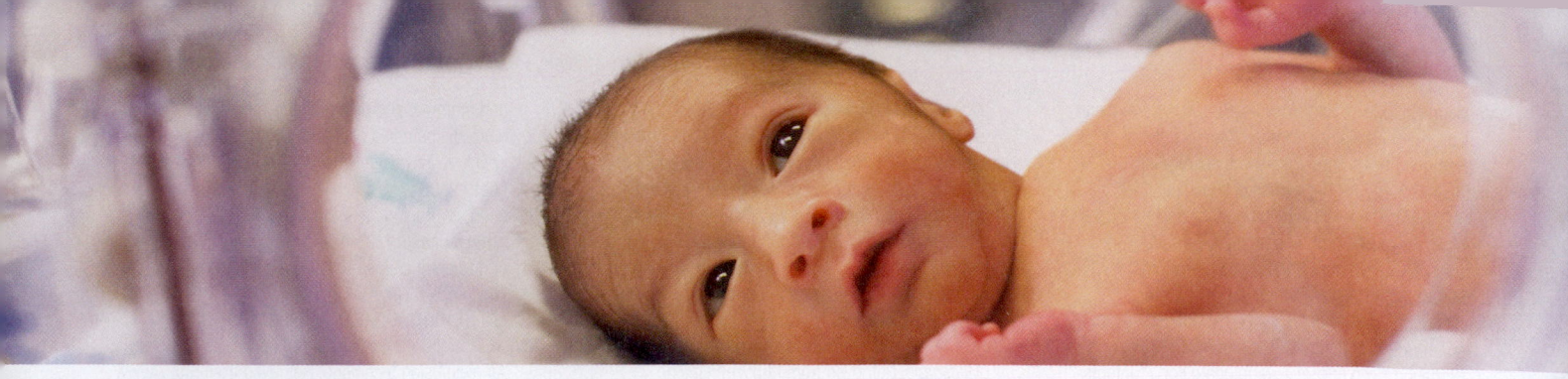

Chapter 21
Childbirth at Risk: Labor-Related Complications

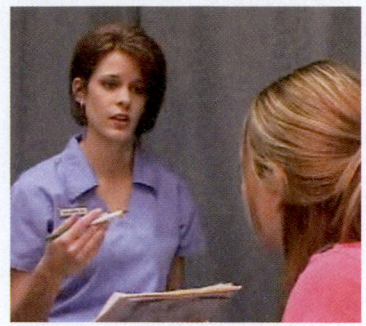

I am very conscientious about making sure that I cover "unexpected outcomes" in my childbirth preparation classes. Although everyone hopes and anticipates that labor and birth will proceed normally, unfortunately it sometimes doesn't. At those times, when the family is anxious or afraid, maybe somewhere in the back of their minds is a little seed of reassurance because we have already talked about problems a little.

—Labor/Delivery Nurse and Childbirth Educator (CBE)

⌄ Learning Outcomes

21.1 Compare tachysystolic and hypotonic labor patterns, including risks, clinical therapy, and nursing management.

21.2 Describe the risks and clinical therapy in determining the community-based and hospital-based nursing management of postterm pregnancy on the childbearing family.

21.3 Relate the various types of fetal malposition and malpresentation, risks, and clinical therapy to the nursing management for each.

21.4 Explain the identification, risks, and clinical therapy in determining the nursing management of the woman and fetus at risk for macrosomia.

21.5 Relate the maternal implications, clinical therapy, prenatal history, and conditions that may be associated with nonreassuring fetal status to the nursing care of the mother and fetus.

21.6 Describe the nursing care for the mother and fetus with a prolapsed umbilical cord.

21.7 Summarize the identification, maternal and fetal/neonatal implications, clinical therapy, and nursing management of women with amniotic fluid embolus.

21.8 Explain the types of cephalopelvic disproportion, its maternal and fetal/neonatal implications, and clinical therapy in determining the nursing management of the woman.

21.9 Identify common complications of the third and fourth stages of labor.

21.10 Explain the etiology, diagnosis, and phases of grief in determining the nursing management of the family experiencing perinatal loss.

Successful completion of a pregnancy requires the harmonious functioning of the five critical factors discussed in Chapter 16: the birth passage, the fetus, the relationship between the passage and the fetus, the forces of labor, and psychosocial considerations. Disruptions in any of these components may cause **dystocia**, which is abnormal or difficult labor. This chapter discusses the most common of these disruptions.

Care of the Woman With Dystocia Related to Dysfunctional Uterine Contractions

Dystocia may be caused by a wide variety of problems, the most common of which is dysfunctional (or uncoordinated) uterine contractions. These uncoordinated contractions result in a prolonged labor. Contractions that result in a more normal progression of labor tend to be moderate to strong when palpated and occur regularly (two to four contractions in 10 minutes in early labor and four to five per 10 minutes in later phases). Dysfunctional contractions are typically irregular in strength, timing, or both. These irregular uterine contractions are not effective in producing dilatation or effacement. Figure 21–1 depicts normal, tachysystolic, and hypotonic uterine contraction patterns.

Tachysystolic Labor Patterns

In tachysystolic (also called *hypertonic*) labor patterns (Figure 21–1B), ineffective uterine contractions of poor quality occur in the latent phase of labor, and the resting tone of the myometrium (uterine muscle) increases. Contractions usually become more frequent, but their intensity may decrease. The contractions are painful but ineffective in the dilatation and effacement of the cervix, and a prolonged latent phase may result. These prolonged contractions can result in fetal hypoxia.

Clinical Tip

To determine if the fetal heart rate (FHR) is reassuring, the following components should be present: a baseline FHR of 110 to 160 beats/min, presence of variability, spontaneous accelerations, and absence of decelerations.

RISKS OF TACHYSYSTOLIC LABOR

Maternal risks of tachysystolic labor include:

- Increased discomfort caused by uterine muscle cell anoxia
- Fatigue as the pattern continues and no labor progress results
- Frustration and stress on coping abilities
- Dehydration and increased incidence of infection if labor is prolonged

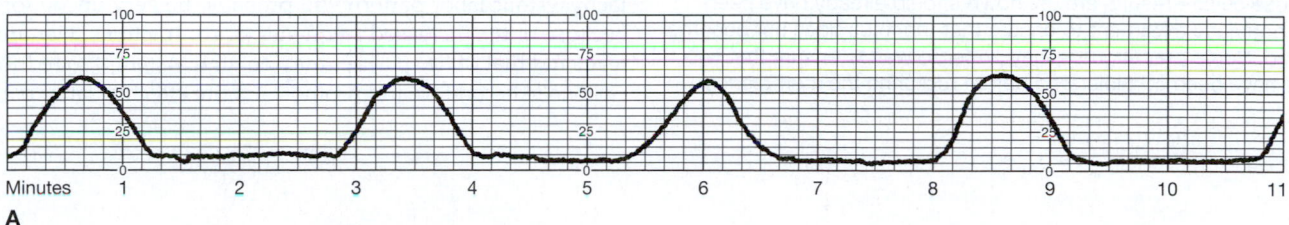

A

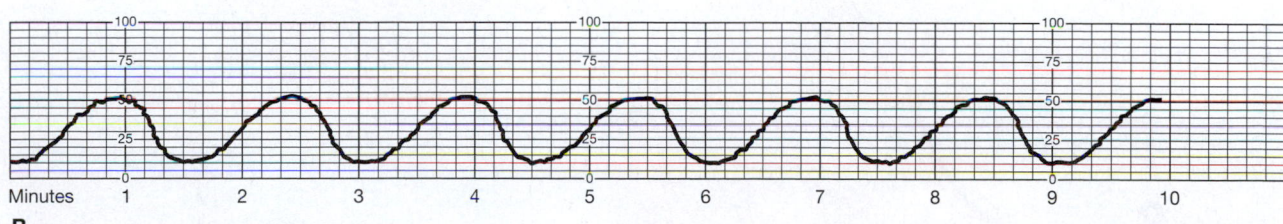

B

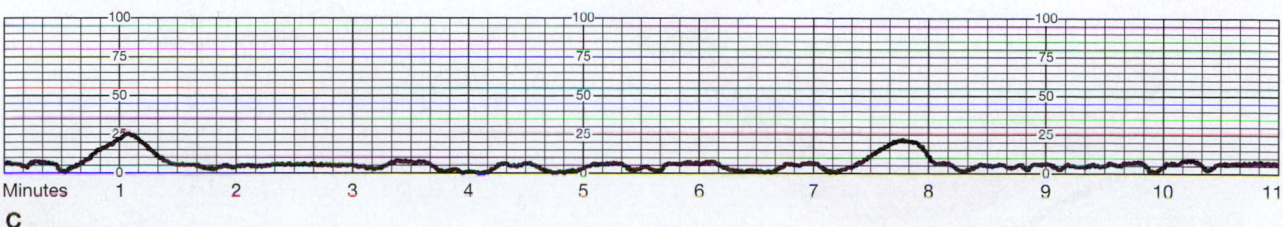

C

Figure 21–1 Comparison of labor patterns. A. Normal uterine contraction pattern. In this example, contraction frequency is every 3 minutes; duration is 60 seconds. The baseline resting tone is below 10 mmHg. B. Tachysystolic uterine contraction pattern. Note that the contraction frequency is every 1.5 minutes, duration is 90.0 seconds. The baseline resting tone is 10 mmHg. C. Hypotonic uterine contraction pattern. In this example, the contraction frequency is every 7 minutes (with some uterine activity between contractions), duration is 50 seconds, and intensity increases approximately 25 mmHg during contractions.

Fetal/neonatal risks include:

- Nonreassuring fetal status caused by contractions and increased resting tone interfering with the uteroplacental exchange of gases and nutrients
- Prolonged pressure on the fetal head, which may result in cephalohematoma, caput succedaneum, or excessive molding (Figure 21–2)

CLINICAL THERAPY

Management of tachysystolic labor may include bedrest and sedation to promote relaxation and reduce pain. Often pharmacologic intervention to promote sedation will stop these contractions. If the tachysystolic pattern continues and develops into a prolonged latent phase, oxytocin (Pitocin) infusion or amniotomy may be considered. An amniotomy can help a normal labor progress because of pressure on the cervix. Oxytocin can be used to strengthen existing contractions and lead to a more productive pattern (see Chapter 22). These methods are instituted only after cephalopelvic disproportion (CPD) and fetal malpresentation have been ruled out. If the maternal pelvic diameters are less than average, if the fetus is particularly large, or if the fetus is in a malpresentation or malposition, CPD is said to be present. In such cases, labor is not stimulated because vaginal birth is not possible. Instead, a cesarean birth will be performed.

Clinical Tip

When an amniotomy is used to augment labor, women who are group B streptococcus (GBS) positive, who have not had a culture, or whose culture results are unknown should already have been given antibiotic treatment to ensure that the fetus does not become infected. Some practitioners may prefer to wait to ensure that two doses have been administered before rupturing the membranes.

Nursing Management

For the Woman Experiencing Tachysystolic Labor

Nursing Assessment and Diagnosis

As part of the labor assessment, evaluate the intensity of the uterine contractions, the woman's perception of discomfort experienced, and the degree of cervical change. Note whether anxiety is negatively affecting labor progress. Evidence of increasing frustration and discouragement on the part of the mother and her partner may indicate the need to provide some additional information or reassurance.

Nursing diagnoses that may apply to the woman in tachysystolic labor include the following (NANDA-I © 2014):

- *Fatigue* related to inability to relax and rest secondary to a hypertonic labor pattern
- *Pain, Acute,* related to the woman's inability to relax secondary to tachysystolic uterine contractions
- *Coping, Ineffective,* related to ineffectiveness of breathing techniques to relieve discomfort
- *Anxiety* related to slow labor progress

Nursing Plan and Implementation

A key nursing responsibility is to provide comfort and support to the laboring woman and her partner. The woman experiencing a tachysystolic labor pattern will probably be very uncomfortable because of the increased frequency of contractions. Her anxiety level and that of her partner may be high. Attempt to reduce the woman's discomfort and promote a more effective labor pattern.

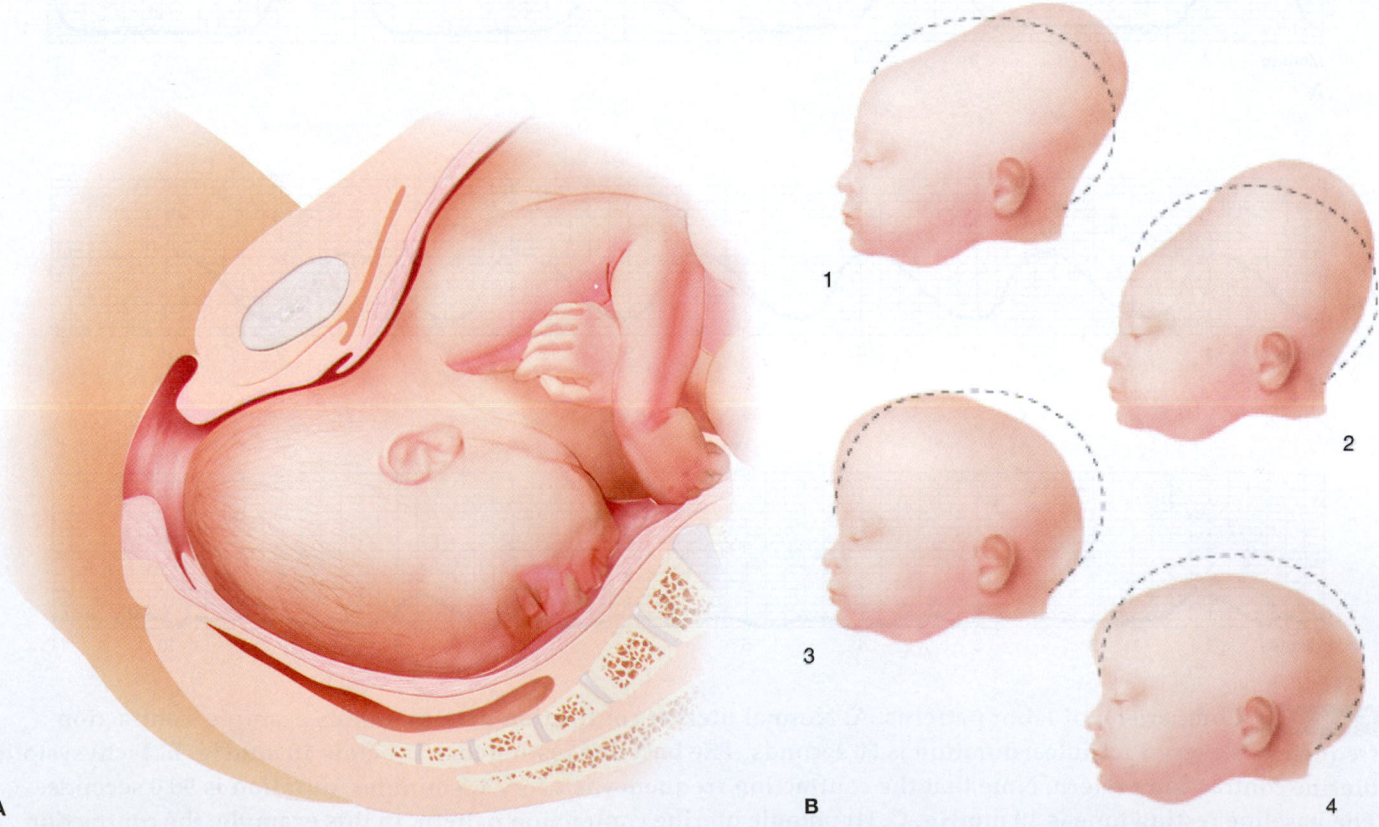

A   B   4

Figure 21–2 Effects of labor on the fetal head. A. Caput succedaneum formation. The presenting portion of the scalp area is encircled by the cervix during labor, causing swelling of the soft tissue. B. Molding of the fetal head in cephalic presentations: (1) occiput anterior, (2) occiput posterior, (3) brow, (4) face.

Suggest supportive measures such as a change of position: left lateral side-lying, high Fowler, on her knees in the bed with her arms up around the top of the bed while it is in high Fowler, rocking in a rocking chair, sitting up, and walking. Soothing measures, such as a quiet environment, use of music the woman finds calming, back rub, therapeutic touch, and visualization, and comfort measures, such as mouth care, change of linens, effleurage, and relaxation exercises, may also be helpful. The use of tub baths or a warm shower can help promote comfort and uterine relaxation. If sedation is ordered, ensure that the environment is conducive to relaxation. The labor partner may also need assistance in helping the woman cope. Your calm, understanding approach offers the woman and her partner further support. Providing information about the cause of the tachysystolic labor pattern and assuring the woman that she is not overreacting to the situation are important nursing actions.

Some women may request pain medication during this time period. For many women, the administration of a pain medication can assist with relaxation, promote rest, and allow them to reestablish coping mechanisms. For a complete guide to pain medication during labor, see Chapter 19.

Client education is key for the woman experiencing tachysystolic labor. She needs information about the dysfunctional labor pattern and the possible implications for her and her baby. Information will help relieve anxiety and thereby increase relaxation and comfort. Take time to explain treatment options and offer opportunities to ask questions.

Evaluation

Anticipated outcomes of nursing care include the following:

- The woman states she has increased comfort and decreased anxiety.
- The woman and her partner verbalize they are able to cope with the labor.
- The woman experiences a more effective labor pattern.
- The woman rates her pain as less than 3 on a 1 to 10 pain scale.

Hypotonic Labor Patterns

A hypotonic labor pattern usually develops in the active phase of labor, after labor has been well established. Hypotonic labor is characterized by fewer than two to three contractions in a 10-minute period (see Figure 21–1C). The contractions may be of low intensity and are characterized as causing minimal discomfort. Hypotonic labor may occur when the uterus is overstretched from a twin gestation, or in the presence of a large fetus, hydramnios, fetal malposition, prematurity, or grand multiparity. Bladder or bowel distention and CPD may also be associated with this pattern.

Clinical Reasoning Fetal Heart Rate Tracing

A fetal heart rate (FHR) tracing demonstrates the following: baseline heart rate of 140 with variability of 6 to 10 beats/min. When you compare the FHR with the uterine contractions, you note that there is a slowing of the FHR at the time of the contraction and that the FHR tracing looks like the contraction curve, but it is upside down.

Based on this tracing, what would you do?

RISKS OF HYPOTONIC LABOR

Maternal implications of hypotonic labor patterns include the following risks:

- Maternal exhaustion
- Stress on coping abilities
- Postpartum hemorrhage from insufficient uterine contractions following birth
- Intrauterine infection if labor is prolonged

Fetal/neonatal implications include the following risks:

- Nonreassuring fetal status caused by prolonged labor pattern
- Fetal sepsis from pathogens that ascend from the birth canal

CLINICAL THERAPY

The goals of therapy are to improve the quality of the uterine contractions while ensuring a safe outcome for the woman and her baby. Uterine contractions can be stimulated in several ways including the use of oxytocin (Pitocin), amniotomy, or stimulation of the nipples, which causes the release of endogenous oxytocin. Before initiating treatment for hypotonic labor, the physician/CNM validates the adequacy of pelvic measurements and establishes gestational age to ensure the fetus has reached maturity. After CPD, fetal malpresentation, and fetal immaturity have been ruled out, oxytocin (Pitocin) may be given intravenously via an infusion pump to improve the quality of uterine contractions. Intravenous fluid is useful to maintain adequate hydration and prevent maternal exhaustion. Amniotomy may be used to stimulate the labor process. An amniotomy is used to allow the presenting part to directly apply pressure on the cervix and promote effacement and dilatation. The application of an electric breast pump or manual stimulation of the nipples may help strengthen uterine contractions, and is an excellent starting point for women who want an unmedicated birth.

Some physicians support the use of **active management of labor (AMOL)**, a process whereby labor is managed from the beginning with client education, identifying true labor by strict definition, amniotomy, timed cervical examinations to determine abnormal labor patterns, and augmentation of labor with high-dose intravenous (IV) administration of oxytocin (Pitocin) if a specified level of progress is not met. Other components of AMOL include strict identification of fetal compromise, one-to-one nursing care, and peer review of operative births. Often, the individualized nursing care and peer review are not carried out as strictly as the other components. Opponents argue that the use of AMOL may increase the incidence of infection (because of frequent vaginal examinations) and necessitates the use of additional interventions.

An improvement in the quality of uterine contractions is demonstrated by changes in the cervical examination and a more active labor pattern. If the labor pattern does not become effective or if other complications develop, further interventions, including cesarean birth, may be necessary.

Nursing Management

For the Woman Experiencing Hypotonic Labor

Nursing Assessment and Diagnosis

Assessment of contractions (for frequency, intensity, and duration), maternal vital signs, and fetal heart rate provides the data to evaluate maternal–fetal status. Be alert for signs and symptoms of infection and dehydration.

Nursing diagnoses that may apply to the woman in hypotonic labor include the following (NANDA-I © 2014):

- *Pain, Acute,* related to uterine contractions secondary to dysfunctional labor
- *Coping, Ineffective,* related to unanticipated discomfort and slow progress in labor
- *Fatigue* related to prolonged labor and discomfort

Nursing Plan and Implementation

Nursing measures to promote maternal–fetal physical well-being include frequent monitoring of contractions, maternal vital signs, and fetal heart rate (FHR). If amniotic membranes are ruptured, the nurse assesses for the presence of meconium (dark green or black stool expelled from the fetal large intestine). The presence of meconium in the amniotic fluid makes close observation of fetal status more critical because it often indicates that the fetus is experiencing some form of stress. An intake and output record provides a way to determine maternal hydration or dehydration. The woman should be encouraged to void every 2 hours, and her bladder should be checked for distention. Because labor may be prolonged, the nurse must continue to monitor the woman and the fetus for signs of infection (elevated temperature, chills, foul-smelling amniotic fluid, and fetal tachycardia). Vaginal examinations should be kept to a minimum to decrease the risk of introducing an infection.

Women experiencing a hypotonic labor pattern require emotional support. A warm, caring approach is coupled with techniques to reduce anxiety and discomfort.

The teaching plan needs to include information regarding the dysfunctional labor process and implications for the mother and the baby. Disadvantages of and alternatives to treatment also need to be discussed and understood.

Evaluation

Anticipated outcomes of nursing care include the following:

- The woman maintains comfort during labor.
- The woman states that she understands the type of labor pattern that is occurring and the treatment plan.

Care of the Woman With Postterm Pregnancy

A **postterm pregnancy** is one that extends more than 294 days or 42 weeks past the first day of the last menstrual period. It is important to distinguish between the term *postdate,* which means that the pregnancy has gone beyond the estimated date of birth (EDB), and *postterm,* which indicates that the pregnancy has gone at least 1 day beyond 42 complete weeks from the last menstrual period. The incidence of postterm pregnancies is approximately 10% (Norwitz, 2015). The majority of postterm pregnancies are actually incorrectly dated pregnancies. The cause of true postterm pregnancy is unknown, but it seems to occur more frequently in primigravidas and in women with a past history of postterm pregnancies, especially women who were postdates themselves (Norwitz, 2015).

Risks of Prolonged Pregnancy

Maternal risks associated with prolonged pregnancy include the following (Norwitz, 2015):

- Probable labor induction
- Increased risk of dystocia

- Increased risk for large-for-gestational-age (LGA) newborn
- Increased incidence of forceps-assisted or vacuum-assisted birth
- Increased psychologic stress as the due date passes and concern for the baby increases
- Increased risk of infection
- Increased risk of severe perineal trauma related to macrosomia
- Double the risk of cesarean birth
- Increased risk of hemorrhage
- Increased risk of thromboembolitic disease

Fetal risks include the following:

- Decreased perfusion from the placenta
- Oligohydramnios (decreased amount of amniotic fluid), which increases the risk of cord compression
- Meconium aspiration (aspiration of meconium-stained amniotic fluid by the fetus at the time of birth), which is more likely if oligohydramnios and thick meconium are present
- Low Apgar scores
- Sudden infant death syndrome (SIDS); risk for death of the infant in the first year of life
- Neonatal acidemia
- Orthopedic or neurologic injury
- Fetal encephalopathy
- Cerebral palsy
- Fetal demise
- Stillbirth

Some fetuses continue to grow beyond the 42nd week of pregnancy and can be excessively large at birth (macrosomia). The macrosomic fetus is at risk for birth trauma associated with shoulder dystocia. In other cases, the intrauterine environment becomes unfavorable for growth, and at birth the baby has lost muscle mass and subcutaneous fat resulting in an intrauterine growth restriction (IUGR) that occurs as a result of uteroplacental insufficiency. This is known as *postmaturity* or *dysmaturity syndrome,* and is frequently associated with oligohydramnios, meconium aspiration, and short-term neonatal complications (Norwitz, 2015). The small-for-gestational-age (SGA) fetus is at risk for nonreassuring fetal status during labor because there is frequently associated oligohydramnios.

Clinical Therapy

When the 40th week of gestation is completed and birth has not occurred, most practitioners begin using the non-stress test (NST) and biophysical profile (BPP), modified BPP (especially the amniotic fluid volume portion of the BPP), or contraction stress test (CST) as assessment tools. These tests may be done two times a week to help evaluate fetal well-being (Caughey, 2013). If at any time the fetal assessment tests indicate a problem, interventions are initiated to accomplish the birth.

Clinical Tip

A reduction in amniotic fluid regardless of other testing considerations on a BPP warrants immediate induction or birth.

EVIDENCE-BASED PRACTICE | Management of Postterm Pregnancy

Clinical Question

What interventions are recommended for postterm pregnancy (42 weeks or longer) to minimize maternal and neonatal morbidity?

The Evidence

Postterm pregnancy of 42 weeks or longer is associated with both maternal and neonatal morbidity and mortality. Neonatal seizures, meconium aspiration syndrome, and low Apgar scores have all been observed at higher rates among postterm babies. Mothers are at risk as well; perineal laceration, infection, postpartum hemorrhage, and surgical birth are all higher among mothers of postmature neonates. The Association of Obstetricians and Gynecologists (ACOG) produced practice guidelines based on a systematic review to determine the interventions that were effective in reducing maternal and fetal mortality and morbidity. More than 60 studies involving thousands of women were included in this rigorous review, which provides the strongest level of evidence.

The authors found the accurate dating of pregnancy helped limit unnecessary interventions for postterm pregnancy. Membrane sweeping, which involves the manual separation of the membranes from the lower uterine segment during a pelvic examination with a dilated cervix, was effective in reducing the number of pregnancies that went beyond 41 weeks' gestation (ACOG, 2014b). However, this procedure causes vaginal bleeding and significant discomfort for the mother, and there are significant contraindications. Antepartum fetal testing was not associated with a reduction in perinatal morbidity and mortality, but was found to be helpful in determining fetal distress when initiated between 41 and 42 weeks. No particular fetal testing method was found to be superior. Induction of labor in the 42nd week is recommended, given evidence of an increase in perinatal morbidity and mortality after the 42nd week has passed. Mothers with conservative, watchful waiting during the 42nd week had a higher rate of surgical births than those with labor induction.

Best Practice

Careful dating of pregnancy helps reduce the risk of unnecessary induction of labor for postterm pregnancy. Pregnancies that continue past the 42nd week are associated with increased perinatal morbidity and mortality, and induction of labor is recommended for these mothers. Membrane sweeping performed by a clinician can be effective, but mothers should be counseled that the procedure is uncomfortable and associated with vaginal bleeding.

Clinical Reasoning

What should be included in the teaching plan for mothers considering membrane sweeping for a postterm pregnancy? How should a mother be counseled who is expecting conservative treatment of a pregnancy lasting longer than 42 weeks?

Nursing Management

For the Woman With Postterm Pregnancy

Nursing Assessment and Diagnosis

When the woman is admitted into the birthing area, ongoing assessments of fetal well-being begin as soon as the postterm condition has been verified. Identify reassuring FHR characteristics and evaluate for the presence of nonreassuring patterns, such as nonperiodic variable decelerations (which are associated with cord compression or oligohydramnios), so that corrective actions can be taken. When the amniotic membranes rupture, assess the fluid for meconium. In addition, assess the woman's knowledge about the condition, implications for her baby, risks, and possible interventions.

Nursing diagnoses that may apply to the woman with postterm pregnancy include the following (NANDA-I © 2015):

- *Knowledge, Deficient,* related to lack of information about postterm pregnancy
- *Fear* related to the unknown outcome for the baby
- *Coping, Ineffective,* related to anxiety about the status of the baby

Nursing Plan and Implementation

If the woman has not been assessing fetal movement every day, teach her how to do so. It is vital to stress the importance of identifying inadequate fetal movement and immediately contacting her healthcare provider. (See Chapter 13 for further discussion of techniques to detect fetal movement.)

Client education about postterm pregnancy is another important nursing responsibility. Address the implications and associated risks for the baby, as well as possible treatment plans. The woman and her partner need opportunities to ask questions and clarify information.

HOSPITAL-BASED NURSING CARE

Promotion of fetal well-being requires careful assessment of the response of the fetus during labor. If oligohydramnios exists, a continuous FHR tracing is obtained and evaluated frequently. Some facilities may choose to use continuous monitoring on any fetus that is postterm because of the increased incidence of oligohydramnios. Variable decelerations are often associated with oligohydramnios, because the decreased amount of fluid allows compression of the umbilical cord. If the fetus is macrosomic, careful assessment of labor progress (contraction characteristics, progressive cervical dilatation, and fetal descent) is also needed.

Emotional support is a key nursing intervention for women with pregnancies that extend past the due date. Women experiencing postterm pregnancy frequently feel increased stress and anxiety and have difficulty coping. Women are also uncomfortable and have difficulty sleeping, resting, or obtaining a comfortable position. Many women are emotionally prepared for the duration of 40 weeks; however, after that period women may become discouraged, anxious, and irritable. Encouragement, support, and recognition of the woman's anxiety are helpful strategies.

Evaluation

Anticipated outcomes of nursing care include the following:

- The woman has knowledge about the postterm pregnancy.
- The woman and her partner feel supported and able to cope with the postterm pregnancy.
- Fetal status is maintained, any abnormalities are quickly identified, and supportive measures are initiated.

Care of the Woman and Fetus at Risk Because of Fetal Malposition

Malposition refers to any position that is not right occiput anterior (ROA), occiput anterior (OA), or left occiput anterior (LOA). The *occiput-posterior (OP)* position is the most common fetal malposition. When the fetus is OP, the occiput of the fetal head is directed toward the back of the maternal pelvis. During labor, 95% of OP fetuses rotate to an OA position. (Refer to Figure 16–9 and Figure 17–3 to review categories of fetal position.)

A variation of OP called the **persistent occiput-posterior (POP) position** occurs in less than 10% of unmedicated labors. In this case the fetus enters the birth canal, descends, and is born in the OP position. Lack of rotation can be caused by poor contractions, abnormal flexion of the head, incomplete rotation, inadequate maternal pushing efforts usually related to epidural anesthesia, fetal anomalies, or a large fetus. Labor may be prolonged; however, most POP fetuses are born without the aid of forceps or a vacuum. Epidural use has been associated with malpositioning (Caughey, Sharshiner, & Cheng, 2015).

Risks of Fetal Malposition

Maternal risks related to the persistent occiput-posterior position include the following:

- Risk of third- or fourth-degree perineal lacerations during birth
- Risk of extension of a midline episiotomy
- Risk of cesarean section birth
- Risk of prolonged birth
- Risk of perinatal morbidity

Fetal implications may include an increased mortality risk if labor is prolonged or additional interventions such as forceps-assisted, vacuum-assisted, or cesarean birth are required.

Clinical Therapy

Clinical treatment focuses on close monitoring of maternal and fetal status and labor progress to determine whether vaginal or cesarean birth is the safer birth method. A cesarean birth is chosen if maternal or fetal problems make a vaginal birth unwise or if cephalopelvic disproportion (CPD) is present.

Although the majority of POP fetuses are born vaginally, in some cases forceps-assisted or vacuum-assisted births may be necessary. The forceps can be used to deliver the fetus while it is still in the OP position or to rotate the occiput to an anterior position (called Scanzoni maneuver). A rotation from LOP or ROP position to an anterior position may also be accomplished with a vacuum-assistance device. (See Chapter 22 for further discussion of forceps and vacuum.) Manual rotation during the first stage of labor is not recommended. In the second stage of labor, manual rotation has been associated with lower rates of cesarean birth and maternal blood loss (Aiken, Aiken, Alberry, et al., 2015). No adverse neonatal effects have been noted.

Nursing Management

For the Laboring Woman With the Fetus in Occiput-Posterior Position

Nursing Assessment and Diagnosis

Signs and symptoms of a persistent occiput-posterior position include complaints of intense back pain by the laboring woman, a dysfunctional labor pattern, hypotonic labor (the fetal head does not put adequate pressure on the cervix), arrest of dilatation, or arrest of fetal descent. The back pain is caused by the fetal occiput compressing the sacral nerves. Further assessment may reveal a depression in the maternal abdomen above the symphysis. FHR is typically heard far laterally on the abdomen, and on vaginal examination the physician/CNM finds the wide, diamond-shaped anterior fontanelle in the anterior portion of the pelvis. This fontanelle may be difficult to feel because of molding of the fetal head.

Nursing diagnoses that may apply to women with persistent occiput-posterior position include the following (NANDA-I © 2014):

- *Pain, Acute,* related to back discomfort secondary to the OP position
- *Coping, Ineffective,* related to unanticipated discomfort and slow progress in labor

Nursing Plan and Implementation

Changing maternal posture has been used for many years to enhance rotation of OP or occiput-transverse (OT) to OA. A number of position changes may be tried. For instance, the woman may be asked to lie on one side and then asked to move to the other side as the fetus begins to rotate. This side-lying position may promote rotation; it also enables the support person to apply counterpressure on the sacral area to decrease discomfort. A knee–chest position provides a downward slant to the vaginal canal, directing the fetal head downward on descent. A hands-and-knees position is often effective in rotating the fetus. In addition to maintaining a hands-and-knees position on the bed, the woman may try pelvic rocking, and the support person may firmly stroke the abdomen. The stroking begins over the fetal back and swings around to the other side of the abdomen. After the fetus has rotated, the woman lies in a Sims position on the side opposite the fetal back.

Some studies have shown success with the physician/ CNM manually rotating the head during labor. Manual rotation done before complete dilatation was associated with a higher failure rate and an increase in perinatal mortality. Inability to manually rotate the fetus was associated with a higher cesarean birth rate (Aiken et al., 2015).

Evaluation

Anticipated outcomes of nursing care include the following:

- The woman's discomfort is decreased.
- The coping abilities of the woman and her partner are strengthened.
- Birth occurs without maternal or fetal complications.

Care of the Woman and Fetus at Risk Because of Fetal Malpresentation

In a normal presentation, the occiput is the presenting part (Figure 21–3A). Fetal malpresentations include brow, face, breech, shoulder (transverse lie), and compound presentation. With a face or chin presentation, an internal scalp electrode should not be used.

Brow Presentation

In a brow presentation, the forehead of the fetus becomes the presenting part. In the military (sinciput) presentation, the fetal head is between flexion and extension (Figure 21–3B), whereas in the occipitomental presentation, the fetal head enters the birth canal with the widest diameter of the head (approximately 13.5 cm [5.3 in.]) foremost (Figure 21–3C).

The brow presentation occurs more often in multiparas than in nulliparas and is thought to be caused by lax abdominal and pelvic musculature. Grand multiparous women have a greater risk. Brow presentations can also occur in cases of cephalopelvic disproportion (CPD) or pelvic contracture and in premature fetuses. Premature rupture of membranes precedes 27% of brow presentations (Talaulikar & Arulkumaran, 2015). Many brow presentations spontaneously convert to face or occipital presentations. Brow presentations are the least common types of abnormal presentations; they are typically not diagnosed until labor and occur in about 1 in 700 to 1 in 1500 births (Talaulikar & Arulkumaran, 2015).

RISKS OF BROW PRESENTATION

Maternal implications of brow presentation include increased risk of the following:

- Longer labor caused by ineffective contractions and slow or arrested fetal descent

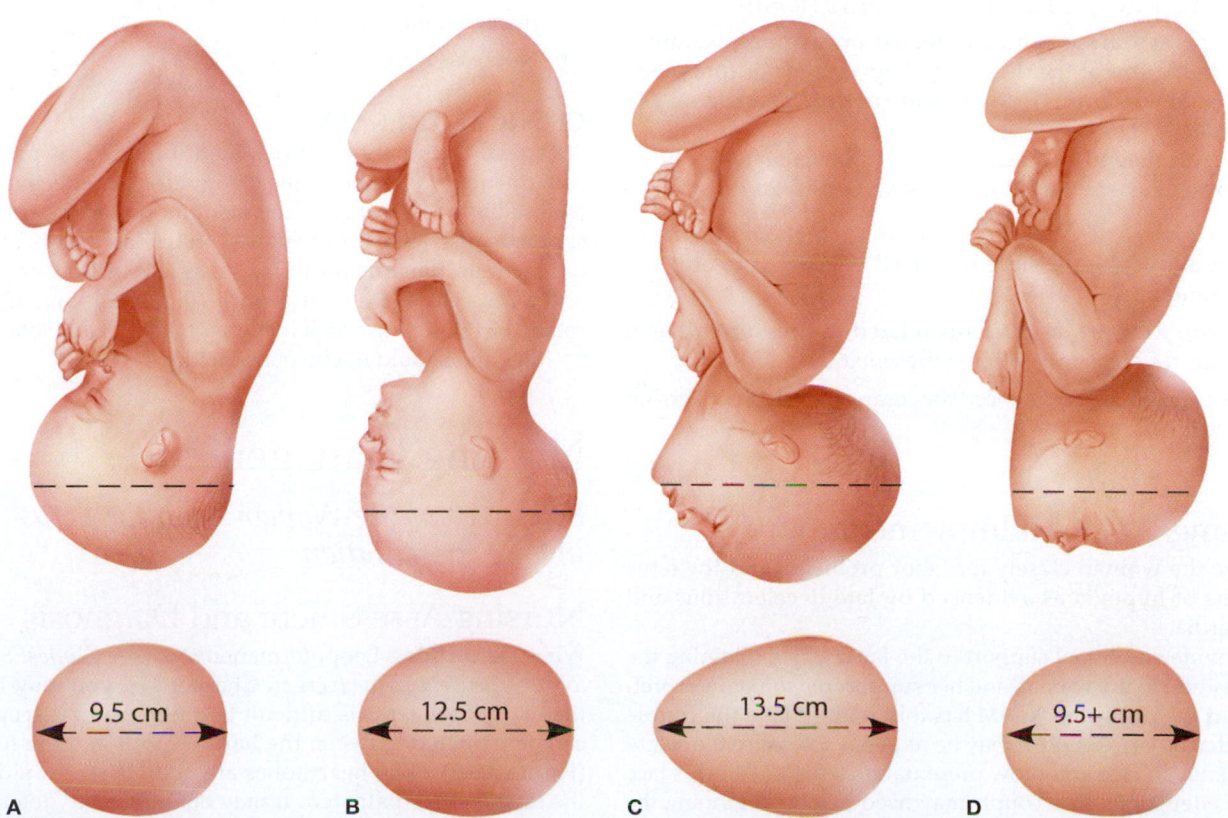

Figure 21–3 Types of cephalic presentations. A. The occiput is the presenting part because the head is flexed and the fetal chin is against the chest. The largest anteroposterior (AP) diameter that presents and passes through the pelvis is approximately 9.5 cm. B. Military (sinciput) presentation. The head is neither flexed nor extended. The presenting AP diameter is approximately 12.5 cm. C. Brow (occipitomental) presentation. The largest diameter of the fetal head (approximately 13.5 cm) presents in this situation. D. Face presentation. The AP diameter is 9.5 cm.

- Dysfunctional labor patterns
- Cesarean birth if brow presentation persists or if the fetus is large

Fetal/neonatal risks include increased mortality because of cerebral and neck compression and damage to the trachea and larynx. In addition, facial edema, bruising, and exaggerated molding of the newborn's head may be observed.

CLINICAL THERAPY

If a brow presentation fails to convert to occipital or face presentation, cesarean birth is indicated in most cases (Talaulikar & Arulkumaran, 2015). If a vaginal birth is attempted, typically in a multiparous woman or with a very small fetus, the woman is closely monitored for CPD, caput succedaneum, facial edema, and nonreassuring fetal status. Attempts to convert brow presentations via manual attempt, forceps, or vacuum are contraindicated, as is the use of oxytocin. Scalp electrodes should not be placed when the fetus is in a brow presentation (Talaulikar & Arulkumaran, 2015). Attempts to facilitate birth using oxytocin can result in a dystocia.

Nursing Management

For the Laboring Woman With the Fetus in Brow Presentation

Nursing Assessment and Diagnosis

A brow presentation can be detected on vaginal examination by palpation of the diamond-shaped anterior fontanelle on one side and orbital ridges and root of the nose on the other side.

Nursing diagnoses that may apply to a woman with a brow presentation include the following (NANDA-I © 2014:

- *Knowledge, Deficient*, related to lack of information about the possible maternal–fetal effects of brow presentation
- *Injury, Risk for,* to the fetus related to pressure on fetal structures secondary to brow presentation
- *Fear* related to sudden need for cesarean birth if conversion does not occur

Nursing Plan and Implementation

Observe the woman closely for labor problems and the fetus for signs of hypoxia as evidenced by late decelerations and bradycardia.

Provide emotional support to the family by explaining the fetal position to the woman and her support person or interpreting what the physician/CNM has told them. Make the couple aware that a cesarean birth may be required to ensure the safety of the fetus. In face and brow presentations, the newborn's face may be edematous. The couple may need help in beginning the attachment process because of the newborn's facial appearance. After the baby is inspected for any abnormalities, assure the couple that the facial edema is only temporary and will subside in 3 or 4 days and that the molding will be much less visible in a few days (even though completion of the process takes several weeks).

Evaluation

Anticipated outcomes of nursing care include the following:

- The woman and her partner understand the implications and associated problems of brow presentation.
- The mother and her baby have a safe labor and birth.

Face Presentation

In a face presentation, the face of the fetus is the presenting part (Figure 21–3D and Figure 21–4). The fetal head is hyperextended even more than in the brow presentation. Face presentation occurs most frequently in fetuses weighing more than 4000 grams (8.8 lb). The incidence of face presentation is 0.14% of live births (Tapisiz, Aytan, Altinbas, et al., 2014).

RISKS OF FACE PRESENTATION

Maternal risks related to face presentation include the following:

- Increased risk of cephalopelvic disproportion (CPD)
- Prolonged labor
- Increased risk of infection (with prolonged labor)
- Cesarean birth if fetal chin is posterior (mentum posterior)

Fetal/neonatal risks include the following:

- Cephalohematoma of the face
- Facial edema
- Laryngeal and tracheal edema
- Pronounced molding of the head
- Increased intrapartum deaths
- Nonreassuring fetal status

CLINICAL THERAPY

A vaginal birth may be anticipated if no CPD is present, the chin (mentum) is anterior, the labor pattern is effective, and the fetal status is reassuring. Many mentum posterior presentations spontaneously convert to anterior in the late stages of labor. If the mentum remains posterior, a vaginal birth is not possible and a cesarean birth is necessary (Figure 21–5). Attempts to rotate the fetus often result in higher maternal and fetal morbidity rates and should not be performed.

Nursing Management

For the Laboring Woman With the Fetus in Face Presentation

Nursing Assessment and Diagnosis

When performing Leopold maneuvers (see *Clinical Skill: Performing Leopold Maneuvers* in Chapter 17), you may find that the back of the fetus is difficult to outline, and a deep furrow can be palpated between the hard occiput and the fetal back (Figure 21–6). Fetal heart tones are audible on the side where the fetal feet are palpated. It may be difficult to determine by vaginal examination whether a breech or a face is presenting, especially if facial edema is already present. During the vaginal examination, palpation of the saddle of the nose and the gums should be attempted. When assessing engagement, remember that the face has to be deep within the pelvis before the biparietal diameters have entered the inlet.

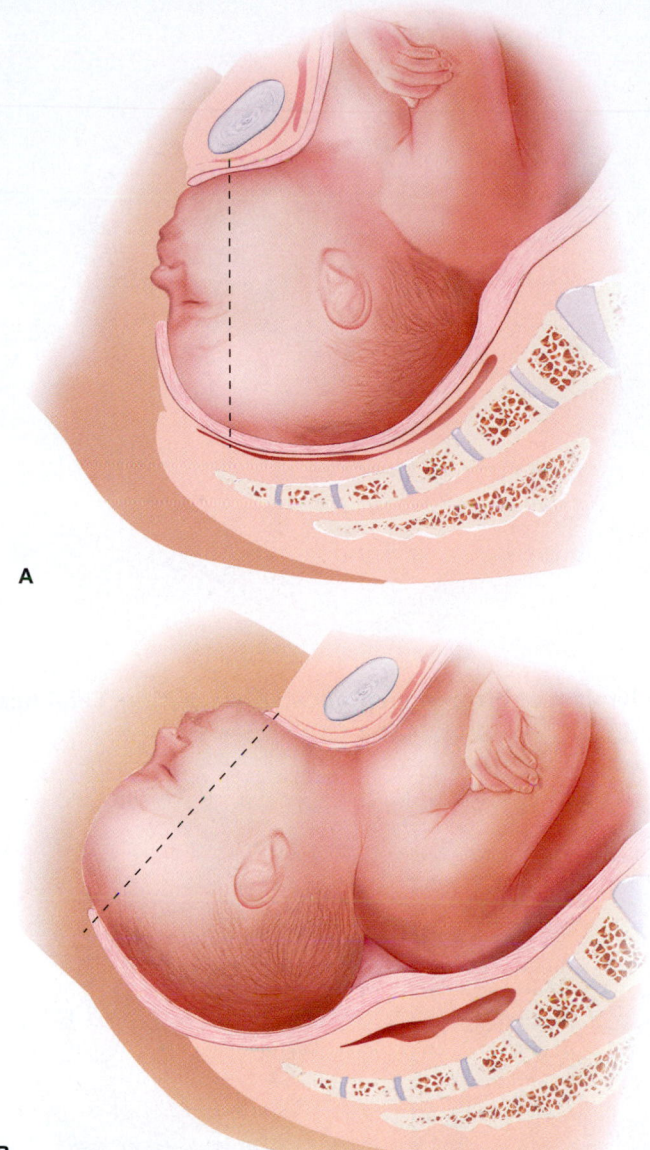

Figure 21–4 Face presentation. Mechanism of birth in mentoanterior position. A. The submentobregmatic diameter at the outlet. B. The fetal head is born by movement of flexion.

Nursing diagnoses that may apply to the woman with a fetus in face presentation include the following (NANDA-I © 2014):

- *Fear* related to unknown outcome of the labor and a possible instrument-assisted or cesarean birth
- *Injury, Risk for,* to the newborn's face related to edema secondary to the birth process

Nursing Plan and Implementation

Nursing interventions are the same as those indicated for the brow presentation.

Evaluation

Anticipated outcomes of nursing care include the following:

- The woman and her partner understand the implications and associated problems of face presentation.
- The mother and her baby have a safe labor and birth.

Breech Presentation

The exact cause of breech presentation (Figure 21–7) is unknown. This malpresentation occurs in about 4% to 5% of labors and is frequently associated with preterm birth, corneal placenta positioning, hydramnios, multiple gestation, uterine anomalies (such as bicornuate uterus), and fetal anomalies (especially anencephaly and hydrocephaly). Fetuses with term breech presentations, regardless of mode of birth, have poorer long-term neurodevelopmental scores (Hofmeyr, 2015).

RISKS OF BREECH PRESENTATION

The maternal implication of breech presentation is a likelihood of cesarean birth. When a vaginal birth is attempted, there is a higher incidence of episiotomy use, perineal trauma, and lacerations. Fetal/neonatal implications for vaginal births of breech fetuses include (Berhan & Haileamlak, 2015):

- Higher perinatal morbidity and mortality rates
- Increased risk of prolapsed cord, especially in incomplete breeches, because space is available between the cervix and the presenting part

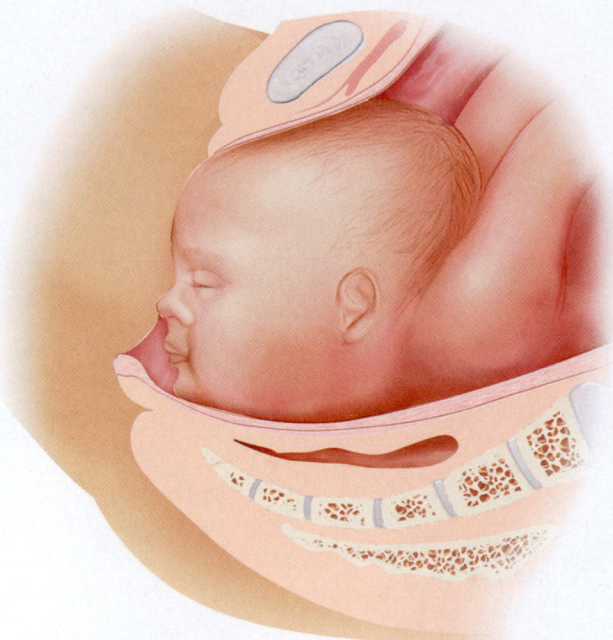

Figure 21–5 Face presentation. Mechanism of birth in mentoposterior position. Fetal head is unable to extend farther. The face becomes impacted.

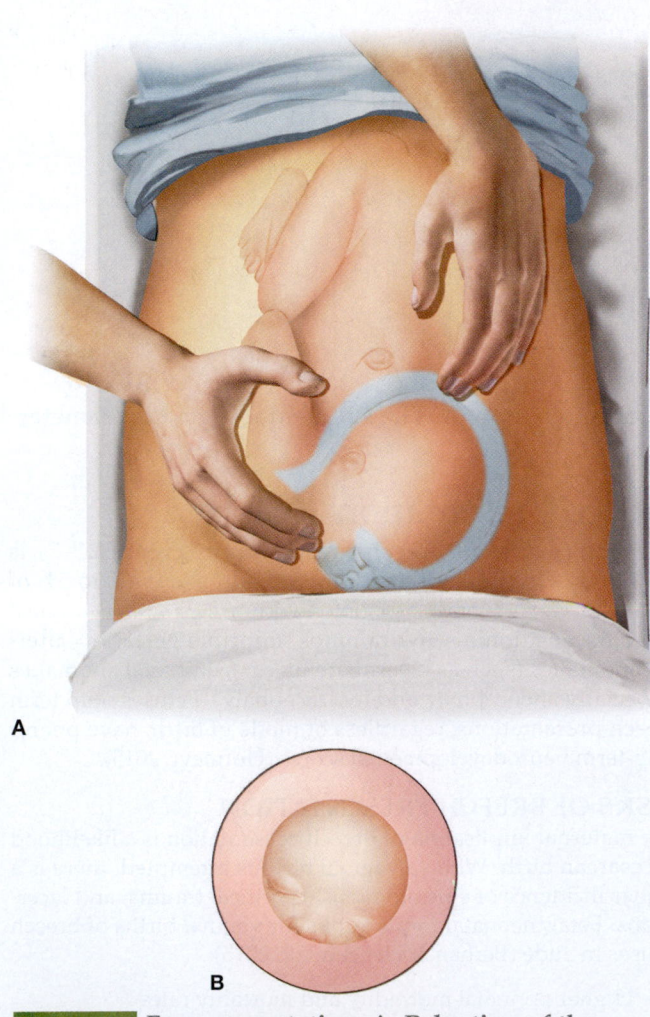

Figure 21–6 Face presentation. A. Palpation of the maternal abdomen with the fetus in right mentum posterior (RMP) position. B. Vaginal examination may permit palpation of facial features of the fetus.

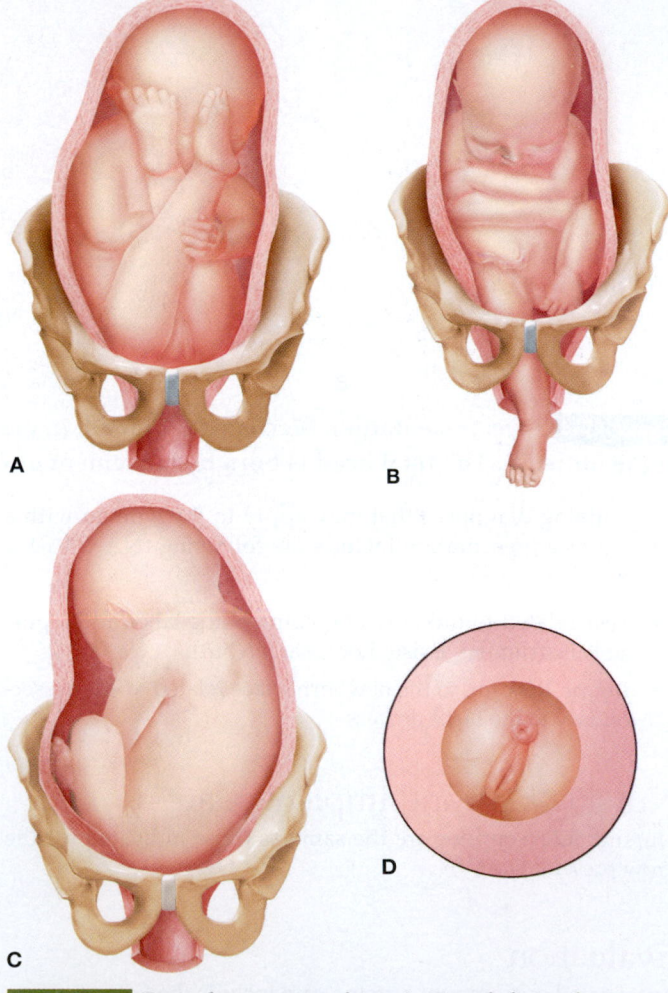

Figure 21–7 Breech presentation. A. Frank breech. B. Incomplete (footling) breech. C. Complete breech in left sacral anterior (LSA) position. D. On vaginal examination, the nurse may feel the anal sphincter. The tissue of the fetal buttocks feels soft.

- Increased risk of cervical spinal cord injuries caused by hyperextension of the fetal head
- Increased brachial plexus injuries
- Increased neurological morbidity
- Increased risk of asphyxia and nonreassuring fetal status
- Increased risk of dystocia
- Increased risk of birth trauma
- Increases in neonatal morbidity and mortality
- Apgar scores less than 7 at 5 minutes
- Neonatal asphyxia

CLINICAL THERAPY

Current clinical therapy is directed toward converting the breech presentation to a cephalic presentation before the beginning of labor. Perinatal mortality and morbidity is two- to five-fold higher in planned vaginal than in planned caesarean birth (Berhan & Haileamlak, 2015). Breech presentations are 16 times more likely to result in intrapartum fetal death (Cunningham et al., 2014). Some physicians attempt an *external cephalic version (ECV)* at 36 to 38 weeks' gestation as long as the woman is not in labor. Other methods to turn a breech fetus to a cephalic presentation include placing headphones on the lower abdomen and playing music or the mother's voice to encourage the baby to move toward the sounds and out of the breech position. Certain chiropractic techniques have also been used to facilitate version as well. The American College of Obstetricians & Gynecologists currently recommends that breech presentations be born via planned cesarean because of the significant increase in complications associated with breech vaginal births (Cunningham et al., 2014). (See Chapter 22 for discussion of external version.) Although there is current discussion for the use of vaginal birth in certain circumstances, the risk remains higher for adverse events, and the practice is rare in contemporary obstetrics.

Box 21–1 **Moxibustion to Promote Version in Breech Presentations**

Traditional Chinese medicine uses the herb mugwort in the form of moxa to promote version in a breech presentation. Moxa is a system of treatment, often combined with acupuncture, in which an herb is dried, rolled into cones (like incense cones), and placed on certain meridian points of the body. The moxa is then lit and allowed to burn close to the skin; hence the "bustion" component of the name. The heat and pungency of mugwort stimulate the point, and it is believed that the energy moves through the body and increases fetal activity.

The meridian point that is used in moxibustion to promote version in breech presentation is acupoint BL 67, located beside the outer corner of the fifth toenail. Treatment may take from 7 days to 2 weeks. There is limited evidence suggesting that moxibustion is an effective modality in managing breech presentations; however, when combined with acupuncture and postural techniques (knee–chest position), the incidence of version increases (Coyle, Smith, & Peat, 2012).

Nursing Management

For the Laboring Woman With the Fetus in Breech Presentation

Nursing Assessment and Diagnosis

Frequently you may be the first to recognize a breech presentation. On palpation you may feel the firm fetal head in the uterine fundus and the wider sacrum in the lower part of the abdomen. If the sacrum has not descended, ballottement causes the entire fetal body to move. Furthermore, fetal heart rate (FHR) is usually auscultated above the umbilicus. Passage of meconium into the amniotic fluid caused by compression of the fetal intestinal tract is common.

If membranes are ruptured, be particularly alert for a prolapsed umbilical cord, especially in footling breeches, because there is space between the cervix and presenting part through which the cord can slip. If the baby is small and the membranes rupture, the danger is even greater. The risk of a prolapsed umbilical cord is one reason why any woman with ruptured membranes should not ambulate until a full assessment, including vaginal examination, has been performed.

Nursing diagnoses that may apply to a woman with a breech presentation include the following (NANDA-I © 2014):

- *Gas Exchange, Impaired,* in the fetus related to interruption in umbilical blood flow secondary to compression of the cord
- *Knowledge, Deficient,* related to lack of information about the implications and associated complications of breech presentation for the mother and the fetus
- *Injury, Risk for,* to the fetus related to possible prolapsed umbilical cord, birth trauma, intrapartum asphyxia, or fetal spinal cord injuries

Nursing Plan and Implementation

During labor, promote maternal–fetal physical well-being by frequently assessing fetal and maternal status. Because the fetus is at increased risk for prolapse of the cord, agency protocols may call for continuous fetal monitoring. If the head is not completely engaged, continuous monitoring is warranted and the woman should maintain complete bedrest. Provide teaching and information about the breech presentation and the nursing care needed.

Most breech vaginal births are performed on multiparous women with a proven pelvis (prior birth of a normal or large size fetus without difficulty) who present in active labor with an unknown breech presentation. Multiparous women who receive care from a healthcare provider experienced in vaginal breech births have the best outcomes when vaginal breech births are performed (Shashidhar, Shashirekha, Bandamma, et al., 2015). Assist with the vaginal birth by including Piper forceps (used to guide the after-coming fetal head) in the birth table setup. You may assist the physician if forceps are needed for the birth. If the family and physician/CNM decide on a cesarean birth, assist as with any cesarean birth. Breech births commonly occur in the operating room with a "double setup" in place. If difficulties arise with the attempted vaginal birth, the room is already prepared for a cesarean birth and the procedure can be performed quickly.

Evaluation

Anticipated outcomes of nursing care include the following:

- The woman and her partner understand the implications and associated problems of breech presentation.
- Major complications are recognized early and corrective measures are instituted.
- The mother and baby have a safe labor and birth.

Transverse Lie (Shoulder Presentation) of a Single Fetus

A transverse lie occurs in approximately 1 in 300 term births (Strauss, 2015). Maternal conditions associated with a transverse lie are multiple gestation, grand multiparity with relaxed uterine muscles, uterine fibroids, prior uterine surgery, preterm fetus, excessive amniotic fluid, placenta previa, and contracted pelvis (Figure 21–8). Fetuses with abnormalities are more likely to present as a transverse lie. These may include chromosomal (autosomal trisomy) and structural abnormalities (hydrocephalus), as well as syndromes of multiple effects (fetal alcohol syndrome) (Global Library of Women's Medicine, 2015).

The management of shoulder presentation depends on the gestational age. If discovered before term, the management is expectant (watchful), because some fetuses change presentation without intervention. When a shoulder presentation is still evident at 37 completed weeks of gestation, an external cephalic version (ECV) attempt (followed, if successful, by induction of labor) is recommended, because of the associated risk of prolapsed cord. If the ECV is unsuccessful, a cesarean birth should be performed before the onset of spontaneous labor.

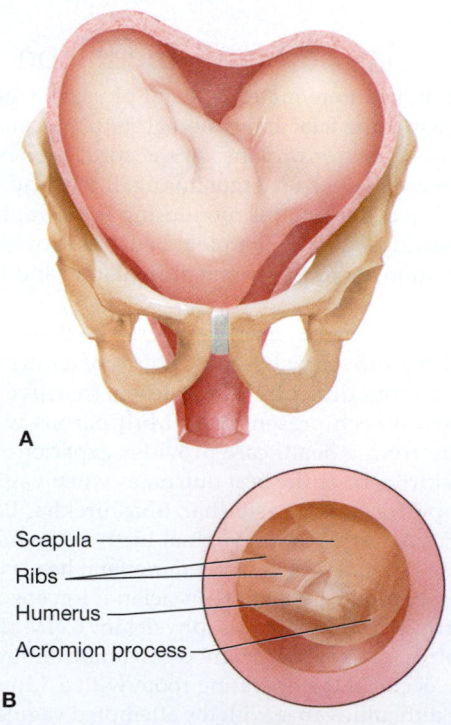

A

Scapula —
Ribs —
Humerus —
Acromion process —

B

Figure 21–8 Transverse lie. A. Shoulder presentation. **B. On vaginal examination, the nurse may feel the acromion process as the fetal presenting part.**

Nursing Management

You may be able to identify a transverse lie by inspection and palpation of the abdomen, by auscultation of FHR, and by vaginal examination. On inspection, the woman's abdomen appears widest from side to side as a result of the long axis of the baby's body lying parallel to the ground and across the mother's uterus.

On palpation no fetal part is felt in the fundal portion of the uterus or above the symphysis. The head may be palpated on one side and the breech on the other. Fetal heart rate is usually auscultated just below the midline of the umbilicus. On vaginal examination, if a presenting part is palpated, it is the ridged thorax or possibly an arm that is compressed against the chest.

Assist in the interpretation of the fetal presentation and provide information and support to the couple. Assess maternal and fetal status frequently and prepare the woman for a cesarean birth (see Chapter 22). An ultrasound examination can be performed to confirm the diagnosis when multiple gestation or maternal obesity interferes with diagnosis.

Compound Presentation

A compound presentation is one in which there are two presenting parts, such as the occiput and the fetal hand or the complete breech and the fetal hand. Most compound presentations resolve themselves spontaneously, but others require additional manipulation at birth. Risk factors include low birth weight, hydramnios, multiple gestation, large maternal pelvis, and lack of engagement with ruptured membranes. Some medical procedures can increase the risk, such as artificial rupture of membranes without a presenting part completely engaged and external cephalic version, in which a fetal part may inadvertently be trapped within the pelvis. Compound presentations occur in 1 in 700 to 1 in 1000 births (Cormier, 2015).

Clinical Tip

If a fetus converts to a transverse lie later in the pregnancy, the women may report greater ease of breathing, a reduction of heartburn, and less pressure on her bladder.

Care of the Woman and Fetus at Risk for Macrosomia

Fetal **macrosomia** is defined as a newborn weight of more than 4000 to 4500 g (8.8 to 9.9 lb) at birth. It is estimated that 10% of neonates in the United States have a birth weight more than 4000 grams while an additional 1% are in excess of 4500 grams (Jazayeri, 2015). The condition is more common with excessive maternal weight gain in pregnancy, maternal obesity, maternal diabetes, mothers with a previous newborn who weighed more than 4000 g, Hispanic ethnicity, genetic tendencies, greater maternal and paternal height and weight, male sex, hydramnios, and prolonged gestation (Jazayeri, 2015).

Risks of Macrosomia

Maternal implications of macrosomia include increased risk of cephalopelvic disproportion (CPD), dysfunctional labor, prolonged labor, soft tissue laceration during vaginal birth, postpartum hemorrhage, puerperium infection, and possible cesarean birth.

The most significant complication for the fetus/neonate with macrosomia is intrapartum and neonatal death. Shoulder dystocia, an obstetric emergency in which, after the birth of the head, the anterior shoulder fails to deliver either spontaneously or with gentle traction (unresolved shoulder dystocia can lead to fetal death) is also a significant risk factor. Other risks include upper brachial plexus injury, permanent nerve damage, fractured clavicle, meconium aspiration, asphyxia, hypoglycemia, hypocalcemia, electrolyte imbalances, polycythemia, and hyperbilirubinemia. Fetuses with suspected macrosomia are also at risk for preterm induced birth based on estimated fetal weight.

In addition, babies who are macrosomic at birth are more likely to become obese in childhood and adolescence. These children are also at risk to develop diabetes in later life (Jazayeri, 2015).

Clinical Therapy

The occurrence of maternal and fetal problems associated with excessively large newborns may be lessened somewhat by identifying macrosomia before the onset of labor. If a large fetus is suspected, the maternal pelvis should be evaluated carefully. Fetal size can be estimated by palpating the crown-to-rump length of the fetus in utero and by ultrasound. Clinical studies have demonstrated that palpation and ultrasound provide equally effective assessments of fetal weight. When the uterus appears excessively large, either hydramnios, an oversized fetus, or a multiple gestation must be considered as the possible cause. If any of these conditions is suspected, evaluation of the etiology should include ultrasonography. Abdominal measurements have also been used in some studies. Of women whose abdominal circumferences measured greater than 35 cm within 2 weeks of their due dates, 90% gave birth to a baby that weighed more than 4000 grams (8.8 lb) (Jazayeri, 2015).

When fetal weight is estimated to be 4500 g or more, a cesarean birth is usually planned. The best method of birth for an estimated fetal weight of 4000 to 4500 g is debated. The discussion centers primarily on the incidence of shoulder dystocia during vaginal birth and the difficulty in accurately estimating the fetal weight. Unexpected shoulder dystocia during vaginal birth can be a grave problem.

SAFETY ALERT!

As an emergency measure, the physician/CNM may ask the nurse to assist the woman into the McRoberts maneuver (sharp flexion of the thighs toward the hips and abdomen) or to apply gentle suprapubic pressure in an attempt to aid in the birth of the fetal shoulders. Fundal pressure should never be used because it can further wedge the anterior shoulder under the symphysis pubis.

Nursing Management

Assist in identifying women who are at risk for carrying a large fetus or those who exhibit signs of macrosomia. Because these women are prime candidates for dystocia and its complications, frequently assess the fetal heart rate (FHR) for indications of nonreassuring fetal status and evaluate the rates of cervical dilatation and fetal descent.

The fetal monitor is applied for continuous fetal evaluation. Early decelerations (caused by fetal head compression) could mean size disproportion at the bony inlet. Any sign of labor dysfunction or nonreassuring fetal status is reported to the physician/CNM immediately. Lack of fetal descent is another indicator that should alert you to the possibility that the baby is too large for a vaginal birth.

Provide support for the laboring woman and her partner and information about the implications of macrosomia and possible associated problems.

Inspect macrosomic newborns after birth for cephalohematoma, Erb palsy, and fractured clavicles. Inform the nursery staff of any problems so that the newborn is observed closely for cerebral, neurologic, and motor problems.

In a woman with a macrosomic fetus, the uterus has been stretched farther than it would have been with an average size fetus. After birth the overstretched uterus may not contract well (uterine atony) and will feel boggy (soft). In this case, uterine hemorrhage is likely. The fundus of the uterus is massaged to stimulate contraction, and IV or IM oxytocin (Pitocin) may be needed. Maternal vital signs are closely monitored for deviations suggestive of shock.

SAFETY ALERT!

Methergine is sometimes prescribed for women with ongoing uterine atony and can aid in reducing postpartum hemorrhage. Methergine is contraindicated in women with any type of hypertensive disorder. Monitor the woman's blood pressure closely prior to administration.

Care of the Woman and Fetus in the Presence of Nonreassuring Fetal Status

When the oxygen supply is insufficient to meet the physiologic needs of the fetus, a nonreassuring fetal status may result. This status may be transient or chronic, and may be prompted by a variety of factors. The most common are cord compression and uteroplacental insufficiency, possibly caused by preexisting maternal or fetal disease or placental abnormalities. If the resulting hypoxia persists and metabolic acidosis occurs, the situation could cause permanent damage to, or be life threatening for, the fetus.

Early signs of nonreassuring fetal status are variations from the normal heart rate pattern and decreased fetal movement. Meconium-stained amniotic fluid and the presence of ominous fetal heart rate (FHR) patterns, such as persistent late decelerations (regardless of the depth of deceleration), persistent severe variable decelerations (especially if the return to baseline is prolonged), and prolonged decelerations are signs of nonreassuring fetal status. Meconium-stained fluid can be determined only after the membranes have ruptured. Other signs of nonreassuring fetal status include tachycardia, bradycardia, and loss of variability. When these patterns are detected, **intrauterine resuscitation** (corrective measures used to optimize the oxygen exchange within the maternal–fetal circulation) should be started without delay. Treatment of maternal hypotension involves having the woman turn to a left lateral position (right lateral may also be tried), beginning an intravenous infusion or increasing the flow rate if an infusion is already in place, or, if cord prolapse is suspected, having the woman assume a knee–chest position. The nurse should have the woman maintain position changes that result in an increase in the FHR and perform a vaginal examination to attempt to detect a prolapsed cord. If a prolapsed cord is discovered, the examiner applies pressure to the presenting part to relieve the additional pressure on the cord. Uterine activity can be decreased by discontinuing intravenous oxytocin (Pitocin) administration or administering a tocolytic agent (such as terbutaline) to decrease contraction frequency and intensity. Oxygen is also administered to the woman via facial mask.

Caregivers can obtain additional information about the condition of the fetus by performing fetal scalp stimulation or fetal acoustical stimulation (see Chapter 17 for more information about these tests). See Table 21–1 for management of nonreassuring fetal status.

Maternal Implications

Indications of a nonreassuring fetal status greatly increase the psychologic stress of a laboring woman and her family members and may even put the woman at risk for posttraumatic stress disorder (PTSD). Professional staff members may become so involved in assessing fetal status and initiating corrective measures that they fail to provide the woman and her partner with explanations and emotional support. It is imperative to offer both. In many instances, if birth is not imminent, the woman must undergo cesarean birth. This method of birth may be a source of fear and of frustration, too, if the couple had prepared for a shared vaginal birth experience.

Clinical Therapy

Treatment centers on improving the blood flow to the fetus by correcting maternal hypotension, decreasing the intensity and

---

TABLE 21–1 Management of Nonreassuring Fetal Status

- Recognize pattern changes that are indicative of nonreassuring fetal status such as:
  - Deep, repetitive variable decelerations
  - Prolonged decelerations
  - Ongoing late decelerations
- Begin intrauterine resuscitation measures:
  - Change maternal position.
  - Correct maternal hypotension.
  - Discontinue oxytocin (Pitocin).
  - Administer medications, such as terbutaline, to decrease uterine activity.
  - Increase intravenous fluid rate or begin IV immediately if not already established.
  - Assess for prolapsed cord via vaginal examination.
- If abnormal patterns resolve, continue with continuous electronic fetal monitoring.
- If abnormal patterns do not resolve and vaginal birth is imminent, proceed with vaginal birth as quickly as possible.
- If birth is not imminent and bradycardia persists, or if a scalp pH level is less than 7.20, a cesarean birth is indicated.
- If these tests are reassuring, cautious assessments can continue every 15 minutes until birth occurs.
- If testing becomes nonreassuring, a cesarean should be performed.

---

frequency of contractions if present, providing IV fluids to the woman as needed, administering oxygen, and gathering further information about fetal status. Fetal response to intrauterine resuscitation measures dictates subsequent actions.

Nursing Management

Review the woman's prenatal history and note the presence of any conditions (such as preeclampsia, diabetes, renal disease, intrauterine growth restriction [IUGR]) that may be associated with decreased uteroplacental–fetal blood flow. When the membranes rupture, assess the FHR immediately and note the characteristics of the amniotic fluid. As labor progresses, be especially alert for suspicious changes in the FHR. At all times, encourage and support maternal positioning that maximizes uteroplacental–fetal blood flow.

Care of the Woman and Fetus With a Prolapsed Umbilical Cord

A **prolapsed umbilical cord** results when the umbilical cord precedes the fetal presenting part. The incidence of prolapsed cord occurs in 1.4 to 6.2 of 1000 births (Bradley & Hollbrook, 2013). When this occurs, pressure is placed on the umbilical cord as it is trapped between the presenting part and the maternal pelvis. Consequently the vessels carrying blood to and from the fetus are compressed (Figure 21–9). Prolapse of the cord may occur with rupture of the membranes if the presenting part is not well engaged in the pelvis. Risk factors include small fetus, multiple gestation, prematurity, abnormal fetal lie, grand multiparity, fetal abnormalities, and interventions such as amniotomy, fetal scalp or intrauterine pressure catheter placement, or external version.

Maternal Implications

Although a prolapsed cord does not directly precipitate physical alterations in the woman, her immediate concern for the baby creates enormous stress. The woman may need to deal with some unusual interventions, a cesarean birth, and, in some circumstances, the death of her baby.

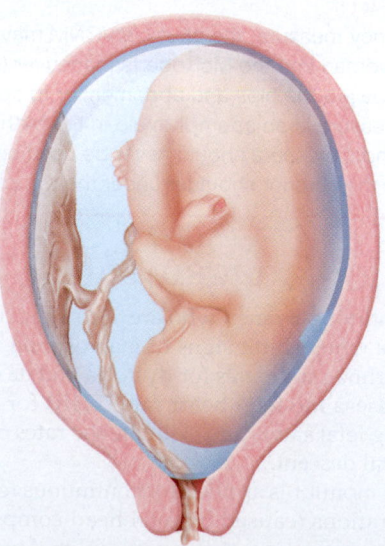

Figure 21–9 Prolapse of the umbilical cord.

Fetal/Neonatal Implications

Compression of the cord results in decreased blood flow and leads to nonreassuring fetal status. If labor is under way, the cord is compressed further with each contraction. If the pressure on the cord is not relieved, the fetus will die.

Clinical Therapy

Preventing the occurrence of prolapse of the cord is the preferred medical approach. A laboring woman with a confirmed rupture of membranes will be kept horizontal, usually in bed, until the fetal head is well engaged and the risk of a prolapse is significantly decreased. If a prolapse occurs, relieving the compression on the cord is critical to fetal outcome. The medical and nursing team must work together to facilitate birth.

Bedrest is indicated for all laboring women with a history of ruptured membranes, until engagement with no cord prolapse has been documented. Furthermore, with spontaneous rupture of membranes or amniotomy, the fetal heart rate (FHR) should be auscultated for at least a full minute and at the beginning and end of contractions for several contractions. If fetal bradycardia is detected on auscultation, a vaginal examination is performed to rule out cord prolapse. In the presence of cord prolapse, electronic monitor tracings show severe, moderate, or prolonged variable decelerations with baseline bradycardia.

If a loop of cord is discovered, the examiner's gloved fingers must remain in the vagina to provide firm pressure on the fetal head (to relieve compression) until the physician/CNM arrives. This is a lifesaving measure. The mother is given oxygen via face mask, and the FHR is monitored to determine whether the cord compression is adequately relieved.

The force of gravity can be employed to relieve umbilical cord compression. The woman assumes the knee–chest position (Figure 21–10) or the bed is adjusted to the Trendelenburg position, and the woman is transported to the birthing or operating room in this position. The nurse must remember that the cord may be occultly prolapsed with an actual loop extending into the vagina or lying alongside the presenting part. It may be pulsating strongly or so weakly that it is difficult to determine on palpation of the cord whether the fetus is alive.

Nursing Management

Because there are few outward signs of cord prolapse, each pregnant woman is advised to call her physician/CNM when the membranes rupture and to go to the office, clinic, or birthing facility. A sterile vaginal examination determines if there is danger of cord prolapse. If the presenting part is well engaged, the risk of cord prolapse is minimal, and the woman may ambulate

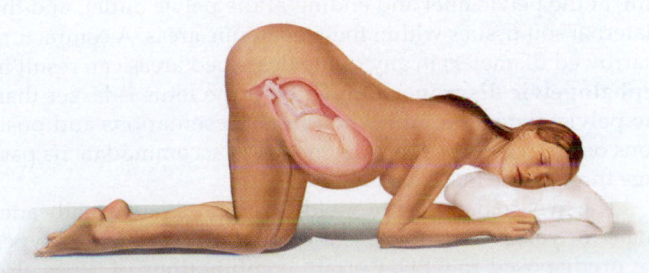

Figure 21–10 The knee–chest position is used to relieve cord compression during cord prolapse emergency.

as desired. If the presenting part is not well engaged, bedrest is recommended to prevent cord prolapse.

Because cord prolapse can be associated with fetal death, some physicians/CNMs insist that bedrest be maintained after rupture of membranes regardless of fetal engagement. This can lead to conflict if the laboring woman and her partner do not hold the same opinions. You can ease this situation by assisting communication between the physician/CNM and the couple.

During labor, any alteration of the FHR or the presence of meconium in the amniotic fluid indicates the need to assess for cord prolapse. Vaginal birth is possible with prolapsed cord if the cervix is completely dilated and pelvic measurements are adequate. In order for a vaginal birth to be attempted, birth should be imminent. In most cases, a vaginal birth is performed only if it results in a shorter time period than the preparations would take for a cesarean birth. Vacuum extraction may also be considered to facilitate a vaginal birth.

If these conditions are not present, cesarean birth is the method of choice. The woman is transported to the operating room, and the examiner continues to relieve the pressure on the cord until the baby is born.

Care of the Woman and Fetus at Risk Because of Anaphylactoid Syndrome of Pregnancy

In the presence of a small tear in the amnion or chorion high in the uterus, a small amount of amniotic fluid may leak into the chorionic plate and enter the maternal system as **amniotic fluid embolism syndrome**, a condition called **anaphylactoid syndrome of pregnancy**. While the syndrome is rare, occurring in only 1 to 12 cases per 100,000 births, the results can be catastrophic for both the mother and the fetus. Although this is a rare labor complication it has an 80% mortality rate and represents 5% to 10% of maternal morbidity in the United States (Moore, 2015). It is estimated that 50% of women die within the first hour after occurrence and survivors have a 50% risk of developing disseminated intravascular coagulation (DIC); nearly all of the women who survive will require a blood transfusion (Moore, 2015).

In anaphylactoid syndrome of pregnancy, amniotic fluid enters at areas of placental separation or cervical tears. Under pressure from the contracting uterus, the fluid is driven into the maternal circulation and then the maternal lungs. The more debris in the amniotic fluid (such as meconium), the greater the maternal problems. This condition frequently occurs during or after the birth when the woman has had a difficult, rapid labor. Other risk factors include advanced maternal age (more commonly after the age of 39), cesarean and instrumental delivery, placenta previa and abruption, grand multiparity (more than 5 live births or stillbirths), cervical lacerations, nonreassuring fetal status, eclampsia, medical induction of labor, Black race, and maternal cerebrovascular disorders and cardiac disease (Baldisseri, 2015).

Maternal Implications

The woman with anaphylactoid syndrome of pregnancy experiences a sudden onset of respiratory distress, circulatory collapse, acute hemorrhage, and cor pulmonale as the embolism blocks the vessels of the lungs. She exhibits dyspnea and cyanosis leading to hemorrhagic shock and coma. Birth must be facilitated immediately to obtain a live fetus.

Clinical Therapy

Any woman exhibiting chest pain, dyspnea, cyanosis, frothy sputum, tachycardia, hypotension, and massive hemorrhage requires the cooperation of every member of the healthcare team if her life is to be saved. Medical interventions are supportive. Recovery is contingent on return of the mother's cardiovascular and respiratory stability. If necessary, a cesarean birth is performed.

Nursing Management

In the absence of the physician/CNM, administer oxygen under positive pressure until medical help arrives. Quickly establish an intravenous line. If respiratory and cardiac arrest occurs, immediately initiate cardiopulmonary resuscitation (CPR). Call the anesthesiologist immediately.

Clinical Tip

When anaphylactoid syndrome is expected, quickly call for additional nursing staff because it is likely a code will be called. Extra staff can prepare intravenous lines, assist with CPR, monitor fetal heart tones, obtain the crash cart, and prepare for emergency cesarean birth.

Ready the equipment necessary for blood transfusion and for the insertion of the central venous pressure (CVP) line. As the blood volume is replaced, using fresh whole blood to provide clotting factors, frequently monitor the CVP. In the presence of cor pulmonale, fluid overload could easily occur.

Care of the Woman With a Uterine Rupture

Uterine rupture is a nonsurgical disruption of the uterine cavity that occurs in 1 in 1,146 woman (0.07%) (Nahum, 2015). A complete rupture is one in which the endometrium, myometrium, and serosa have separated. An incomplete or partial rupture occurs when one but not all of the layers have disrupted. The extent of the maternal and fetal distress is typically proportional to the degree of rupture. Only 13% of uterine ruptures occur in women who have not had uterine surgery (Smith & Wax, 2015). Rupture preceding labor is rare but does occur. Uterine rupture can also occur as a result of uterine manipulation (such as a version), operative vaginal delivery, abdominal trauma, certain congenital uterine disorders (Ehlers-Danlos type IV), interval of births less than 18 months, postpartum fever during a previous cesarean birth, failed trial of labor after cesarean section in subsequent pregnancy, or a one-layer closure performed with a previous cesarean birth (Smith & Wax, 2015).

Clinical Therapy

Uterine rupture can be diagnosed only after a surgical incision, but suspected uterine rupture is based on maternal and fetal symptoms. If the rupture occurs and vaginal bleeding is present, a pad count is performed. Preparations for a cesarean birth, anesthesiology services, and neonatology services are indicated. Maternal and neonatal resuscitation should be anticipated.

Nursing Management

For the Woman With a Uterine Rupture

Nursing Assessment and Diagnosis

A nonreassuring fetal heart rate (FHR) is the earliest warning sign of a possible uterine rupture. It can be associated with variable or late decelerations followed by a bradycardia. Upon palpation, there may be loss of a fetal station. Maternal symptoms include constant abdominal pain, uterine tenderness, change in uterine shape, cessation of contractions, hematuria, and signs of shock.

Nursing Plan and Implementation

When a nonreassuring pattern is identified, the physician/ CNM is immediately contacted. Women with a previous cesarean or uterine rupture are at greatest risk. Maternal and fetal signs should be assessed. Leopold maneuvers and maternal vital signs should be obtained. Prepare for an emergency birth and ensure that the anesthesiology and neonatal care providers are called. Blood should be typed and matched for possible transfusion. An additional 18-gauge line should be placed. During the surgery, the degree of rupture is assessed and the repair is made if possible. Women who are hemodynamically unstable may require a hysterectomy.

Nursing diagnoses include the following (NANDA-I © 2014):

- *Gas Exchange, Impaired,* in the fetus related to decreased blood flow secondary to uterine rupture
- *Gas Exchange, Impaired,* in the mother related to decreased blood flow secondary to uterine rupture
- *Fear* related to unknown outcome
- *Anxiety* related to emergency procedures and unknown fetal outcome
- *Coping, Ineffective,* due to emergent situation secondary to uterine rupture

Evaluation

- The mother remains hemodynamically stable throughout emergency cesarean birth.
- The fetus retains optimal oxygenation until a safe birth is achieved.

Care of the Woman With Cephalopelvic Disproportion

The birth passage includes the maternal bony pelvis, beginning at the pelvic inlet and ending at the pelvic outlet, and the maternal soft tissues within these anatomic areas. A contracture (narrowed diameter) in any of the described areas can result in **cephalopelvic disproportion (CPD)** if the fetus is larger than the pelvic diameters. Abnormal fetal presentations and positions occur in CPD as the fetus moves to accommodate its passage through the maternal pelvis.

The gynecoid and anthropoid pelvic types are usually adequate for vertex birth, but the android and platypelloid types are predisposed to CPD. Certain combinations of types also can result in pelvic diameters inadequate for vertex birth. (See Figure 16–1 for a comparison of pelvic types and Table 16-2 for their implications for childbirth.)

Types of Contractures

The pelvic inlet is contracted if the shortest anterior-posterior diameter is less than 10 cm (3.9 in.) or the greatest transverse diameter is less than 12 cm (4.7 in.). The anterior-posterior diameter may be approximated by measuring the diagonal conjugate, which in the contracted inlet is less than 11.5 cm (4.5 in.). Clinical pelvimetry, a learned skill, is used to determine the smallest anterior-posterior diameter through which the fetal head must pass. X-rays are no longer performed on a pregnant woman to determine the adequacy of her pelvis. Soft-tissue dystocia can occur as a result of fibroids, Bandl ring, stool, or a full bladder. Anomalies of the reproductive tract can also affect a woman's ability to have a vaginal birth.

The treatment goal is to allow the natural forces of labor to push the biparietal diameter of the fetal head beyond the potential interspinous obstruction. Although forceps may be used, they cause difficulty because pulling on the head destroys flexion, and the space is further diminished. A bulging perineum and crowning indicate that the obstruction has been passed.

An interischial tuberous diameter of less than 8 cm (3.1 in.) constitutes an outlet contracture. Outlet and midpelvic contractures frequently occur simultaneously. Whether vaginal birth can occur depends on the woman's interischial tuberous diameters and the fetal posterosagittal diameter.

Women With Special Needs Cephalopelvic Disproportion

Women with certain birth defects are prone to cephalopelvic disproportion (CPD), making a cesarean birth the only choice for birth. Women with dwarfism have platypelloid pelvises which are not compatible with vaginal birth. The physician caring for a woman with dwarfism should consult with another physician with experience in performing cesarean births on this population because some women's pelvic anatomy may have slight deviations.

Maternal Implications

Labor is prolonged in the presence of CPD. Membrane rupture can result from the force of the unequally distributed contractions being exerted on the fetal membranes. In obstructed labor, in which the fetus cannot descend, uterine rupture can occur. With delayed descent, necrosis of maternal soft tissues can result from pressure exerted by the fetal head. Eventually, necrosis can cause fistulas from the vagina to other nearby structures. Difficult, forceps-assisted births can also result in damage to maternal soft tissue.

Fetal/Neonatal Implications

If the membranes rupture and the fetal head has not entered the inlet, there is a danger of cord prolapse. Excessive molding of the fetal head can result. Traumatic, forceps-assisted birth can damage the fetal skull and central nervous system. Facial bruising, facial nerve trauma, and damage to the eye sockets can also occur.

Clinical Therapy

Fetopelvic relationships can be assessed by comparing pelvic measurements obtained by a manual examination before labor. An estimated weight of the fetus can be obtained by ultrasound measurements.

When the pelvic diameters are borderline or questionable, a trial of labor (TOL) may be advised. In this process, the woman continues to labor and careful, frequent assessments of cervical dilatation and fetal descent are made. Internal uterine and fetal scalp electrode monitoring may be used to more accurately assess uterine and fetal status. As long as there is continued progress, the TOL continues. Oxytocin should be used only if CPD is not suspected. When CPD is suspected, oxytocin should be discontinued. If progress ceases, the decision for a cesarean birth is made.

Nursing Management

The adequacy of the maternal pelvis for a vaginal birth should be assessed both during and before labor. During the intrapartum assessment, the size of the fetus and its presentation, position, and lie must also be considered. (See Chapter 17 for intrapartum assessment techniques.)

Suspect CPD when labor is prolonged, cervical dilatation and effacement are slow, and engagement of the presenting part is delayed. The couple may need support in coping with the stresses of this complicated labor. Keep the couple informed of what is happening and explain the procedures being used.

Nursing actions during the TOL are similar to care during any labor except that cervical dilatation and fetal descent are assessed more frequently. Both contractions and the fetus should be monitored continuously. Report any signs of nonreassuring fetal status to the physician/CNM immediately.

The mother may be positioned in a variety of ways to increase the pelvic diameters. Sitting or squatting increases the outlet diameters and may be effective when there is failure of or slow fetal descent. Changing from one side to the other or maintaining a hands-and-knees position may assist the fetus in the occiput-posterior position to change to an occiput-anterior position. The mother may instinctively want to assume one of these positions. If not, encourage a change of position.

Care of the Woman With a Complication of the Third or Fourth Stage of Labor

Common complications of the third and fourth stages of labor include retained placenta, lacerations, and placenta accreta.

Retained Placenta

Retention of the placenta beyond 30 minutes after birth is termed **retained placenta**. It occurs in one per 100 to 300 vaginal births (Urner, Zimmermann, & Krafft, 2014). Postpartum hemorrhage may be excessive. If placenta expulsion does not occur, manual removal of the placenta by the physician/CNM is attempted. In women who do not have an epidural in place, intravenous sedation or administration of intravenous pain medication may be required. Failure to retrieve the placenta via manual removal usually necessitates surgical removal by curettage. If the woman does not have an epidural in place, the procedure can be performed under general anesthesia. Retained placenta may be a symptom of an accreta, increta, or percreta (to be discussed shortly).

Lacerations

Lacerations of the cervix or vagina may be indicated when bright-red vaginal bleeding persists in the presence of a well-contracted uterus. "Instrumental delivery, nulliparity, persistent posterior orientation and increased birth weight are independently associated with severe perineal lacerations. Restrictive use of mediolateral episiotomy protects against severe perineal lacerations especially in case of instrumental delivery" (Schmitz, Alberti, Andriss, et al., 2014, p. 11).

Vaginal and perineal lacerations are often categorized in terms of degree, as follows:

- First-degree laceration is a superficial tear limited to the fourchette, perineal skin, and vaginal mucous membrane.
- Second-degree laceration involves the perineal skin, vaginal mucous membrane, underlying fascia, and muscles of the perineal body; it may extend upward on one or both sides of the vagina.
- Third-degree laceration extends through the perineal skin, vaginal mucous membranes, and perineal body and involves the anal sphincter.
- Fourth-degree laceration is the same as third degree but extends through the rectal mucosa to the lumen of the rectum; it may be called a third-degree laceration with a rectal wall extension.

Placenta Accreta

The chorionic villi attach directly to the myometrium of the uterus in *placenta accreta*. Two other types of placental adherence are *placenta increta*, in which the myometrium is invaded, and *placenta percreta*, in which the myometrium is penetrated. The adherence itself may be total, partial, or focal, depending on the amount of placental involvement. The incidence of placenta accreta is 14.4 per 10,000 births (Creanga, Bateman, Butwick, et al., 2015). It is the most common type of adherent placenta types. Major risk factors include placenta previa and a previous uterine incision. Other risk factors include maternal age more than 30 years, non-Hispanic Black race, presence of medical conditions, previous uterine surgery, and birth occurring at an urban, teaching, or larger hospital (Creanga et al., 2015). Risk increases as the number of cesarean births increase.

The primary complication with placenta accreta is maternal hemorrhage and failure of the placenta to separate following birth of the baby. Twenty-nine percent of all hysterectomies performed after birth are related to adherent placenta disorders (Creanga et al., 2015). The need for a hysterectomy depends on the amount and depth of involvement.

Care of the Family Experiencing Perinatal Loss

Perinatal loss is death of a fetus or neonate from the time of conception through the end of the newborn period 28 days after birth. Spontaneous abortion (miscarriage) in the antepartum period is discussed in Chapter 15; this section discusses intrauterine fetal death (IUFD) after 20 weeks' gestation, often referred to as *stillbirth* or *fetal demise*. Maternal death is any death that occurs during pregnancy or within 42 days of the termination of a pregnancy.

Common Causes of Perinatal Loss

The *perinatal mortality rate (PMR)* is defined by the National Center for Health Statistics as late fetal deaths (over 28 gestational weeks) and neonatal deaths that occur before 7 days (Gregory, MacDorman, & Martin, 2014). Perinatal deaths may be related to fetal, maternal, or placental factors or may have no apparent cause.

KEY FACTS TO REMEMBER
Factors Associated With Perinatal Loss

Fetal Factors

- Chromosomal disorders
- Congenital malformations/birth defects
- Anencephaly, open neural tube defects, isolated hydrocephalus, congenital heart defects
- Nonimmune hydrops fetalis
- Infections
- Complications of multiple gestations
- Intrauterine growth restriction
- Asphyxia
- Cord accidents

Maternal Factors

- Prolonged pregnancy
- Diabetes
- Chronic hypertension
- Preeclampsia/eclampsia
- Advanced maternal age (>40 years)
- Non-Hispanic Black race
- Nulliparity
- Obesity
- Hereditary thrombophilias
- Antiphospholipid syndrome
- Systemic lupus erythematosus
- Thyroid disorders
- Cholestasis of pregnancy
- Uterine rupture
- Rh disease
- Presence of certain infections (e.g., syphilis, malaria)
- Use of certain medications (e.g., antipsychotics, antiepileptic drugs)
- Substance abuse
- Smoking

Placental and Other Factors

- Placenta previa
- Abruptio placentae
- Cord accident
- Unknown factors

Perinatal loss has declined as a result of early diagnosis of congenital anomalies and advances in genetic testing techniques. Although the incidence is extremely low, certain diagnostic testing options can contribute to fetal deaths, including amniocentesis and chorionic villus sampling (CVS). Pregnancies conceived by in vitro fertilization have higher rates of pregnancy complications and loss; multiple gestations related to infertility treatments have a lower rate of loss because these procedures commonly result in dichorionic twins. Monochorionic twins, which are most often conceived naturally, have a higher incidence of loss (Burgess, Unal, Nietert, et al., 2014).

In developing countries, infection plays a significant role in fetal mortality. These may include:

- *Escherichia coli*
- Group B streptococci
- *Ureaplasma urealyticum*
- Parvovirus
- Coxsackievirus
- *Toxoplasma gondii*
- *Listeria monocytogenes*
- Leptospirosis
- Q fever
- Lyme disease

Maternal Physiologic Implications

The greatest maternal risk occurs when there is prolonged retention of the deceased fetus. These may include (Patel, Thaker, Shah, et al., 2014):

- Disseminated intravascular coagulation (DIC)
- Infection
- Endometritis
- Sepsis
- Acute renal failure
- Maternal death

Induction is commonly scheduled immediately upon diagnosis but may be delayed if the mother refuses or if it is a multiple gestation. When delays occur, fibrinogen levels are monitored weekly or biweekly to identify progressive coagulopathy. In cases of fetal death in the presence of a multiple gestation, coagulation labs may be obtained. DIC rarely occurs in cases of multiple gestations where the remaining fetus(es) are allowed to grow and mature (Jain & Purohit, 2014).

Clinical Therapy

Fetal loss may present as an absence of fetal activity. Diagnosis of IUFD is confirmed by visualization of the fetal heart with absence of heart action on ultrasound. Some practitioners routinely have a second opinion with a follow-up ultrasound to verify the diagnosis. In most cases, spontaneous labor begins within 2 weeks of fetal death without medical intervention. Because complications increase with delayed birth and identification of the cause of death becomes more difficult the longer pregnancy continues, labor is typically induced as soon as possible.

Most women with a fetal demise will select a time to schedule an induction. Most women will elect for an induction immediately, although some women may wish to arrange for family members or other support persons to be present, which may necessitate a brief waiting period. The mode of induction

is dependent on the gestational age, cervical readiness, and the type of incision if a cesarean was previously performed (American College of Obstetricians & Gynecologists [ACOG], 2014a). In women who have had previous cesarean births, a trial of labor is favored unless unusual circumstances exist (ACOG, 2014a).

Women with an unfavorable cervix may be given misoprostol or, if a second trimester dilatation and extraction is planned, laminaria tents. *Laminaria tents* are made from the stems of brown seaweed, which are cut, shaped, dried, sterilized, and packaged in specific sizes. Laminaria tents work by drawing water out of the cervical tissue, allowing the cervix to soften and dilate, and are most commonly used in preterm gestations. Sagiv and colleagues (2015) compared the efficiency of misoprostol and laminaria tents and found both were equally effective. Laminaria tents were associated with more pain and discomfort at the time of placement while misoprostol was associated with more side effects. Both may be placed before surgical procedures or inductions of labor. Transcervical Foley catheter placement or oxytocin (Pitocin) induction can also be used in women with an unfavorable cervix.

Postbirth Evaluation

Identifying the causative factor of fetal loss assists many families in progressing through the grieving process. Postmortem examination or studies can provide information related to the cause of the fetal death and risk of reoccurrence, and assist with future preconception counseling, prenatal screening procedures, and pregnancy management, as well as provide closure for the couple (ACOG, 2014a). The types of studies and tests performed depend on the parents' past history, medical history, pregnancy course, appearance of the fetus, and the couple's preferences for the testing. Fetal, maternal, and placental testing are performed (Table 21–2).

A visual inspection of the baby determines obvious defects or abnormalities. The placenta and membranes are inspected. The umbilical cord should be inspected for true knots, a velamentous insertion, lack of Wharton jelly, or a short cord to determine if a cord accident was the cause. An autopsy is the best mechanism to determine the cause of death; however, in the event that the parents decline an autopsy, magnetic resonance imaging can also provide detailed information (ACOG, 2014a).

Phases of Grief

Grief is an individual's total response to a loss, including physical symptoms, thoughts, feelings, functional limitations, and spiritual reactions. It may be manifested by certain behaviors and rituals of **mourning**, such as weeping or visiting a gravesite, which help the person experience, accept, and adjust to the loss. The period of adjustment to loss is known as **bereavement**.

Grief and mourning were first described by Kubler-Ross (1969) as five stages that characterize the grief process. Wright (2015), a critical care nurse with a special interest in grief, expanded the Kubler-Ross Model as follows:

- Shock/denial
- Pain/guilt
- Anger/bargaining
- Depression/reflection/loneliness
- The upward turn
- Reconstruction/working through
- Acceptance/hope

The grieving process is entirely variable and dependent on many factors. It may be nonlinear and represents a process that encompasses the need of the griever to remain connected to the

TABLE 21–2 Tests to Determine Cause of Fetal Loss

FETAL TESTING	MATERNAL TESTING	PLACENTAL TESTING
Fetal blood tests and X-rays	Random sugar/hemoglobin	Placental studies (IgG and IgM if specific infections suspected)
Fetal ultrasound	A1C	Pathology
Autopsy or MRI	CBC with platelet count	
Fetal cultures (IgG and IgM if specific infections suspected)	Rh testing	
Chromosomal studies (if indicated)	Kleihauer-Betke test	
	Abnormal antibody testing (lupus anticoagulant, anticardiolipin antibodies)	
	TSH levels	
	Infectious disease testing (rubella, syphilis, malaria, toxoplasmosis, cytomegalovirus, human parvovirus 19)	
	Hereditary thrombophilia testing	
	Toxicology testing	
	Protein S & C activity	

deceased, while simultaneously finding a way to exist without the child (Wright, 2015).

Maternal Death

Maternal death is defined by the World Health Organization (WHO) as "the death of a woman while pregnant or within 42 days of termination of pregnancy, irrespective of the duration and the site of the pregnancy, from any cause related to or aggravated by the pregnancy or its management, but not from accidental or incidental causes" (2015). The most common causes of maternal death are hemorrhage, hypertensive disorders, embolism, infection, and preexisting chronic conditions, such as diabetes and cardiovascular disease. Obesity is also becoming a significant factor in maternal deaths because of the medical conditions that result. The national maternal mortality rate has remained at 14 deaths per 100,000 live births since 2011 (World Health Organization, 2015). While they have been excluded from the definition of maternal death, some researchers have noted that maternal deaths related to homicide (and intimate partner or family violence) and suicide represent a small but significant number of deaths that occur during the pregnancy and postpartum period (Pallodino, Singh, Campbell, et al., 2012).

For the spouse or partner, the death is shocking and traumatic, despite known medical problems. Because the death has occurred in what is typically an expectedly joyous event, profound grief and shock are common. The grieving process is complicated by a number of factors (such as possibly caring for the newborn while grieving the deceased partner) and too comprehensive a topic for this text. Initial grief reactions may be extremely intense. As long as safety is sustained, the father/partner and family should be supported as they express their grief. Interactions should be brief and direct, such as offering tissues, and straightforward condolences (i.e., "I'm so sorry this is happening to you"). As with all losses, it is important to resist offering explanations or platitudes, which may prove harmful.

For the staff, a maternal death on the perinatal unit can be traumatic as well. When a death occurs on any unit, there are individual as well as group reactions to the event. The individual nurses involved may experience feelings of shock, sadness, anger, guilt, and other grief-associated reactions. The unit as a whole may experience feelings of inadequacy, anger, guilt, confusion, and sadness. For the nurses directly involved, the father/partner and family must still be cared for, and for everyone on the unit, nursing care continues.

It is important for obstetric nurses in situations of loss to be provided with adequate support within the work environment (Rondinelli, Long, Seelinger, et al., 2015). Staff members need the opportunity to express their feelings in a safe environment. Interventions for staff may include professional debriefing, professional counseling when needed, and the use of peer support. A model of peer training in which nurses comfortable with caring for bereaved families act as peer mentors for less experienced nurses or for nurses who are uncomfortable caring for families with a perinatal loss can provide a foundation for staff growth. Nurses need to take care of their own grief reactions and allow time for personal healing. Focusing on the positive aspects of the situation where they exist (such as personal kindness shown to the mother before the death, or to the family in the aftermath) is an important step in the healing process as well as reflecting objectively on those things out of one's personal control (the mother's underlying medical issues or unforeseen complications). The idea, as with the loss of a baby, is to eventually memorialize the event with a balanced perspective, recognizing where personal effectiveness as well as limitations exist and learning to live with them, both personally and professionally.

Professionalism in Practice Bereavement Certification

Several organizations offer bereavement certification that focuses on perinatal loss and the needs of families during this difficult event. Ideally, each hospital should have a certified on-call specialist who can be brought in to meet the needs of families during the grief process.

Nursing Management

For the Family Experiencing Perinatal Death

Nursing Assessment and Diagnosis

Cessation of fetal movement is frequently the first indication of fetal death, followed by a gradual decrease in the signs and symptoms of pregnancy. Fetal heart tones are absent, and fetal movement is no longer palpable. Once fetal demise has been established, assess the family members' ability to adapt to their loss. At that time, you may discuss previous losses and perceived coping abilities. Identifying social supports and resources is also important.

Perinatal loss may also occur during labor or birth as a result of an intrapartum complication, such as an unresolved shoulder dystocia, prolapsed umbilical cord, abruptio placentae, or other complication. In such emergency situations, healthcare team members often focus on the physical needs of the mother and an attempt to save the fetus's life. The family may not be aware that a perinatal death has occurred until the baby is delivered. Thus, the parents are faced with the sudden and completely unanticipated death of their baby. The most common reaction is protest or disbelief. Although the physician/CNM informs the family of the death, the nurse continues one-on-one care with the family, providing both physical and emotional support throughout this crucial period. Support the grief process and identify parental wishes to spend time with the newborn. It is important to explain that men and women experience grief differently and that sometimes these differences can result in relationship issues. Some grief reactions may be associated with posttraumatic stress, depression, anxiety, and sleeping disorders and warrant professional intervention. Predictors for adverse grief responses include lack of social support, marital or relationship difficulties, absence of surviving children, or ambivalence regarding the pregnancy (Kersting & Wagner, 2012).

Nursing diagnoses that may apply include the following (NANDA-I © 2014):

- *Grieving* related to imminent loss of a child
- *Coping: Family, Compromised,* related to death of a child/ unresolved feelings regarding perinatal loss
- *Family Processes, Interrupted,* related to fetal demise
- *Hopelessness* related to sudden, unexpected fetal loss
- *Spiritual Distress, Risk for,* related to intense suffering secondary to unexpected fetal loss

Nursing Plan and Implementation

Most facilities have an established holistic, family-centered protocol to follow in the event of perinatal death that includes notification of staff prior to the family's arrival to prevent inappropriate remarks. Many facilities have a symbol, such as a card with a leaf, a heart, or a cluster of flowers, which is placed on the mother's door so that all staff members are aware of the loss (Figure 21–11).

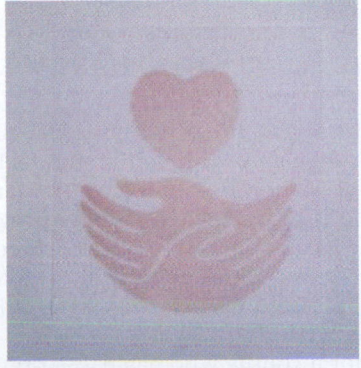

Figure 21–11 Door card.

SOURCE: Share Pregnancy & Infant Loss Support, Inc.

PREPARING THE FAMILY FOR THE BIRTH

On arrival at the facility, the family should be placed in a private room, preferably away from laboring women. Avoidance of prolonged waiting with other expectant parents or visitors waiting for news from other women in labor is optimal.

Provide the couple with privacy in a supportive environment that includes providing an explanation about procedures and obtaining information regarding their personal preferences for the birth. Encourage questions and answer them clearly and straightforwardly. It is not uncommon for the same questions to be asked repeatedly as a part of the initial grief process. Stay with the family to provide support and prevent isolation but be acutely aware of cues that privacy is desired. Some couples may want outside support, such as family members, friends, or a spiritual leader, to be present during the labor. It is your responsibility to facilitate the couple's wishes.

When possible, the same nurse should provide care so that a therapeutic relationship can be established. Arrange for other members of the interdisciplinary team to interact with the family, including a grief counselor, social worker, neonatologist, chaplain, genetic counselor, and other professionals needed to provide holistic care.

Explain details of the plan of care and the availability of anesthesia and analgesia whenever the woman desires. Facilitate the participation of the woman and her partner in the labor and birth process to whatever extent they wish to participate.

It is important to remember that in contrast to a typical birth experience, the birth of a stillborn baby marks both the beginning and the end. For this reason, it is imperative that the couple and family have all wishes and preferences respected. The family may be overwhelmed and may have difficulty making decisions in this period. Assist the couple to explore their feelings and help them to make decisions about who is present and what rituals will occur during and following the birth. Examples of birth preferences include:

- Use of music, dimmed lighting, or other environmental preferences
- Laboring or birthing in a specific position
- Having the baby placed on the mother's chest immediately after birth
- Allowing the mother or father to assist in the birth or cut the umbilical cord
- Including other family members or friends at the birth
- Establishing opportunities for other children in the family to be involved

Sometimes couples worry that others may view their preferences as "strange" or "wrong." Reassure the family that it is their experience and that there are no right or wrong feelings or wishes. Culture diversity will play a vital role in how the couple responds or reacts during the birthing process.

The couple may have waves of overwhelming grief, disbelief, or sadness. Encourage the couple to experience the grief that they feel. It is not uncommon for one partner to attempt to put on a "brave front," feeling that by showing grief, he or she will make the other partner feel worse. Encourage partners to express their emotions freely to the extent they are able. Help them understand that they may each experience different feelings.

SUPPORTING THE FAMILY IN VIEWING THE STILLBORN BABY

Advocates of seeing the stillborn baby believe that viewing assists in dispelling denial and enables the couple to progress to the next step in the grieving process. If they choose to see their stillborn baby, prepare the couple for what they will see by saying, "She is going to feel cold," "He is going to be blue," or other appropriate statements. When known, use the baby's name. Babies are often wrapped in a blanket to cover birth defects when the parents first view them. Most parents will eventually remove the covering to inspect their baby; however, applying a covering allows them time to adjust to the appearance at their own pace.

Some parents may elect to bathe or dress their stillborn; support them in their choice. Some couples may want other family members, friends, or their other children to see the baby. Act as an advocate to ensure the family's wishes are respected.

PROVIDING DISCHARGE CARE

Most facilities prepare a remembrance box or package for the family to take home. This typically consists of a photograph taken of the baby or the family, a card with the baby's footprints, a crib card, an identification band, a lock of hair, and possibly a blanket or clothing worn by the baby. In the event that the couple declines the package, it is common for the hospital to retain these items for a specific period of time.

After the birth, the couple can be given the option of an early discharge (as early as 6 to 8 hours after the birth). Discharge focuses on the physical considerations and adaptation of the mother. Provide the mother with postpartum directions for follow-up care, written materials, and a phone number for questions. The woman should also be given information on her milk coming in and interventions to follow to decrease the discomfort associated with engorgement.

Additional information should be given on the grief process (Figure 21–12). Prepare the couple to return home by stressing that others may not know what to say, and that even loved ones may make inappropriate comments because they do not know how to respond to grief and loss. This can prepare the couple for the reactions of others. If there are siblings, each will usually progress through age-appropriate grieving. Provide the parents with information about normal mourning reactions, both psychologic and physiologic.

FACILITATING THE FAMILY'S GRIEF WORK

During the pregnancy, the couple has already begun the attachment process, which now must be terminated through the grieving process. Facilitating the family's grief work is thus a critical nursing intervention—one that requires skill, sensitivity, and compassion.

Families are routinely referred for counseling services with a perinatal specialist to assist the couple with grieving. Concerns about future pregnancies are common and appropriate; referrals to genetic counselors, religious support persons, and social service agencies should be provided. Scheduled follow-up phone calls to assess the family's functioning and progress with grief work are typically performed by the nurse who provided care during the birth. During these phone calls, information and emotional support can be given and additional resources can be identified.

Clinical Tip

Families should be encouraged to implement cultural, religious, or social customs to assist them in grieving and mourning. Advise the family that certain upcoming milestones, such as holidays, future birthdays, baby showers, Mother's Day, Father's Day, and other social events, may trigger their grief. The family can better cope with these events if they are adequately prepared.

REFERRING THE FAMILY TO COMMUNITY SERVICES

Most facilities have an established protocol for families experiencing perinatal loss. Community support groups that focus on perinatal loss can provide resources and an important support network. Specialized groups, such as those focused on early pregnancy loss, stillbirth, and perinatal loss associated with specific congenital anomalies, allow families the opportunity to interact with peers who have lost babies under similar circumstances. Provide the group name, contact person (if possible), and phone number. Various books written by mothers who have lost children are available in bookstores and are valuable resources for grieving parents.

Internet technology has allowed large numbers of individuals to share resources and information, and participate in online support groups. Internet resources can be effective for all families and may be the only resources available for families in rural underserved areas.

CARE OF THE COUPLE WHO HAS EXPERIENCED LOSS IN A PREVIOUS PREGNANCY

Couples who have had a previous perinatal loss typically enter a subsequent pregnancy with conflicting feelings and may experience ambivalence, fear, and anxiety. Many times, their past experience is relived when another pregnancy occurs. Some couples conceive soon after a loss, whereas others wait years. Some couples enter a subsequent pregnancy with grief work largely completed whereas others are still experiencing unresolved grief.

In caring for a couple who has had a previous loss, you need to be kind, compassionate, and patient. Provide information and clear explanations of all prenatal information. Referrals to a genetic counselor or perinatologist may be indicated.

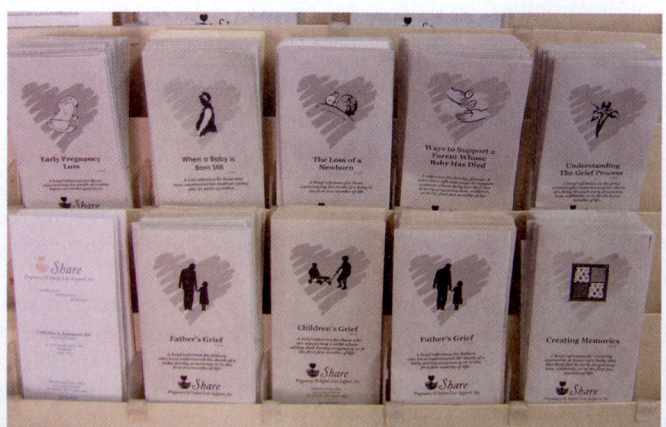

Figure 21–12 Bereavement literature.

SOURCE: Share Pregnancy & Infant Loss Support, Inc.

If unresolved grief issues are present or the family experiences extreme anxiety, counseling may be beneficial.

Interventions to decrease anxiety should be performed, including early ultrasound to verify the presence of the fetal heart. Some women may be fearful when first-trimester pregnancy symptoms begin to resolve. Women with a previous loss typically receive additional antepartum testing including ultrasounds that can be used to provide reassurance and assess fetal growth and development, placental functioning, and cord variations; non-stress testing and biophysical profiles are performed weekly after 32 weeks' gestation. Fetal kick counts should be initiated at 28 weeks. Women with a previous loss should undergo an induction at 39 weeks' gestation or once lung maturity has been established via amniocentesis because placental functioning can decline in postdate pregnancies. Great anxiety and stress are common in these mothers even after the birth of a healthy baby and postpartum and nursery nurses should provide ongoing assessment and support to these families.

Evaluation

Anticipated outcomes of nursing care include the following:

- Family members express their feelings about the death of their baby.
- Family members participate in decision making regarding preferences for the labor, birth, and immediate postpartum period.
- Family members participate in the decision of whether to see their baby and other decisions about the baby.
- The family has resources available for continued support.
- Family members know the community resources available and have names and phone numbers to use if they choose.
- The family is moving into and through the grieving process.

Nursing care of a family experiencing perinatal loss is further described in the accompanying *Nursing Care Plan*.

Nursing Care Plan: For a Family Experiencing Perinatal Loss

1. Nursing Diagnosis: *Coping: Family, Compromised,* related to perinatal loss as evidenced by crying/sadness, irritability/anger, guilt responses, and/or fear (NANDA-I © 2014)

GOAL: The woman will verbalize thoughts and feelings associated with the loss, and understand the factual events surrounding the loss. She will begin to form a trust relationship with the nurse and freely ask for and accept support provided by nursing staff.

INTERVENTION	RATIONALE
• Normalize the experience by assuring parents that there is no right or wrong way to express grief.	• Grief reactions encompass a broad spectrum of thoughts and emotions. Providing a nonjudgmental, supportive environment validates the grief response, thereby establishing a trust relationship, which helps to facilitate a healthy mourning process.
• Crying. Offer tissues while allowing free expression of emotion.	• Crying is a normal reaction to the loss event and offering tissues is a tangible form of acceptance.
• Anger. Avoiding defensiveness, state the obvious and enlist the parent's assistance in exploring possible sources of, and solutions to, their anger.	• Anger as a part of the grief response usually stems from frustration at the circumstances and should not be taken personally. Allowing for the free expression of anger, as well as remaining neutral in responses, will help to defuse the situation. Utilizing a team approach will assist the woman in viewing hospital personnel as partners in care, rather than adversaries.
• Guilt responses. Reframe the event in a reality-based forum, reassuring the parents that they did nothing to precipitate the loss.	• Guilt is a predominant feature of grief following loss, especially in parents experiencing the death of a baby. Reality testing, which involves referencing factual information versus the parents' perceptions of culpability, assists them in coming to the conclusion that they did the best they could in the circumstance.
• Fear. Provide honest, simple explanations of what to expect before, during, and after the loss event.	• Families can cope with extreme situations when they are properly informed in an honest and forthright manner. Maintaining a close presence while providing factual information will help alleviate feelings of fear and isolation. Offering simple choices allows clients to maintain a semblance of control over their circumstances.

Expected Outcomes: The woman and family acknowledge the loss as evidenced by verbalizing an understanding of the factual events surrounding the loss and openly expressing thoughts and feelings regarding the loss in a safe and constructive manner. The woman and family begin to form a trust relationship as evidenced by freely asking for and accepting support provided by nursing staff, and relating to the nurse in an environment of acceptance.

Focus Your Study

- A tachysystolic labor pattern is characterized by painful contractions that are not effective in effacing and dilating the cervix. It usually leads to a prolonged latent phase.

- Hypotonic labor patterns begin normally and then progress to infrequent, less intense contractions.

- Postterm pregnancy is one that extends more than 294 days or 42 weeks past the first day of the last menstrual period.

- The occiput-posterior position of the fetus during labor prolongs the labor process, causes severe back discomfort in the laboring woman, and predisposes her to vaginal and perineal trauma and lacerations during birth.

- The types of fetal malpresentations include face, brow, breech, shoulder, and compound.

- A fetus or newborn weighing more than 4000 g is termed macrosomic. Problems with a fetus this size may occur during labor, birth, and the early neonatal period.

- Multiple-gestation pregnancies carry an increased risk of pregnancy-related complications.

- Nonreassuring fetal status is indicated by persistent late decelerations, persistent severe variable decelerations, and prolonged decelerations. If nonreassuring fetal status is recognized and treated appropriately, the fetus may not experience permanent damage.

- Prolapsed umbilical cord results when the umbilical cord precedes the fetal presenting part. This places pressure on the umbilical cord and diminishes blood flow to the fetus.

- Anaphylactoid syndrome of pregnancy is an extremely rare event that occurs when a bolus of amniotic fluid enters the maternal circulation and then the maternal lungs. The maternal mortality rate is very high with this complication.

- Uterine rupture is a nonsurgical disruption of the uterine cavity and is an obstetric emergency requiring prompt and immediate intervention.

- Hydramnios occurs when more than 2000 mL of amniotic fluid is contained within the amniotic membranes. Hydramnios is associated with fetal malformations that affect fetal swallowing and with maternal diabetes mellitus, Rh sensitization, and multiple-gestation pregnancies.

- Oligohydramnios is present when there is a severely reduced volume of amniotic fluid. It is associated with intrauterine growth restriction (IUGR), postmaturity, and fetal renal or urinary malfunctions. The fetus is more likely to experience variable decelerations because the amniotic fluid is insufficient to keep pressure off the umbilical cord.

- Cephalopelvic disproportion (CPD) occurs when there is a narrowed diameter in the maternal pelvis. The narrowed diameter is called a contracture and may occur in the pelvic inlet, the midpelvis, or the outlet. If pelvic measurements are borderline, a trial of labor may be attempted. Failure of cervical dilatation or fetal descent necessitates a cesarean birth.

- Third- and fourth-stage complications usually involve hemorrhage. The causes of hemorrhage include retained placenta, lacerations of the birth canal or cervix, and placenta accreta.

- Perinatal loss poses a major nursing challenge to provide support and care for the parents.

Clinical Reasoning in Action

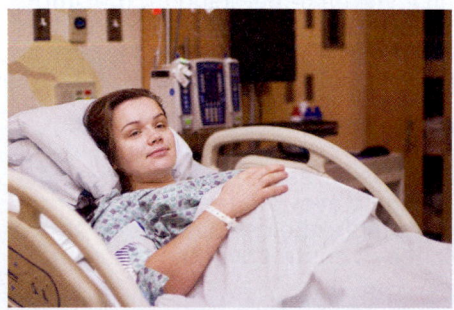

SOURCE: Mikhail Tchkheidze/Shutterstock.

June Dice, a 25-year-old G3, P1011, is admitted to you in labor and delivery at 38 weeks with a moderate amount of dark red vaginal bleeding. June's prenatal history is significant for late prenatal care (20 weeks' gestation by ultrasound) and cocaine abuse. An ultrasound is done upon admission that demonstrates a marginal placental abruption. You place June on the fetal monitor and observe a fetal heart rate baseline of 146 to 155 with accelerations to 166 with fetal movement. There are occasional mild variable decelerations with a quick return to baseline. Contraction pattern is interpreted as an irritable uterus. An intravenous infusion with Ringer lactate is started with a #18 intracath. June's vital signs are within normal limits. Her hematocrit is 29%. You assist the physician with a vaginal examination to rupture membranes and insert a fetal scalp electrode and intrauterine pressure catheter. A small amount of light yellow-green amniotic fluid is observed. The exam shows June is 4 cm dilated, 50% effaced, vertex at −1 station. You follow protocol and start an oxytocin-induction/augmentation. June is asking why oxytocin is needed.

1. Explain the goal of labor induction/augmentation in response to June's question.

2. Explain potential risk factors associated with oxytocin induction of labor.

3. You observe a nonreassuring fetal heart rate of 144 to 150 with decreased variability, and persistent late decelerations with each contraction. What interventions would you immediately take?

4. What supportive actions are taken to decrease the risk of hypofibrinogenemia?

5. What complications might be present in the newborn at birth?

References

Aiken, A. R., Aiken, C. E., Alberry, M. S., Brockelsby, J. C., & Scott, J. G. (2015). Management of fetal malposition in the second stage of labor: A propensity score analysis. *American Journal of Obstetrics and Gynecology, 212*(3), 355–e1. doi:10.1016/j.ajog.2014.10.023

American College of Obstetricians & Gynecologists (ACOG). (2014a). *Management of stillbirth* (Practice Bulletin No. 120). Washington, DC: Author.

American College of Obstetricians and Gynecologists. (2014b). Practice bulletin: Management of late-term and postterm pregnancies. *Clinical Management Guidelines for Obstetrician-Gynecologists, 124*(2), Part 1, 390–395.

Baldisseri, M. R. (2015). Amniotic fluid embolism syndrome. Up-to-Date. Retrieved from http://www.uptodate.com/contents/amniotic-fluid-embolism-syndrome

Berhan, Y., & Haileamlak, A. (2015).The risks of planned vaginal breech delivery versus planned Caesarean section for term breech birth: A meta-analysis including observational studies. *BJOG: An International Journal of Obstetrics & Gynaecology, 123*(1). doi:10.1111/1471-0528.13524

Bradley, D., & Hollbrook, T. (2013). Umbilical cord prolapse. *Contemporary OB/GYN.* Retrieved from http://contemporaryobgyn.modernmedicine.com/contemporary-obgyn/content/tags/bradley-holbrook-md/umbilical-cord-prolapse?page=full

Burgess, J. L., Unal, E. R., Nietert, P. J., & Newman, R. B. (2014). Risk of late-preterm stillbirth and neonatal morbidity for monochorionic and dichorionic twins. *American Journal of Obstetrics and Gynecology, 210*(6), 578–e1. doi:10.1016/j.ajog.2014.03.003

Caughey, A. B. (2013). Postterm pregnancy. *eMedicine.* Retrieved from http://emedicine.medscape.com/article/261369-overview#aw2aab6b6

Caughey, A. B., Sharshiner, R., & Cheng, Y. W. (2015). Fetal malposition: Impact and management. *Clinical Obstetrics and Gynecology, 58*(2), 241–245. doi:10.1097/GRF.0000000000000106

Cormier, C. M. (2015). *Management of the fetus with a compound presentation.* Retrieved from http://www.uptodate.com/contents/management-of-the-fetus-with-compound-presentation

Coyle, M. E., Smith, C. A., & Peat, B. (2012). Cephalic version by moxibustion for breech presentation. *Cochrane Database of Systematic Reviews,* Issue 5. Art. No.: CD003928. doi:10.1002/14651858.CD003928.pub3

Creanga, A. A., Bateman, B. T., Butwick, A. J., & Raleigh, L. (2014). Morbidity associated with cesarean delivery in the United States: Is placenta accreta an increasingly important contributor? *American Journal of Obstetrics & Gynecology, 213*(3), 384.e1–384.e11. doi:10.1016/j.ajog.2015.05.002

Cunningham, F. G., Leveno, K. J., Bloom, S. L., Spong, C. Y., Dashe, J. S., Hoffman, B. L., . . . Sheffield, J. S. (2014). *Williams obstetrics* (24th.). New York, NY: McGraw-Hill.

Global Library of Women's Medicine. (2015). *Abnormal fetal lie and presentation.* Retrieved from http://www.glowm.com/section_view/heading/Abnormal%20Fetal%20Lie%20and%20Presentation/item/135#5771

Gregory, E. C. W., MacDorman, M. F., & Martin, J. A. (2014). Trends in fetal and perinatal mortality in the United States: 2006–2011. *NCHS Data Brief,* 169. Retrieved from http://www.cdc.gov/nchs/data/databriefs/db169.htm

Hofmeyr, G. J. (2015). Breech delivery. In John T. Queenan, Catherine Y. Spong, Charles J. Lockwood (Eds.), *Protocols for high-risk pregnancies: An evidence-based approach* (6th ed., p. 423). Hoboken, NJ: Wiley-Blackwell.

Jain, D., & Purohit, R. C. (2014). Review of twin pregnancies with single fetal death: Management, maternal and fetal outcome. *The Journal of Obstetrics and Gynecology of India, 64*(3), 180–183. doi:10.1007/s13224-013-0500-5

Jazayeri, A. (2015). Macrosomia. *E-Medicine.* Retrieved from http://emedicine.medscape.com/article/262679-overview

Kersting, A., & Wagner, B. (2012). Complicated grief after perinatal loss. *Dialogues Clinical Neuroscience,14*(2), 187–194.

Kubler-Ross, E. (1969). *On death and dying.* New York, NY: Macmillan.

Moore, L. E. (2015). *Amniotic fluid embolism.* Retrieved from http://emedicine.medscape.com/article/253068-overview#a2

Nahum, G. G. (2015). Uterine rupture in pregnancy. *Medscape.* Retrieved from http://reference.medscape.com/article/275854-overview

Norwitz, E. R. (2015). Patient information: Postterm pregnancy. Beyond the Basics. Retrieved from http://www.uptodate.com/contents/postterm-pregnancy-beyond-the-basics

Pallodino, C. L., Singh, V., Campbell, J., Flynn, H., & Gold, K. (2012). Homicide and suicide during the perinatal period: Findings from the National Violent Death Reporting System. *Obstetrics & Gynecology, 118*(5), 1056–1063. doi:10.1097/AOG.0b013e31823294da

Patel, S., Thaker, R., Shah, P., & Majumder, S. (2014). Study of causes and complications of intra uterine fetal death (IUFD). *International Journal of Reproduction, Contraception, Obstetrics and Gynecology, 3*(4), 931–935. doi:10.5455/2320-1770.ijrcog20141211

Rondinelli, J., Long, K., Seelinger, C., Crawford, C. L., & Valdez, R. (2015). Factors related to nurse comfort when caring for families experiencing perinatal loss: Evidence for bereavement program enhancement. *Journal for Nurses in Professional Development, 31*(3), 158–163. doi: 10.1097/NND.0000000000000163

Sagiv, R., Mizrachi, Y., Glickman, H., Kerner, R., Keidar, R., Bar, J., & Golan, A. (2015). Laminaria vs. vaginal misoprostol for cervical preparation before second-trimester surgical abortion: A randomized clinical trial. *Contraception, 91*(5), 406–411. 1doi:10.1016/j.contraception.2015.01.018

Schmitz, T., Alberti, C., Andriss, B., Moutafoff, C., Oury, J. F., & Sibony, O. (2014). Identification of women at high risk for severe perineal lacerations. *European Journal of Obstetrics & Gynecology and Reproductive Biology, 182,* 11–15. doi:10.1016/j.ejogrb.2014.08.031

Shashidhar, T. G., Shashirekha, S. R., Bandamma, N., Nivedita, S. K., & Raj, S. (2015). Clinical study of the mode of delivery and perinatal outcome in breech delivery. *Indian Journal of Public Health Research & Development, 6*(3), 17–21.

Smith, J. F., & Wax, J. R. (2015). Rupture of the unscarred uterus. Up-to-Date. Retrieved from http://www.uptodate.com/contents/rupture-of-the-unscarred-uterus

Strauss, R. A. (2015). Transverse lie. Up-to-Date. Retrieved from http://www.uptodate.com/contents/transverse-fetal-lie

Talaulikar, V. S., & Arulkumaran, S. (2015). Malpositions and malpresentations of the fetal head. *Obstetrics, Gynaecology & Reproductive Medicine, 25*(6), 152–159. doi:10.1016/j.ogrm.2015.03.004

Tapisiz, O. L., Aytan, H., Altinbas, S. K., Arman, F., Tuncay, G., Besli, M., . . . & Danişman, N. (2014). Face presentation at term: A forgotten issue. *Journal of Obstetrics and Gynaecology Research, 40*(6), 1573–1577. doi:10.1111/jog.12369

Urner, F., Zimmermann, R., & Krafft, A. (2014). Manual removal of the placenta after vaginal delivery: An unsolved problem in obstetrics. *Journal of Pregnancy,* Volume 2014. doi:10.1155/2014/274651

World Health Organization. (2015). *Maternal mortality.* Retrieved from http://www.who.int/mediacentre/factsheets/fs348/en/index.html

Wright, J. (2015). *7 stages of grief: Through the process and back to life.* Retrieved from http://www.recover-from-grief.com/7-stages-of-grief.html

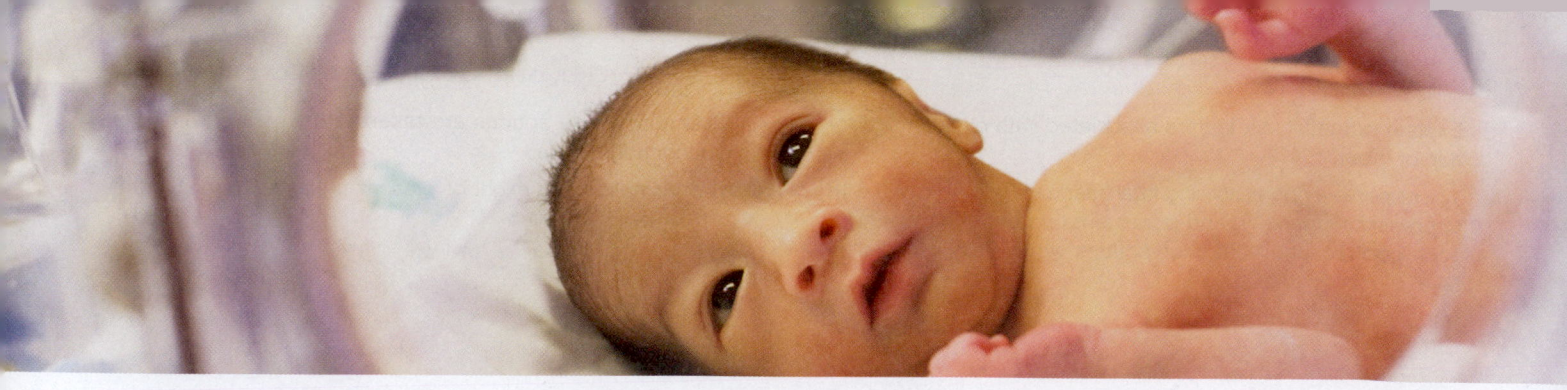

Chapter 22
Birth-Related Procedures

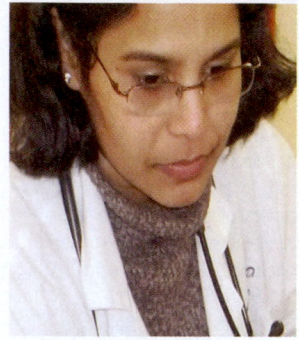

Labor and birth today are remarkably safe for both the mother and her baby. With all of our advanced technology, we in health care have the ability to make enormous strides toward our outcome goals. But the bigger challenge is to do all of that and still honor the truly life-changing, miraculous nature of the birth experience.

—Labor and Delivery RNC

⌄ Learning Outcomes

22.1 Explain the methods, purpose, criteria, and contraindications of external version in determining nursing management.

22.2 Explain the indications, the contraindications, labor readiness, and methods in determining the nursing management for women during labor induction.

22.3 Describe the use of amniotomy and the nursing management of the woman and fetus.

22.4 Describe the indications for amnioinfusion and the nursing care of the woman during amnioinfusion.

22.5 Delineate the measures to prevent episiotomy, factors that predispose women to needing an episiotomy, and types of episiotomy in determining the nursing management.

22.6 Explain the indications, maternal and neonatal risks, and nursing management during forceps-assisted birth.

22.7 Describe the nursing management of the woman and newborn during vacuum-assisted birth.

22.8 Explain the indications for cesarean birth, impact on the family unit, preparation and teaching needs, and associated nursing care.

22.9 Examine the risks, guidelines, and nursing care of the woman undergoing vaginal birth following cesarean birth.

Most births occur without the need for operative obstetric intervention. In some instances, however, procedures are necessary to maintain the safety of the woman and the fetus. The most common of these procedures are version, cervical ripening, induction of labor, amniotomy, amnioinfusion, episiotomy, forceps- or vacuum-assisted birth, cesarean birth, and vaginal birth following a previous cesarean birth.

Generally, women are aware of the possible need for an obstetric procedure during their labor and birth. However, some women expect to have a "natural" experience and feel disappointed, angry, or even guilty when an unanticipated procedure is needed. This conflict between expectation and the need for intervention presents a challenge to maternity nurses. The nurse provides information regarding any procedure to help the woman and her partner understand what is proposed, the anticipated benefits and possible risks, and any alternatives.

Care of the Woman During Version

Version, or turning of the fetus, is a procedure used to change the fetal presentation by abdominal or intrauterine manipulation. The most common type of version is **external cephalic version (ECV)**, in which the fetus is changed from a breech to a cephalic presentation by external manipulation of the maternal abdomen (Figure 22–1). The use of ECV has dramatically decreased as it is estimated that 90% of breech presentations are born via cesarean birth. The increased rates of cesarean births are directly related to reluctance to perform external cephalic versions (ECV) by either mothers or practitioners, failure of ECVs, women's preference for a cesarean birth in the presence of a breech presentation, or practitioners' clinical judgment or inexperience with the procedure (Berhan & Haileamlak, 2016).

Criteria for External Version

If breech or shoulder presentation (transverse lie) is detected in the later weeks of pregnancy, an external version may be attempted. Before the external version is begun, an ultrasound is used to locate the placenta and to confirm fetal presentation.

The following criteria should be met before performing external version:

- The pregnancy is at 36 or more weeks of gestation. A version may result in complications that require immediate birth by cesarean.

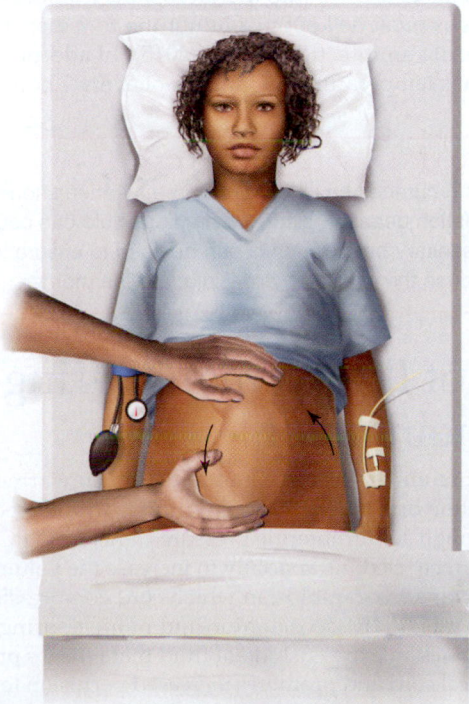

Figure 22–1 External (or cephalic) version of the fetus. A new technique involves applying pressure to the fetal head and buttocks so that the fetus completes a "backward flip" or "forward roll."

- A non-stress test (NST), obtained immediately before performing the version, is reactive. A reactive NST indicates fetal well-being.
- The fetal breech is not engaged. Once the presenting part is engaged it is difficult, if not impossible, to do a version.

Contraindications for External Version

Evidenced-based contraindications include the following (Berhan & Haileamlak, 2016):

- History of placental abruption or suspected placental abruption
- Severe preeclampsia
- Nonreassuring fetal status

Complications based on expert opinion include the following (Berhan & Haileamlak, 2016):

- Amniotic fluid alterations, including rupture of membranes, oligohydramnios, or hydramnios
- Placenta previa or vasa previa
- Previous cesarean birth or other significant uterine surgery
- Multiple gestations
- Fetal abnormalities, such as intrauterine growth restriction (IUGR) or nuchal cord

Before the ECV begins, an intravenous line may be established to administer medications in case of difficulty. The woman may receive tocolytics to relax the uterus. Some physicians may also order regional anesthesia for the procedure. Both tocolytics and regional anesthesia have been associated with higher success rates and fewer cesarean births (Berhan & Haileamlak, 2016). Ultrasound is frequently used to provide information about the fetal position and placental location. The version is discontinued in the presence of severe maternal pain or significant fetal bradycardia or decelerations.

Clinical Tip

Because the ECV procedure can be uncomfortable, encourage the woman to take slow, deep breaths. Using distraction and speaking in a calm, reassuring voice can help decrease fear and anxiety.

Nursing Management

On admission begin a thorough assessment by verifying that there are no contraindications to the version procedure. Maternal vital signs and a reactive non-stress test (NST) are obtained. This initial assessment period provides an ideal time for educating the woman and her partner and for addressing their concerns. They can be encouraged to express their understanding and expectations of the procedure. At the same time, the possibility of failure of the ECV; the slight risk of vaginal bleeding or spontaneous rupture of membranes; or the need for a cesarean birth if the FHR becomes nonreassuring should also be discussed. Explaining what will occur in any of these circumstances will better prepare the woman and her partner if intervention becomes necessary. Although the physician is ultimately responsible for obtaining informed consent, it is also your role to ensure that the woman understands the procedure and has the opportunity to ask questions and voice her concerns or fears.

Place an intravenous (IV) line before beginning the procedure to maintain IV access in case of a complication. Throughout the procedure, continue to monitor maternal blood pressure, pulse, and comfort level frequently (because the mother may experience pain during the procedure). Fetal well-being is ascertained before, intermittently during, and for (at least) 30 minutes following the procedure, using electronic fetal monitoring (EFM), ultrasound, or both. Also assess maternal–fetal response to the tocolytic. If an epidural catheter was placed for anesthesia purposes, remove the catheter prior to discharge. Provide aftercare instructions, which should include maternal monitoring for contractions, fetal movement (fetal kick counts), and signs of complications from the procedure.

Care of the Woman During Amniotomy

Amniotomy is the *artificial rupture of the amniotic membranes (AROM)*. It is probably the most common invasive procedure in obstetrics. Because the amniotomy requires that an instrument, called an amniohook, be inserted through the cervix, at least 2 cm (0.8 in.) of cervical dilatation is required. Amniotomy is thought to manipulate both hormones and mechanical factors to stimulate labor. Upon rupturing of the membranes, natural prostaglandins are released that stimulate uterine contractions. The escape of amniotic fluid allows the presenting part to descend and place direct pressure on the cervix, thus resulting in an acceleration of dilatation. Amniotomy can be performed during the first stage of labor and has been associated with a reduced length of labor in the first stage (World Health Organization [WHO], 2015). Hiersch and colleagues (2015) found that myometrial activity increased after amniotomy

Some clinicians combine amniotomy with oxytocin infusion to increase uterine contractions (WHO, 2015). Routine use of amniotomy in early labor is not generally recommended because of the increased risk of possible complications, including risk of infection and cesarean birth. Amniotomy is appropriate for use when inadequate contractions are the cause of failure to progress (WHO, 2015).

Amniotomy may also be performed for placement of an internal fetal heart monitoring electrode or an intrauterine pressure catheter. Routine use of internal monitoring devices is not recommended as they increase the risk of infection. Use of internal monitoring is contraindicated in women who are HIV positive as it increases the risk of vertical transmission to the fetus (WHO, 2015). Amniotomy also enables the nurse to assess the color and composition of amniotic fluid. Amniotomy performed when the presenting part is not well applied to the cervix increases the risk of umbilical cord prolapse (see Chapter 21 for discussion of umbilical cord prolapse).

SAFETY ALERT!
The fetal head should be engaged prior to rupturing the membranes to prevent a possible prolapsed umbilical cord, a situation in which the umbilical cord slips through the cervical opening ahead of the presenting part. This constitutes an obstetric emergency and can be avoided by using strict criteria before an amniotomy is performed.

Amniotomy Procedure

While performing a vaginal examination, the physician/CNM introduces an amniohook into the vagina and makes a small tear in the amniotic membrane, which allows amniotic fluid to escape.

Clinical Tip
Before the AROM procedure, place several layers of disposable pads under the woman's buttocks and a folded towel between the woman's legs. The towel readily absorbs the fluid released during the procedure and prevents soiling of the bed linens. After the procedure, remove the towel as well as all layers of absorbent pads that have been soiled. Several clean absorbent pads should be placed under the woman's buttocks because amniotic fluid will continue to leak from the vagina. These actions increase the woman's comfort.

Nursing Management

Explain the AROM procedure to the woman and then assess fetal presentation, position, and station, because amniotomy is usually delayed until engagement has occurred. Provide information regarding the expected effects of the amniotomy, explaining that amniotic fluid is constantly produced and that the woman will not experience a "dry birth." Ask the woman to assume a semireclining position and drape her to provide privacy. The fetal heart rate (FHR) is assessed just before and immediately after the amniotomy, and the two FHR assessments are compared. If there are marked changes, check for prolapse of the cord. Inspect the amniotic fluid for amount, color, odor, and the presence of meconium or blood. While wearing disposable gloves, cleanse and dry the perineal area and change the underpads as needed. Because there is now an open pathway for organisms to ascend into the uterus, the number of vaginal examinations must be kept to a minimum to reduce the chance of introducing an infection (WHO, 2015). In addition, monitor the woman's temperature a minimum of every 2 hours.

SAFETY ALERT!
Once the membranes have been ruptured, women should use care with ambulation because dispelled amniotic fluid can cause a fall hazard. A sanitary pad or a chux can be used to ensure floors stay dry and reduce the risk of physical injury to the mother.

Care of the Woman During Amnioinfusion

Amnioinfusion (AI) is a technique by which warmed, sterile normal saline or Ringer lactate solution is introduced into the uterus through an intrauterine pressure catheter (IUPC). Amnioinfusion can be used intrapartally to increase the volume of fluid in cases of oligohydramnios, in which cord compression causes fetal heart rate (FHR) deceleration and nonreassuring fetal status. It provides an extra cushion of fluid that relieves pressure on the umbilical cord and promotes increased perfusion to the fetus.

Nursing Management

Assess the FHR monitoring strip to detect fetal heart rate patterns associated with cord compression. If suspected, assist the laboring woman to another position and initiate intrapartum resuscitation. If intrapartum resuscitation does not restore the FHR, an amnioinfusion may be considered.

Help administer the AI; assess the woman's vital signs, pain level, and contraction status; and monitor the fetal heart rate by continuous electronic fetal monitoring (EFM). Provide ongoing information and reassurance to the laboring woman and her partner and answer questions as they arise. Comfort measures and positioning are vital because the woman is now on bedrest. Frequent changing of disposable underpads and perineal care are also needed because of the constant leakage of fluid from the vagina. Ensure that fluids that are infused into the uterus are being adequately expelled. Fluid expulsion is evaluated by counting sanitary pads and visual observation during perineal care.

Care of the Woman During Cervical Ripening

Cervical ripening is the softening and effacing of the cervix. Women with unfavorable cervixes that need induction for medical indications have much higher rates of successful vaginal births when prostaglandin agents are used and are administered prior to oxytocin. Prostaglandin E1 (PGE1) (misoprostol) or Prostaglandin E2 (GE2) (Prepidil or Cervidil) may be used for the pregnant woman who is at term or late preterm in cases where there is a medical, obstetric, or fetal indication for immediate birth, including fetal demise. Mechanical dilatation is another method that can be used to facilitate cervical ripening.

Prostaglandin Agents

A commonly used ripening agent is Prepidil gel, which contains 0.5 mg dinoprostone, a prostaglandin E_2 (PGE$_2$) agent. It is placed either intracervically or intravaginally; both placement sites yield comparable outcomes (Goldberg, 2015). Prepidil is packaged as a 3 g gel/0.5 mg dinoprostone and can be administered every 6 hours with a maximum of 3 doses in a 24 hour period (Goldberg, 2015)

A similar agent, Cervidil, is packaged as a 2-cm (0.8-in.) square vaginal mesh releasing 10 mg of dinoprostone at a rate of 0.3 mg/hr over 12 hours. In a study by Zeng and colleagues (2015), women who received the Cervidil vaginal insert had more vaginal births within 24 hours of administration, shorter hospitalizations, and a lower incidence of postpartum hemorrhage compared to women who received the prostaglandin gel.

Women who receive prostaglandin agents have lower requirements for oxytocin (Pitocin) during labor induction (Zeng et al., 2015). Prostaglandin agents are used when labor induction is indicated, but not emergent, such as for maternal gestational diabetes, preeclampsia, or large-for-gestational-age (LGA) fetuses, or for births that are late-term (41 0/7 weeks to 41 6/7 weeks) or post-date (> 42 0/7 weeks) that warrant birth occurring in the near future. Current recommendations by ACOG concludes that "Induction of labor between 41 0/7 and 42 0/7 weeks *can be* considered" and "Induction of labor after 42 0/7 weeks and by 42 6/7 weeks of gestation *is recommended*, given evidence of an increase in perinatal morbidity and mortality" (ACOG, 2014, para 4). For example, a woman who is at 42 weeks' gestation but has a very unfavorable cervix may be given prostaglandin gel to ripen her cervix before an oxytocin (Pitocin) induction is scheduled.

Prostaglandin gel is administered in a hospital setting where women can be monitored for approximately 2 hours (depending on agency protocol) after administration of the medication. The woman is then sent home and an induction is scheduled in the near future. Complications such as hypersystole and nonreassuring fetal status typically occur in the first hour after administration and peak at 4 hours. If the fetal heart rate remains unchanged during the initial 2-hour assessment and uterine activity has not become regular, the woman may be discharged once appropriate follow-up instructions and warning signs have been provided (Zeng et al., 2015).

Women receiving the Cervidil vaginal insert are observed in the hospital setting and have continuous fetal monitoring while the insert is in place. The woman should remain recumbent for 2 hours after administration. The insert should be removed immediately if uterine hypersystole or nonreassuring fetal status occurs. A beta-adrenergic agent should also be administered if hyperstimulation occurs (Forest Pharmaceuticals, 2016).

Misoprostol (Cytotec)

Misoprostol (Cytotec) is a synthetic PGE$_1$ analogue that can be used to soften and ripen the cervix and to induce labor. Oral and sublingual administration was commonly used in the past, but due to increased efficacy, vaginal administration is now the preferred method. Cytotec is approved by the U.S. Food and Drug Administration (FDA) for prevention of peptic ulcer disease along with labeling for indication of cervical ripening and induction (ACOG, 2015a).

Misoprostol (Cytotec) has been found to be more effective for cervical ripening and labor induction than either oxytocin or prostaglandin agents. Misoprostol (Cytotec) has several advantages over other pharmacological methods including birth within 24 hours of administration and lower cesarean birth rates. When it is compared with women who have been induced using prostaglandin agents or oxytocin, the adverse outcomes do not differ among the three methods (ACOG, 2015a). Most adverse perinatal outcomes have been associated with doses beyond the recommended 25 mcg. Guidelines for misoprostol (Cytotec) induction include the following (ACOG, 2015a):

- The initial dosage should be 25 mcg.
- Recurrent administration should not exceed dosing intervals of more than 3 to 6 hours.
- Oxytocin (Pitocin) should not be administered less than 4 hours after the last misoprostol (Cytotec) dose.
- Misoprostol should only be administered where the uterine activity and fetal heart rate (FHR) can be monitored continuously for an initial observation period.
- Misoprostol (Cytotec) is contraindicated in women with a previous cesarean birth or in women with previous uterine surgery due to risk of uterine rupture.

Other Methods of Cervical Ripening

Transcervical Balloon Catheter. Transcervical balloon catheter insertion is a mechanical method that uses a Foley catheter balloon placed in the uterus to induce cervical ripening and dilatation. The Foley catheter is inserted through the cervix into the lower uterine segment and is then filled with 30 mL to 50 mL of sterile water resulting in direct pressure, which causes stress in the lower uterine segment and probably the local production of prostaglandins. Advantages of the balloon catheter include higher vaginal birth rates and lower rates of hypersystolic labor when combined with PGE$_2$ gel (Goldberg, 2015). Balloon catheter placement is often combined with other methods, including saline infusion, which has not been associated with any increased risk of chorioamnioitis (Goldberg, 2015).

Low-Dose Oxytocin. Low-dose administration of intravenous oxytocin has been used as a means of cervical ripening. The dosage is typically increased by 1 to 4 mu/min and may be more appropriate for fetuses with risk factors for labor intolerance, although this approach is less common than the prostaglandin agents (Goldberg, 2015).

Laminaria. The use of laminaria in contemporary practice is mainly reserved for women with fetal demise. Laminaria sticks or tents are made from dried seaweed under the brand names of Dilapan and Lamicel. The agent works by water absorption and is a form of mechanical dilatation. Laminaria work in the same manner as the transcervical balloon catheter in that it results in mechanical dilatation (Goldberg, 2015).

Nursing Management

Physicians/CNMs and birthing room nurses who have had special education and training may administer agents for cervical ripening. Provide the woman and her support person(s) information about the procedure and answer any questions. Assess baseline maternal vital signs and apply an electronic fetal monitor. The electronic fetal monitoring (EFM) tracing should indicate minimal or absent uterine activity, a reassuring fetal heart rate (FHR) pattern, and a reactive non-stress test (NST). If uterine contractions are not occurring regularly, the ripening agent is inserted into the vagina. Prepidil can be administered every 6 hours. If prescribed, Misoprostol (Cytotec) is administered every 3 to 6 hours until adequate cervical change occurs (ACOG, 2015a). Instruct the woman to empty her bladder prior to insertion. After insertion she should lie supine with a right hip wedge for a specified time (usually at least 1 hour). The woman can then assume any comfortable position. As discussed previously, monitor the woman for uterine hypersystole and FHR abnormalities (changes in baseline rate, variability, presence of decelerations) for at least 2 hours following insertion. During administration of PGE$_2$, if nausea and vomiting are present or contractions occur more frequently than every 2 minutes (and/or last longer than 75 seconds), the gel is removed.

Care of the Woman During Labor Induction

The American College of Obstetricians and Gynecologists (2015a) defines **labor induction** as the stimulation of uterine contractions before the spontaneous onset of labor, with or without ruptured fetal membranes, for the purpose of accomplishing birth. Induction may be indicated in the presence of the following (ACOG, 2015a):

- Diabetes mellitus
- Renal disease
- Preeclampsia–eclampsia
- Chronic pulmonary disease
- Premature rupture of membranes (PROM)
- Chorioamnionitis
- Postterm gestation greater than 42 weeks
- Mild abruptio placentae without evidence of nonreassuring fetal status
- Intrauterine fetal demise (IUFD)
- Intrauterine fetal growth restriction (IUGR)
- Alloimmunization
- Oligohydramnios
- Nonreassuring fetal status
- Nonreassuring antepartum testing
- Fetal macrosomia

Relative indications include chronic hypertension, systemic lupus erythematosus, gestational diabetes, hypercoagulation disorders, cholestasis of pregnancy, polyhydramnios, fetal anomalies requiring specialized neonatal care, previous stillbirth, and late-term gestation (Dögl , Vanky, & Heimstad, 2016).

All contraindications to spontaneous labor and vaginal birth are contraindications to the induction of labor. Maternal contraindications include but are not limited to the following (Dögl et al., 2016):

- Client refusal
- Placenta previa or vasa previa
- Transverse fetal lie
- Prior classic uterine incision (or any vertical incision in the upper portion of the uterus)
- Active genital herpes infection
- Umbilical cord prolapse
- Absolute cephalopelvic disproportion
- Previous ruptured uterus

Relative contraindications include cervical carcinoma; malpresentation, such as breech; and funic presentation. A **funic presentation** is when the umbilical cord is interposed between the cervix and the presenting part. It can be located by clinical evaluation or by ultrasound (Macones, 2015).

Healthy People 2020

(MICH-6) Reduce maternal illness and complications due to pregnancy (complications during hospitalized labor and delivery)

Labor Readiness

Before induction is attempted, appropriate assessment must indicate that both the woman and the fetus are ready for the onset of labor. This includes evaluation of fetal maturity and cervical readiness.

FETAL MATURITY

The gestational age of the fetus is best evaluated by accurate maternal menstrual dating and early ultrasounds. Amniotic fluid studies also provide valuable information in assessing fetal lung maturity (see Chapter 13).

CERVICAL READINESS

The findings on vaginal examination help determine whether cervical changes favorable for induction have occurred. Bishop (1964) developed a prelabor scoring system that is helpful in predicting the potential success of induction (Table 22–1). Components evaluated are cervical dilatation, effacement, consistency, and position, as well as the station of the fetal presenting part. A score of 0, 1, 2, or 3 is given to each assessed characteristic. The higher the total score for all the criteria, the more likely it is that labor will occur. The lower the total score, the higher the failure rate. A favorable cervix is the most important criterion for a successful induction (Macones, 2015). The presence of a cervix that is anterior, soft, 50% effaced, and dilated at least 2 cm (0.8 in.), with the fetal head at −1 to +1 station or lower (Bishop score of 8 or 9), is favorable for successful induction (Macones, 2015). If the cervix is unfavorable, a method of cervical ripening may be tried.

Methods of Inducing Labor

When the cervix is favorable, the most frequently used methods of induction are amniotomy (discussed previously), stripping the amniotic membranes, intravenous oxytocin (Pitocin) infusion, and complementary methods.

STRIPPING THE MEMBRANES

A nonpharmacologic method of induction is stripping (or sweeping) the amniotic membranes. The practitioner inserts a gloved finger into the internal os and rotates it 360 degrees twice, separating the amniotic membranes that are lying against the lower uterine segment. This is thought to release prostaglandins that stimulate uterine contractions. The procedure is usually uncomfortable and can result in cramping, uterine contractions, and vaginal bleeding. Stripping of membranes has been shown to be safe for GBS positive women; however, there is a lack of research in HIV positive women; therefore, it should be considered a contraindication in women with HIV/AIDS (Heilman & Susherebe, 2015).

TABLE 22–1 Prelabor Status Evaluation Scoring System

FACTOR	ASSIGNED VALUE: BISHOP SCORE			
	0	1	2	3
Cervical dilatation	Closed	1–2 cm	3–4 cm	5 cm or more
Cervical effacement	0%–30%	40%–50%	60%–70%	80% or more
Fetal station	−3	−2	−1, 0	+1, or lower
Cervical consistency	Firm	Moderate	Soft	
Cervical position	Posterior	Midposition	Anterior	

Source: Data from Bishop, E. H. (1964). Pelvic scoring for elective inductions. *Obstetrics & Gynecology, 24,* 266.

OXYTOCIN (PITOCIN) INFUSION

Administration of oxytocin (Pitocin) is an effective method of initiating uterine contractions to induce labor and may also be used to enhance ineffective contractions (*labor augmentation*). A primary line of 1000 mL of electrolyte solution (e.g., lactated Ringer solution) is started intravenously. Ten units of oxytocin (Pitocin) are added to a secondary line of intravenous (IV) fluid so the resulting mixture will contain 10 milliunits/mL of oxytocin (Pitocin) (1 milliunit/min, or 6 mL/hr), and the prescribed dose can be calculated easily. After the primary infusion is started, the oxytocin (Pitocin) solution is piggybacked into the primary tubing port closest to the catheter insertion. The infusion is then administered using an infusion pump to control the flow rate precisely. The rate of infusion is based on physician/CNM orders and hospital protocol. Changes to the infusion rate are determined by assessment of the contraction pattern and fetal response. The goal for induction is to achieve stable contractions every 2 to 3 minutes that last 40 to 60 seconds. The uterus should relax to full baseline resting tone between each contraction. Progress is determined by changes in the effacement and dilatation of the cervix and station of the presenting part.

Oxytocin (Pitocin) induction is not without some associated risks, including hyperstimulation of the uterus, resulting in uterine contractions that are too frequent or too intense, with an increased resting tone. Hypersystole may lead to a reduction in placental perfusion and may increase the risk of nonreassuring fetal status. Other risks include uterine rupture, water intoxication, fetal hypoxia, and in rare circumstances, fetal death (Wilson, Shannon, & Shields, 2015).

> ### Clinical Reasoning Determining Infusion Rate
>
> Wendy Johnson, a G2P1, is undergoing an oxytocin (Pitocin) infusion to induce her labor. Wendy has been receiving the medication via infusion pump for 4 hours and currently is receiving 6 milliunits/min (36 mL/hr). You have just completed your assessments and found the following: BP 120/80, pulse 80, respirations 16; contractions every 3 minutes lasting 60 seconds and of strong intensity; the FHR baseline is 144 to 150 with average variability; and cervical dilatation is 6 cm (2.4 in.).
>
> *Will you continue the same infusion rate, increase the rate, or decrease the rate?*

COMPLEMENTARY AND ALTERNATIVE THERAPIES

The use of complementary and alternative therapies has risen dramatically over the last decade. It is estimated that 37% of pregnant women and 28% of postpartum women use alternative therapies during the perinatal period (Birdee, Kemper, Rothman, et al., 2014). In addition to the medical (allopathic) methods just discussed, a variety of more natural, noninvasive methods to initiate contractions may also be used. These methods include sexual intercourse; nipple or breast stimulation with breast pump or manual stimulation; the use of herbs or homeopathic agents; castor oil or enemas; acupuncture and acupressure; chiropractic manipulation; and mechanical dilatation of the cervix with transcervical balloon catheters (Birdee et al., 2014). The cautions and contraindications are the same as those for medical induction of labor. Although castor oil has been used for many years it has not been frequently studied as a method of labor induction. The mechanism by which castor oil stimulates uterine contractions is not understood. Some practitioners consider it to be an old-fashioned, nonuseful substance, whereas others have noted that it is especially effective for primigravidas.

In addition to allopathic techniques, complementary and alternative therapies can be effective, although some have not undergone rigorous scientific research. Many healthcare practitioners and their clients desire a more natural approach and methods when possible. It is important for the provider to have knowledge and education in these options prior to recommending them to women. It is important for nursing students, nurses, and clients to be aware of all aspects of pregnancy care.

Clinical Tip

Many women research complementary and alternative therapies and utilize them without consulting their healthcare provider. It is important to ask women at each visit about new medications and the use of any complementary and alternative therapies.

Sexual intercourse is a logical method of inducing cervical ripening and uterine contractions; female orgasm stimulates contractions, and male ejaculate is a rich source of prostaglandins. Penetration during intercourse can also stimulate the lower uterine segment and cause uterine contractions. In addition, breast and nipple stimulation produces endogenous oxytocin, which in turn stimulates the uterus to contract.

Box 22–1 **Evening Primrose Oil to Facilitate the Onset of Labor**

Evening primrose oil is a natural substance that is extracted from the plant's seeds. It has been widely used for centuries by midwives as a means of softening the cervix, vagina, and perineum to facilitate the onset of labor. Evening primrose oil contains a fatty acid called gamma linolenic acid, which is converted into a prostaglandin compound that is commonly used but has been shown to be associated with adverse outcomes (Dante, Bellei, Neri, et al., 2014). Prostaglandins play a key role in ripening the cervix so that labor can begin. Women can be advised to begin evening primrose oil supplementation during the 36th week of pregnancy. The recommended dose is 2500 mg per day taken either orally or vaginally until birth. Side effects are rare but can include headaches, nausea, or skin rashes. Women who experience side effects should be counseled to discontinue the supplement unless advised otherwise by their physician (Dante et al., 2014).

Nursing Management

Aspects to address during teaching about induction of labor include the purpose, the procedure itself, nursing care that will be provided, assessments, comfort measures, and a review of breathing techniques that may be used during labor. Regardless of the induction method used, close observation and accurate, ongoing assessments are mandatory to provide safe, optimal care for both woman and fetus. A qualified clinician should be readily accessible to manage any complications that may occur.

As contractions are established, vaginal examinations are done to evaluate cervical dilatation, effacement, and station. The frequency of vaginal examinations primarily depends on the woman's parity, her comfort level, and the strength of her contractions. If evaluating the need for analgesia, a vaginal examination should be performed to avoid giving the medication too early and increasing the risk of prolonging labor. This examination also helps identify advanced dilatation and imminent birth.

Pitocin induction protocols recommend obtaining baseline data (maternal temperature, pulse, respirations, blood pressure, pain level), a 20- to 30-minute electronic fetal monitoring (EFM) recording demonstrating a reassuring fetal heart rate (FHR), a reactive non-stress test (NST), and the contraction status before the induction is started. The fetal monitor is used to provide continuous data.

Before each increase of the Pitocin infusion rate, assess the following:

- Maternal blood pressure, pulse, respirations, temperature, and pain level
- Contraction status including frequency, duration, intensity, and resting tone
- FHR baseline, variability, and reactivity, noting the presence of accelerations, any decelerations, or bradycardia

For additional information about nursing interventions when oxytocin (Pitocin) is being used, see *Nursing Care Plan: For Induction of Labor*.

Care of the Woman During an Episiotomy

An **episiotomy** is a surgical incision of the perineal body to enlarge the outlet. Historically, episiotomy was thought to reduce the risk of lacerations caused by overstretching of perineal tissues. Current research has shown that the routine use of episiotomies can increase blood loss, pain in the postpartum period, fourth-degree perineal lacerations, infection, dyspareunia, perineal trauma, fecal incontinence, and anovaginal and rectovaginal fistulas. Women who receive episiotomies also have a higher incidence of deep lacerations in future births and prolonged healing time (Ettore, Torrisi, & Ferraro, 2016).

Factors That Predispose Women to Episiotomy

Overall factors that place a woman at increased risk for episiotomy are primigravid status, macrosomia, occiput-posterior position, use of forceps or vacuum extractor, nonreassuring fetal status with a lack of fetal heart rate (FHR) returning to baseline after the contraction ceases, presumed or actual shoulder dystocia, maternal exhaustion, and practitioner's routine use of the procedure (Ettore et al., 2016).

Preventive Measures

Following are some general tips to help reduce the incidence of routine episiotomies:

- Perineal massage with lubricant during pregnancy
- Delaying pushing in second stage until strong maternal urge occurs

Nursing Care Plan: For Induction of Labor

1. *Nursing Diagnosis: Injury, Risk for,* related to tachysystole of uterus caused by induction of labor (NANDA-I © 2014)

GOAL: Progression of labor without difficulty or complications

INTERVENTION	RATIONALE
• Obtain a baseline for maternal blood pressure, pulse, respirations, temperature, and pain level.	• Oxytocin (Pitocin) induction can affect the cardiovascular system. Blood pressure may initially be decreased. If the induction is prolonged the blood pressure (BP) may increase by 30%. Respirations can become elevated because of pain sensation, anxiety, or physiologic causes. Temperature is obtained to monitor for infection. The pain level is assessed continuously to determine if pain medication is warranted or changes in vital signs are caused by maternal discomfort.
• Place client on external fetal monitor for 20 min to obtain a baseline for fetal heart rate (FHR) and variability.	• Assesses for fetal well-being. Normal FHR ranges from 110–160 beats/min. Variability measuring three to five fluctuations in 1 minute is documented as average. Continuous electronic fetal monitoring (EFM) is performed during an oxytocin induction.
• Perform non-stress test.	• A non-stress test is performed to assess the fetal heart rate in response to fetal movement. Accelerations of FHR with fetal movement may indicate the fetus has adequate oxygenation and an intact central nervous system. A reactive non-stress test indicates there were at least two accelerations of 15 beats/min above baseline, lasting 15 sec in a 20-min period.
• Insert IV line and begin primary infusion with 1000 mL of electrolyte solution.	• An electrolyte solution such as lactated Ringer is used for the primary solution. A primary IV allows continuous intravenous access and fluid infusion in the event the oxytocin drip needs to be discontinued.
• Piggyback oxytocin solution into primary IV tubing, via pump, in the port closest to the IV insertion site.	• Oxytocin is mixed in 1000 mL of an electrolyte solution (usually 5% dextrose in lactated Ringer solution) and piggybacked to main IV line. A pump is used to ensure dosage accuracy.
• Begin oxytocin infusion per agency protocol.	• The rate to be used is determined by physician/CNM orders or agency protocol.
• Monitor infusion pump and connections.	• This ensures adequate dosing. Early identification of problems with the infusion site, the piggyback connection, or flow rate will minimize effects on uterine contractions and FHR. If a problem is found, correct and restart infusion at the beginning dose.
• Monitor and evaluate maternal BP and pulse before each increase in the oxytocin infusion rate.	• Prolonged inductions may increase the blood pressure by 30%. The oxytocin infusion rate should not be advanced if maternal hypertension or hypotension is present or if there are any radical changes in pulse rate.
• Evaluate urine output.	• There is an antidiuretic effect with dosages of oxytocin above 20 milliunits/min. This level decreases free water exchange in the kidneys, thereby markedly decreasing urine output.
• Evaluate and document FHR before each increase in oxytocin infusion rate.	• During oxytocin infusion, FHR should range between 110 and 160 beats/min. Tachysystole of the maternal uterus may cause nonreassuring fetal status. Fetal bradycardia may occur along with a decrease in variability, leading to fetal hypoxia. Fetal tachycardia may also occur. If persistent fetal bradycardia or fetal tachycardia occurs, the oxytocin is discontinued.
• Evaluate and document contraction pattern before each increase of the oxytocin infusion rate.	• Contractions every 2–3 min, lasting 40–60 sec with moderate intensity, are considered adequate. Cervical dilatation progresses an average of 1.2 cm/hr to 1.5 cm/hr (0.5 in./hr to 0.6 in./hr) during the active phase of labor.
• Increase oxytocin infusion dosage until adequate contractions are achieved or the maximum dose per agency protocol is reached.	• Oxytocin may be increased every 20–40 min until an adequate contraction pattern is achieved.

(continued)

Nursing Care Plan: For Induction of Labor (*continued*)

INTERVENTION	RATIONALE
• Evaluate contraction frequency, duration, and intensity before increasing the infusion rate. Discontinue oxytocin infusion and infuse primary solution if signs of tachysystole of the uterus are detected.	• Signs of tachysystole include contraction frequency more than 2 min, duration exceeding 60 sec, and increased resting tone. Tachysystole of the uterus puts the client at risk for abruptio placentae and uterine rupture.
• Initiate treatment measures to reverse the effects of oxytocin infusion if fetal tachycardia or bradycardia occurs.	• When the FHR falls outside the normal range (110–160 beats/min), treatment measures should be initiated. To reverse the effects of oxytocin, immediately discontinue oxytocin, infuse primary solution, administer oxygen by tight face mask at 8–10 L/min, place client in side-lying position, and notify physician/CNM.

Expected Outcome: Contractions will increase in frequency, duration, and intensity. An increase in cervical dilatation, effacement, and intensity will be achieved. The uterus will remain soft between contractions.

- Spontaneous pushing during labor (without instruction for prolonged breath holding)
- Maternal choice to change position during second stage while discouraging lithotomy or recumbent positions
- Warm or hot compresses on the perineum
- Encouraging a gradual expulsion of the baby at the time of birth by encouraging the mother to "push, take a breath, push, take a breath" thereby easing the baby out slowly (controlled crowning).

Clinical Tip

Pregnant women should be encouraged to perform perineal massage to increase pliability and flexibility of the perineal muscles. Kegel exercises and dorsiflexion of the legs are pelvic floor muscle training measures to prevent urinary/anal incontinence.

Episiotomy Procedure

The two types of episiotomy are midline and mediolateral (Figure 22–2). Just before birth, when approximately 3 to 4 cm (1.2 to 1.6 in.) of the fetal head is visible during a contraction, the episiotomy is performed using sharp scissors with rounded points (Macones, 2015). The midline incision begins at the bottom center of the perineal body and extends straight down the midline to the fibers of the rectal sphincter. The mediolateral incision, which is rarely used, begins in the midline of the posterior fourchette and extends at a 45-degree angle downward to the right or left.

The episiotomy is usually performed with regional or local anesthesia but may be done without anesthesia in emergency situations. It is generally proposed that as crowning occurs, the distention of the tissues causes numbing. Repair of the episiotomy (episiorrhaphy) and repair of any lacerations are completed during the period after the birth of the newborn and either before or after expulsion of the placenta. Some practitioners routinely wait to do repairs until the placenta has been delivered in case complications occur and manual exploration of the uterus is indicated. Adequate anesthesia must be given for the repair.

Clinical Tip

Although it is no longer recommended, some practitioners continue routinely to perform episiotomy. Therefore, nurses should provide information about episiotomy and encourage women to talk to their practitioner about the incidence of its use within the practice. Encourage women who are opposed to an episiotomy to discuss their objection to the procedure with their healthcare provider at a prenatal visit before the onset of labor. Advise women that episiotomies are sometimes indicated, such as in cases of severe fetal nonreassuring status, macrosomia, instrument-assisted births, or an unresolving shoulder dystocia.

Nursing Management

Support the woman during the episiotomy and the repair; sensations of pressure, pulling, or tugging are common. In the absence of adequate anesthesia, pain may occur. Placing a hand on the woman's shoulder and talking with her can provide comfort and distraction from the repair process. The woman can also be distracted by allowing her to hold her newborn during this time; however, supervision is needed to ensure newborn safety. Advocate for the mother to receive pain medication if the pain is more than she can handle. At all times the woman needs to be the one who decides whether the amount of discomfort she is experiencing is tolerable. She should never be told, "This doesn't hurt." She is the person experiencing the discomfort and her evaluation needs to be respected.

The type of episiotomy is recorded on the birth record. This information should also be included in the medical record so that adequate assessments can be made and relief measures instituted by subsequent caregivers.

Comfort measures may begin immediately after birth with the application of an ice pack to the perineum. For optimal effect the ice pack should be applied for 20 to 30 minutes and removed for at least 20 minutes before being reapplied. Assess the perineal tissues frequently to prevent injury from the ice pack. Inspect the episiotomy site every 15 minutes during the first hour after the birth for redness, swelling, tenderness, bruising, and hematomas. As part of postpartum care, provide the mother with instructions in perineal hygiene, self-care, and comfort measures.

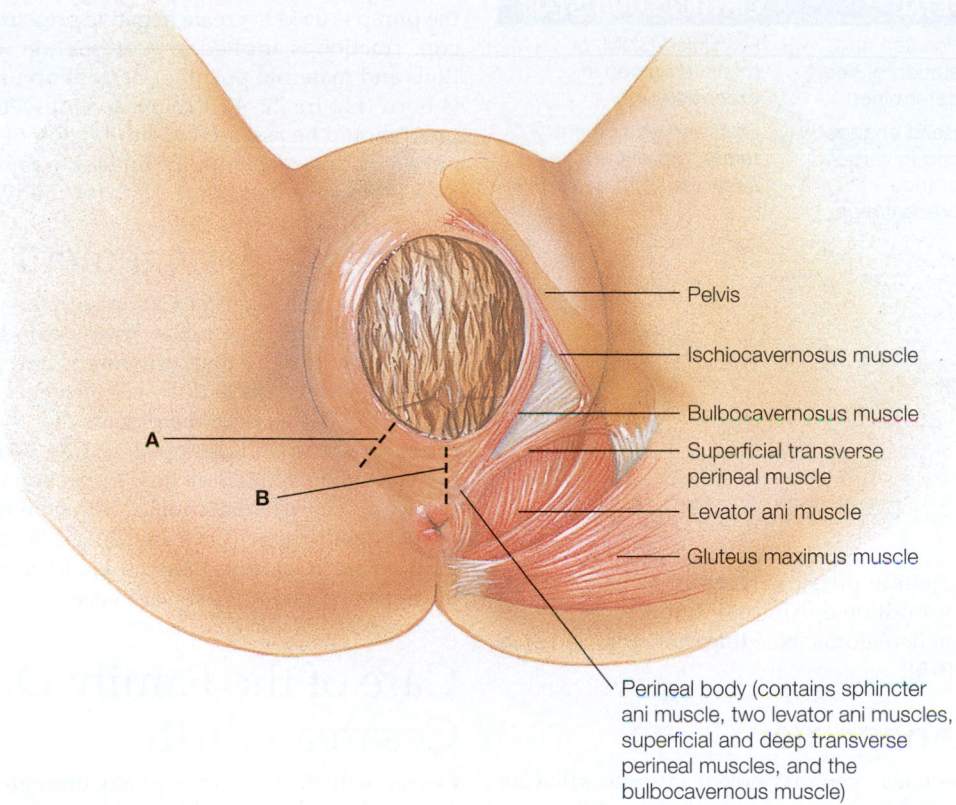

- Pelvis
- Ischiocavernosus muscle
- Bulbocavernosus muscle
- Superficial transverse perineal muscle
- Levator ani muscle
- Gluteus maximus muscle
- Perineal body (contains sphincter ani muscle, two levator ani muscles, superficial and deep transverse perineal muscles, and the bulbocavernous muscle)

Figure 22–2 The two most common types of episiotomies are midline and mediolateral. A. Right mediolateral. B. Midline.

It is important to recognize that perineal pain continues for a period of time and may be significant. This pain should not be discounted; women with prolonged perineal pain are at greater risk for inflammation, sexual dysfunction, breastfeeding difficulties, stress, and postpartum depression (Dunn, Paul, Ware, et al., 2015). Provide ongoing assessment for these complications.

Care of the Woman During Forceps-Assisted Birth

Forceps are surgical instruments designed to assist in the birth of a fetus by providing either traction or the means to rotate the fetal head to an occiput-anterior position. In medical literature and practice, **forceps-assisted birth** is also known as *instrumental delivery* or *operative vaginal delivery*. The use of forceps is rare in modern obstetrics, with only 1% of deliveries being accomplished with forceps. This significant reduction has led to a reduction in trained obstetricians that are able to teach or perform the procedures; therefore, its use is likely to continue to decline. Three categories of forceps application exist:

1. Outlet forceps are applied when the fetal skull has reached the perineum, the fetal scalp is visible, and the sagittal suture is not more than 45 degrees from the midline.

2. Low forceps are applied when the leading edge (presenting part) of the fetal skull is at a station of +2 or more.

3. Midforceps are applied when the fetal head is engaged.

Indications for Forceps-Assisted Birth

Forceps may be indicated in the presence of any condition that threatens the mother or the fetus and when immediate birth is indicated. Maternal conditions include cardiac or pulmonary disease, infection, inability of the mother to maintain effective pushing efforts, and history of spontaneous pneumothorax. Fetal conditions include premature placental separation, prolapsed umbilical cord when complete dilatation has been reached and fetal head is engaged, and nonreassuring fetal status (Ross, 2015). Forceps may be used to shorten the second stage of labor and assist the woman's pushing effort. Table 22–2 lists the conditions that must be met before forceps are used.

Neonatal and Maternal Risks

Newborn complications may include ecchymosis or facial edema, facial lacerations, and brachial plexus (Ross, 2015). Caput succedaneum or cephalohematoma (entrapped hemorrhage) with subsequent hyperbilirubinemia may occur, as may transient facial paralysis. Although rare, cerebral hemorrhages, fractures, brain damage, and fetal death have also been reported (Ross, 2015).

TABLE 22–2 Conditions for Use of Forceps

MATERNAL	FETAL	BIRTHING UNIT/STAFF
Consent for procedure obtained	Position and station of head determined	Physician/CNM, or midwife trained in procedure
Type of pelvis determined	Head engaged and in vertex or face presentation	Staff and equipment ready to provide a cesarean birth if needed
No degree of cephalopelvic disproportion present		
Cervix completely dilated		
Membranes ruptured		
Bladder empty		
Anesthesia given		

Source: Data from Cunningham, F. G., Leveno, K. J., Bloom, S. L., Spong, C.Y., Dashe, J. S., Hoffman, B. L., . . . Sheffield, J. S. (2014). *Williams obstetrics* (24th ed.). New York, NY: McGraw-Hill.

Maternal risks include possible lacerations of the birth canal; extensions of a midline episiotomy into the anus; vulvar or perineal edema, hematoma, bleeding, bruising, and anal incontinence (Ross, 2015).

Nursing Management

By using ongoing assessment, you may note the variables that are associated with an increased rate of instrument-assisted or operative birth. Nursing care measures should be focused on decreasing risk factors, such as changing position of the woman, ambulation, use of breast/nipple stimulation or an electric breast pump, and frequent bladder emptying in the presence of labor dystocia. Fetal heart rate (FHR) abnormalities may be improved by position changes, increased fluid intake, and/or adequate oxygen exchange.

If a forceps-assisted birth is required, explain the procedure to the woman. Inform her that she should feel only pressure during the procedure, and if pain occurs, she should notify you immediately so additional regional anesthesia can be provided. Encourage breathing techniques that help prevent pushing during application of the forceps. Monitor contractions and alert the physician when one is present so that traction can be applied. The woman needs to push with each contraction as traction is applied. The combined efforts of maternal pushing and traction from the forceps help with expulsion of the fetus (Figure 22–3). Traction is applied only during an actual contraction. Mild transient bradycardia may occur secondary to head compression.

Immediately following birth, assess the newborn for facial edema, bruising, caput succedaneum, cephalohematoma, lacerations, eye injuries, excessive molding, and any signs of cerebral edema. In the fourth stage, assess the woman for perineal swelling, bruising, hematoma, excessive bleeding, and hemorrhage. In the postpartum period it is important to assess for signs of infection. Provide an opportunity for questions and reiterate explanations provided as necessary.

Care of the Woman During Vacuum-Assisted Birth

Vacuum-assisted birth is an obstetric procedure used to facilitate the birth of a fetus by applying suction to the fetal head. The vacuum extractor is composed of a soft suction cup attached to a suction bottle (pump) by tubing. The suction cup, which comes in various sizes, is placed against the fetal occiput, and the pump is used to create negative pressure (suction) inside the cup. Traction is applied in coordination with uterine contractions and maternal pushing, descent occurs, and the fetal head is born (Figure 22–4). Progressive descent with the first two pulls should be assessed. Continuation of the procedure without noted descent should be limited to prevent cephalohematomas, brain injury, and fetal death (O'Grady, 2015).

Nursing Management

Provide ongoing communication with the woman and her partner regarding the procedure, assess pain level, and advise the woman that if more than pressure is felt, pain medication can be provided. Assess FHR by continuous electronic fetal monitoring (EFM). Reassure the parents that the caput (chignon) on the baby's head will disappear within 2 to 3 days. Assessment of the newborn should include inspection and continued observation for cephalohematomas, intracerebral hemorrhage, and retinal hemorrhage (O'Grady, 2015). Because babies born via vacuum are at increased risk for jaundice, careful assessment of the newborn's skin color is also needed.

Care of the Family During Cesarean Birth

Cesarean birth, the birth of a baby through abdominal and uterine incisions, was historically used as a last resort in attempting to save the fetus of a dying woman. Over time, reductions in perinatal morbidity and mortality rates associated with cesarean births led to a rise in the proportion of cesarean births. In 2014, the United States cesarean birth rate was 32.2%, down from the highest peak of 32.9% in 2009 (Centers for Disease Control & Prevention [CDC], 2016).

In the United States, the number of cesarean births is linked to a rise in repeat cesarean births due to concerns regarding the risk of uterine rupture with a trial of labor after cesarean (TOLAC), even though the risk is relatively rare. Cesarean birth on request (or demand) is now considered an acceptable option for primigravida women, although it is estimated that they only account for 1% to 3% of cesarean births annually (Norwitz, 2016). This trend was spurred by multiple variables including fear of pain, wish to avoid fetal adverse outcomes, prevention of pelvic floor damage, and convenience of either the parents or the physician (Norwitz, 2016).

Cesarean birth on request is associated with a reduction in maternal hemorrhage risk, but has been associated with increased neonatal respiratory problems, longer hospitalizations, risk of preterm birth due to errors in due date calculations, and an increase in complications in subsequent pregnancies, including placenta implantation problems and uterine rupture (Norwitz, 2016). Many other factors have contributed to the rise in the cesarean birth rate, including an increased use of epidural anesthesia, maternal age more than 35 years, failed inductions, decline in vaginal breech deliveries, decreases in operative vaginal deliveries, increased repeat cesarean rates, reduced vaginal birth after cesarean birth rates, increased scheduling of cesarean births for personal convenience, policy statements from professional organizations encouraging cesarean birth, political pressure from malpractice insurance carriers who attempt to dictate practice standards, and fear of litigation (Norwitz, 2016).

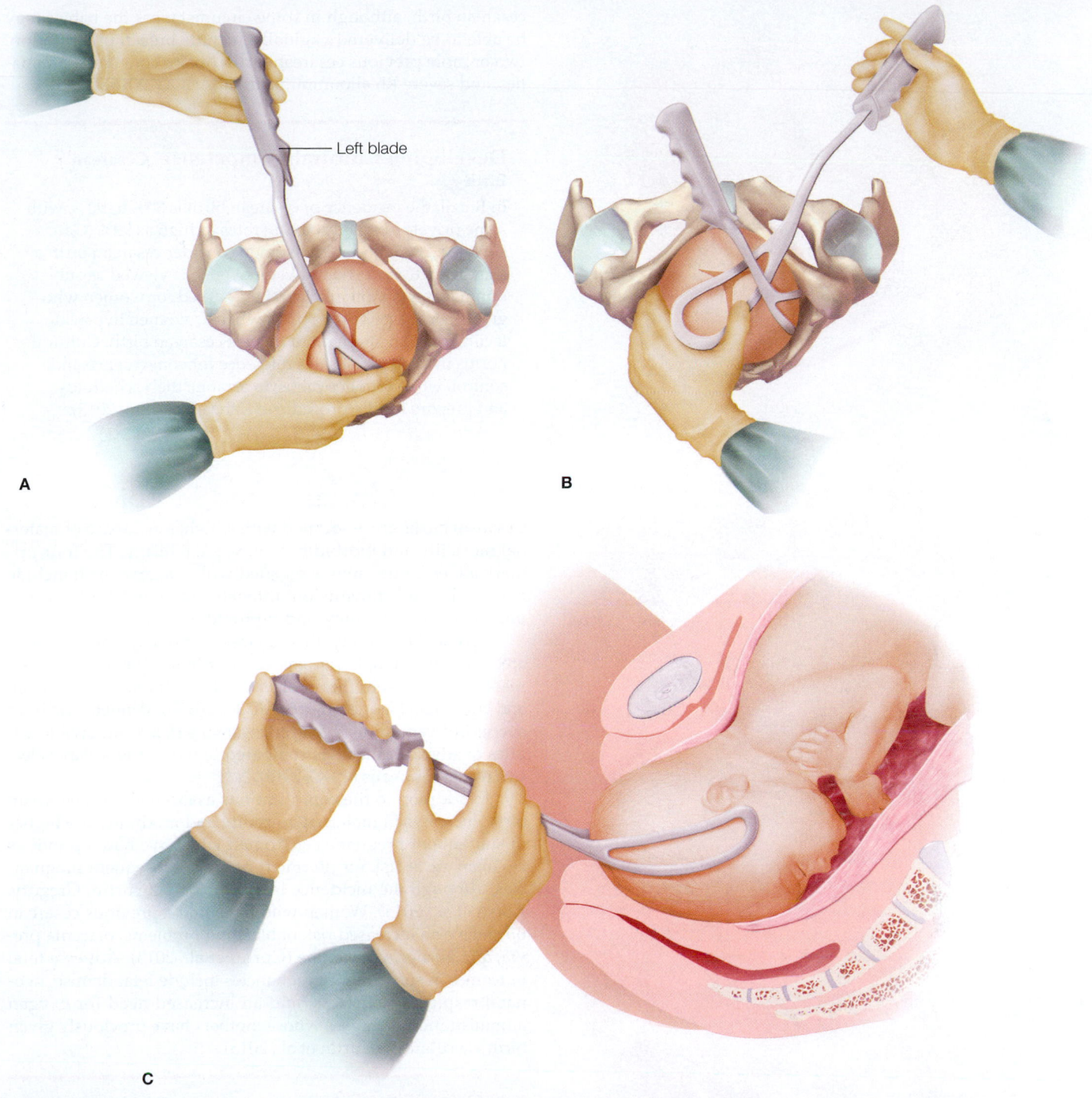

Left blade

A

B

C

Figure 22–3 Application of forceps in occiput-anterior (OA) position. A. The left blade is inserted along the left side wall of the pelvis over the parietal bone. B. The right blade is inserted along the right side wall of the pelvis over the parietal bone. C. With correct placement of the blades, the handles lock easily. During uterine contractions, traction is applied to the forceps in a downward and outward direction to follow the birth canal.

Indications

Commonly accepted indications for cesarean birth include complete placenta previa, cephalopelvic disproportion, placental abruption, active genital herpes, umbilical cord prolapse, failure to progress in labor, nonreassuring fetal status, previous classical incision on the uterus (either previous cesarean birth or myomectomy), more than one previous cesarean birth, benign and malignant tumors that obstruct the birth canal, and cervical cerclage. Certain maternal medical conditions including cardiac disorders; severe maternal respiratory disease; central nervous system disorders that increase intracranial pressure; mechanical vaginal obstruction, such as an ovarian mass or lower uterine segment fibroids; and severe mental illness that results in an altered state of consciousness are all contraindications to a vaginal birth and warrant a cesarean birth (Cunningham et al., 2014). Other indications that are now commonly associated with

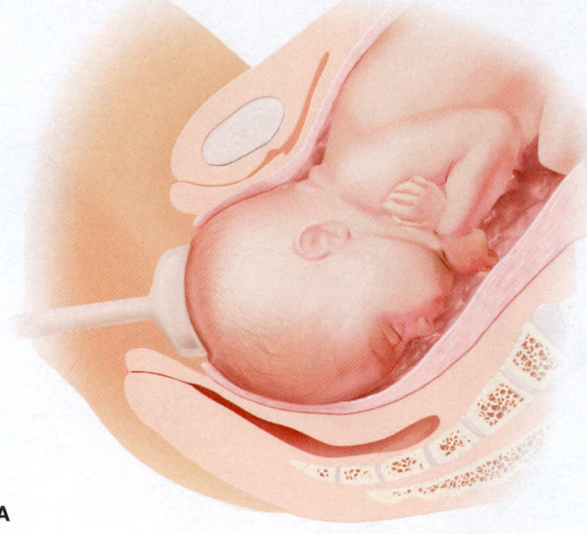

A

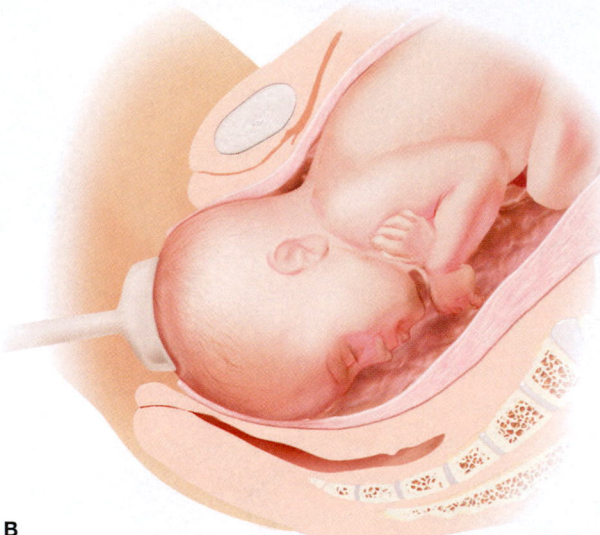

B

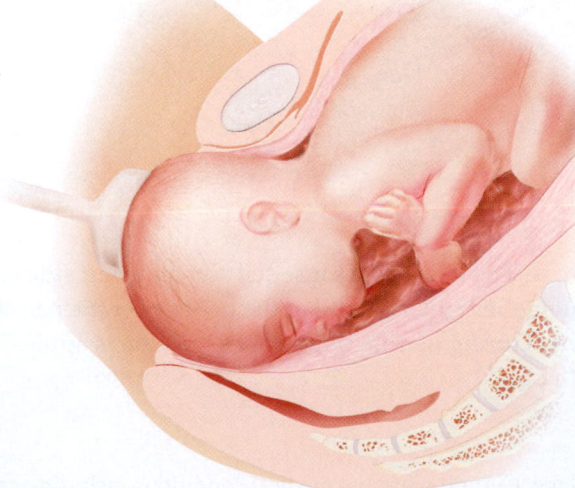

C

Figure 22–4 Vacuum extractor traction. **A.** The cup is placed on the fetal occiput, creating suction. Traction is applied in a downward and outward direction. **B.** Traction continues in a downward direction as the fetal head begins to emerge from the vagina. **C.** Traction is maintained to lift the fetal head out of the vagina.

cesarean birth, although in some circumstances the babies may be able to be delivered vaginally, include breech presentation, two or more previous cesarean births, major congenital anomalies, and severe Rh alloimmunization (ACOG, 2015b).

Maternal Mortality and Morbidity

Cesarean births are associated with a higher incidence of maternal mortality and morbidity than vaginal births. The four primary adverse outcomes associated with cesarean birth include maternal blood transfusion, intensive care (ICU) admission, unplanned hysterectomy, and ruptured uterus.

Perinatal morbidity after cesarean birth may also be associated with infection, hypertensive disorders, adverse anesthesia reactions, deep vein thrombosis (DVT), pulmonary embolism, and bowel and bladder injury (ACOG, 2015b). Women who have successful vaginal births after cesareans (VBACs) have lower rates of adverse outcomes compared to women who have elective repeat cesareans (CDC, 2016).

In addition to the complications associated with cesarean birth, increases in maternal mortality and morbidity are higher in subsequent pregnancies. Women who have had a previous cesarean are at risk for uterine rupture in subsequent pregnancies, although the incidence is 0.3% to 0.7% (Curtin, Gregory, Korst, et al., 2015). Women who have had a previous cesarean birth have an increased risk of bleeding problems, placenta previa, and abruptio placentae (Curtin et al., 2015). Adverse fetal outcomes in subsequent pregnancies include fetal demise, neonatal respiratory distress, and an increased need for oxygen administration in fetuses whose mothers have previously given birth via cesarean (Curtin et al., 2015).

Healthy People 2020

(MICH-7.1) Reduce cesarean births among low-risk (full-term, singleton, and vertex presentation) women

(MICH 7.2) Reduce cesarean birth among low-risk women giving birth with a prior cesarean birth

Skin Incisions

The skin incision for a cesarean birth is either transverse (Pfannenstiel) or vertical and is not indicative of the type of incision made into the uterus. The transverse incision (Figure 22–5) is made across the lowest and narrowest part of the abdomen. Because the incision is made just below the pubic hairline, it is almost invisible after healing. The limitation of this type of skin incision is that it does not allow for extension of the incision if needed. This incision is used when there is not an emergent need for birth, such

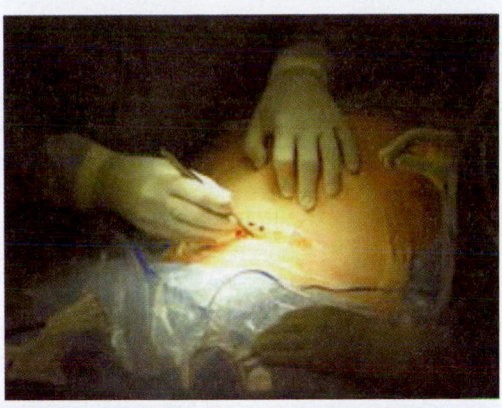

Figure 22–5 Transverse skin incision for a cesarean birth.

SOURCE: Wilson Garcia and The Valley Hospital, Ridgewood, NJ.

as failure to progress, unknown breech presentation, or cephalopelvic disproportion (CPD) with no maternal or fetal stress. This type of incision is typically preferred by women for cosmetic reasons but does require more time to make and repair.

The vertical incision is made between the navel and the symphysis pubis and is typically reserved for emergent situations, such as nonreassuring fetal status when rapid birth is indicated. It is also used in preterm or macrosomic neonates, or when the woman is significantly obese (Cunningham et al., 2014). Time factors, client preference, previous vertical skin incision, or physician preference determines the type of skin incision.

Uterine Incisions

The type of uterine incision depends on the need for the cesarean. The choice of incision affects the woman's opportunity for a subsequent vaginal birth and her risks of a ruptured uterine scar with a subsequent pregnancy.

The two major locations of uterine incisions are in the lower uterine segment and in the upper segment of the uterine corpus. The lower uterine segment incision most commonly used is a transverse incision (Figure 22–6). The classic incision is

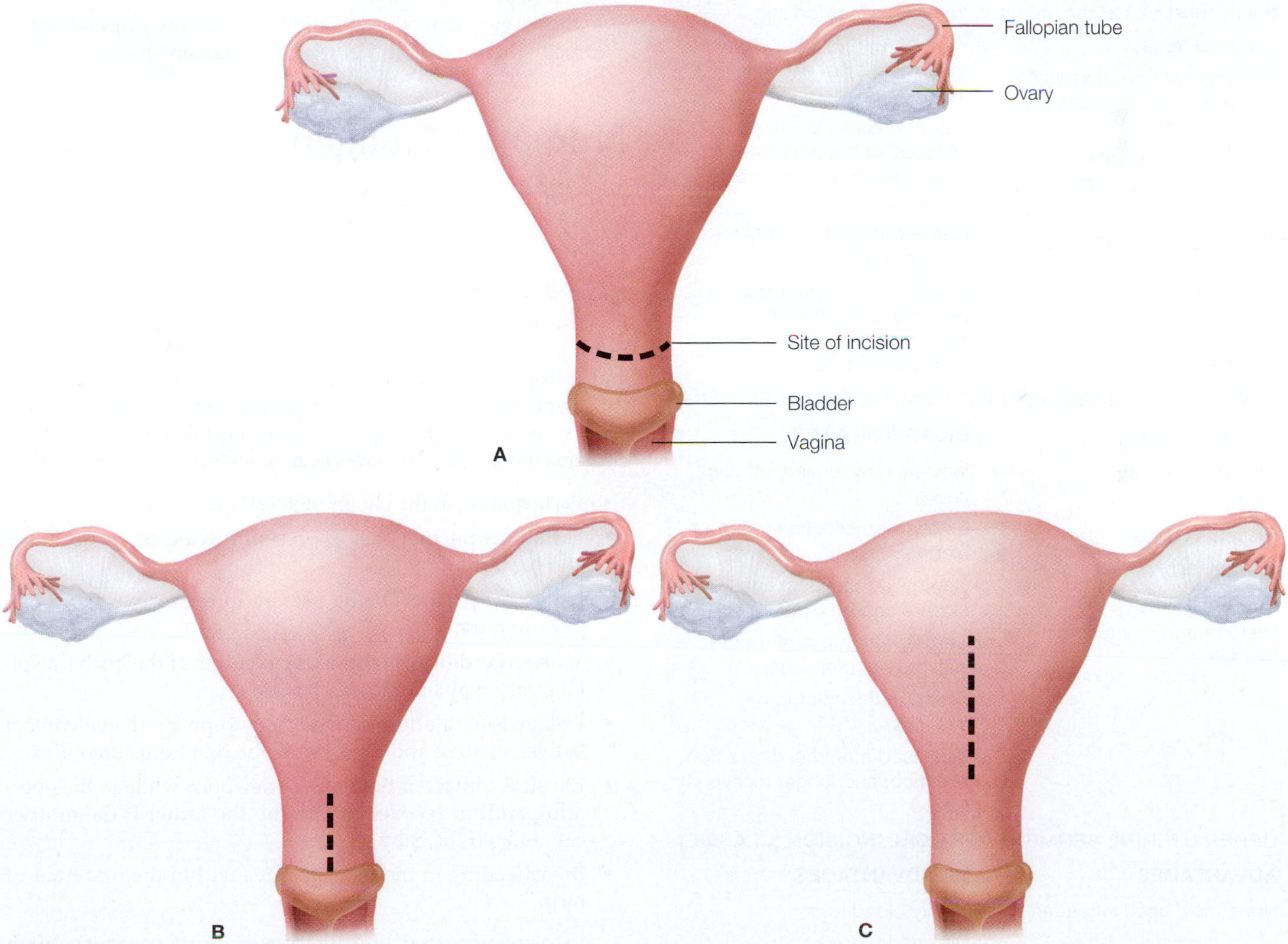

Fallopian tube

Ovary

Site of incision

Bladder

Vagina

A

B

C

Figure 22–6 Uterine incisions for a cesarean birth. **A.** This transverse incision in the lower uterine segment is called a Kerr incision. **B.** The Sellheim incision is a vertical incision in the lower uterine segment. **C.** This view illustrates the classic uterine incision that is done in the body (corpus) of the uterus. The classic incision was commonly done in the past and is associated with increased risk of uterine rupture in subsequent pregnancies and labor.

a vertical incision made into the upper uterine segment and is no longer used.

See Table 22–3 for a comparison of the advantages and disadvantages of three types of uterine incisions.

Analgesia and Anesthesia

There is no perfect anesthesia for cesarean birth. Each has its advantages, disadvantages, possible risks, and side effects. Goals for analgesia and anesthesia administration include safety, comfort, and emotional satisfaction for the woman (see Chapter 19 for an in-depth discussion of pharmacological pain management during labor and childbirth).

TABLE 22–3 Types of Uterine Incisions for Cesarean Birth

LOWER UTERINE SEGMENT TRANSVERSE INCISION (KERR) (MOST COMMONLY USED)	
ADVANTAGES	**DISADVANTAGES**
Less blood loss because it is the thinnest part of the uterus	Takes longer to make a transverse incision and complete the repair
Easier to repair	Extension is not possible if needed
Requires minimal dissection of the bladder from underlying myometrium	Size of incision is limited because of the presence of major vessels on either side of the uterus
Less chance of adherence of bowel or omentum to the incision line	Can extend laterally into the uterine vessels
Area is less likely to rupture during subsequent pregnancies	Incision may stretch and become a thin sheath, causing problems in subsequent labors

LOWER UTERINE SEGMENT VERTICAL INCISION (SELLHEIM)	
ADVANTAGES	**DISADVANTAGES**
Preferred for:	Incision may extend into the cervix
Multiple gestation	Extensive dissection of the bladder
Placenta previa	
Nonreassuring fetal status	Controlling bleeding and closure can be difficult
Abnormal presentation	Carries a high risk of rupture with subsequent labor
Preterm and macrosomic fetuses	Future births need to be cesarean
	Increased maternal discomfort, infection, and longer recovery period

UPPER UTERINE SEGMENT VERTICAL INCISION (CLASSIC)	
ADVANTAGES	**DISADVANTAGES**
None; now used infrequently	Heavy blood loss
	Difficult to repair
	Increased risk of uterine rupture with subsequent pregnancy

Source: Data from Cunningham, F. G., Leveno, K. J., Bloom, S. L., Spong, C.Y., Dashe, J. S., Hoffman, B. L., . . . Sheffield, J. S. (2014). *Williams obstetrics* (24th ed.). NewYork, NY: McGraw-Hill.

KEY FACTS TO REMEMBER
Cesarean Birth

- Cesarean births account for more than one third of all births in the United States.
- A cesarean birth is performed via a surgical incision into the uterine cavity to give birth to the baby.
- Cesarean births have higher morbidity and mortality rates for the mother than vaginal births.
- Cesarean births result in a higher blood loss than vaginal births.

Women With Special Needs Dwarfism
in Childbearing Women

There are over 200 types of dwarfism that may impact childbearing women. Women with dwarfism are at risk for alterations in ambulation as the center of gravity changes. Because of their pelvic bone anatomy, these women are unable to have a vaginal birth. Women with dwarfism should be scheduled for an elective cesarean birth at 39 gestational weeks. Should spontaneous labor occur prior to the surgery date, they should be advised to proceed directly to the birthing facility for a cesarean birth.

Nursing Management

For the Woman Undergoing a Cesarean Birth

Preparation for Cesarean Birth

Because one of every three births is a cesarean, education should be an integral part of all prenatal education. Pregnant women and their partners should be encouraged to discuss the possibility of a cesarean birth with their physicians/CNMs and at the same time discuss their specific needs and desires under those circumstances. Their preferences may include the following:

- Participating in the choice of anesthetic
- Father (or partner) being present during the procedures and/or birth
- Father (or partner) being present in the recovery or post-partum room
- Video recording and/or taking pictures of the birth (hospital policy may limit these options)
- Delayed instillation of eye drops to promote eye contact between parent and newborn in the first hours after birth
- Physical contact or holding the newborn while in the operating and/or recovery room (by the father if the mother cannot hold the baby)
- Breastfeeding in the recovery area within the first hour of birth

Information that couples need about cesarean birth includes the following:

- Preparatory procedures to expect
- Description of the operating suite and the personnel who will be present

- Types of anesthesia for birth and analgesia available postpartum
- Sensations that may be experienced
- Roles of partner/family members
- Interaction with newborn
- Immediate recovery phase
- Postpartum phase

Preparing the woman and her family for birth involves more than the procedures of establishing an intravenous (IV) line, instilling a urinary indwelling catheter, and performing an abdominal prep. As discussed previously, good communication skills are essential in preparing the woman and her support person. The use of therapeutic touch and direct eye contact (if culturally acceptable and possible) assist the woman in maintaining a sense of control and lessen anxiety.

If the cesarean birth is scheduled and not an emergency, you have ample time for preoperative teaching. The context in which this information is relayed should be birth oriented rather than surgery oriented and should be conveyed in a positive manner. This provides an opportunity for the woman to express her concerns, ask questions, and develop a relationship with you.

Much like previous opinions on intake in labor, controversy exists regarding oral intake in women undergoing an elective cesarean birth. Many proponents note that women undergoing an emergency cesarean birth often have been given liquids during labor. Ghorashi and colleagues (2014) randomized 411 women who had been fasting since midnight prior to an elective cesarean birth into two groups. The experimental group was given 150 mL fluid prior to the cesarean while the control group remained NPO. Both groups had one incidence of regurgitation. None of the women experienced aspiration. To reduce potential aspiration of gastric contents, many physicians order antacids to be administered within 30 minutes of surgery.

An IV line is started with a large-bore needle to permit blood administration if it becomes necessary. Epidural or spinal anesthesia is almost always used. You may assist with the procedure, monitor blood pressure and pulse, and continue electronic fetal monitoring (EFM). Perform an abdominal and perineal prep and insert an indwelling catheter to prevent bladder distention. Give any preoperative medication. Notify the neonatal provider regarding attendance at the birth. Prepare for the newborn's needs by turning on the radiant warmer and assembling and testing the resuscitation equipment. Ensure that the proper equipment for the fetus's gestational age and probable birth weight is available. Turn on oxygen and preheat blankets under the warmer. Ready other items such as identification bands, cord clamp, and hat.

Assist in positioning the woman on the operating table. Assess fetal heart rate (FHR) before surgery and during preparation because fetal hypoxia can result from the supine position. Adjust the operating room table so it slants slightly to one side or place a hip wedge (folded blanket or towels) under the right hip to tip the uterus slightly and reduce compression of blood vessels. The uterus should be displaced 15 degrees from the midline; this helps relieve the pressure of the heavy uterus on the vena cava and lessens the incidence of vena cava compression and maternal supine hypotension. Confirm that suction is in working order. Position the urine collection bag under the operating table to obtain proper drainage. Continue auscultation or EFM of the fetal heart rate until immediately before the procedure. Perform a last-minute check to ensure that any internal monitoring equipment has been removed.

Continue to provide reassurance and describe the various procedures being performed along with a rationale to ease anxiety and give the woman a sense of control.

Clinical Tip

Women undergoing elective cesarean birth can be taught many aspects of postoperative teaching before their birth experience. Important components of client education that can be emphasized before birth include dealing with postoperative discomfort, splinting the incision to decrease pain, frequent deep breathing and coughing, and the importance of early ambulation. Women who receive this information before the birth are more apt to remember it when it is reviewed in the early postpartum period.

Preparation for Repeat Cesarean Birth

Women with a previous cesarean birth should undergo a labor and birth history with their healthcare provider to weigh the risks and benefits for birth. When a couple is anticipating a repeat cesarean birth, they have a general understanding of what will occur, which can help them make informed choices about their birth experience. Couples who have had previous negative experiences need an opportunity to describe what they felt. Encourage them to identify what they would like to be different and to list options that would make the experience more positive. Reassure those who have already had positive experiences that their needs and desires will be met in a similar manner. In addition, provide an opportunity to discuss any fears or anxieties. Emphasize the positive aspects of a repeat cesarean birth. For women who previously labored and then had an unexpected cesarean birth, the experience may be perceived as negative. Positive aspects that should be emphasized include participation in selecting the birth date, lack of fatigue related to labor, ability to prepare and make arrangements for other children, and ability for other family members or friends to be present at the hospital during or immediately after birth if desired by the couple.

Preparation for Emergency Cesarean Birth

When the need for an emergency cesarean birth occurs, it is imperative that caregivers use their most effective communication skills in supporting the couple and describing what to expect. Explain to them that certain requests may warrant an immediate response, but you will provide them with information and answer questions as soon as you can. If time permits, providing them with information of what will occur during the next few hours helps to reduce anxiety and increase knowledge. Asking them "What questions or concerns do you have about the decision?" gives them an opportunity for clarification. Prepare the woman in stages, giving her information and the rationale for interventions before beginning any procedure when possible. It is essential to tell the woman (1) what is going to happen, (2) why it is being done, and (3) what sensations she may experience. This allows the woman to be informed and to consent to the procedure, which gives her a sense of control and reduces her feelings of helplessness.

Supporting the Father or Partner

Every effort should be made to include the father or partner in the birth experience. When attending the cesarean birth, the father/partner wears protective coverings similar to those worn by others in the operating suite. A stool can be placed beside the woman's head so that the father/partner can sit nearby to provide physical touch, visual contact, and verbal reassurance.

To promote the participation of the father/partner who chooses not to be in the operating suite, do the following:

- Encourage the father/partner to enter the nursery area with the newborn for the initial assessment.
- Involve the father/partner in postpartum care in the recovery room.

In some emergency circumstances, a support person may not be permitted in the operating room. Some facilities have policies that prohibit a support person from being in the operating room if the woman requires general anesthesia or if an emergency birth is being performed. In these situations, the support person should receive a thorough explanation of what is happening and why, be advised when the staff will return to provide information, know the expected length of time for the procedure, and be reassured that the mother is receiving the care she and the baby need. Because this exclusion is stressful for family members, staff should try to provide information as soon as possible after providing emergency care to the mother.

Immediate Postnatal Recovery Period

After the birth, assess the Apgar score and complete the same initial assessment and identification procedures used for vaginal births. Place identification bands on the newborn and the mother (as well as the father/partner, if present) before removing the baby from the operating room. Make every effort to assist the parents in bonding with their baby. If the mother is awake, free one of her arms so she can touch and stroke the baby. The newborn may be placed on the mother's chest or held in an *en face* position. If physical contact is not possible, provide a running narrative so the mother knows what is happening with her baby. Assist the anesthesia provider with raising the mother's head so she can see her baby immediately after birth. Encourage the parents to talk to the baby, and allow the father/partner to hold the baby until moved to the nursery.

Clinical Tip

Promote maternal–newborn attachment by allowing the mother to hold or nurse the baby during this time period. If the baby has been moved to a separate area, such as the nursery, encourage maternal participation by allowing the father/partner to visit the baby and report back to the mother. The father/partner can take digital pictures or bring back the blanket that was used to wrap up the baby immediately after the birth. Frequent updates from the nurse such as "Your baby is doing just fine" provide reassurance to the mother if separation is needed.

Assess the mother's vital signs every 5 minutes until they are stable, then every 15 minutes for an hour, then every 30 minutes until she is discharged to the postpartum unit. Remain with the woman until she is stable.

Evaluate the dressing and perineal pad every 15 minutes for at least an hour. The fundus should be gently palpated to determine whether it is remaining firm; it may be palpated by placing a hand to support the incision. Intravenous oxytocin (Pitocin) is usually administered to promote the contractility of the uterine musculature. If the woman has been under general anesthesia, position her on her side to facilitate drainage of secretions, turn her, and assist her with coughing and deep breathing every 2 hours for at least 24 hours. If she has received a spinal or epidural anesthetic, check the level of anesthesia every 15 minutes until full sensation has returned. It is important to monitor intake and output, to ensure that the urinary catheter is draining properly, and to observe the urine for a bloody tinge, which could mean surgical trauma to the bladder. Administer as needed any medication the physician has prescribed to relieve the mother's pain and nausea. Some women may have an epidural catheter remain in place. Inspect the site to ensure the dressing is in place and that the catheter appears in the correct position.

Care of the Woman Undergoing Trial of Labor After Cesarean (TOLAC) and Vaginal Birth After Cesarean (VBAC)

After an alarming trend in escalating cesarean birth rates, there was a movement for women to be counseled regarding options for a *trial of labor after cesarean (TOLAC)* and attempt **vaginal birth after cesarean (VBAC)**. TOLAC is a desirable option for women with nonrecurring indications for a cesarean (such as umbilical cord prolapse, breech, placenta previa, or nonreassuring fetal status).

Women who have previously had a vaginal birth, have had one previous cesarean (and in some cases two), and have no medical, obstetric, or fetal contraindications for vaginal birth are excellent candidates for a TOLAC. While women with a previous vaginal birth and women who present in spontaneous labor have the highest success rates, women should be counseled on all birthing options. The average VBAC success rate is 60% to 80% (ACOG, 2015b). The ACOG (2015b) guidelines state that the following aspects are encouraging when considering a TOLAC:

- No contraindications for vaginal birth
- A woman with one or two previous cesarean births and a low transverse uterine incision
- A clinically adequate pelvis based on clinical pelvimetry or prior vaginal birth
- A woman with one previous cesarean birth with an undocumented uterine scar unless there is a high suspicion there was a classic incision performed previously
- Absence of other uterine scars or history of previous uterine rupture

Risks associated with failed VBAC births are hemorrhage, need for blood products, ICU admission, uterine scar separation or uterine rupture, hysterectomy, surgical injuries, neonatal death, neurologic complications, and maternal death. Note that these complications occur as a result of a uterine rupture. The incidence of uterine rupture is 0.9% of all TOLACs (ACOG, 2015b). Women who go into spontaneous labor have a much lower incidence of uterine rupture than those who are given oxytocin (Pitocin) for induction or augmentation (ACOG, 2015b). Prostaglandin agents should not be used in women attempting a VBAC because of the increased risk of uterine rupture. The incidence of uterine rupture in women who receive a prostaglandin agent is as high as 2.25%, which is a 15.6-fold increase when prostaglandins are administered (ACOG, 2015b).

Conservative policies, such as awaiting spontaneous labor, prohibiting the use of prostaglandin agents, and avoiding elective inductions, can assist in reducing the incidence of uterine rupture. See the Concept Map: TOLAC.

Women who have a successful VBAC have lower incidences of infection, less blood loss, fewer blood transfusions, and shorter hospital stays. Healthcare costs are considerably lower for women who have a VBAC than for those who have a repeat cesarean birth (ACOG, 2015b). After a woman has had one successful VBAC, the risks of neonatal and maternal complications are low in subsequent attempts. An increasing number of VBACs are associated with greater VBAC success (ACOG, 2015b). Avoidance of repeat cesarean births is advocated for women who wish to have subsequent pregnancies because this reduces maternal and fetal morbidity and mortality in women desiring more children.

Research shows that there are some factors that decrease the odds of a successful VBAC. These include recurrent indication for the initial cesarean, advanced maternal age, non-White ethnicity, gestational age greater than 40 weeks, maternal obesity, preeclampsia, shortened interval between pregnancies, and macrosomia (ACOG, 2015b).

Nursing Management

The nursing care of a woman undergoing VBAC varies according to institutional protocols. Generally, an intravenous infusion of fluids is started, continuous electronic fetal monitoring (EFM) is used, and clear fluids may be taken. A woman at higher risk may require additional precautionary measures, such as internal monitoring after the membranes have ruptured. Care must be taken to ensure that the woman and her partner feel safe but not unduly restricted by the VBAC status.

Supportive and comfort measures are very important. The woman may be excited about this opportunity to experience labor and vaginal birth, or she may be hesitant and frightened about the possibility of complications. Your presence is important in providing information and encouragement for the laboring woman and her partner.

Concept Map

Medical Diagnoses: Failure to Progress in Labor, Trial of Labor After Cesarean (TOLAC)

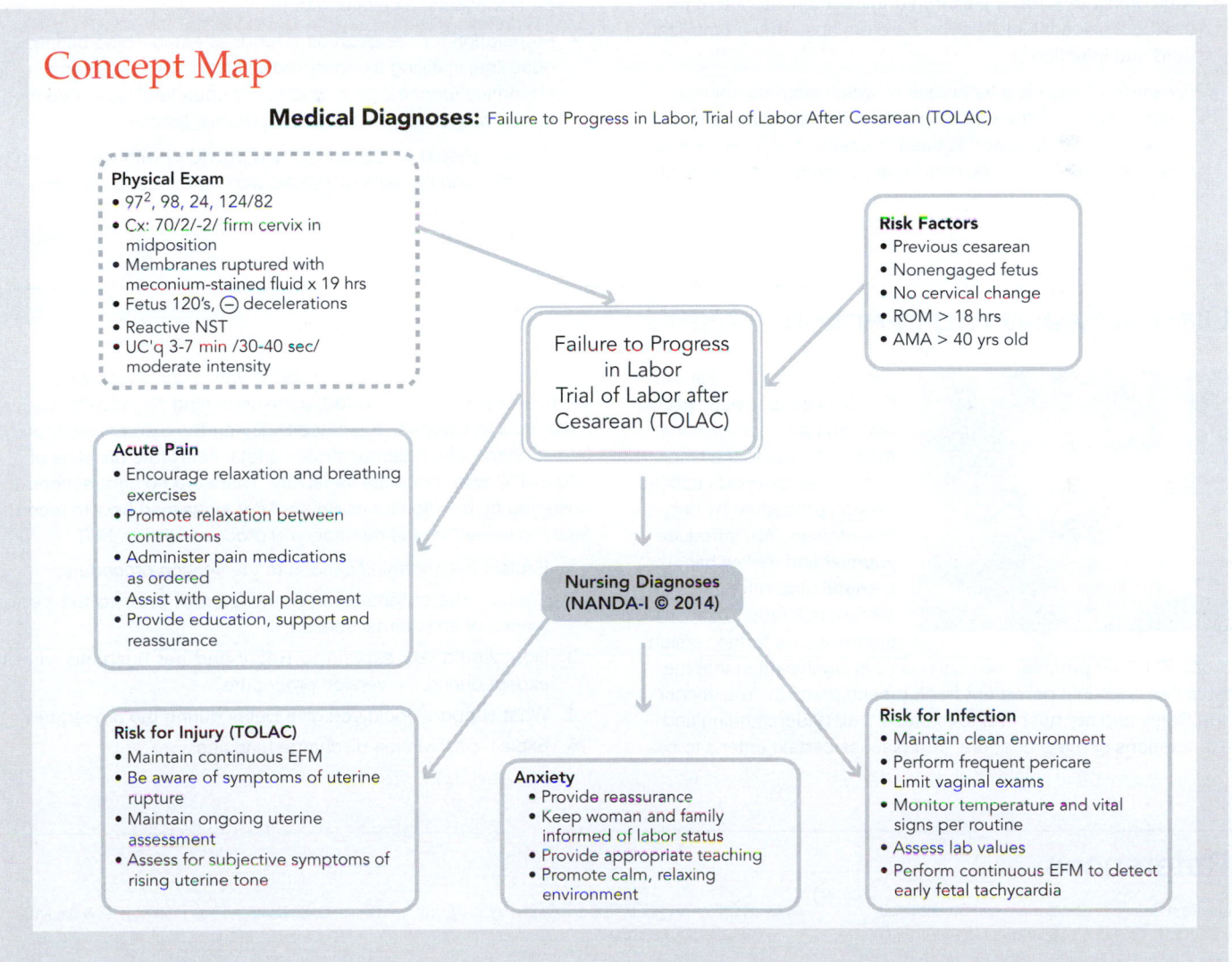

Physical Exam
- 97^2, 98, 24, 124/82
- Cx: 70/2/-2/ firm cervix in midposition
- Membranes ruptured with meconium-stained fluid x 19 hrs
- Fetus 120's, ⊖ decelerations
- Reactive NST
- UC'q 3-7 min /30-40 sec/ moderate intensity

Risk Factors
- Previous cesarean
- Nonengaged fetus
- No cervical change
- ROM > 18 hrs
- AMA > 40 yrs old

Failure to Progress in Labor Trial of Labor after Cesarean (TOLAC)

Acute Pain
- Encourage relaxation and breathing exercises
- Promote relaxation between contractions
- Administer pain medications as ordered
- Assist with epidural placement
- Provide education, support and reassurance

Nursing Diagnoses (NANDA-I © 2014)

Risk for Injury (TOLAC)
- Maintain continuous EFM
- Be aware of symptoms of uterine rupture
- Maintain ongoing uterine assessment
- Assess for subjective symptoms of rising uterine tone

Anxiety
- Provide reassurance
- Keep woman and family informed of labor status
- Provide appropriate teaching
- Promote calm, relaxing environment

Risk for Infection
- Maintain clean environment
- Perform frequent pericare
- Limit vaginal exams
- Monitor temperature and vital signs per routine
- Assess lab values
- Perform continuous EFM to detect early fetal tachycardia

Focus Your Study

- An external (or cephalic) version may be done after 36 weeks' gestation to change a breech presentation to a cephalic presentation. Benefits of the version are that a lower risk vaginal birth may be anticipated. The version is accomplished with the use of tocolytics to relax the uterus.

- Prostaglandin E_1, E_2, low-dose oxytocin (Pitocin), transcervical balloon catheter, or laminaria (in cases of fetal death) may be used to soften and efface the cervix, a process called *cervical ripening*.

- Labor is induced for many reasons. The medical (allopathic) methods include amniotomy, stripping the membranes, and intravenous Pitocin infusion. Nursing responsibilities are heightened during an induced labor.

- Amniotomy (AROM) is performed to augment labor and evaluate the amniotic fluid. The risks are prolapse of the umbilical cord and infection.

- An amnioinfusion is a technique in which warmed solution is introduced into the uterine cavity during the intrapartum period. An amnioinfusion is used in cases of oligohydramnios when nonreassuring fetal heart rate patterns related to cord compression occur.

- An episiotomy is an incision made to enlarge the outlet just before birth of the fetus.

- Forceps-assisted birth can be accomplished using outlet, low, or midforceps. Outlet forceps are the most common and are associated with the least maternal–fetal complications.

- A vacuum extractor is a soft, pliable cup attached to suction that can be applied to the fetal head and used in much the same way as forceps.

- The U.S. cesarean birth rate accounts for one third of all births. Cesarean births rose sharply as trends for repeat cesarean births rose. Maternal cesarean upon request accounts for only 1% to 3% of all cesareans. The nurse has a vital role in providing information, support, and encouragement to the couple participating in a cesarean birth.

- Preparation for cesarean birth requires establishing an intravenous line, instilling a urinary indwelling catheter, performing an abdominal/perineal prep, and continuous fetal heart rate monitoring, as well as providing preoperative teaching.

- Women should be supported and provided with information on the risks and benefits of TOLAC and repeat cesarean birth.

Clinical Reasoning in Action

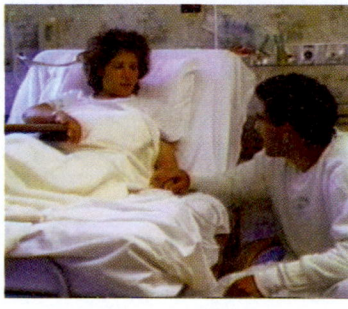

Betsy Jones, a 28-year-old G1P0, is at 39 weeks' gestation. She and her husband present to you in the labor suite for an external cephalic version procedure by her obstetrician. You introduce yourself and review her prenatal record for any significant risk factors or contraindications to the version procedure. Her prenatal medical record is significant in that the fetus has been in a persistent frank breech position. You encourage Betsy and her husband to express their understanding and expectations of the procedure. You discuss certain criteria to be met prior to the procedure and obtain vital signs as follows: T 98.8°F, P 88, R 14, BP 110/80, urine screening negative for sugar, albumin, and ketones. You place Betsy on the external electronic fetal monitor, which demonstrates a fetal heart rate baseline of 140 to 152 with moderate variability. There are no contractions observed by the monitor or Betsy. After explaining how to record fetal movement on the monitor, you proceed with an NST.

1. Explain the contraindications to the version procedure.

2. Discuss the criteria that should be met prior to the performance of an external version.

3. How would you explain to Betsy and her husband what to expect during the version procedure?

4. What support would you give Betsy during the procedure?

5. Explain postversion discharge teaching.

References

American College of Obstetricians and Gynecologists (ACOG). (2014). *Management of late-term and post-term pregnancies.* (Practice Bulletin No. 146). Washington, DC: ACOG.

American College of Obstetricians and Gynecologists (ACOG). (2015a). *Induction of labor.* (Practice Bulletin 107). Washington, DC: Author.

American College of Obstetricians and Gynecologists (ACOG). (2015b). *Vaginal birth after previous cesarean delivery.* (Practice Bulletin No. 115). Washington, DC: Author.

Berhan, Y., & Haileamlak, A. (2016). The risks of planned vaginal breech delivery versus planned caesarean section for term breech birth: A meta-analysis including observational studies. *BJOG: An International Journal of Obstetrics & Gynaecology, 123*(1), 49–57.

Birdee, G. S., Kemper, K. J., Rothman, R., & Gardiner, P. (2014). Use of complementary and alternative medicine during pregnancy and the postpartum period: An analysis of the National Health Interview Survey. *Journal of Women's Health, 23*(10), 824–829. doi: 10.1089/jwh.2013.4568.

Bishop, E. H. (1964). Pelvic scoring for elective inductions. *Obstetrics and Gynecology, 24,* 266.

Centers for Disease Control & Prevention (CDC). (2016). *Birth: Method of delivery. Fast-stats*. Retrieved from http://www.cdc.gov/nchs/fastats/delivery.htm

Cunningham, F. G., Leveno, K. J., Bloom, S. L., Spong, C. Y., Dashe, J. S., Hoffman, B. L., . . . Sheffield, J. S. (2014). *Williams obstetrics* (24th ed.). New York, NY: McGraw-Hill.

Curtin, S. C., Gregory, K. D., Korst, L. A., & Uddin, S. F. G. (2015). Maternal morbidity for vaginal and cesarean deliveries according to previous cesarean history: New birth certificate data: 2013. *National Vital Statistics Reports, 64*(4), 1–42. Retrieved from http://www.cdc.gov/nchs/data/nvsr/nvsr64/nvsr64_04.pdf

Dante, G., Bellei, G., Neri, I., & Facchinetti, F. (2014). Herbal therapies in pregnancy: What works? *Current Opinions in Obstetrics & Gynecology, 26*(2), 83–91. doi: 10.1097/GCO.0000000000000052.

Dögl, M., Vanky, E., & Heimstad, R. (2016). Changes in induction methods have not influenced cesarean section rates among women with induced labor. *Acta Obstetrics Gynecology Scandinavia, 95*, 112–115. doi:10.1111/aogs.12809

Dunn, A. B., Paul, S., Ware, L. Z., & Corwin, E. J. (2015). Perineal injury during childbirth increases risk of postpartum depressive symptoms and inflammatory markers. *Journal of Midwifery & Women's Health, 60*(4), 428–436. doi: 10.1111/jmwh.12294

Ettore, G., Torrisi, G., & Ferraro, S. (2016). Perineal care during pregnancy, delivery, and postpartum. In *Childbirth-related pelvic floor dysfunction*. New York, NY: Springer International Publishing.

Forest Pharmaceuticals. (2016). *Cervidil dinoprostone 10 mg vaginal insert*. St. Louis, MO: Author.

Garcia-Navvaro, L. (2015). C-Sections deliver cachet for wealthy Brazilian women. National Public Radio. Retrieved from http://www.npr.org/2013/05/12/182915406/c-sections-deliver-cachet-for-wealthy-brazilian-women

Ghorashi, Z., Ashori, V., Aminzadeh, F., & Mokhtari, M. (2014). The effects of oral fluid intake an hour before cesarean section on regurgitation incidence. *Iranian Journal of Nurse Midwifery Research, 19*(4), 439–442.

Goldberg, A. E. (2015). Cervical ripening. E-medicine. Retrieved from http://emedicine.medscape.com/article/263311-overview#a6

Heilman, E., & Susherebe, E. (2015). Amniotic membrane sweeping. *Seminars in Perinatology, 39*(6), 466–470. doi:10.1053/j.semperi.2015.07.010

Hiersch, L., Rosen, H., Salzer, L., Avarim, A., Ben-Harough, A., & Yogev, Y. (2015). Does artificial rupturing of membranes in the active phase of labor enhance myometrial electrical activity? *The Journal of Maternal-Fetal & Neonatal Medicine, 28*(5), 515–518. doi:10.3109/14767058.2014.92743

Macones, G. (2015). *Management of labor and delivery* (2nd ed.). Oxford, UK: Wiley-Blackwell.

Norwitz, E. R. (2016). Cesarean delivery upon request. Up-to-Date. Retrieved from http://www.uptodate.com/contents/cesarean-delivery-on-maternal-request

O'Grady, J. P. (2015). Vacuum extraction. Medscape. Retrieved from http://emedicine.medscape.com/article/271175-overview

Ross, M. G., (2015). Forceps delivery and management. *E-Medicine*. Retrieved from http://emedicine.medscape.com/article/263603-treatment#d11

Wilson, B. A., Shannon, M. T., & Shields, K. M. (Eds.). (2015). *Nursing drug guide: 2016*. Upper Saddle River, NJ: Prentice Hall.

World Health Organization (WHO). (2015). *Recommendations for augmentation of labor*. Retrieved from http://apps.who.int/iris/bitstream/10665/174001/1/WHO_RHR_15.05_eng.pdf

Zeng, X., Zhang, Y., Tian, Q., Xue, Y., Sun, R., Zheng, W., & An, R. (2015). Efficiency of dinoprostone insert for cervical ripening and induction of labor in women of full-term pregnancy compared with dinoprostone gel: A meta-analysis. *Drug Discoveries & Therapeutics, 9*(3), 165–172. Retrieved from http://doi.org/10.5582/ddt.2015.01033

Chapter 23
The Physiologic Responses of the Newborn to Birth

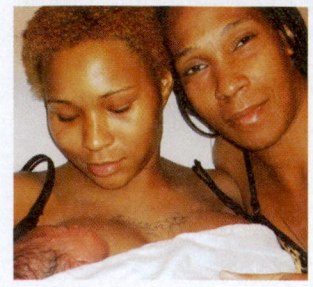

I had been a nurse for nine years when my youngest sister asked me to be her labor coach. I thought I remembered my maternity nursing rotation, but it is so different when it is family. My sister was great, however, and my niece was active and beautiful. I was struck by the reality that the transition babies must make to the world is simply staggering. You know, I love the work I do as a nurse, but this experience vividly reminded me that nursing is about life and death, joy and suffering, and everything in between.

—Hospice Nurse

⌄ Learning Outcomes

23.1 Explain the respiratory and cardiovascular changes that occur during the newborn's transition to extrauterine life and during stabilization in determining the nursing care of the newborn.

23.2 Identify the differences in fetal and adult hemoglobin and why this is important in the transition to extrauterine life.

23.3 Relate the process of thermogenesis in the newborn and the major mechanisms of heat loss to the challenge of maintaining newborn thermal stability.

23.4 Explain the steps involved in conjugation and excretion of bilirubin in the newborn.

23.5 Identify the reasons why a newborn may develop hyperbilirubinemia (jaundice) and the nursing interventions that can decrease the probability or severity of jaundice.

23.6 Delineate the functional abilities of the newborn's gastrointestinal tract and liver.

23.7 Relate the development of the newborn's kidneys to the newborn's ability to maintain fluid and electrolyte balance.

23.8 Describe basic newborn immunologic response.

23.9 Explain the physiologic and behavioral characteristics of newborn neurologic function, patterns of behavior during the periods of reactivity, and possible nursing interventions.

23.10 Describe the normal sensory-perceptual abilities and behavioral states seen in the newborn period.

The newborn period is the time from birth through the 28th day of life. During this period, the newborn adjusts from intrauterine to extrauterine life. This transition from fetus to newborn is the most complex physiologic adaptation that occurs in the human experience and involves virtually every organ system of the body (Graves & Haley, 2013). The nurse needs to be knowledgeable about a newborn's normal physiologic and behavioral adaptations and be able to recognize alterations from normal transition. The first 6 hours of life, in which the newborn stabilizes respiratory and circulatory functions, are called **neonatal transition**.

Respiratory Adaptations

To begin life as a separate being, the newborn must immediately establish respiratory functioning and ventilation. Adequate respiratory gas exchange in conjunction with marked circulatory changes are radical and rapid changes crucial to successful transition to extrauterine life.

Intrauterine Factors Supporting Respiratory Function

Even before the significant respiratory events occur at birth, certain intrauterine factors also enhance the newborn's ability to breathe. Adequate fetal lung development allows the newborn to expand his or her lungs and exchange oxygen and carbon dioxide gases. Even before birth the fetus practices breathing movements, which allows the neonate to breathe immediately after birth.

FETAL LUNG DEVELOPMENT

The respiratory system is in an ongoing state of development during fetal life, and lung development continues into early childhood. During the first 20 weeks' gestation, development is limited to the differentiation of pulmonary, vascular, and lymphatic structures. From 20 to 28 weeks, alveolar ducts begin to appear, followed by primitive alveoli. During this time, the alveolar epithelial cells begin to differentiate into type I cells (structures necessary for gas exchange) and type II cells (structures that provide for the synthesis and storage of surfactant). **Surfactant**, a lipoprotein that coats the inner surfaces of the alveoli, is composed of surface-active phospholipids (lecithin and sphingomyelin), which are critical for alveolar stability.

At 28 to 32 weeks' gestation, the number of type II cells increases further, and surfactant is produced by a more stable cellular pathway. It peaks at 35 weeks' gestation and remains high until term, paralleling late fetal lung development. At this time, the lungs are structurally developed enough to permit maintenance of lung expansion and adequate exchange of gases at birth. The neonate born before the lecithin/sphingomyelin (L/S) ratio is 2:1 will have varying degrees of respiratory distress. (See discussion of L/S ratio in Chapter 13.)

FETAL BREATHING MOVEMENTS

During intrauterine development, the lungs are filled with fetal lung fluid produced by the pulmonary epithelium, which stretches the lung tissue and stimulates growth of alveoli. Production and maintenance of a normal volume of fetal lung fluid are essential for normal lung growth (Fraser, 2014). Through intermittent **fetal breathing movements (FBM)**, the fetus practices respiration and develops the chest wall muscles and the diaphragm, as well as regulates lung fluid volume and resultant lung growth.

Fetal Circulation

In utero, the placenta is the organ of gas exchange. The low vascular resistance of the placenta and the high vascular resistance of the fluid-filled lungs result in shunts characteristic of fetal circulation. From the placenta, highly oxygenated blood (oxygen saturation of 65% to 70%) flows through the umbilical vein. A small amount of blood perfuses the liver, with the majority of blood volume flowing through the inferior vena cava and to the right atrium. Because of intracardiac streaming, blood is preferentially directed from the right atrium across the **foramen ovale (FO)** (an opening in the septum between the atria) into the left atrium, the left ventricle, and the ascending aorta (Fraser, 2014). This results in better oxygenated fetal blood directed to the mycocardium and the fetal brain.

A smaller volume of blood enters the right ventricle and is pumped through the pulmonary artery. Because pulmonary vascular resistance is very high because of the fluid-filled fetal lungs, more than 60% of right ventricular output bypasses the lung and flows through the **ductus arteriosus (DA)** (a tubular connection between the pulmonary artery and the descending aorta) into the descending aorta (Fraser, 2014). This mixing of well-oxygenated and poorly oxygenated blood results in an oxygen saturation of 45% in the blood that perfuses the lower part of the body. Vascular resistance of the placenta is low; approximately 50% of the combined ventricular cardiac output flows through the umbilical arteries to the placenta, where it releases carbon dioxide and waste products and collects oxygen and nutrients (Berger, 2012). Therefore, in fetal circulation the right and left ventricles function together, in parallel, rather than sequentially (one after the other), to perfuse the fetal body and the placenta. See Table 23–1.

TABLE 23–1 Fetal and Neonatal Circulation

SYSTEM	FETAL	NEONATAL
Pulmonary blood vessels	Constricted, with very little blood flow; lungs not expanded	Vasodilation and increased blood flow; lungs expanded; increased oxygen stimulates vasodilation.
Systemic blood vessels	Dilated, with low resistance; blood mostly in placenta	Arterial pressure rises because of loss of placenta; increased systemic blood volume and resistance.
Ductus arteriosus	Large, with no tone; blood flow from pulmonary artery to aorta	Reversal of blood flow; now from aorta to pulmonary artery because of increased left atrial pressure. Ductus is sensitive to increased oxygen and body chemicals and begins to constrict.
Foramen ovale	Patent, with increased blood flow from right atrium to left atrium	Increased pressure in left atrium attempts to reverse blood flow and shuts one-way valve.

Cardiopulmonary Adaptations

Marked changes occur in the cardiopulmonary system at birth. During late gestation, lung fluid secretion decreases. The onset of labor stimulates the production of catecholamines and other hormones, causing fetal pulmonary epithelial cells to begin reabsorption of fluid from the alveolar spaces (Fraser, 2014). With birth, the change in the sensory environment from the warm, dark womb to the brightly lighted, cold delivery room is an important stimulus for the initiation of breathing (Van Woudenberg, Wills, & Rubarth, 2012). The cold stimulates skin sensory receptors, and the newborn responds with rhythmic respirations. A number of physical and sensory influences help to sustain respiration after birth. They include the numerous tactile, auditory, visual, and painful stimuli of birth and the normal handling after delivery. Joint movement results in enhanced proprioceptor stimulation to the respiratory center. Thoroughly drying and then placing the newborn in skin-to-skin contact with the mother provides stimulation in a comforting way, as well as decreases heat loss.

The neonate's first breaths of air initiate a sequence of events that empties the airways of fluid, establishes volume and function of the newborn's lungs, and causes fetal circulation to convert to neonatal circulation. The initial first breaths generate a high negative pressure, driving fluid from the lungs and filling the alveoli with air. As the lungs expand and are exposed to higher concentrations of oxygen (room air), pulmonary vascular resistance falls, causing pulmonary vasodilation and increased blood flow to the lungs. Figure 23–1 summarizes the initiation of respiration.

When the umbilical cord is clamped, the low-resistance placenta is excluded from circulation; cessation of blood flow through the umbilical vein facilitates collapse of the *ductus venosus (DV)*, and the systemic vascular resistance increases. Thus the fetal pulmonary to systemic pressure relationships are reversed, and systemic pressure becomes greater than pulmonary pressure. These pressure changes cause the foramen ovale to close. As pressure in the pulmonary artery decreases and pressure in the aorta increases, the shunt across the ductus arteriosus reverses to left to right and constricts, leading to closure in the first few days of life. This closure of fetal shunts establishes the serial arterial–venous circulation indicative of neonatal circulation. See Figure 23–2.

In summary, the four major cardiopulmonary actions of **cardiopulmonary adaptation** (Figure 23–3) are as follows:

1. *Increased systemic vascular resistance and decreased pulmonary vascular resistance.* With the loss of the low-resistance placenta, systemic vascular resistance increases, resulting in greater systemic pressure. At the same time, lung expansion and exposure to high oxygen concentrations increase pulmonary blood flow and dilate pulmonary blood vessels. The combination of vasodilation and increased pulmonary blood flow decreases pulmonary vascular resistance. As the pulmonary vascular beds open, the systemic vascular pressure increases, enhancing perfusion of the other body systems.

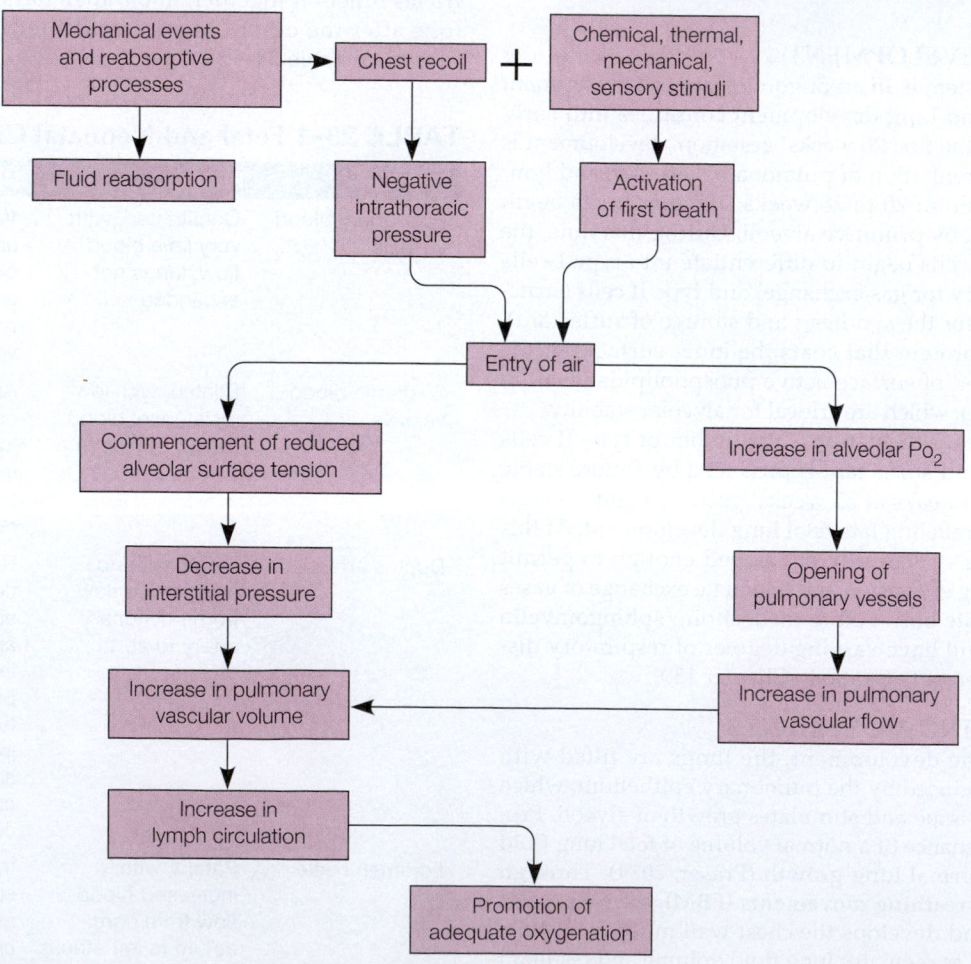

Figure 23–1 Initiation of respiration in the newborn.

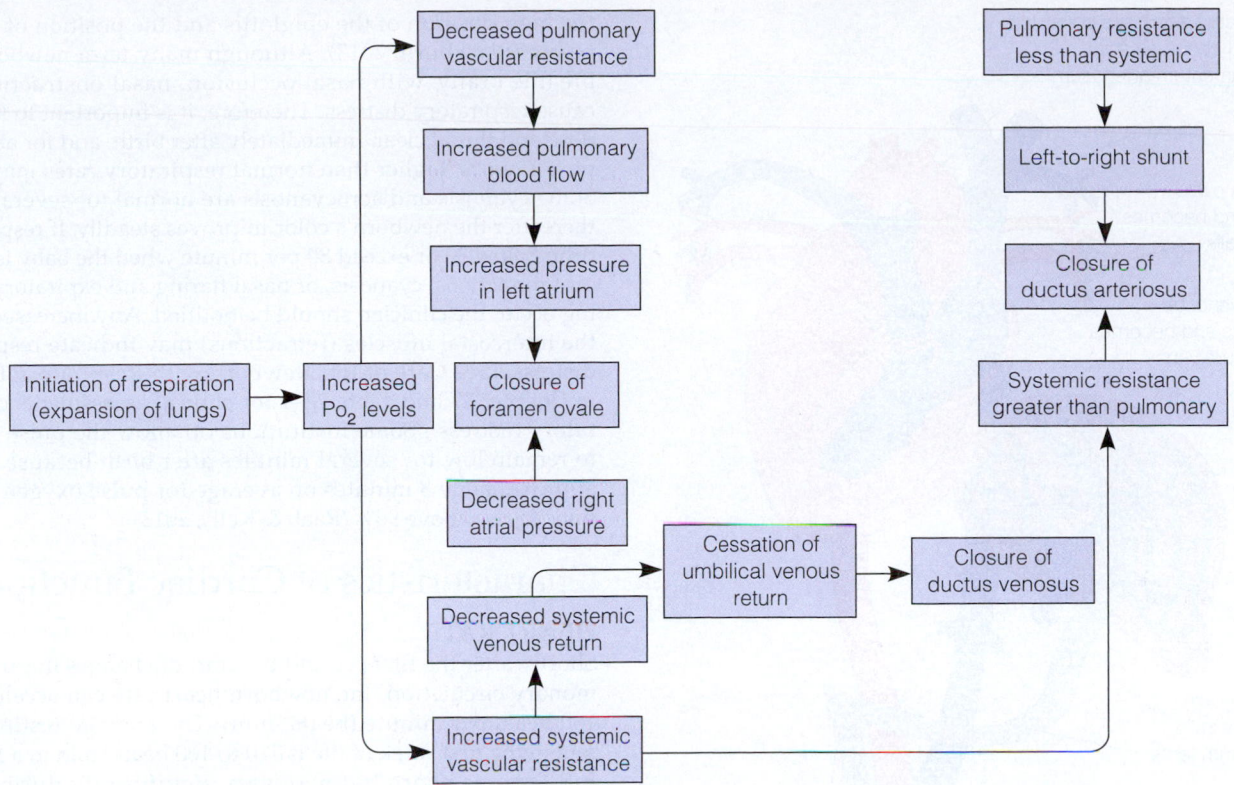

Figure 23–2 Transitional circulation: conversion from fetal to neonatal circulation.

2. *Closure of the foramen ovale.* Closure of the foramen ovale is a function of changing arterial pressures. In utero, pressure is greater in the right atrium, and the foramen ovale is open after birth, shunting blood from the right atrium to the left. The decreased pulmonary vascular resistance and the decreased umbilical venous return to the right atrium also cause a decrease in right atrial pressure. The pressure gradients across the atria are now reversed, with left atrial pressure greater; this causes the foramen ovale to functionally close 1 to 2 hours after birth. Anatomic closure of the foramen ovale occurs within 30 months (Berger, 2012).

3. *Closure of the ductus arteriosus.* Initial elevation of the systemic vascular pressure above the pulmonary vascular pressure increases pulmonary blood flow by reversing the flow through the ductus arteriosus. Blood now flows from the aorta into the pulmonary artery. An increase in blood PO_2 triggers the ductus arteriosus to constrict. In utero the placenta produces prostaglandin E_2 (PGE_2), which causes ductus vasodilation. With the loss of the placenta and increased pulmonary blood flow, PGE_2 levels drop, leaving the active constriction by PO_2 unopposed. Functional closure of the ductus arteriosus in the well newborn starts within 18 hours after birth; fibrosis or anatomic closure occurs within 2 to 3 weeks after birth (Fraser, 2014).

4. *Closure of the ductus venosus.* Closure of the ductus venosus is related to mechanical pressure changes that result from severing the cord, redistribution of blood, and cardiac output. Closure of the ductus venosus forces perfusion of the liver. Fibrosis or anatomic closure of the ductus venosus occurs within 2 months, at which time it becomes known as the ligamentum venosum.

Clinical Tip

Gentle physical contact by thoroughly drying the newborn and placing the baby in skin-to-skin contact with the mother's chest and abdomen is emphasized when using external stimulation means for the first breaths. These actions will also decrease heat loss and promote mother–newborn bonding.

Maintaining Respiratory Function

The ability of the lungs to maintain oxygenation and ventilation (the exchange of oxygen and carbon dioxide) is influenced by such factors as *lung compliance* and *airway resistance*. Lung compliance is influenced by the elastic recoil of the lung tissue and anatomic differences in the newborn. The newborn has a relatively large heart and mediastinal structures that reduce available lung space. Also, the newborn chest is equipped with weak intercostal muscles and a rigid rib cage with horizontal ribs and a high diaphragm, which restricts the space available for lung expansion. The large abdomen further encroaches on the high diaphragm to decrease lung space. Another factor that limits ventilation is airway resistance, which depends on the radii, length, and number of airways. Airway resistance is increased in the newborn when compared with adults.

Characteristics of Newborn Respiration

The normal newborn respiratory rate is 30 to 80 breaths per minute. Initial respirations may be largely diaphragmatic, shallow, and irregular in depth and rhythm. The abdomen's movements are synchronous with the chest movements. Breathing patterns in newborns can be irregular and variable. Periodic breathing

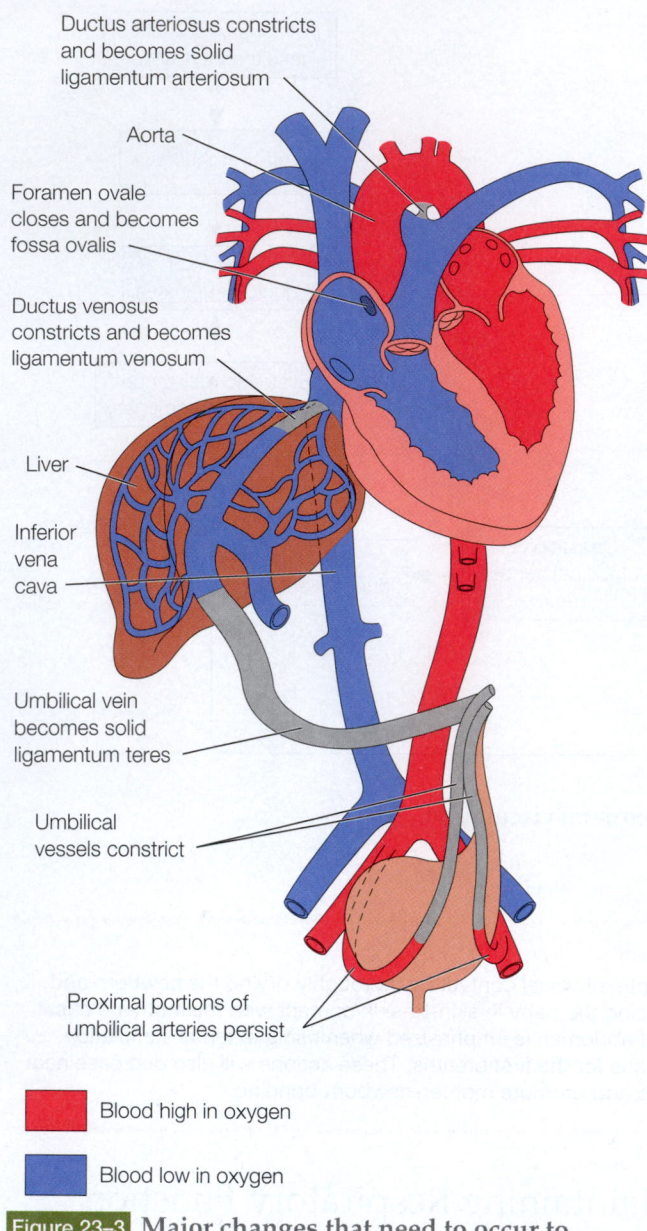

Ductus arteriosus constricts and becomes solid ligamentum arteriosum

Aorta

Foramen ovale closes and becomes fossa ovalis

Ductus venosus constricts and becomes ligamentum venosum

Liver

Inferior vena cava

Umbilical vein becomes solid ligamentum teres

Umbilical vessels constrict

Proximal portions of umbilical arteries persist

■ Blood high in oxygen

■ Blood low in oxygen

Figure 23–3 Major changes that need to occur to complete the transition to neonatal circulation.

the high position of the epiglottis and the position of the soft palate (Blackburn, 2013). Although many term newborns can breathe orally, with nasal occlusion, nasal obstructions can cause respiratory distress. Therefore, it is important to keep the nose and throat clear. Immediately after birth, and for about the next 2 hours, higher than normal respiratory rates may occur. Some cyanosis and acrocyanosis are normal for several hours; thereafter the newborn's color improves steadily. If respirations drop below 30 or exceed 80 per minute when the baby is at rest, or if retractions, cyanosis, or nasal flaring and expiratory grunting occur, the clinician should be notified. Any increased use of the intercostal muscles (retractions) may indicate respiratory distress. (See Care of the Newborn with Respiratory Distress in Chapter 27 and Table 27–1 for clinical assessments of respiratory distress.) Some institutions do allow the pulse oxygen to remain low for several minutes after birth because it takes approximately 8 minutes on average for pulse oxygen saturations to rise above 90% (Raab & Kelly, 2013).

Characteristics of Cardiac Function

HEART RATE
Shortly after the first cry and the start of changes in cardiopulmonary circulation, the newborn heart rate can accelerate to 180 beats per minute (beats/min). The average resting heart rate in the first week of life is 110 to 160 beats/min in a healthy, full-term newborn but may vary significantly during deep sleep or active awake states. In the full-term newborn, the heart rate may drop to 80 to100 beats/min during deep sleep (Van Woudenberg et al., 2012).

Apical pulse rates should be obtained by auscultation (Figure 23–4) for a full minute, preferably when the newborn is asleep. The heart rate should be evaluated for abnormal rhythms or beats. Peripheral pulses of all extremities should also be evaluated to detect any inequalities or unusual characteristics. While radial pulses are usually readily found, pedal pulses may be difficult to palpate in the newborn. Additionally, brachial and femoral pulses are usually easily palpated in the well newborn.

BLOOD PRESSURE
Blood pressure tends to be highest immediately after birth and then descends to its lowest level at about 3 hours of age. By days 4 to 6, the blood pressure rises and plateaus at a level approximately the same as the initial level. Blood pressure is sensitive

is common in preterm newborns, but can also be seen in term babies. **Periodic breathing** is defined as "pauses in respiratory movements that last for up to 20 seconds alternating with breathing" (Blackburn, 2013). Periodic breathing is rarely associated with differences in skin color or heart rate changes, and it has no prognostic significance. Tactile or other sensory stimulation increases the inspired oxygen and converts periodic breathing patterns to normal breathing patterns during neonatal transition. With deep sleep, the pattern is reasonably regular. Periodic breathing occurs with rapid-eye-movement (REM) sleep, and grossly irregular breathing is evident with motor activity, sucking, and crying. Cessation of breathing lasting more than 20 seconds is defined as *apnea* and is abnormal in term newborns. Apnea may or may not be associated with changes in skin color or heart rate (drop below 100 beats per minute). Apnea always needs to be further evaluated.

Newborns tend to be obligatory nose breathers because the nasal route is the primary route of air entry. This is because of

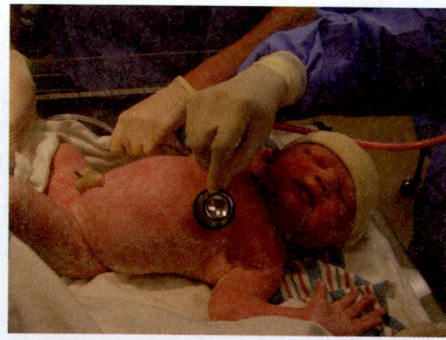

Figure 23–4 Apical pulse rates should be obtained by auscultation for a full minute, preferably when the newborn is asleep.

SOURCE: Wilson Garcia.

to the changes in blood volume that occur in the transition to newborn circulation (Figure 23–5). Peripheral perfusion pressure is a particularly sensitive indicator of the newborn's ability to compensate for alterations in blood volume before changes in blood pressure. Capillary refill should be less than 2 to 3 seconds when the skin is blanched.

Blood pressure (BP) values during the first 12 hours of life vary with the birth weight and gestational age. The average mean BP is 42 to 60 mmHg in the full-term, resting newborn over 3 kg (6.6 lb) during the first 12 hours of life (Gomella, 2013). In the preterm newborn, the average BP varies according to weight. Crying may cause an elevation of 20 mmHg in both the systolic and the diastolic blood pressure; thus accuracy is more likely in the quiet newborn. The measurement of blood pressure is best accomplished by using the Doppler technique with a size- and weight-appropriate cuff over the brachial artery. Four point extremity BP assessment is warranted in the presence of any cardiovascular symptoms (tachycardia, persistent murmur, abnormal pulses, poor perfusion, or abnormal precordial activity). Blood pressure in the lower extremities is usually higher than that in the upper extremities.

CARDIAC MURMURS

Cardiac murmurs are produced by turbulent blood flow. Murmurs may be heard when blood flows across an abnormal valve or across a stenosed valve, when there is an atrial or ventricular septal defect, or when there is increased flow across a normal valve.

Murmurs are often present in the initial newborn period as transition from fetal to neonatal circulation occurs. These murmurs heard in the transition period (first 48 hours of life) should be followed up (Blackburn, 2013). They usually involve incomplete closure of the ductus arteriosus or foramen ovale. Soft murmurs may be heard as the pulmonary branch arteries increase their blood flow from 7% to 50% of the combined ventricular output during transition, causing a physiologic peripheral pulmonary stenosis. Clicks may normally be heard at the lower left sternal border as the great vessels dilate to accommodate systolic blood flow in the first few hours of life. Hearing a murmur is often the most common means of recognizing cardiac disease. Because of the current practice of early discharge, murmurs associated with ventricular septal defect and patent ductus arteriosus often are not picked up until the first well-baby checkup at 4 to 6 weeks of age. Thus newborns with serious cardiac anomalies may not be identified until weeks after discharge from the birthing facility.

CARDIAC WORKLOAD

Before birth the right ventricle does approximately two thirds of the cardiac work, resulting in increased size and thickness of the right ventricle at birth. After birth the left ventricle must assume a larger share of the cardiac workload, and it progressively increases in size and thickness. This may explain why right-sided heart defects are better tolerated than left-sided ones and why left-sided defects rapidly become symptomatic after birth.

Hematopoietic System

Birth brings dramatic changes in circulation and oxygenation, which affect hematopoiesis. The mean hemoglobin level in cord blood at term is 17 g/dL (Gomella, 2013). Normally the hemoglobin and hematocrit values rise in the first several hours after birth because of the movement of plasma from intravascular to the extravascular space. By 3 to 5 days after birth, nucleated red blood cells are normally no longer found in the blood of term or preterm newborns, but may be present in marked elevated numbers in the presence of hemolysis or hypoxic stress (Diab & Luchtman-Jones, 2015).

Oxygen Transport

The transportation of oxygen to the peripheral tissues depends on the type of hemoglobin in the red blood cells. In the fetus and newborn, a variety of hemoglobins exist, the most significant being fetal hemoglobin (HbF) and adult hemoglobin (HbA). Approximately 70% to 90% of the hemoglobin in the fetus and newborn is of the fetal variety. The greatest difference between HbF and HbA relates to the transport of oxygen and release of it to tissues.

Because HbF has a greater affinity for oxygen than does HbA, the oxygen saturation in the newborn's blood is greater than in the adult's, but the amount of oxygen available to the tissues is less. This situation is beneficial prenatally, because the fetus must maintain adequate oxygen uptake in the presence of very low oxygen tension (umbilical venous PO_2 cannot exceed the uterine venous PO_2). Because of this high concentration of oxygen in the blood, hypoxia in the newborn is particularly difficult to recognize. Clinical manifestations of cyanosis do not appear until low blood levels of oxygen are present.

In addition, alkalosis (increased pH) and hypothermia can result in less oxygen being available to the body tissues, whereas acidosis, hypercarbia, and hyperthermia can result in less oxygen being bound to hemoglobin and more oxygen being released to the body tissues.

In the first days of life, hemoglobin may rise 1 to 2 g/dL above fetal levels as a result of placental transfusion, low oral fluid intake, and diminished extracellular fluid volume. The fetal hemoglobin concentration in blood decreases after birth by approximately 3% per week and is less than 5% to 8% of total hemoglobin by 6 months of age (Bagwell, 2014). The hemoglobin level declines progressively during the first 2 months of life. This initial decline in hemoglobin creates a phenomenon known as **physiologic anemia of the newborn**. The lowest hemoglobin level is reached at about 3 months of age and is called the *physiologic nadir*. The newborn usually tolerates this physiologic state without any clinical difficulties. Hemoglobin values fall mainly from a decrease in red cell mass

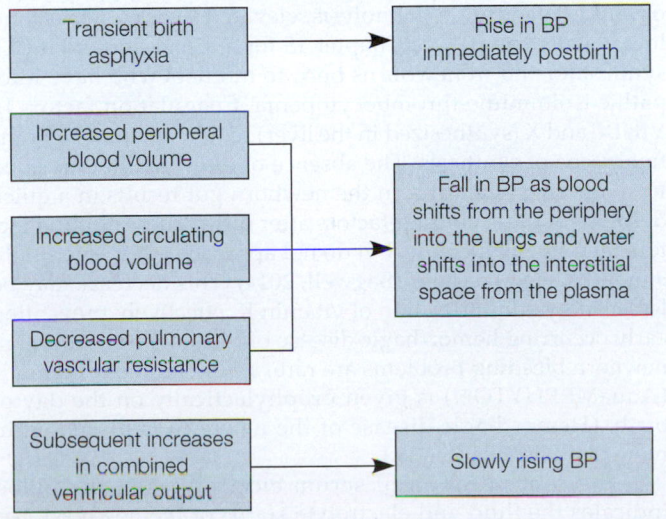

Figure 23–5 Response of blood pressure (BP) to neonatal changes in blood volume.

rather than from the diluting effect of increasing plasma volume. The fact that red cell survival is lower in newborns than in adults, and that red cell production is less, also contributes to this anemia. Neonatal red blood cells (RBCs) have a life span of 60 to 70 days, approximately two thirds the life span of adult RBCs (Bagwell, 2014). Erythropoiesis resumes normally when levels of erythropoietin rise in response to low hemoglobin levels and tissue oxygen needs (Bagwell, 2014). Once erythropoiesis resumes, iron stores will be used to produce new RBCs. Most newborns require supplemental iron to maintain adequate iron stores.

Leukocytosis is a normal finding, because the stress of birth stimulates increased production of neutrophils during the first few days of life. Neutrophils then decrease to 35% of the total leukocyte count by 2 weeks of age. Lymphocytes play a role in antibody formation and eventually become the predominant type of leukocyte and the total white blood cell count falls.

The platelet count of the newborn is comparable to adult values. A number of maternally administered pharmacologic agents have been implicated in hematologic abnormalities of the fetus or newborn. Therefore, obtaining an accurate maternal history, including medications, is important.

Blood volume is approximately 85 ml/kg of body weight for a term newborn (Diab & Luchtman-Jones, 2015). For example, a 3.6-kg (8-lb) newborn has a blood volume of 306 mL. Blood volume varies based on the amount of placental transfusion received during the delivery of the placenta, as well as other factors, including the following:

- *Gestational age.* There appears to be a positive association among gestational age, RBC numbers, and hemoglobin concentration.

- *Prenatal and/or perinatal hemorrhage.* Significant prenatal or perinatal bleeding decreases the hematocrit level and causes hypovolemia.

- *The site of the blood sample.* Hemoglobin and hematocrit levels are significantly higher in capillary blood than in venous blood. Sluggish peripheral blood flow creates RBC stasis, thereby increasing RBC concentration in the capillaries. Consequently, blood samples taken from venous blood sites are more accurate than those from capillary sites.

Delayed Cord Clamping

In utero, the fetus's blood flows through the umbilical cord to and from the fetus and the placenta, bringing oxygen and nutrition to the fetus from the mother's blood. If the umbilical cord is left unclamped for a short period of time after birth, some of the blood from the placenta passes to the newborn (this is called placental transfusion) to increase the neonate's blood volume and improve blood flow to the newborn's organs (Katheria, Truong, Cousins, et al., 2015). For many years, the standard of care has included immediate clamping of the umbilical cord at birth. The World Health Organization was the first to recommend delayed cord clamping as a standard for all newborns at birth. Although many randomized control trials of term and preterm newborns have evaluated the benefits and risks of immediate umbilical cord clamping versus delayed umbilical cord clamping, generally defined as umbilical cord clamping performed 30 to 60 seconds after birth, the ideal timing for umbilical cord clamping has not yet been established and continues to be a subject of controversy and debate (American College of Obstetricians and Gynecologists [ACOG], 2014).

Physiologic studies in term newborns have demonstrated that placental blood is rapidly transferred into the newborn via the uninterrupted umbilical cord in a stepwise fashion over the initial seconds after birth. Approximately 80 mL of blood is transferred by 1 minute after birth, reaching approximately 100 mL at 3 minutes after birth (ACOG, 2014). Providing babies with additional blood through delayed umbilical cord clamping may facilitate transition from fetal to neonatal circulation (Katheria et al., 2015). Reviews of multiple clinical trials found that delayed umbilical cord clamping had both positive and negative effects on neonatal outcomes. Newborns in the delayed umbilical cord clamping group had significantly higher levels of hemoglobin compared with newborns in the immediate umbilical cord clamping group. Newborns in the delayed umbilical cord clamping group also had higher ferritin levels until 6 months of age and fewer suffered from iron deficiency anemia (Raju, 2013). However, a significant increase was noted in the need for phototherapy for jaundice in the delayed umbilical cord clamping group.

The benefits of delayed umbilical cord clamping for the preterm newborn are much more compelling. Clinical trials in preterm newborns found that delaying umbilical cord clamping was associated with fewer babies who required blood transfusion for anemia and/or low blood pressure. Also, a significant reduction in the incidence of intraventricular hemorrhage and less risk of necrotizing enterocolitis (a severe infection in the bowel) were found in neonates in the delayed umbilical cord clamping group (ACOG, 2014; Katheria et al., 2015). These effects may be related to an improvement in the circulating neonatal blood volume and better control of blood pressure following placental transfusion. However, there are some legitimate arguments for clamping the umbilical cord soon after birth. Maternal emergency and concern that delayed umbilical cord clamping could hinder the timely initiation of resuscitation for the asphyxiated neonate or one with cardiopulmonary failure are valid reasons for immediate umbilical cord clamping (Raju, 2013).

Coagulation

The platelet count of the newborn is comparable to adult values; however, the newborn may have transient diminished platelet function. Transient neonatal thrombocytopenia may occur in newborns born to mothers with severe hypertension or HELLP syndrome (hemolysis, elevated liver enzymes, and low platelet count) (see Chapter 15 for a discussion of HELLP syndrome) and in newborns born to mothers who have idiopathic isoimmune thrombocytopenia. Coagulation factors II, VII, IX, and X (synthesized in the liver) require vitamin K for the final steps of synthesis. The absence of intestinal flora needed to synthesize vitamin K in the newborn gut results in a quick decrease of these clotting factors after birth. These clotting factors then slowly increase, but do not approach adult levels until 9 months of age or later (Bagwell, 2014). This decrease may be lessened by administration of vitamin K, effectively preventing early occurring hemorrhagic disease of the newborn. Although newborn bleeding problems are rare, an injection of vitamin K (AquaMEPHYTON) is given prophylactically on the day of birth. (Hemorrhagic disease of the newborn is discussed in more depth in Chapter 26.)

The concentration of serum electrolytes in the blood indicates the fluid and electrolyte status of the newborn. See Table 23–2 for normal term newborn cord blood values and cord blood gas values.

TABLE 23–2 Normal Term Newborn Cord Blood and Cord Blood Gas Values

LABORATORY DATA	NORMAL RANGE
Cord Blood Values	
Hemoglobin	14–20 g/dL
Hematocrit	43%–63%
WBC	10,000–30,000/mm³
WBC differential	
Neutrophils	40%–80%
Lymphocytes	20%–40%
Monocytes	3%–10%
Platelets	150,000–350,000/mm³
Reticulocytes	3%–7%
Sodium	127–144 mEq/L
Potassium	3.4–9.9 mEq/L
Chloride	103–111 mEq/L
Bicarbonate	18–23 mEq/L
Carbon dioxide	13–27 mmol/L
Calcium	8.2–111 mg/dL
Glucose	45–96 mg/dL
Total protein	4.8–7.3 g/dL
Cord Blood Gas Values	
Venous Blood Gas	
pH	7.25–7.35
PO_2	2–32 mmHg
PCO_2	40–50 mmHg
Base Excess	± 0–5
HCO_3	22
Arterial Blood Gas	
pH	7.14–7.4
PO_2	16–20 mmHg
PCO_2	32–68 mmHg
Base Excess	± 0–10
HCO_3	15–26.8

Source: Data from Fanaroff, A. A., & Martin, R. J. (Eds.). (2015). *Neonatal-perinatal medicine* (10th ed.). St. Louis, MO: Mosby.

Temperature Regulation

Temperature regulation is the maintenance of thermal balance by the loss of heat to the environment at a rate equal to heat production. Newborns are *homeothermic*; they attempt to stabilize their internal (core) body temperatures within a narrow range in spite of significant temperature variations in their environment. Thermoregulation in the newborn is closely related to the rate of metabolism and oxygen consumption. Within a specific environmental temperature range, called the **neutral thermal environment (NTE)** zone, the rates of oxygen consumption and metabolism are minimal, and internal body temperature is maintained because of thermal balance (Blackburn, 2013). The normal newborn requires higher environmental temperatures than adults do to maintain a thermoneutral environment.

Several newborn characteristics affect the establishment of thermal stability:

- Heat transfer from neonatal organs to skin surface is increased compared to transfer in adults because of the neonate's decreased subcutaneous fat and large body surface to weight ratio.
- Neonates rely on nonshivering thermogenesis for heat production via metabolism of brown adipose tissue.
- Blood vessels in the newborn are closer to the skin than those of an adult. Therefore, the circulating blood is influenced by changes in environmental temperature and in turn influences the hypothalamic temperature-regulating center.
- The flexed posture of the term newborn decreases the surface area exposed to the environment, thereby reducing heat loss.

A table listing neutral thermal environmental temperatures gives a recommended temperature range depending on the weight and age of the newborn. Generally speaking, the smaller babies in each weight group will require a temperature in the higher portion of the temperature range. Within each time range, the younger the baby, the higher the temperature required. For example, the preterm or small-for-gestational-age (SGA) newborn has less adipose tissue and is hypoflexed, and therefore requires higher environmental temperatures to achieve a thermal neutral environment. Larger, well-insulated newborns may be able to cope with lower environmental temperatures. If the environmental temperature falls below the lower limits of the NTE, the newborn responds with increased oxygen consumption and metabolism, which results in greater heat production and decreased weight gain and growth. Prolonged exposure to the cold may result in depleted glycogen stores and acidosis. Oxygen consumption also increases if the environmental temperature is above the NTE.

Heat Loss

A newborn is at a distinct disadvantage in maintaining a normal temperature. With a large body surface in relation to mass and a limited amount of insulating subcutaneous fat, the full-term newborn loses about four times the heat of an adult. The newborn's poor thermal stability is primarily because of excessive heat loss rather than impaired heat production. Because of the risk of hypothermia and possible cold stress, minimizing heat loss in the newborn after birth is essential. (See Initial Care of the Newborn in Chapter 18 and *Clinical Skill: Thermoregulation of the Newborn* in Chapter 25 for nursing measures.)

Two major routes of heat loss are from the internal core of the body to the body surface and from the external surface to the environment. Usually the core temperature is higher than the skin temperature, resulting in continuous transfer or conduction of heat to the surface. The greater the difference in temperature between core and skin, the more rapidly heat transfers. The transfer is accomplished through an increase in oxygen consumption, depletion of glycogen stores, and metabolization of brown fat. Heat loss from the body surface to the environment takes place in four ways—by convection, radiation, evaporation, and conduction (Figure 23–6).

- **Convection** is the loss of heat from the warm body surface to the cooler air currents. Air-conditioned rooms, air currents with a temperature below the newborn's skin temperature, oxygen by mask, and removal from an incubator for procedures increase convective heat loss in the newborn. The amount of heat transferred depends on the velocity of the moving air, the temperature difference between the air and the baby's skin, and the proportion of body surface area exposed.

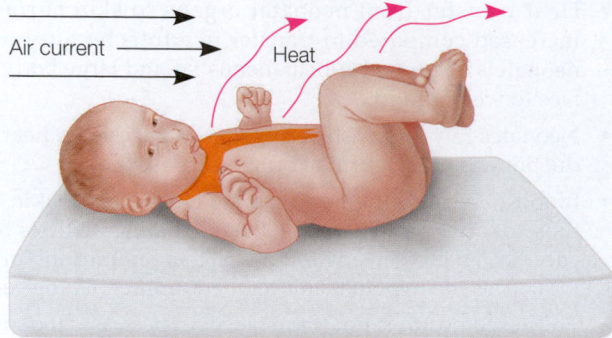

A. Convection

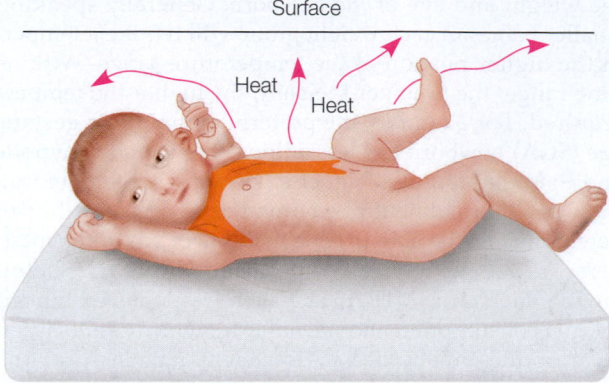

B. Radiation

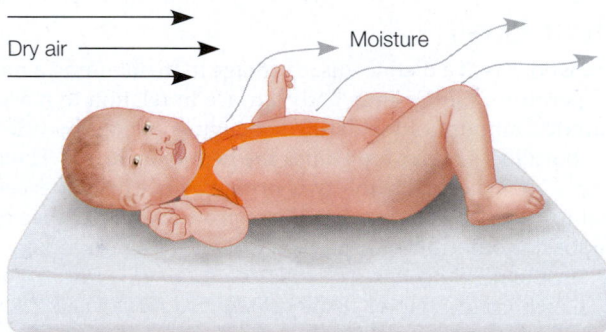

C. Evaporation

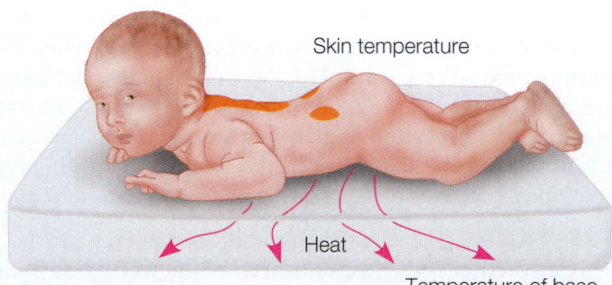

D. Conduction

Figure 23–6 Methods of heat loss. A. Convection. B. Radiation. C. Evaporation. D. Conduction. The distribution of brown adipose tissue (brown fat) in the newborn is shown in the shaded areas.

- **Radiation** losses occur when heat transfers from the heated body surface to cooler surfaces and objects not in direct contact with the body. The walls of a room or of an incubator are potential causes of heat loss by radiation, even if the ambient temperature of the incubator is within the thermal neutral range for that newborn. Placing cold objects (such as ice for blood gases) onto the incubator or near the baby in the radiant warmer will increase radiant losses.

- **Evaporation** is the loss of heat incurred when water is converted to a vapor. The newborn is particularly prone to lose heat by evaporation immediately after birth (when the baby is wet with amniotic fluid), and during baths; thus drying the newborn is critical. Evaporation accounts for 25% of heat loss immediately after delivery (Blackburn, 2013). Evaporation also occurs from expired air from the respiratory tract. Radiant warming beds and bank photo-therapy lights also accentuate evaporative loss.

- **Conduction** is the loss of heat to a cooler surface by direct skin contact. Chilled hands, cool scales, cold examination tables, and cold stethoscopes can cause loss of heat by conduction. Even if objects are warmed to the incubator temperature, the temperature difference between the baby's core temperature and the ambient temperature may be significant. This difference results in heat transfer.

Once the newborn has been dried after birth, the highest losses of heat generally result from radiation and convection. The baby can respond to the cooler environmental temperature with adequate peripheral vasoconstriction, but this mechanism is not entirely effective because of the minimal amount of fat insulation present, the large body surface, and ongoing thermal conduction. Because of these factors, minimizing the baby's heat loss and preventing hypothermia are imperative. Most hospitalized newborns are weighed daily. Placing unclothed newborns on a cold scale can induce heat loss. Therefore the undressed newborn should be examined in a warm environment with an external heat source such as a radiant warmer. (See Care of the Newborn With Cold Stress in Chapter 27 for nursing measures to prevent hypothermia.)

Clinical Tip

Bath time is when many newborns experience cold stress. To minimize the risk, always bathe newborns in a warm room, gather all supplies prior to beginning the bath, and prewarm soaps or shampoos. Dry them with warmed blankets and dress immediately. The baby's head accounts for a large portion of body surface area and has great capacity for heat loss, so placing a hat on the newborn is an effective way to minimize heat loss. Placing newborns skin-to-skin with mother after bathing is a good way to help them rewarm and maintain body temperature.

Most hospitalized newborns are weighed daily. Placing unclothed babies on a cold scale can induce heat loss. A safer and more developmentally beneficial way to weigh a baby is by doing a "swaddled weight." Place blankets, diaper, hat, and clothing on the scale before calibrating the scale to zero. Then you will be able to dress and swaddle the baby for weighing and the scale will reflect only the baby's weight.

Heat Production (Thermogenesis)

When exposed to a cool environment, the newborn requires additional heat. The newborn has several physiologic mechanisms that increase heat production, or **thermogenesis**.

These mechanisms include increased basal metabolic rate, muscular activity, and chemical thermogenesis (also called *non-shivering thermogenesis [NST]*).

Nonshivering thermogenesis is an important mechanism of heat production unique to the newborn. It occurs when skin receptors perceive a drop in the environmental temperature and, in response, transmit sensations to stimulate the sympathetic nervous system. NST uses the newborn's stores of **brown adipose tissue (BAT)** (also called brown fat) to provide heat. It first appears in the fetus at about 26 to 28 weeks' gestation and continues to increase until 3 to 5 weeks after the birth of a term newborn, unless the fat is depleted by cold stress (Blackburn, 2013). Brown fat is deposited in the midscapular area, around the neck, and in the axillas, with deeper placement around the trachea, esophagus, abdominal aorta, kidneys, and adrenal glands (see Figure 23–6). BAT receives its name from the dark color caused by its enriched blood supply, dense cellular content, and abundant nerve endings. These characteristics of brown fat cells promote rapid metabolism, heat generation, and heat transfer to the peripheral circulation. The large numbers of brown fat cells increase the speed with which triglycerides are metabolized to produce heat but cause increased oxygen consumption and caloric output in the already compromised newborn.

Shivering, a form of muscular activity common in the cold adult, is rarely seen in the newborn. If the newborn shivers, it means the newborn's metabolic rate has already doubled. The extra muscular activity does little to produce needed heat.

Thermographic studies of newborns exposed to cold show an increase in the skin heat produced over the newborn's brown fat deposits between 1 and 14 days of age. If a baby is SGA, intrauterine growth restricted (IUGR), or premature, his or her brown fat stores will be inadequate to produce sufficient heat. If the brown fat supply has been depleted, the metabolic response to cold will be limited or lacking.

An increase in basal metabolism as a result of hypothermia results in an increase in oxygen consumption. A decrease in the environmental temperature of 2°C, from 33° to 31°C, is a drop sufficient to double the oxygen consumption of a term newborn. Keeping the normal newborn warm promotes normal oxygen requirements, whereas chilling can cause the newborn to show signs of respiratory distress.

When exposed to cold, the normal term newborn is usually able to cope with the increase in oxygen requirements, but the preterm newborn may be unable to increase ventilation to the necessary level of oxygen consumption. Because oxidation of fatty acids depends on the availability of oxygen, glucose, and adenosine triphosphate (ATP), the newborn's ability to generate heat can be altered by pathologic events such as hypoxia, acidosis, and hypoglycemia or by medication that blocks the release of norepinephrine. The effect of certain drugs such as meperidine (Demerol) may also prevent metabolism of brown fat. Newborn hypothermia prolongs and also potentiates the effects of many analgesic and anesthetic drugs in the newborn.

Response to Heat

Sweating is the term newborn's usual initial response to hyperthermia. The newborn sweat glands have limited function until after the fourth week of extrauterine life; heat is lost through peripheral vasodilation and evaporation of insensible water loss. Vasodilation caused by overheating predisposes the baby to hypotension. The term newborn will be flaccid and assume a position of extension to facilitate heat loss. Oxygen consumption

and metabolic rate also increase in response to hyperthermia. Severe hyperthermia can lead to death or to gross brain damage if the baby survives.

Developing Cultural Competence Newborn Baths in Jordan

In Jordan, the birth of a male baby is a much celebrated event. The newborn is bathed daily during the first week of life. During the final bath, salt is added to the water to help the newborn's skin adjust to the external environment and protect it from changes in the weather.

Hepatic Adaptations

The liver performs many essential functions, including the production of bile, regulation of plasma proteins and glucose, coagulation, and the biotransformation of drugs and toxins. It is relatively large and occupies about 40% of the abdominal cavity. The neonate has less than 20% of the hepatocytes that are present in the adult liver, and liver growth continues after birth until it reaches its mature size.

Iron Storage and Red Blood Cell Production

Iron is an essential micronutrient that plays a significant role in critical cellular functions in all organ systems. The serum iron level in umbilical cord blood is elevated compared to maternal levels (Diab & Luchtman-Jones, 2015). As red blood cells (RBCs) are destroyed after birth, the iron is stored in the liver until needed for new RBC production. Newborn iron stores are determined by total body hemoglobin content and length of gestation. The term newborn has about 270 mg of iron at birth, and about 140 to 170 mg of this amount is in the hemoglobin. If the mother's iron intake has been adequate, enough iron will be stored to last until the newborn is about 5 months of age. After about 6 months of age, foods containing iron or iron supplements must be given to prevent anemia.

Healthy People 2020

(NWS-21) Reduce iron deficiency among young children and females of childbearing age

Carbohydrate Metabolism

At term, the newborn's cord blood glucose level is 15 mg/dL lower than maternal blood glucose level. Newborn carbohydrate reserves are relatively low. One third of this reserve is in the form of liver glycogen. Newborn glycogen stores are twice those of the adult. The newborn enters an energy crunch at the time of birth, with the removal of the maternal glucose supply and the increased energy expenditure associated with the birth process and extrauterine life. Fuel sources are consumed at a faster rate because of the work of breathing, loss of heat when exposed to cold, activity, and activation of muscle tone. By secreting glucagon and suppressing insulin release, the newborn gradually mobilizes glucose to meet his or her energy needs. Thus, even if a healthy term newborn is not fed soon after birth, blood glucose levels rise at 3 to 4 hours of age

(Cloherty, Eichenwald, Hansen, et al., 2012). However, hepatic glycogen is rapidly depleted if feeding is not established early. The nurse may assess the glucose level on admission if risk factors are present or per agency protocol (see Care of the Newborn with Hypoglycemia in Chapter 27).

Conjugation of Bilirubin

In the body, the breakdown of the heme portion of hemoglobin causes the production of bilirubin. Conjugation, or the changing of bilirubin into an excretable form, is the conversion of the yellow lipid-soluble pigment (unconjugated, indirect) into water-soluble pigment (excretable, direct). Unconjugated bilirubin is fat soluble, has a propensity for fatty tissues, is not in an excretable form, and is a potential toxin. **Total bilirubin** is the sum of conjugated (direct) and unconjugated (indirect) bilirubin.

Fetal unconjugated bilirubin crosses the placenta to be excreted, so the fetus does not need to conjugate bilirubin. Total bilirubin at birth is usually less than 3 mg/dL unless an abnormal hemolytic process has been present in utero. After birth the newborn's liver must begin to conjugate bilirubin. This produces a normal rise in serum bilirubin levels in the first few days of life.

The unconjugated bilirubin formed, after RBCs are destroyed, is transported in the blood bound to albumin. The bilirubin is transferred into the hepatocytes and bound to intracellular proteins. These proteins determine the amount of bilirubin held in a liver cell for processing and consequently determine the amount of bilirubin uptake into the liver. The activity of uridine-diphospho glucuronosyltransferase (UDPGT) enzyme results in the attachment of unconjugated bilirubin to glucuronic acid (a product of liver glycogen), producing bilirubin glucuronides (conjugated, direct bilirubin). Direct (water-soluble) bilirubin is excreted into the tiny bile ducts, then into the common duct and duodenum. The conjugated (direct) bilirubin then progresses down the intestines, where bacteria transform it into urobilinogen (urine bilirubin) and stercobilinogen. Stercobilinogen is not reabsorbed but is excreted as a yellow-brown pigment in the stools.

Even after the bilirubin has been conjugated and bound, it can be changed back to unconjugated bilirubin via the enterohepatic circulation. In the intestines β-D-glucuronidase enzyme acts to split off (deconjugate) the bilirubin from glucuronic acid if it has not first been acted on by gut bacteria to produce urobilinogen; the free bilirubin is reabsorbed through the intestinal wall and brought back to the liver via portal vein circulation. This recycling of the bilirubin and decreased ability to clear bilirubin from the system are prevalent in babies with very high β-D-glucuronidase activity levels, those who are exclusively breastfed, and those with delayed bacterial colonization of the gut (such as with the use of antibiotics) and further increase the newborn's susceptibility to jaundice. The longer the direct bilirubin remains in the newborn's gut, the greater chance it has of becoming deconjugated. Because of this, babies who establish gut motility and active stooling through early and frequent feedings are less likely to develop physiologic jaundice. Conjugation of bilirubin in newborns is depicted in Figure 23–7.

The newborn liver has relatively less glucuronyl transferase activity in the first few weeks of life than an adult liver. This reduction in hepatic activity, along with a relatively large bilirubin load, decreases the liver's ability to conjugate bilirubin and increases susceptibility to jaundice. Jaundice (icterus) is the yellowish coloration of the skin and the sclera caused by the presence of bilirubin in elevated concentrations. *Hyperbilirubinemia* is an elevated total serum bilirubin level.

Abnormal values differ by gestational age, days of life, and presence of risk factors.

Physiologic Jaundice

Physiologic jaundice (nonpathologic unconjugated hyperbilirubinemia) develops in more than 60% of term newborns and 80% of preterm neonates. It is visible when the serum bilirubin concentration is greater than 6 to 7 mg/dL on about the second or third day (Blackburn, 2013). Usually bilirubin levels increase soon after birth because of increased bilirubin production and/or delayed bilirubin elimination, as well as by a unique neonatal phenomenon of enterohepatic recirculation of bilirubin. However, by the end of the first week of life the bilirubin levels decline. Peak bilirubin levels are reached between days 3 and 5 in the full-term newborn and between days 5 and 7 in the preterm newborn. This condition does not have a pathologic basis, but rather is a normal biologic response of the newborn. Note that these values are established for European and American White newborns. Chinese, Japanese, Korean, and Native American newborns have considerably higher bilirubin levels that are not as apparent and that persist for longer periods with no apparent ill effects (Blackburn, 2013). Because of the shorter life span of fetal RBCs, newborns have a 2 to 3 times greater production or breakdown of bilirubin. Bruising from the delivery process can also increase the amount of bilirubin to be handled by the liver. The low volume and inadequate caloric intake of the newborn's initial feedings increase reabsorption of bilirubin and are further aggravated by decreased gastrointestinal activity characteristic of the early postnatal period. Enterohepatic recirculation of bilirubin is the deconjugation and reabsorption of bilirubin that occurs in the bowel. The signs of physiologic jaundice appear *after* the first 24 hours postnatally. This differentiates physiologic jaundice from pathologic jaundice (see Chapter 27), which is clinically seen at birth or within the first 24 hours of postnatal life.

In some newborns the rise of bilirubin continues or accelerates. Thus unmonitored and untreated severe hyperbilirubinemia may progress to excessive levels that are associated with bilirubin neurotoxicity (kernicterus). All newborns should be routinely monitored for the development of jaundice, and nurseries should have protocols for the assessment of jaundice. Visual inspection is no longer considered an accurate method by itself; a combination of universal total serum bilirubin (TSB) and transcutaneous bilirubin (TcB) measurements along with a risk score is the preferred method of assessment (Muchowski, 2014). The newborn develops jaundice in cephalocaudal progression, meaning that jaundice is first seen in the face and then travels down the trunk.

Several newborn care procedures will decrease the probability of high bilirubin levels:

- Maintain the newborn's skin temperature at 36.5°C (97.8°F) or above, because cold stress results in acidosis. Acidosis in turn decreases available serum albumin-binding sites, weakens albumin-binding powers, and causes elevated unconjugated bilirubin levels.

- Monitor stool for amount and characteristics. Bilirubin is eliminated in the feces; inadequate stooling may result in reabsorption and recycling of bilirubin. Encourage early breastfeeding because the laxative effect of colostrum increases excretion of meconium and transitional stool.

- Encourage early feedings to promote intestinal elimination and bacterial colonization and provide caloric intake necessary for formation of hepatic binding proteins.

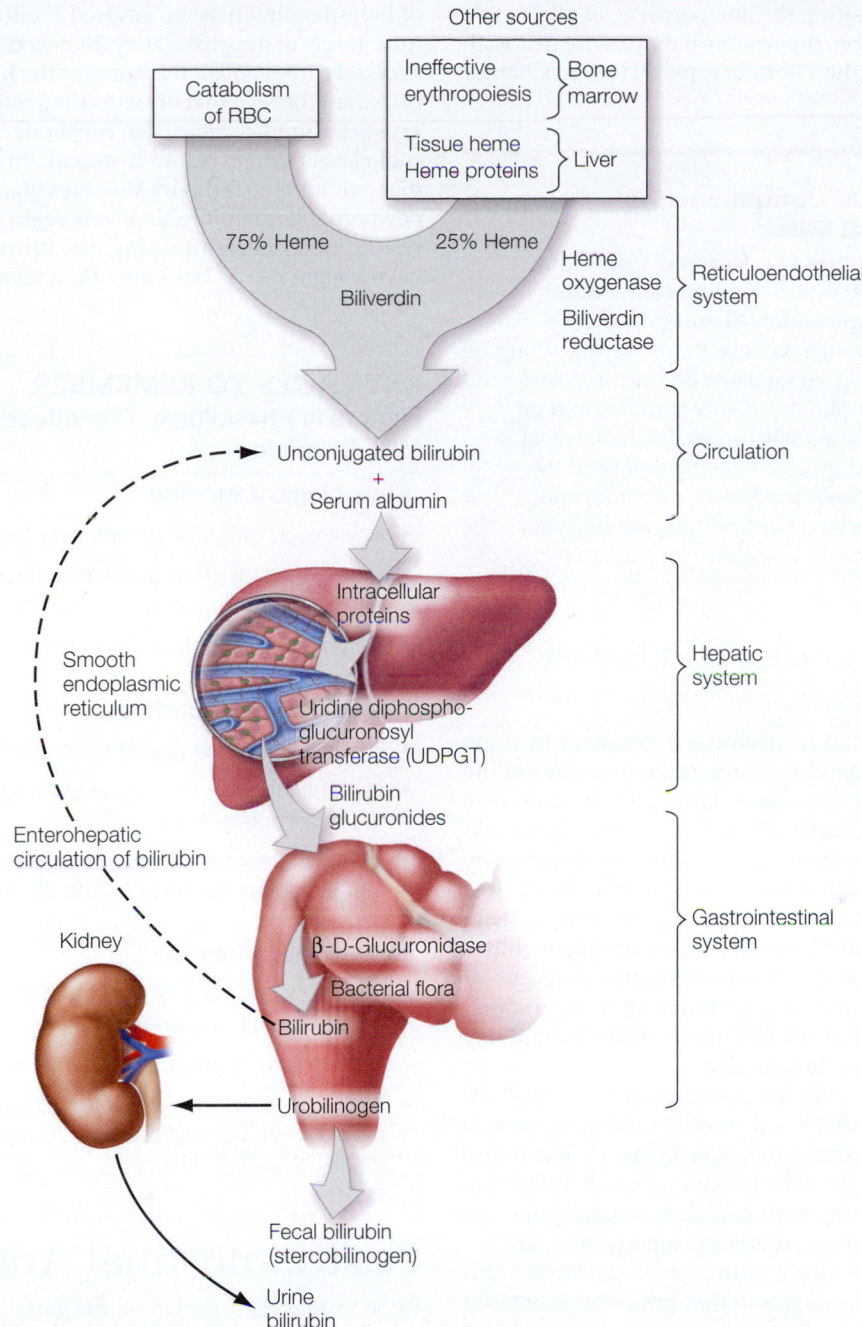

Other sources

| Ineffective erythropoiesis | Bone marrow |
| Tissue heme Heme proteins | Liver |

Catabolism of RBC

75% Heme   25% Heme

Biliverdin

Heme oxygenase

Biliverdin reductase

Reticuloendothelial system

Unconjugated bilirubin + Serum albumin

Circulation

Intracellular proteins

Smooth endoplasmic reticulum

Uridine diphospho-glucuronosyl transferase (UDPGT)

Bilirubin glucuronides

Hepatic system

Enterohepatic circulation of bilirubin

Kidney

β-D-Glucuronidase

Bacterial flora

Bilirubin

Gastrointestinal system

Urobilinogen

Fecal bilirubin (stercobilinogen)

Urine bilirubin

Figure 23–7 Conjugation of bilirubin in newborns.

Absence of jaundice, however, is not an indication of absence of hyperbilirubinemia. Therefore, screening using hour-specific bilirubin measurement and clinical risk factors can identify neonates who are likely to develop severe hyperbilirubinemia. Predischarge bilirubin screening identifies neonates with bilirubin levels higher than the 75th percentile for age in hours. Clinical risk factors for severe hyperbilirubinemia include exclusive and insufficient breast milk feedings, family history of neonatal jaundice, bruising, assisted delivery with vacuum or forceps, cephalohematoma, Asian ethnicity, maternal age (>25 years), male gender, and gestational age. (See Chapter 27 for more information.)

If jaundice becomes apparent, nursing care is directed toward keeping the newborn well hydrated and promoting intestinal elimination. For specific nursing management and therapies, see *Nursing Care Plan: For the Newborn with Hyperbilirubinemia* in Chapter 27.

Physiologic jaundice may be very upsetting to parents; they require emotional support and thorough explanation of the condition. If the baby is placed under phototherapy, a few additional days of hospitalization may be required, which may also be disturbing to parents. They can be encouraged to provide for the emotional needs of their newborn by continuing to feed, hold, and caress the baby. If the mother is discharged, the parents are encouraged to return for feedings and to telephone or visit whenever they wish. In many instances, the mother, especially if she is breastfeeding, may elect to remain hospitalized with her newborn; the nurse should support this decision. If insurance limitations make this unrealistic, it may be possible to find an empty room for the discharged mother and her family to use while visiting the newborn. As an alternative to continued hospitalization, the newborn may be treated with home phototherapy. (See the Phototherapy section in Chapter 27 for more information.)

Developing Cultural Competence Interpreting Illness Through Cultural Beliefs

Cultural beliefs lead mothers to interpret illness within their cultural framework, especially when left without clear and understood explanations (Lauderdale, 2012). For example, some Latina women believe that showing strong maternal emotions during pregnancy and during breastfeeding can be detrimental. They blame jaundice in their newborn on "bili" associated with anger. Such maternal reactions can be lessened by careful explanations to the mothers about the diagnosis, prognosis, duration, and management options for jaundice and the possibility for recurrence.

Breastfeeding Jaundice and Breast Milk Jaundice

Breastfeeding is implicated in prolonged jaundice in some newborns. *Breastfeeding jaundice* occurs in the first days of life in 12.9% of breastfeeding newborns having a bilirubin level greater than 12mg/dL (Gomella, 2013). It appears to be associated with poor feeding practices and not with any abnormality in milk composition (Hardy, D'Agata, & McGrath, 2016). It is related to inadequate fluid intake with some element of dehydration. Prevention of early breastfeeding jaundice includes encouraging frequent (every 2 to 3 hours) breastfeeding, avoiding supplementation, and accessing maternal lactation counseling. Breastfeeding jaundice is self-limiting; it peaks around day 3 as enteral intake increases, then resolves.

Breast milk jaundice occurs in approximately 2% to 4% of term newborns with onset at 4 to 7 days of life (Riley, Spencer, & Prater, 2014). The exact mechanism of true breast milk jaundice is unknown, but it is thought to be because of unidentified factors in breast milk interfering with bilirubin metabolism causing an exaggerated physiologic jaundice (Cloherty et al., 2012).

In contrast to breastfeeding jaundice, breast milk jaundice is related to a milk composition that promotes increased bilirubin reabsorption from the intestine. Some women's breast milk contains several times the normal concentration of certain free fatty acids. These free fatty acids may compete with bilirubin for binding sites on albumin and inhibit the conjugation of bilirubin or increase lipase activity, which disrupts the RBC membrane. Increased lipase activity enhances absorption of bile across the gastrointestinal tract membrane, thereby increasing the enterohepatic circulation of bilirubin.

Clinical Tip

Encourage and support mothers who desire to breastfeed their babies. Assist and instruct them on how to pump and express milk during the interrupted breastfeeding period. Reassure them that nothing is wrong with their milk or mothering abilities.

Newborns with breastfeeding jaundice appear well, and at this time, development of kernicterus (toxic levels of bilirubin in the brain) has not been documented. Temporary cessation of breastfeeding may be advised if bilirubin reaches presumed toxic levels of approximately 20 mg/dL or if the interruption is necessary to establish the cause of the hyperbilirubinemia. Most physicians believe that breastfeeding may be resumed once other causes of jaundice have been ruled out and as long as serum bilirubin levels remain below 20 mg/dL. In cases of breast milk jaundice, within 24 to 36 hours after breastfeeding is discontinued, the newborn's serum bilirubin levels begin to fall dramatically. With resumption of breastfeeding, the bilirubin concentration may have a slight rise of 2 to 3 mg/dL, with a subsequent decline.

KEY FACTS TO REMEMBER
Factors in Physiologic, Breastfeeding, and Breast Milk Jaundice

Physiologic Jaundice

- Physiologic jaundice occurs after the first 24 hours of life.
- During the first week of life, bilirubin should not exceed 13 mg/dL. Some pediatricians allow levels up to 15 mg/dL.
- Bilirubin levels peak at 3 to 5 days in term newborns.

Breastfeeding Jaundice

- Bilirubin levels rise after the first 24 hours of age.
- Peaks on third or fourth day of life and declines through first month to normal levels.
- Incidence can be decreased by increasing the number of breastfeeding episodes to 8 to 12 in 24 hours.

Breast Milk Jaundice

- Bilirubin levels begin to rise after the first week of life when mature breast milk comes in.
- Peak of 5 to 10 mg/dL is reached at 2 to 3 weeks of age.
- It may be necessary to interrupt breastfeeding for a short period when bilirubin reaches 20 mg/dL.

Gastrointestinal Adaptations

By 36 to 38 weeks' gestation, the gastrointestinal system is adequately mature, with enzymatic activity and the ability to transport nutrients.

Digestion and Absorption

The full-term newborn has sufficient intestinal and pancreatic enzymes to digest most simple carbohydrates, proteins, and fats. The carbohydrates requiring digestion in the newborn are usually disaccharides (lactose, maltose, sucrose), which are split into monosaccharides (galactose, fructose, and glucose) by the enzymes of the intestinal mucosa. Lactose is the primary carbohydrate in the breastfeeding newborn and is generally easily digested and well absorbed. The only enzyme lacking is pancreatic amylase, which remains relatively deficient during the first few months of life. Newborns have trouble digesting starches (changing more complex carbohydrates into maltose), so they should not eat solids until after the first 6 months of life.

Although proteins require more digestion than carbohydrates, they are well digested and absorbed from the newborn intestine. The newborn digests and absorbs fats less efficiently because of the minimal activity of the pancreatic enzyme lipase. The newborn excretes about 10% to 20% of the dietary fat intake, compared with 10% for the adult. The newborn absorbs the fat in breast milk more completely than the fat in cows' milk, because breast milk consists of more medium-chain triglycerides and contains lipase.(See Chapter 25 for further discussion of newborn nutrition.)

Healthy People 2020

(MICH-21) Increase the proportion of infants who are breastfed

The fetal gastrointestinal tract is sterile. Microbes begin to establish as soon as the neonate's oral mucosa is exposed to the environment. The gastrointestinal microbiota is important in the development of immune tolerance to allergens. The mode of delivery sets the pattern of gastrointestinal tract colonization. Babies born by vaginal delivery become colonized by microbes present in the birth canal and mother's gastrointestinal tract, whereas babies born by cesarean section are initially colonized by skin flora (Sim, Powell, Shaw, et al., 2012). The establishment and type of feeding are major factors influencing the composition of gastrointestinal tract microbes. Formula-fed babies have elevated levels of the bacteria *Clostridia* and *Bacteroides,* while the microbiota of breastfed babies has abundant *Bifidobacteria* because of natural prebiotics in human breast milk (Sim et al., 2012). Breast milk confers significant anti-infective benefits.

By birth, the newborn has experienced swallowing, gastric emptying, and intestinal propulsion. In utero, fetal swallowing is accompanied by gastric emptying and peristalsis of the fetal intestinal tract. By the end of gestation, peristalsis becomes much more active in preparation for extrauterine life. Fetal peristalsis is also stimulated by anoxia, causing the expulsion of meconium into the amniotic fluid in postterm fetuses.

Air enters the stomach immediately after birth. The small intestine is filled with air within 2 to 12 hours and the large bowel within 24 hours. The salivary glands are immature at birth, and the newborn produces little saliva until about age 3 months. The newborn's stomach has a capacity of about 50 to 60 mL. It empties intermittently, starting within a few minutes of the beginning of a feeding and ending 2 to 4 hours after feeding. Bowel sounds are present within the first 30 to 60 minutes of birth and the newborn can successfully feed during this time. The newborn's gastric pH becomes less acidic about a week after birth and remains less acidic than that of adults for the next 2 to 3 months.

The cardiac sphincter is immature, as is neural control of the stomach, so some regurgitation may be noted in the newborn period. Regurgitation of the first few feedings during the first day or two of life can usually be lessened by avoiding overfeeding and by burping the newborn well during and after the feeding.

When no other signs and symptoms are evident, vomiting is limited and ceases within the first few days of life. Continuous vomiting or regurgitation should be observed closely. If the newborn has swallowed bloody or purulent amniotic fluid, lavage of the stomach may be indicated in the term newborn to relieve the problem. Bilious vomiting is abnormal and must be evaluated thoroughly because it might represent a condition that warrants prompt surgical intervention.

Adequate digestion and absorption are essential for newborn growth and development. If optimal nutritional support is available, postnatal growth should parallel intrauterine growth; that is, after 30 weeks' gestation, the fetus gains 30.0 g (1.05 oz) per day and adds 1.2 cm (0.5 in.) to body length daily. To gain weight at the intrauterine rate, the term newborn requires 120 cal/kg/day. Following birth, caloric intake is often insufficient for weight gain until the newborn is 5 to 10 days old. During this time, there may be a weight loss of 5% to 10% in term newborns. A shift of intracellular water to extracellular space and insensible water loss account for the 5% to 10% weight loss; thus failure to lose weight when caloric intake is inadequate may indicate fluid retention.

Clinical Reasoning   Newborn Weight Loss

Jonathon Sykes is a 5-day-old term male baby who has returned to the hospital for a lactation visit. Jonathon's birth weight was 3260 grams (7.2 lb) and his current weight is 2963 grams (6.5 lb). The lactation nurse is worried about this weight loss and shares her concerns with Jonathon's mother.

What would you tell Jonathon's mother about his weight loss since birth? What are other questions you might ask Jonathon's mother about his daily habits? Based on his birth weight, what is the appropriate number of kilocalories that Jonathon needs in order to grow?

Elimination

Term newborns usually pass meconium within 8 to 24 hours of life and almost always within 48 hours. **Meconium** is formed in utero from the amniotic fluid and its constituents, intestinal secretions, and shed mucosal cells. It is recognized by its thick, tarry black or dark green appearance. Transitional (thin brown to green) stools consisting of part meconium and part fecal material are passed for the next day or two, and then the stools become entirely fecal. Generally the stools of a breastfed newborn are pale yellow (but may be pasty green); they are more liquid and more frequent than those of formula-fed newborns, whose stools are paler and often the consistency of peanut butter (see Figure 25–24). Frequency of bowel movement varies but ranges from one every 2 to 3 days to as many as 10 daily. Totally breastfed newborns often progress to stools that occur every 5 to 7 days. Mothers should be counseled that the newborn is not constipated as long as the bowel movement remains soft.

KEY FACTS TO REMEMBER
Physiologic Adaptations to Extrauterine Life

- Periodic breathing may be present.
- Desired axillary temperature of 36.5° to 37.5°C (97.7° to 99.5°F) stabilizes 4 to 6 hours after birth for term newborn (Cloherty et al., 2012).
- Desired blood glucose level reaches 60 to 70 mg/dL by third postnatal day.
- Stools progress from (for detailed discussion see Chapter 25):
  - Meconium (thick, tarry, black; meconium plug may be expelled)
  - Transitional stools (thin, brown to green)
  - Breastfed newborns (yellow-gold, soft, or mushy)
  - Formula-fed newborns (pale yellow, formed, and pasty)

Urinary Tract Adaptations

Kidney Development and Function

In utero the placenta is the organ responsible for fluid and electrolyte homeostasis. After birth the kidney assumes the role of regulation. The kidney is structurally developed with a full complement of functioning nephrons by 34 to 36 weeks of gestation.

Glomerular filtration occurs as blood passes through the capillaries and plasma is filtered through the glomerular capillary walls. Filtrate is collected in the Bowman space and the tubules, where composition is modified until it is excreted as urine. Glomerular filtration rate (GFR) doubles in the first 2 weeks of life in term neonates to 30 to 40 mL/minute (Parker, 2014). The neonate's ability to dilute urine is fully developed, but concentrating ability is limited (Parker, 2014). A major function of the kidney is to maintain osmolality of extracellular fluid within the narrow range compatible with optimal cellular function. The ability to concentrate urine fully is attained by 3 months of age. Feeding practices may affect the osmolarity of the urine but have limited effect on concentration of the urine.

Characteristics of Newborn Urinary Function

Many newborns void immediately after birth, and the voiding frequently goes unnoticed. Among normal newborns, 90% void by 24 hours after birth and 99% void by 48 hours after birth (Cloherty et al., 2012). A newborn who has not voided by 48 hours should be assessed for adequacy of fluid intake, bladder distention, restlessness, and symptoms of pain. The appropriate clinical personnel should be notified if indicated.

The initial bladder volume is 6 to 44 mL of urine. Unless edema is present, normal urinary output is often limited, and the voidings are scanty until fluid intake increases. (The fluid of edema is eliminated by the kidneys, so newborns with edema have a much higher urinary output.) The first 2 days postnatally, the newborn voids two to six times daily, with a urine output of 15 mL/kg/day. The newborn subsequently voids 5 to 25 times every 24 hours, with a volume of 25 mL/kg/day. Observation and documentation of adequate output is necessary given the large number of term newborns who have early hospital discharge.

Following the first voiding, the newborn's urine frequently appears cloudy (because of mucus content) and has a high specific gravity, which decreases as fluid intake increases. Occasionally pink stains ("brick dust spots") appear on the diaper. These are caused by urates and are innocuous. Blood may occasionally be observed on the diapers of female newborns. This *pseudomenstruation* is related to the withdrawal of maternal hormones. Males may have bloody spotting from a circumcision if performed. In the absence of apparent causes for bleeding, the clinician should be notified. During early infancy, normal urine is straw colored and almost odorless, although odor occurs when certain drugs are given, metabolic disorders exist, or infection is present. Table 23–3 contains urinalysis values for the normal newborn.

Immunologic Adaptations

Neonatal defense against infections in utero or after delivery is dependent on maternal immunity because neonates lack immunologic memory and often have slower capacities to develop

TABLE 23–3 Newborn Urinalysis Values

Protein: <5–10 mg/dL
WBC: <2–3/hpf
RBC: 0
Casts: 0
Bacteria: 0
Color: pale yellow

immune responses (Futata, Fusaro, de Brito, et al., 2012). Maternal–fetal infection transmission (transplacental, perinatal, postnatal) is a major cause of morbidity and mortality in newborns. Limitations in the newborn's inflammatory response result in failure to recognize, localize, and destroy invasive bacteria. Thus the signs and symptoms of infection are often subtle and nonspecific in the newborn. The newborn also has a poor hypothalamic response to pyrogens; therefore fever is not a reliable indicator of infection. In the neonatal period, hypothermia is a more reliable sign of infection (Futata et al., 2012).

Nonspecific immune mechanisms include phagocytosis, inflammatory response, complement, and coagulation. These nonspecific immune mechanisms function without prior exposure, can be identified early in gestation, and reach functional development at 32 to 33 weeks' gestation.

The specific immune responses consist of cell-mediated (T cell) and humoral (B cell) systems. The maturation of specific immune responses begins in utero at about 7 to 12 weeks' gestation. The newborn's immune system has a decreased ability to develop effective antibody responses. Humoral immunity is a specific antibody-mediated response that functions most effectively if there has been recent exposure.

Of the three major types of immunoglobulins that are primarily involved in immunity—IgG, IgA, and IgM—only IgG crosses the placenta. The pregnant woman forms antibodies in response to illness or immunization. This process is called **active acquired immunity**. When IgG antibodies are transferred to the fetus in utero, **passive acquired immunity** results, because the fetus does not produce the antibodies itself. IgG antibodies are very active against bacterial toxins.

Because the maternal immunoglobulin is transferred primarily during the third trimester, preterm newborns (especially those born before 34 weeks' gestation) may be more susceptible to infection. In general, newborns have maternally induced immunity to tetanus, diphtheria, smallpox, measles, mumps, poliomyelitis, and a variety of other bacterial and viral diseases. The period of resistance varies: Immunity against common viral infections such as measles may last 4 to 8 months, whereas immunity to certain bacteria may disappear within 4 to 8 weeks. It is customary to begin the majority of routine immunizations at 2 months of age so that the infant can develop active acquired immunity. Some immunizations for specific viruses (such as hepatitis B) are even given in the first day after birth. (For discussion of newborn immunization, see Chapter 25.)

IgM antibodies are produced in response to blood group antigens, gram-negative enteric organisms, and some viruses in the expectant mother. Because IgM does not normally cross the placenta, most or all of it is produced by the fetus beginning at 10 to 15 weeks' gestation. Elevated levels of IgM at birth may indicate placental leaks or, more commonly, antigenic stimulation in utero. Consequently, elevations suggest that the newborn was exposed to an intrauterine infection such as syphilis or TORCH syndrome (toxoplasmosis, rubella, cytomegalovirus, herpesvirus hominis type 2 infection). (For further discussion of intrauterine infections, see Chapter 15.) The lack of available maternal IgM in the newborn also accounts for the susceptibility to gram-negative enteric organisms such as *Escherichia coli*.

IgA immunoglobins appear to provide protection mainly on secreting surfaces such as the respiratory tract, gastrointestinal tract, and eyes. Serum IgA does not cross the placenta and is not normally produced by the fetus in utero. Unlike the other immunoglobulins, IgA is not affected by gastric action. Colostrum, the forerunner of breast milk, is very high in the secretory form of IgA. Consequently it may be of significance in providing some passive immunity to the baby of a breastfeeding mother. Newborns begin to produce secretory IgA in their intestinal mucosa about 4 weeks after birth.

Neurologic Adaptations

The newborn's brain is about one quarter the size of an adult's, and myelination of nerve fibers is incomplete. Unlike the cardiovascular and respiratory systems, which undergo tremendous changes at birth, the nervous system is minimally influenced by the actual birth process. Because many biochemical and histologic changes have yet to occur in the newborn's brain, the postnatal period is considered a time of risk with regard to the development of the brain and nervous system. For neurologic development—including development of intellect—to proceed, the brain and other nervous system structures must mature in an orderly, unhampered fashion. (For discussion of cranial nerves, see Chapter 24.)

Intrauterine Environment Influence on Newborn Behavior

Newborns respond to and interact with the environment in a predictable pattern of behavior that is somewhat shaped by their intrauterine experience. This intrauterine experience is affected by intrinsic factors such as maternal nutrition and external factors such as the mother's physical environment. Depending on the newborn's intrauterine experience and individual temperament, neonatal behavioral responses to different stresses vary. Some newborns react quietly to stimulation, others become overreactive and tense, and some may exhibit a combination of the two.

Factors such as exposure to intense auditory stimuli in utero can eventually be manifested in the behavior of the newborn. For example, the fetal heart rate (FHR) initially increases when the pregnant woman is exposed to auditory stimuli, but repetition of the stimuli leads to decreased FHR. Thus the newborn who was exposed to intense noise during fetal life is significantly less reactive to loud sounds postnatally.

Characteristics of Newborn Neurologic Function

Normal newborns are usually in a position of partially flexed extremities with the legs near the abdomen. When awake, the newborn may exhibit purposeless, uncoordinated bilateral movements of the extremities. The organization and quality of the newborn's motor activity are influenced by a number of factors, including the following (Nugent, 2013):

- Sleep–alert states
- Presence of environmental stimuli, such as heat, light, cold, and noise

- Conditions causing a chemical imbalance, such as hypoglycemia
- Hydration status
- State of health
- Recovery from the stress of labor and birth

The newborn's body growth progresses in a cephalocaudal (head-to-toe), proximal-distal fashion. The newborn is somewhat hypertonic; that is, there is resistance to extending the elbow and knee joints. Muscle tone should be symmetrical. Diminished muscle tone and flaccidity may indicate neurologic dysfunction.

Reflexes, including the Moro, grasping, Babinski, rooting, and sucking reflexes, are characteristic of neurologic integrity. (For discussion of reflexes see Chapter 24.) Complex behavioral patterns reflect the newborn's neurologic maturation and integration. Newborns who can bring their hands to their mouths may be demonstrating motor coordination as well as a self-quieting technique, thus increasing the complexity of the behavioral response. **Self-quieting ability** is the ability of newborns to use their own resources to quiet and comfort themselves.

Habituation is the newborn's ability to process and respond to complex stimulation. For example, when a bright light is flashed into the newborn's eyes, the initial response is blinking, constriction of the pupil, and perhaps a slight startle reaction. However, with repeated stimulation, the newborn's responses gradually diminish and disappear. The capacity to ignore repetitious disturbing stimuli is a newborn defense mechanism that readily allows the newborn to shut out overwhelming and disturbing stimuli. Sensory abilities include visual, auditory, olfactory, taste, and tactile capacities.

Periods of Reactivity

The baby usually shows a predictable pattern of behavior during the first several hours after birth, characterized by two **periods of reactivity** separated by a sleep phase.

FIRST PERIOD OF REACTIVITY

The first period of reactivity lasts approximately 30 minutes after birth. During this period the newborn is awake and active and may appear hungry and have a strong sucking reflex. This is an optimal period for parent–newborn bonding as well as a natural opportunity to initiate breastfeeding if the mother has chosen it. Bursts of random, diffuse movements alternating with relative immobility may occur. Respirations are rapid, as high as 80 breaths per minute, and there may be retraction of the chest, transient flaring of the nares, and grunting. The heart rate is rapid, and the rhythm may be irregular. Bowel sounds are usually absent.

PERIOD OF INACTIVITY TO SLEEP PHASE

After approximately half an hour the newborn's activity gradually diminishes, and the heart rate and respirations decrease as the newborn enters the sleep phase. The sleep phase may last from a few minutes to 2 to 4 hours. During this period, the newborn will be difficult to awaken and will show no interest in sucking. Bowel sounds become audible, and cardiac and respiratory rates return to baseline values.

SECOND PERIOD OF REACTIVITY

During the second period of reactivity, the newborn is again awake and alert. This period lasts 4 to 6 hours in the normal newborn. Physiologic responses are variable during this stage. The heart and respiratory rates increase; however, the nurse must be alert for apneic periods, which may cause a drop in the heart rate and oxygen level (desaturation). The newborn is stimulated to continue breathing during such times. The newborn may develop rapid color changes and become mildly cyanotic or mottled during these fluctuations. Production of respiratory and gastric mucus increases, and the newborn responds by gagging, choking, and regurgitating.

SAFETY ALERT!

Because newborns are often unable to handle oral secretions effectively enough to protect their airway, parents must be instructed in the proper use of the bulb syringe. The bulb syringe used correctly creates mild suction for removal of oral and nasal secretions. Overuse or vigorous use of the bulb syringe causes unnecessary trauma and inflammation of the small nasal airways, resulting in swelling and partial airway obstruction. (See *Clinical Skill: Performing Nasal Pharyngeal Suctioning* in Chapter 18.)

Continued close observation and intervention may be required to maintain a clear airway during this period of reactivity. The gastrointestinal tract becomes more active. The newborn often passes the first meconium stool and may also have an initial voiding. The newborn will indicate readiness for feeding by such behaviors as sucking, rooting, and swallowing. If feeding was not initiated in the first period of reactivity, it is done at this time. (See Newborn Feeding in Chapter 25 for further discussion of the first feeding.)

Behavioral States of the Newborn

The behavior of the newborn can be divided into two categories, the sleep state and the awake or alert state (McGrath & Vittner, 2015; Gardner, Goldson, & Hernandez, 2016). These postnatal behavioral states are similar to those that have been identified during pregnancy. Subcategories are identified under each major category.

SLEEP STATES

The sleep states are as follows:

1. **Deep or quiet sleep.** Deep sleep is characterized by closed eyes with no eye movements; regular, even breathing; and jerky motions or startles at regular intervals. Behavioral responses to external stimuli are likely to be delayed. Startles are rapidly suppressed, and changes in state are not likely to occur. Heart rate may range from 100 to 120 beats per minute.

2. **Active or light sleep (rapid-eye-movement [REM] sleep).** The baby has irregular respirations; eyes closed, with REM; irregular sucking motions; minimal activity; and irregular but smooth movement of the extremities. Environmental and internal stimuli may initiate a startle reaction and a change of state.

Newborn sleep cycles have been recognized and defined according to duration. The length of the sleep cycle depends on the age of the newborn. At term, REM active sleep and quiet sleep occur in intervals of 50 to 60 minutes (Gardner et al., 2016). About 45% to 50% of the newborn's total sleep is active sleep, 35% to 45% is quiet sleep, and 10% is transitional between these two periods. Growth hormone secretion depends on regular sleep patterns. Any disturbance of the sleep–wake cycle can result in irregular spikes of growth hormone. REM sleep stimulates the highest peaks of growth hormone and the growth of the neural system. Over a period of time, the newborn's sleep–wake patterns become diurnal; that is, the newborn sleeps at night and stays awake during the day. (See Assessment of Neurologic Status in Chapter 24 for a short discussion of Brazelton's assessment of newborn states.)

ALERT STATES

In the first 30 to 60 minutes after birth, many newborns display a quiet alert state, characteristic of the first period of reactivity (Figure 23–8). Nurses should use these alert states to encourage bonding and breastfeeding. These periods of alertness tend to be short the first 2 days after birth to allow the baby to recover from the birth process. Subsequent alert states are of choice or of necessity (Gardner et al., 2016). The newborn's increasing choice of wakefulness indicates a maturing capacity to achieve and maintain consciousness. Heat, cold, and hunger are but a few of the stimuli that can cause wakefulness by necessity. Once the disturbing stimuli are removed, the baby tends to fall back asleep.

The following are subcategories of the alert state (Gardner et al., 2016):

1. *Drowsy or semidozing.* The behaviors common to the drowsy state are open or closed eyes; fluttering eyelids; semidozing appearance; and slow, regular movements of the extremities. Mild startles may be noted from time to time. Although the reaction to a sensory stimulus is delayed, a change of state often results.

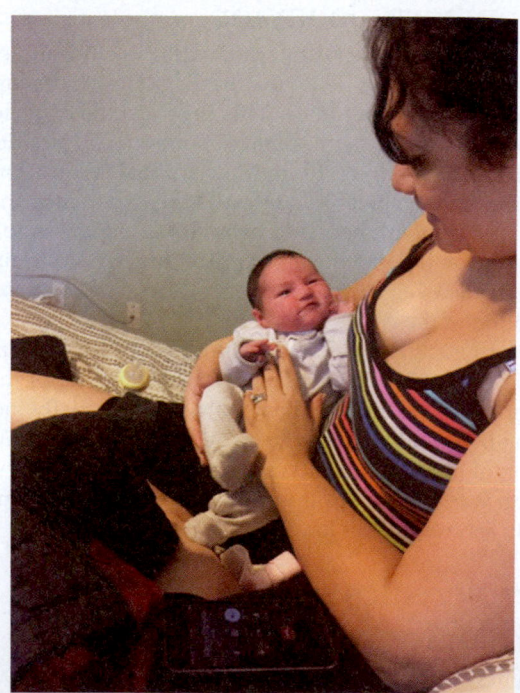

Figure 23–8 Mother and newborn baby gaze at each other. This quiet, alert state is the optimum state for interaction.

SOURCE: Craig London.

2. *Quiet alert.* The newborn is alert and follows and fixates on attractive objects, faces, or auditory stimuli. Motor activity is minimal, and the response to external stimuli is delayed.

3. *Active alert.* The eyes are open and motor activity is quite intense, with thrusting movements of the extremities. Environmental stimuli increase startles or motor activity, but individual reactions are difficult to distinguish because of the generally high activity level.

4. *Crying.* Intense crying is accompanied by jerky motor movements. Crying serves several purposes for the newborn. It may be a distraction from disturbing stimuli such as hunger and pain. Fussiness often allows the newborn to discharge energy and reorganize behavior. Most important, crying elicits an appropriate response of help from the parents. See Crying in Chapter 29 for calming techniques the nurse can teach parents.

Clinical Tip

While the mother–newborn couplet is in the hospital, the nurse has a perfect opportunity to teach parents techniques to deal with newborn/infant crying and fussiness. Most important, it is necessary for parents and caregivers to know that for the first several months crying is the only means of communication available to the baby and usually signifies unmet needs.

Sensory Capacities of the Newborn

VISUAL CAPACITY

Orientation is the newborn's ability to be alert to, to follow, and to fixate on appealing and attractive complex visual stimuli. The newborn prefers the human face and eyes and high-contrast objects and patterns. The newborn is nearsighted and has best vision at a distance of 8 to 15 inches. As the face or object comes into the line of vision, the newborn responds with bright, wide eyes, still limbs, and fixed staring. The intense visual involvement may last several minutes, during which time the newborn is able to follow the stimulus from side to side (Figure 23–9).

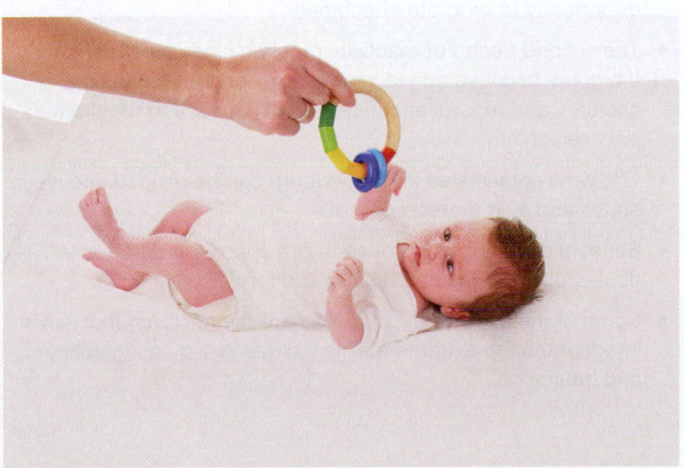

Figure 23–9 Newborn in active alert state turning his head to follow an object.

The newborn uses this sensory capacity to become familiar with family, friends, and surroundings.

AUDITORY CAPACITY

The newborn responds to auditory stimulation with a definite, organized behavior repertoire. The stimulus used to assess auditory response should be selected to match the state of the newborn. A rattle is appropriate for light sleep, a voice for an awake state, and a clap for deep sleep. As the newborn hears the sound, the cardiac rate rises, and a minimal startle reflex may be seen. If the sound is appealing, the newborn will become alert and search for the site of the auditory stimulus. Newborns prefer the sound of the human voice to nonhuman sounds and have very acute hearing immediately after birth. The newborn's hearing should be evaluated prior to discharge. (See Chapter 25 for discussion of newborn hearing screening tests).

Healthy People 2020

(ENT-VSL-1) Increase the proportion of newborns who are screened for hearing loss by no later than age 1 month, have audiologic evaluation by age 3 months, and are enrolled in appropriate intervention services no later than age 6 months

OLFACTORY CAPACITY

Newborns can select their mother by smell rapidly, and can differentiate their mother by smell within the first week of life (Lehtonen, 2015). Newborns are able to distinguish their mothers' breast pads from those of other mothers at just 1 week postnatally and will turn preferentially toward the mother's odor.

TASTE AND SUCKING

Newborns respond differently to varying tastes. They can distinguish between sweet and sour at 3 days of age. Sugar, for example, increases sucking. Newborns fed with a rubber nipple versus the breast also show sucking pattern variations. When breastfeeding, the newborn sucks in bursts, with frequent regular pauses. The bottle-fed newborn tends to suck at a regular rate, with infrequent pauses.

When awake and hungry, the newborn displays rapid searching motions in response to the rooting reflex. Once feeding begins, the newborn establishes a sucking pattern according to the method of feeding. Finger sucking happens not only postnatally, but also in utero. The newborn frequently uses nonnutritive sucking as a self-quieting activity, which assists in the development of self-regulation.

TACTILE CAPACITY

The newborn is very sensitive to being touched, cuddled, and held; thus touch may be the most important of all the senses. Often a mother's first response to an upset or crying newborn is touching or holding. Swaddling, placing a hand on the abdomen, or holding the arms to prevent a startle reflex are other methods of soothing the newborn. The settled newborn is then able to attend to and interact with the environment. Touch is also used to rouse drowsy babies, making them more alert for feeding.

Focus Your Study

- Newborn respiration is initiated primarily by chemical and mechanical events in association with thermal and sensory stimulation.

- The production of surfactant is crucial to keeping the lungs expanded during expiration by reducing alveolar surface tension.

- Onset of respirations stimulates cardiovascular changes: Air enters the lungs; oxygen content rises in alveoli and stimulates relaxation of pulmonary arteries. This leads to a decrease in pulmonary vascular resistance, which allows complete vascular flow to the lungs. With increased oxygenated pulmonary blood flow and loss of the placenta, systemic blood flow increases and the foramen ovale and ductus arteriosus begin to close.

- The newborn is an obligatory nose breather. Respirations change from being primarily shallow, irregular, and diaphragmatic to synchronous abdominal and chest breathing.

- Normal respiratory rate is 30 to 60 beats per minute.

- The status of the cardiopulmonary system may be measured by evaluating the heart rate, blood pressure, and presence or absence of murmurs. The normal heart rate is 80 to 160 beats per minute.

- Oxygen transport in the newborn is significantly affected by the presence of greater amounts of HbF (fetal hemoglobin) than HbA (adult hemoglobin); HbF holds oxygen more easily but releases it to the body tissues only at low PO_2 levels.

- Blood values in the newborn are modified by several factors, such as the site of the blood sample, gestational age, prenatal and/or perinatal hemorrhage, and the timing of the clamping of the umbilical cord.

- The newborn is considered to have established thermoregulation when oxygen consumption and metabolic activity are minimal.

- Evaporation is the primary heat loss mechanism in newborns who are wet from amniotic fluid or a bath. In addition, excessive heat loss occurs from radiation and convection, because of the newborn's larger surface area compared with weight, and from thermal conduction, because of the marked difference between core temperature and skin temperature.

- The primary source of heat production in the cold-stressed newborn is brown adipose tissue.

- By secreting glucagon and suppressing insulin release, newborns gradually mobilize glucose to meet their energy needs.

- Blood glucose levels should reach a steady state by 3 hours of age.

- The newborn's liver plays a crucial role in iron storage, carbohydrate metabolism, conjugation of bilirubin, and coagulation.

- Jaundice (icterus) is the yellowish coloration of the skin and the sclera. It may develop because of accelerated destruction of fetal RBCs, impaired conjugation of bilirubin, and increased bilirubin reabsorption from the intestinal tract.

- The newborn possesses the ability to digest and absorb nutrients necessary for growth and development but has trouble digesting starches.

- The newborn's stools change from meconium (thick, tarry, dark green) to transitional stools (thin, brown-to-green), and then to the distinct forms for either breastfed newborns (yellow-gold, soft, or mushy) or formula-fed newborns (pale yellow, formed, and pasty). Most newborns pass their first stool within 24 to 48 hours of birth.

- The newborn's kidneys are characterized by a decreased rate of glomerular flow, limited tubular reabsorption, limited excretion of solutes, and limited ability to concentrate urine. Most newborns void within 24 hours of birth.

- The immune system in the newborn is not fully activated until it begins to produce its own immunity at about 4 weeks of age. The newborn does possess some immunologic abilities and has passive immunity from the mother, lasting from 4 weeks to 8 months.

- Neurologic and sensory-perceptual functioning in the newborn is evident from the newborn's interaction with the environment, presence of synchronized motor activity, and well-developed sensory capacities.

- The first period of reactivity lasts for 30 minutes after birth. The newborn is alert and hungry at this time, making this a natural opportunity to promote attachment.

- The second period of reactivity requires close monitoring by the nurse because apnea, decreased heart rate, gagging, choking, and regurgitation are likely to occur and require nursing intervention.

- The behavioral states in the newborn can be divided into sleep states and alert states.

- Sensory development proceeds in a specific order: tactile/vestibular, olfactory/gustatory, and auditory/visual.

- Some of the behavioral capabilities of the newborn that assist in adaptation to extrauterine life include self-quieting ability and habitation.

Clinical Reasoning in Action

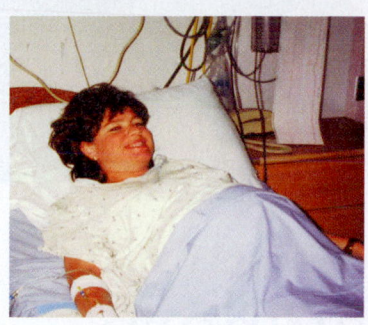

Sandra Dee, a 21-year-old, G1P0, at 36 weeks' gestation, has been in labor for the last 12 hours and is fully dilated with caput visible on the perineum. The fetal heart rate is 148 to 152 with early deceleration down to 142 with contraction and pushing. Her contractions are 4 to 5 minutes apart and of good quality. Sandra's mother and sister are present for the birth. Her prenatal record shows no significant pregnancy problems or complications, and her vital signs have been stable within normal limits. Sandra has received two doses of Stadol for a total of 2 mg IV for pain relief during her labor. The last dose was given 2 hours ago. You assist with the vaginal birth of a live baby without an episiotomy. You observe the gender and the time as the midwife places the newborn girl on the mother's abdomen, suctions out the baby's mouth and nose, and proceeds to clamp the cord. You dry the baby and stimulate her to breathe, remove the wet blanket and replace it with a dry one, and place the baby skin-to-skin on the mother's chest. You assess the need for resuscitation. The baby has a lusty cry spontaneously less than 30 seconds after birth. You palpate the cord, obtaining a heart rate of 120, and observe that the baby's chest and face are pink, and the legs and arms are flexed with open fists.

1. Explain the changes that must occur in the newborn's cardiopulmonary system at birth.
2. What criteria do you look for when you assess the newborn for adequate cardiopulmonary adaptation at birth?
3. What steps do you take to maintain a neutral thermal environment at birth?
4. Sandra plans to breastfeed. When would you initiate the first feeding?
5. Discuss nursing actions that can decrease the probability of high bilirubin levels in the newborn.

References

American College of Obstetricians and Gynecologists (ACOG). (2012, reaffirmed 2014). Timing of umbilical cord clamping after birth. *Committee on Obstetric Practice, 120*(6).

Bagwell, G. A. (2014). Hematologic system. In C. Kenner & J. W. Lott (Eds.), *Comprehensive neonatal nursing care* (5th ed., pp. 334–375). New York, NY: Springer.

Berger, T. M. (2012). Neonatal resuscitation: Foetal physiology and pathophysiological aspects. *European Journal of Anaesthesiology, 29*, 362–370.

Blackburn, S. T. (2013). *Maternal, fetal, & neonatal physiology: A clinical perspective* (4th ed.). St. Louis, MO: Saunders.

Cloherty, J. R., Eichenwald, E. C., Hansen, A. R., & Stark, A. R. (2012). *Manual of neonatal care* (7th ed.). Philadelphia, PA: Lippincott Williams & Wilkins.

Diab, Y. & Luchtman-Jones, L., (2015). The blood and hematopoietic system. In R. J. Martin, A. A. Fanaroff, & M. C. Walsh (Eds.), *Fanaroff & Martin's neonatal-perinatal medicine* (10th ed., pp. 1294–1343). St. Louis, MO: Elsevier-Mosby.

Fraser, D. (2014). Newborn adaptation to extrauterine life. In K. R. Simpson & P. A. Creehan (Eds.). *Perinatal Nursing* (4th ed., pp.581–596). Philadelphia, PA: Lippincott Williams & Wilkins

Futata, E. A., Fusaro, A. E., de Brito, C. A., & Sato, M. N. (2012). The neonatal immune system: Immunomodulation of infections in early life. *Expert Reviews: Anti-Infective Therapies 10*(3), 289–298.

Gardner, S. L., Goldson, E., & Hernandez, J. A. (2016). The neonate and the environment: Impact on development. In S. L. Gardner, B. S. Carter, M. Enzman-Hines, & J. A. Hernandez (Eds.), *Merenstein & Gardner's handbook of neonatal intensive care* (7th ed., pp. 262–314). St. Louis, MO: Elsevier.

Gomella, T. L. (Ed.). (2013). *Neonatology: Management, procedures, on-call problems, diseases, and drugs* (7th ed.). New York, NY: McGraw-Hill Education.

Graves, B. W., & Haley, M. M. (2013). Newborn transition. *Journal of Midwifery & Women's Health, 58* (6), 662–670.

Hardy, W., D'Agata, A., & McGrath, J. M. (2016). The infant at risk. In S. Mattson & J. E. Smith (Eds.), *Core curriculum for maternal-newborn nursing* (5th ed., pp. 363–416). St. Louis, MO: Saunders.

Katheria, A. C., Truong, G., Cousins, L., Oshiro, B., & Finer, N. N. (2015). Umbilical cord milking versus delayed cord clamping in preterm infants. *Pediatrics 136* (1), 61–69. doi:10.1542/peds.2015-0368

Lauderdale, J. (2012). Transcultural perspectives in childbearing. In M. M. Andrews & J. S. Boyle (Eds.), *Transcultural concepts in nursing care* (6th ed., pp. 91–122). Philadelphia, PA: Wolters Kluwer/ Lippincott Williams & Wilkins.

Lehtonen, L., (2015). Assessment and optimization of neurobehavioral development in preterm infant. In R. J. Martin, A. A. Fanaroff, & M. C. Walsh (Eds.), *Fanaroff & Martin's neonatal-perinatal medicine* (10th ed., pp. 1001–1017). St. Louis, MO: Elsevier-Mosby.

McGrath, J. M., & Vittner, D. (2015). Behavioral assessment. In E. P. Tappero & M. E. Honeyfield (Eds.), *Physical assessment of the newborn* (5th ed., pp. 193–219). Petaluma, CA: NICU INK.

Muchowski, K. E. (2014). Evaluation and treatment of neonatal hyperbilirubinemia. *American Family Physician, 89*(11), 873–878.

Nugent, J. K. (2013). The competent newborn and the neonatal behavioral assessment scale: T. Berry Brazelton's legacy. *Journal of Child and Adolescent Psychiatric Nursing 26*(3), 173–179.

Parker, L. A. (2014). Genitourinary system. In C. Kenner & J. W. Lott (Eds.), *Comprehensive neonatal nursing care* (5th ed., pp. 472–507). New York, NY: Springer.

Raab, E. L., & Kelly, L. K. (2013). Normal newborn assessment & care. In A. H. Decherney, L. Nathan, N. Laufer, & A. S. Roman (Eds.), *Current diagnosis & treatment: Obstetrics & gynecology* (11th ed., pp. 181–189). New York, NY: McGraw-Hill.

Raju, T. N. (2013). Timing of umbilical cord clamping after birth for optimizing placental transfusion. *Current Opinions in Pediatrics, 25,* 180–187.

Riley, C., Spencer, B., & Prater, L. S. (2014). Normal term newborn. In C. Kenner & J. W. Lott (Eds.), *Comprehensive neonatal nursing care* (5th ed., pp. 113–132). New York, NY: Springer.

Sim, K., Powell, E., Shaw, A. G., McClure, Z., Bangham, M., & Kroll, J. S. (2012). The neonatal gastrointestinal microbiota: The foundation of future health? *Archives of Diseases of Children: Fetal Neonatal Edition, 98*(4), F362–F364.

Van Woudenberg, C. D., Wills, C. A., & Rubarth, L. B. (2012). Newborn transition to extrauterine life. *Neonatal Network, 31*(5), 317–322.

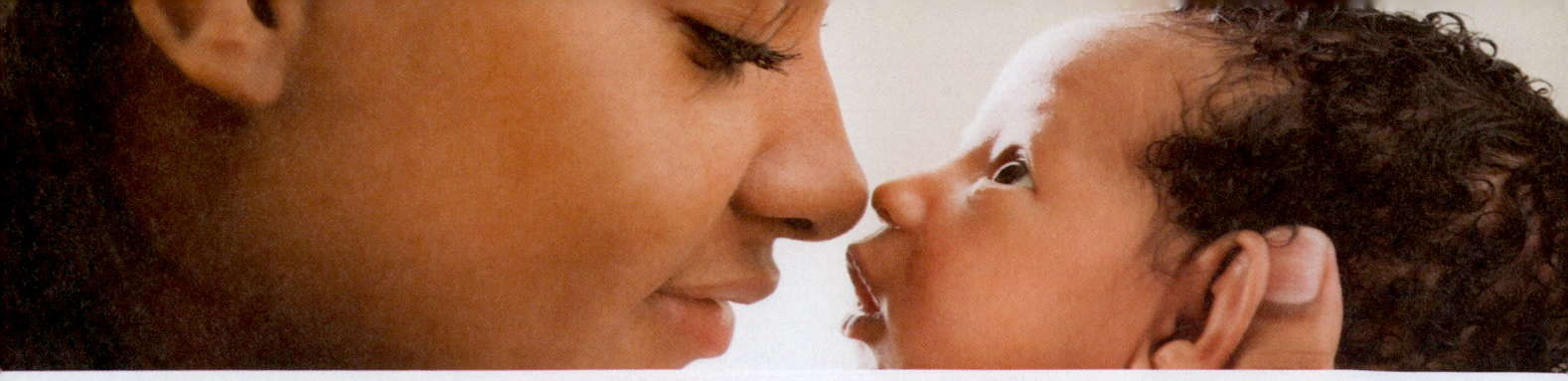

Chapter 24
Nursing Assessment of the Newborn

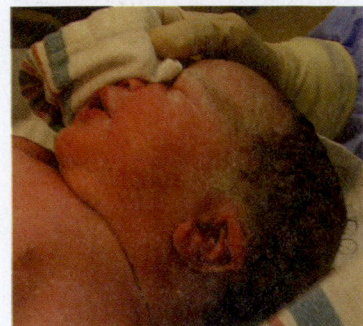

Each time I do a newborn's first bath I am struck anew by the magic of human life. It is one of my favorite parts of the day.

—Newborn Nursery Nurse

Learning Outcomes

24.1 Describe the physical and neuromuscular maturity characteristics assessed to determine the gestational age of the newborn.

24.2 Summarize the components of a systematic physical newborn assessment and the significance of normal variations and abnormal findings and possible nursing responses.

24.3 Describe the components of a newborn neurologic/neuromuscular assessment.

24.4 Describe the components of the newborn behavioral assessment.

24.5 Identify the reflexes that may be present at birth.

24.6 Compare the normal behavioral characteristics of the newborn with the normal variations that may be present.

24.7 Describe how to use the assessment procedure and results of the newborn physical, neurologic, and behavioral assessments to teach and involve parents in the care of the newborn.

Newborns communicate their needs primarily by behavior. Because nurses are the most consistent professional observers of newborns, they can translate this behavior into information about an individual newborn's condition and respond with appropriate nursing interventions. This chapter focuses on the assessment of the newborn and the interpretation of these findings.

Assessment of the newborn is a continuous process designed to evaluate development and adjustments to extrauterine life. In the birth setting, the Apgar scoring procedure and careful observation form the basis of assessment and are correlated with information such as the following:

• Maternal prenatal care history
• Birthing history

• Maternal analgesia and anesthesia
• Complications of labor or birth
• Treatment instituted immediately after birth, in conjunction with determination of clinical gestational age
• Consideration of the classification of newborns by weight and gestational age and by neonatal mortality risk
• Physical examination of the newborn

The nurse incorporates data from these sources with the assessment findings during the first 1 to 4 hours after birth to formulate a plan for nursing interventions.

The various newborn assessments and the data obtained from them are valuable only to the degree to which they are shared with the parents. The parents must be included in the assessment process from the moment of their child's birth. The *Apgar score* and its meaning should be explained immediately to the family (see discussion of Apgar score in Chapter 18). As soon as possible, the parents should take part in the physical and behavioral assessments as well.

The nurse encourages the parents to identify the unique behavioral characteristics of their newborn and to learn nurturing activities. Attachment is promoted when parents have an opportunity to explore their newborn in private and identify individual physical and behavioral characteristics. The nurse's supportive responses to parents' questions and observations are essential throughout the assessment process. The newborn physical examination is the beginning of newborn health surveillance and health education for the newborn's family that continues into the community setting.

Timing of Newborn Assessments

During the first 24 hours of life, the newborn makes the critical transition from intrauterine to extrauterine life. The risk of mortality and morbidity is statistically high during this period. Assessment of the newborn is essential to ensure that the transition proceeds successfully.

The major time periods for assessments of newborns while they are in the birth facility are as follows:

- *Delivery room disposition.* The first assessment is done in the birthing area immediately after birth to determine the need for resuscitation or other interventions. The stable newborn should stay with the family after birth to initiate early attachment. The newborn with complications is usually taken to the special nursery for further evaluation and intervention.
- *Nursery or couplet care admission examination.* A second assessment may be done by the nursery nurse as part of routine admission procedures. During this assessment, the nurse carries out a brief physical examination to estimate gestational age and evaluate the newborn's adaptation to extrauterine life. No later than 2 hours after birth, the admitting nursery nurse should evaluate the newborn's status and any problems that place the newborn at risk.
- *Discharge examination.* A certified nurse-midwife (CNM), healthcare provider, or nurse practitioner will carry out a discharge examination. It includes a well-baby admission examination, a behavioral assessment, and additional information from the baby's stay in the birthing unit to assess if the newborn is ready for routine care at home. A complete physical examination is done to detect any emerging or potential problems. When the birthing center stay is short, a combination admission–discharge examination is appropriate.

This chapter presents the procedures for estimating gestational age and performing the complete physical examination and behavioral assessment.Chapter 18 discusses the immediate postbirth assessment. Chapter 25 describes the brief assessment performed during the first 4 hours of life.

Estimation of Gestational Age

The nurse must establish the newborn's gestational age in the first 4 hours after birth so that careful attention can be given to age-related problems. Traditionally, a newborn's gestational age was determined from the date of the pregnant woman's last menstrual period. However, this method was accurate only 75% to 85% of the time. Because of the problems that develop with the preterm newborn or the newborn whose weight is inappropriate for gestational age, a more accurate system was developed to postnatally evaluate the newborn. Once learned, the procedure can be done in a few minutes.

SAFETY ALERT!

It is essential for the nurse to wear gloves when assessing the newborn in these early hours after birth and before the first bath until amniotic fluid, vaginal secretions, and blood on the skin are removed.

Clinical **gestational age assessment tools** have two components: external physical characteristics and neurologic or neuromuscular development. Physical characteristics generally include the following:

- Sole creases
- Amount of breast tissue
- Amount of lanugo
- Cartilaginous development of the ear
- Testicular descent and scrotal rugae in the male
- Labial development in the female

These are objective clinical criteria that are not influenced by labor and birth and do not change significantly within the first 12 hours after birth.

Neurologic examination facilitates assessment of functional or physiologic maturation in addition to physical development. A variety of factors can affect the newborn's nervous system during the first 24 hours of life; neurologic evaluation findings based on reflexes or assessments dependent on the higher brain centers may not be reliable. If the neurologic findings drastically deviate from the gestational age derived by evaluation of external characteristics, a second assessment is done in 24 hours.

The neurologic assessment components (excluding reflexes) can aid in assessing the gestational age of newborns of less than 34 weeks' gestation. Between 26 and 34 weeks, neurologic changes are significant, whereas significant physical changes are less evident.

Ballard et al. (1991) developed the *estimation of gestational age by maturity rating,* a simplified version of the well-researched *Dubowitz tool.* The Ballard tool omits some of the neuromuscular tone assessments, such as leg recoil, which are difficult to assess in very ill newborns or those on respirators. In the Ballard tool, each physical and neuromuscular finding is given a value, and the total score is matched to a gestational age. The maximum score on the Ballard tool is 50, which corresponds to a gestational age of 44 weeks.

For example, on completion of a gestational assessment of a 1-hour-old newborn, the nurse gives a score of 3 to all the physical characteristics, for a total of 18, and gives a score of 3 to all neuromuscular assessments, for a total of 18. The physical characteristics score of 18 is added to the neurologic score of 18 for a total score of 36, which correlates with 38+ weeks' gestation. Because all newborns vary slightly in the development of physical characteristics and maturation of neurologic function, scores usually vary instead of all being 3, as in this example.

Postnatal gestational age assessment tools can overestimate preterm newborns of less than 28 weeks' gestational age and underestimate postterm newborns of more than 43 weeks' gestation. Ballard et al. (1991), in the **New Ballard Score (NBS)**, added criteria for more accurate assessment of the gestational age of newborns between 20 and 28 weeks' gestation and less than 1500 g (3.3 lb). They suggest that the assessments should be made within 12 hours of birth to optimize accuracy, especially in newborns of less than 26 weeks' gestational age. Also the Ballard assessment may be overstimulating to newborns of less than 27 weeks' gestation (Cavaliere & Sansoucie, 2014). Some maternal conditions, such as preeclampsia, diabetes, and maternal analgesia and anesthesia, may affect certain gestational assessment components and warrant further evaluation. Maternal diabetes, although it appears to accelerate fetal physical growth, seems to retard maturation. Maternal hypertension states, which retard fetal physical growth, seem to speed maturation.

Newborns of women with preeclampsia on magnesium sulfate may have a poor correlation with the neuromuscular criteria involving active muscle tone and edema. Maternal analgesia and anesthesia may cause respiratory depression. Babies with respiratory distress syndrome (RDS) tend to be flaccid and edematous and to assume a "froglike" posture (see Chapter 27 for care of the newborn with RDS). These characteristics affect the scoring of the neuromuscular components of the assessment tool used. The NBS gestational age assessment tool will be used throughout the chapter to demonstrate the assessment of the physical and neuromuscular criteria associated with gestational age.

Assessment of Physical Maturity Characteristics

The nurse first evaluates observable characteristics without disturbing the baby. Selected physical characteristics common to the Ballard gestational assessment tools are presented here in the order in which they might be most effectively evaluated:

1. *Resting posture,* although a neuromuscular component, should be assessed as the baby lies undisturbed on a flat surface (Figure 24–1).

2. *Skin* in the preterm newborn appears thin and transparent, with veins prominent over the abdomen early in gestation. As the newborn approaches term, the skin appears opaque because of increased subcutaneous tissue. Disappearance of the protective vernix caseosa promotes skin desquamation; this is commonly seen in postmature newborns (babies of more than 42 weeks' gestational age) and those showing signs of placental insufficiency (see Chapter 26 for care of the postterm newborn).

3. **Lanugo,** a fine hair covering, decreases as gestational age increases. The amount of lanugo is greatest at 28 to 30 weeks. It is most abundant over the back (particularly between the scapulae), although it will also be noted over the face, legs, and arms. Lanugo disappears first from the face and then from the trunk and extremities (Figure 24–2).

4. *Sole (plantar) creases* are reliable indicators of gestational age in the first 12 hours of life. Later the skin of the foot begins drying, and superficial creases appear. Development of sole creases begins at the top (anterior) portion of the sole and, as gestation progresses, proceeds to the heel (Figure 24–3). Peeling may also occur. Plantar creases vary with race. In newborns of Black descent, sole creases may be less developed at term.

5. The nurse inspects the *areolae* and gently palpates the *breast bud tissue* by applying the forefinger and middle finger to the breast area and measuring the tissue between them in centimeters or millimeters (Figure 24–4). At term gestation, the tissue measures between 0.5 and 1 cm (5 and 10 mm).

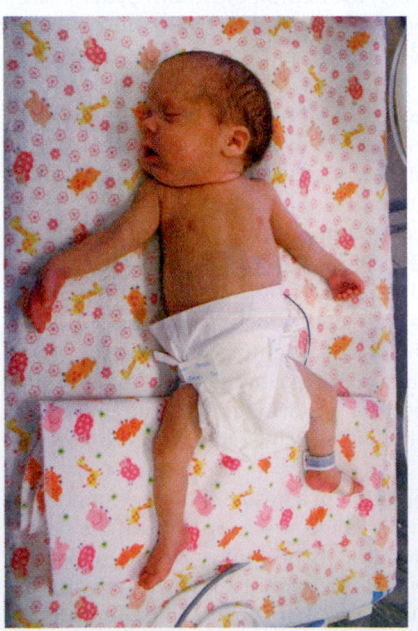
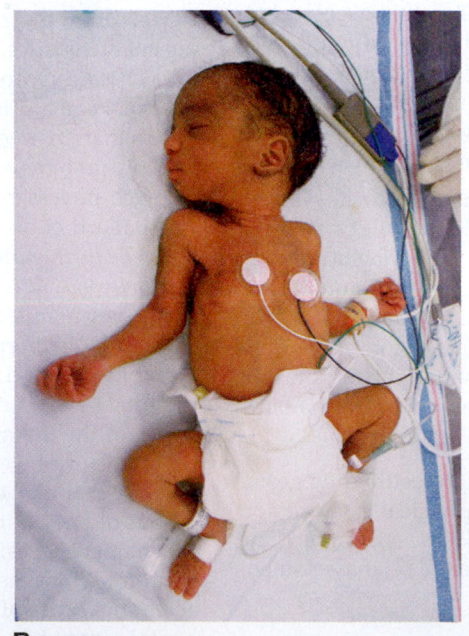
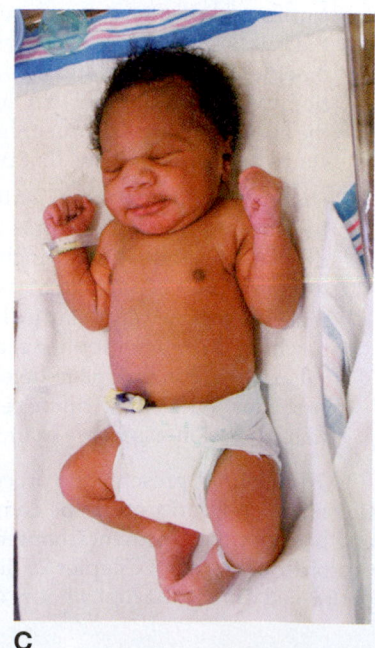

A   B   C

Figure 24–1 Resting posture. A. Newborn exhibits beginning of flexion of the thigh. The gestational age is approximately 31 weeks. Note the extension of the upper extremities. Score 1 or 2. B. Newborn exhibits stronger flexion of the arms, hips, and thighs. The gestational age is approximately 35 weeks. Score 3. C. The full-term newborn exhibits hypertonic flexion of all extremities. Score 4.

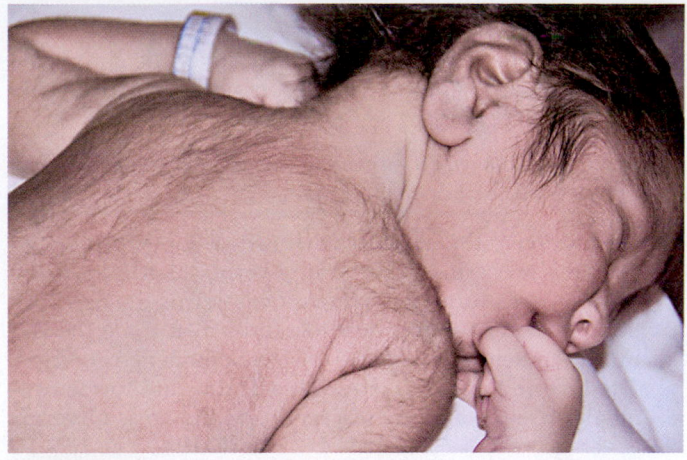

Figure 24–2 Lanugo.

SOURCE: Vanessa Howell, RN, MSN.

During the assessment, the nipple should not be grasped firmly because skin and subcutaneous tissue will prevent accurate estimation of size. The nurse must do this procedure gently to avoid causing trauma to the breast tissue.

As gestation progresses, the breast bud and areola enlarge. However, a large breast engorgement can occur as a result of specific conditions other than advanced gestational age or the effects of maternal hormones on the baby. In the large-for-gestational-age (LGA) newborn, accelerated development of breast tissue is a reflection of subcutaneous fat deposits. Small-for-gestational-age (SGA), term, or postterm newborns may have used subcutaneous fat (which would have been deposited as breast tissue) to survive in utero; as a result, their lack of breast tissue may indicate a gestational age of 34 to 35 weeks, even though other factors indicate a term or postterm newborn (Cloherty, Eichenwald, Hansen, & Stark, 2012).

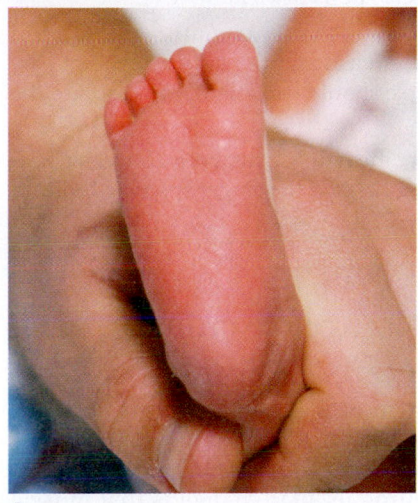

A

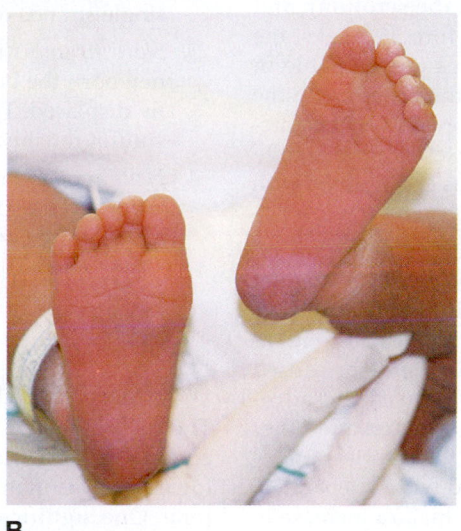

B

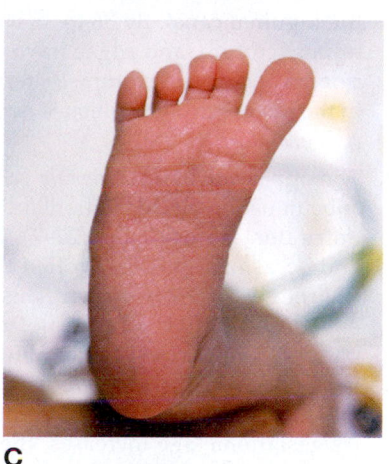

C

Figure 24–3 Sole creases. A. Newborn has a few sole creases on the anterior portion of the foot. Note the slick heel. Score 2. The gestational age is approximately 35 weeks. B. Newborn has a deeper network of sole creases on the anterior two thirds of the sole. Note the slick heel. Score 3. The gestational age is approximately 37 weeks. C. The full-term newborn has deep sole creases down to and including the heel as the skin loses fluid and dries after birth. Score 4. Sole (plantar) creases can be seen even in preterm newborns.

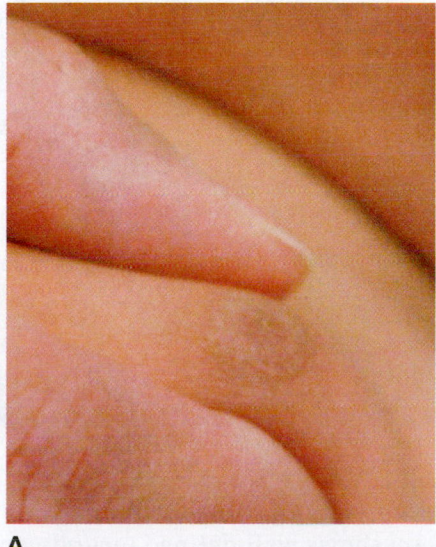

A

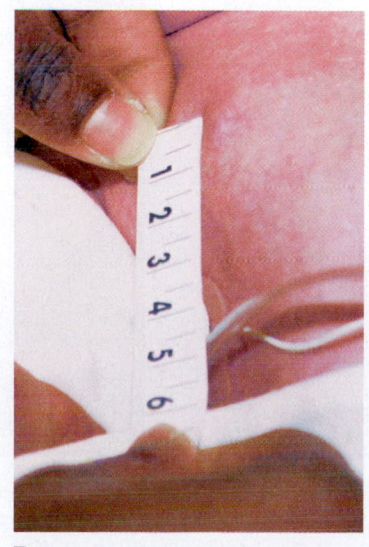

B

Figure 24–4 Breast tissue. A. Newborn has a visible raised area greater than 0.75 cm (0.3 in.) diameter. Score 3. The gestational age is 38 weeks. B. Gently compress the tissue between the middle and index fingers and measure the tissue in centimeters or millimeters. Absence of or decreased breast tissue often indicates premature or small-for-gestational-age (SGA) newborn.

6. *Ear form and cartilage distribution* develop with gestational age. The cartilage gives the ear its shape and substance (Figure 24–5). In a newborn of less than 34 weeks' gestation, the ear is relatively shapeless and flat; it has little cartilage, so the ear folds over on itself and remains folded. By approximately 36 weeks' gestation, some cartilage and incurving of the upper pinna are present, and the pinna springs back slowly when folded. (The nurse tests this response by holding the top and bottom of the pinna together with the forefinger and thumb and then releasing them or by folding the pinna of the ear forward against the side of the head, releasing it and observing the response.) By term, the newborn's pinna is firm, stands away from the head, and springs back quickly from the folding.

7. *Male genitals* are evaluated for size of the scrotal sac, presence of rugae (wrinkles and ridges in the scrotum), and descent of the testes (Figure 24–6). Before 36 weeks, the scrotum has few rugae, and the testes are palpable in the inguinal canal. By 36 to 38 weeks, the testes are in the upper scrotum, and rugae have developed over the anterior portion of the scrotum. By term, the testes are generally in the lower scrotum, which is pendulous and covered with rugae.

8. The appearance of the *female genitals* depends in part on subcutaneous fat deposition and therefore relates to fetal nutritional status (Figure 24–7). The clitoris varies in size, and occasionally is so swollen that it is difficult to identify the sex of the newborn. This swelling may be caused by adrenogenital syndrome, which causes the adrenals to secrete excessive amounts of androgen and other hormones. At 30 to 32 weeks' gestation, the clitoris is prominent, and the labia majora are small and widely separated. As gestational age increases, the labia majora increase in size. At 36 to 40 weeks, they nearly cover the clitoris. At 40 weeks and beyond, the labia majora cover the labia minora and clitoris.

Other physical characteristics assessed by some gestational age scoring tools include the following:

1. *Vernix* covers the preterm newborn. The postterm newborn has no vernix. After noting vernix distribution, the birthing area nurse (wearing gloves) dries the newborn to prevent evaporative heat loss, thus disturbing the vernix and potentially altering this gestational age criterion. The birthing area nurse must communicate to the neonatal nurse the amount of vernix and the areas of vernix coverage.

2. *Hair* of the preterm newborn has the consistency of matted wool or fur and lies in bunches rather than in the silky, single strands of the term newborn's hair.

3. *Skull firmness* increases as the fetus matures. In a term newborn the bones are hard, and the sutures are not easily displaced. The nurse should not attempt to displace the sutures forcibly.

4. *Nails* appear and cover the nail bed at about 20 weeks' gestation. Nails extending beyond the fingertips may indicate a postterm newborn.

Assessment of Neuromuscular Maturity Characteristics

The central nervous system of the fetus matures at a fairly constant rate. Tests have been designed to evaluate neurologic status as manifested by development of neuromuscular tone. One significant neuromuscular change is that muscle

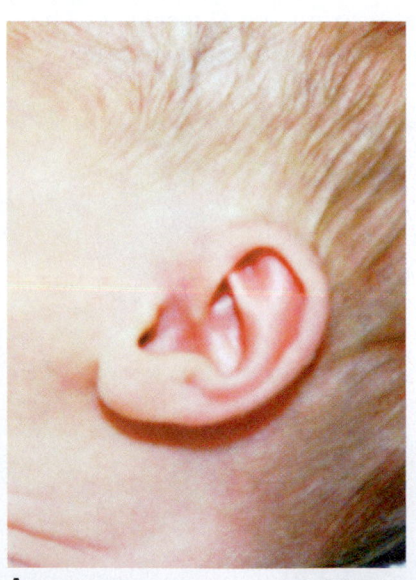
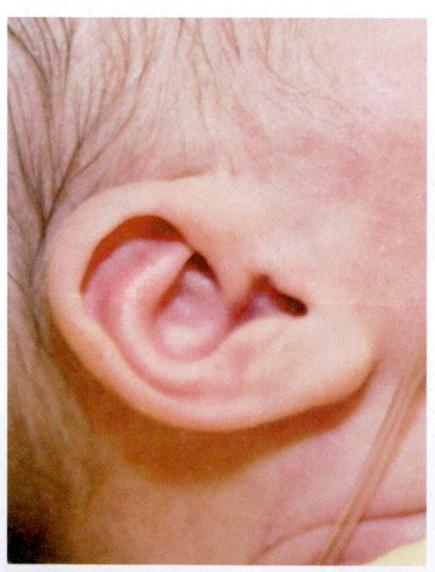
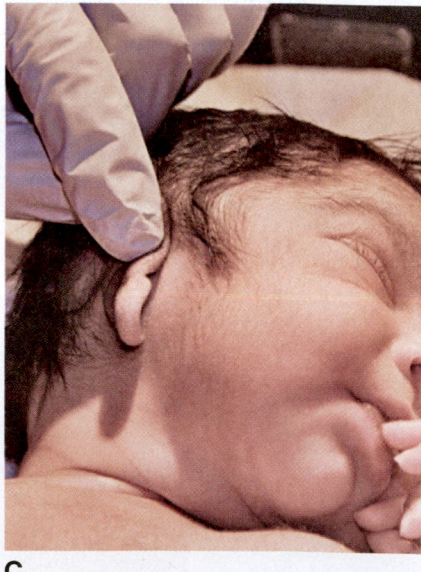

A   B   C

Figure 24–5 Ear form and cartilage. **A.** The ear of the newborn at approximately 36 weeks' gestation shows incurving of the upper two thirds of the pinna. Score 2. **B.** Newborn at term shows well-defined incurving of the entire pinna. Score 3. **C.** The pinna is folded toward the face and released. If the auricle stays in the position in which it is pressed or returns slowly to its original position, it usually means the gestational age is less than 38 weeks.

SOURCE: C. Vanessa Howell, RN, MSN.

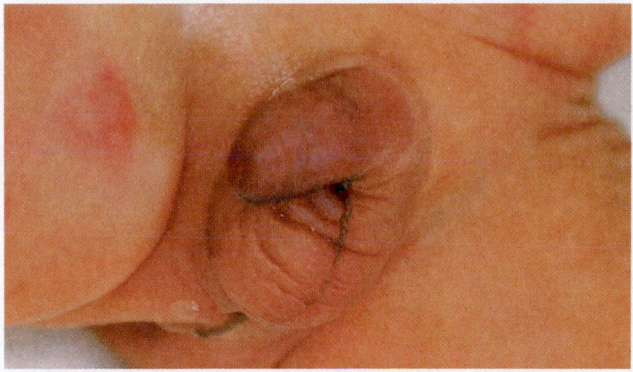
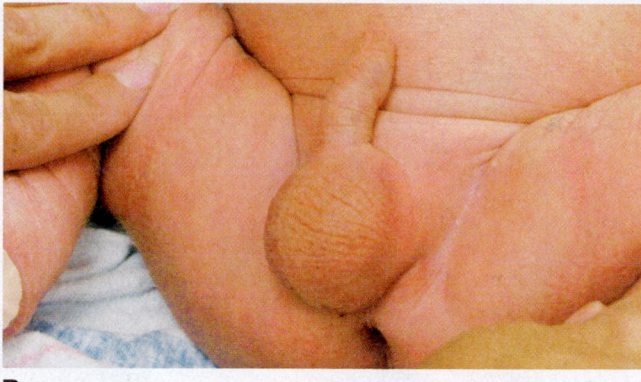

A   **B**

Figure 24–6 Male genitals. A. Preterm newborn's testes are not within the scrotum. The scrotal surface has few rugae. Score 2. B. Term newborn's testes are generally fully descended. The entire surface of the scrotum is covered by rugae. Score 3.

tone progresses from extensor tone to flexor tone and from the lower to the upper extremities as the neurologic system matures in a *caudocephalad* (tail-to-head) progression. The neuromuscular evaluation requires more manipulation and disturbances than the physical evaluation of the newborn. The neuromuscular evaluation is best performed when the newborn has stabilized.

1. The *square window sign* is elicited by gently flexing the newborn's hand toward the ventral forearm until resistance is felt. The angle formed at the wrist is measured (Figure 24–8).
2. *Recoil* is a test of flexion development. Because flexion first develops in the lower extremities, recoil is first tested in the legs. The nurse places the newborn on the back on a

flat surface. With a hand on the newborn's knees, the nurse places the baby's legs in flexion, then extends them parallel to each other and flat on the surface. The response to this maneuver is recoil of the newborn's legs. According to gestational age, they may not move or they may return slowly or quickly to the flexed position. Preterm newborns have less muscle tone than term newborns, so preterm newborns have less recoil.

Arm recoil is tested by flexion at the elbow and extension of the arms at the newborn's side. While the baby is in the supine position, the nurse completely flexes both elbows, holds them in this position for 5 seconds, extends the arms at the baby's side, and releases them. On release, the elbows of a full-term newborn form an angle of less than 90 degrees and rapidly recoil back to a

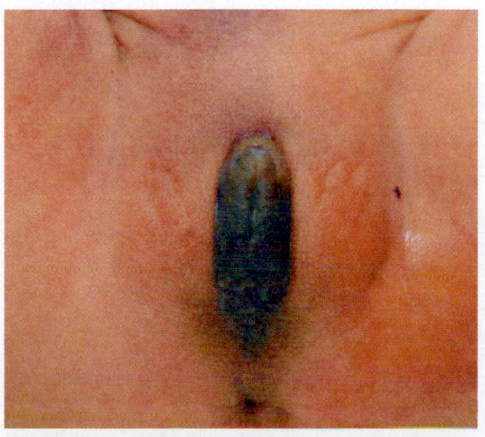
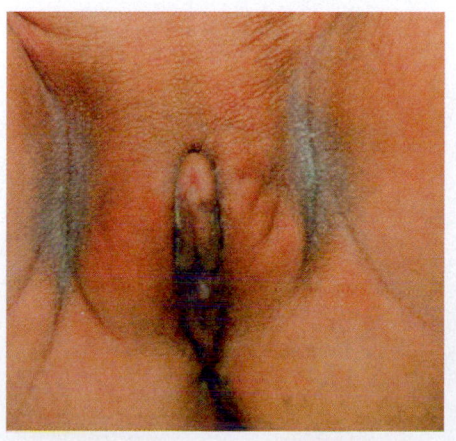
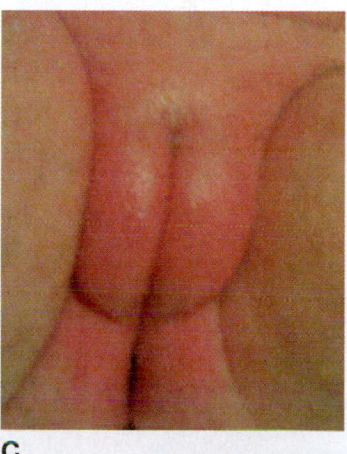

A   **B**   **C**

Figure 24–7 Female genitals. A. Newborn has a prominent clitoris. The labia majora are widely separated, and the labia minora, viewed laterally, would protrude beyond the labia majora. Score 1. The gestational age is 30 to 36 weeks. B. The clitoris is still visible. The labia minora are now covered by the larger labia majora. Score 2. The gestational age is 36 to 40 weeks. C. The term newborn has well-developed, large labia majora that cover both clitoris and labia minora. Score 3. The labia minora is often dark in some ethnic and racial groups of newborns.

SOURCE: C. Christine Mescolotto.

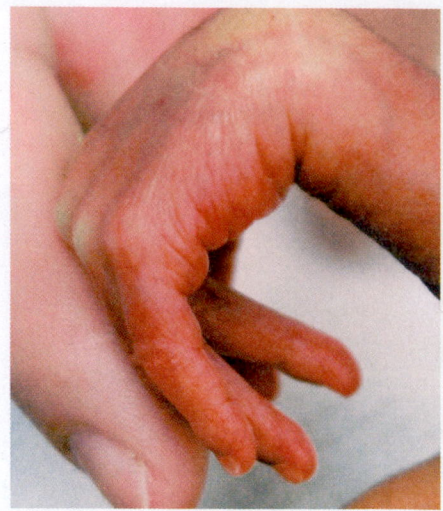
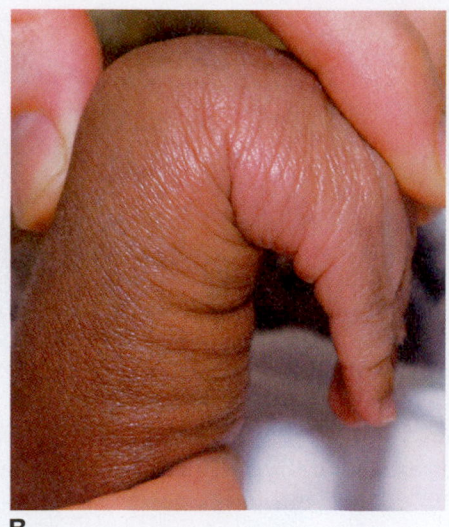
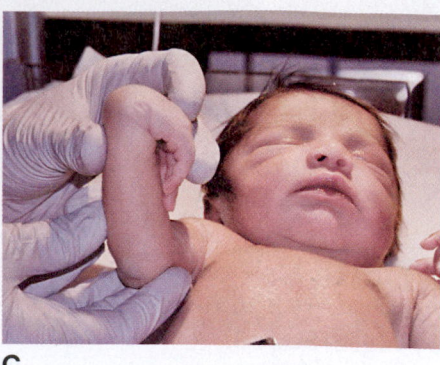

A   B   C

Figure 24–8 Square window sign. A. This angle is 90 degrees and suggests an immature newborn of 28 to 32 weeks' gestation. Score 0. B. A 30- to 40-degree angle is commonly found in newborns from 38 to 40 weeks' gestation. Score 2 to 3. C. A 0- to 15-degree angle occurs in newborns from 40 to 42 weeks' gestation. Score 4.

SOURCE: C. Vanessa Howell, RN, MSN.

flexed position. The elbows of a preterm newborn have slower recoil time and form an angle greater than 90 degrees. Arm recoil is also slower in healthy but fatigued newborns after birth; therefore arm recoil is best elicited after the first hour of birth, when the baby has had time to recover from the stress of the birth. The deep sleep state also decreases the arm recoil response. Assessment of arm recoil should be bilateral to rule out brachial palsy.

3. The *popliteal angle* (degree of knee flexion) is determined with the newborn flat on the back. The thigh is flexed on the abdomen and chest, and the nurse places the index finger of the other hand behind the newborn's ankle to extend the lower leg until resistance is met. The angle formed is

then measured. Results vary from no resistance in the very immature newborn to an 80-degree angle in the term newborn.

4. The *scarf sign* is elicited by placing the newborn supine and drawing an arm across the chest toward the newborn's opposite shoulder until resistance is met. The location of the elbow is then noted in relation to the midline of the chest (Figure 24–9). A preterm newborn's elbow will cross the midline of the chest, whereas a full-term newborn's elbow will not cross midline.

5. The *heel-to-ear extension* is performed by placing the newborn in a supine position and then gently drawing the foot toward the ear on the same side until resistance is felt. The

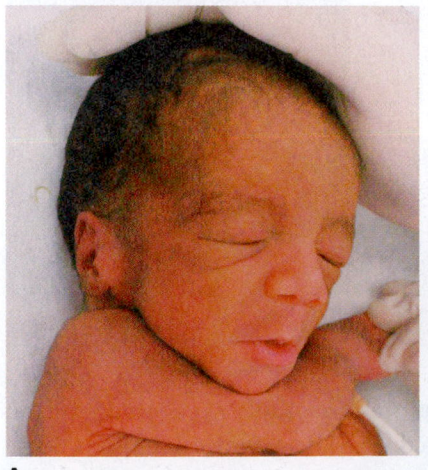
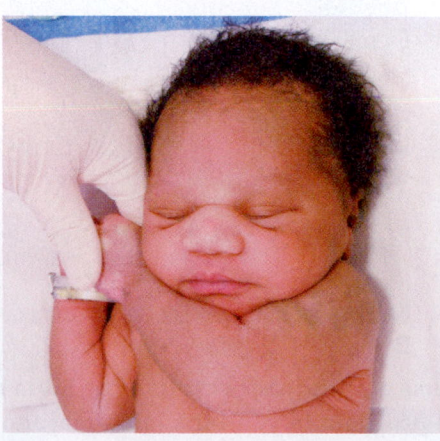
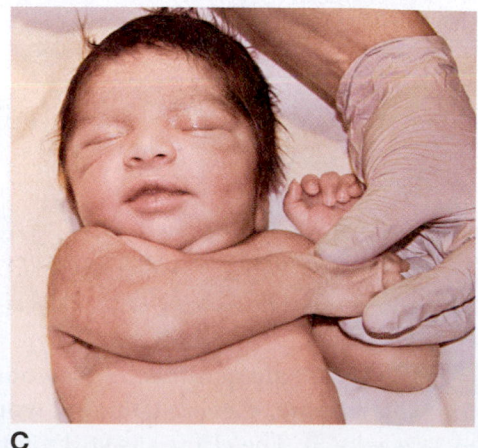

A   B   C

Figure 24–9 Scarf sign. A. No resistance is noted until after 30 weeks' gestation. The elbow can be readily moved past the midline. Score 1. B. The elbow is at midline at 36 to 40 weeks' gestation. Score 2. C. Beyond 40 weeks' gestation, the elbow will not reach the midline. Score 4.

SOURCE: C. Vanessa Howell, RN, MSN.

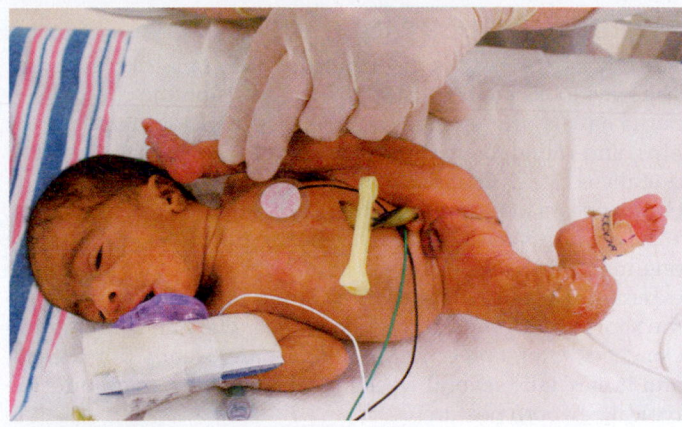

Figure 24–10 Heel to ear. No resistance. Leg fully extended. Score 0.

nurse should allow the knee to bend during the test. It is important to hold the buttocks down to keep from rolling the baby. Both the proximity of the foot to the ear and the degree of knee extension are assessed. A preterm, immature newborn's leg will remain straight and the foot will go to the ear or beyond (Figure 24–10). With advancing gestational age, the newborn demonstrates increasing resistance to this maneuver. Maneuvers involving the lower extremities of newborns who had frank breech presentation should be delayed to allow for resolution of leg positioning.

6. *Ankle dorsiflexion* is determined by flexing the ankle on the shin. The nurse uses a thumb to push on the sole of the newborn's foot while the fingers support the back of the leg. Then the angle formed by the foot and the interior leg is measured (Figure 24–11). Intrauterine position and congenital deformities can influence this sign.

7. *Head lag* (neck flexor) is measured by pulling the newborn to a sitting position and noting the degree of head lag. Total

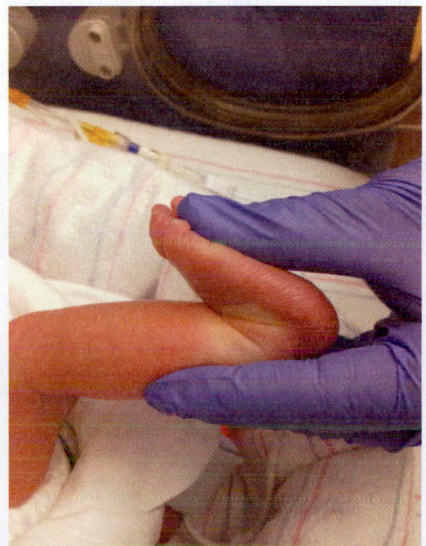

Figure 24–11 Ankle dorsiflexion. A 45-degree angle indicates 32 to 36 weeks' gestation.

SOURCE: Carol Harrigan, RNC, MSN, NNP-BC.

lag is common in newborns up to 34 weeks' gestation. Full-term newborns can support their heads momentarily.

8. *Ventral suspension* (horizontal position) is evaluated by holding the newborn prone on the nurse's hand. The position of the head and back and the degree of flexion in the arms and legs are noted. Some flexion of arms and legs indicates 36 to 38 weeks' gestation; fully flexed extremities, with head and back even, are characteristic of a term newborn.

9. *Major reflexes* such as sucking, rooting, grasping, Moro, tonic neck, and others are evaluated during the newborn examination. These reflexes are discussed later in the chapter.

A supplementary method for estimating gestational age (done by the healthcare provider) is to view the vascular network of the cornea with an ophthalmoscope. The nurse should delay administration of prophylactic eye ointment until after this vascular eye examination is done. The amount of vascularity present over the surface of the lens assists in identifying newborns of 27 through 34 weeks' gestational age.

When the gestational age determination and birth weight are considered together, the newborn can be identified as one whose growth is:

- *Small for gestational age (SGA)* (below the 10th percentile)
- *Appropriate for gestational age (AGA)*
- *Large for gestational age (LGA)* (above the 90th percentile).

This determination (Figure 24–12) enables the nurse to anticipate possible physiologic problems. The information is used in conjunction with a complete physical examination, to establish a plan of care appropriate for the individual newborn. For example, an SGA or LGA newborn often requires frequent

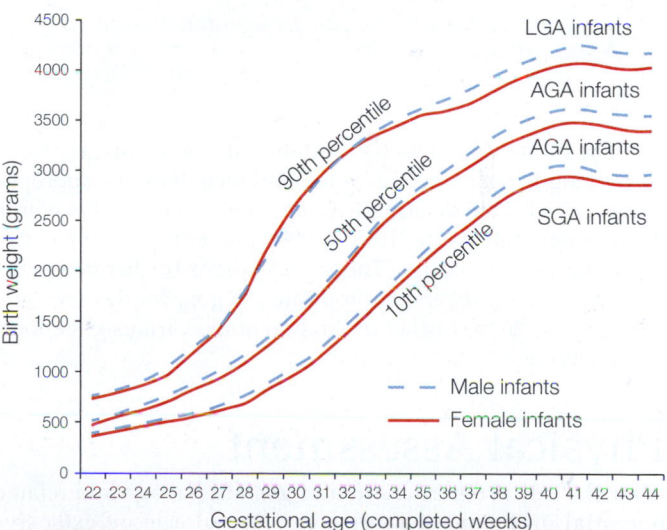

Figure 24–12 Select reference percentiles for birth weight at each gestational age from 22 to 44 completed weeks for male and female singleton infants: 10th, 50th, and 90th percentiles. Data from 3,423,215 male and 3,267,502 female infants in the 1999–2000 U.S. Natality datasets.

SOURCE: Oken, E., Kleinman, K. P., Rich-Edwards, J., & Gillman, M. W. (2003). A nearly continuous measure of birth weight for gestational age using a United States national reference. *BMC Pediatrics, 3*, 6. Retrieved from http://www.biomedcentral.com/1471-2431/3/6© 2003 Oken et al; licensee BioMed Central Ltd. This is an Open Access article: verbatim copying and redistribution of this article are permitted in all media for any purpose, provided this notice is preserved along with the article's original URL.

glucose monitoring and early feedings. (See Chapter 26 for more complete discussions of these categories and the potential problems associated with them.)

Healthy People 2020

(MICH–8) Reduce low birth weight (LBW) and very low birth weight (VLBW)

Clinical Reasoning Determining Gestational Age

A nurse has completed the gestational assessment on newborn Travis Bell, who weighs 3000 g (6.6 lb) and is 48 cm (18.9 in.) long with a head circumference of 33 cm (13 in.). His Apgar scores were 8 at 1 minute and 9 at 5 minutes. Other assessment data include skin dry and cracking with pale areas and rare veins, no lanugo, sole creases covering the entire sole, raised areola 3 mm (0.125 in.), well-curved pinna soft with ready recoil, and testes descended with moderate rugae. Reflex data include square window at 0 degree, arm recoil 100 degree, popliteal angle 100 degree, scarf sign yield elbow will not reach midline, heel to ear 90 degree, and posture fully flexed. The parents express concerns over his small size.

What are the newborn's physical maturity score and neuromuscular maturity score?

Interpret the newborn's combined scores of neuromuscular and physical maturity.

Determine if the newborn is small for gestational age (SGA), appropriate for gestational age (AGA), or large for gestational age (LGA).

What should the nurse tell the parents regarding their concern over his small size?

The nurse also plots the gestational age against the newborn's length, head circumference, and weight on the appropriate growth chart to determine if these measurements fall within the average range—the 10th to 90th percentile for the corresponding gestational age. These correlations further document the level of maturity and appropriate category for the newborn. (See Chapter 26 for further discussion of the various gestational age newborns.)

Physical Assessment

After the initial determination of gestational age and related potential problems, the nurse carries out a more extensive physical assessment in a warm, well-lit area that is free of drafts. Completing the physical assessment in the presence of the parents provides an opportunity to acquaint them with their unique newborn. The examination is performed in a systematic, head-to-toe manner, and all findings are recorded. When assessing the physical and neurologic status of the newborn, the nurse should first consider general appearance and then proceed to specific areas.

Assessment Guide: Newborn Physical Assessment at the end of this chapter outlines how to systematically assess the newborn. Normal findings, alterations, and related causes are presented and correlated with suggested nursing responses. The findings are typical for a full-term newborn.

General Appearance

The newborn's head is disproportionately large for the body. The neck looks short because the chin rests on the chest. Newborns have a prominent abdomen, sloping shoulders, narrow hips, and rounded chests. The center of the baby's body is the umbilicus rather than the symphysis pubis as in the adult. The body appears long and the extremities short.

Newborns tend to stay in a flexed position similar to the one maintained in utero and will offer resistance when the extremities are straightened. This flexed position contributes to the short appearance of the extremities. The hands are tightly clenched. After a breech birth, the feet are usually dorsiflexed, and it may take several weeks for the newborn to assume the typical newborn posture.

Weight and Measurements

The normal full-term White newborn has an average birth weight of 3405 g (7 lb, 8 oz). Newborns of African, Asian, or Hispanic descent are usually somewhat smaller at term. Other factors that influence weight are age and size of parents, health of mother (smoking and malnutrition decrease birth weight), and the interval between pregnancies (short intervals, such as every year, result in lower birth weights). After the first week, and for the first 6 months, the newborn's weight increases about 198 g (7 oz) weekly.

Approximately 70% to 75% of the newborn's body weight is water. During the initial newborn period (the first 3 or 4 days), term newborns have a physiologic weight loss of about 5% to 10% because of fluid shifts. This weight loss may reach 15% for preterm newborns. Large babies also tend to lose more weight because of greater fluid loss in proportion to birth weight. If weight loss is greater than 10%, clinical reappraisal is indicated. Factors contributing to weight loss include insufficient fluid intake resulting from delayed breastfeeding or a slow adjustment to the formula, increased volume of meconium excreted, urination, and dehydration or consistent chilling (because of nonshivering thermogenesis).

The length of the normal newborn is difficult to measure because the legs are flexed and tensed. To measure length, the nurse should place newborns flat on their backs with their legs extended as much as possible (Figure 24–13). The average length is 50 cm (20 in.), and the range is 46 to 56 cm (18 to 22 in.). The newborn will grow approximately 2.5 cm (1 in.) a month for the next 6 months. This is the period of most rapid growth.

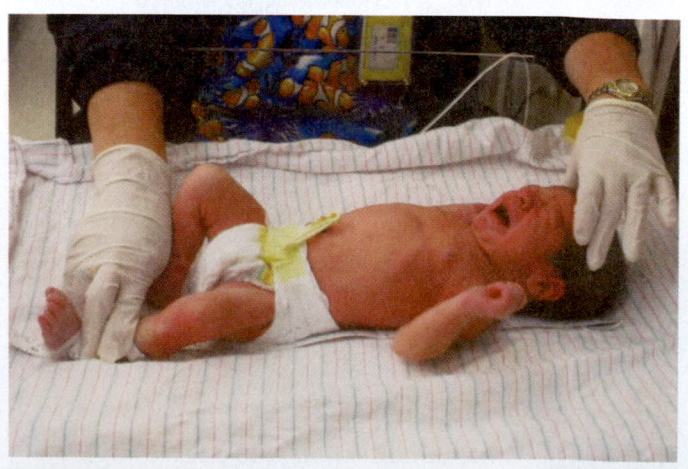

Figure 24–13 Measuring the length of the newborn.

SOURCE: Vanessa Howell, RNC, MSN.

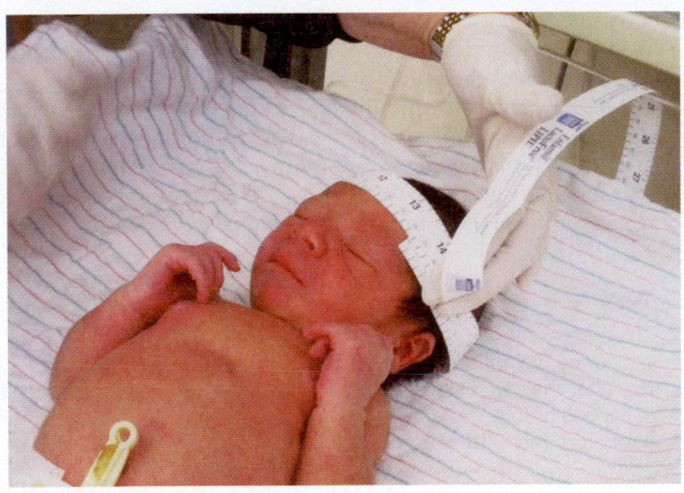

A

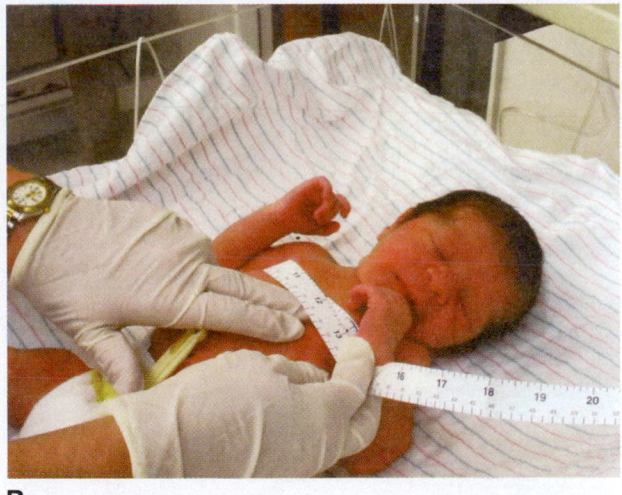

B

Figure 24–14 A. Measuring the head circumference of the newborn. B. Measuring the chest circumference of the newborn.

SOURCE: Vanessa Howell, RNC, MSN.

At birth the newborn's head is one fourth the size of an adult's head, with a circumference (biparietal diameter) of 32 to 37 cm (12.5 to 14.5 in.). For accurate measurement, the nurse places the tape over the most prominent part of the occiput and brings it just above the eyebrows (Figure 24–14A). The circumference of the newborn's head is approximately 2 cm (0.8 in.) greater than the circumference of the newborn's chest at birth, and will remain in this proportion for the next few months. (Factors that alter this measurement are discussed in the section titled Head later in the chapter.) It is best to take another head circumference on the second day if the newborn experienced significant head molding or developed a caput from the birth process.

The average circumference of the chest is 32 cm (12.5 in.) and it ranges from 30 to 35 cm (12 to 14 in.). Chest measurements are taken with the tape measure placed at the lower edge of the scapulas and brought around anteriorly, directly over the nipple line (Figure 24–14B). The abdominal circumference, or girth, may also be measured at this time, by placing the tape around the newborn's abdomen at the level of the umbilicus, with the bottom edge of the tape at the top edge of the umbilicus.

KEY FACTS TO REMEMBER
Newborn Measurements

Measurement	Average	Range	Growth
Weight (Weight is influenced by a variety of factors, and maternal age and size. Physiologic weight loss 5% to 10% for term newborns, up to 15% for preterm newborns.)	3405 g (7 lb, 8 oz)	2500–4000 g (5 lb, 8 oz–8 lb, 13 oz)	198 g (7 oz) per week for first 6 months
Length	50 cm (20 in.)	46–56 cm (18–22 in.)	2.5 cm (1 in.) per month for first 6 months
Head circumference (Approximately 2 cm [0.8 in.] larger than chest circumference)	33–35 cm (13–14 in.)	32.0–37.0 cm (12.5–14.5 in.)	
Chest circumference	32.0 cm (12.5 in.)	30–35 cm (12–14 in.)	

Temperature

Initial assessment of the newborn's temperature is critical. In utero, the temperature of the fetus is about the same as, or slightly higher than, the mother's temperature. When babies enter the outside world, their temperature can suddenly drop as a result of exposure to cold drafts and the skin's heat loss mechanisms.

If no heat conservation measures are started, the normal term newborn's deep body temperature falls 0.1°C (0.2°F) per minute; skin temperature drops 0.3°C (0.5°F) per minute. Skin temperature markedly decreases within 10 minutes after exposure to room air. The temperature should stabilize within 8 to 12 hours. Temperature is monitored when the newborn is admitted to the birthing unit and at least every 30 minutes until the newborn's status has remained stable for 2 hours (American Academy of Pediatrics [AAP] Committee on Fetus and Newborn & American College of Obstetricians and Gynecologists [ACOG], 2012).

Thereafter, the nurse should assess temperature at least once every 8 hours, or according to institutional policy. In newborns who have been exposed to group B hemolytic streptococcus, more frequent temperature monitoring may be required. (See Chapter 23 for a discussion of the physiology of temperature regulation.)

Temperature can be assessed by the axillary skin method, using a continuous skin probe, or via the rectal route. Axillary temperature reflects body (core) temperature and the body's compensatory response to the thermal environment. In preterm and term newborns, there is less than 0.1°C (0.2°F) difference in temperatures between the two sites and the axillary method is preferred. Axillary temperature ranges from 36.4° to 37.2°C (97.5° to 99°F) (Figure 24–15). Keep in mind that axillary temperatures can be misleading, because the friction caused by apposition of the inner arm skin and upper chest wall and the nearness of brown fat to the probe may elevate the temperature.

Skin temperature is measured most accurately by means of continuous skin probe, especially for small newborns or newborns maintained in incubators or under radiant warmers. Normal skin temperature is 36° to 36.4°C (96.8° to 97.5°F). Continuous assessment of skin temperature allows time for initiation of interventions before a more serious fall in core temperature occurs (Figure 24–16).

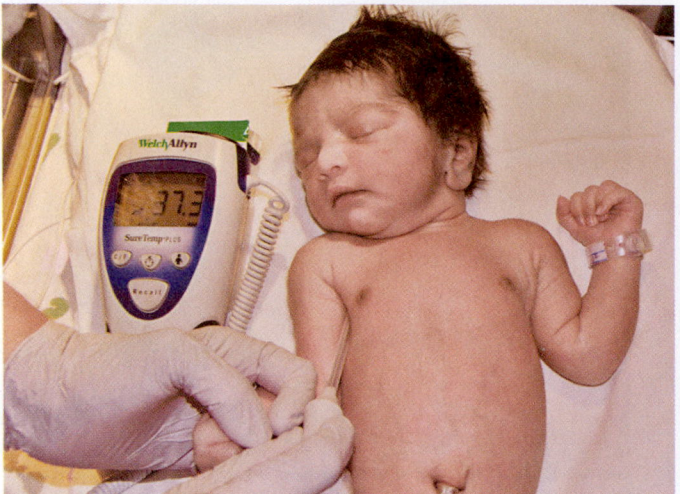

Figure 24–15 Axillary temperature measurement. The newborn's arm should be tightly but gently pressed against the thermometer and the newborn's side, as illustrated.

SOURCE: Vanessa Howell, RN, MSN.

Rectal temperature is assumed to be the closest approximation to core temperature, but the accuracy of this method depends on the depth to which the thermometer is inserted. Normal rectal temperature is 36.6° to 37.2°C (97.8° to 99°F). The rectal route is recommended as a routine method, unless temperature is taken with a digital or electronic thermometer (American Academy of Pediatrics [AAP], 2013).

Temperature instability, a deviation of more than 1°C (2°F) from one reading to the next, or a subnormal temperature may indicate an infection. In contrast to an elevated temperature in older children, an increased temperature in a newborn may indicate a reaction to too many coverings, too hot a room, or dehydration. Dehydration, which tends to increase body temperature, occurs in newborns whose feedings have been delayed for any reason. Newborns may respond to overheating

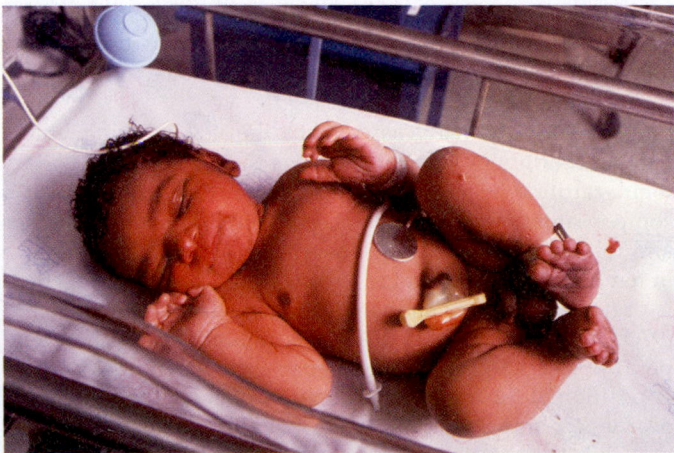

Figure 24–16 Temperature monitoring for the newborn. A skin thermal sensor is placed on the newborn's abdomen, upper thigh, or arm and secured with porous tape or a foil-covered foam pad.

SOURCE: © Tom McCarthy/PhotoEdit.

(a temperature greater than 37.5°C [99.5°F]) after 35 to 40 minutes of exposure (Blackburn, 2013). The perspiration appears initially on the head and face and then on the chest.

Many newborns initially cannot perspire, so they increase their respiratory and heart rates, which increases oxygen consumption. Whether the initial temperature is elevated or subnormal, the newborn must have a stable temperature per agency protocol prior to leaving the nursery.

Clinical Tip

Measuring weight and height often aggravates newborns and may alter their vital signs. For better accuracy, take the newborn's vital signs before weighing and measuring. In addition, assess the respiratory rate and heart rate before taking the temperature.

Skin Characteristics

Although the newborn's skin color varies with genetic background, all healthy newborns have a pink tinge to their skin. The ruddy hue results from increased red blood cell concentrations in the blood vessels and limited subcutaneous fat deposits.

Skin pigmentation is slight in the newborn period, so color changes may be seen even in darker-skinned babies. White newborns have a pinkish-red skin tone a few hours after birth, and newborns of African descent have a skin color that is reddish-brown to pale pink perhaps tinged with yellow or red. Hispanic and Asian newborns can have a pink or rosy red to olive or yellow skin tone. Skin pigmentation deepens over time; therefore, variations in skin color indicating illness are more difficult to evaluate in African American and Asian newborns (Cloherty et al., 2012). A newborn who is cyanotic at rest and pink only with crying may have *choanal atresia* (congenital blockage of the passageway between the nose and the pharynx). If crying increases the cyanosis, heart or lung problems should be suspected. Very pale newborns may be anemic or have hypovolemia (low BP) and should be evaluated for these problems.

Acrocyanosis (bluish discoloration of the hands and feet) may be present in the first 2 to 6 hours after birth but can be normal for up to 24 hours (Figure 24–17). This condition is caused by poor peripheral circulation, which results in vasomotor instability and capillary stasis, especially when the baby is exposed to cold. Therefore, blue hands and nails are a poor

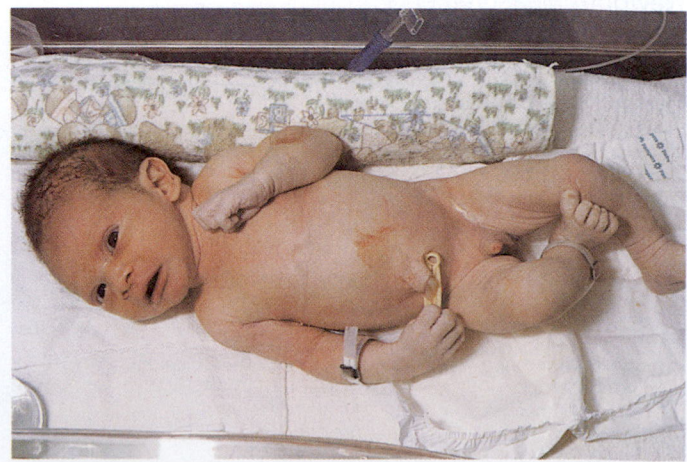

Figure 24–17 Acrocyanosis.

indicator of decreased oxygenation in a newborn. If the central circulation is adequate, the blood supply should return quickly (2 to 3 seconds) to the extremity after the skin is blanched with a finger. The face and mucous membranes should be assessed for pinkness reflecting adequate oxygenation. Further oxygenation assessment is needed if signs of respiratory distress are observed. Pulse oximetry can be obtained.

Developing Cultural Competence Keeping Newborns Warm

In the Latino and other cultures, parents may be overly concerned about keeping their newborn warm. Parents should be informed that overdressing babies while they are sleeping is related to a higher risk of sudden infant death syndrome (SIDS) and that bundling them excessively can be uncomfortable and lead to heat rash.

Mottling (lacy pattern of dilated blood vessels under the skin) occurs as a result of general circulation fluctuations. It may last several hours to several weeks or may come and go periodically. Mottling may be related to chilling or to prolonged apnea, sepsis, or hypothyroidism.

Harlequin sign (clown) color change is occasionally noted: A deep red color develops over one side of the newborn's body while the other side remains pale, so that the skin resembles a clown's suit. This color change results from a vasomotor disturbance in which blood vessels on one side dilate while the vessels on the other side constrict (Gomella, 2013). It usually lasts from 1 to 20 minutes. Affected newborns may have single or multiple episodes, but they are transient and clinically insignificant. The nurse should document each occurrence.

Jaundice is first detectable on the face (where skin overlies cartilage) and the mucous membranes of the mouth. It has a head-to-toe progression and regresses in the opposite direction (Cloherty et al., 2012). Evaluation and determination of the cause of jaundice must be initiated immediately to prevent possibly serious sequelae. The jaundice may be related to hematomas, immature liver function, or poor feeding or may be caused by blood incompatibility, oxytocin (Pitocin) augmentation or induction, or a severe hemolysis process. Any jaundice noted before a newborn is 24 hours of age should be reported to the healthcare provider or neonatal nurse practitioner. Breastfeeding is a possible cause of late-onset jaundice. See *Clinical Skill: Assessing Jaundice in the Newborn*. (For discussion of various types of jaundice see Chapter 23, and for a detailed discussion of causes and treatment for jaundice, see Chapter 27.)

Clinical Skill 24–1
Assessing Jaundice in the Newborn

NURSING ACTION

Preparation

- Wash hands.
- Assemble equipment.

Equipment and Supplies

- Transcutaneous bilimeter

Procedure

1. Observe newborn in a well-lit room or near a window during daylight hours. Baby should be specifically checked for jaundice at least twice a shift or with every assessment.

2. Blanch skin on forehead, sternum, or gum line with digital pressure for 1 second and release. Observe for underlying yellow tinge to skin. If jaundice is observed on the sternum, also check palms and soles, and blanch skin below the knee. Another area to assess for jaundice is the sclera (whites of the eyes) or the inner aspect of the cheek in darker-skinned newborns.

Rationale: Progression of jaundice is head to toe (cephalocaudal progression). Jaundice is first seen in the face and neck when levels reach 4 to 8 mg/dL. Jaundice can be seen on palmar and plantar surfaces at levels greater than 15 mg/dL. Visual assessment is often an inaccurate predictor of bilirubin levels. Jaundice regresses in the opposite direction.

3. If the newborn appears jaundiced, a total serum bilirubin or a transcutaneous bilirubin (TcB) level should be checked. TcB levels are monitored with a transcutaneous bilimeter. The device should be used according to manufacturer directions and calibrated as directed. The TcB measurement is obtained from the forehead or the sternum and plotted on a nomogram. A total serum bilirubin (TSB) level is still required when treatment with phototherapy or an exchange transfusion is being considered.

Rationale: A transcutaneous or total serum bilirubin level should be checked on all newborns who appear jaundiced in the first 24 hours of life. A TcB is as reliable as a TSB in most instances and is less invasive. The hour specific nomogram recommended by the AAP provides guidelines for initiating phototherapy in hospitalized newborns of 35 weeks or greater gestational age. Full-term newborns receive phototherapy for bilirubin levels > 12 mg/dl. The recommended treatment levels for premature newborns are dependent on postnatal age, weight, and contributing factors.

4. Assessment of jaundice risk requires gathering information about hydration status to include how the newborn is being fed, feeding tolerance, amount of urine and stool, and weight. Hemoglobin (Hgb) and hematocrit (Hct) levels are also helpful.

Rationale: Newborns who are not eating well are more prone to hyperbilirubinemia. Babies born at high altitude develop higher levels of bilirubin than babies born at sea level (related to elevated hematocrit and hypoxemia).

5. The nurse assesses the newborn for early signs of bilirubin encephalopathy, which include poor feeding, hypotonia, and lethargy.

6. Document any physical findings and TcB levels, and report jaundice to the primary care practitioner.

Erythema toxicum is an eruption of lesions in the area surrounding a hair follicle that are firm, vary in size from 1 to 3 mm, and consist of a white or pale yellow papule or pustule with an erythematous base. It is often called "newborn rash" or "flea bite" dermatitis. The rash may appear suddenly, usually over the trunk and diaper area, and is frequently widespread (Figure 24–18). The lesions do not appear on the palms of the hands or the soles of the feet. The peak incidence is at 24 to 48 hours of life. The condition rarely presents at birth or after 5 days of life. The cause is unknown, and no treatment is necessary. Some clinicians believe it may be caused by irritation from clothing. The lesions disappear in a few hours or days. If a maculopapular rash (eruption consisting of both macules and papules) appears, a smear of the aspirated papule will show numerous eosinophils on staining; no bacteria will be cultured.

Milia, which are exposed sebaceous glands, appear as raised white spots on the face, especially across the nose (Figure 24–19). No treatment is necessary, because they will clear spontaneously within the first month. Newborns of African heritage have a similar condition called *transient neonatal pustular melanosis.*

Skin turgor is assessed to determine hydration status and the presence of any infectious processes. The usual places to assess skin turgor are over the abdomen, the forearm, or the thigh. Skin should be elastic and should return rapidly to its original shape.

Vernix caseosa, a whitish, cheeselike substance, covers the fetus while in utero and lubricates the skin of the newborn. The skin of the term or postterm newborn has less vernix and is frequently dry; peeling is common, especially on the hands and feet.

Forceps marks may be present after a vaginal birth. The newborn may have reddened areas over the cheeks and jaws. It is important to reassure the parents that these marks will disappear, usually within 1 or 2 days. Transient facial paralysis resulting from forceps pressure is a rare complication. Vacuum extractor suction marks (abrasions or ecchymosis) on the vertex of the scalp may be seen when vacuum extractors are used to assist with the birth (Gleason & Devaskar, 2012). These are benign and do not indicate any underlying brain lesions.

Sucking blisters (vesicles or bullae) may appear on the lips, fingers, or hands of newborns as a result of vigorous sucking, either in utero or after birth. These sucking blisters (Figure 24–20) may be intact or ruptured and require no treatment.

Birthmarks

Telangiectatic nevi (stork bites) appear as pale pink or red spots and are frequently found on the eyelids, nose, lower occipital bone, and nape of the neck (Figure 24–21). These lesions are common in newborns with light complexions and are more noticeable during periods of crying. These areas have no clinical significance and usually fade by the second birthday.

Congenital dermal melanocytes, also called *Mongolian blue spots,* are macular areas of bluish black or gray-blue pigmentation usually on the dorsal area and the buttocks, but may be anywhere on the body (Figure 24–22). They are common in newborns of Asian, Hispanic, and African descent and other dark-skin races and can be seen in 1% to 9% of Whites. They gradually fade during the first or second year of life. They may be mistaken for bruises and should be documented in the newborn's medical record.

Nevus flammeus (port-wine stain) is a capillary angioma directly below the epidermis. It is a nonelevated,

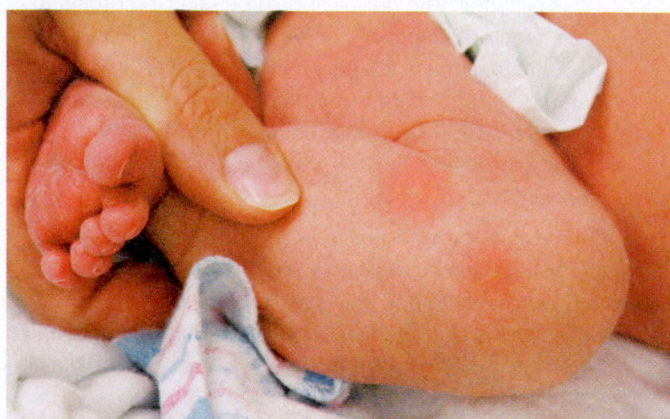

Figure 24–18 Erythema toxicum on leg.

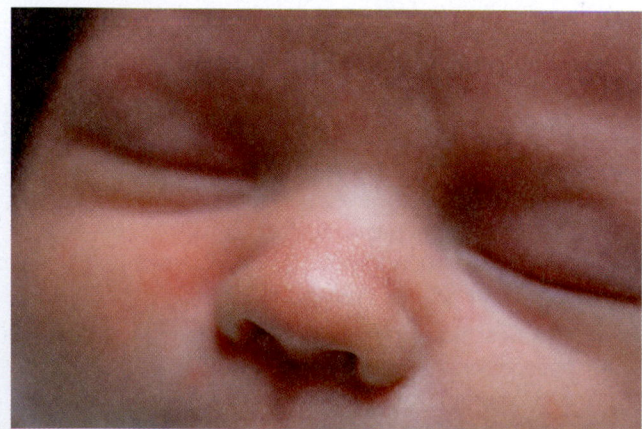

Figure 24–19 **Facial milia over bridge of nose.**
SOURCE: © Jack Sullivan/Alamy.

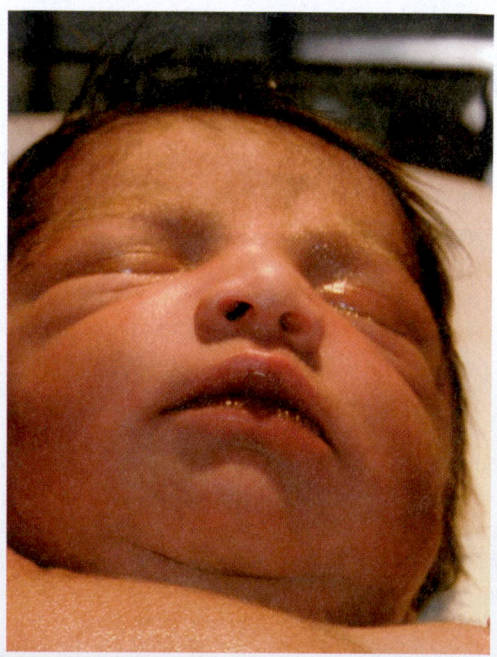

Figure 24–20 Sucking blister in middle of upper lip.
SOURCE: Vanessa Howell, RN, MSN.

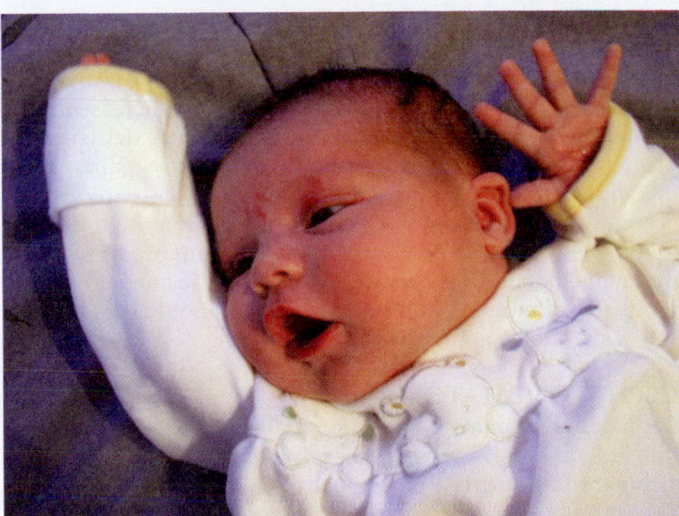

Figure 24–21 Stork bites over left eyelid and near right eyebrow.

SOURCE: Anne Garcia.

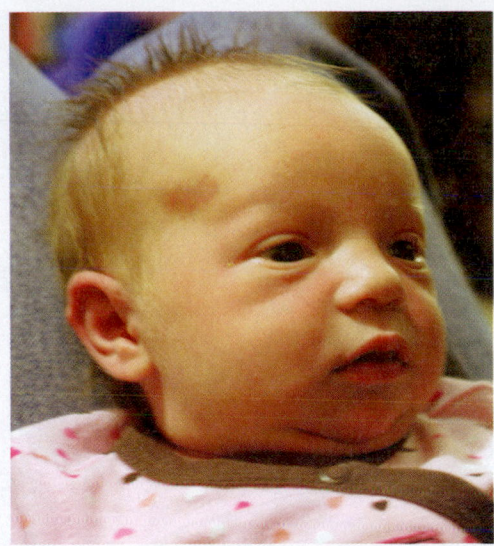

Figure 24–23 Port-wine stain over temple area.

SOURCE: Alyssa Torres.

sharply demarcated, red-to-purple area of dense capillaries (Figure 24–23). In newborns of African descent, it may appear as a purple-black stain. The size and shape vary, but it commonly appears on the face. It does not grow in size, does not fade with time, and does not blanch as a rule. If convulsions and other neurologic problems accompany the nevus flammeus, the clinical picture is suggestive of *Sturge-Weber syndrome,* with involvement of the fifth cranial nerve (the ophthalmic branch of the trigeminal nerve).

Nevus vasculosus (strawberry mark) is a capillary hemangioma. It consists of newly formed and enlarged capillaries in the dermal and subdermal layers. It is a raised, clearly delineated, dark red, rough-surfaced birthmark commonly found in the head region. Such marks usually grow (often rapidly) starting during the second or third week of life and may not reach their full size until about 6 months of age (Witt, 2015). They begin to shrink and start to resolve spontaneously several weeks to months after they reach peak growth. A pale purple or gray spot on the surface of the hemangioma signals the start of resolution. The best cosmetic effect is achieved when the lesions are allowed to resolve spontaneously.

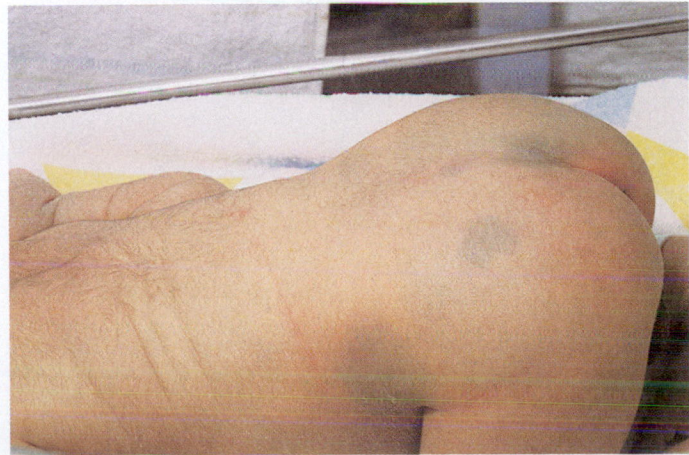

Figure 24–22 Mongolian blue spots.

Head

The newborn's head is large (approximately one fourth of the body size), with soft, pliable skull bones. For most term newborns, the occipital-frontal circumference (OFC) is 32 cm to 37 cm (12.6 in. to 14.6 in.). The head may appear asymmetrical in the newborn who has had a vertex birth. This asymmetry, called **molding**, is caused by the overriding of the cranial bones during labor and birth (Figure 24–24). The degree of molding varies with the amount and length of pressure exerted on the head. Within a few days after birth, the overriding usually diminishes and the suture lines become palpable; therefore a second measurement is indicated a few days after birth. Any extreme differences in head size may indicate microcephaly (abnormally small head) or *hydrocephalus* (an abnormal buildup of fluid in the brain), which can result in an enlarged head. Variations in the shape, size, or appearance of the head measurements may be caused by *craniosynostosis* (premature closure of the cranial sutures), which will need to be corrected through surgery to allow brain growth, and *plagiocephaly* (unilateral closure of coronal or lamboidal suture). The asymmetry may be caused by pressure on the fetal head during gestation (Johnson, 2015).

Two *fontanelles* ("soft spots") may be palpated on the newborn's head. Fontanelles, which are openings at the juncture of the cranial bones, can be measured with the fingers. Accurate measurement necessitates that the examiner's finger be measured in centimeters. The assessment should be carried out with

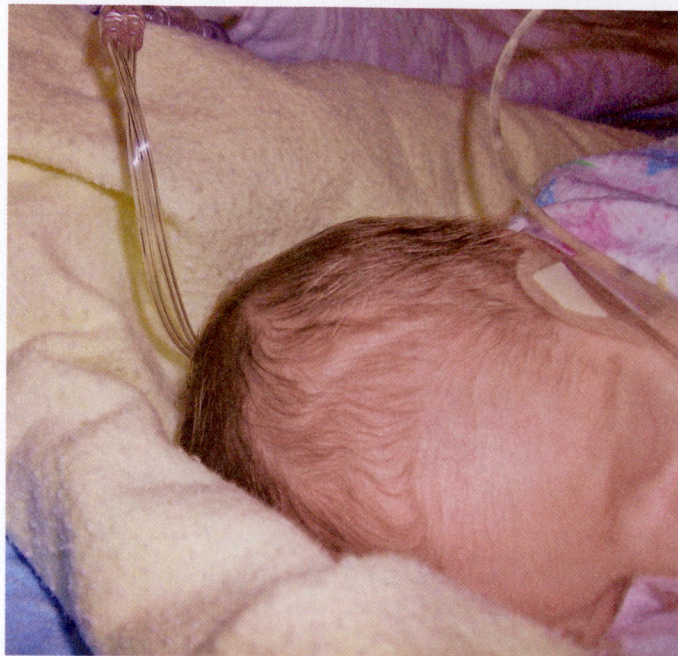

Figure 24–24 Overlapped cranial bones produce a visible ridge in a premature newborn. Easily visible overlapping does not occur often in term newborns.

SOURCE: Vanessa Howell, RN, MSN.

the newborn in a sitting position and not crying. The *diamond-shaped anterior fontanelle* is approximately 3 to 4 cm (1.2 to1.6 in.) long by 2 to 3 cm (0.79 to 1.2 in.) wide. It is located at the juncture of the frontal and parietal bones. The *posterior fontanelle*, smaller and triangular, is formed by the parietal bones and the occipital bone and is 0.5 by 1.0 cm. Because of molding, the fontanelles are smaller immediately after birth than several days later. The anterior fontanelle closes within 18 months, whereas the posterior fontanelle closes within 8 to 12 weeks.

The fontanelles are a useful indicator of the newborn's condition. The anterior fontanelle may swell when the newborn cries or passes a stool or may pulsate with the heartbeat, which is normal. A bulging fontanelle usually signifies increased intracranial pressure; a depressed fontanelle indicates dehydration. The sutures between the cranial bones should be palpated for the amount of overlapping. In newborns whose growth has been restricted, the sutures may be wider than normal, and the fontanelles may also be larger because of impaired growth of the cranial bones. In addition to inspecting the newborn's head for degree of molding and size, the nurse should evaluate it for soft tissue edema and bruising.

CEPHALOHEMATOMA

Cephalohematoma is a collection of blood resulting from ruptured blood vessels between the surface of a cranial bone (usually parietal) and the periosteal membrane (Figure 24–25). The scalp in these areas feels loose and slightly edematous. These areas emerge as defined hematomas between the first and second day. Although external pressure may cause the mass to fluctuate, it does not increase in size when the newborn cries. Cephalohematomas may be unilateral or bilateral and do not cross suture lines. They are relatively common in vertex births and may disappear within 2 weeks to 3 months. They may be associated with physiologic jaundice, because extra red blood cells are being destroyed within the cephalohematoma. A large cephalohematoma can lead to anemia and hypotension.

CAPUT SUCCEDANEUM

Caput succedaneum is a localized, easily identifiable, soft area of the scalp, generally resulting from a long and difficult labor or vacuum extraction (Figure 24–26). The sustained pressure of the presenting part against the cervix results in compression of local blood vessels, and venous return is slowed. Slowed venous return in turn causes an increase in tissue fluids, edematous swelling, and occasional bleeding under the periosteum. The caput may vary from a small area to a severely elongated head. The fluid in the caput is reabsorbed within 12 hours to a

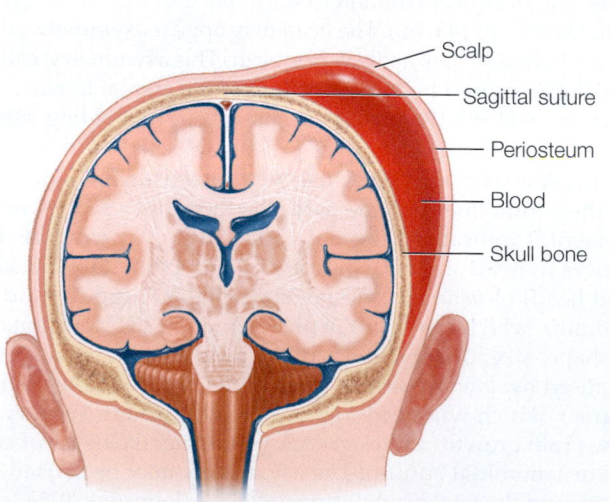

Scalp
Sagittal suture
Periosteum
Blood
Skull bone

A

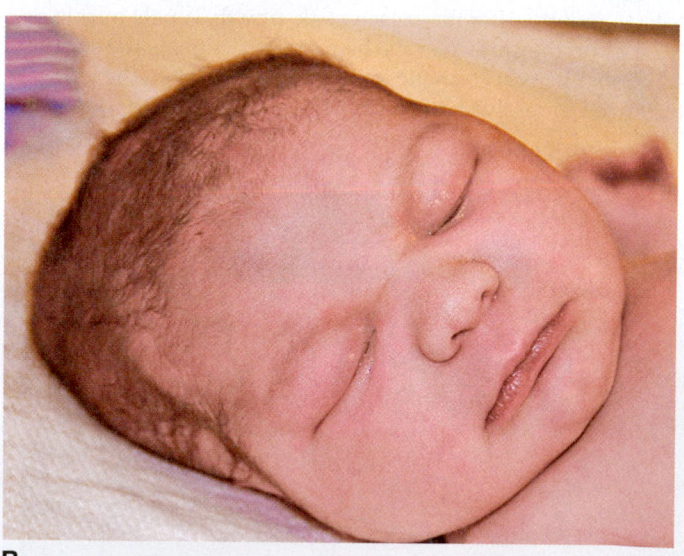

B

Figure 24–25 A. Cephalohematoma is a collection of blood between the surface of a cranial bone and the periosteal membrane. B. This is a cephalohematoma over the right parietal bone.

SOURCE: B: Vanessa Howell, RN, MSN.

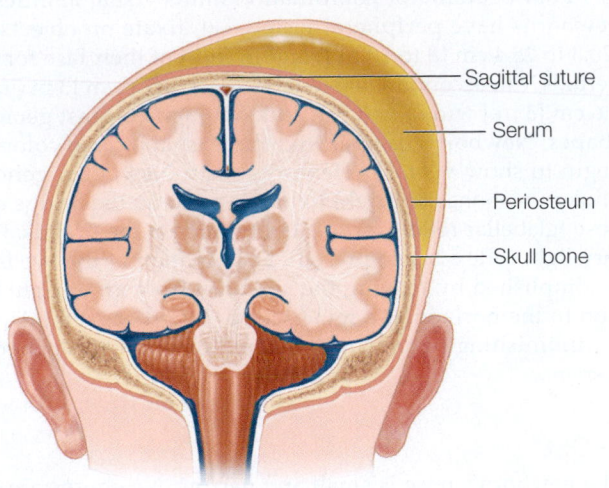

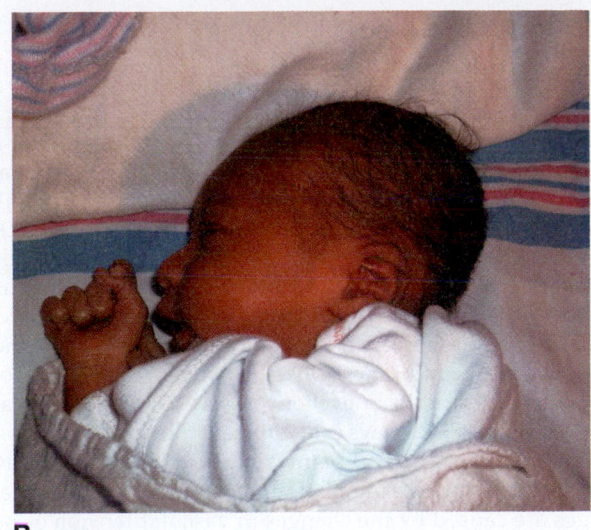

A

B

Figure 24–26 A. Caput succedaneum is a collection of fluid (serum) under the scalp. B. Newborn with caput succedaneum.

SOURCE: Michele Davidson.

few days after birth. Caputs resulting from vacuum extractors are sharply outlined, circular areas up to 2 cm (0.8 in.) thick. They disappear more slowly than naturally occurring edema.

See Table 24–1 for ways to distinguish between cephalohematoma and caput succedaneum.

Hair

The term newborn's hair is smooth with texture variations depending on ethnic background. Scalp hair is usually high over the eyebrows. Assessment of the newborn's hair characteristics such as color, quantity, texture, hairlines, direction of growth, and hair whorls can identify genetic, metabolic, and neurologic disorders (Johnson, 2015). For example, coarse, brittle, and dry hair may indicate hypothyroidism.

Face

The newborn's face is well designed to help the newborn suckle. Sucking (fat) pads are located in the cheeks. The chin is recessed, and the nose is flattened. The lips are sensitive to touch, and the sucking reflex is easily initiated. Symmetry of the eyes, nose, and ears is evaluated. Facial movement symmetry should be assessed to determine the presence of facial palsy. Facial paralysis appears when the newborn cries; the affected side is immobile, and the palpebral (eyelid) fissure widens (Figure 24–27). Paralysis may result from forceps-assisted birth

or pressure on the facial nerve from the maternal pelvis during birth. Facial paralysis usually disappears within a few days to 3 weeks, although in some cases it may be permanent.

Eyes

The eyes of the newborn of northern European descent are a blue-gray or slate blue-gray color. Dark-skinned newborns tend to have dark eyes at birth. Scleral color tends to be bluish white because of the relative thinness of the sclera. A blue sclera is associated with osteogenesis imperfecta. The newborn's eye color is usually established at approximately 3 months, although it may change any time up to 1 year.

The eyes should be checked for size, equality of pupil size, reaction of pupils to light, blink reflex to light, and edema and inflammation of the eyelids. The eyelids are usually edematous

TABLE 24–1 Comparison of Cephalohematoma and Caput Succedaneum

CEPHALOHEMATOMA	CAPUT SUCCEDANEUM
Collection of blood between cranial (usually parietal) bone and periosteal membrane	Collection of fluid, edematous swelling of the scalp
Does not cross suture lines	Crosses suture lines
Appears between first and second day	Present at birth or shortly thereafter
Disappears after 2 to 3 weeks or may take months	Reabsorbed within 12 hours or a few days after birth

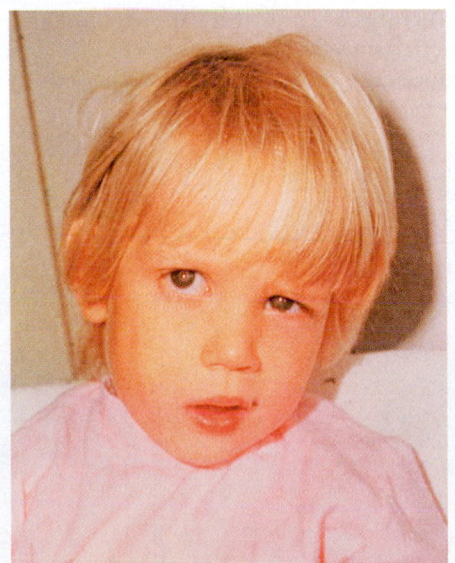

Figure 24–27 Facial paralysis that occurred during birth. Paralysis of the left side of the toddler's face from injury to the left facial nerve.

SOURCE: Science Source.

during the first few days of life because of the pressure associated with birth.

Erythromycin and tetracycline (in some agencies) are used prophylactically instead of silver nitrate and usually do not cause chemical irritation of the eye. The instillation of silver nitrate drops in the newborn's eyes may cause edema, and **chemical conjunctivitis** may appear a few hours after instillation, but it disappears in 1 to 2 days (Cloherty et al., 2012). If infectious conjunctivitis exists, the newborn has the same purulent (greenish yellow) discharge exudate as in chemical conjunctivitis, but it is caused by gonococci, *Chlamydia*, staphylococci, or a variety of gram-negative bacteria. It requires treatment with ophthalmic antibiotics. Onset is usually after the second day. Edema of the orbits or eyelids may persist for several days, until the newborn's kidneys can eliminate the fluid.

Small **subconjunctival hemorrhages** appear in about 10% of newborns and are commonly found on the sclera. These hemorrhages are caused by the changes in vascular tension or ocular pressure during birth. They will remain for a few weeks and are of no pathologic significance. Parents need reassurance that the newborn is not bleeding from within the eye and that vision will not be impaired.

The newborn may demonstrate transient strabismus caused by poor neuromuscular control of eye muscles (Figure 24–28). It gradually regresses in 3 to 4 months. The "doll's eye" phenomenon is also present for about 10 days after birth. As the newborn's head position is changed to the left and then to the right, the eyes move to the opposite direction. "Doll's eye" results from underdeveloped integration of head–eye coordination.

The nurse should observe the newborn's pupils for opacities or whiteness and for the absence of a normal red retinal reflex. Red retinal reflex is a red-orange flash of color observed when an ophthalmoscope light reflects off the retina. In a newborn with dark skin color, the retina may appear paler or more grayish. Absence of red reflex occurs with cataracts. Congenital cataracts should be suspected in newborns of mothers with a history of rubella, cytomegalic inclusion disease, or syphilis. Brushfield spots (black or white spots on the periphery of the iris) can be associated with trisomy 21 (Johnson, 2015).

The cry of the newborn is commonly tearless because the lacrimal structures are immature at birth and are not usually fully functional until the second month of life. However, some babies produce tears during the newborn period.

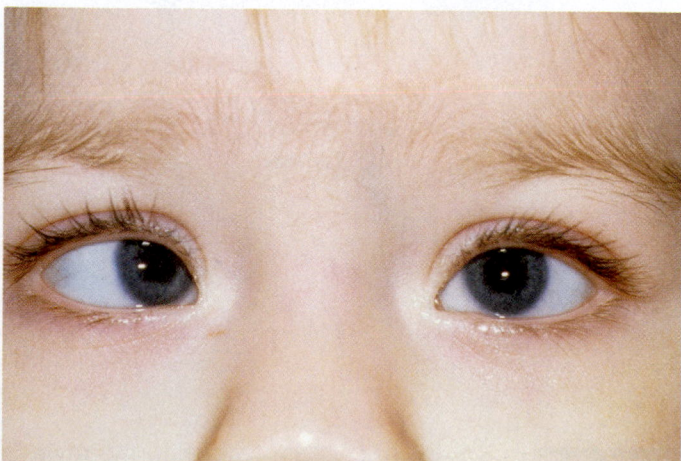

Figure 24–28 Transient strabismus in the newborn may be due to poor neuromuscular control.

SOURCE: Biophoto Associates/Science Source.

Poor oculomotor coordination limits visual abilities, but newborns have peripheral vision, can fixate on objects near (20.3 to 25.4 cm [8 to 10 in.]) and in front of their face for short periods, can accommodate to large objects (7.6 cm [3 in.] tall by 7.6 cm [3 in.] wide), and can seek out high-contrast geometric shapes. Newborns can perceive faces, shapes, and colors and begin to show visual preferences early. Newborns generally blink in response to bright lights, to a tap on the bridge of the nose (glabellar reflex), or to a light touch on the eyelids. Pupillary light reflex is also present. Examination of the eye is best accomplished by rocking the newborn from an upright position to the horizontal a few times or by other methods, such as diminishing overhead lights, which elicit an opened-eye response.

Nose

The newborn's nose is small and narrow. Newborns are characteristically nose breathers for the first few months of life and generally remove obstructions by sneezing. The nose is patent if the newborn breathes easily with the mouth closed. If respiratory difficulty occurs, the nurse checks for choanal atresia (congenital blockage of the passageway between nose and pharynx). This can be done by observing the newborn feeding because newborns are obligatory nose breathers, or by gently occluding each of the nares (Caveliere & Sansoucie, 2014).

The newborn has the ability to smell after the nasal passages have been cleared of amniotic fluid and mucus. Newborns demonstrate this ability by the search for milk. Newborns turn their heads toward a milk source, whether bottle or breast. Newborns react to strong odors, such as alcohol, by turning their heads away or blinking.

Mouth

The lips of the newborn should be pink, and a touch on the lips should produce sucking motions. Saliva is normally scant. The taste buds develop before birth, and the newborn can easily discriminate between sweet and bitter flavors.

The easiest way to examine the mouth completely is to stimulate newborns to cry by gently depressing their tongue, thereby causing them to open the mouth fully. It is extremely important to examine the entire mouth to check for a cleft palate, which can be present even in the absence of a cleft lip. The examiner moves an unpowdered gloved index finger along the hard and soft palates to feel for any openings (Figure 24–29).

Occasionally, an examination of the gums will reveal *precocious teeth* over the area where the lower central incisor will erupt. If they appear loose, they should be removed to prevent aspiration. Gray-white lesions (inclusion cysts) on the gums may be confused with teeth. On the hard palate and gum margins, **Epstein's pearls**, small glistening white specks (keratin-containing cysts) that feel hard to the touch, are often present. They usually disappear in a few weeks and are of no significance. **Thrush** may appear as white patches that look like milk curds adhering to the mucous membranes, and bleeding may occur when patches are removed. Thrush is caused by *Candida albicans*, often acquired from an infected vaginal tract during birth, antibiotic use, or poor hand washing when the mother handles her newborn. Thrush is treated with a preparation of nystatin (Mycostatin). The mother should also be treated at the same time.

A newborn may have a ridge of frenulum tissue attached to the underside of the tongue at varying lengths from its base, causing a heart shape at the tip of the tongue. "Clipping the

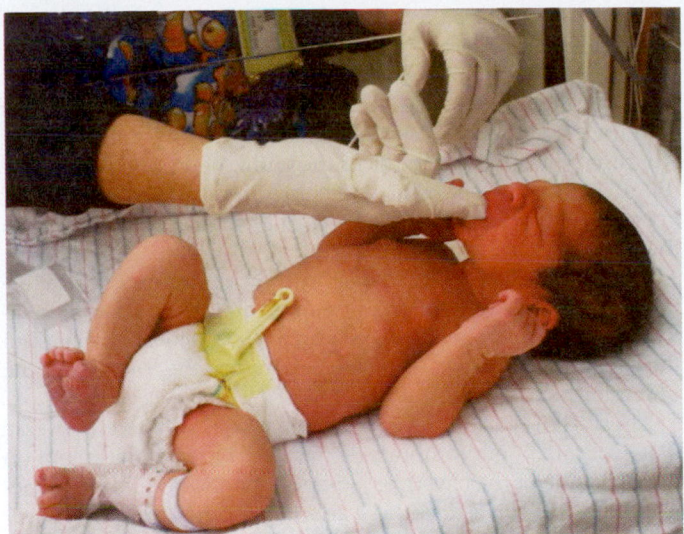

Figure 24–29 The nurse inserts a gloved index finger into the newborn's mouth and feels for any openings along the hard and soft palates.

NOTE: Gloves or a finger cot are always worn to examine the palate.
SOURCE: Vanessa Howell, RNC, MSN.

tongue," or cutting the ridge of tissue, is not usually recommended unless the newborn has trouble feeding. In this case, the healthcare provider would perform a *frenotomy*. This ridge does not affect speech or eating, but cutting creates an entry for infection. Transient nerve paralysis resulting from birth trauma may be manifested by asymmetrical mouth movements when the newborn cries or by difficulty with sucking and feeding.

Ears

The ears of the newborn are soft and pliable and should recoil readily when folded and released. In the normal newborn, the top of the ear (pinna) should be parallel to the outer and inner canthus of the eye. The ears should be inspected for shape, size, firmness of cartilage, and position. *Low-set ears* are characteristic of many syndromes and may indicate chromosomal abnormalities (especially trisomies 13 and 18), intellectual disability, and internal organ abnormalities, especially bilateral renal agenesis as a result of embryologic developmental deviations (Figure 24–30). *Preauricular skin tags* may be present just in

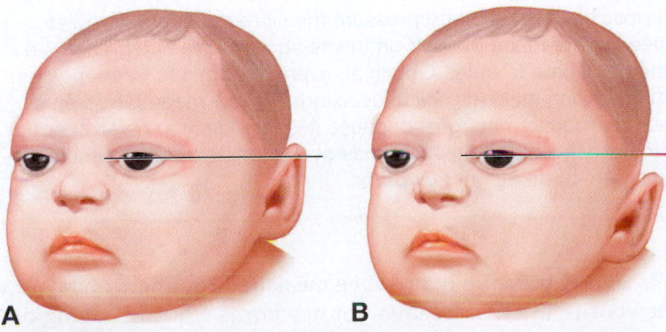

A   **B**

Figure 24–30 The position of the external ear may be assessed by drawing a line across the inner and outer canthus of the eye to the insertion of the ear. A. Normal position. B. True low-set position.

front of the ear. Visualization of the tympanic membrane is not usually done soon after birth because blood and vernix block the ear canal.

Following the first cry, the newborn's hearing becomes acute as mucus from the middle ear is absorbed, the eustachian tube becomes aerated, and the tympanic membrane becomes visible. The newborn's hearing initially can be evaluated by noting the baby's response to loud or moderately loud noises that are not accompanied by vibrations. The sleeping newborn should stir or awaken in response to nearby sounds. (This is not a very accurate test, but it may alert the examiner to a possible problem.) The newborn can discriminate the individual characteristics of the human voice and is especially sensitive to sound levels within the normal conversational range. The newborn in a noisy nursery may habituate to the sounds and not stir unless the sound is sudden or much louder than usual.

The AAP has endorsed universal newborn hearing screening (UNHS) before discharge from the birthing unit as the standard of care (AAP & ACOG, 2012; Johnson, 2015). See Chapter 25 for further discussion.

Neck

A short neck, creased with skin folds, is characteristic of the normal newborn. Because muscle tone is not well developed, the neck cannot support the full weight of the head, which rotates freely. The head lags considerably when the newborn is pulled from a supine to a sitting position, but the prone newborn is able to raise the head slightly. The neck is palpated for masses and the presence of lymph nodes and is inspected for webbing. Adequacy of range of motion and neck muscle function is determined by moving the head in all directions while supporting the newborn to prevent injury. Injury to the sternocleidomastoid muscle (congenital torticollis) must be considered in the presence of neck rigidity.

The nurse evaluates the clavicles for evidence of fractures, which occasionally occur during difficult births or in newborns with broad shoulders. The normal clavicle is straight. If fractured, a lump and a grating sensation (crepitus) during movements may be palpated along the course of the side of the break. The nurse also elicits the Moro reflex (see Table 24–2) to evaluate bilateral equal movement of the arms. If the clavicle is fractured, the response will be demonstrated only on the unaffected side.

Chest

The thorax is cylindric and symmetric at birth, and the ribs are flexible. The general appearance of the chest should be assessed. A protrusion at the lower end of the sternum, called the xiphoid cartilage, is frequently seen. It is under the skin and will become less apparent after several weeks as adipose tissue accumulates.

Engorged breasts occur frequently in both male and female newborns. This condition, which occurs by the third day, is a result of maternal hormonal influences and may last up to 2 weeks (Figure 24–31). A whitish secretion from the nipples may also be noted. The newborn's breast should not be massaged or squeezed, because this may cause a breast abscess. Supernumerary nipples are occasionally noted below and medial to the true nipples. These harmless pink or brown (in dark-skinned newborns) spots vary in size and do not contain glandular tissue. Accessory nipples can be differentiated from pigmented nevi (mole) by placing the fingertips alongside the accessory nipple and pulling the adjacent tissue laterally. The accessory nipple will appear dimpled.

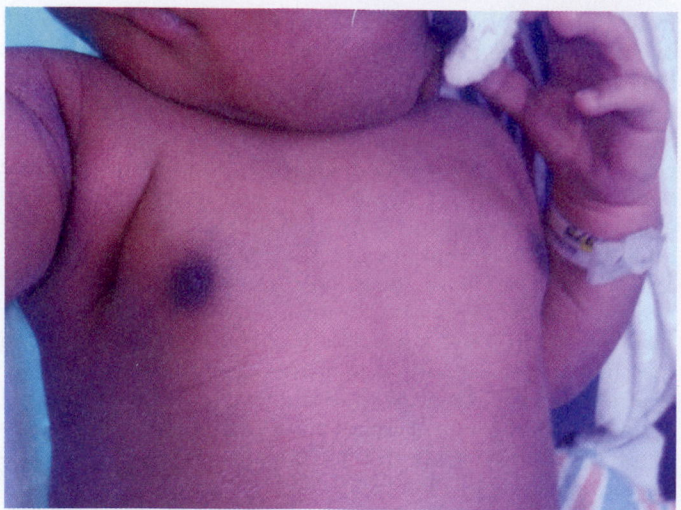

Figure 24–31 Breast hypertrophy.
SOURCE: Michele Davidson.

Cry

The newborn's cry should be strong, lusty, and of medium pitch. A high-pitched, shrill cry is abnormal and may indicate neurologic disorders or hypoglycemia. Periods of crying usually vary in length after consoling measures are used. Babies' cries are an important method of communication and alert caregivers to changes in their conditions and needs.

Clinical Tip

Vital sign assessments are most accurate if the newborn is at rest, so measure pulse and respirations first if the baby is quiet. To soothe a crying baby, try placing your moistened gloved finger in the baby's mouth, and then complete your assessment while the baby suckles.

Respiration

Normal breathing for a term newborn is 30 to 60 respirations per minute and is predominantly diaphragmatic, with associated rising and falling of the abdomen during inspiration and expiration. The nurse should note any signs of respiratory distress, nasal flaring, intercostal or xiphoid retraction, expiratory grunt or sigh, seesaw respirations, or tachypnea (greater than 60 breaths per minute). Hyperextension (chest appears high) or hypoextension (chest appears low) of the anteroposterior diameter of the chest should also be noted. Both the anterior and the posterior chest are auscultated. Some breath sounds are heard best when the newborn is crying, but localizing and identifying breath sounds are difficult in the newborn. Upper airway noises and bowel sounds can be heard over the chest wall, making auscultation difficult. Because sounds may be transmitted from the unaffected lung to the affected lung, the absence of breath sounds may not be diagnosed. Air entry may be noisy in the first couple of hours until lung fluid resolves, especially after cesarean births. Brief periods of apnea (episodic breathing) occur, but no color or heart rate changes occur in healthy, term newborns. Sepsis should be suspected in full-term newborns experiencing apneic episodes.

Heart

Heart rates can be as rapid as 200 beats per minute (beats/min) in newborns and fluctuate a great deal, especially if the baby moves or is startled. The normal range is 110 to 160 beats/min.

The heart is examined for rate and rhythm, position of the apical impulse, and heart sound intensity. Dysrhythmias should be evaluated by the healthcare provider.

The pulse rate is variable and is influenced by physical activity, crying, state of wakefulness, and body temperature. Auscultation is performed over the entire heart region (precordium), below the left axilla, and below the scapula. *Apical pulse rates are obtained by auscultation for a full minute,* preferably when the newborn is asleep.

The placement of the heart in the chest should be determined when the newborn is in a quiet state. The heart is relatively large at birth and is located mid to left chest and high in the chest, with its apex somewhere between the fourth and the fifth intercostal spaces.

A shift of heart tones in the mediastinal area to either side may indicate pneumothorax, dextrocardia (heart placement on the right side of the chest), or a diaphragmatic hernia. The experienced nurse can detect these and many other problems early with a stethoscope. The nurse should auscultate heart sounds using both the bell and the diaphragm of the stethoscope. Normally, the heart beat has a "toc tic" sound. A slur or slushing sound (usually after the first sound) may indicate a *murmur*. Although 90% of all murmurs are transient and are considered normal, they should be monitored closely by a healthcare provider. Many murmurs are secondary to closing of the patent ductus arteriosus or patent foramen ovale, which should close 1 to 2 days after birth. See Chapter 26 for discussion of congenital heart defects.

Peripheral pulses (brachial, femoral, pedal) are also evaluated to detect any lags or unusual characteristics. Brachial pulses are palpated bilaterally for equality and compared with the femoral pulses. Femoral pulses are palpated by applying gentle pressure with the middle finger over the femoral canal (Figure 24–32). Decreased or absent femoral pulses may indicate coarctation of the aorta or hypovolemia and require additional evaluation. A wide difference in blood pressure between the upper and lower extremities also indicates coarctation of the aorta.

The measurement of blood pressure is best accomplished by using a noninvasive blood pressure device (Figure 24–33). If a blood pressure cuff is used, the newborn's extremities must be immobilized during the assessment, and the cuff should cover two thirds of the upper arm or upper leg. Movement, crying, and inappropriate cuff size can give inaccurate measurements of the blood pressure.

Clinical Tip

If possible, obtain blood pressure measurements during quiet sleep state. Place the cuff on the newborn's arm or leg and give the baby time to quiet. Obtain an average of two to three measurements when making clinical decisions. Follow mean blood pressure to monitor changes, because it is less likely to be erroneous. Noninvasive blood pressure may overestimate blood pressure in very low-birth-weight newborns.

Blood pressure may not be measured routinely on healthy newborns, but it is essential for newborns who are having distress, are premature, or are suspected of having a cardiac anomaly, renal disease, or clinical signs of hypotension (Vargo, 2015). Newborns who have birth asphyxia and are on ventilators have significantly lower systolic and diastolic blood pressures than healthy newborns. If a cardiac anomaly is suspected, blood pressure is measured in all four extremities. At birth, systolic values usually range from 70 to 50 mmHg and diastolic values from 45 to 30 mmHg. By the 10th day of life, blood pressure rises to 90/50 mmHg. See *Key Facts to Remember: Newborn Vital Signs*.

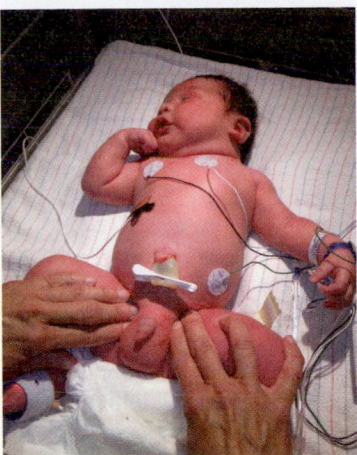

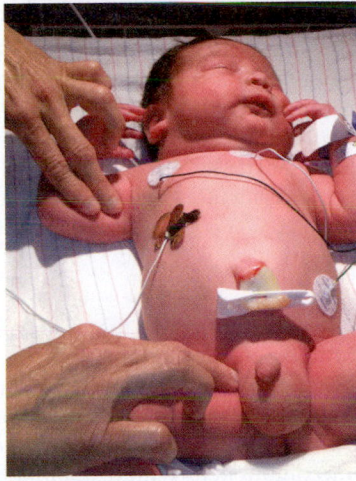

KEY FACTS TO REMEMBER
Newborn Vital Signs

Pulse

110 to 160 beats/min

During sleep as low as 80 beats/min; if crying, up to 180 beats/min (Gomella, 2013)

Apical pulse counted for 1 full minute

Respirations

30 to 60 respirations/minute

Predominantly diaphragmatic but synchronous with abdominal movements

Respirations are counted for 1 full minute

Blood Pressure

70–50/45–30 mmHg at birth

90/50 mmHg at day 10

Temperature

Normal range: 36.5° to 37.5°C (97.7° to 99.4°F)

Axillary: 36.4° to 37.2°C (97.5° to 99°F)

Skin: 36° to 36.5°C (96.8° to 97.7°F)

Rectal: 36.6° to 37.2°C (97.8° to 99°F)

Figure 24–32 A. Bilaterally palpate the femoral arteries for rate and intensity of the pulses. Press fingertip gently at the groin as shown. B. Compare the femoral pulses to the brachial pulses by palpating the pulses simultaneously for comparison of rate and intensity.
SOURCE: Carol Harrigan, RNC, MSN, NNP.

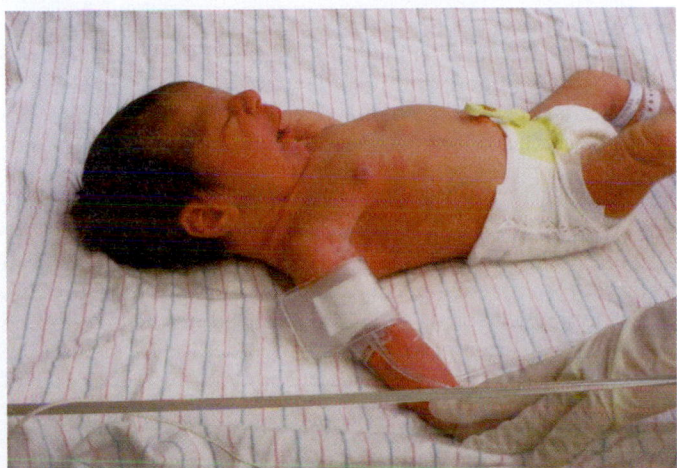

Figure 24–33 Blood pressure measurement using noninvasive Dinamap and Doppler blood pressure devices. The cuff can be applied to either the newborn's upper arm or the thigh.
SOURCE: Vanessa Howell, RNC, MSN.

Abdomen

The nurse can learn a great deal about the newborn's abdomen without disturbing the baby. The abdomen should be cylindrical, protrude slightly, and move with respiration. A certain amount of laxness of the abdominal muscles is normal. A scaphoid (hollow-shaped) appearance suggests the absence of abdominal contents, often seen in diaphragmatic hernias. No cyanosis should be present, and few if any blood vessels should be apparent to the eye. There should be no gross distention or bulging. The more distended the abdomen, the tighter the skin becomes, with engorged vessels appearing. Distention is the first sign of many gastrointestinal abnormalities.

Before palpation of the abdomen, the nurse should auscultate for the presence or absence of bowel sounds in all four quadrants. Bowel sounds may be present by 1 hour after birth. Palpation can cause a transient decrease in bowel sound intensity.

Abdominal palpation should be done systematically. The nurse palpates each of the four abdominal quadrants and moves in a clockwise direction until all four quadrants have been palpated for softness, tenderness, and the presence of masses. The nurse should place one hand under the back for support during palpation.

Umbilical Cord

Initially the umbilical cord is white and gelatinous in appearance, with the two umbilical arteries and one umbilical vein readily apparent. Because a single umbilical artery is frequently associated with congenital anomalies, the nurse should count the vessels during the newborn assessment. The cord begins drying within 1 or 2 hours of birth and is shriveled and blackened by the second or third day. Care of the umbilical cord is discussed in Chapter 25.

Cord bleeding is abnormal and may result from tension on the cord or clamp. Foul-smelling drainage is also abnormal and is generally caused by infection, which requires immediate treatment to prevent septicemia. Serous or serosanguineous drainage that continues after the cord falls off may indicate a granuloma. It appears as a small red button deep in the umbilicus without any central depression or lumen. If the newborn has a patent urachus (abnormal connection between the umbilicus and the bladder), moistness or draining urine may be apparent at the base of the cord. Another umbilical cord anomaly that can occur is umbilical cord hernia and associated patent omphalomesenteric duct (Figure 24–34). Umbilical hernias are more common in babies of African American descent than in White babies (Goodwin, 2015). The umbilical hernias usually close spontaneously by 2 years of age.

> ### Developing Cultural Competence   Native Americans and Umbilical Cord Care
> In the Woodland Indian tribe, upon birth, the umbilical cord is tied and a small piece is saved. This section of the umbilical cord is sewn into a diamond-shaped deerskin pocket. The pocket is hung over the baby's crib to provide protection.

Genitals

FEMALE NEWBORNS
The nurse examines the labia majora, labia minora, and clitoris and notes the size of each as appropriate for gestational age. A vaginal tag or hymenal tag is often evident and will usually disappear in a few weeks. During the first week of life, the female newborn may have a vaginal discharge composed of thick, whitish mucus. This discharge, which can become tinged with blood, is called **pseudomenstruation** and is caused by the withdrawal of maternal hormones. *Smegma*, a white, cheeselike substance, is often present between the labia. Removing it may traumatize tender tissue.

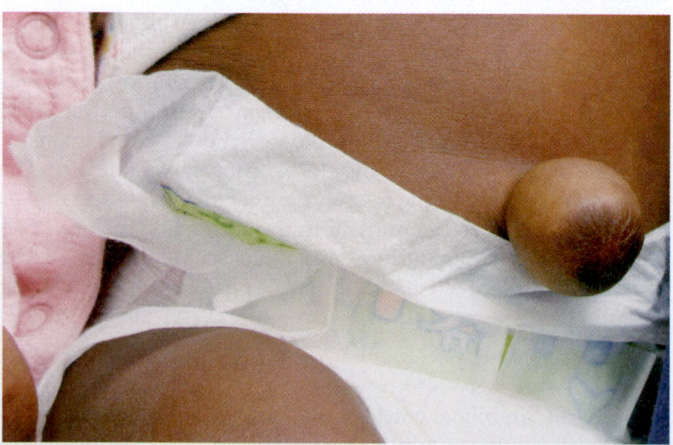

Figure 24–34 Umbilical hernia.

MALE NEWBORNS
The nurse inspects the penis to determine whether the urinary orifice is correctly positioned. *Hypospadias* occurs when the urinary meatus is located on the ventral surface of the penis, whereas in *epispadius,* the meatus is on the dorsal surface of the glans. Hypospadias occurs most commonly among people of Western European descent. *Phimosis* is a condition in which the opening of the foreskin (prepuce) is small and the foreskin cannot be pulled back over the glans at all. This condition may interfere with urination, so the adequacy of the urinary stream should be evaluated.

The scrotum is inspected for size and symmetry. Scrotal color variations are especially prominent in African American, Indian, and Hispanic newborns (Cloherty et al., 2012). The scrotum should be palpated to verify the presence of both testes and to rule out *cryptorchidism* (failure of testes to descend). The testes are palpated separately between the thumb and forefinger, with the thumb and forefinger of the other hand placed together over the inguinal canal. Scrotal edema and discoloration are common in breech births. *Hydrocele* (a collection of fluid surrounding the testes in the scrotum) is common in newborns and should be identified. It usually resolves without intervention. The presence of a discolored or dusky scrotum and solid testis should raise the suspicion of testicular torsion and should be reported immediately.

Anus

The anal area is inspected to verify that it is patent and has no fissure. Imperforate anus and rectal atresia may be ruled out by observation. Digital examination, if necessary, is done by a healthcare provider or nurse practitioner. The nurse also notes the passage of the first meconium stool. Atresia of the gastrointestinal tract or meconium ileus with resultant obstruction must be considered if the newborn does not pass meconium in the first 24 hours of life.

Extremities

Extremities are examined for gross deformities, extra digits or webbing, clubfoot, and range of motion. Normal newborn extremities appear short, are generally flexible, and move symmetrically.

ARMS AND HANDS
Nails extend beyond the fingertips in term newborns. The nurse should count fingers and toes. *Polydactyly* is the presence of extra digits on either the hands or the feet. *Syndactyly* refers to fusion (webbing) of fingers or toes. This condition can be hereditary or associated with trisomy 21. The hands are inspected for normal palmar creases. A single palmar crease is frequently present in children with Down syndrome (trisomy 21).

Brachial palsy, paralysis of portions of the arm, results from trauma to the brachial plexus during a difficult birth. It occurs commonly when strong traction is exerted on the head of the newborn in an attempt to deliver a shoulder lodged behind the symphysis pubis in the presence of shoulder dystocia. Brachial palsy may also occur during a breech birth if an arm becomes trapped over the head and traction is exerted.

The portion of the arm affected is determined by the nerves damaged. **Erb-Duchenne paralysis (Erb palsy)** involves damage to the upper arm (fifth and sixth cervical nerves) and is the most common type. Injury to the eighth cervical and first thoracic nerve roots and the *lower portion* of the plexus produces the relatively rare lower arm injury. The *whole-arm type* results from damage to the entire plexus.

With Erb-Duchenne paralysis the newborn's arm lies limply at the side. The elbow is held in extension, with the forearm pronated. The newborn is unable to elevate the arm, and the Moro reflex cannot be elicited on the affected side. Lower arm injury causes paralysis of the hand and wrist; complete paralysis of the limb occurs with the whole-arm type.

The degree of nerve damage resulting from the trauma and hemorrhage within the nerve sheath determines recovery. Complete recovery occurs within a few months with minimal trauma. Moderate trauma may result in partial paralysis. Recovery is unlikely with severe trauma, and muscle wasting may develop.

Clinical Tip

Always examine more closely any newborn who is reluctant to move an extremity. Fractures are often asymptomatic in the newborn; paralytic injuries are characterized by immobility of an extremity. A fractured clavicle should be suspected when it is noted that the newborn is moving only one arm.

LEGS AND FEET

The legs of the newborn should be of equal length and with symmetrical skin folds. However, they may assume a fetal posture similar to the position in utero, and it may take several days for the legs and feet to relax into a normal position. The nurse should assess for asymmetry of inner thigh folds, limited hip abduction, and the Allis sign (an indication of fracture in the neck of the femur in which a finger easily sinks into the relaxed fascia between the great trochanter and the iliac crest) (Figure 24–35A).

To evaluate for hip dislocation or hip instability, the Ortolani and Barlow maneuvers are performed. The nurse (or more commonly, the healthcare provider or nurse practitioner) performs the **Barlow maneuver** (Figure 24–35B) to rule out the possibility of developmental dysplastic hip, also called congenital hip dysplasia (hip dislocatability). The examiner grasps and adducts the newborn's thigh and applies gentle downward pressure. Dislocation can be felt as the femoral head slips out of the acetabulum (Figure 24–35C).

The **Ortolani maneuver** (Figure 24–35D) should be performed with the newborn relaxed and quiet on a firm surface. With hips and knees flexed at a 90-degree angle, the examiner grasps the newborn's thigh with the middle finger over the greater trochanter and lifts the thigh to bring the femoral head from its posterior position toward the acetabulum. With gentle abduction of the thigh, the femoral head is returned to the acetabulum and the examiner feels a sense of reduction or a "clunk" as the femoral head returns, confirming the diagnosis of an unstable or dislocatable hip.

The feet are then examined for evidence of a talipes deformity (clubfoot). Intrauterine position frequently causes the feet to appear to turn inward (Figure 24–36); this is termed a *"positional" clubfoot.* If the feet can easily be returned to the midline by manipulation, no treatment is indicated and the nurse teaches range-of-motion exercises to the family. Further evaluation is indicated when the foot will not turn to a midline position or align readily. This is considered the most severe type of "true clubfoot," or talipes equinovarus.

Back

With the newborn prone, the nurse examines the back. The spine should appear straight and flat, because the lumbar and sacral curves do not develop until the newborn begins to sit.

The base of the spine is examined for a dermal sinus. A nevus pilosus ("hairy nerve") is occasionally found at the base of the spine in newborns. It is significant because it is frequently associated with spina bifida. A pilonidal dimple should be examined to ascertain that there is no connection to the spinal canal.

Assessment of Neurologic Status

The nurse should begin the neurologic examination with a period of observation, noting the general physical characteristics and behaviors of the newborn. Important behaviors to assess are the *state of alertness, resting posture, cry,* and *quality of muscle tone and motor activity.*

The usual position of the newborn is with partially flexed extremities, with the legs abducted to the abdomen. When awake, the newborn may exhibit purposeless, uncoordinated bilateral movements of the extremities. If these movements are absent, minimal, or obviously asymmetrical, neurologic dysfunction should be suspected. Eye movements are observable during the first few days of life. An alert newborn is able to fixate on faces and brightly colored objects. Shining a bright light in the newborn's eyes elicits the blinking response.

The nurse evaluates muscle tone by moving various parts of the body while the head of the newborn is in a neutral position. The newborn is somewhat hypertonic; that is, there should be resistance to extending the elbow and knee joints. Muscle tone should be symmetrical. Diminished muscle tone and flaccidity require further evaluation.

Tremors or jitteriness (tremor-like movements) in the full-term newborn must be evaluated to differentiate the tremors from convulsions. Tremors may also be related to hypoglycemia, hypocalcemia, or substance withdrawal. Environmental stimuli may initiate tremors. Jitteriness may be distinguished from tonic–clonic seizure activity because it usually can be stopped by the newborn's sucking on the extremity or by the nurse's holding or flexing the involved extremity. A fine jumping of the muscle is likely to be a central nervous system (CNS) disorder and requires further evaluation. Newborn seizures may consist of no more than chewing or swallowing movements, deviations of the eyes, rigidity, or flaccidity because of CNS immaturity. In contrast to tremors, seizures are not usually initiated by stimuli, and cannot be stopped by holding.

Specific deep tendon reflexes can be elicited in the newborn but have limited value unless they are obviously asymmetric. The knee jerk is typically brisk; a normal ankle clonus may involve three or four beats. Plantar flexion is present.

The immature CNS of the newborn is characterized by a variety of reflexes. Because the newborn's movements are uncoordinated, methods of communication are limited, and control of bodily functions is restricted, the reflexes serve a variety of purposes. Some aid in feeding (rooting, sucking) and may not be very active if the newborn has eaten recently, and some stimulate human interaction (grasping). In addition, newborns can *blink, gag, yawn, cough, sneeze,* and *draw back from pain* (protective reflexes). They can even move a little on their own. When placed on their stomachs, they push up and try to crawl (prone crawl). The absence of or a variance in the response requires motor function evaluation by a specialist. Absence of the *plantar grasp reflex* and the *Galant (truncal incurvation) reflex* requires neurologic evaluation. The most common reflexes found in the normal newborn are shown in Table 24–2.

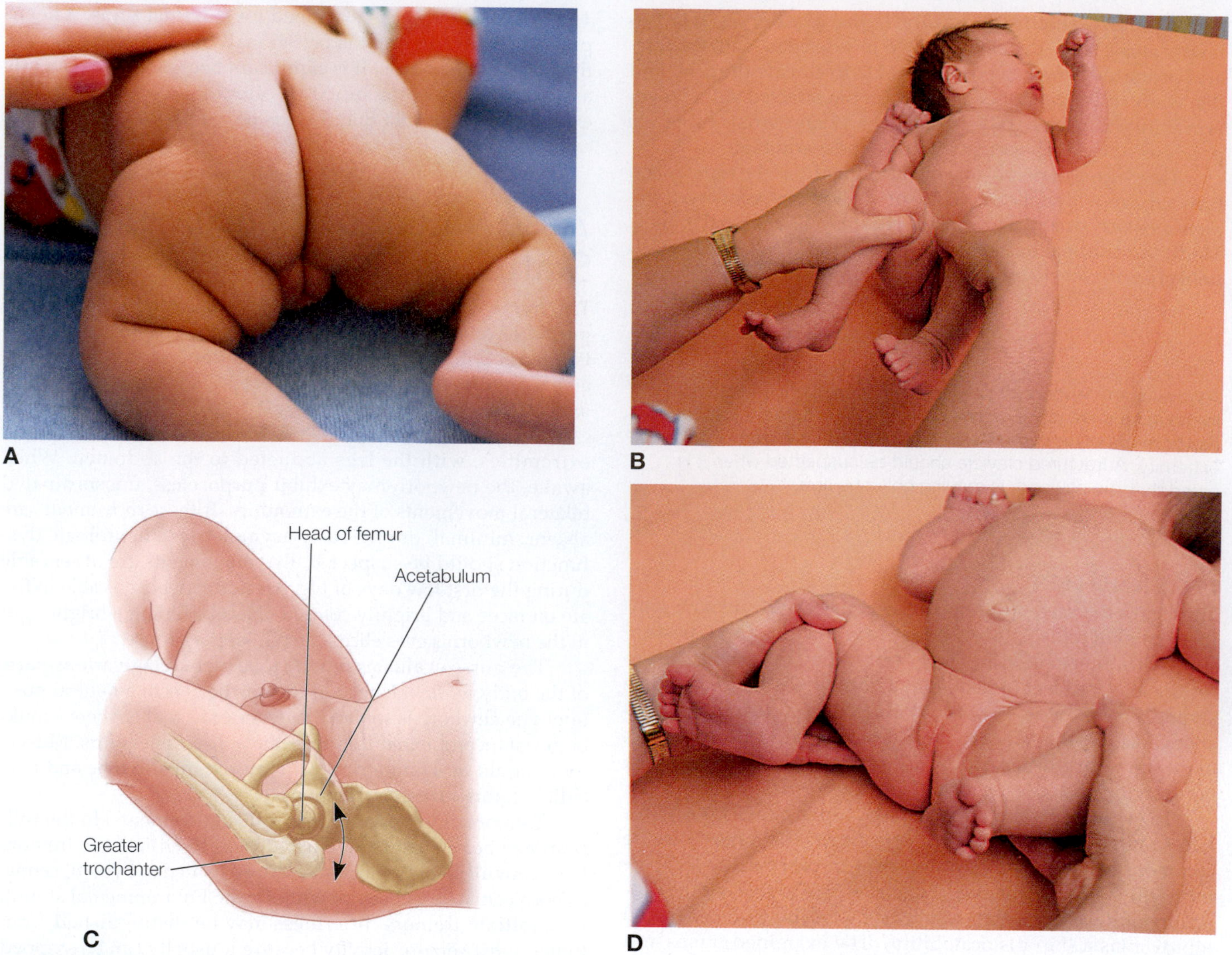

Figure 24–35 A. The asymmetry of gluteal and thigh fat folds seen in a newborn with left developmental dysplasia of the hip. B. The Barlow (dislocation) maneuver. Baby's thigh is grasped and adducted (placed together) with gentle downward pressure. C. Dislocation is palpable as femoral head slips out of acetabulum. D. The Ortolani maneuver puts downward pressure on the hip and then inward rotation. If the hip is dislocated, this maneuver will force the femoral head back into the acetabular rim with a noticeable "clunk."

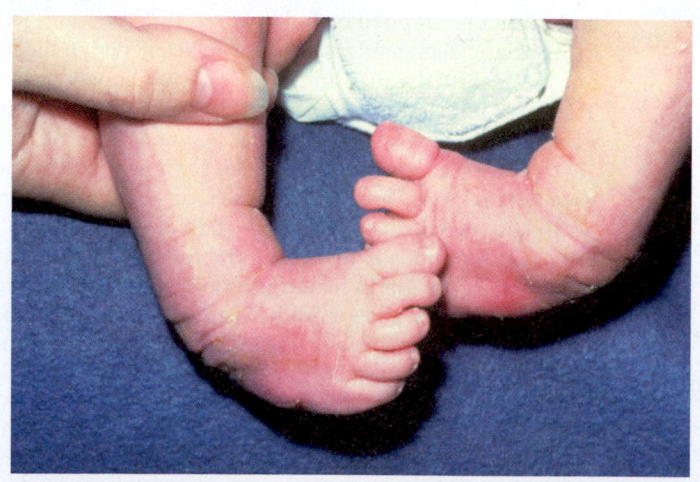

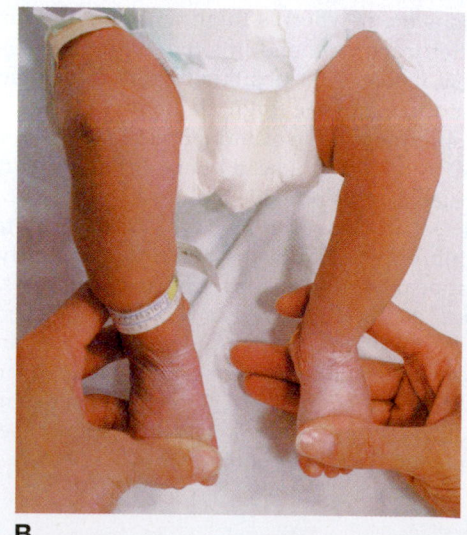

Figure 24–36 A. Unilateral talipes equinovarus (clubfoot). B. To determine the presence of clubfoot, the nurse moves the foot to the midline. Resistance indicates true clubfoot.

SOURCE: A. Jim Stevenson/Science Source.

TABLE 24–2 Common Newborn Reflexes

Tonic neck reflex (fencer position). Elicited when the newborn is supine and the head is turned to one side. In response, the extremities on the same side straighten, whereas on the opposite side they flex. This reflex may not be seen during the early newborn period, but once it appears it persists until about the third month.

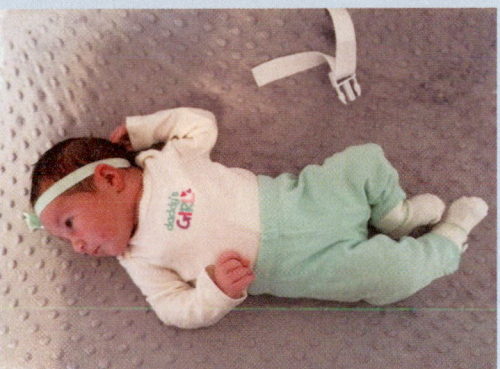

Tonic neck reflex.
Source: Craig London.

Moro reflex. Elicited when the newborn is startled by a loud noise or lifted slightly above the crib and then suddenly lowered. In response, the newborn straightens arms and hands outward while the knees flex. Slowly the arms return to the chest, as in an embrace. The fingers spread, forming a C, and the newborn may cry. This reflex may persist until about 6 months of age.

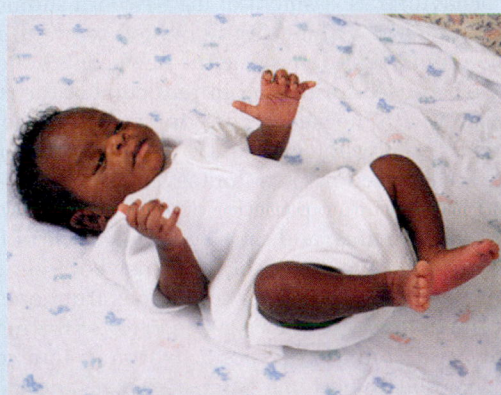

Moro reflex.

Stepping reflex. When held upright with one foot touching a flat surface, the newborn puts one foot in front of the other and "walks" (*stepping reflex*). This reflex is more pronounced at birth and is lost in 4–8 weeks.

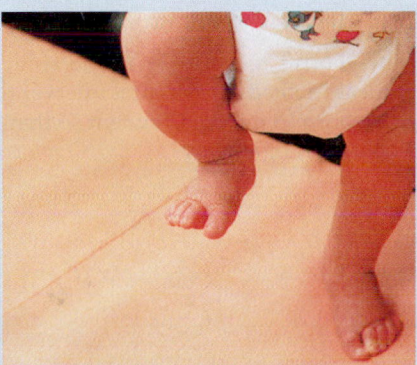

Stepping reflex.

Palmar grasping reflex. Elicited by stimulating the newborn's palm with a finger or an object; the newborn grasps and holds the object or finger firmly enough to be lifted momentarily from the crib.

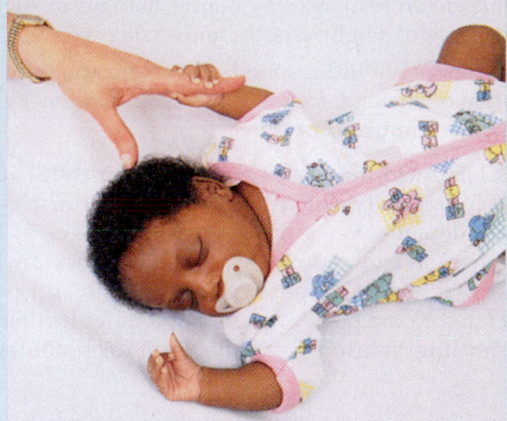

Palmar grasping reflex.

Rooting reflex. Elicited when the side of the newborn's mouth or cheek is touched. In response, the newborn turns toward that side and opens the lips to suck (if not fed recently).

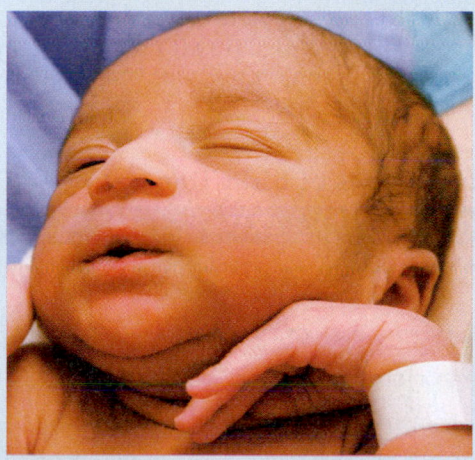

Rooting reflex.

Sucking reflex. Elicited when an object is placed in the newborn's mouth or anything touches the lips. Newborns suck even while sleeping; this is called *nonnutritive sucking*, and it can have a quieting effect on the baby. Disappears by 12 months.

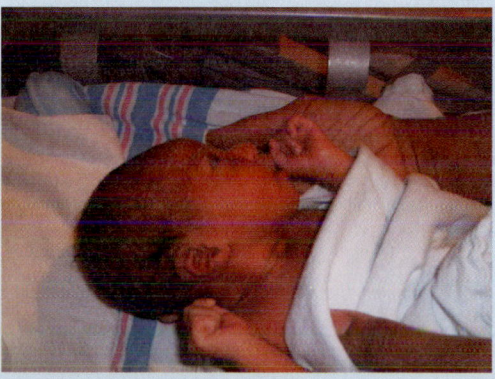

Sucking reflex.
SOURCE: Michele Davidson.

The nurse uses the following steps to assess CNS integration:

1. Insert a gloved finger into the newborn's mouth to elicit a sucking reflex.

2. As soon as the newborn is sucking vigorously, assess hearing and vision responses by noting changes in sucking in the presence of a light, a rattle, and a voice.

3. The newborn should respond to such stimuli with a brief cessation of sucking, followed by continuous sucking with repetitious stimulation.

This CNS integration examination demonstrates auditory and visual integrity as well as the ability to perform complex behavioral interactions. As healthcare providers carry out the newborn physical and neurologic assessment, they are always on the alert to recognize possible alterations and possible injuries related to the birth process that require further investigation and intervention. See Table 24–3 for potential birth injuries.

The Brazelton Neonatal Behavioral Assessment Scale

The **Brazelton Neonatal Behavioral Assessment Scale** attempts to identify the newborn's repertoire of behavioral responses to the environment and also documents the neurologic adequacy and capabilities. (For a complete discussion of all test items and maneuvers, see Nugent, 2013.) It provides a way for the healthcare provider, in conjunction with the parents (primary

TABLE 24–3 Types of Birth Trauma

CLASSIFICATION	EXAMPLES
Soft-tissue injuries	Lacerations, abrasions, bruising, fat necrosis
Skull injuries	Cephalohematoma, fractures*
Scalp laceration/abscess	Fetal scalp electrode
Intracranial hemorrhage	Subdural, subarachnoid
Eye injuries	Subconjunctival and retinal hemorrhages*
Bone fractures	Clavicle, humerus, femur, facial bones*
Nasal injuries	Dislocation, fracture*
Dislocations	Hip
Cranial nerve injuries	Phrenic nerve, recurrent laryngeal nerve (vocal cord paralysis), Horner syndrome, facial nerve*, brachial plexus*

*Most common birth injuries seen in newborns.

Clinical Reasoning Newborn Behavior

Maria Reyes, a 19-year-old G2 (now P2) mother, delivered a 40 weeks' gestation female newborn 24 hours ago. The newborn examination was normal. Mrs. Reyes says she has noticed that the baby cries more than her first child did and seems to require holding for longer periods of time after feeding before "quieting down." She is concerned that there is something she is doing wrong and wants to know when her newborn will start to act like her first baby.

What should you discuss with her about newborn behavior?

caregivers), to identify and understand the individual newborn's states, temperament, capabilities, and individual behavior patterns. Families learn which responses, interventions, or activities best meet the special needs of their newborn, and this understanding fosters positive attachment experiences.

Because the first few days after birth are a period of behavioral disorganization, the complete assessment should be done on the third day after birth. The nurse should make every effort to elicit the best response. This may be accomplished by repeating tests at different times or by testing during situations that facilitate the best possible response, such as when the parents are holding, cuddling, rocking, and/or singing to their baby.

The behavioral assessment of the newborn should be carried out initially in a quiet, dimly lighted room, if possible. The nurse should first determine the newborn's state of consciousness, because scoring and introduction of the test items are correlated with the sleep or waking state. The newborn's state depends on physiologic variables, such as the amount of time from the last feeding, positioning, environmental temperature, and health status; presence of such external stimuli as noises and bright lights; and the sleep–wake cycle of the newborn. An important characteristic of the newborn period is the pattern of states, as well as the transitions from one state to another. The pattern of states is a predictor of the newborn's receptivity and ability to respond to stimuli in a cognitive manner. Babies learn best in a quiet, alert state and in an environment that is supportive and protective and that provides appropriate stimuli.

The nurse should observe the newborn's sleep–wake patterns (as discussed in Chapter 23), including the rapidity with which the newborn moves from one state to another, the ability to be consoled, and the ability to diminish the impact of disturbing stimuli. The following questions may provide the nurse with a framework for assessment:

- Does the newborn's response style and ability to adapt to stimuli indicate a need for parental interventions that will alert the newborn to the environment so that the baby can grow socially and cognitively?

- Are parental interventions necessary to lessen the outside stimuli, as in the case of the baby who responds to sensory input with intensity?
- Can the baby control the amount of sensory input that will be experienced?

The behaviors, and the sleep–wake states in which they are assessed, are categorized as follows:

- *Habituation.* The nurse assesses the newborn's ability to diminish or shut down innate responses to specific repeated stimuli, such as a rattle, bell, light, or pinprick to heel.
- *Orientation to inanimate and animate visual and auditory assessment stimuli.* The nurse observes how often and where the newborn attends to auditory and visual stimuli. Orientation to the environment is determined by an ability to respond to clues given by others and by a natural ability to fix on and follow a visual object horizontally and vertically. This capacity and parental appreciation of it are important for positive communication between newborn and parents; the parents' visual (*en face*) and auditory (soft, continuous voice) presence stimulates their newborn to orient to them. Inability or lack of response may indicate visual or auditory problems. It is important for parents to know that their newborn can turn to voices soon after birth or by 3 days of age and can become alert at different times with a varying degree of intensity in response to sounds.
- *Motor activity.* Several components are evaluated. Motor tone of the newborn is assessed in the most characteristic state of responsiveness. This summary assessment includes overall use of tone as the newborn responds to being handled—whether during spontaneous activity, prone placement, or horizontal holding—and overall assessment of body tone as the newborn reacts to all stimuli.
- *Variations.* Frequency of alert states, state changes, color changes (throughout all states as examination progresses), activity, and peaks of excitement are assessed.
- *Self-quieting activity.* This assessment is based on how often, how quickly, and how effectively newborns can use their resources to quiet and console themselves when upset or distressed. Considered in this assessment are such self-consolatory activities as putting hand to mouth, sucking on a fist or the tongue, and attuning to an object or sound (Figure 24–37). The newborn's need for outside consolation must also be considered (e.g., seeing a face; being rocked, held, or dressed; using a pacifier; being swaddled).

Newborns with neurologic impairment are unable to use self-quieting activities and require more frequent comforting from caregivers when stimulated. For example, drug-positive newborns often exhibit abnormal sleep and feeding patterns and irritability. Swaddling newborns is

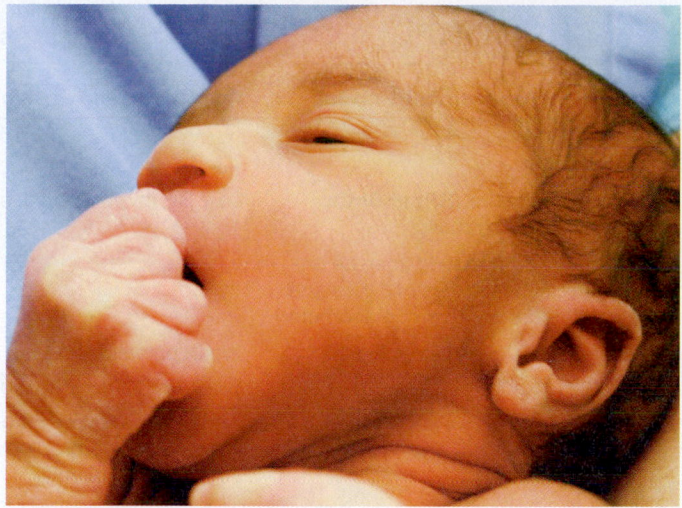

Figure 24–37 The newborn can bring hand to mouth as a self-soothing activity.

one way to provide comfort and security. Swaddling also helps the newborn organize and control his body movements and behaviors. Blanket swaddling should be loose and should allow the newborn easy hand to mouth access to promote self-soothing abilities. Tight swaddling, "straitjacket" techniques with arms at sides, is not comforting and may further agitate the newborn.

- *Cuddliness or social behaviors.* This area encompasses the newborn's need for, and response to, being held. Also considered is how often the newborn smiles. These behaviors influence the couple's self-esteem and feelings of acceptance or rejection. Cuddling also appears to be an indicator of personality. Cuddlers appear to enjoy, accept, and seek physical contact; are easier to placate; sleep more; and form earlier and more intense attachments. Noncuddlers are active, are restless, have accelerated motor development, and are intolerant of physical restraint. Smiling, even as a grimace reflex, greatly influences parent–newborn feedback. Parents identify this response as positive.

Newborn Physical Assessment Guide

Review the *Newborn Physical Assessment Guide* for systematically assessing the newborn. Normal findings, alterations, and related causes are presented and correlated with suggested nursing responses. The findings are typical for a full-term newborn.

ASSESSMENT GUIDE | Newborn Physical Assessment

Physical Assessment/Normal Findings	Alterations and Possible Causes*	Nursing Responses to Data†
Vital Signs		
Blood Pressure (BP) at Birth: 70–50/ 45–30 mm Hg	Low BP (hypovolemia, shock)	Monitor BP in all cases of distress, prematurity, or suspected anomaly.
Day 10: 90/50 mmHg (may be unable to measure diastolic pressure with standard sphygmomanometer)		Low BP: Refer to healthcare provider immediately so measures to improve circulation are begun.
Pulse: 110–160 beats/min (if asleep, as low as 70 beats/min; if crying, up to 180 beats/min)	Weak pulse (decreased cardiac output)	Assess skin perfusion by blanching (capillary refill test: normal < 3 seconds).
	Bradycardia (severe asphyxia)	Correlate finding with BP assessments; refer to healthcare provider.
	Tachycardia (over 160 beats/min at rest) (infection, CNS problems, arrhythmia, stress, hypovolemia)	Carry out neurologic and thermoregulation assessments.
		Check BP and hematocrit (Hct).
Respirations: 30–60 breaths/min		
Synchronization of chest and abdominal movements	Tachypnea (pneumonia, respiratory distress syndrome [RDS])	Identify sleep–wake state; correlate with respiratory pattern.
Diaphragmatic and abdominal breathing	Rapid, shallow breathing (hypermagnesemia caused by large doses given to mothers with preeclampsia)	Evaluate for all signs of respiratory distress; report findings to healthcare provider.
	Respirations below 30 breaths/minute (maternal anesthesia or analgesia)	
Transient tachypnea	Expiratory grunting, subcostal and substernal retractions; flaring of nares (respiratory distress); apnea (cold stress, respiratory disorder)	Evaluate for cold stress. Report findings to healthcare provider/neonatal nurse practitioner.
Crying: Strong and lusty		
Moderate tone and pitch	High pitched, shrill (neurologic disorder, hypoglycemia)	Discuss newborn's use of cry for communication.
Cries vary in length from 3 to 7 minutes after consoling measures are used.	Weak or absent (CNS disorder, laryngeal problem)	Assess and record abnormal cries.
	Inconsolable crying (GI discomforts, feeding intolerances)	Reduce environmental noises.
Temperature: Axilla 36.4°–37.2°C (97.5°–99°F)	Elevated temperature (room too warm, too much clothing or too many covers, dehydration, sepsis, brain damage)	Notify healthcare provider of elevation or drop.
	Subnormal temperature (brainstem involvement, cold, sepsis)	Counsel parents on possible causes of elevated or low temperatures, appropriate home care measures, when to call healthcare provider.
Heavier newborns tend to have higher body temperatures.	Swings of more than 2°F from one reading to the next or subnormal temperature (infection)	Teach parents how to take rectal and/or axillary temperature; assess parents' information regarding use of thermometer; provide teaching as needed.
Weight: 2500–4000 g (5 lb, 8 oz–8 lb, 13 oz)	Less than 2748 g (less than 6 lb) = SGA or preterm newborn	Plot weight and gestational age on growth chart to identify high-risk newborns.
	Greater than 4050 g (greater than 9 lb) = LGA or newborns of mothers with diabetes	Ascertain body build of parents. Counsel parents regarding appropriate caloric intake.
Within first 3 to 4 days, normal weight loss of 5% to 10%	Loss greater than 15% (low fluid intake, loss of meconium and urine, feeding difficulties, diabetes insipidus)	Notify healthcare provider of net losses or gains.
Large babies tend to lose more because of greater fluid loss in proportion to birth weight (except newborns of mothers with diabetes).		Calculate fluid intake and losses from all sources (insensible water loss, radiant warmers, and phototherapy lights). Weigh daily and before discharge.

Physical Assessment/Normal Findings	Alterations and Possible Causes*	Nursing Responses to Data†
Length: 46–56 cm (18–22 in.) Grows 10 cm (3.9 in.) during first 3 months	Less than 45 cm (17.7 in.) (congenital dwarf) Short/long bones proximally (achondroplasia) Short/long bones distally (Ellis-van Creveld syndrome)	Assess for other signs of dwarfism. Determine other signs of skeletal system adequacy. Plot progress at subsequent well-baby visits.
Posture		
Body usually flexed, hands may be tightly clenched, neck appears short as chin rests on chest	Only extension noted, inability to move from midline (trauma, hypoxia, immaturity)	Record spontaneity of motor activity and symmetry of movements.
In breech presentations, feet are usually dorsiflexed.	Constant motion (maternal caffeine intake or drug withdrawal)	If parents express concern about newborn's movement patterns, reassure and evaluate further if appropriate.
Skin		
Color: Color consistent with genetic background	Pallor of face, conjunctiva (anemia, hypothermia, anoxia)	Discuss with parents common skin color variations to allay fears. Skin color can vary widely in newborns of African descent.
Newborns of European descent: pink-tinged or ruddy color over face, trunk, extremities	Beefy red (hypoglycemia, immature vasomotor reflexes, polycythemia)	Document extent and time of occurrence of color change.
Newborns of African or Native American descent: pale pink with yellow or red tinge		
Newborns of Asian descent: pink or rosy red to yellow tinge		
Common variations: acrocyanosis, circumoral cyanosis, Mongolian spots, or harlequin color change	Meconium staining (nonreassuring fetal status) Jaundice (hemolytic reaction from blood incompatibility within first 24 hours, sepsis)	Obtain hemoglobin (Hb) and Hct values, obtain bilirubin levels. Assess for respiratory difficulty and temperature instability. Differentiate between physiologic and pathologic jaundice.
Mottled when undressed	Cyanosis (choanal atresia, CNS damage or trauma, respiratory or cardiac problem, cold stress)	Assess degree of (central or peripheral) cyanosis and possible causes; refer to healthcare provider.
Minor bruising: over buttocks in breech presentation and over eyes and forehead in facial presentations		Discuss with parents cause and course of minor bruising related to labor and birth.
Texture: Smooth, soft, flexible, may have dry, peeling hands and feet	Generalized cracked or peeling skin (SGA or postterm; blood incompatibility; metabolic, kidney dysfunction)	Report to healthcare provider.
	Seborrheic dermatitis (cradle cap) Absence of vernix (postmature) Yellow vernix (meconium staining)	Instruct parents to shampoo the scalp and anterior fontanelle areas daily with soap; rinse well; avoid use of oil.
Turgor: Elastic, returns to normal shape after pinching	Maintains tent shape (dehydration)	Assess for other signs and symptoms of dehydration.
Pigmentation: Clear; milia across bridge of nose, forehead, or chin will disappear within a few weeks		Advise parents not to pinch or prick these pimplelike areas.
Café-au-lait spots (one or two)	Six or more (neurologic disorder such as von Recklinghausen disease, cutaneous neurofibromatosis)	If there are six or more café-au-lait spots, refer for genetic and neurologic consult.
Mongolian blue spots common over dorsal area and buttocks in dark-skinned newborns		Assure parents of normalcy of this pigmentation; it will fade in first year or two.

(continued)

Physical Assessment/Normal Findings	Alterations and Possible Causes*	Nursing Responses to Data†
Erythema toxicum	Impetigo (group A ß-hemolytic strep-tococcus or *Staphylococcus aureus* infection)	If impetigo occurs, instruct parents about hand washing and linen precautions during home care.
Telangiectatic nevi	Hemangiomas:	Collaborate with healthcare provider.
	Nevus flammeus (port-wine stain)	Counsel parents about birthmark's progression to allay misconceptions.
	Nevus vascularis (strawberry hemangioma)	Record size and shape of hemangiomas.
	Cavernous hemangiomas	Refer for follow-up at well-baby clinic.
Rashes	Rashes (infection)	Assess location and type of rash (macular, papular, vesicular).
		Obtain history of onset, prenatal history, and related signs and symptoms.
Petechiae of head or neck (breech presentation, cord around neck)	Generalized petechiae (clotting abnormalities)	Determine cause; advise parents if further health care is needed.

Head

Physical Assessment/Normal Findings	Alterations and Possible Causes*	Nursing Responses to Data†
General appearance, size, movement	Asymmetric, flattened occiput on either side of the head (plagiocephaly)	Instruct parents to change newborn's positions frequently when awake; needs to spend "tummy time." Newborns should be placed supine for sleep per "safe to sleep" guidelines (see Chapter 25).
Round, symmetric, and moves easily from left to right and up and down; soft and pliable	Head held at angle (torticollis)	
	Unable to move head side to side (neurologic trauma)	Determine adequacy of all neurologic signs.
Circumference 32–37 cm (12.5–14.5 in.); 2 cm (0.8in.) greater than chest circumference	Extreme differences in size may be micro-encephaly (Cornelia de Lange syndrome, cytomegalic inclusion disease [CID], rubella, toxoplasmosis, chromosomal abnormalities), hydrocephalus (meningo-myelocele, achondroplasia), anencephaly (neural tube defect)	Measure circumference from occiput to fron-tal area using metal or paper tape. Measure chest circumference using metal or paper tape and compare to head circumference.
Head one fourth of body size		Record measurements on growth chart.
	Head is 3 cm (1.2 in.) or more larger than chest circumference (preterm, hydro-cephalus)	Reevaluate at well-baby visits.
Common Variations: Molding	Cephalohematoma (trauma during birth, may persist up to 3 months)	Evaluate neurologic response.
Breech and cesarean newborns' heads are round and well shaped	Caput succedaneum (long labor and birth; disappears in 1 week)	Observe for hyperbilirubinemia. Check Hct.
		Reassure parents regarding common mani-festations caused by birth process and when they should disappear.
Fontanelles: Palpation of juncture of cranial bones	Overlapping of anterior fontanelle (mal-nourished or preterm newborn)	Discuss normal closure times with parents and care of "soft spots" to allay misconcep-tions.
Anterior fontanelle: 3–4 cm (1.2–1.6 in.) long by 2–3 cm (0.8–1.2 in.) wide, diamond shaped	Premature closure of sutures (craniosyn-ostosis)	Refer to healthcare provider.
Posterior fontanelle: 1–2 cm (0.4–0.8 in.) at birth, triangle shaped	Late closure (hydrocephalus)	Observe for signs and symptoms of hydro-cephalus.
Slight pulsation	Moderate to severe pulsation (vascular problems)	Refer to healthcare provider.
Moderate bulging noted with cry-ing, stooling, or pulsations with heartbeat	Constant bulging (increased intracranial pressure, meningitis)	Report to healthcare provider.
		Evaluate neurologic status.
	Sunken (dehydration)	Evaluate hydration status.

Hair

Physical Assessment/Normal Findings	Alterations and Possible Causes*	Nursing Responses to Data†
Texture: Smooth with fine texture variations (Note: Variations depend on ethnic background.)	Coarse, brittle, dry hair (hypothyroidism)	Instruct parents regarding routine care of hair and scalp.
	White forelock (Waardenburg syndrome)	

Physical Assessment/Normal Findings	Alterations and Possible Causes*	Nursing Responses to Data†
Distribution: Scalp hair high over eyebrows (In some ethnicities the hairline begins mid-forehead and extends down back of neck.)	Low forehead and posterior hairlines may indicate chromosomal disorders	Assess for other signs of chromosomal aberrations. Refer to healthcare provider.
Face		
Symmetric movement of all facial features, normal hairline, eyebrows and eyelashes present		Assess and record symmetry of all parts, shape, regularity of features, sameness or differences in features.
Spacing of Features: Eyes at same level, nostrils equal size, cheeks full, and sucking pads present	Eyes wide apart—ocular hypertelorism (Apert syndrome, cri-du-chat, Turner syndrome)	Observe for other signs and symptoms indicative of disease states or chromosomal aberrations.
Lips equal on both sides of midline	Abnormal face (Down syndrome, cretinism, gargoylism)	
Chin recedes when compared with other bones of face	Abnormally small jaw—micrognathia (Pierre Robin syndrome, Treacher Collins syndrome)	Maintain airway; do not position supine. Initiate surgical consultation and referral.
Movement: Makes facial grimaces	Inability to suck, grimace, and close eyelids (cranial nerve injury)	Initiate neurologic assessment and consultation.
Symmetric when resting and crying	Asymmetry (paralysis of facial cranial nerve)	Assess and record symmetry of all parts, shape, regularity of features, and sameness or differences in features.
Eyes		
General placement and appearance:	Gross nystagmus (damage to third, fourth, and sixth cranial nerves)	
Bright and clear; even placement; slight nystagmus (involuntary cyclical eye movements)		
Concomitant strabismus	Constant and fixed strabismus	Reassure parents that strabismus is considered normal up to 6 months.
Move in all directions		
Blue or slate blue-gray in White newborns	Lack of pigmentation (albinism)	Discuss with parents any necessary eye precautions.
Brown color at birth in dark-skinned newborns	Brushfield spots (a light or white speckling of the outer two thirds of the iris) may indicate Down syndrome	Assess for other signs of Down syndrome. Discuss with parents that permanent eye color is usually established by 3 months of age.
Eyelids: Positioned above pupils but within iris, no drooping	Elevation of (hydrocephalus) or retraction of upper lid (hyperthyroidism)	Assess for signs of hydrocephalus and hyperthyroidism.
	"Sunset sign" lid elevation and downward gaze (hydrocephalus), ptosis (congenital or paralysis of oculomotor muscle)	Evaluate interference with vision in subsequent well-baby visits.
Eyes on parallel plane	Upward slant of eyes in non-Asians (Down syndrome)	Assess for other signs of Down syndrome.
Epicanthal folds in Asians and 20% of newborns of northern European descent	Epicanthal folds (Down syndrome, cri-du-chat syndrome)	
Movement: Blink reflex in response to light stimulus. Eyes open wide in dimly lighted room	Blink absent (CNS injury, cranial nerve damage)	Evaluate neurologic status. Refer to healthcare provider.
Inspection: Edematous for first few days of life, resulting from birth; no lumps or redness	Purulent drainage (infection); infectious conjunctivitis (gonococcus, chlamydia, staphylococcus, or gram- negative organisms)	Initiate good hand washing. Refer to healthcare provider. Evaluate newborn for seborrheic dermatitis; scales can be removed easily.
	Marginal blepharitis (lid edges red, crusted, scaly)	
Cornea: Clear	Ulceration (herpes infection); large cornea or corneas of unequal size (congenital glaucoma)	Refer to ophthalmologist.

(continued)

ASSESSMENT GUIDE | Newborn Physical Assessment (*continued*)

Physical Assessment/Normal Findings	Alterations and Possible Causes*	Nursing Responses to Data†
Corneal reflex present	Clouding, opacity of lens (cataract)	Assess for other manifestations of congenital herpes; institute nursing care measures.
Sclera: May appear bluish in newborn, then white; slightly brownish color frequent in newborns of African descent	True blue sclera (osteogenesis imperfecta)	Refer to healthcare provider.
Pupils: Pupils equal in size, round, and react to light by accommodation	Anisocoria—unequal pupils (CNS damage)	Refer for neurologic examination.
	Dilation or constriction (intracranial damage) retinoblastoma, glaucoma	
	Pupils nonreactive to light or accommodation (brain injury)	
Slight nystagmus in newborn who has not learned to focus	Nystagmus (labyrinthine disturbance, CNS disorder)	
Pupil light reflex demonstrated at birth or by 3 weeks of age	Lack of reflex (damage to cranial nerve, CNS injury)	
Conjunctiva: Chemical conjunctivitis	Pale color (anemia)	Obtain Hct and Hgb. Reassure parents that chemical conjunctivitis will subside in 1 to 2 days and subconjunctival hemorrhage will disappear in a few weeks.
Subconjunctival hemorrhage		
Palpebral conjunctiva (red but not hyperemic)	Inflammation or edema (infection, blocked tear duct)	
Vision: 20/200	Cataracts (congenital infection)	Record any questions about visual acuity, and initiate follow-up evaluation at first well-baby checkup.
Tracks moving object to midline		
Fixed focus on objects at a distance of about 20.3–25.4 cm (8–10 in.); may be difficult to evaluate in newborn		
Prefers faces, geometric designs, and black and white to colors		
Lashes and Lacrimal Glands: Presence of lashes (lashes may be absent in preterm newborns)	No lashes on inner two thirds of lid (Treacher Collins syndrome); bushy lashes (Hurler syndrome); long lashes (Cornelia de Lange syndrome)	
Cry commonly tearless	Excessive tearing (plugged lacrimal duct, natal narcotic withdrawal), glaucoma	Demonstrate to parents how to milk blocked tear duct.
		Refer to ophthalmologist if tearing is excessive before third month of life.
Nose		
Appearance of external nasal aspects: May appear flattened as a result of birth process	Continued flat or broad bridge of nose (Down syndrome)	Arrange consultation with specialist.
		May be normal racial variation—Asian or African ancestry.
Small and narrow in midline, even placement in relationship to eyes and mouth	Low bridge of nose, beaklike nose (Apert syndrome, Treacher Collins syndrome)	Initiate evaluation of chromosomal abnormalities.
	Upturned (Cornelia de Lange syndrome)	
Patent nares bilaterally (nose breathers)	Blockage of nares (mucus and/or secretions), choanal atresia	Inspect for obstruction of nares.
Sneezing common to clear nasal passages	Flaring nares (respiratory distress)	Maintain oral airway until surgical correction is made.
Responds to odors, may smell breast milk	No response to stimulating odors	Inspect for obstruction of nares.
Mouth		
Function of Facial, Hypoglossal, Glossopharyngeal, and Vagus Nerves: Symmetry of movement and strength	Mouth draws to one side (transient seventh cranial nerve paralysis caused by pressure in utero or trauma during birth, congenital paralysis)	Initiate neurologic consultation.
		Administer artificial tears if eye on affected side of face is unable to close.
	Fishlike shape (Treacher Collins syndrome)	

Physical Assessment/Normal Findings	Alterations and Possible Causes*	Nursing Responses to Data†
Presence of gag, swallowing, reflexes coordinated with sucking reflex	Suppressed or absent reflexes	Evaluate other neurologic functions of these nerves.
Adequate salivation		
Palate (soft and hard): Hard palate dome shaped	High-steepled palate (Treacher Collins syndrome), bifid uvula (congenital anomaly)	Assess for other congenital anomalies.
Uvula midline with symmetrical movement of soft palate		
Palate intact, sucks well when stimulated	Clefts in either hard or soft palate (polygenic disorder)	Initiate a surgical consultation referral.
Epithelial (Epstein) pearls appear on mucosa		Assure parents that these are normal and will disappear at 2 or 3 months of age.
Esophagus patent, some drooling common in newborn	Excessive drooling or bubbling (esophageal atresia)	Test for patency of esophagus.
Tongue: Free moving in all directions, midline	Lack of movement or asymmetric movement (neurologic damage)	Further assess neurologic functions.
	Tongue-tied (ridge of frenulum tissue attached to the underside of the tongue [tip of tongue is heart shaped])	Cutting the ridge of tissue is not recommended because it can create an entry for infection.
	Fasciculations (fine tremors)	Test reflex elevation of tongue when depressed with tongue blade.
	Spinal muscular atrophy	
Pink color, smooth to rough texture, noncoated	Deviations from midline (cranial nerve damage)	Check for signs of weakness or deviation.
	White cheesy coating (thrush)	Differentiate between thrush and milk curds by wiping patches: if white patches don't come off easily, it is thrush.
	Tongue has deep ridges.	Reassure parents that tongue pattern may change from day to day.
Tongue proportional to mouth	Large tongue with short frenulum (cretinism, trisomy 21, other syndromes)	Evaluate in well-baby clinic to assess development delays. Initiate referrals.
Ears		
External Ear: Without lesions, cysts, or nodules	Nodules, cysts, or sinus tracts in front of ear	Evaluate characteristics of lesions.
	Adherent earlobes	
	Low-set ears (genetic anomaly or syndrome)	Counsel parents to clean external ear with washcloth only; discourage use of cotton-tip applicators.
	Preauricular skin tags	Refer to healthcare provider for ligation.
Hearing: Eustachian tubes are cleared with first cry		
Attends to sounds; sudden or loud noise elicits Moro reflex	No response to sound stimuli (deafness)	Test for Moro reflex.
Neck		
Appearance: Short, straight, creased with skin folds	Abnormally short neck (Turner syndrome)	Report findings to healthcare provider.
	Arching or inability to flex neck (meningitis, congenital anomaly)	
Posterior neck lacks loose extra folds of skin	Webbing of neck (Turner syndrome, Down syndrome, trisomy 18)	Assess for other signs of the syndromes.
Clavicles: Straight and intact	Knot or lump on clavicle (fracture during difficult birth)	Obtain detailed labor and birth history; apply figure-8 bandage. Consider oral analgesics.
Moro reflex elicitable	Unilateral Moro reflex response on unaffected side (fracture of clavicle, brachial palsy, Erb-Duchenne paralysis)	Collaborate with healthcare provider.

(continued)

Physical Assessment/Normal Findings	Alterations and Possible Causes*	Nursing Responses to Data†
Symmetric shoulders	Hypoplasia	
Chest		
Appearance and Size: Circumference: 32.5 cm (12.8 in.), 1–2 cm (0.4–0.8 in.) less than head		Measure at level of nipples after exhalation.
Wider than it is long		
Normal shape without depressed or prominent sternum	Funnel chest (congenital or associated with Marfan syndrome)	Determine adequacy of other respiratory and circulatory signs.
Lower end of sternum (xiphoid cartilage) may be protruding; is less apparent after several weeks	Continued protrusion of xiphoid cartilage (Marfan syndrome, "pigeon chest")	Assess for other signs and symptoms of various syndromes.
Sternum 8 cm (3.1 in.) long	Barrel chest	
Expansion and retraction:		
Bilateral expansion	Unequal chest expansion (pneumonia, pneumothorax, respiratory distress)	Assess respiratory effort regularity, flaring of nares, difficulty on both inspiration and expiration.
No intercostal, subcostal, or supra-costal retractions	Retractions (respiratory distress)	
	See-saw respirations (respiratory distress)	
Auscultation: Breath sounds are louder in newborns than in adults because there is less subcutaneous tissue to muffle transmission	Decreased breath sounds (decreased respiratory activity, atelectasis, pneumothorax)	Obtain transillumination. Record findings and consult healthcare provider.
Chest and axillae clear on crying	Increased breath sounds (resolving pneumonia or in cesarean births)	Perform assessment and report positive findings to healthcare provider.
Bronchial breath sounds (heard where trachea and bronchi are closest to chest wall, above sternum and between scapulae):		
Bronchial sounds bilaterally Air entry clear Rales may indicate normal newborn atelectasis Cough reflex absent at birth, appears in 2 or more days	Adventitious or abnormal sounds (respiratory disease or distress)	Evaluate color for pallor or cyanosis. Report to healthcare provider.
Breasts: Flat with symmetric nipples	Lack of breast tissue (preterm or SGA)	
Breast tissue diameter 5 cm (2 in.) or more at term	Discharge	Evaluate for infection.
Distance between nipples 8 cm (3.1 in.)	Breast abscesses	
Breast engorgement occurs on third day of life; liquid discharge may be expressed in term newborns	Enlargement	Reassure parents of normality of breast engorgement.
Nipples	Supernumerary nipples	No intervention is necessary.
	Dark-colored nipples	
Heart		
Auscultation: Location: lies horizontally, with left border extending to left of midclavicle		
Regular rhythm and rate	Arrhythmia (anoxia), tachycardia, bradycardia	Refer all arrhythmia and gallop rhythms. Initiate cardiac evaluation.
Determination of point of maximal impulse (PMI)	Malpositioning (enlargement, abnormal placement, pneumothorax, dextrocardia, diaphragmatic hernia)	
Usually lateral to midclavicular line at third or fourth intercostal space		

Physical Assessment/Normal Findings	Alterations and Possible Causes*	Nursing Responses to Data†
Functional murmurs No thrills	Location of murmurs (possible congenital cardiac anomaly)	Evaluate murmur: location, timing, and duration; observe for accompanying cardiac pathology symptoms; ascertain family history.
Horizontal groove at diaphragm shows flaring of rib cage to mild degree.	Inadequacy of respiratory movement Marked rib flaring (vitamin D deficiency)	Initiate cardiopulmonary evaluation; assess pulses and BPs in all four extremities for equality and quality.
Abdomen		
Appearance: Cylindrical with some protrusion, appears large in relation to pelvis, some laxness of abdominal muscles	Distention, shiny abdomen with engorged vessels (gastrointestinal abnormalities, infection, congenital megacolon)	Examine abdomen thoroughly for mass or organomegaly. Measure abdominal girth.
No cyanosis, few vessels seen	Scaphoid abdominal appearance (diaphragmatic hernia)	Report deviations of abdominal size.
Diastasis recti—common in newborns of African descent		
	Increased or decreased peristalsis (duodenal stenosis, small bowel obstruction)	Assess other signs and symptoms of obstruction.
	Localized flank bulging (enlarged kidneys, ascites, or absent abdominal muscles)	Refer to healthcare provider.
Umbilicus: No protrusion of umbilicus (protrusion of umbilicus common in newborns of African descent)	Umbilical hernia Patent urachus (congenital malformation)	Measure umbilical hernia by palpating the opening and record; it should close by 1 year of age; if not, refer to healthcare provider.
Bluish white color	Omphalocele (covered defect) Gastroschisis (uncovered defect)	Cover omphalocele and gastroschisis with sterile, moist dressing or plastic sterile bag.
Cutis navel (umbilical cord projects), granulation tissue present in navel	Redness or exudate around cord (infection) Yellow discoloration (hemolytic disease, meconium staining)	Instruct parents on cord care and hygiene.
Two arteries and one vein apparent	Single umbilical artery (congenital anomalies)	Refer anomalies to healthcare provider.
Begins drying 1 to 2 hours after birth		
No bleeding	Discharge or oozing of blood from the cord	
Auscultation of All Four Quadrants: Soft bowel sounds heard shortly after birth every 10 to 30 seconds	Bowel sounds in chest (diaphragmatic hernia) Absence of bowel sounds Hyperperistalsis (intestinal obstruction)	Collaborate with healthcare provider. Assess for other signs of dehydration and/or infection.
Femoral Pulses: Palpable, equal bilateral	Absent or diminished femoral pulses (coarctation of aorta)	Monitor BP in upper and lower extremities.
Inguinal Area: No bulges along inguinal area	Inguinal hernia	Initiate referral.
No inguinal lymph nodes felt		Continue follow-up in well-baby clinic.
Bladder: Percusses 1 to 4 cm (0.4 to 1.6 in.) above symphysis	Failure to void within 24 to 48 hours after birth	Check whether baby voided at birth.
Should void within 24 hours after birth, if not at time of birth	Exposure of bladder mucosa (exstrophy of bladder)	Cover exstrophy with sterile moist gauze Consult with clinician.
Urine—inoffensive, mild odor	Foul odor (infection)	Obtain urine specimen if infection is suspected.
Genitals		
Gender clearly delineated	Ambiguous genitals	Refer for genetic consultation.

(continued)

ASSESSMENT GUIDE | Newborn Physical Assessment (*continued*)

Physical Assessment/Normal Findings	Alterations and Possible Causes*	Nursing Responses to Data†
MALE		
Penis: Slender in appearance, about 2.5 cm (1 in.) long, 1 cm (0.4 in.) wide at birth	Micropenis (congenital anomaly) Meatal atresia	Observe and record first voiding.
Normal urinary orifice, urethral meatus at tip of penis	Hypospadias, epispadias	Collaborate with healthcare provider in presence of abnormality. Delay circumcision.
Noninflamed urethral opening	Urethritis (infection)	Palpate for enlarged inguinal lymph nodes and record painful urination.
Foreskin adheres to glans	Ulceration of meatal opening (infection, inflammation)	Evaluate whether ulcer is because of diaper rash; counsel regarding care.
Uncircumcised foreskin tight for 2 to 3 months	Phimosis—if still tight after 3 months	Instruct parents on how to care for uncircumcised penis.
Circumcised		Teach parents how to care for circumcision. Check for voiding after procedure and evaluation for excessive bleeding
Erectile tissue present		
Scrotum: Skin loose and hanging or tight and small; extensive rugae and normal size	Large scrotum containing fluid (hydrocele) Red, shiny scrotal skin (orchitis)	Shine a light through scrotum (transilluminate) to verify diagnosis.
Normal skin color		
Scrotal discoloration common in breech	Minimal rugae, small scrotum	Assess for prematurity.
Testes: Descended by birth; not consistently found in scrotum	Undescended testes (cryptorchidism)	If testes cannot be felt in scrotum, gently palpate femoral, inguinal, perineal, and abdominal areas for presence.
Testes size 1.5 to 2 cm (0.6 to 0.8 in.) at birth	Enlarged testes (tumor) Small testes (Klinefelter syndrome or adrenal hyperplasia)	Refer and collaborate with healthcare provider for further diagnostic studies.
FEMALE		
Mons: Normal skin color, area pigmented in dark-skinned newborns		
Labia majora cover labia minora in term and postterm newborns; symmetric size appropriate for gestational age	Hematoma, lesions (trauma) Labia minora prominent	Evaluate for recent trauma. Assess for prematurity.
Clitoris: Normally large in newborn Edema and bruising in breech birth	Hypertrophy (hermaphroditism)	Refer for genetic workup.
Vagina: Urinary meatus and vaginal orifice visible (0.5 cm [0.2 in.] circumference)	Inflammation; erythema and discharge (urethritis) Congenital absence of vagina	Collect urine specimen for laboratory examination. Refer to healthcare provider.
Discharge; smegma under labia	Foul-smelling discharge (infection)	Collect data and further evaluate reason for discharge.
Bloody or mucoid discharge	Excessive vaginal bleeding (blood coagulation defect)	
Buttocks and Anus		
Buttocks symmetric	Pilonidal dimple	Examine for possible sinus. Instruct parents about cleansing this area.
Anus patent and passage of meconium within 24 to 48 hours after birth	Imperforate anus, rectal atresia (congenital gastrointestinal defect)	Evaluate extent of problems. Initiate surgical consultation.

Physical Assessment/Normal Findings	Alterations and Possible Causes*	Nursing Responses to Data†
No fissures, tears, or skin tags	Fissures	Perform digital examination to ascertain patency if patency uncertain.
Extremities and Trunk		
Short and generally flexed, extremities move symmetrically through range of motion but lack full extension	Unilateral or absence of movement (spinal cord involvement) Fetal position continued or limp (anoxia)	Review birth record to assess possible cause.
All joints move spontaneously; good muscle tone of flexor type, birth to 2 months	Spasticity when newborn begins using extensors (cerebral palsy)	Collaborate with healthcare provider.
Arms: Equal in length	Brachial palsy (difficult birth)	Report to clinician.
Bilateral movement	Erb-Duchenne paralysis	
Flexed when quiet	Muscle weakness, fractured clavicle	
	Absence of limb or change of size (phocomelia, amelia)	
Hands: Normal number of fingers	Polydactyly (Ellis-van Creveld syndrome) Syndactyly—one limb (developmental anomaly); both limbs (genetic component)	Report to clinician.
Normal palmar crease	Single palmar crease (trisomy 21)	Refer for genetic workup.
Normal size hands	Short fingers and broad hand (Hurler syndrome)	Evaluate for history of distress in utero.
Nails present and extend beyond fingertips in term newborn	Cyanosis and clubbing (cardiac anomalies)	Carry out cardiac and respiratory assessments.
	Nails long or yellow stained (postterm)	Check pulse oximetry.
Spine: C-shaped spine	Spina bifida occulta (nevus pilosus)	Evaluate extent of neurologic damage; initiate care of spinal opening.
Flat and straight when prone	Dermal sinus	
Slight lumbar lordosis	Myelomeningocele	
Easily flexed and intact when palpated	Head lag; limp, floppy trunk (neurologic problems)	
At least half of back devoid of lanugo		
Full-term newborn in ventral suspension should hold head at 45-degree angle, back straight		Elicit reflex to assess degree of involvement.
Hips: No sign of instability	Sensation of abnormal movement, jerk, or snap of hip dislocation	Healthcare provider or nurse practitioner examines all newborns for dislocated hip before discharge from birthing center.
Hips abduct to more than 60 degrees	Limited abduction (developmental dysplasia of hip)	If this is suspected, refer to orthopedist for further evaluation. Reassess at well-baby visits.
Inguinal and Buttock Skin Creases: Symmetric inguinal and buttock creases	Asymmetry (dislocated hips)	Refer to orthopedist for evaluation. Counsel parents regarding symptoms of concern, and discuss therapy.
Legs: Legs equal in length	Shortened leg (dislocated hips)	Refer to orthopedist for evaluation.
Legs shorter than arms at birth	Lack of leg movement (fractures, spinal defects)	Counsel parents regarding symptoms of concern, and discuss therapy.
Feet: Foot is in straight line	Talipes equinovarus (true clubfoot)	Discuss differences between positional and true clubfoot with parents.
Positional clubfoot—based on position in utero		Teach parents passive manipulation of foot. Refer to orthopedist if not corrected by 3 months of age.

(continued)

ASSESSMENT GUIDE | Newborn Physical Assessment (*continued*)

Physical Assessment/Normal Findings	Alterations and Possible Causes*	Nursing Responses to Data†
Fat pads and creases on soles of feet	Incomplete sole creases in first 24 hours of life (premature)	
Talipes planus (flat feet) normal under 3 years of age		Reassure parents that flat feet are normal in newborns.
Neuromuscular		
Motor Function: Symmetric movement and strength in all extremities	Limp, flaccid, or hypertonic (CNS disorders, infection, dehydration, fracture)	Appraise newborn's posture and motor functions by observing activities and motor characteristics.
May be jerky or have brief twitching	Tremors (hypoglycemia, hypocalcemia, infection, neurologic damage)	Evaluate for electrolyte imbalance, hypoglycemia, and neurologic functioning.
Head lag not over 45 degrees	Delayed or abnormal development (preterm, neurologic involvement)	
Neck control adequate to maintain head erect briefly	Asymmetry of tone or strength (neurologic damage)	Refer for genetic evaluation.

Possible causes of alterations are identified in parentheses.

†This column provides guidelines for further assessment and initial nursing interventions.*

Focus Your Study

- A perinatal history, determination of gestational age, physical examination, and behavior assessment form the basis of a complete newborn assessment.

- The common physical characteristics included in the gestational age assessment are skin, lanugo, sole (plantar) creases, breast tissue and size, ear form and cartilage, and genitalia.

- The neuromuscular components of gestational age scoring tools are usually posture, square window sign, popliteal angle, arm recoil, heel-to-ear extension, and scarf sign.

- By assessing the physical and neuromuscular components specified in a gestational age tool, the nurse can determine the gestational age of the newborn.

- After determining the gestational age of the baby, the nurse can assess how the newborn will make the transition to extrauterine life and anticipate potential physiologic problems.

- The nurse identifies the newborn as small for gestational age (SGA), appropriate for gestational age (AGA), or large for gestational age (LGA), and prioritizes individual needs.

- Normal newborn measurements are as follows: weight range, 2500 to 4000 g (5 lb, 8 oz to 8 lb, 13 oz), with weight dependent on maternal size and age; length range, 46 to 56 cm (18 to 22 in.); and head circumference range, 32 to 37 cm (12.5 to 14.5 in.)—approximately 2 cm (0.8 in.) larger than the chest circumference.

- Normal ranges for vital signs assessed in the newborn are as follows: heart rate, 110 to 160 beats per minute; respirations, 30 to 60 respirations per minute; blood pressure at birth, 70–50/45–30 mmHg; axillary temperature, 36.4° to 37.2°C (97.5° to 99°F); skin temperature, 36° to 36.5°C (96.8° to 97.7°F); rectal temperature, 36.6° to 37.2°C (97.8° to 99°F).

- The newborn should have a head that appears large for its body, a prominent abdomen, sloping shoulders, narrow hips, and a rounded chest. The body appears long and the extremities short. Newborns tend to stay in a flexed position and will resist straightening of the extremities. Hands remain clenched.

- Neurologic assessment characteristics include state of alertness, resting position, muscle tone, cry, and motor activity.

- Neuromuscular assessment characteristics include symmetric movements and strength of all extremities, head lag less than 45 degrees, and ability to hold head erect briefly.

- Commonly elicited newborn reflexes are tonic neck, grasping, Moro, rooting, stepping, sucking, and blink.

- Newborn behavioral abilities include habituation, orientation to visual and auditory stimuli, motor activity, cuddliness, and self-quieting activity.

- An important role of the nurse during the physical and behavioral assessments of the newborn is to teach parents about their newborn and involve them in their baby's care. This involvement facilitates the parents' identification of their newborn's uniqueness and allays their concerns.

Clinical Reasoning in Action

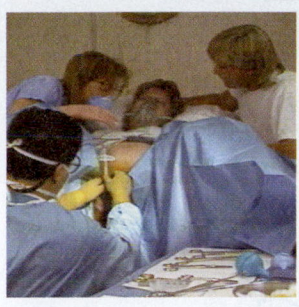

Susan Pine, a 21-year-old G2, now P1011, delivers a 39 2/7-weeks' gestation female newborn. The vaginal birth is assisted with a vacuum extractor. The prenatal record is significant for an increase of maternal blood pressure to 140/90 mmHg on the day of birth. Susan is treated with magnesium sulfate during her labor and has an epidural analgesia for the pain of labor. The baby's Apgar is 8 and 9 at 1 and 5 minutes, and she has been admitted to the newborn nursery. The newborn's admission examination is normal except for a 2-cm (0.8 in.) round caput

succedaneum. Now, 8 hours later, the baby's condition is stable and she needs to be bottle-fed. You take her to her mother's room where you observe that Susan does not reach out to take her from you. She seems unsure when handling her baby. Susan asks you about the swelling on her baby's head and wonders if it will ever go away.

1. How would you explain the cause of Susan's baby's caput succedaneum?

2. Compare the difference between a cephalohematoma and caput succedaneum.

3. Explore with Susan her baby's reflexes and state of alertness.

4. Susan asks you how she will know what her baby needs. How would you respond?

References

American Academy of Pediatrics. (2013). *How to take a child's temperature*. Retrieved from http://www.healthychildren.org/English/health-issues/conditions/fever/Pages/How-to-Take-a-Childs-Temperature.aspx

American Academy of Pediatrics (AAP) Committee on Fetus and Newborn & American College of Obstetricians and Gynecologists (ACOG) Committee on Obstetrics. (2012). *Guidelines for perinatal care* (7th ed.). Evanston, IL: Author.

Ballard, J. L., Khoury, J. C., Wedig, K., Wang, L., Eilers-Walsman, B. L., & Lipp, R. (1991). New Ballard score, expanded to include extremely premature infants. *Journal of Pediatrics, 119*(3), 417–423.

Blackburn, S. T. (2013). *Maternal, fetal, neonatal physiology: A clinical perspective* (4th ed.). London, UK: MacKeith.

Cavaliere, T. A., & Sansoucie, D. A. (2014). Assessment of the newborn and infant. In C. Kenner & J. W. Lott (Eds.). *Comprehensive neonatal nursing care.*(5th ed., pp. 71–112). New York, NY: Springer.

Cloherty, J. P., Eichenwald, E. C., Hansen, A. R., & Stark, A. R. (2012). *Manual of neonatal care* (7th ed.). Philadelphia, PA: Lippincott Williams & Wilkins.

Gleason, C. A., & Devaskar, S. U. (2012). *Avery's diseases of the newborn.* (9th ed.) St. Louis, MO: Elsevier Saunders.

Gomella, T. L. (Ed.) (2013). *Neonatology: Management, procedures, on-call problems, diseases, and drugs* (7th ed.). New York, NY: McGraw-Hill Education.

Goodwin, M. (2015). Abdomen assessment. In E. P. Tappero & M. E. Honeyfield (Eds.), *Physical assessment of the newborn.* (5th ed., pp. 111–120). Petaluma, CA: NICU Ink.

Johnson, P. (2015). Head, eyes, ears, nose, mouth, and neck assessment. In E. P. Tappero & M. E. Honeyfield (Eds.), *Physical assessment of the newborn.* (5th ed., pp. 61–78). Petaluma, CA: NICU Ink.

Nugent, J. K. (2013). The competent newborn and the neonatal behavioral assessment scale: T Berry Brazelton's legacy. *Journal of Child and Adolescent Psychiatric Nursing 26*(3), 173–179.

Vargo, L. (2015). Cardiovascular assessment. In E. P. Tappero & M. E. Honeyfield (Eds.), *Physical assessment of the newborn.* (5th ed., pp. 93–110). Petaluma, CA: NICU Ink.

Witt, C. (2015). Skin assessment. In E. P. Tappero & M. E. Honeyfield (Eds.), *Physical assessment of the newborn.* (5th ed., pp. 45–60). Petaluma, CA: NICU Ink.

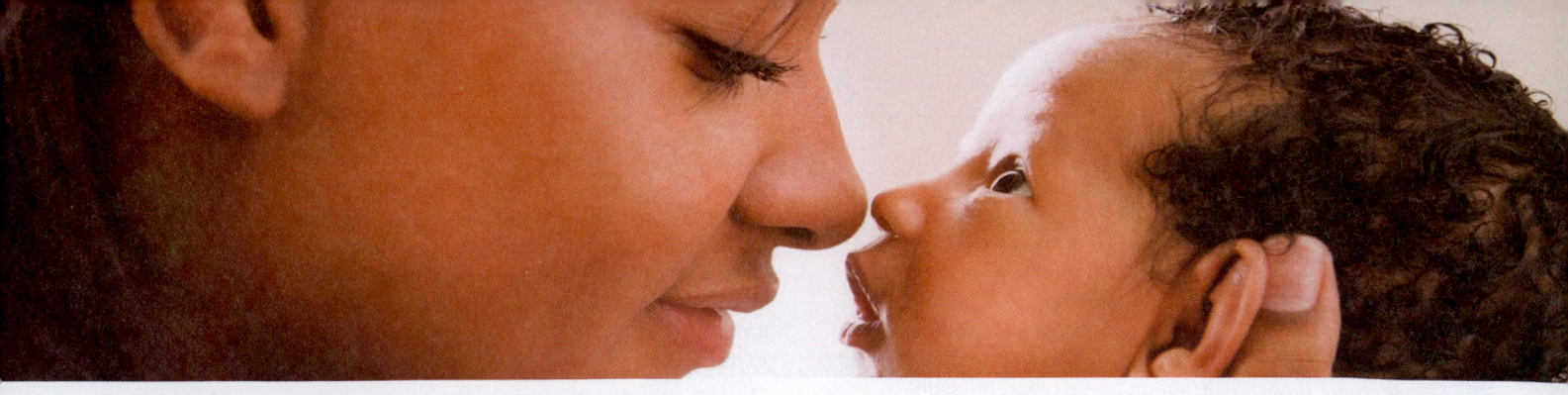

Chapter 25

The Normal Newborn: Needs, Care, and Feeding

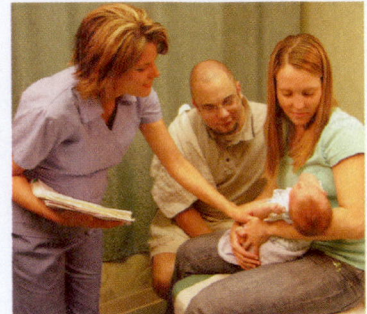

I've been a postpartum nurse for about 6 years. A large part of my job involves teaching or enhancing parenting skills. I get enormous satisfaction out of watching a hesitant dad change his newborn for the first time or helping a mother breastfeed this baby, when she wasn't able to with her last one. I only wish I had more time to spend with each family.

—Mother–Baby Nurse

⌄ Learning Outcomes

25.1 Summarize essential information to be obtained about a newborn's birth experience and immediate postnatal period.

25.2 Explain how the physiologic and behavioral responses of the newborn during the first 4 hours after birth (admission and transitional period) determine the nursing care of the newborn.

25.3 Identify activities that should be included in a daily care plan for a normal newborn.

25.4 Explain the advantages and disadvantages of breastfeeding and formula-feeding in determining the nursing care of both mother/family and newborn.

25.5 Formulate guidelines for helping both breast- and formula-feeding mothers to feed their newborns successfully in hospital and community-based settings.

25.6 Describe the influence of cultural values on newborn care, especially feeding practices.

25.7 Identify the safety needs of the newborn in the birthing unit and at home.

25.8 Describe the common concerns of families regarding their newborn.

25.9 Identify opportunities to individualize parent teaching and enhance each parent's abilities and confidence while providing newborn care in the birthing unit.

At the moment of birth, numerous physiologic adaptations begin to take place in the newborn's body. Because of these dramatic changes, newborns require close observation to determine how smoothly they are making the transition to extrauterine life. Newborns also require specific care that enhances their chances of making the transition successfully.

The two broad goals of nursing care during this period are the following:

1. Promote the physical well-being of the newborn by providing comprehensive care to the newborn while in the mother–baby unit.

2. Support the establishment of a well-functioning family unit by teaching family members how to care for their new baby and support their efforts so that they feel confident and competent.

Thus the nurse must be knowledgeable about necessary family adjustments as well as the healthcare needs of the newborn. It is important that the family return home confident, knowing that they have the support, information, and skills to care for their newborn. Equally important is the need for each member of the family to begin a unique relationship with the newborn. The cultural and social expectations of individual families and communities affect the ways in which normal newborn care is carried out.

The previous two chapters presented an informational database of the physiologic and behavioral changes occurring in the newborn and the pertinent nursing assessments that are needed. This chapter discusses nursing management while the newborn is in the birthing unit and feeding methods for the full-term, healthy newborn.

Admission and the First 4 Hours of Life

Immediately after birth, the baby is formally admitted to the healthcare facility.

Nursing Management

For the Newborn During Admission and the First 4 Hours of Life

Nursing Assessment and Diagnosis

Before the birth of the baby, review the prenatal record of the mother for information concerning possible risk factors for the newborn. These include infectious disease screening results, drug or alcohol use by the mother, gestational diabetes, and any other data determined to be of use in anticipating the needs of the newborn. In addition, review the birth record for prolonged rupture of membranes, instrument or vacuum delivery, use of narcotic analgesia, presence of meconium, and any other data that may impact the newborn's ability to successfully transition to the extrauterine environment.

During the first hours after birth, a preliminary physical examination will be conducted, including an assessment of the newborn's physiologic adaptations. In many birthing units, the nurse performs and documents the initial head-to-toe physical assessment during the first hour of transition. The nurse is responsible for notifying the healthcare provider of any deviations from normal. A complete physical examination is also performed later by the healthcare provider, within the first 24 hours after birth and within 24 hours before discharge. This can be accomplished with one physical examination (see Chapter 24) (American Academy of Pediatrics [AAP] Committee on Fetus and Newborn & American College of Obstetricians and Gynecologists [ACOG] Committee on Obstetrics (AAP & AOG), 2012).

Nursing diagnoses are based on an analysis of the assessment findings. Physiologic alterations of the newborn form the basis of many nursing diagnoses, as does the family members' incorporation of them in caring for their newborn. Nursing diagnoses that may apply to newborns include the following (NANDA-I © 2014):

- *Airway Clearance, Ineffective,* related to presence of mucus and retained lung fluid

- *Body Temperature: Imbalanced, Risk for,* related to evaporative, radiant, conductive, and convective heat losses
- *Pain, Acute,* related to heel sticks for glucose or hematocrit tests, vitamin K injection, or hepatitis B immunization

As discussed in Chapter 23, the newborn's physiologic adaptation to extrauterine life occurs rapidly and all body systems are affected. Therefore, many of these nursing diagnoses and associated interventions must be identified and implemented in a very short period of time.

Planning and Implementation

INITIATING ADMISSION PROCEDURES

If the initial assessment, which must be performed within 2 hours after birth, indicates that the newborn is not at risk physiologically, you can perform many of the routine admission procedures in the presence of the parents in the birthing area. Some care measures indicated by the assessment findings may be performed by you or by the family members under your guidance in an effort to educate and support the family. Other interventions may be delayed until the newborn has been transferred to an observational nursery.

First check and confirm the newborn's identification with the mother's identification and then obtain and record all significant information. The essential data to be recorded in the newborn's medical record are as follows:

1. *Condition of the newborn.* Pertinent information includes the newborn's Apgar scores at 1 and 5 minutes, any resuscitative measures required in the birthing area, physical examination, vital signs, voidings, and passing of meconium. Complications to be noted are excessive mucus, delayed spontaneous respirations or responsiveness, abnormal number of cord vessels, and obvious physical abnormalities.

2. *Labor and birth record.* A copy of the labor and birth record should be placed in the newborn's medical record or be accessible on the computer. The record contains the significant data about the birth—for example, duration, course, and status of mother and fetus throughout labor and birth and any analgesia or anesthesia administered to the mother. Take particular care to note any variation or difficulties, such as prolonged rupture of membranes, abnormal fetal position, presence or absence of meconium-stained amniotic fluid, signs of nonreassuring fetal heart rate during labor, nuchal cord (cord around the newborn's neck at birth), precipitous birth, use of forceps or vacuum extraction assisted device, maternal analgesics and anesthesia received within 1 hour before birth, and administration of antibiotics during labor.

3. *Antepartum history.* Preexisting maternal conditions or any maternal problems that may have compromised the fetus in utero, such as preeclampsia, spotting, illness, recent infections (evidence of chorioamnionitis), blood type, rubella status, serology results, hepatitis B screen results, colonization with group B streptococci, recent exposure to infectious disease, HIV status, or a history of maternal substance abuse, are of immediate concern in newborn assessment. The medical record should also include information about maternal age, estimated date of delivery (EDD), previous pregnancies, and presence of any congenital anomalies. An HIV serology test should be encouraged and performed according to state law (AAP & ACOG, 2012).

4. *Parent–newborn interaction information.* Note the parents' interactions with their newborn and their desires regarding care, such as rooming in, circumcision, and the type of feeding. Information about other children in the home, available support systems, interactional patterns within each family unit, situations that compromise lactation (breast surgery, previous lactation failure), and any high-risk circumstances (adolescent mother, domestic violence, history of child abuse) helps in providing comprehensive care (AAP & ACOG, 2012).

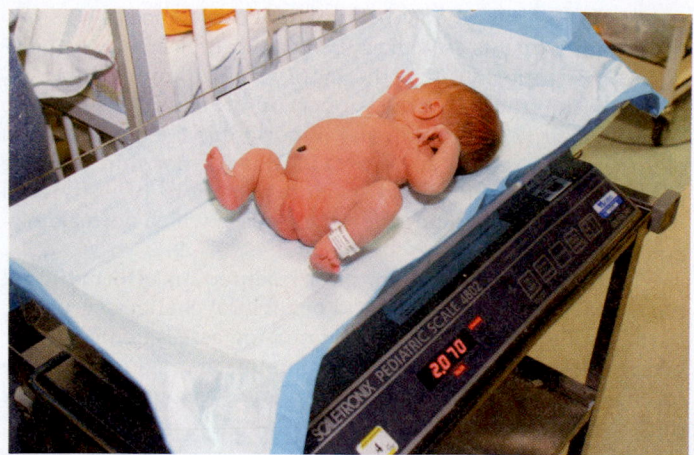

Figure 25–1 Weighing of newborn: The scale is cleaned and balanced before each weighing, with the protective pad in place.

Developing Cultural Competence   Newborn Naming in Kenya

In Kenya, the naming of a child is an important event. Names are commonly selected to mirror important or current events. For example, a baby who is born while traveling may be given a name that means "wanderer" or "traveler." Other names may be chosen after a relative who is among the "living-dead" (deceased). It is believed that this results in a partial reincarnation of that relative, especially if the child has characteristics in common with that individual. It is also believed there is a connection between newborns and the spirit world.

In some parts of the country, the name is chosen when the child is crying. Different names of the living or dead are called, and if the child stops crying when a particular name is called, that becomes the child's given name. In some areas, the name is given on the third day and is marked by a celebration with feasting and rejoicing. On the fourth day, the father of the child commonly hangs an iron necklace on the child's neck. It is at this time that the newborn is considered a full human being and the connection with the spirit world is lost.

As part of the admission procedure, weigh the newborn in both kilograms and pounds and ounces. In the United States, parents understand weight best when it is stated in pounds and ounces (Figure 25–1). Clean the scale, cover it, and set it to zero each time a newborn is weighed to prevent cross-infection. Remove all clothing and blankets for accurate weight and do the weighing under a warmer light to avoid heat loss from conduction.

Measure the newborn, recording the measurements in both centimeters and inches. The three routine measurements are length, head circumference, and chest circumference. In some facilities, abdominal girth may also be measured (see Table 24–1: Newborn Measurements). Rapidly assess the baby's color, muscle tone, alertness, and general state. Remember that the first period of reactivity may have concluded, and the baby may be in the sleep-inactive phase, which makes the newborn hard to arouse. Do basic assessments for estimating gestational age and complete the physical assessment (see *Assessment Guide: Newborn Physical Assessment* in Chapter 24).

In addition to obtaining vital signs, perform a hematocrit and blood glucose evaluation on at-risk newborns or as clinically indicated (such as for small-for-gestational-age [SGA] or large-for-gestational-age [LGA] newborns, or if the newborn is jittery). These procedures may be done on admission or within the first 2 hours after birth (AAP & ACOG, 2012). (See *Clinical Skill: Performing a Heel Stick on a Newborn* in Chapter 27.)

MAINTAINING A CLEAR AIRWAY AND STABLE VITAL SIGNS

Be sure that free flow oxygen is readily available. Position the newborn in a supine position (or on the side, if the baby has copious secretions). If necessary, use a bulb syringe or DeLee wall suction (see Figure 18-7; also see *Clinical Skill: Performing Nasal Pharyngeal Suctioning* in Chapter 18) to remove mucus from the stomach to help prevent possible aspiration. When possible, this procedure should be delayed for 10 to 15 minutes after birth to reduce the potential for severe vasovagal reflex apnea.

In the absence of any newborn distress, continue with the admission by taking the newborn's vital signs (see *Key Facts to Remember: Newborn Vital Signs* in Chapter 24). The initial temperature is taken by the axillary method. A wider range of normal exists for axillary temperature, specifically 36.4° to 37.2°C (97.5° to 99°F).

Once the initial temperature is taken, monitor the core temperature either by obtaining axillary temperatures at intervals or by placing a skin sensor on the newborn for continuous reading. The vital signs for a healthy term newborn should be monitored at least every 30 minutes until the newborn's condition has remained stable for 2 hours (AAP & ACOG, 2012). The newborn's respirations may be irregular yet still be normal. Brief periods of apnea, lasting only 5 to 10 seconds with no color or heart rate changes, are considered normal. The normal pulse range is 110 to 160 beats per minute (beats/min), and the normal respiratory range is 30 to 60 respirations per minute.

MAINTAINING A NEUTRAL THERMAL ENVIRONMENT

A neutral thermal environment is essential to minimize the newborn's need for increased oxygen consumption and use of calories to maintain body heat in the optimal range of 36.4° to 37.2°C (97.5° to 99°F). If the newborn becomes hypothermic, the body's response can lead to metabolic acidosis, hypoxia, and shock. See *Clinical Skill: Thermoregulation of the Newborn.*

A neutral thermal environment is best achieved by performing the newborn assessment and interventions with the newborn unclothed and under a radiant warmer. The radiant warmer's thermostat is controlled by the thermal skin sensor taped to the newborn's abdomen, upper thigh, or arm

Clinical Skill 25–1
Thermoregulation of the Newborn

NURSING ACTION

Preparation

- Prewarm the incubator or radiant warmer. Make sure warm towels and/or lightweight blankets are available.
- Maintain the temperature of the birthing room at 22°C (71°F), with a relative humidity of 60% to 65%.

Rationale: The change from a warm, moist intrauterine environment to a cool, dry, drafty environment stresses the newborn's immature thermoregulation system.

Equipment and Supplies

- Prewarmed towels or blankets
- Stocking cap
- Servocontrol probe
- T-shirt and diaper
- Open crib

Procedure: Clean Gloves

1. Don gloves.

Rationale: Gloves are worn whenever there is the possibility of contact with body fluids—in this case, a newborn wet with amniotic fluid, vernix, and maternal blood.

2. Place the newborn under the radiant warmer. Wipe the newborn free of blood, fluid, and excess vernix, especially from the head, using prewarmed towels.

Rationale: The radiant warmer creates a heat-gaining environment. Drying is important to prevent the loss of body heat through evaporation.

3. If the newborn is stable, wrap him or her in a prewarmed blanket, apply a stocking cap, and carry the baby to the mother. The mother and her partner/support person can hold and enjoy the newborn together. Alternatively, carry the newborn wrapped to the mother, loosen the blanket, and place the baby skin-to-skin on the mother's chest under a warmed blanket.

Rationale: Use of a prewarmed blanket reduces convection heat loss and facilitates maternal–newborn contact without compromising the newborn's thermoregulation. A snug cap can be fashioned from a piece of stockinette to help reduce heat loss from the head. Skin-to-skin contact with the mother or father/partner helps maintain the newborn's temperature.

4. After the newborn has spent time with the parents, return him or her to the radiant warmer and apply a diaper. Leave the newborn uncovered (except for the cap and diaper) under the radiant warmer.

Rationale: Radiant heat warms the outer skin surface, so the skin needs to be exposed.

5. Tape a servocontrol probe on the newborn's anterior abdominal wall, with the metal side next to the skin. Do not place it over the ribs. Secure the probe with porous tape or a foil-covered aluminum heat deflector patch.

6. Turn the heater to servocontrol mode so that the abdominal skin is maintained at 36.0° to 36.5°C (96.8° to 97.7°F).

7. Monitor the newborn's axillary and skin probe temperatures per agency protocol.

Rationale: The temperature indicator on the radiant warmer continually displays the newborn's probe temperature. The axillary temperature is checked to ensure that the machine is accurately recording the newborn's temperature.

8. When the newborn's axillary temperature reaches 37°C (98.6°F), add a T-shirt, double-wrap the baby (two blankets), and place the newborn in an open crib.

9. Recheck the newborn's temperature in 1 hour and regularly thereafter according to agency policy.

Rationale: It is important to monitor the newborn's ability to maintain his or her own thermoregulation.

10. If the newborn's temperature drops below 36.1°C (97°F), rewarm the baby gradually. Place the newborn (unclothed except for a diaper) under the radiant warmer with a servocontrol probe on the anterior abdominal wall.

Rationale: Rapid heating can lead to hyperthermia, which is associated with apnea, insensible water loss, and increased metabolic rate.

11. Recheck the newborn's temperature in 30 minutes, then hourly.

12. When the temperature reaches 37°C (98.6°F), dress the newborn, remove him or her from the radiant warmer, double-wrap, and place in an open crib. Check the temperature hourly until stable, then regularly according to agency policy.

Note: A newborn who repeatedly requires rewarming should be observed for other signs and symptoms of illness and a healthcare provider notified, because it may warrant screening for infection.

and can give a reading closely correlated with the mean body temperature (see Figure 24–16). The sensor indicates when the newborn's temperature exceeds or falls below the acceptable temperature range. Be aware that leaning over the newborn may block the radiant heat waves from reaching the newborn (Blackburn, 2013).

In light of early discharge practices (12 to 48 hours), healthy term newborns can be safely bathed immediately after the admission assessment is completed. The Association of Women's Health, Obstetrics and Neonatal Nurses (AWHONN) (2013) recommends washing off only the blood and fluid with the first bath and massaging the vernix into the skin. The baby is bathed while still under the radiant warmer; bathing may be done in the parents' room and by the parents. Bathing the newborn offers an excellent opportunity for teaching and welcoming parents' involvement in the care of their newborn. If there is any doubt regarding the newborn's condition, a sponge bath may be given when the baby's temperature is normal and vital signs are stable (about 2 to 4 hours after birth), when the baby's condition dictates, or when the parents wish to give the first bath.

Recheck the newborn's temperature after the bath and, if it is stable, dress him or her in a shirt, diaper, and cap; wrap the baby; and place the newborn in an open crib at room temperature. If the newborn's axillary temperature is below 36.5°C (97.7°F), return the newborn to the radiant warmer or place the newborn skin-to-skin with the mother to rewarm and promote early bonding and breastfeeding. The rewarming process should be gradual to prevent hyperthermia. (See Chapter 24 for information about temperature assessment and instability and see *Key Facts to Remember: Maintenance of Stable Newborn Temperature*.)

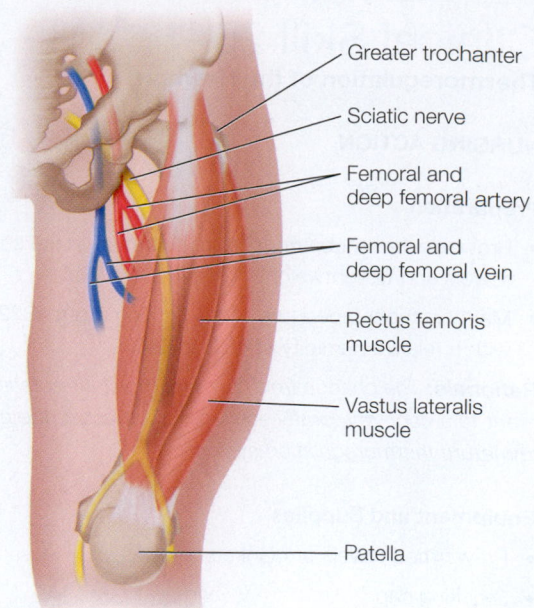

Figure 25–2 Injection site. The middle third of the vastus lateralis muscle is the preferred site for intramuscular injection in the newborn.

KEY FACTS TO REMEMBER
Maintenance of Stable Newborn Temperature

Take action to help the newborn maintain a stable temperature:

- Keep the newborn's clothing and bedding dry.
- Double-wrap the newborn and put on a stocking cap.
- Use the radiant warmer during procedures.
- Reduce the newborn's exposure to drafts.
- Warm objects that will be in contact with the newborn (e.g., stethoscope, blankets).
- Encourage the mother to snuggle with the newborn under blankets or to breastfeed with a hat and a light cover on the baby.

Neonatal side effects can be pain and edema at the injection site. Allergic reactions, such as rash and urticaria, may also occur. Nursing consideration should include the following:

- Protect drug from light.
- Give vitamin K_1 before circumcision procedure.
- Observe for signs of local inflammation.

PREVENTING VITAMIN K DEFICIENCY BLEEDING

A prophylactic injection of phytonadione vitamin K_1 (Aqua-MEPHYTON) is recommended to prevent vitamin K deficiency bleeding (VKDB) and hemorrhage, which can occur because of low prothrombin levels in the first few days of life. The potential for hemorrhage is considered to result from the absence of gut bacterial flora, which influences the production of vitamin K_1 in the newborn (see Coagulation in Chapter 23 for further discussion). Current recommendations underscore the need for treatment in newborns who are exclusively breastfed (Blackburn, 2013). Vitamin K injection can be delayed up to 6 hours after birth (Marcewicz, 2014). It is often given in the labor and delivery unit before transfer to the newborn nursery.

A one-time-only prophylactic dose of 0.5 to 1.0 mg is given intramuscularly in the middle third of the vastus lateralis muscle, located in the lateral aspect of the thigh (Figure 25–2). Before injecting, thoroughly clean the newborn's skin site for the injection with a small alcohol swab. Use a 25–gauge, 5/8-in. needle for the injection (Figure 25–3). If the mother received anticoagulants during pregnancy, an additional dose may be ordered by the healthcare provider and is given 6 to 8 hours after the first injection.

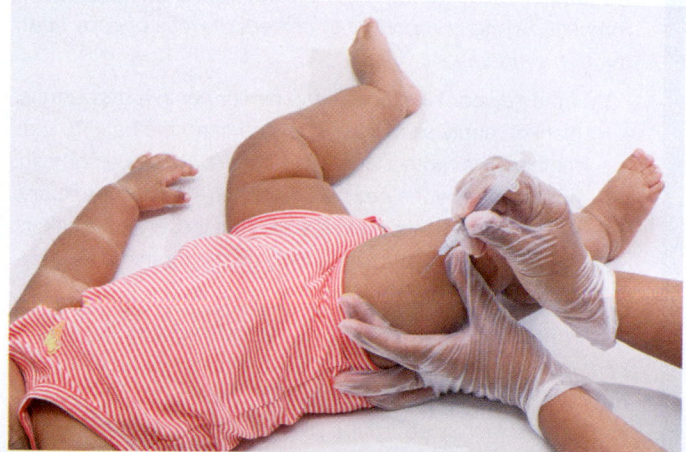

Figure 25–3 Procedure for vitamin K injection. Cleanse area thoroughly with alcohol swab and allow skin to dry. Bunch the tissue of the upper outer thigh (vastus lateralis muscle) and quickly insert a 25–gauge, 5/8–in. needle at a 90–degree angle to the thigh. Slowly inject the solution to distribute the medication evenly and minimize the baby's discomfort. Remove the needle and gently massage the site with an alcohol swab.

SOURCE: © Marlon Lopez/Shutterstock.

- Observe for bleeding (usually occurs on second or third day). Bleeding may be seen as generalized ecchymoses or bleeding from umbilical cord, circumcision site, nose, or gastrointestinal tract. Results of serial prothrombin time (PT) and international normalized ratio (INR) should be assessed.

PREVENTING EYE INFECTION

Another nursing responsibility is administering the legally required prophylactic eye treatment for *Neisseria gonorrhoeae*, which may have infected the newborn of an infected mother during the birth process. A variety of topical agents appear to be equally effective. Ophthalmic ointments that are used include 0.5% erythromycin (Ilotycin Ophthalmic), 1% tetracycline, or per agency protocol. All are also effective against chlamydia, which has a higher incidence rate of infection than gonorrhea.

Successful eye prophylaxis requires that the medication be instilled into the lower conjunctival sac of each eye (Figure 25–4). After administration, gently close the eye and manipulate to ensure the spread of ointment (Wilson, Shannon, & Shields, 2015). It is instilled only once in each eye (AAP & ACOG, 2012). The ointment may be administered in the birthing area or, alternatively, 1 hour later in the nursery so that eye contact between newborn and parent is facilitated and the bonding process immediately after birth is not interrupted.

Nursing considerations include the following:

- Use standard precautions before instillation to prevent introduction of bacteria if the baby has not been bathed yet.
- Do not irrigate the eyes after instillation. Use a new tube or single-use container for ophthalmic ointment administration shortly after birth. Excess ointment may be wiped away after 1 minute.
- Observe for hypersensitivity.
- Teach parents about the need for eye prophylaxis. Educate parents regarding side effects and signs that need to be reported to the healthcare provider.

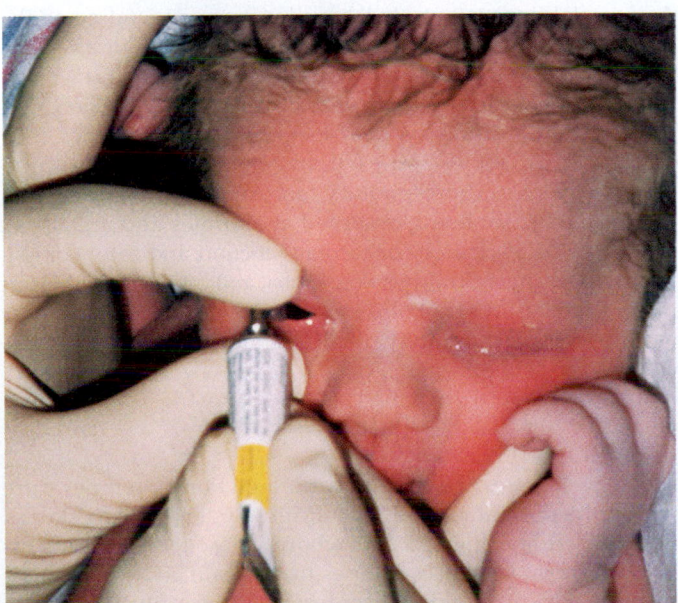

Figure 25–4 Ophthalmic ointment. Retract the lower eyelid outward to instill a 1/4-in. (1 cm) long strand of ointment from a single-dose tube along the lower conjunctival surface. Make sure that the tip of the tube does not touch the eye.

Eye prophylaxis medications can cause chemical conjunctivitis, which gives the newborn some discomfort and may interfere with the ability to focus on the parents' faces. The resulting edema, inflammation, and discharge may cause concern if the parents have not been informed that the side effects will clear in 24 to 48 hours and that this prophylactic eye treatment is necessary for the newborn's well-being.

EARLY ASSESSMENT OF NEONATAL DISTRESS

During the first 24 hours of life, be constantly alert for signs of distress. If the newborn is with the parents during this period, take extra care to teach them how to maintain their newborn's temperature, recognize the hallmarks of newborn distress, and respond immediately to signs of respiratory problems. The parents must learn to observe the newborn for changes in color or activity, grunting or "sighing" sounds with breathing, rapid breathing with chest retractions, or facial grimacing. Their interventions include nasal and oral suctioning with a bulb syringe, positioning, and vigorous fingertip stroking of the newborn's spine to stimulate respiratory activity if necessary. You must be available immediately if the newborn develops distress. See *Key Facts to Remember: Signs of Newborn Distress*.

KEY FACTS TO REMEMBER
Signs of Newborn Distress

- Respiratory changes
  - Increased respiratory rate (more than 60/minute) or difficult respirations
  - Grunting
  - Sternal, substernal, intercostal retractions
  - Nasal flaring
  - Excessive mucus
- Color change
  - Cyanosis (central: skin, lips, tongue)
  - Pallor
  - Mottling
  - Plethora (ruddy skin)
- Abdominal distention or mass
- Vomiting of bile-stained material
- Absence of meconium elimination within 48 hours of birth
- Absence of urine elimination more than 24 hours after birth
- Temperature instability (hypothermia or hyperthermia)
- Jitteriness, irritability, or abnormal movements
- Difficulty in wakening; signs of lethargy or hypotonicity
- Weight change greater than 10% loss of weight from birthweight

Source: Data from AAP & ACOG (2012).

A common cause of neonatal distress is early-onset group B streptococcal (GBS) disease. Infected mothers transmit GBS infection to their newborns during labor and birth; thus it is recommended that at-risk mothers receive intrapartum antimicrobial prophylaxis (IAP) for GBS disease. All newborns of mothers identified as at risk should be assessed and observed for signs and symptoms of sepsis (see Chapter 15 for discussion of maternal care and Chapter 27 for discussion of newborn care).

FACILITATING EARLY PARENT–NEWBORN ATTACHMENT

To facilitate **parent–newborn attachment**, eye-to-eye contact between the parents and their newborn is extremely important during the early hours after birth when the newborn is in the first period of reactivity. The newborn is alert during this time, the eyes are wide open, and the baby often makes direct eye contact with human faces within optimal range for visual acuity (7 to 8 in.). It is theorized that this eye contact is an important foundation in establishing attachment in human relationships (Klaus & Klaus, 1985). Consequently, administration of the prophylactic eye medication is often delayed, but no more than 1 hour, to provide an opportunity for a period of eye contact between parents and their newborn, thus facilitating the attachment process (AAP & ACOG, 2012). Parents who cannot be with their newborns in this first period because of maternal or neonatal distress may need reassurance that the bonding process can proceed normally as soon as both mother and baby are stable.

Another situation that can facilitate attachment is the interactive bath. While bathing their newborn for the first time, parents attend closely to their baby's behavior. In this way, the newborn becomes an active participant and parents are drawn into an interaction with their newborn. During this time, you may interpret the newborn's behavior for the parents, model ways to respond to the behavior, and support parental strategies for doing so.

Evaluation

When evaluating the nursing care provided during the period immediately after birth, the nurse may anticipate the following outcomes:

- The newborn's adaptation to extrauterine life is successful as demonstrated by all vitals within acceptable parameters.
- The newborn's physiologic and psychologic integrity is supported.
- Positive interactions between parent and newborn will be supported.

The Newborn Following Transition

Once a healthy newborn has demonstrated successful adaptation to extrauterine life, he or she needs appropriate observations for the first 6 to 12 hours after birth and the remainder of the stay in the birthing facility.

Nursing Management

For the Newborn Following Transition

Nursing Assessment and Diagnosis

Examples of nursing diagnoses that may apply during daily care of the newborn include the following (NANDA-I © 2014):

- *Breathing Pattern, Ineffective*, related to periodic breathing
- *Nutrition, Imbalanced: Less than Body Requirements*, related to limited nutritional and fluid intake and increased caloric expenditure
- *Urinary Elimination, Impaired*, related to meatal edema secondary to circumcision
- *Infection, Risk for*, related to umbilical cord healing, circumcision site, immature immune system, or potential birth trauma (forceps or vacuum extraction birth)
- *Knowledge, Readiness for Enhanced*, related to information about basic newborn care, male circumcision, and breastfeeding and/or formula-feeding
- *Family Processes, Readiness for Enhanced*, related to integration of newborn into family or demands of newborn care and feeding

Planning and Implementation

MAINTAINING CARDIOPULMONARY FUNCTION

Assess vital signs every 6 to 8 hours or more, depending on the newborn's status. The newborn should be placed on the back (supine) for sleeping. A bulb syringe is kept within easy reach should the newborn need oral–nasal suctioning. If the newborn has respiratory difficulty, clear the airway. Vigorous fingertip stroking of the baby's spine will frequently stimulate respiratory activity. A cardiorespiratory monitor can be used on newborns that are not being observed at all times and are at risk for decreased respiratory or cardiac function. Indicators of risk are pallor, cyanosis, ruddy color, apnea, and other signs of instability. Changes in skin color may indicate the need for closer assessment of temperature, cardiopulmonary status, hematocrit, glucose, and bilirubin levels.

MAINTAINING A NEUTRAL THERMAL ENVIRONMENT

Make every effort to maintain the newborn's temperature within the normal range by continuing interventions started in the first 4-hour period. A newborn whose temperature falls below optimal level uses calories to maintain body heat rather than for growth. Chilling also decreases the affinity of serum albumin for bilirubin, thereby increasing the likelihood of newborn jaundice. In addition, it increases oxygen use and may cause respiratory distress. An overheated newborn will increase activity and respiratory rate in an attempt to cool the body. Both measures deplete caloric reserves, and the increased respiratory rate leads to increased insensible fluid loss (Blackburn, 2013).

Clinical Reasoning Maintaining the Newborn's Temperature

John Fredricks, the father of a newborn less than a day old, has the baby lying supine and wearing only a diaper. When you suggest that the baby may need more covering, he responds: "He doesn't like all that stuff on. After all, he's been naked until now."

What actions and teaching are appropriate in this situation?

PROMOTING ADEQUATE HYDRATION AND NUTRITIONAL STATUS

Record caloric and fluid intake and enhance adequate hydration by maintaining a neutral thermal environment and offering early and frequent feedings. Early feedings promote gastric emptying and increase peristalsis, thereby decreasing the potential for hyperbilirubinemia by decreasing the amount of time fecal material is in contact with enzyme β-glucuronidase in the small intestine. This enzyme frees the bilirubin from the feces, allowing it to be reabsorbed into the vascular system (see Chapter 27 for a detailed discussion of hyperbilirubinemia).

Record voiding and stooling patterns. The first voiding should occur within 24 hours and the first passage of stool within 48 hours. When these do not occur, continue the normal observation routine while assessing for abdominal distention, bowel sounds, hydration, fluid intake, and temperature stability.

Newborns should be weighed at the same time each day for accurate comparisons and should be kept warm during the weighing. A weight loss of up to 10% for term newborns is considered within normal limits during the first week of life (Cloherty, Eichenwald, Hansen, et al., 2012). This weight loss is the result of limited intake, loss of excess extracellular fluid, and passage of meconium. Tell the parents about the expected weight loss, the reason for it, and the expectations for regaining the birth weight. Birth weight is usually regained by 2 weeks if feedings are adequate.

Excessive handling can cause an increase in the newborn's metabolic rate and caloric use and cause fatigue. Be alert to the newborn's subtle cues of fatigue, including a decrease in muscle tension and activity in the extremities and neck, as well as loss of eye contact, which may be manifested by fluttering or closure of the eyelids. Quickly cease stimulation when signs of fatigue appear. Demonstrate to parents the need to be aware of newborn cues and to wait for periods of alertness for contact and stimulation. Assess the woman's comfort and latching-on techniques if she is breastfeeding, or assess the bottle-feeding techniques. Breastfeeding and formula-feeding the newborn are discussed in detail later in this chapter.

PROMOTING SKIN INTEGRITY

Newborn skin care, including bathing, is important for the health and appearance of the individual newborn and for infection control within the nursery. Ongoing skin care involves cleansing the buttock and perianal areas with fresh water and cotton or a mild soap and water with diaper changes. If commercial baby wipes are used, those without alcohol should be selected. Perfume- and latex-free wipes are also available.

The umbilical cord is assessed for signs of bleeding or infection. Removal of the cord clamp within 24 to 48 hours of birth reduces the chance of tension injury to the area. Keeping

the umbilical stump clean and allowing it to air dry without the routine application of topical agents can reduce the chance for infection (AWHONN, 2013) (Figure 25–5).

Many types of routine cord care are practiced, including the use of air-drying, triple dye, an antimicrobial agent such as bacitracin, or application of 70% alcohol to the cord stump, but should not be encouraged (AWHONN, 2013). These practices are largely based on tradition rather than evidence-based findings. The skin absorption and toxicity of triple-dye agents in newborns have not been carefully studied. No single method of umbilical cord care has been proven to be superior in preventing umbilical cord colonization of microorganisms and infection (omphalitis) (AWHONN, 2013). Folding the diaper down to avoid covering the cord stump can prevent contamination of the area and promote drying. Cord care per agency policy is your responsibility. The cord should look dark and dry up before falling off (Figure 25–6). It is also your responsibility to instruct parents in caring for the cord and observing for signs and symptoms of infection after discharge, such as foul smell, redness and greenish yellow drainage,

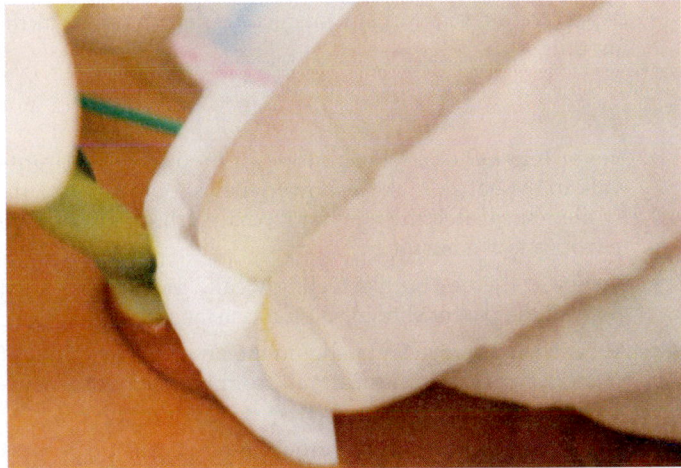

Figure 25–5 Routine umbilical cord care. The umbilical cord base is carefully cleansed.

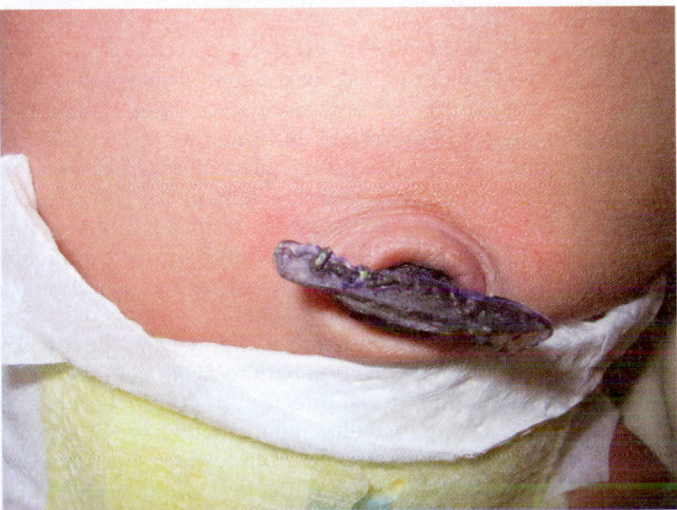

Figure 25–6 The umbilical cord looks dark and dries up prior to falling off.

localized heat and tenderness, or bright red bleeding or if the area remains unhealed 2 to 3 days after the cord stump has sloughed off.

PROMOTING SAFETY

The threat of abduction requires that hospitals have active programs to prevent such an event (Fraser, 2014). Be aware of these policies and follow them rigorously. Informing parents of their role in this process is part of a comprehensive safety plan. Parental measures to prevent abduction and promote newborn safety include the following:

Security

- Check that identification bands are in place as the parents care for their baby and, if missing, ask that they be replaced immediately.

- If an electronically tagged band is used, keep the baby within the bounds of the system and notify the staff if the band becomes loose or comes off.

- Allow only people with proper birthing unit identification to remove the baby from the room. If parents do not know the staff person, they should call the nurse for assistance.

- Report the presence of any suspicious people on the birthing unit.

Safety

- Never leave the newborn alone in the room. If parents walk in the halls or take a shower, they should have a family member watch the newborn, or they should return the newborn to the nursery.

- Never lift the newborn if feeling weak, faint, or unsteady. Instead, the parent should call for assistance.

- Always keep an eye and hand on the newborn when out of the crib, because babies can fall from beds and other surfaces if left alone.

- Protect from infection, even though newborns do possess some immunity. All caregivers should practice good hand washing before and after giving care. Parents should ask visitors to leave if they have any of the following: cold, diarrhea, discharge from sores, or contagious disease. Security monitoring devices should be sterilized after use to prevent transmission of infection.

PREVENTING COMPLICATIONS

Newborns are at continued risk for the complications of hemorrhage, late-onset cardiac symptoms, and infection. Pallor may be an early sign of hemorrhage and must be reported to the healthcare provider. The newborn is placed on a cardiorespiratory monitor to permit continuous assessment. Several newborn conditions put newborns at risk for hemorrhage. Cyanosis that is not relieved by oxygen administration requires emergency intervention, may indicate a congenital cardiac condition or shock, and requires ongoing assessment.

It is recommended that nursing staff gown and glove when handling a newborn until the first bath to avoid contamination by blood and amniotic fluids. Infection in the nursery is best prevented by requiring that all personnel who have direct contact with newborns scrub for 2 to 3 minutes from the fingertips up to and including the elbows at the beginning of each shift. The hands must also be washed with soap and rubbed vigorously for 15 seconds, or a topical antimicrobial applied, before and after contact with every newborn and after touching any

soiled surface such as the floor or one's hair or face. Instruct parents to practice good hand washing and/or use of an antiseptic hand cleaner before touching the newborn. Emphasize that anyone holding the baby should practice good hand washing, even after the family returns home. In some clinical settings family members are asked to wear gowns (preferably disposable) over their street clothes during their contact with newborns. These are good opportunities to reinforce the efficacy of hand washing in preventing the spread of infection.

Jaundice occurs in most newborns. Most jaundice is benign, but because of the potential toxicity of bilirubin, newborns must be monitored to identify those who might develop severe hyperbilirubinemia and, in rare cases, acute bilirubin encephalopathy or kernicterus (see Chapter 27 for more detailed discussion) (AAP & ACOG, 2012). Current recommendations include obtaining a total serum bilirubin level in any newborn who is visibly jaundiced in the first 24 hours of life, and obtaining either a serum or a transcutaneous bilirubin level before discharge. Nomograms for evaluating risk factors based on bilirubin levels and age of newborn are available (see Chapter 24).

CIRCUMCISION

Circumcision is a surgical procedure in which the prepuce, an epithelial layer covering the tip of the penis, is separated from the glans penis and excised. This permits exposure of the glans for easier cleaning.

Scientific evidence demonstrates that the preventive health benefits of elective circumcision of newborn males outweigh the risks of this procedure (Healthy Children, 2015g). The 2012 AAP policy statement, however, reaffirmed that it does not recommend *routine* circumcision but acknowledges that medical indications for circumcision still exist (AAP, 2012a).

Circumcision *should not be performed* if the newborn is premature or compromised, has a known bleeding problem, or is born with a genitourinary defect such as hypospadias or epispadias, which may necessitate the use of the foreskin in future surgical repairs.

Parents will need to weigh medical information in the context of their own religious, ethical, and cultural beliefs and practices, as it is the parents who must ultimately decide whether circumcision is in the best interests of their child (Healthy Children, 2015g). To ensure informed consent, parents should be informed during the prenatal period about possible long-term medical effects of circumcision and non-circumcision. Parents must be knowledgeable about the potential risks and outcomes of circumcision. Hemorrhage, infection, difficulty in voiding, separation of the edges of the circumcision, discomfort, and restlessness are early potential problems (Cloherty et al., 2012). You can allay parents' anxiety by sharing information and allowing them to express their concerns.

Circumcision Care

The procedure is performed when the newborn is well stabilized and has received an initial physical examination by a healthcare provider. Before a circumcision, ensure that the healthcare provider has explained the procedure, determine whether the parents have any further questions about the procedure, and verify that the circumcision permit is signed. As with any surgical procedure, the newborn's identification band should be checked to verify his identity before the procedure begins. Gather the equipment and prepare the newborn by removing the diaper and placing him on a padded circumcision board or some other type of restraint, but restraining only the legs. These restraint measures along with the application of warm blankets to the upper body increase comfort during the procedure. In Jewish circumcision ceremonies, the baby is held by the father or godfather and given wine before the procedure.

A variety of devices (Gomco clamp, Plastibell, Mogen clamp) are used for circumcision (Figures 25–7 and 25–8), and all produce minimal bleeding. Therefore, make special note of newborns with a family history of bleeding disorders or with mothers who took anticoagulants, including aspirin, prenatally. During the procedure, assess the newborn's response.

One important consideration is pain experienced by the newborn. The 2012 AAP policy recommends that acceptable methods of analgesia (dorsal penile nerve block [DPNB], subcutaneous ring block, and eutectic mixture of local anesthetics [EMLA] cream) be used during circumcision to decrease procedural pain (Cloherty et al., 2012). The DPNB and subcutaneous ring block are the most effective options. The use of sucrose pacifiers has also been studied. Indications are that a combination of methods is most effective in reducing pain during circumcision (AAP & ACOG, 2012).

During the procedure, provide comfort measures such as swaddling, lightly stroking the newborn's head, providing a pacifier for nonnutritive sucking, and talking to him. Following

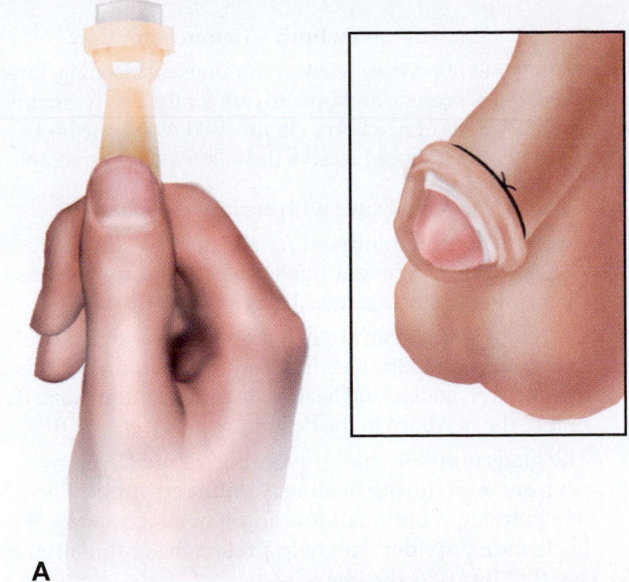

A

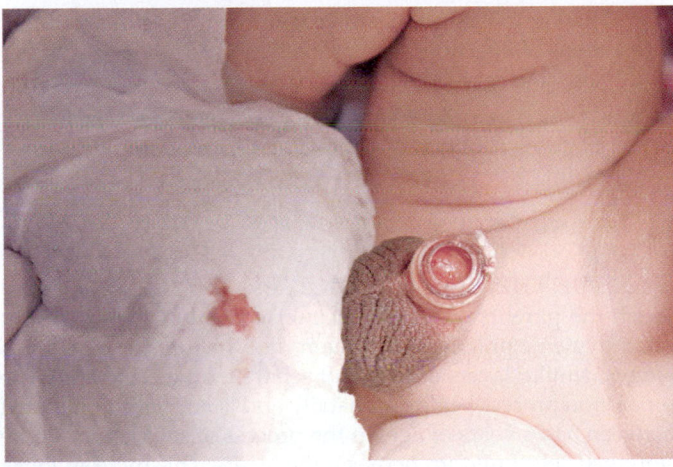

B

Figure 25–8 Circumcision using the Plastibell. A. The bell is fitted over the glans. A suture is tied around the bell's rim and the excess prepuce is cut away. The plastic rim remains in place for 3 to 4 days until healing occurs. The bell may be allowed to fall off; it is removed if still in place after 8 days. B. Plastibell.

SOURCE: B. Vanessa Howell, RN, MSN.

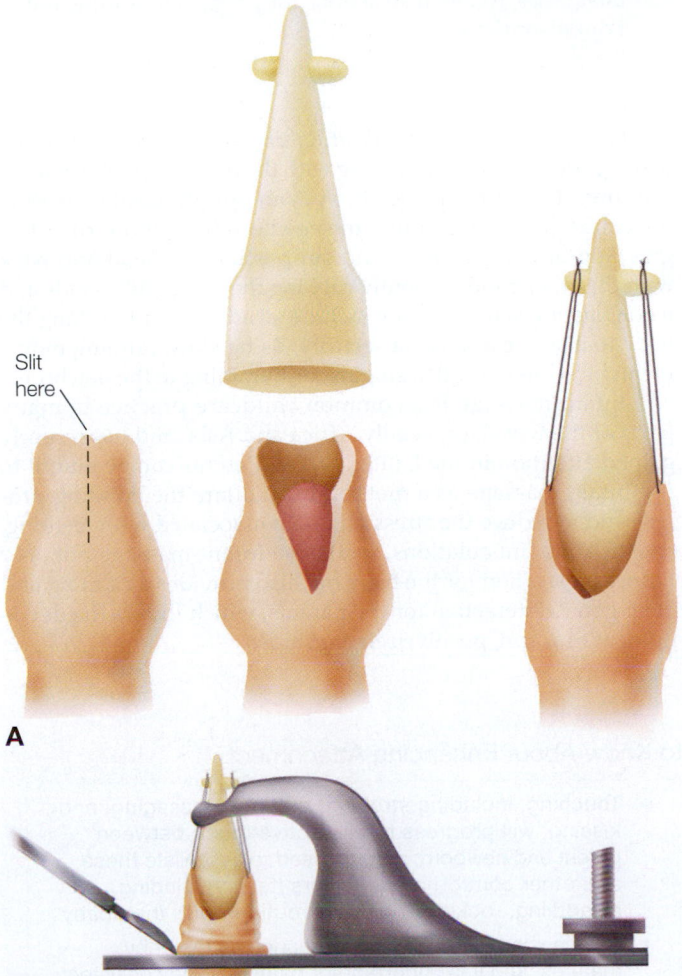

Slit here

A

B

Figure 25–7 Circumcision using the Yellen or Gomco clamp. A. The prepuce is drawn over the cone and B. the clamp is applied. Pressure is maintained for 3 to 4 minutes, and then excess prepuce is cut away.

the circumcision, the baby should be held and comforted by you or a family member. Be alert to any behavioral cues that these measures are overstimulating the newborn instead of comforting him. Such cues include turning away of the head, increased generalized body movement, skin color changes, hyperalertness, and hiccupping.

Ideally, assess the circumcision every 30 minutes for at least 2 hours following the procedure. It is important to observe the first voiding after a circumcision to evaluate for urinary obstruction related to penile injury or edema. If the Plastibell is used, provide information to the parents about normal appearance and how to observe for infection. Inform them that the Plastibell should fall off within 8 days. If it remains on after 8 days, they should consult with the newborn's healthcare provider. Though no ointments or creams should be used while the bell remains, application of petroleum ointment may protect granulation tissue afterward (AWHONN, 2013).

Health Promotion · Newborn Circumcision Care

Teach family members how to assess for unusual bleeding, how to respond if it is present, and how to care for the newly circumcised penis. Parents of newborns circumcised with a method other than Plastibell should receive the following information:

- Clean with warm water with each diaper change.
- Apply petroleum ointment for the next few diaper changes to help prevent further bleeding and to protect the healing tissue afterward (Figure 25–9).
- If bleeding does occur, apply light pressure with a sterile gauze pad to stop the bleeding within a short time. If this is not effective, contact the healthcare provider immediately, or take the newborn to the healthcare provider.
- The glans normally has granulation tissue (a yellowish film) on it during healing. Continued application of a petroleum ointment (or ointment suggested by the healthcare provider) can help protect the granulation tissue that forms as the glans heals.
- Report to the healthcare provider any signs or symptoms of infection, such as increasing swelling, pus drainage, and cessation of urination.
- When diapering, ensure that the diaper is not too loose (causing rubbing with movement), or too tight (causing pain).

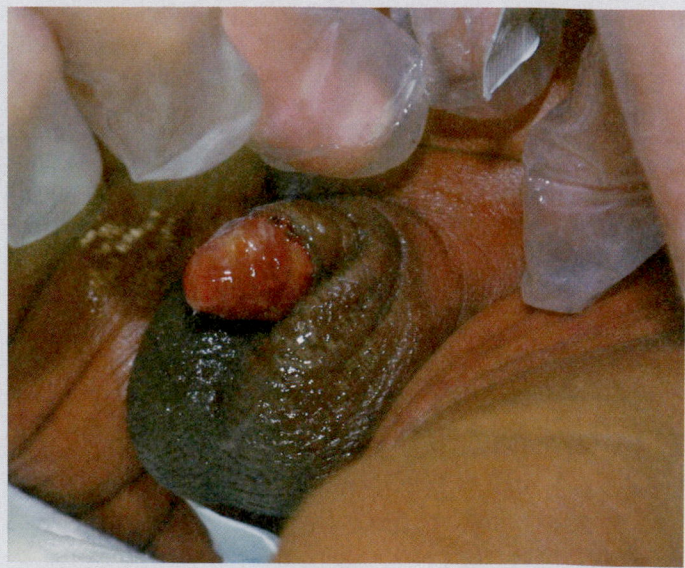

Figure 25–9 Following circumcision, petroleum ointment may be applied to the site for the next few diaper changes.

- If the newborn's healthcare provider recommends oral analgesics, follow instructions for proper measuring and administration.

CARE OF THE UNCIRCUMCISED NEWBORN

Teach the parents of an uncircumcised male newborn about good hygienic practices. Tell them that the foreskin and glans are two similar layers of cells that separate from each other. The separation process begins prenatally and is normally completed between 3 to 5 years of age. In the process of separation, sterile sloughed cells build up between the layers. This buildup looks similar to the smegma secreted after puberty, and it is harmless. Occasionally during the daily bath, the parent can gently test for retraction. If retraction has occurred, daily gentle washing of the glans with soap and water is sufficient to maintain adequate cleanliness. The parents should teach the child to incorporate this practice into his daily self-care activities. Most uncircumcised males have no difficulty doing so.

ENHANCING PARENT–NEWBORN ATTACHMENT

Encourage parent–newborn attachment by involving all family members with the new member of the family. (For specific interventions see Chapter 18 and Chapter 29 and *Teaching Highlights: What Parents Need to Know About Enhancing Attachment*.) Discuss waking activities such as talking with the newborn while making eye contact, holding the newborn in an upright position (sitting or standing), gently bending the newborn back and forth while grasping under the knees and supporting the head and back with the other hand, or gently rubbing the newborn's hands and feet. Quieting activities may include swaddling or bundling the baby to increase a sense of security; using slow, calming movements; and talking softly, singing, or humming to the newborn.

Infant massage is a common childcare practice in many parts of the world, especially Africa and Asia, and has recently gained attention in the United States. Parents can be taught to use infant massage as a method to facilitate the bonding process and to reduce the stress and pain associated with teething, constipation, inoculations, and colic. Infant massage not only induces relaxation for the baby but also provides a calming and "feel-good" interaction for the parents, which fosters the development of warm, positive relationships.

TEACHING HIGHLIGHTS | What Parents Need to Know About Enhancing Attachment

- Information on the periods of reactivity, expected newborn responses, and normal newborn physical characteristics.
- The gradual developmental nature of the bonding process and the reciprocal interactive nature of the process.
- The newborn's capabilities for interaction such as nonverbal communication abilities. Nonverbal communications include movement, gaze, touch, facial expressions, and vocalizations—including crying. Eye contact is considered one of the cardinal factors in developing newborn–parent attachment and will be integrated with touching and vocal behaviors.

- Touching, including stroking, patting, massaging, and kissing, will progress to interactive touch between parent and newborn; parents need to assimilate these and other comforting behaviors (talking, singing, swaddling, rocking) into daily routines with their baby.
- The newborn's behaviors will change as the baby matures, and it is important for parents to be consistent in response to their baby's cues and needs.
- Information about pamphlets, videos, and support groups in the community.

Caring for newborns in the birthing setting and fostering parent–newborn attachment means that the nurse will have contact with parents from a wide variety of racial, religious, and cultural backgrounds. Although it may not be possible to be conversant with all cultures, the nurse can demonstrate cultural competence with both colleagues and parents. The nurse must be sensitive to the cultural beliefs and values of the family and be aware of cultural variations in newborn care such as naming the newborn, giving compliments about the newborn, and using good luck charms (see *Developing Cultural Competence: Examples of Cultural Beliefs and Practices Regarding Baby Care*).

EVALUATION

When evaluating the nursing care provided during the newborn period, the following outcomes may be anticipated:

- The baby's physiologic and psychologic integrity is supported by maintaining stable vital signs and interactions based on normal newborn behaviors.
- The newborn feeding pattern will be satisfactorily established.
- The parents express understanding of the bonding process and display attachment behaviors.

Newborn Feeding

Early nutrition has a significant impact on the present and future health and well-being of the newborn because this is a period of rapid growth and brain development. Good nutrition fosters physical growth and helps maintain a healthy immune system. In addition, newborn feeding is an important component of newborn socialization that promotes cognitive and emotional development.

The newborn's diet must supply all the nutrients required by the body in the proper quantities to meet the newborn's rapid rate of physical and neurologic growth and development. A newborn's diet should provide adequate hydration and sufficient calories and must include protein, carbohydrates, fat, vitamins, and minerals. Exclusive breast milk and/or iron-fortified 20-calorie/ounce formula are sufficient as sole sources of nutrition to meet the dietary needs of the baby from birth up to 6 months of age. Complementary solid foods are introduced in the second half of the first year, and the infant continues to receive breast milk and/or formula until at least 12 months of age (AAP, 2012b).

Developing Cultural Competence Examples of Cultural Beliefs and Practices Regarding Baby Care*

Umbilical Cord

- People of Latin American or Filipino cultural background may use an abdominal binder or bellyband to protect against dirt, injury, and umbilical hernia. They may also apply oils to the stump of the cord or tape metal to the umbilicus to ward off evil spirits (Purnell, 2013).
- People of northern European ancestry may expect a sterile cutting of the cord at birth. They may allow the stump to air-dry and discard the cord once it falls off.
- Chinese and some Latin American parents cauterize the stump with a hot flame, hot coal, or the like (Smith, 2009).
- In Kenya and Iran, women may express colostrum onto the cord stump (Smith, 2009).
- In Ecuador, the cord stump is left long in girls to prevent a small uterus and problems with childbirth (Smith, 2009).

Parent–Newborn Contact

- People of Asian ancestry may pick up the baby as soon as it cries, or they may carry the baby at all times.
- Several native North American nations' people, notably the Navajos, may use cradle boards, so the newborn can feel secure and be with family even during work (Woodring & Andrews, 2012).
- The Muslim father traditionally calls praise to Allah in the newborn's right ear and cleans the baby after birth (Purnell, 2013).

Circumcision

- People of Muslim and Jewish ancestry practice circumcision as a religious ritual (Purnell, 2013).
- Many native people of Africa and Australia practice circumcision as a puberty rite.
- Native Americans and people of Asian and Latin American cultures rarely perform circumcision (Lipson & Dibble, 2008).

Health and Illness

- Some people from Latin American cultural backgrounds may believe that touching the face or head of a baby when admiring it will ward off the "evil eye." They also may not cut the baby's nails to avoid nearsightedness and instead put mittens on the baby's hands to prevent scratching. They also may believe that fat babies are healthy (Woodring & Andrews, 2012).
- Some people of Asian heritage may not allow anyone to touch the baby's head without asking permission.
- Some Orthodox Jews believe that saying the baby's name before the formal naming ceremony will harm the baby.
- Asians and Haitians may delay naming their newborns until after the confinement month (Purnell, 2013).
- Some people of Vietnamese ancestry believe that cutting a baby's hair or nails will cause illness.

*Note: The information given here is meant only to provide examples of the behaviors that may be found within certain cultures. Not all members of a culture practice the behaviors described.

KEY FACTS TO REMEMBER
Newborn Caloric and Fluid Needs

- Caloric intake: 45.5 to 52.5 kcal/lb/day or 100 to 115 kcal/kg/day
- Fluid requirements: 64 to 73 mL/lb/day or 140 to 160 mL/kg/day

Growth Rates

Breastfed and formula-fed babies have different growth rates. This is understandable because the compositions of breast milk and formula are different. Most healthcare providers (as well as formula company representatives) consider breastfeeding to be the "gold standard" for neonatal nutrition and the basis from which to compare nutritional outcomes (Baker, 2016).

It is normal for both breastfed and formula-fed newborns to lose weight in the first 3 to 4 days of life. Newborns lose weight with the passage of meconium and because their fluid intake is normally low in the first few days while transitioning to enteral feedings, especially among breastfed newborns. This loss is normal and does not result in dehydration, because newborns can draw on their extracellular water reserves. Newborns should begin gaining weight by day of life 5 or sooner and should be at or above birth weight by 10 to 14 days of age.

Formula-fed newborns tend to regain their birth weight earlier than breastfed newborns because the formula-fed newborn has a greater fluid intake early on. The breastfeeding newborn's fluid intake depends on the mother's milk supply and breastfeeding efficiency. If a baby has a weight loss of 10% or greater, then an evaluation, intervention, and follow-up weight check are indicated to make certain that the newborn receives sufficient fluid and calories and to determine if the feeding problem is resolved.

Growth rates for breastfed and formula-fed newborns are somewhat different once feedings have been established. Exclusively breastfed infants have the same or slightly higher weight gain than their formula-fed and mixed-fed peers in the first 3 to 4 months. Thereafter, formula-fed and mixed-fed infants have a greater weight gain pattern compared with breastfed infants. This characteristic weight gain pattern results in a leaner body build in the breastfed group by the latter half of the first year of life (Baker, 2016). Measurements of length and head circumference are the same for both groups. An infant typically grows 2.5 cm (1 in.) per month in the first 6 months, and then 1.3 cm (0.5 in.) for the next 6 months. Length is a greater indicator of growth than is weight. Weight gain in the first few weeks is about 1 oz/day (or about half a pound per week). Infants generally double their birth weight by 5 months, triple their birth weight by 1 year of age, and quadruple their birth weight by 2 years (Baker, 2016). Growth charts for tracking an infant's weight, length, and head circumference can be downloaded from the Centers for Disease Control and Prevention (CDC) website.

Choice of Feeding: Breast Versus Formula

Feeding their newborn is an exciting, satisfying, but often worrisome task for parents. Meeting this essential need of their new child helps parents strengthen their attachment to their child and fosters their self-images as nurturers and providers, yet carries great responsibility. Whether a woman chooses to breastfeed or formula-feed, she can adequately meet her newborn's needs. As questions about feeding arise, the nurse works with the woman to help her develop skill in her chosen method. In

---

EVIDENCE-BASED PRACTICE | Increasing Breastfeeding Rates

Clinical Question
Is telephone consultation effective in increasing breastfeeding rates, especially among low-income and underserved mothers?

The Evidence
Despite widespread evidence about the benefits of breastfeeding for both mother and baby, breastfeeding rates remain relatively low. National data show that less than half of babies born in the United States are fed any breast milk at 6 months of age and only 16% of babies at this age are exclusively breastfed. Babies who are breastfed have stronger immune systems, lower risk of allergies, fewer dental caries, and reduced incidence of sudden infant death syndrome. Support for breastfeeding is an important perinatal effort. This researcher undertook a systematic review of the literature to determine evidence-based strategies for enhancing breastfeeding that could be delivered efficiently and with low cost via telephone consultation. The studies reviewed included samples of more than 500 mothers. This type of structured review of randomized trials forms the strongest evidence for practice.

An effective strategy for low-income and underserved mothers used scheduled telephone support provided by lactation consultants. Weekly telephone consultation for the first 3 postnatal months was effective in increasing breastfeeding rates and

duration (Flannery, 2014). Monthly telephone consultation from 3 to 6 months was effective in sustaining the effect. The types of telephone consultation that were most effective were anticipatory guidance, education, and empowerment. The review also reported that the use of a lactation consultant was desirable but not imperative; peer counseling and support was effective in encouraging mothers to breastfeed for a longer duration. Services provided by either group increased breastfeeding rates by 27% to 34%. Women in these studies reported that the credentials of the counselors were not as important as their approach; mothers wanted counseling from someone they trusted, who entered into a dialogue rather than a lecture, and who offered information that was not confusing or conflicting. The advantage of telephone consultation was the lack of geographic boundaries; one of the studies in the review focused exclusively on rural mothers and found the effects were similar to those women who had access to urban services.

Best Practice
Telephone consultation that involves supportive communication, an authentic dialogue, and accurate information provided routinely during the postnatal period can increase the rate and duration of breastfeeding. This type of consultation is effective for low-income and rural mothers as well as those in urban areas.

every interaction, it is the nurse's responsibility to support the parents and promote the family's sense of confidence.

The mother usually decides to breastfeed or formula-feed by the 6th month of pregnancy and often even before conception. However, she may not make her final decision until admission to the birth center. The decision is often influenced by relatives, especially the baby's father and maternal grandmother (Janke, 2014), by friends, and by social customs rather than being based on knowledge about the nutritional and psychologic needs of the mother and her newborn.

Once the parents have made an informed choice of feeding method, the nurse's primary responsibilities are to support the family's decision and to help the family achieve a positive result. No woman should be made to feel either inadequate or superior because of her choice in feeding. There are advantages and disadvantages to breastfeeding and bottle-feeding, but positive bonds in parent–child relationships can be developed with either method.

Breastfeeding

Breast Milk Production

The female breast is divided into 15 to 20 lobes, separated from one another by fat and connective tissue, and interspersed with blood vessels, lymphatic vessels, and nerves. These lobes are subdivided into connected lobules composed of small units called *alveoli* where milk is synthesized by the alveolar secretory epithelium. The lobules have a system of lactiferous ducts that join larger ducts and eventually open onto the nipple surface. Mothers are often surprised to see milk coming out of multiple nipple pores when they express their milk. See Figure 25–10 to view the anatomy of the breast.

Health Promotion *Healthy People 2020* **Objectives for Exclusive Breastfeeding**

The goals of the *Healthy People 2020* national health promotion and disease prevention program state that at least 82% of all mothers will initiate breastfeeding, at least 61% will continue to breastfeed until their infants are 6 months old, and at least 34% will continue to breastfeed until their infants are 12 months old. The *Healthy People 2020* objective for exclusive breastfeeding at 3 months is 46%; the current rate is 33.6%. The *Healthy People 2020* objective for exclusive breastfeeding at 6 months is 26%; the current rate is 14.1% (U.S. Breastfeeding Committee, 2011). It is the healthcare provider's responsibility to provide the parents with accurate information about the distinct advantages of breastfeeding to the mother and baby.

Physiologic and Endocrine Control of Lactogenesis

During pregnancy, increased levels of estrogen stimulate breast duct proliferation and development, and elevated progesterone levels promote the development of lobules and alveoli in preparation for lactation. Prolactin levels rise from approximately 10 ng/mL prepregnancy to 200 ng/mL at term. However, lactation is suppressed during pregnancy by elevated progesterone levels secreted by the placenta. Once the placenta is expelled at birth, progesterone levels fall and the inhibition is removed, triggering milk production. This occurs whether the mother has breast stimulation or not. However, if by the third or fourth day breast stimulation is not occurring, prolactin levels begin to drop.

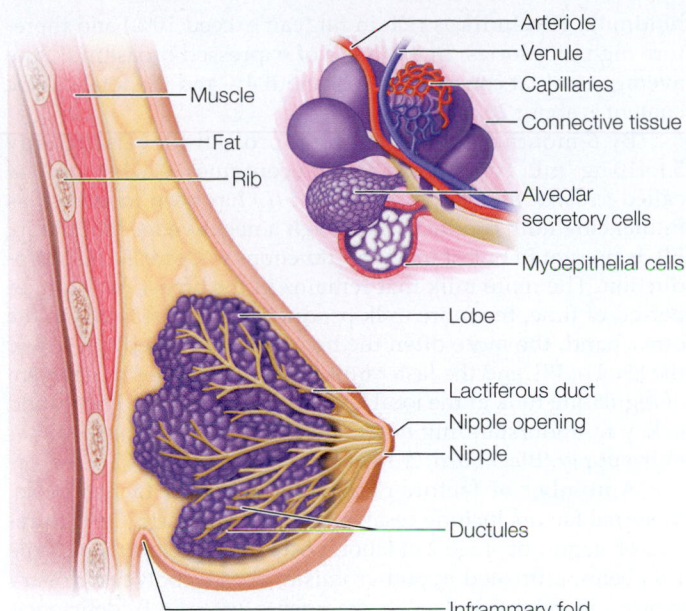

Figure 25–10 Anatomy of the breast.

Initially, lactation is under endocrine control. The hormone **prolactin** is released from the anterior pituitary in response to breast stimulation from suckling or the use of a breast pump. Prolactin levels double each time the baby suckles at the breast, regardless of the age of the baby or duration of lactation. Prolactin stimulates the milk-secreting cells in the alveoli to produce milk, then rapidly drops back to baseline. If more than approximately 3 hours occur between stimulation, prolactin levels begin to drop below baseline. To reverse the overall decline in prolactin level, the mother can be encouraged to stimulate her breasts more frequently (e.g., every 1.5 to 2 hours). Mothers should be strongly encouraged to stimulate their breasts frequently if their babies are not effective feeders or if they are separated from their babies. Prolactin receptors are established during the first 2 weeks postpartum in response to frequency of breast stimulation (Walker, 2016). Inadequate development of prolactin receptors during this time is likely to negatively impact the mother's long-term milk volume. By 2 weeks (14 days) postpartum, prolactin levels will be back to prepregnancy levels and milk production will cease if stimulation of the breasts by breastfeeding or pumping does not occur (Walker, 2016).

The milk that flows from the breast at the start of a feeding or pumping session is called **foremilk**. The foremilk is watery milk high in protein and lactose and low in fat (1% to 2%). This milk has trickled down from the alveoli between feedings to fill the lactiferous ducts. It is low-fat milk because the fat globules made in the alveoli stick to each other and to the walls of the alveoli and do not trickle down.

In addition to prolactin release, stretching of the nipple and compression of the areola signal the hypothalamus to trigger the posterior pituitary gland to release oxytocin.

Oxytocin acts on the myoepithelial cells surrounding the alveoli in the breast tissue to contract, ejecting milk, including the fat globules present, into the ducts. This process is called the *milk ejection reflex*, better known in lay terms as the **let-down reflex** or *let-down response*. The average initial let-down response occurs about 2 minutes after a baby begins to suckle, and there will be 4 to 10 let-down responses during a feeding session. The milk that flows during let-down is called

Labels for Figure 25–10:
Arteriole
Venule
Capillaries
Connective tissue
Muscle
Fat
Rib
Alveolar secretory cells
Myoepithelial cells
Lobe
Lactiferous duct
Nipple opening
Nipple
Ductules
Inframmary fold

hindmilk. **Hindmilk** is rich in fat (can exceed 10%) and therefore high in calories. In a sample of expressed breast milk, the average total fat concentration is about 4% and the total caloric content is about 20 calories/ounce.

By 6 months of breastfeeding, prolactin levels are only 5 to 10 ng/mL, yet milk production continues. A whey protein called *feedback inhibitor of lactation (FIL)* has been identified as influencing milk production through a negative feedback loop. FIL is present in breast milk and functions to decrease milk production. The more milk that remains in the breast for a longer period of time, the more milk production is decreased. On the other hand, the more often the breasts are emptied, the lower the level of FIL and the faster milk is produced. This mechanism of regulating milk at the local level is called *autocrine control* and is key to understanding how a mother maintains or loses her milk supply (Blackburn, 2013).

A number of factors can delay or impair lactogenesis. Maternal factors include cesarean birth, primiparity, long duration of stage 1 or stage 2 of labor, postpartum hemorrhage, type 1 diabetes, untreated hypothyroidism, obesity, polycystic ovary syndrome, retained placenta fragments, vitamin B_6 deficiency, history of previous breast surgery, insufficient glandular breast tissue, and significant stress (Janke, 2014; Morrison & Wambach, 2016). Other factors that can interfere with breastfeeding include smoking and use of alcohol, as well as some prescription and over-the-counter medications (e.g., antihistamines, combined birth control pills). One of the most important factors that influences breast milk production and the success of breastfeeding is the regular emptying of the breast. Therefore, mothers who opt to give their baby a bottle—and who do not pump to replace the feeding—are putting breastfeeding success in jeopardy.

STAGES OF HUMAN MILK

During the establishment of lactation there are three stages of human milk: colostrum, transitional milk, and mature milk.

Colostrum is the initial milk that begins to be secreted during midpregnancy and is immediately available to the baby at birth. The volume of colostrum is small, and this encourages the newborn to nurse frequently, helping to stimulate milk production. No supplementation with other fluids is necessary unless there is a medical indication. Colostrum is a thick, creamy yellowish fluid with concentrated amounts of protein, fat-soluble vitamins, and minerals, and it has lower amounts of fat and lactose compared with mature milk. It also contains antioxidants and high levels of lactoferrin and secretory IgA. It promotes the establishment of *Lactobacillus bifidus* flora in the digestive tract, which helps to protect the newborn from disease and illness. Colostrum also has a laxative effect on the newborn, which helps the baby pass meconium stools, which in turn helps decrease hyperbilirubinemia.

The onset of copious milk secretion begins between 32 and 96 hours postpartum. For most women this is observed on day 3. Laypeople refer to this as the milk "coming in," and it is called **transitional milk**. Transitional milk has qualities intermediate to colostrum and mature milk but may look indistinguishable from colostrum. It is still light yellow in color but is more copious than colostrum and contains more fat, lactose, water-soluble vitamins, and calories. See Figure 25–11 to view a picture of transitional milk. By day 5, most mothers are producing about 16 oz/day (Riordan, 2016).

Mature milk is white or slightly blue-tinged in color. It is present by 2 weeks postpartum and continues thereafter until lactation ceases. Mature milk contains about 13% solids (carbohydrates, proteins, and fats) and 87% water. Although mature human milk appears similar to skim cow's milk and

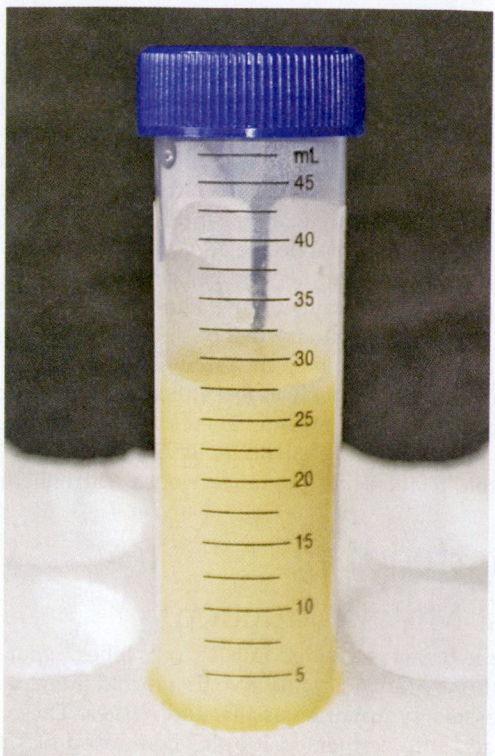

Figure 25–11 Transitional human milk.
SOURCE: Brigitte Hall, RNC, MSN, IBCLC.

may cause mothers to question whether their milk is "rich enough," mothers should be reassured that this is the normal appearance of mature human milk and that it provides the baby with all the necessary nutrients. Although gradual changes in composition do occur continuously over periods of weeks to accommodate the needs of the growing newborn, in general the composition of mature milk is fairly consistent with the exception of the fat content as noted previously. Milk production continues to increase slowly over the first month. By 6 months postpartum a mother produces about 27 oz (800 mL) per day (Blackburn, 2013).

Advantages of Breast Milk

In their breastfeeding policy statement, the American Academy of Pediatrics recommends exclusive breastfeeding as the preferred feeding for all newborns/infants, with a few exceptions, for the first 6 months and continued breastfeeding during the introduction of solids until the infant is 12 months old or older, as desired (AAP, 2012b). There is overwhelming scientific evidence that shows that breastfeeding provides newborns and infants with specific nutritional, immunologic, and psychosocial advantages over formula-feeding (AAP & ACOG, 2012b).

NUTRITIONAL ADVANTAGES

Human milk provides optimum nutrition for the human baby because it is species specific. The macronutrients such as protein, fat, and carbohydrates (lactose) are synthesized by the mother in the alveoli of the breasts by specialized secretory cells. Micronutrient elements such as vitamins and minerals derive from the circulating maternal plasma. There are more than 200 distinct components in breast milk, with more remaining to be identified (Riordan, 2016).

Additional health advantages for breastfed babies include reduced risk of developing type 1 or type 2 diabetes mellitus, lymphoma, leukemia, Hodgkin disease, obesity, hypercholesterolemia, and asthma. There are health benefits to the breastfeeding mother as well; when breastfeeding is initiated immediately after delivery, there is decreased risk for postpartum bleeding and more rapid uterine involution. Research has also shown that breastfeeding offers a protective function against premenopausal breast cancer and ovarian cancer and may be associated with a decrease in type 2 diabetes, rheumatoid arthritis, and hypertension (Healthy Children, 2015a).

IMMUNOLOGIC ADVANTAGES

The immunologic advantages of breast milk include varying degrees of protection from respiratory tract and gastrointestinal tract infections, necrotizing enterocolitis, urinary tract infections, otitis media, bacterial meningitis, bacteremia, and allergies (Healthy Children, 2015b). Transplacental passage of maternal immunoglobulin gradually diminishes over the first 6 months of life until the infant can begin to produce his or her own immunoglobulins. Human milk-derived immunologic protection helps supplement this protection.

Secretory IgA, an immunoglobulin present in colostrum and breast milk, has antiviral, antibacterial, and antigenic-inhibiting properties, specifically across mucosal surfaces such as the intestinal tract. Secretory IgA plays a role in decreasing the permeability of the small intestine to help prevent large protein molecules from triggering an allergic response. Other constituents of colostrum and breast milk that act to inhibit the growth of bacteria or viruses are *Lactobacillus bifidus*, lysozymes, lactoperoxidase, lactoferrin, transferrin, and various immunoglobulins.

All babies should receive vaccination following a schedule as recommended by the Centers for Disease Control and Prevention (CDC) (CDC, 2015b). The current vaccination schedule can be viewed online at the CDC website for Breastfeeding Resources (CDC, 2015b). Mothers may worry that their antibodies will inactivate the live poliovirus. But breastfeeding does not adversely affect immunization and is not a contraindication for any vaccine. Some mothers also wonder if it is safe for them to receive vaccinations while they are breastfeeding. Mothers should be reassured that most vaccines can safely be taken during the lactation period (Sachs & AAP Committee on Drugs, 2013).

PSYCHOSOCIAL BENEFITS OF BREASTFEEDING

The psychosocial advantages of breastfeeding include increased self-esteem, enhanced bonding, and a decrease in stress for the mother and baby.

A mother's self-esteem is increased in knowing that she has provided the perfect food for her baby and provided protection with her own antibodies. For many mothers breastfeeding takes effort, understanding, and an emotional commitment to endure the demands of this lifestyle choice. The mother's sense of accomplishment in being able to satisfy her baby's needs for nourishment and comfort can be a tremendous source of personal satisfaction. Also breastfeeding can provide the baby with a fresh, clean, naturally warm source of nutrition. Women who breastfeed, by its nature, have close contact with their babies. Newborns are very responsive to touch, and it is vital for the baby's emotional well-being. The tactile stimulation associated with breastfeeding can communicate warmth, closeness, comfort, and the opportunity to learn each other's behavioral cues and needs. From the release of prolactin and oxytocin while breastfeeding, mothers may feel more affectionate toward their newborns, have improved let-down response, and breastfeed more frequently and for longer periods of time (Healthy Children, 2015a). See Table 25–1 for a comparison of breastfeeding and formula-feeding.

POTENTIAL DISADVANTAGES TO BREASTFEEDING

The following is a list of sometimes cited potential disadvantages to breastfeeding:

- *Pain with breastfeeding.* Breastfeeding is a natural process but requires a certain knowledge base that formerly was passed along from generation to generation. With the decline in the extended family structure, this source of knowledge and assistance is often missing for the new mother. Nipple tenderness is the most common source of discomfort and is usually related to improper positioning and/or not obtaining a proper attachment of the baby on the breast. Pain can also be related to engorgement or infection. Breastfeeding with proper technique should not hurt and these mothers should be encouraged to seek assistance from a knowledgeable person skilled in lactation.

- *Leaking milk.* Some women will leak milk when their breasts are full and it is nearly time to breastfeed again or whenever they experience letdown, which can be triggered by hearing, seeing, or even thinking of their baby. If this causes concern to the mother, she can be instructed on how to apply gentle pressure directly over her nipple for a minute or so to stop the leaking momentarily. The mother can wear nursing pads inside her bra (with instructions to change wet pads frequently). Mothers should be given reassurance that this problem diminishes over time.

- *Embarrassment.* Some mothers feel uncomfortable about breastfeeding because they are modest or may feel embarrassed because our society views breasts as sexual objects and/or an unfriendly social environment makes it difficult to breastfeed in public. This is not an easy issue to overcome. Some mothers will feel more confident after learning how to breastfeed discreetly while in public.

- *Stress.* Many mothers feel a lot of stress juggling work or school and the demands of home life. Some mothers cite this reason for wanting to wean. There are options to suggest for this concern. Mothers can learn about "double pumping" to save time. A double electric breast pump allows the mother to pump both breasts simultaneously, which cuts the pumping time in half. If a mother struggles to keep up her milk supply, she can try taking an herbal supplement to give her milk supply a boost, unless contraindicated for her. Finally, it is still preferable to decrease the frequency of pumping rather than quitting altogether, if that makes things more manageable for the mother. Babies who get some breast milk are still receiving more of the benefits of breast milk than babies who do not receive any breast milk.

- *Unequal feeding responsibilities/fathers or partners left out.* Some parents want feedings to be a shared responsibility.

Healthy People 2020

(MICH-21) Increase the proportion of infants who are ever breastfed

TABLE 25–1 Comparison of Breastfeeding and Formula-Feeding

BREASTFEEDING	FORMULA (IRON-ENRICHED)-FEEDING
NUTRITION	
Species specific. An ideal balance of nutrients, efficiently absorbed. High bioavailability of iron leaves less iron for bacterial growth, cell injury.	Derived from bovine milk and/or plant sources. Lower bioavailability of nutrients requires higher concentrations in milk. Additives may cause intolerance.
Higher levels of essential fatty acids, lactose, cystine, and cholesterol, necessary for brain and nerve growth.	Still missing numerous ingredients. Formulas do not contain cholesterol. Soy and hydrolysate formulas do not contain lactose. Docosahexaenoic (DHA) and arachidonic (ARA) now added.
Composition varies according to gestational age and stage of lactation, meeting changing nutritional needs.	Nutritional value not varied. Nutritional adequacy depends on proper preparation/dilution.
Long-term decreased incidence of diabetes, cancer, obesity, asthma.	
Contains unsaturated fats.	Contains saturated fats.
Babies determine the volume of milk consumed.	Parents or healthcare provider determine the volume consumed. Overfeeding may occur if caregiver is determined that baby empty bottle.
Frequency of feeding is determined by cues from the baby. May feed more frequently as milk digestion is faster.	Frequency of feeding is determined by cues from the baby. May feed less frequently as milk digestion is slower.
IMMUNOLOGIC PROPERTIES	
Contains immunoglobulins, enzymes, and leukocytes that protect against pathogens. Nutrients promote growth of *Lactobacillus*, protective bacteria. Lower rates of urinary tract infections, otitis media, and other infectious diseases.	No anti-infective properties. Formula is linked to an increased incidence of gastrointestinal and respiratory tract infections.
Anti-infective properties present in the milk permit longer storage duration.	Potential for bacterial contamination exists during preparation and storage.
Breast milk is hypoallergenic, with minimal risk of protein allergy/intolerance.	Cow's milk protein allergy relatively common.
MATERNAL HEALTH	
Faster return to prepregnancy weight.	Provides nutrition when breast milk not available because of maternal illness, medication/drug use, or lactation failure (breast surgery, endocrine disease) or if not chosen as a feeding choice.
Breastfeeding associated with lower risk of breast, ovarian cancer.	
PSYCHOSOCIAL ASPECTS	
Skin-to-skin contact enhances bonding.	Both parents can participate in positive parent–baby interaction during feeding.
Hormones of lactation promote maternal feelings and sense of well-being.	Father/partner can assume feeding responsibilities. Mothers can receive more rest in the beginning because others can assume feeding responsibilities.
The value system of modern society can create barriers to successful breastfeeding.	
Some mothers may feel ashamed or embarrassed.	
Breastfeeding after returning to work may be difficult.	
COST	
Healthy diet for mother.	Hypoallergenic formula is more expensive than standard formula. Cost approximately $1400/year.
Savings for infant medical costs: approximately $400 average in first year of life.	
Ancillary costs: nursing pads, nursing bras.	Ancillary costs: bottles or bottle liners, nipples, cleaning costs.
A breast pump may be needed.	
Refrigeration is necessary for storing expressed milk.	Refrigeration is needed if preparing more than one bottle at a time.
CONVENIENCE	
Milk is always the perfect temperature. No preparation time is needed.	Formula must be purchased commercially. Preparation is time consuming. Less convenient for traveling or for night feedings.
The mother must be available to feed or will need to provide expressed milk to be given in her absence.	Mother need not be present—anyone can feed the baby.
If she misses a feeding, the mother must express milk to maintain lactation.	
The mother may experience slight discomfort in the early days of lactation.	

The parents should be informed that it is advisable for the father/partner to wait to bottle-feed the baby with expressed breast milk until after the milk supply and breastfeeding are established, generally when their baby is about 3 to 4 weeks old. In the meantime, the father/partner can be encouraged to be supportive of the breastfeeding mother, to have a lot of skin-to-skin contact with the baby, and to share the responsibilities of all other aspects of baby care (e.g., bathing, dressing, diapering, burping, rocking).

- *Diet restriction.* Some mothers think that they have to give up eating certain foods when they breastfeed. This is generally not true. Most mothers can still eat all the foods they are accustomed to eating. Mothers do need to restrict alcohol intake and keep caffeine to a minimum. In the uncommon case where a baby has intolerance or allergy symptoms, the mother should consult with a lactation consultant or the baby's healthcare provider to help her work through this complication.

- *Limited hormonal birth control options.* Some mothers think that they cannot use a hormonal method of birth control while breastfeeding. Mothers should be informed that using birth control pills containing progesterone and estrogen can cause a decrease in milk volume and may affect the quality of breast milk. It is preferred that the mother who wants to use a hormonal birth control method consider using the progestin-only pill (e.g., Micronor, Nor-QD, Aygestin, or Norlutate); receive Depo-Provera, a progestin-only injection administered every 90 days; or have a progestin-only implant. Although progestin-only hormonal birth control is compatible with lactation, it is recommended that the mother wait 6 weeks before taking the hormonal medication to ensure a good milk supply (AAP, 2012b). Mothers can be reassured that barrier methods of birth control and natural family planning do not interfere with lactation at all and are good options to consider as well.

- *Vaginal dryness associated with breastfeeding.* Some mothers experience vaginal dryness related to a low level of estrogen while lactating. This is only a temporary side effect. A water-based lubricant such as K-Y jelly or Astroglide can be used during intercourse until the woman weans and estrogen levels increase again.

MEDICATIONS

Mothers can be reassured that most prescription and over-the-counter medications are safe for the breastfeeding baby. Medications taken by the breastfeeding mother may penetrate human milk to some degree. This is the primary reason that mothers cite for discontinuing breastfeeding. Having a basic understanding of the kinetics of drug entry into human milk, as well as factors influencing its availability to the baby (bioavailability), may help the nursing mother to continue safely breastfeeding her baby.

It should be noted that (1) most drugs penetrate into human milk, (2) almost all medications appear in only small amounts in human milk (usually less than 1% of the maternal dosage), and (3) very few drugs are contraindicated for breastfeeding women (Briggs & Freeman, 2015; Hale, 2014; Sachs & AAP Committee on Drugs, 2013).

The healthcare provider should consider the following when prescribing a medication (Sachs & AAP Committee on Drugs, 2013):

- Mother's need for the medication
- Drug's potential effect on milk production

- Amount of drug excreted into the milk
- Extent of oral absorption of the drug by the baby
- Drug's potential adverse effects to the baby
- Baby's age and health

The properties of a drug influence its passage into breast milk, as does the amount of the drug taken, the frequency and route of administration, and the timing of the dose in relationship to infant feeding. The drug's effects are influenced by the baby's age, the feeding frequency, the volume of milk taken, and the degree of absorption through the gastrointestinal tract. LactMed is a database that has current data on individual medications.

SAFETY ALERT!

The mother should be advised to inform her healthcare provider and her baby's healthcare provider that she is breastfeeding when a drug is prescribed for her.

Five adjustments should be made when administering drugs to a nursing mother to decrease the effects of the medication on the baby (Blackburn, 2013):

1. Avoid long-acting forms of drugs. The baby may have difficulty metabolizing and excreting them, and accumulation may be a problem.

2. Consider absorption rates and peak blood levels in scheduling the administration of the drugs. Less of the drug crosses into the milk if the baby is fed before the mother is given the oral medication.

3. Use preparations that can be given at longer intervals (once versus three to four times per day).

4. Select the drug that shows the least tendency to pass into breast milk when alternatives are available.

5. Use single-symptom drugs versus multisymptom drugs (e.g., a decongestant for allergy rather than a multisymptom drug, especially because liquid forms may contain alcohol).

CONTRAINDICATIONS

In some instances breastfeeding is or may be contraindicated:

- Mother is HIV positive or has AIDS and is counseled against breastfeeding, except in countries where the risk of neonatal death from diarrhea and other disease (excluding AIDS) is high (Janke, 2014; Morrison & Wambach, 2016).

- Mother has active, untreated tuberculosis, has varicella, is HTLV1-positive (human T-cell leukemia virus type 1), or has another illness, on a case-by-case basis.

- Mother has active herpes on her breast—the baby may still feed on the unaffected side only until the lesion has healed.

- Mother uses illicit drugs (e.g., cocaine, heroin) or is an alcoholic; however, AAP (2012b) allows breastfeeding when the mother is taking methadone as part of a drug withdrawal program.

- Mother smokes, posing health risks to herself and potential secondhand exposure risks to her baby. Research shows that smoking by breastfeeding mothers can significantly alter the sleep–wake cycles of babies, causing them to sleep less, and also affects milk flavor. The fat content of a smoker's breast milk is lower than that of nonsmokers; the fat content is essential for newborn/infant growth (Morrison & Wambach, 2016). Maternal smoking can result in breast milk concentrations of nicotine of 1.5 to 3 times the maternal plasma concentration. However, babies who receive breast milk from mothers who smoke are healthier than babies who receive formula and live in a household with smokers. Mothers who smoke cigarettes can breastfeed. To minimize effects on the baby, mothers should time their smoking to immediately *after* breastfeeding and should not smoke in the same room the baby is in (AAP & ACOG, 2012). Smoking has been associated with an increase in respiratory infections and allergies as well as being a considerable risk factor for low milk supply and poor weight gain in the newborn/infant (AAP, 2012b; Morrison & Wambach, 2016). Mothers who smoke are also at greater risk for breast abscess and breast periductal inflammation (Morrison & Wambach, 2016).

- Mother takes specific medications (e.g., radioactive isotopes, antimetabolites chemotherapy drugs). A mother with a diagnosis of breast cancer should not breastfeed so that she can begin treatment immediately (Janke, 2014).

- Baby has galactosemia.

POTENTIAL PROBLEMS IN BREASTFEEDING

Because mothers are discharged from the birthing unit before breastfeeding is well established, they are frequently alone when they encounter changes in the breastfeeding process. Many women stop nursing if the situations they encounter seem to pose problems. Nurses can offer anticipatory guidance regarding common breastfeeding phenomena and provide resources such as seeking help from a lactation specialist and contact information for lactation support groups for the woman's use after discharge. (See Chapter 29 for a detailed discussion of self-care measures the nurse can suggest to a woman with a breastfeeding problem after discharge from the birthing unit.)

Timing of Newborn Feedings

The timing of newborn feedings is ideally determined by physiologic and behavioral cues rather than a set schedule.

INITIATING THE FIRST FEEDING

If there are no complications at the birth and the mother is not overly sedated, the baby may be placed on the mother's chest after birth. This skin-to-skin contact after birth helps the baby maintain body temperature, helps with self-regulation, increases maternal oxytocin levels, helps the mother to notice subtle feeding cues, and promotes bonding (Figure 25–12).

The nurse should assess for active bowel sounds, absence of abdominal distention, and a lusty cry that quiets and is replaced with rooting and sucking behaviors when a stimulus is placed near the lips. These signs indicate that the newborn is hungry and physically ready to tolerate the initial feeding.

Throughout the first 2 hours after birth, but especially during the first hour of life, the baby is usually alert and ready to breastfeed. This first feeding should not be forced. Some babies are content just licking the nipple or nuzzling up against the breast initially. Early breastfeeding can enhance maternal–newborn bonding and facilitate release of oxytocin, which helps contract the uterus, expelling the placenta and decreasing the risk of postpartum hemorrhage. For the newborn it provides the

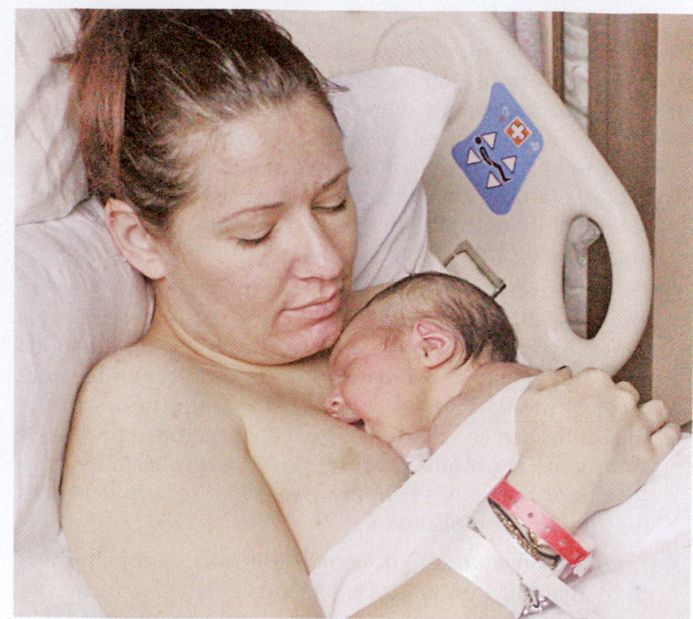

Figure 25–12 **Mother and newborn skin-to-skin.**
SOURCE: Brigitte Hall, RNC, MSN, IBCLC.

immunologic protection of colostrum; it also begins to stimulate further maternal milk production, helping prevent later feeding difficulties. Mothers who choose to breastfeed their newborns should be encouraged to put the baby to the breast during the first period of reactivity. This practice should be encouraged because successful, long-term breastfeeding during infancy appears to be related to beginning breast feedings in the first few hours of life. Sleep–wake states affect feeding behavior and need to be considered when evaluating the newborn's sucking ability.

If the mother plans to bottle-feed, she and her newborn can still enjoy skin-to-skin contact initially. Formula-feedings are not typically initiated in the birthing room. Bottle-fed newborns are offered formula as soon as they show an interest or feeding cues, or per agency policy. For both breastfed and formula-fed babies, early feeding enhances maternal–newborn attachment; stimulates peristalsis, which helps to eliminate the by-products of bilirubin conjugation, thus decreasing the risk of jaundice; helps prevent hypoglycemia; and promotes the passage of meconium.

Assessment of the newborn's physiologic status is a primary and ongoing concern to the nurse throughout the first feeding. Extreme fatigue coupled with tachypnea, dusky color, and diaphoresis while feeding is most likely symptomatic for respiratory and/or cardiac problems or, rarely, esophageal anomalies (see Chapter 26). Findings associated with esophageal anomalies include maternal polyhydramnios and increased oral mucus in the baby.

Although the nurse is always on the alert for any complications, keep in mind that it is not unusual for healthy newborns to regurgitate a small amount of mucus, fluid, or milk shortly after feeding, or to develop hiccups. Most babies have "wet burps" at some point and virtually all have some degree of reflux. Holding the baby upright on the parent's chest for 15 to 20 minutes after a feeding and not placing the baby in a car seat or swing (which increases abdominal pressure) for that time can help decrease the incidence of reflux. Once the newborn is tolerating feeding, the baby's normal position after feeding should be on the back.

ESTABLISHING A FEEDING PATTERN

An "on-demand" feeding program facilitates each baby's own rhythm and helps a new mother establish lactation. Unrestricted feedings are best accomplished by hospitals that provide mother–baby rooming-in practices on a 24-hour basis. When the father/partner is able to room in with the mother and new baby, it allows both parents to participate and learn how to care for their baby; this has been shown to be important in the development of the family relationship. Having the father/partner room in also allows the mother with a cesarean delivery to keep her baby at the bedside. When mothers and babies are not separated after birth, parents are better able to respond to their babies' needs more quickly than the nursery staff may be able to, resulting in less newborn crying, natural feeding intervals, and an adequate number of feedings in a 24-hour period.

Following the initial alert period (approximately the first 2 hours after birth), the newborn typically falls into a deep sleep for several hours. Mothers should be encouraged to rest during this time too. Upon awakening, the newborn will likely want to nurse frequently, alternating between relatively short periods of light sleep and quiet wakefulness. As wakefulness and interest in nursing increase, the baby will often cluster 5 to 10 feeding episodes over 2 to 3 hours (Riordan, 2016). The mother may misinterpret "cluster feedings" in the first few days of life to mean that her newborn is not satisfied because she is not producing enough milk. The nurse should take this opportunity to reinforce the mother's perception that the baby wants additional milk, but point out that cluster feeding is a normal and necessary pattern to stimulate the mother's milk production. Formula supplementation is not indicated and will actually delay milk production.

Some healthy newborns are uninterested in nursing and just want to sleep for the first few days after birth. This pattern is noted in babies whose mothers have had a difficult labor, a prolonged pushing stage during delivery, or medication (especially multiple dosing) for labor pain or for a cesarean birth.

Late-preterm newborns (babies born between 34 0/7 and 36 6/7 weeks' gestation) also tend to be very sleepy for the first few days, much more so than full-term newborns (Spong, 2013). In addition, newborn boys who have undergone a circumcision procedure often become very sleepy after surgery. These sleepy babies are at risk of losing an excessive amount of weight, becoming dehydrated, and developing exaggerated jaundice in just a few days after birth. In addition, the mother may develop pathologic engorgement if her baby does not wake up to breastfeed frequently and effectively during this time.

To avoid these complications, parents can be taught techniques to wake their sleepy baby whenever the newborn shows signs of being in the light state-of-sleep cycle. With a little help, the baby may be gently aroused to breastfeed. One method is to remove the blanket and clothing so that the baby is wearing only a diaper and T-shirt. Babies feed better when they are not bundled, and they can actually achieve a better attachment without the bulk of extra clothing and blankets in the way. If the room is too cool for the newborn to feed in just a diaper and T-shirt, have the mother apply a blanket over the top of her baby *after* the baby has attached to the breast. Another technique is to undo and check the baby's diaper. Sitting the baby in a burping position and gently "walking" fingers along the back will usually arouse the baby. Parents should also be encouraged to talk or sing to their baby while trying these techniques to further arouse their baby from sleep.

If the newborn falls asleep after the first few suckles, encourage the mother to use tactile stimulation while the newborn is still attached to the breast. The mother can also be encouraged to use breast compression or breast massage while the baby is breastfeeding to keep milk trickling into the baby's mouth until the breast is stimulated to release the milk. If this is not sufficient to keep the baby actively feeding, suggest that the mother remove the baby from the breast momentarily and try to burp the baby. The newborn may not actually burp but the burping technique may help wake the baby.

Clinical Tip

With a sleepy baby, remove the blanket, encourage lots of skin-to-skin contact between mother and baby, and have the mother rest with her baby near her breast so that the baby can feel and smell the breast. Encourage the mother to watch for feeding cues, such as hand-to-mouth activity, fluttering eyelids, vocalization (but not necessarily crying), and mouthing activities.

A newborn's feeding pattern may change again when the mother's breasts become fuller. Mothers' breasts begin to look and feel noticeably heavier between the second and the fourth day postpartum. When milk production has noticeably increased, the "cluster feeding" pattern ceases until the newborn has the first growth spurt at about 2 weeks of age. Now a newborn generally feeds every 1.5 to 3 hours around the clock, about 8 to 12 feedings per day. Feeding intervals are counted from the time of the start of one feeding to the start of the next feeding. During this engorgement phase of lactation some babies may struggle initially with latch-on, especially if the mother allows greater than 3 hours to lapse between feedings. If the newborn is not breastfeeding often or effectively enough to soften the breasts, then the breasts may become quite firm and the mother's nipple may become less pliable; this can lead to a shallow latch attachment and sore nipples. If this occurs, the mother can try to express some milk to soften her areola before latching her baby. When her baby breastfeeds on this fuller-than-usual breast, it is not uncommon for the baby to want to feed only on just the one side. This feeding pattern usually does not last long either. Within days the baby will be back to feeding at both breasts again.

Formula-fed newborns generally sleep longer at a stretch and awaken to feed every 3 to 4 hours, typically feeding only 6 to 8 times per day. To compensate for sleeping longer between feedings, formula-fed babies feed a larger volume at each feeding.

Regardless of whether a mother is breastfeeding or formula-feeding her newborn, many parents are distressed by their baby's erratic feeding pattern. Parents need to be informed about normal newborn/infant feeding and sleeping patterns and be aware that these patterns vary among babies and change over days, weeks, and months according to the baby's growth and development. In the beginning, the "average" newborn sleeps a total of 16 hours a day. Newborns wake to feed and generally fall back to sleep within an hour.

Satiety behaviors are the same for formula-fed babies as for breastfed babies. These behaviors include longer pauses toward the end of the feeding and noticeable total body relaxation (the baby lies limp with hands down at the side and unclenched). The baby may also release the mother's nipple or the bottle nipple, and may fall asleep. If a baby is satiated and content following feedings, is meeting daily output expectations, and is gaining weight as expected, then feedings are going well.

On the other hand, if a breastfeeding baby awakens shortly after feeding and is exhibiting feeding cues, this baby should be offered the breast again regardless of when the last feeding occurred. The newborn may be cluster feeding or may not have fed efficiently at the previous feeding. Pacifier use in response to this early waking is especially inappropriate. The pacifier needlessly postpones the feeding, which is indicated based on hunger cues and can have a negative consequence for the mother's milk supply and the baby's weight. The American Academy of Pediatrics recommends waiting to introduce a pacifier in the breastfeeding newborn until breastfeeding is well established: generally when the baby is 3 to 4 weeks old. A formula-feeding baby can be offered a pacifier any time after birth, which is thought to help reduce the risk for sudden infant death syndrome (SIDS) (Healthy Children, 2015e).

Both breastfed and formula-fed newborns experience growth spurts at certain times and require increased feeding. The breastfeeding mother may meet these increased demands by nursing more frequently to increase her milk supply. It takes about 72 hours for the milk supply to increase adequately to meet the new demand. A slight increase in feedings meets the formula-fed baby's needs. Once the formula-feeding baby appears satiated, the baby should not be forced to continue to feed in order to the finish the bottle.

SAFETY ALERT!

Parents should be instructed never to put honey or corn syrup on their baby's pacifier to encourage the baby to accept it. Honey and possibly corn syrup may be contaminated with *Clostridium botulinum*, a bacterium that causes infantile botulism. Botulism is rare, but when it occurs it causes serious illness.

Nourishing her newborn is a major concern of the new mother. Her feelings of success or failure may influence her self-concept as she assumes her maternal role. With proper instruction, support, and encouragement from professionals, breastfeeding becomes a source of pleasure and satisfaction to both the mother and the baby.

Cultural Considerations in Newborn Feeding

Healthcare professionals can learn about an individual client's cultural background by engaging in discussions with the client and asking questions in a sensitive and respectful way. This provides opportunity to validate healthy practices and to exert a positive influence on other matters (Callister, 2014). An occasion for this kind of dialogue might arise during interactions with a new mother who may have misconceptions about breastfeeding. For example, if a new mother says she heard that getting upset or angry will spoil her milk, you can point out that this belief likely stems from the correct observation that breastfeeding babies can sense maternal tension (which also may delay let-down) and may therefore act fussy as well, appearing to behave as if they were getting "spoiled milk." Then reassure the mother that there is no evidence that the milk composition itself is changed. This will allow you to focus on the real issues of bonding and relaxation technique. Simply understanding what is really going on may help the mother to be more relaxed.

Whenever possible, it is best to have a female translator who is not a family member present to interpret for a mother. For Muslim women, it is culturally unacceptable for them to speak about intimate matters in front of their families. Therefore, it would be inappropriate to ask the new mother's husband or one of her children to be her interpreter. Even among those who speak English, language barriers and miscommunications still exist, due in

part to words having different meanings to people of different cultures. It is important to give enough explanation to ensure that the mother clearly understands the information provided. These are but a few of the numerous cultural influences related to feeding. (See *Developing Cultural Competence: Breastfeeding in Other Cultures*.) When nurses are faced with a newborn/infant care practice different from the ones to which they are accustomed, they need to evaluate the effect of the practice. Different practices are not necessarily inferior. The nurse should intervene only if the practice is actually harmful to the mother or baby.

Breastfeeding in public is another frequently expressed concern that can create a barrier to achieving *Healthy People 2020* breastfeeding goals. Although people agree that breastfeeding is the most natural and healthy way to feed a baby, mothers feel conflicted because in the United States breast exposure is often viewed in a sexual context and this may lead to disapproval of attempts to breastfeed in public. Public places are incorporating "mother rooms" to provide a comfortable, private area for the nursing mother. There is no state

---

Developing Cultural Competence Breastfeeding in Other Cultures

Among traditional societies around the world, weaning from the breast occurs when a child is between 2 and 4 years of age. Some people of African ancestry may wean their babies after they begin to walk.

Some women of Asian heritage may breastfeed their babies for the first 1 to 2 years of life. Many women of Cambodian heritage practice breastfeeding on demand without restriction, or, if formula-feeding, provide a "comfort bottle" in between feedings (Lipson & Dibble, 2008).

Chinese women go through a 30-day period of home confinement ("doing the month" [*zuo yue zij*] following delivery, during which they are not permitted to bathe or wash their hair (Callister, 2014). This is a centuries-old tradition to nurture the mother back to her prenatal state and intended to keep her body warm to ward off *fong* (flatulence) and other future health ailments. A *Pui Yuet* (companion) is hired to provide total care for the mother and newborn. The Pui Yuet will cook traditional confinement foods daily (provide "heating foods" and avoid "cooling foods"). Most foods must be cooked in sesame oil and old ginger. The mother drinks hot herbal tea with her meals and is not permitted to drink any water because it is thought to cause water retention (Callister, 2014).

Muslim women generally breastfeed until their children are 2 years of age. This is encouraged in the Koran. Although Muslim women do not breastfeed in public, they will breastfeed in front of family members and relatives as long as the breast is not exposed (Ott, Al-Khadhuri, & Al-Junaibi, 2003).

People of Iranian heritage may breastfeed female babies longer than male babies.

Some Asians, Cambodians, Latin Americans, Eastern Europeans, and Native Americans may delay breastfeeding because they believe colostrum is "bad" (Wambach, 2016; Callister, 2014). Haitian mothers may believe that "strong emotions" spoil breast milk, and that thick breast milk causes skin rashes and thin milk results in diarrhea (Callister, 2014; Purnell, 2013).

To increase breastmilk production, Ethiopian women eat a special diet of milk and warm oat and honey gruel, Arab women eat lentil soup, and Korean women eat a special seaweed soup with beef broth (Callister, 2014; Purnell, 2013).

Professionalism in Practice Breastfeeding Promotion Legislation

It is important to be a patient advocate and be involved in legislative initiatives on the national and local levels. The Breastfeeding Promotion Act of 2009 was enacted into law on March 23, 2010, and acts to protect breastfeeding in the workplace by providing five provisions. These include:

Title I: Amending the Civil Rights Act of 1964 to protect lactating women from being fired or discriminated against in the workplace.

Title II: Giving tax incentives to businesses that establish a private space in the workplace for their employees to breastfeed or express their milk. Employers can also receive tax credits for supplying breastfeeding equipment and providing lactation consultation services for their employees.

Title III: Establishing set standards for breast pumps to ensure that they are safe and effective.

Title IV: Expanding the Internal Revenue Code definition of "medical care" to include breastfeeding equipment and lactation services as tax-deductible for families.

Title V: Requiring employers with 50 or more employees to provide lactating employees break time and a private area to express their milk.

In addition, the U. S. Department of Labor (2011) enacted the Fair Labor Standards Act: Break Time for Nursing Mothers provision.

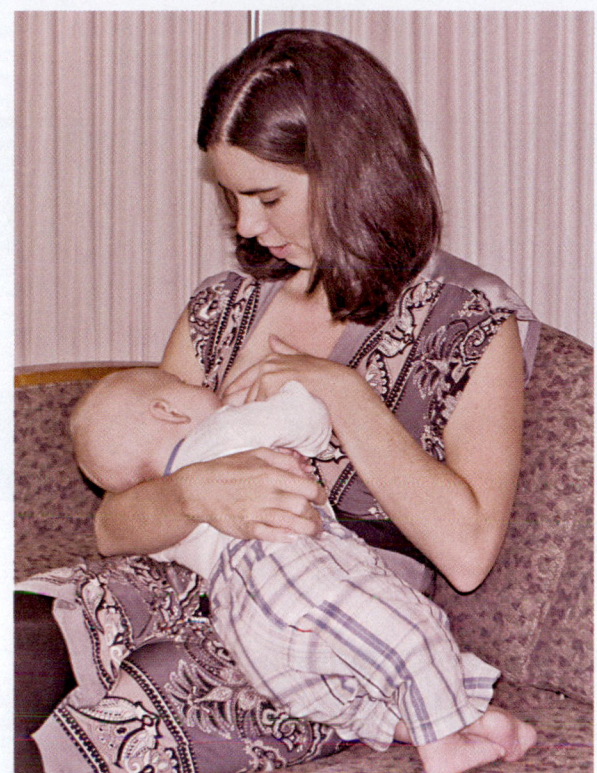

Figure 25–13 **Breastfeeding discreetly.**

SOURCE: Brigitte Hall, RNC, MSN, IBCLC.

that prohibits breastfeeding in a public place, and currently 49 states, the District of Columbia, and the Virgin Islands have created laws that specify that a woman is permitted to breastfeed in any location in which she is authorized to be (National Conference of State Legislatures, 2015). Mothers may also be taught how to breastfeed discreetly in public. This is often taught at breastfeeding classes or mother-to-mother support group meetings. See Figure 25–13 to observe a mother discreetly breastfeeding. Some mothers may prefer a baby blanket or shawl to drape over their chests, which will provide more coverage. Finally, mothers who prefer not to breastfeed even discreetly in public can be encouraged to at least pump their breasts and feed the expressed milk in a bottle so they have the option of getting out of the house.

Breastfeeding Technique

BREASTFEEDING POSITIONS AND LATCHING ON

Breastfeeding is not instinctive, it is learned. It is a natural process, but it takes "know-how." Ideally, each breastfeeding mother should have a breastfeeding evaluation to determine any knowledge deficits, acknowledge any concerns, provide instructions, and assist with breastfeeding.

Positioning. There are many breastfeeding positions, but only the four classic breastfeeding positions will be discussed here: (1) modified cradle position, (2) cradle position, (3) football (or clutch) hold position, and (4) side-lying position (Figures 25–14 through 25–17). After a mother has fed using one position, she can be encouraged to try a different position when she

offers her second breast. Alternating positions facilitates drainage of the breasts and changes the pressure points on the breast. This will provide some relief to the mother with sore nipples. In addition to the classic positions, "laid-back" breastfeeding is being advocated. This concept is based on biologic nursing (BN), a mother-centered approach, and purports that women can find the best position for themselves because breastfeeding initiation is intrinsic for both mother and baby (La Leche League International, 2013).

Clinical Tip

Regardless of the feeding position, encourage the mother to support her baby's head with her hand at the base of the baby's neck or upper back. This allows for the baby's head to extend slightly back so the baby leads chin first during attachment. If lined up "nose to nipple" to start with, then the baby will attach to the breast with the lower jaw first. This technique will allow for a deeper latch attachment and a pleasant breastfeeding experience.

Latching On. It is important to have the mother and baby positioned properly in order to achieve an optimal attachment. If, for example, the newborn is lying flat on the back (supine position) to feed, then the baby can obtain only a shallow latch (not attached far back onto the areola). The baby's shoulder becomes an obstacle, putting distance between the baby's mouth and the mother's breast. Anything that contributes to

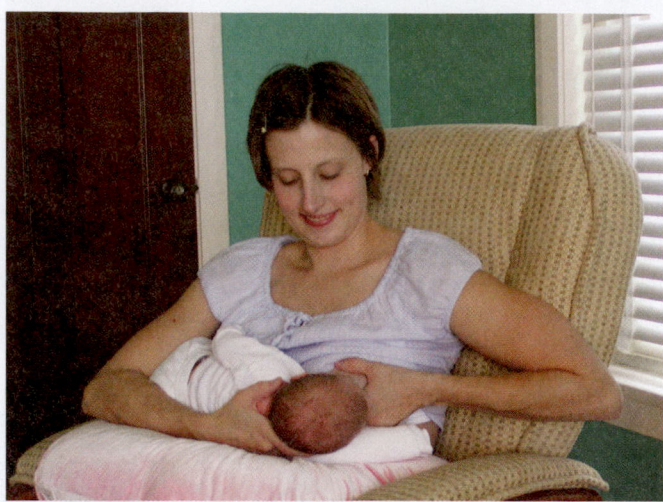

Figure 25–14 Modified cradle position.

SOURCE: Brigitte Hall, RNC, MSN, IBCLC.

- Have the mother sit comfortably in upright position using good body alignment. Use pillows for support (may use Boppy, body pillow, or standard bed pillows). Lap pillow should help bring the baby up to breast level so the mother does not lean over baby.
- Place the baby on the mother's lap and turn the baby's entire body toward the mother (the baby is in side-lying position). Position the baby's body so that the baby's nose lines up to the nipple. Maintain the baby's body in a horizontal alignment.
- To feed at left breast, the mother supports the baby's head with her right hand at nape of the baby's neck (allow head to slightly lag back); the mother's right thumb by the baby's left ear, and right forefinger near the baby's right ear.
- With the mother's free left hand, she can offer her left breast.

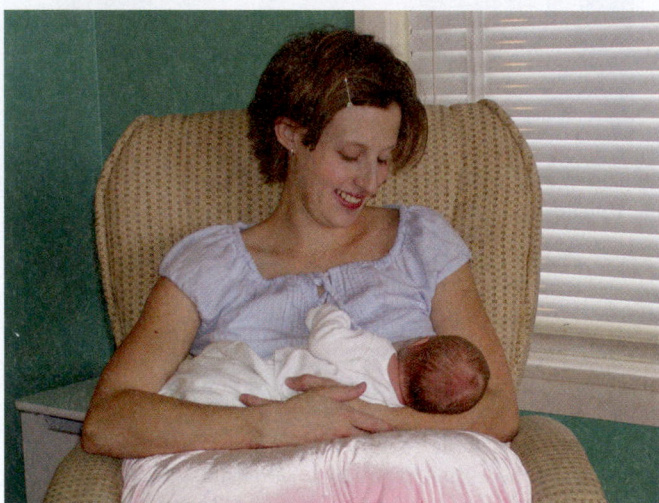

Figure 25–15 Cradle position.

SOURCE: Brigitte Hall, RNC, MSN, IBCLC.

- Have the mother sit comfortably in upright position using good body alignment. Use pillows for support (may use Boppy, body pillow, or standard bed pillows). Lap pillow should help bring the baby up to breast level so the mother does not lean over the baby.
- Place the baby on the mother's lap and turn the baby's entire body toward the mother (the baby is in side-lying position). Position the baby's body so that the baby's nose lines up to the nipple. Maintain the baby's body in a horizontal alignment.
- If feeding from the left breast, have the mother cradle the baby's head near the crook of her left arm while supporting her baby's body with her left forearm.
- With the mother's free right hand, she can offer her left breast.

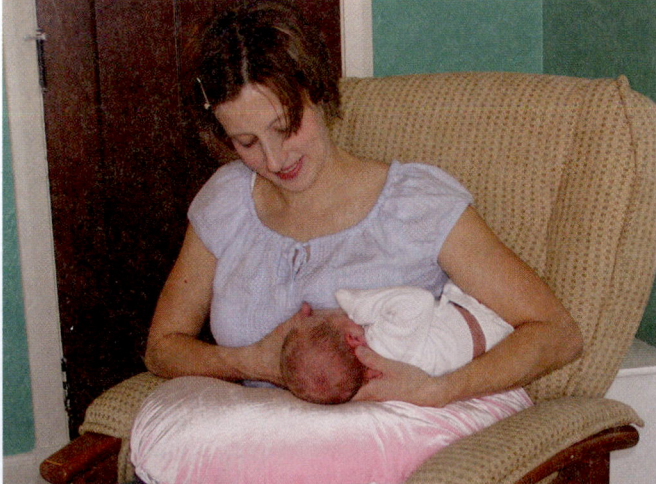

Figure 25–16 Football hold position.

SOURCE: Brigitte Hall, RNC, MSN, IBCLC.

- Have the mother sit comfortably and use pillows to raise the baby's body to breast level. If using a Boppy and the Boppy is in "normal" position on the mother's lap, turn it counterclockwise slightly (if feeding at left breast) to provide extended support for the baby's body resting along the mother's left side and near the back of the mother's chair.
- If feeding at left breast, place the baby on the left side of the mother's body, heading the baby into position feet first. The baby's bottom should rest on the pillow near the mother's left elbow.
- Turn the baby slightly on her side so that she faces the breast.
- The mother's left arm clutches the baby's body close to the mother's body. The baby's body should feel securely tucked in under the mother's left arm.
- Have the mother support the baby's head with her left hand. With the mother's free right hand, she can offer her breast. (Good position for the mother with c-section.)

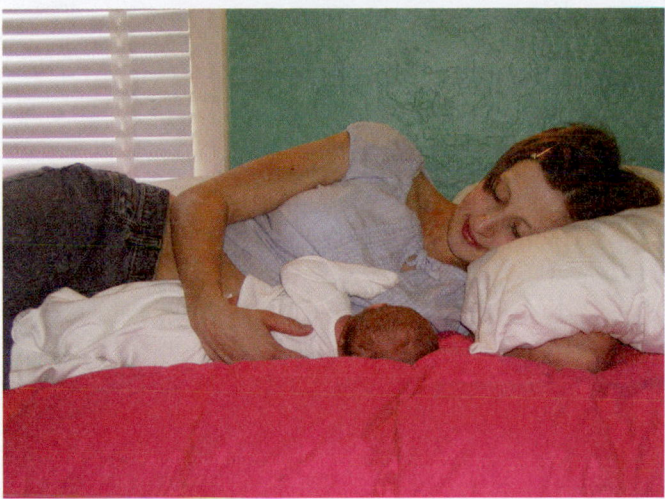

Figure 25–17 Side-lying position.
SOURCE: Brigitte Hall, RNC, MSN, IBCLC.

- Have the mother rest comfortably lying on her side (left side for this demonstration). Use pillows to support the mother's head and back, and provide support for the mother's hips by placing a pillow between her bent knees.
- Place the baby in side-lying position next to the mother's body. The baby's body should face the mother's body. The baby's nose should line up to the mother's nipple. Place a roll behind the baby's back, if desired.
- With the mother's free right hand, she can offer her left breast. After the baby is securely attached, mom can rest her right hand anywhere that is comfortable for her.

a shallow latch is going to cause sore nipples and other complications. The newborn could have a short lingual frenulum (be "tongue-tied") and not be able to properly cup the breast, resulting in painful, cracked nipples and poor milk transfer. Nipple trauma, although relatively common, is not normal. (See Chapter 29 for a discussion of breastfeeding with inverted or flat nipples.)

The baby needs to attach the lips onto the breast or, more accurately, far back onto the areola, not on the nipple. If the baby attaches just to the nipple, the mother will have sore nipples and pain may inhibit the let-down reflex. To obtain a deep latch, the mother needs to be taught how to elicit the baby's rooting reflex, stimulating the baby to open the mouth as widely as possible (like a big yawn). Once the baby does this, the mother should quickly but gently draw her baby in toward her. During the first few days of life, the newborn typically opens the mouth widely only for a second or so, and then begins to close the mouth again. If the mother misses her chance to get her baby latched on, she needs to simply start over again.

Figures 25–18 through 25–23 demonstrate various positions and techniques used in latching on.

Clinical Tip

As you assist new mothers with breastfeeding, it is important to create a relaxed environment and approach to breastfeeding. Encourage the mother to get into a comfortable position, well supported with pillows. Remind her to bring the baby to her breast rather than leaning forward to the baby.

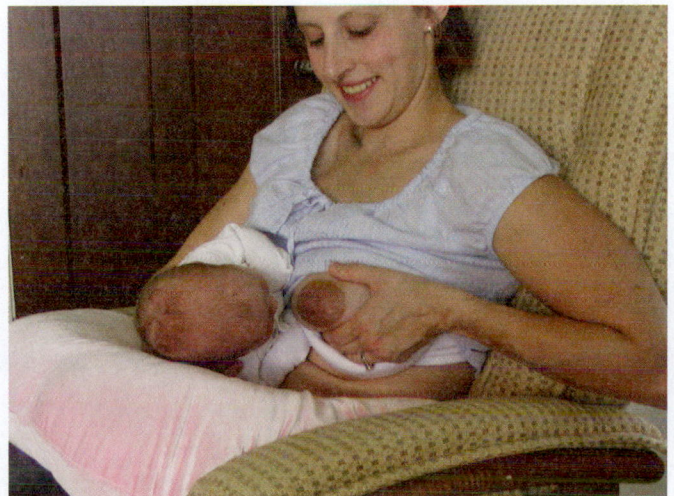

Figure 25–18 C-hold hand position.
SOURCE: Brigitte Hall, RNC, MSN, IBCLC.

To be ready to draw the baby's mouth onto the mother's breast, as soon as the baby opens her mouth widely enough, the mother needs to have her hand supporting her breast in the ready position. She can use various hand holds, but she needs to keep her fingers well behind the areola. One such hand position is called the "C-hold." In this hold, the thumb is placed on top of the breast near 12:00 position and the other four fingers are placed on the underside of the breast near the 6:00 position (depends on mother's hand size and length of fingers). The key point is to keep the fingers at least 1 1/2 inches back from the base of the nipple as the fingers support the breast. Mothers are not often aware of where they place their fingers especially on the underside of the breast. If the fingers are too far forward (too close to the nipple), then the baby cannot grasp a large amount of areola in her mouth and this results in a "shallow" latch. A shallow latch is associated with nipple pain and ineffective drainage of the breast.

An alternate hand hold not shown is a "U-hold" hand position. The thumb and forefinger are near the 3 and 9 position on the breast again with fingers at least 1 1/2 inches back from the base of the nipple; the body of the hand rests on the lower portion of the breast. Using this hand hold, the mother's arm position is down at her side rather than sticking outward as it is when supporting the breast using the C-hold position.

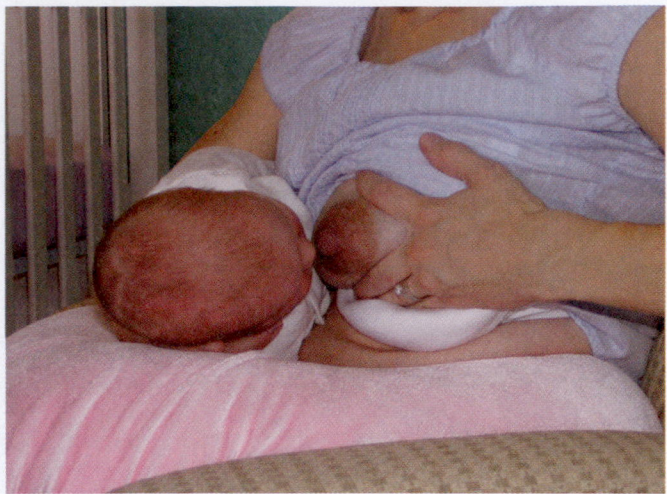

The scissor hold is often discouraged because mothers (especially mothers with small hands) have a difficult time keeping their fingers off the areola or at least 1½ inches back from the base of the areola. Here, the mother is able to support her breast well without letting her fingers encroach onto the areola.

The mother should be instructed to gently support the breast and not press too deeply, which can obstruct the flow of milk through the ducts.

Figure 25–19 Scissor hold hand position.

SOURCE: Brigitte Hall, RNC, MSN, IBCLC.

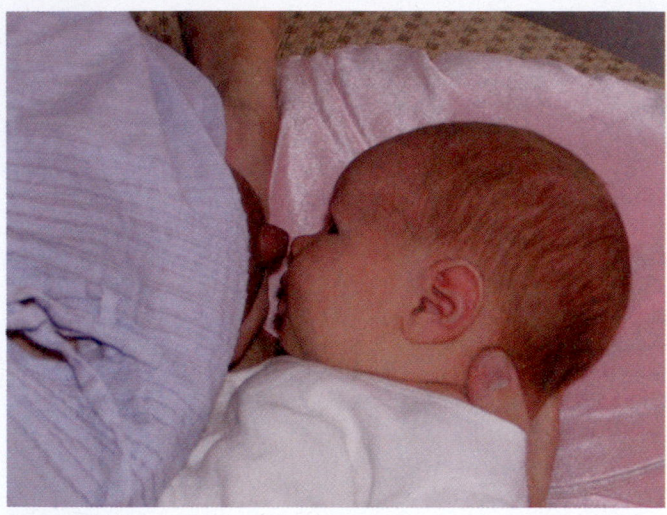

Before eliciting the rooting reflex, it is important to have the baby in good alignment. When the baby opens his mouth to latch on, the goal is to achieve a deep, asymmetric latch attachment. The goal is *not* to center the nipple in the baby's mouth. The rationale for this is to optimize oral-motor function. The jaw is a hinge joint. The upper jaw is immobile; the lower jaw compresses the breast. The breast is efficiently drained if more areola is drawn into the baby's mouth from the inferior aspect of the breast and a smaller amount drawn in from the superior aspect of the areola. Aligning the baby to the mother with baby's nose facing mother's nipple permits the jaw to be in a lower position. The next step is to let the baby drop his head back (head in "sniff position"), so that the baby leads into the breast with the chin.

Figure 25–20 Nose to nipple.

SOURCE: Brigitte Hall, RNC, MSN, IBCLC.

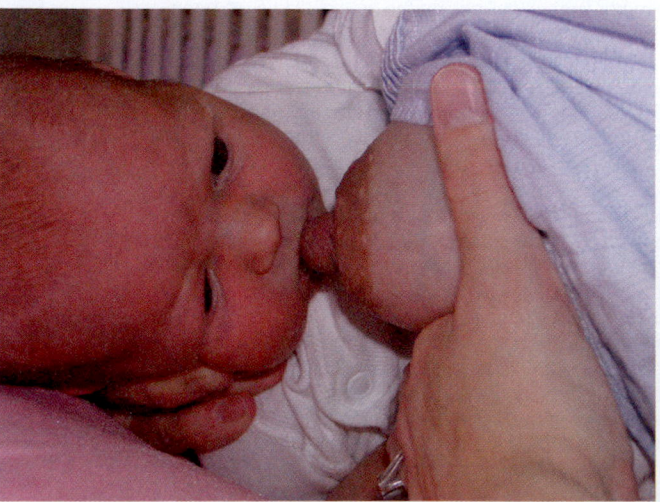

To trigger the rooting reflex, teach the mother to use her nipple to stroke downward in a vertical motion across the middle of baby's lower lip. Initially, the baby may respond by licking or smacking. This is a normal response to the stimulus. Encourage the mother to keep stimulating the baby's lower lip until the baby finally opens his mouth widely. If the baby is not responding at all, then the baby is probably too sleepy and may need help waking up. After trying wake up techniques, the baby may be ready to try breastfeeding again.

Figure 25–21 Initial attempt to elicit the rooting reflex.

SOURCE: Brigitte Hall, RNC, MSN, IBCLC.

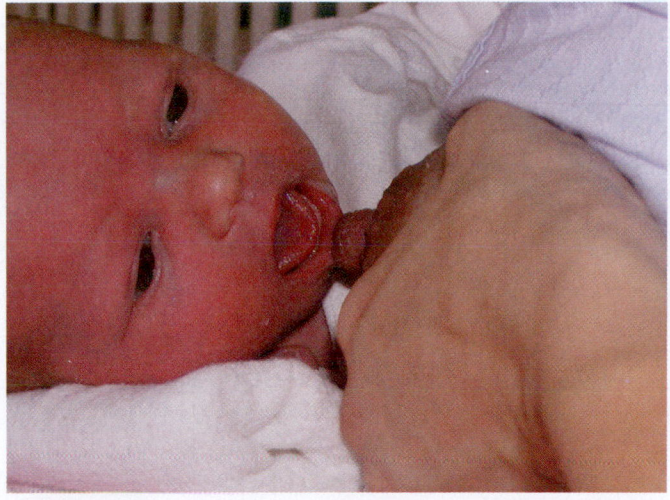

Teach the mother to be patient and wait for the baby's mouth to gape open as widely as possible. Here the baby needs to open the mouth even wider before the mother draws her baby toward the breast. The mother should be encouraged to continue stroking the baby's lip until the baby opens the mouth wider.

Figure 25–22 Continued attempt to elicit the rooting reflex.

SOURCE: Brigitte Hall, RNC, MSN, IBCLC.

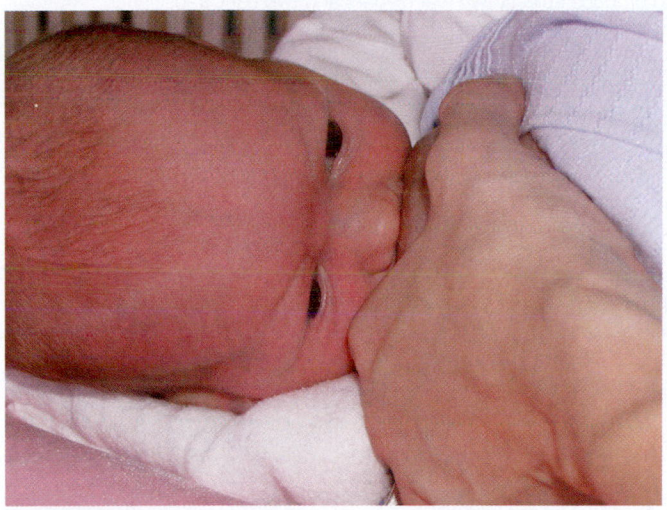

Once the baby has latched onto the breast, the mother should check that the baby is latched-on properly. The baby's chin should be embedded into the mother's breast. The baby's nose should be very close but not actually touching the breast. The nose should be centered. If the mother feels a little pinch on her areola, she can slowly release the hand supporting her breast so she can have a free hand to attempt to move her baby's jaw gently downward. To do this maneuver, the mother needs to place the thumb or forefinger of her free hand (the hand that just released the breast) on the baby's lower jaw (there is a horizontal groove to use as leverage—the groove on the baby's chin is parallel with the baby's lips). With gentle downward pressure the mother should feel relief of any persistent tenderness. This procedure opens the jaw wider and it also helps to roll out the baby's lower lip that may have been inadvertently drawn into the baby's mouth. As the baby begins to suckle, there should be no dimpling of the baby's cheeks and no smacking or clicking noises.

Figure 25–23 Baby is latched on.

SOURCE: Brigitte Hall, RNC, MSN, IBCLC.

BREASTFEEDING ASSESSMENT

During the birthing unit stay, the nurse must carefully monitor the progress of the breastfeeding pair. A systematic assessment of several breastfeeding episodes provides the opportunity to teach the new mother about lactation and the breastfeeding process, provide anticipatory guidance, and evaluate the need for follow-up care after discharge. Criteria for evaluating a breastfeeding session include maternal and newborn cues, latch-on, position, let-down, nipple condition, newborn response, and maternal response. The literature provides various tools to guide the assessment and documentation of the breastfeeding efforts, such as the LATCH Scoring Table.

BREASTFEEDING EFFICIENCY

The mother should be taught to observe the baby for effective, active breastfeeding. The baby should have a rhythmic suckling pattern (the slight pause between jaw compressions on the breast permits the mouth to fill with milk before swallowing). To note if the jaw compressions are strong enough, the mother should observe or feel if there is movement at the bilateral temporomandibular joints located in front of the baby's ears.

The newborn should maintain a rhythmic feeding pattern with only brief pauses (lasting only seconds, not minutes) between spurts of active feeding, with the feeding session typically lasting for 10 to 20 minutes on the first breast. The baby may feed only a few minutes on the second breast or not at all, so the mother should alternate the first breast at the next feeding. The mother should visually observe for swallowing and later, as her milk is abundant, she will hear the baby's swallows. Discourage the mother from watching the clock to determine when the baby needs to switch breast sides but rather encourage her to watch the newborn's feeding pattern to note when active feeding ceases. When satiated, the baby will either pull away from the breast or fall asleep. The newborn will be extremely relaxed at the end of the feeding and will sleep until the next feeding is due (at least an hour). As the baby matures, the feeding intervals will lengthen.

Another indicator of breastfeeding efficiency is softening of the mother's breasts, although this is not a reliable indicator in the first few days postpartum while breast milk volume is low. Within a week, however, this is a good indicator of milk transfer.

The newborn who feeds well will have a characteristic output. See Figure 25–24 for breastfeeding intake and output

- Newborns should breastfeed 8 to 12 times per day and should appear relaxed after feeding.
- Colostrum is all that a newborn needs in the first few days of life in most cases.
- It is normal for a newborn to lose up to 7% of birth weight in the first few days; however, up to 10% weight loss is tolerated if the mother's breasts are full, the baby is observed to breastfeed well, and the baby is not dehydrated.
- Newborns should gain 10 grams/kg/day after the mother's milk supply is abundant (about day 4 of life).
- Newborns should be back to their birth weight by 2 weeks of age.
- Newborn's stool should change in color, consistency, and frequency during the first few days of life. The photo images noted below depict stool color progression. Some babies progress faster to yellow milk stools, as early as day 3.

Day 1

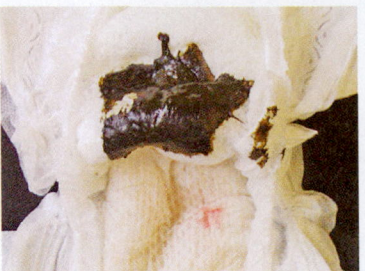

Day 2

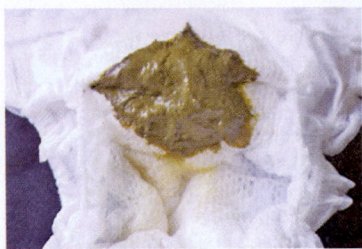

Day 3

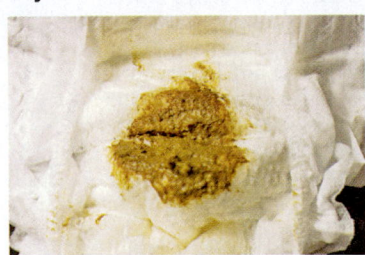

Day 4

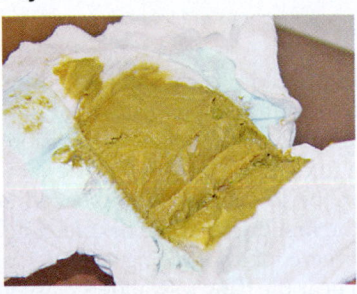

Day 5

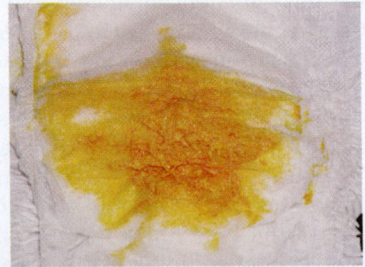

Minimum Output

On day 1, the newborn should produce at least one wet diaper and one meconium stool by 24 hours of age.

Note the pinkish-red "brick dust" appearance on the diaper. The uric acid crystals produced by the kidneys is associated with concentrated urine. A red flag is raised if their presence is continued beyond day 2 or 3 of life.

On day 2, the newborn should produce at least two wet diapers and two early transitional stools in a 24-hour period by 48 hours of age.

On day 3, the newborn should produce at least three wet diapers and three transitional stools in a 24-hour period by 72 hours of age.

When a mother's milk supply is abundant on day 2, some babies will have transitioned to yellow milk stools as early as day 3.

On day 4, the newborn should produce at least four wet diapers and three to four yellow-green transitional stools or yellow milk stools in a 24-hour period by 96 hours of age.

On day 5, the newborn should produce at least five wet diapers and three to four yellow milk stools per day; the stools are typically explosive and have a curdy or seedy appearance.

Hereafter, breastfeeding babies will consistently produce at least six well-saturated wet diapers per day. These newborns will typically continue to produce at least three to four yellow milk stools daily, but may have up to 10 stools per day until they are about a month old. Infants 4 weeks or older may suddenly decrease their stool frequency, even skipping days.

Figure 25–24 **Breastfeeding intake and output expectations.**
SOURCE: Brigitte Hall, RNC, MSN, IBCLC.

expectations. The newborn should also have the characteristic weight loss followed by weight gain pattern discussed earlier in this chapter.

In situations where there is a question regarding milk transfer effectiveness, it can be most reliably measured by obtaining prebreastfeeding and postbreastfeeding weight checks using an accurate infant scale. The difference in preweights and postweights is the amount of milk (each gram increase reflects 1 mL) transferred to the baby and may be useful for assessing breastfeeding efficiency and maternal milk volume.

Women With Special Needs Breastfeeding Assistance

For the woman with upper extremity impairment, breastfeeding may require assistance from a partner or care provider should she choose to breastfeed. Women with limited arm strength or manual dexterity may require wrist supports to maintain a proper latch-on. These women are also more prone to nipple soreness, cracking, and bleeding because if the baby slips off the nipple, it may be difficult to reattach the baby properly. A lactation consultation should be performed with all women with upper extremity limitations.

BOTTLE-FEEDING BREAST MILK (EXPRESSION, PUMPS, STORAGE)

Breast milk is bottle-fed to babies for a variety of reasons. The nurse should evaluate the indications in order to recommend the best technique for the mother and her particular need.

Hand Expression. Some mothers prefer to hand express their milk rather than use a breast pump, and many find that in the immediate postpartum period hand expression of milk may be a more effective method of removing drops of colostrum than using an electric breast pump. Nurses should teach all mothers the skill of hand expressing breast milk because a mother may find herself in a situation without a breast pump and need to relieve herself from engorgement.

To help the mother hand express breast milk, have the mother follow steps 1 through 4 of the pumping instructions provided in Table 25–2. The mother should use the Marmet technique of hand expression described next. The steps are as follows.

1. The mother will position her thumb at the 12:00 position on the top edge of the areola (about 1.0 to 1.5 inches back from the tip of her nipple) and her forefinger and middle finger pads at the 6:00 position on the bottom edge of the areola (about 1.0 to 1.5 inches from the tip of her nipple).

TEACHING HIGHLIGHTS | Successful Breastfeeding Evaluation

A baby is probably getting enough milk if:

- The newborn is nursing at least 8 times in 24 hours.
- In a quiet room, the mother can hear her baby swallow while nursing, once her milk supply has become abundant.
- The mother's breasts appear to soften after breastfeeding.
- The number of wet diapers increases daily by a

minimum of one additional diaper until the fifth day after birth; after day 5, the baby should have six to eight wet diapers daily.

- The newborn's stools are beginning to lighten in color by the third day after birth, or have changed to yellow no later than day 5.

Note: Offering a supplemental bottle is not a reliable indicator because most newborns will take a few ounces even if they are getting enough breast milk.

TABLE 25–2 Pumping Instructions and Storage Guidelines

1. Once a day rinse the breasts with water while bathing or showering. Avoid applying soap directly on the nipples.
2. Wash hands well with soap and water before preparing to pump.
3. Take a few minutes to massage the breasts and relax. Do some slow, deep breathing and think about or look at a picture of your baby. Being relaxed is very important for releasing milk from the breasts. (Stress can inhibit or delay let-down because stress hormones, such as cortisol and epinephrine, can block receptors for let-down.)
4. Sit up straight or lean slightly forward. A pillow placed behind your back may facilitate the slightly tilted forward posture, because gravity aids in the flow of milk from the breasts.
5. For single-sided pumping, pump each breast for 10 to 20 minutes. Some mothers find that they empty their breasts more efficiently if they switch back and forth from one breast to the other as the milk flow diminishes, until they have stimulated each breast for 15 to 20 minutes. The entire pumping session will last 30 to 40 minutes.
6. Pump the expressed milk preferably into glass or plastic bottles. Mothers of healthy babies may also use bottle bags or liners intended for human milk collection and storage; however, note that up to 60% of secretory IgA (SIgA) is lost when milk is stored in these kinds of containers for 48 hours because of the attraction of the antibodies to the polyethylene material used in making the bottle bags or liners (Riordan, 2016). Because of the loss of antibodies that can occur with bottle bags or liners, mothers of premature and fragile babies should especially avoid using these kinds of storage containers. Do not fill milk storage containers more than 3/4 full, because milk expands during freezing.
7. Feed *freshly* expressed breast milk whenever there is a need to give a supplement, when possible. Reserve the stored milk for times when fresh milk is not available (e.g., when separated from baby). Fresh breast milk retains more nutrients than refrigerated or frozen milk, although these are still preferred over formula. Expressed human milk may be stored in the refrigerator for up to 8 days, but if intended to be frozen, this should be done within 48 hours of initial refrigeration. Avoid placing human milk in the freezer door or on the bottom of a self-defrosting freezer because the temperature fluctuates more in those areas.

(continued)

TABLE 25–2 Pumping Instructions and Storage Guidelines (*continued*)

8. Store expressed human milk in volumes the baby is likely to consume at a single feeding or in a volume the baby will consume in a day.
9. Human milk should never be thawed in a microwave oven or placed in a pan and warmed up on the stove. These methods may cause the milk to warm up too hot (and unevenly) and can burn a baby as well as cause heat-sensitive nutrients to be destroyed. Frozen milk can be thawed safely using one of two methods:
   - For a quick thaw, remove the container of frozen milk from the freezer, place the container in a bowl in the sink, and run warm water over it for no longer than 15 minutes. Take care not to immerse the container in water because water may leach into the container of milk, possibly contaminating it and diluting it.
   - For a slow thaw overnight, take the frozen container of milk from the freezer the day before or several hours before it is needed and let it defrost in the refrigerator (not on the kitchen counter) over several hours. The time it takes to defrost depends on the volume in the container. Note that breast milk that has been sitting for a while will normally separate. Figure 25–26 shows breast milk that has separated. To remix it, simply swirl the bottle (avoid vigorous shaking) until the milk is evenly mixed. Make certain that the fat that clings to the wall of the container has mixed into the milk. If the volume in the bottle is more than can be used in one feeding, pour only the amount needed into a clean bottle, and put the rest of the milk immediately back in the refrigerator. Place the feeding bottle in a bowl in the sink and run warm water over it for no longer than 15 minutes. The bottle should remain fairly upright, and the water level in the bowl should remain below the lid of the bottle or milk container to prevent water from inadvertently entering the bottle.
10. Previously frozen thawed breast milk is good in the refrigerator for 24 hours only. It must be used in that time frame or discarded. Thawed milk should never be refrozen.
11. Check the temperature of the milk before feeding it to the baby. Babies will drink milk when the milk temperature is between room temperature and body temperature (roughly 65 to 100 degrees).
12. Any milk left over from a feeding should be discarded within an hour of starting the feeding. The reason for this is that saliva "back washes" into the bottle while nipple feeding, and the saliva contains bacteria that can multiply and potentially make a baby sick.

If positioned correctly, a line between the thumb and fingers will cross the nipple (see Figure 25–25).

2. Next, the mother will stretch her areola back toward her chest wall without lifting her fingers off her breast.
3. Now she should roll her thumb and fingers simultaneously forward. This action compresses the ducts beneath the areola and stimulates the breast to empty both manually and by triggering the let-down reflex.
4. The mother should repeat the sequence multiple times to completely drain her breasts. She should try to maintain a steady rhythm, cycling 45 to 60 times/minute. It is also more effective if the mother repositions her fingers to other positions on the same breast (e.g., 3:00 and 9:00, 1:00 and 7:00, etc.) when the milk flow slows.

It is important that the mother take care to place her hands exactly as directed. She should take care not to traumatize her breasts or nipples. Hand expression should not be painful. Most mothers will need assistance in learning this technique initially.

Reassure the mother that this skill is learned; with practice, she can become an expert at hand expression.

Pump. Although hand expression can be efficient, many mothers will choose to use a mechanical breast pump to express their milk. Not all breast pumps are of the same quality, even within the same category (see Figures 25–27, 25–28, and 25–29 and Table 25–3). Pumps generally cycle from low to high suction at a frequency similar to that of a breastfeeding baby (about 45 to 60 cycles per minute). However, differences in the

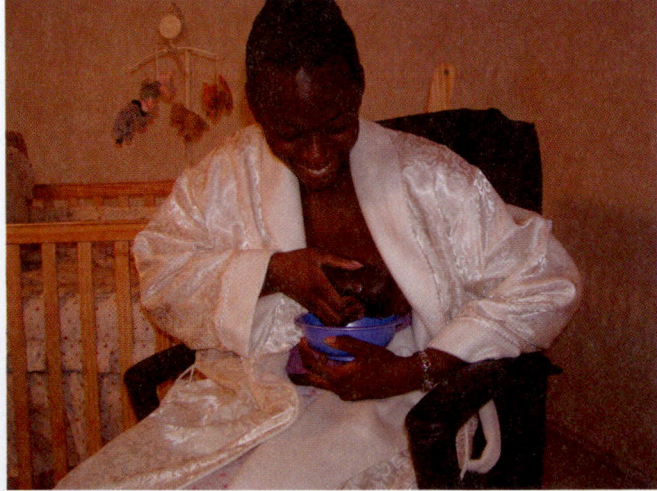

Figure 25–25 Hand expression of breast milk.
SOURCE: Brigitte Hall, RNC, MSN, IBCLC.

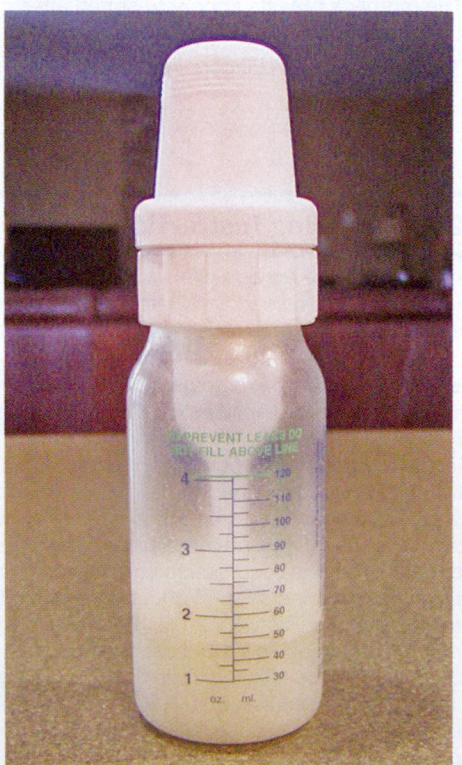

Figure 25–26 Expressed breast milk that has separated.
SOURCE: Brigitte Hall, RNC, MSN, IBCLC.

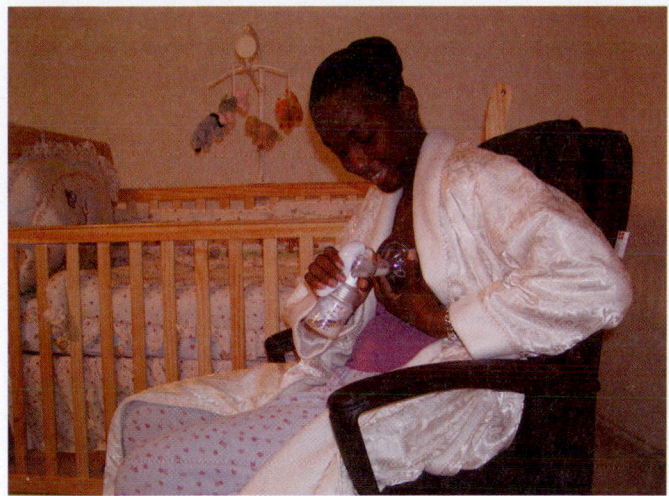

Figure 25–27 **Manual breast pump.**
SOURCE: Brigitte Hall, RNC, MSN, IBCLC.

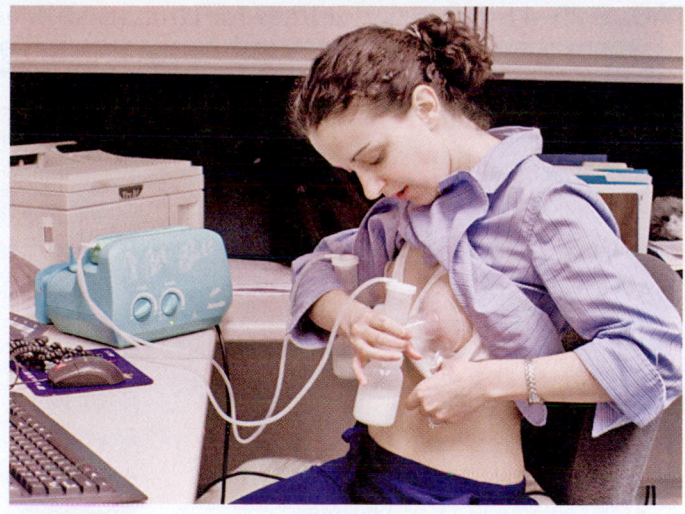

Figure 25–29 **Hospital-grade multiuser breast pump.**
SOURCE: Brigitte Hall, RNC, MSN, IBCLC.

quality of the pump motor or the presence or absence of controls over suction pressure mean that some pumps will generate inadequate pressure or cycle too slowly to be effective, whereas others may exert too high a suction that can cause injury. Breast flange size, proper fit, and comfort are other variables to consider. Some good-quality pumps have multiple flange sizes available to accommodate the various nipple sizes of mothers. Excessive rubbing of the mother's nipple in the flange tunnel can cause discomfort and result in a decreased volume expressed. The nurse should refer the mother to a lactation consultant or other person knowledgeable regarding different breast pumps.

Storing Human Breast Milk.   There are different guidelines for storage of expressed breast milk (EBM) depending on whether the baby is a healthy full-term baby or a premature or sick baby in the hospital. The guidelines in Table 25–4 (which also include storage guidelines for formula) are intended as a resource for the mother of a healthy, full-term baby.

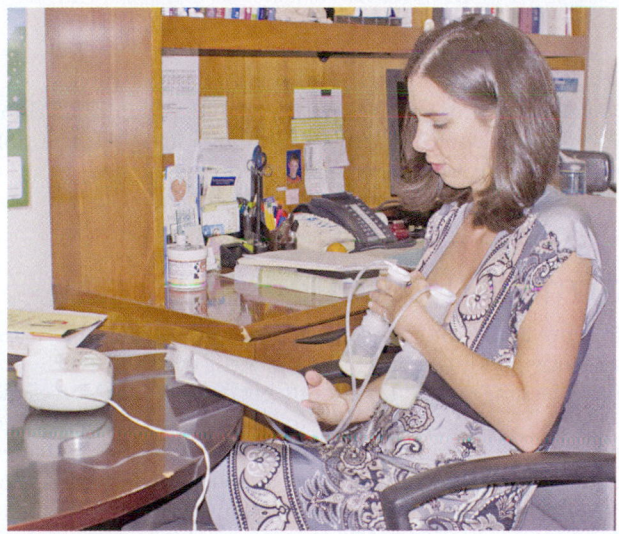

Figure 25–28 **Individual double electric breast pump.**
SOURCE: Brigitte Hall, RNC, MSN, IBCLC.

TABLE 25–3 Types of Breast Pumps and Indications for Use

INDICATION	MANUAL BREAST PUMP (FIGURE 25–27)	SMALL BATTERY/ELECTRIC BREAST PUMP	INDIVIDUAL DOUBLE ELECTRIC BREAST PUMP (FIGURE 25–28)	HOSPITAL-GRADE MULTIUSER DOUBLE ELECTRIC BREAST PUMP (FIGURE 25–29)
A missed feeding	■	◊		
An evening out	■	◊		
Working part-time	■	◊		
Convenience—occasional use	■	◊		
Working full-time			*	*
Premature/hospitalized newborn			■	*
Low milk supply				*
Sore nipples/engorgement			*	*
Latch-on problems/infection				*
Drawing out flattish nipples	■	◊	*	*

■ Good ◊ Better *Best
Source: Adapted from the *Medela Breastfeeding Information Guide Tips and Products.* (2010). Table: Which Breast Pump Is Best for You? (p. 9). McHenry, IL: Medela, Inc.

TABLE 25–4 Storage Guidelines for Human Milk and Formula

MILK	ENVIRONMENT	TIME UNTIL DISCARD
Human milk or formula, opened/reconstituted	Being fed	Finish feed within 1 hour
Fresh human milk	Room temperature 72°–79°F (22.2°–26.0° C)	4 hours
Fresh human milk	Room temperature 66°–72°F (18.1°–22.2°C)	6–10 hours
Fresh human milk	Cooler w/ frozen ice packs 59°F (15°C)	24 hours
Formula, opened/reconstituted	Room temperature	2 hours
Thawed human milk	Refrigerator	24 hours
Formula, opened/reconstituted	Refrigerator	24–48 hours (see label)
Fresh human milk	Refrigerator	8 days
Formula powder, opened can	Room temperature	1 month
Fresh human milk	Freezer	3–4 months
Formula powder, sealed container	Avoid excessive heat	Printed expiration date
Thawed human milk	Freezer	Do not refreeze
Formula	Freezer	Do not freeze

Sources: Data from Human Milk Banking Association of North America (HMBANA). (2011). *Best practice for expressing, storing and handling human milk in hospitals, homes and child care settings* (3rd ed.). Raleigh, NC: Author; Mead-Johnson Nutritionals. (2012); *Pediatric products handbook.* New York, NY: Bristol-Myers Squibb Company; Ross Products Division. (2014). *Pediatric nutritionals product guide.* Columbus, OH: Abbott Laboratories.

SUPPLEMENTARY FORMULA-FEEDING FOR BREASTFED NEWBORNS

Supplementary formula-feedings for the breastfeeding newborn are not routinely recommended. Supplementation should be given only when medically indicated (Janke, 2014). Routine supplements are unnecessary in the early days after birth, and bottle-feeding may cause the newborn to develop an incorrect sucking pattern or may cause the baby to refuse the breast altogether (Riordan, 2016). Early supplementation with formula may contribute to a delay in early maternal milk production, may result in maternal engorgement after the mother's milk production has increased, and may possibly sensitize an at-risk newborn for milk-protein allergy. These types of problems have been implicated in early breastfeeding terminations (Mercer, Teasley, Hopkinson, et al., 2010).

A newborn's refusal to breastfeed after receiving bottles in the early postdelivery period may be related to a phenomenon referred to as *nipple confusion* or, more accurately termed, *nipple preference*. This potential problem occurs because the techniques for breastfeeding and bottle-feeding are different. In breastfeeding, the baby has to open the mouth very wide in order to latch on to the breast. To transfer milk from the mother's breast to the mouth, the baby has to extend the tongue forward, cupping the nipple and drawing the mother's nipple deep into the baby's mouth until the teat reaches the "comfort zone" near the junction of the baby's hard and soft palates. After the baby creates suction from the tongue and cheeks and seals the latch with the lips, then the baby rhythmically compresses the breast with his or her jaw while the tongue moves in an undulating motion to move fluid toward the baby's pharynx before swallowing, in coordination with breathing. On average, it takes a couple of minutes before the breastfeeding mother's milk flow increases during let-down. With bottle-feeding, the baby keeps the tongue retracted and uses the tip of the tongue to block the flow of milk, which otherwise drips continuously by gravity even when suction is not applied. The bottle-feeding baby merely needs to create suction with his or her mouth on the bottle nipple and the fluid easily flows.

At times there are valid medical indications for supplementing a breastfeeding newborn in the early postpartum period. When supplementation is indicated, the first choice is to use the mother's own milk (fresh, previously expressed, or frozen/ thawed). If maternal milk is not available, pasteurized donor milk is the next choice, and then formula (Jones, 2016). Supplementation can be administered using various methods based on the particular situation, parental preference, and agency policy.

Formula-Feeding

With more attention being placed on promoting and assisting breastfeeding mothers, the teaching needs of the mother who is formula-feeding may inadvertently get overlooked. Nurses may assume that families can simply follow the formula preparation instructions on the side of the formula containers. Parents need teaching, counseling, and support. Parents need to learn about the feeding pattern for a formula-feeding newborn, the intake and output expectations, the recommended type of formula for their baby, how to prepare and store formula, what equipment they will need, feeding technique, and safety precautions.

Formula-Feeding Guidelines and Technique

Commercial formulas are available in three forms: powder, concentrate, and ready-to-feed. There are situations in which one formula may be better to use than another, but in general, convenience and cost usually influence the parents' decision.

- *Powdered formula* is the least expensive type of formula. This formula can be made up one bottle at a time, or multiple bottles can be prepared, but they must be used within 24 to 48 hours. Standard powdered formula is made by adding one level scoop of powdered formula to 60 mL (2 oz) of water. Powdered formulas are not sterile. Powdered formula is made from pasteurized liquid that is then freeze-spray dried into a powder; contamination with microorganisms can occur in the final stages of production. Preparation of any newborn/infant formula, but especially powdered formula, requires careful handling to avoid contamination with microorganisms.

- *Formula concentrate* is more expensive than powder but is not as expensive as ready-to-feed formula. Formula concentrate is commercially sterile. This formula must be diluted with an equal part of water. By adding boiled water that has been cooled, the preparer can maintain sterility.

- *Ready-to-feed* formula is the easiest to use because it does not require any mixing; however, this convenience comes at a cost: it is the most expensive formula. It is indicated for use when adequate water is not available, when the baby is immunocompromised and requires commercially sterile (pasteurized) formula, when an inexperienced baby-sitter will be feeding the baby, and for convenience.

Whatever the type of formula chosen, the nurse should underscore the importance of proper preparation and prompt refrigeration. Parents will need to be briefed on safety precautions during formula preparation. A primary concern is proper mixing to reconstitute formula. Parents need clear instructions to avoid unintentional harm to their baby. Parents should be instructed to follow the directions on the formula container label precisely as written. They should know that adding too much water during preparation dilutes the nutrients and caloric density. This contributes to undernourishment, insufficient weight gain, and possibly water intoxication, which can cause hyponatremia and seizures. Not adding enough water concentrates nutrients and calories and can tax a baby's immature kidneys and digestive system as well as cause dehydration. See Table 25–4 for storage guidelines for formula. See *Teaching Highlights: Sanitary and Safety Precautions for Infant Formula.*

Parents also need guidance about what kind of water to use to reconstitute formula (see Table 25–5 to review types of water sources) and should discuss with their baby's healthcare provider whether to boil the water before use. If boiling is used, parents need to be instructed to heat the water until it reaches a rolling boil, to continue to let the water boil for 1 to 2 minutes,

TABLE 25–5 Water Sources for Reconstituting Formula

TYPE	DESCRIPTION
Distilled water	Minerals and most other impurities have been removed. It will not contain any fluoride. An acceptable water source for reconstituting formula.
Filtered tap water	Some minerals and impurities removed during filtration, including fluoride. This is an acceptable water source for reconstituting formula.
Natural mineral water	Comes from protected groundwater and by law cannot be treated. Naturally contains high levels of minerals and sodium and so is not suitable for babies or for reconstituting formula.
Spring water	Comes from a single nonpolluted groundwater source, but unlike natural mineral water, it can be further treated. Because there is no regulation requiring the mineral content to be printed on the bottle label, it is best to avoid this water source for reconstituting formula.
Tap water	Water from the municipal water supply, and regulated by drinking water regulations. It is treated and considered safe for use in reconstituting formula.
Well water	Needs to be tested before use. Higher risk of nitrate poisoning. Untested water is not recommended for use in reconstituting formula.

TEACHING HIGHLIGHTS | Sanitary Precautions and Safety Precautions for Infant Formula

- Check the expiration date on the formula container.
- Ensure good hand washing before preparing formula; never dip into the can without clean hands.
- Clean bottles, nipples, rings, discs, and bottle caps.
  a. Washing in a dishwasher when available (small items and heat-sensitive items on top rack secured in a basket), or
  b. Boiling briefly (1 to 2 minutes) in a pot of water, or
  c. Cleaning using a microwave sterilization kit, or
  d. Cleaning using very warm soapy water and a nipple and bottle brush.
- Inspect and replace bottle nipples as soon as they show wear; worn nipples can break apart and can become a choking hazard.
- Wash the top of the formula container before piercing the lid.
- Shake the liquid formula well before pouring off the desired amount.
- Shake prepared milk that has been sitting in the refrigerator before feeding.
- Allow tap water to run for 1 minute before obtaining water to use for mixing—this helps clear any lead standing in the pipes. Also, always use cold tap water, because warm water tends to contain higher levels of lead.
- Use only the scoop supplied in the can of formula when formula preparation instructions call for a "scoop" of powdered formula. A scoop should not be "packed" and should be leveled off (e.g., with the back of a knife).

- Do not add anything else to the bottle, except under direction of the baby's healthcare provider.
- Warm the milk in a bottle by placing the bottle in a bowl of warm tap water for no longer than 15 minutes. Do not fill the bowl with water higher than the rim of the bottle. (Infants can take cold formula but most newborns will prefer it warm.)
- Allow freshly prepared (unused) formula to sit out at room temperature for no longer than 2 hours; use an insulated pack to transport formula. Milk left over in the bottle after a feeding should be discarded.
- In warm weather, transport reconstituted formula or concentrate from an open can in an insulated pack with frozen gel packs.
- Travel with water and formula separated; carry premeasured water bottles and bottles with premeasured amounts of powdered formula, or carry premeasured commercially prepared formula packets, or have the can of formula available.
- Holding the baby during feeding (even when the infant can hold the bottle) promotes bonding and prevents supine feedings.
- Do not allow the baby to formula-feed in a supine position because this increases the risk of otitis media and dental caries in the older infant.
- Never prop a bottle—this is a choking hazard.
- Allow babies to take what they want and to stop when they want. Overeeding can lead to obesity.

and, most important, to allow the water to cool before using it to reconstitute the formula. Parents should also be instructed not to let the water boil down to a low level in the pan because this can cause minerals in the water to become concentrated.

Use of distilled bottle water and filtered tap water raises concerns with regard to fluoride. The American Academy of Pediatrics recommends that no fluoride supplements be given to a baby before 6 months of age (AAP & ACOG, 2012). Parents should be encouraged to read the labels on bottled water to see if fluoride has been added and to determine if the water source is suitable depending on the baby's age.

BOTTLES AND NIPPLES

Parents often have questions about the kind of bottles and nipples to purchase. Many newly designed bottles are marketed to lessen air intake while the baby feeds. No one particular bottle design is best for all babies. A key point to emphasize to the families is feeding technique. Parents should try to avoid situations in which the baby is crying for a prolonged time. Crying results in increased ingestion of air even before the baby has started feeding. Babies who are very hungry also gulp more air. For these situations, instruct the parents to burp their baby frequently to prevent the baby from having a large emesis (Figure 25–30 and Figure 25–31). The parents may want to pat the baby's back briefly before starting the feeding to calm a crying baby and possibly burp the baby as well. Another tip to avoid excessive ingestion of air is to have the parent hold the baby cradled in his or her arms while bottle-feeding and tilt the bottle at a 45-degree angle in order for fluid to cover the nipple. This prevents the baby from sucking in air and swallowing it. The vented bottle design eliminates the negative effects of a vacuum and channels air through an internal vent system above the milk, avoiding air bubbles in the milk. Figure 25–32 shows a baby bottle-feeding.

Parents will want to consider a slow-flow nipple for all newborns and for older breastfeeding infants learning to formula-feed—over time the baby will graduate to medium-flow and high-flow nipples. Nipples come in different shapes. Generally, nipple shape plays a greater importance for breastfeeding babies receiving expressed breast milk or supplemental formula in a bottle. Breastfed babies transition best going from breast to bottle and back to breast again when using a bottle nipple that has a relatively wide base (to help maintain a wide open latch) and a medium to long nipple length. Another variable to consider is nipple construction. Nipples are generally made from either rubber or silicone. Families with a history of sensitivity to latex are advised to use silicone nipples. Silicone nipples also have less of an odor, which may be an issue for some babies who are breastfed.

To know if a newborn is bottle-feeding well, the nurse needs to observe a bottle-feeding session. Parents should be informed that if the baby is sucking effectively, they should observe bubbles rising in the fluid of standard bottles. (If a family is using vented bottles or bottles with liners that retract as fluid is removed, bubbles will not be detected.) No bubbles will be observed if the parent unintentionally places the bottle nipple under the baby's tongue, preventing the baby from sucking effectively. Some newborns, especially premature babies, raise the tongue to the roof of the mouth and so it is sometimes a challenge to place the nipple on top of the tongue. Newborns who persistently leak milk from the side of the mouth may be getting fluid too quickly. The nurse could suggest using a slower-flowing nipple. If symptoms persist, the baby should have an oral evaluation. The baby could have a short lingual frenulum (be tongue-tied) and not be able to properly cup the tongue under the nipple and channel fluid to the back of the

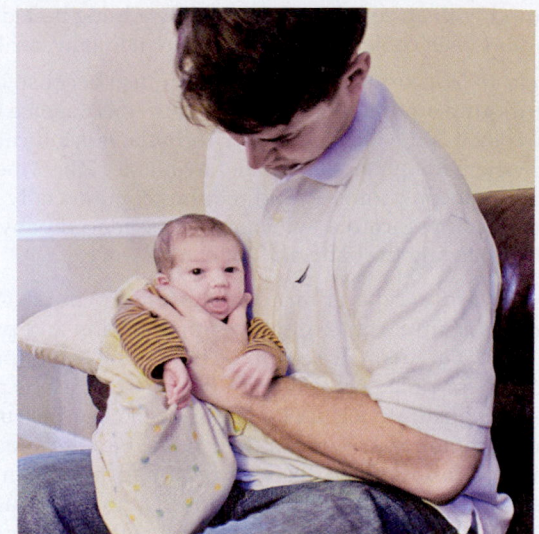

Figure 25–30 Burping baby sitting up on lap.
SOURCE: Brigitte Hall, RNC, MSN, IBCLC.

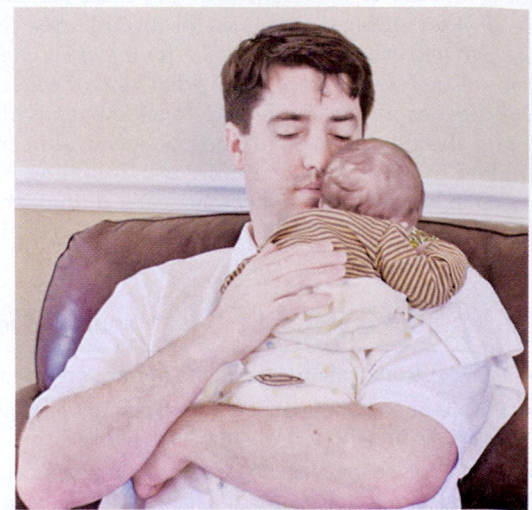

Figure 25–31 Burping baby over the shoulder.
SOURCE: Brigitte Hall, RNC, MSN, IBCLC.

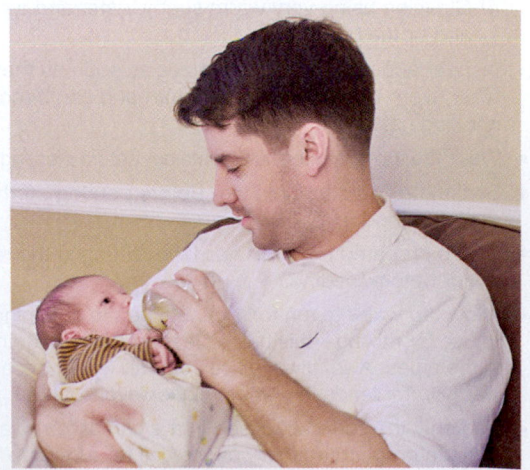

Figure 25–32 Bottle-feeding.
SOURCE: Brigitte Hall, RNC, MSN, IBCLC.

throat, or may have an oral–motor dysfunction and need speech therapy or occupational therapy evaluation.

There is still concern regarding specific chemicals used in the manufacture of plastic baby bottles, the material used in lining formula cans, sippy cups, microwavable containers, and soft plastics such as bisphenol-A (BPA) that could leach from polycarbonate plastic used in the manufacture of some baby bottles and transfer into the baby's milk (U.S. Food and Drug Administration [USFDA], 2016).

SAFETY ALERT!

Parents need to be instructed to read product labels to see if the merchandise they are purchasing is free of potentially harmful chemicals. If product labels do not explicitly state that they are free of these chemicals, then it cannot be assumed they are BPA-free, PVC-free, lead-free, and phthalates-free.

If parents cannot afford to purchase new BPA-free bottles, then encourage them to limit heating the bottles (avoid using the dishwasher and bottle warmers) and to throw out old bottles and nipples with scratches. The harmful chemicals are leached most when the plastic is heated or damaged.

Involving Fathers/Partners

Our traditional view of the family following the birth of a child places most of the attention on the mother and newborn, often-times leaving the father/partner out. Nurses need to recognize this and make every effort to speak to both parents when entering the baby's room. Fathers/partners play a vital role in the family by providing support to the mother and care for their newborn. If a mother has chosen not to breastfeed, the father/partner can be involved with bottle-feedings from the start. However, if the mother is breastfeeding, it is important to ask the father/partner to wait to introduce a bottle until the mother's milk supply and breastfeeding are well established. The father/partner can be encouraged to assist with breastfeeding in the meantime by helping the mother get in position and helping tweak the baby's latch if the mother complains of any discomfort. The father/partner can also massage the mother's breasts during breastfeeding to help stimulate the sleepy baby to feed better and to relieve any engorgement.

The father/partner can help with other aspects too, such as burping the baby, changing diapers, and bathing and comforting the baby. The father/partner can also provide skin-to-skin contact that enhances bonding, provides comfort to the newborn, and calms the baby down before offering the breast. One strategy is to have the father/partner hold the baby vertically on the chest and let the baby suck on a clean finger for a minute or so (see Figure 25–33). These are just a few ways to involve the father/partner after the birth of the baby. These interactions promote family bonding and are important for paternal/maternal role development.

Promotion of Successful Newborn Breastfeeding

With the trend toward earlier discharge from the birthing center, there is limited time for inpatient education. Teaching moments, when they occur, may not be optimal because of the distraction of visitors and the mother's being sleep deprived, uncomfortable, or under the effects of an analgesic. It is important that parents receive verbal and written instructions and community resource information to which they can later refer. (See Chapter 29 for a complete discussion of self-care measures

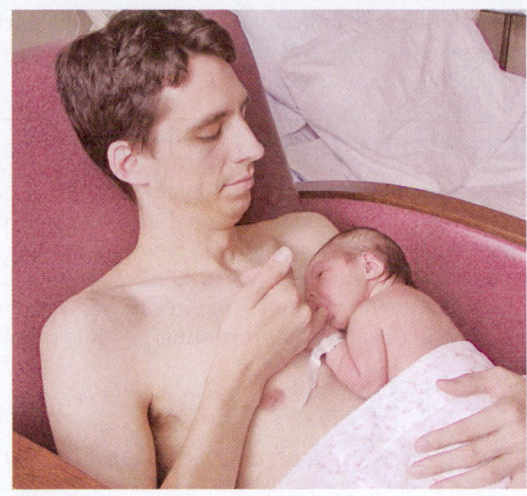

Figure 25–33 Father and newborn skin-to-skin.

SOURCE: Brigitte Hall, RNC, MSN, IBCLC.

the nurse can suggest to a woman with a breastfeeding problem after discharge from the birthing center.)

To promote a supportive hospital environment for breast-feeding, the Baby-Friendly Hospital Initiative recognizes hospitals and birthing centers that offer optimal lactation services and comply with the 10 steps outlined in Table 25–6. Baby-Friendly status is not easy to achieve. One obstacle to achieving Baby-Friendly status, among many, is the requirement that agencies agree to not accept free or low-cost formula. As of March 2016, there were approximately 340 hospitals in the United States with the Baby-Friendly designation, according to an update on the Baby-Friendly Hospital Initiative USA website (Baby-Friendly Hospital Initiative USA, 2016).

Breastfeeding mothers who work outside the home and are supported in their decision tend to breastfeed their babies for longer periods than mothers who work but do not receive support. A baby-friendly workplace needs to be seen as a valuable item in a benefit package offered by a company. Families

TABLE 25–6 Baby-Friendly Requirements

BABY-FRIENDLY 10 STEPS TO SUCCESSFUL BREASTFEEDING
• Have a written breastfeeding policy that is routinely communicated to all healthcare staff.
• Train all healthcare staff in skills necessary to implement this policy.
• Inform all pregnant women about the benefits and management of breastfeeding.
• Help mothers initiate breastfeeding within one hour of birth.
• Show mothers how to breastfeed and maintain lactation, even if they should be separated from their babies.
• Give newborns no food or drink other than breast milk, unless medically indicated.
• Practice rooming in—that is, allow mothers and newborns to remain together 24 hours a day.
• Encourage breastfeeding on demand.
• Give no artificial teats or pacifiers (also called dummies or soothers) to breastfeeding babies.
• Foster the establishment of breastfeeding support groups and refer mothers to them on discharge from the hospital or clinic.

Source: World Health Organization/United Nations Children's Emergency Fund (WHO/UNICEF). (2010). *U.S. committee for UNICEF interim program in the United States to promote the Baby-Friendly ten steps to successful breastfeeding.* Washington, DC: Government Printing Office.

and nurses who believe in breastfeeding need to be part of the solution to breastfeeding and workplace issues by educating employers in their communities.

Preparation for Discharge

Although the adjustment to parenting is a normal process, going home presents a critical transition for the family. The parents become the primary caregivers for the newborn and must provide a nurturing environment in which the emotional and physical needs of the newborn can be met. Nursing interventions focus on promoting health and preventing possible problems.

Nursing Management

For the Newborn in Preparation for Discharge

Nursing Assessment and Diagnosis

When preparing for discharge, assess whether parents have realistic expectations of the newborn's behavior and the depth of their knowledge in caring for their newborn.

Nursing diagnoses that may apply to the newborn's family include the following (NANDA-I © 2014):

- *Parenting, Readiness for Enhanced,* related to appropriate behavioral expectations for the newborn
- *Family Processes, Readiness for Enhanced,* related to integration of newborn into family unit or demands of newborn care and feeding.

Planning and Implementation

PARENT TEACHING

To meet the parents' need for information, the nurse who is responsible for the care of the mother and newborn should assume the primary responsibility for parent education. Nearly every contact with the parents presents an opportunity for sharing information that can facilitate their sense of competence in newborn care. You will need to recognize and respect the many good ways of providing safe care. Unless their care methods are harmful to the newborn, the parents' methods of giving care should be reinforced rather than contradicted.

The information that follows is provided to increase your knowledge of newborn care and can also be used to meet parents' needs for information. If they are new parents, gently teach them by example and provide instructions geared to their needs and previous knowledge about the various aspects of newborn care.

Observe how parents interact with their newborn during feeding and caregiving activities. Even during a short stay, there are opportunities to provide information and observe whether the parents are comfortable with changing the diapers of, wrapping, handling, and feeding their newborn (Figure 25–34). Do both parents get involved in the newborn's care? Is the mother depending on someone else to help her at home? Does the mother give reasons (e.g., "I'm too tired," "My stitches hurt," or "I'll learn later") for not wanting to be involved in her baby's care? As the family provides care, enhance parental confidence by giving them positive feedback. If the parents encounter problems, express confidence in their abilities to master the new skill or information, suggest alternatives, and serve as a role model. All these factors need to be considered when evaluating the educational needs of the parents. Providing mother–baby care and home care instruction on the night shift as well as during the day assists with education needs for early discharge parents.

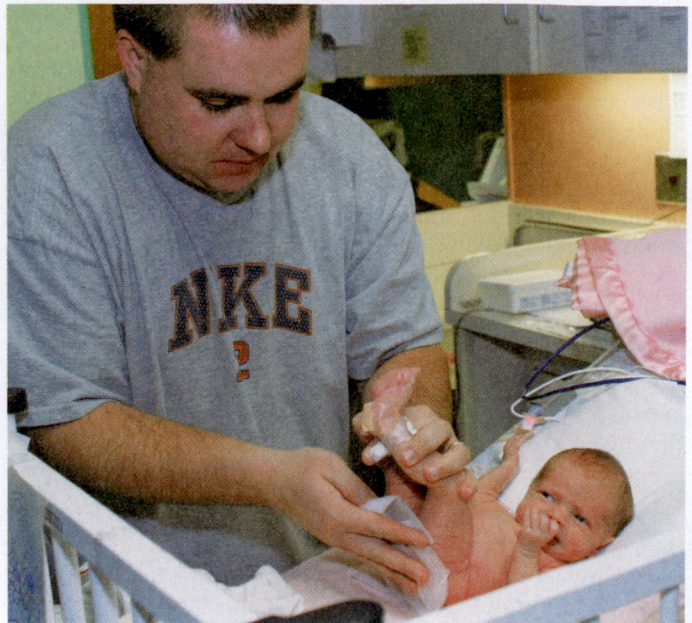

Figure 25–34 A father demonstrates competence and confidence in diapering his newborn daughter.

One-to-one teaching while you are in the mother's room is the most effective educational method, rated as such by both first-time and experienced postpartum parents. With shorter stays, most teaching unfortunately tends to focus on infant feeding and immediate physical care needs of the mother, with limited anticipatory guidance provided in other areas. To address this deficit, see *Teaching Highlights: What to Tell Parents About Newborn Care,* which includes a broad range of information important to share with new parents.

Clinical Tip

For mothers who are hearing impaired, videotapes with information in both spoken and signed formats are most helpful. Birthing centers should have handouts available for families who do not speak English and for the birthing center that does not have interpreters (not family members) or language interpreter phones.

GENERAL INSTRUCTIONS FOR NEWBORN CARE

One of the first concerns of anyone who has not had the experience of picking up a baby is how to do it correctly. The newborn is easily picked up by sliding one hand under the neck and shoulders and the other hand under the buttocks or between the newborn's legs and then gently lifting upward. This technique provides security and support for the head (which the newborn is unable to support until 3 or 4 months of age).

You must be an excellent role model for families in the area of safety. Safety topics include proper positioning of the newborn on the back to sleep and correct use of the bulb syringe. The baby should never be left alone anywhere but in the crib. Remind the mother that while she and her newborn are together in the birthing unit, she should never leave her baby alone for security reasons and because newborns spit up frequently the first day or two after birth. Other newborn safety measures are discussed in detail in Chapter 29.

| TEACHING HIGHLIGHTS | What to Tell Parents About Newborn Care |

Immediate Safety Measures for the Newborn

- Watch for excessive mucus: use a bulb syringe to remove mucus.
- Have baby sleep on the back in a crib or in someone's arms.

Voiding and Stool Characteristics and Patterns

- Urine is straw to amber color without foul smell. Small amounts of uric acid crystals are normal in first days of life (may be mistaken by parents as blood in diaper because of reddish "brick dust" appearance).
- At least 6 to 10 wet diapers a day after the first few days of life.
- Normal progression of stool changes: (1) meconium (thick, tarry, dark green); (2) transitional stools (thin, brown to green); (3a) breastfed baby: yellow gold, soft or mushy stools; (3b) formula-fed baby: pale yellow, formed and pasty stools.
- Only one to two stools a day for formula-fed baby.
- Six to 10 small, loose yellow stools per day or only one stool every few days after breastfeeding is well established (after about 1 month).

Cord Care

- Wash hands with clean water before and after care.
- Keep the cord dry and exposed to air or loosely covered with clean clothes. (If cultural custom demands binding of the abdomen, a sanitary method such as the use of a clean piece of gauze can be recommended.)
- Clean the cord and skin around the base with a cotton swab or cotton ball. Clean two to three times a day or with each diaper change. Touching the cord, applying unclean substances to it, and applying bandages should be avoided. Do not give tub baths until the cord falls off in 7 to 14 days.
- Fold diapers below the umbilical cord to air-dry the cord (contact with wet or soiled diapers slows the drying process and increases the possibility of infection).
- Check the cord each day for any odor, oozing of greenish yellow material, or reddened areas around the cord. Expect tenderness around the cord and darkening and shriveling of the cord. Report to the healthcare provider any signs of infection.
- Normal changes in cord: The cord should look dark and dry up before falling off. A small drop of blood may present when the cord falls off.
- Never pull the cord or attempt to loosen it.

Circumcision Care

- Squeeze water over the circumcision site once a day.
- Rinse the area off with warm water and pat dry.
- Apply a small amount of petroleum jelly (unless a Plastibell is in place) with each diaper change.
- Fasten a diaper over the penis snugly enough so that it does not move and rub the tender glans.
- Because the glans is sensitive, avoid placing baby on the stomach for the first day after the procedure.
- Check for any foul-smelling drainage or bleeding at least once a day.
- Let the Plastibell fall off by itself (about 8 days after circumcision). It should not be pulled off.
- Light, sticky, yellow drainage (part of healing process) may form over the head of the penis.

Uncircumcised Care

- Clean the uncircumcised penis with water during diaper changes and with bath.
- Do not force the foreskin back over the penis; foreskin will retract normally over time (may take 3 to 5 years).

Techniques for Waking Baby

- Loosen clothing, change diaper.
- Hand-express milk onto baby's lips.
- Talk with baby while making eye contact.
- Hold baby in upright position (sitting or standing).
- Have baby do sit-ups (gently and rhythmically bend baby back and forth while grasping the baby under his or her knees and supporting baby's head and back with your other hand).
- Play patty-cake with baby.
- Stimulate the rooting reflex (brush one cheek with a hand or nipple).
- Increase skin contact (gently rub hands and feet).

Techniques for Quieting Baby

- Check for a soiled diaper.
- Hold swaddled baby upright against midchest, supporting the bottom and back of head. Baby can hear heartbeat, feel warmth, and hear your softly spoken words or calming sounds.
- Use slow, calming movements with baby.
- Softly talk, sing, or hum to baby.

Signs of Illness

See *Key Facts to Remember: When Parents Should Call Their Healthcare Provider*

Demonstrating a bath (see Chapter 29), cord care, and temperature assessment is the best way to provide information on these topics to parents.

Demonstrate and review the taking of axillary or tympanic temperatures and discourage the use of mercury thermometers. It is important that families understand the differences and know how to select a thermometer. The newborn's temperature needs to be taken only when signs of illness are present. Advise parents to call their healthcare provider or pediatric nurse practitioner immediately if they observe any signs of illness.

Nasal and Oral Suctioning

Most newborns are obligatory nose breathers for the first months of life. They generally maintain air passage patency by coughing or sneezing. During the first few days of life, however, the newborn has increased mucus, and gentle suctioning with a bulb syringe may be indicated—but only in cases of obvious obstruction. The newborn's mouth should be suctioned first so that there is nothing to aspirate if the newborn gasps when the nose is suctioned (AAP & ACOG, 2012). Demonstrate the use of the bulb syringe in the mouth and nose and have the parents do a return demonstration. The parents should repeat this demonstration of suctioning and cleansing the bulb before discharge so they feel confident in performing the procedure. Care should be taken to apply only gentle suction to prevent nasal bleeding.

To suction the newborn, the bulb syringe is compressed before the tip is placed in the nostril. Take care not to occlude the passageway. The bulb is permitted to re-expand slowly by releasing the compression on the bulb (Figure 25–35). The bulb syringe is removed from the nostril, and drainage is then compressed out of the bulb and onto a tissue. The bulb syringe may also be used in the mouth if the newborn is spitting up and unable to handle the excess secretions. The bulb is compressed, the tip of the bulb syringe is placed about 1 inch to one side of the newborn's mouth, and compression is released. This draws up the excess secretions. The procedure is repeated on the other side of the mouth. The roof of the mouth and the back of the throat are avoided because suction in these areas might stimulate the gag reflex.

The bulb syringe should be washed in warm, soapy water and rinsed in warm water daily and as needed after use. Rinsing with a half-strength white vinegar solution followed by clear water may help to extend the useful life of the bulb syringe by inhibiting bacterial growth. A bulb syringe should always be kept near the newborn. New parents who are inexperienced with babies may fear that the baby will choke and are relieved to know how to take action if such an event occurs. They should

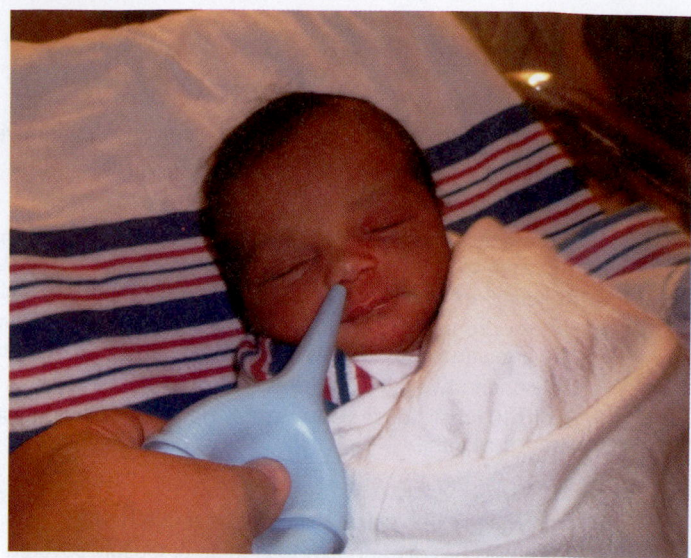

Figure 25–35 Nasal and oral suctioning. The bulb is compressed, the tip is placed in either the mouth or the nose, and the bulb is released.

SOURCE: Michele Davidson.

be advised to turn the newborn's head to the side or hold the newborn with the head down as soon as there is any indication of gagging or vomiting and to use the bulb syringe as needed. (See *Clinical Skill: Performing Nasal Pharyngeal Suctioning* in Chapter 18). Some newborns may have transient edema of the nasal mucosa following suctioning of the airway after birth. Demonstrate the use of normal saline to loosen secretions, and instruct parents in the gentle and moderate use of the bulb syringe to avoid further irritation of the mucous membranes. If parents will be using humidifiers at home, instruct them to follow the manufacturer's cleaning instructions carefully so that molds, spores, and bacteria from a dirty humidifier do not enter the baby's environment.

SAFETY ALERT!
You will find that left-handed people tend to hold the baby over their right shoulder, and right-handed people do the opposite. This keeps the dominant hand free. However, most health personnel wear their name tags on the left side. To avoid scratching the baby's face, wear your name tag on the same side as your dominant hand.

Sleep and Activity

The National Institute of Child Health and Human Development and the American Academy of Pediatrics recommend that healthy term babies be placed on their backs to sleep. Teach parents the importance of following "Safe to Sleep Guidelines" to reduce the incidence of sudden infant death syndrome (SIDS) (Healthy Children, 2015f). No evidence exists that babies need to be placed on their sides initially because of copious or thick secretions. Placing babies on their backs in the newborn period serves to educate parents regarding proper positioning. Studies indicate that parents position their babies in the same positions they observe in the hospital setting, so nurses must demonstrate this behavior to reduce the risk of SIDS. If exceptions are warranted, these should be explained to families so they do not misinterpret what they observe. The placement of babies in a prone position during supervised wakeful play sessions or "tummy time" should be encouraged as well (AAP, 2014). Providing regular periods of tummy time enhances a baby's gross motor skills and upper body strength and reduces the incidence of positional plagiocephaly. Also encourage parents to hold their babies and not allow them to remain in infant carriers for prolonged periods of time.

Healthy People 2020

(MICH-21) Increase the proportion of infants who are put to sleep on their backs

Perhaps nothing is more individual to each baby than the sleep–activity cycle. It is important to recognize the individual variations of each newborn and to assist parents as they develop sensitivity to their baby's communication signals and rhythms of activity and sleep. See Chapter 23 for a detailed discussion of sleep–wake activity.

Car Safety Considerations

Half of the children killed or injured in automobile crashes could have been protected by the use of federally approved car seats. Newborns must go home from the birthing unit in a car seat adapted to fit them (Figure 25–36). Babies should never be placed in the front seat of a car equipped with a passenger-side airbag. The car seat should be positioned to face the rear of the car until the baby is 2 years old, or until they reach maximum height and weight for their seat (Healthy Children, 2015c). Ensure that all parents are knowledgeable about the benefits of child safety seat use and proper installation. Encourage parents to have their infant safety seats checked by local groups trained specifically for that purpose. The Seat Check Initiative provides locations and information about child safety seats.

NEWBORN SCREENING AND IMMUNIZATION PROGRAMS

Before the newborn and mother are discharged from the birthing unit, inform the parents about **newborn screening tests** and tell them when to return to the birthing center or clinic if further tests are needed. Newborn screening tests include the following:

- Blood spot screening, which allows for diagnosis of many disorders that might otherwise go unidentified and untreated in children. The number of disorders screened differs slightly from state to state.
- Hearing screening
- Hyperbilirubinemia screening
- Critical congenital heart disease screening

For information on the specific disorders tested for in your state, you can visit the website of the National Newborn Screening and Genetic Resource Center (Genetics Home Reference, 2015). It is the responsibility of the nursing staff to see that these screening tests are completed by the time of discharge and that the parents understand the need for follow-up tests where indicated (AAP, 2011).

Hearing loss is found in 1 to 3 per 1000 babies in the normal newborn population (Healthy Children, 2015d). Hearing screenings before discharge are now conducted in all 50 states. The recommended initial newborn hearing screening should be accomplished before discharge from the birthing unit with appropriate follow-up if the newborn fails to pass the initial screen in all hospitals providing obstetric services.

Sometimes newborns fail to pass these tests for reasons other than hearing loss. Amniotic fluid in the ear canals is a frequent cause of suboptimal test results. In these cases, babies are retested in a week or two. The current goal is to screen all newborns by 1 month of age, confirm hearing loss with audiologic examination by 3 months of age, and treat with comprehensive early intervention services before 6 months of age (Centers for Disease Control and Prevention [CDC], 2015a). Typically, screening programs use a two-stage screening approach (otoacoustic emissions [OAE] repeated twice, OAE followed by auditory brainstem response [ABR], or automated ABR repeated twice). Families need to be educated about appropriate interpretation of screening test results and appropriate steps for follow-up (Figure 25–37).

Immunization programs against the hepatitis B virus during the newborn period and infancy are in place in many states, at least 20 countries, and high-incidence areas such as American

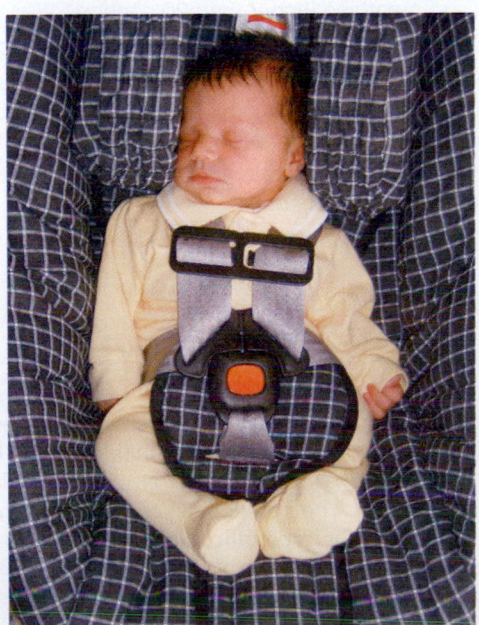

Figure 25–36 An infant car restraint such as this one should be used from birth to about 24 months of age.

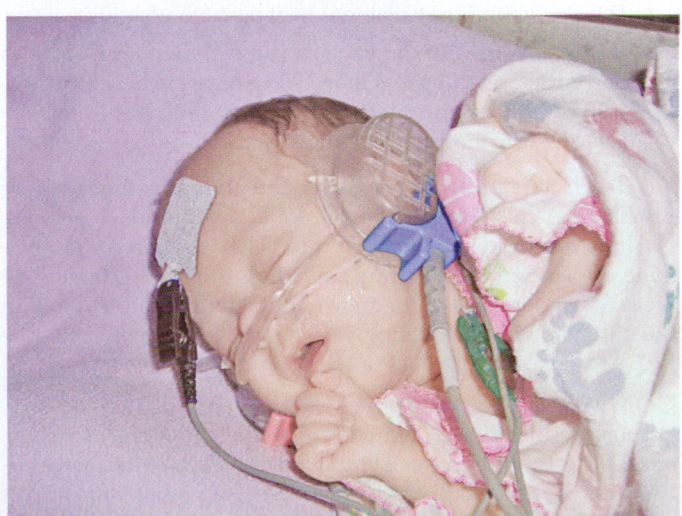

Figure 25–37 Newborn hearing screen.
SOURCE: Vanessa Howell, RN, MSN.

Samoa. Universal vaccination of newborns/infants is recommended. Parents need to be advised whether their birthing center provides newborn hepatitis vaccination so that an adequate follow-up program can be set in motion (AAP & ACOG, 2012). Recombinant hepatitis B vaccine (Engerix-B, Recombivax HB) is used as a prophylactic treatment against all subtypes of hepatitis B virus. It provides passive immunization for newborns of HBsAg-negative and HBsAg-positive mothers. Hepatitis B can be transmitted across the placenta, but most newborns are infected during birth. Delay administration during active infection, as the vaccine will not prevent infection during its incubation period.

The vaccine is produced from baker's yeast and plasmid containing the HBsAg gene. Hepatitis B (thimerosal-free) vaccine contains more than 95% HBsAg protein and is an inactivated (noninfective) product. Newborns of HBsAg-positive mothers should concurrently receive 0.5 mL of hepatitis B immunoglobulin (HBIG) prophylaxis at separate injection sites (CDC, 2015b; Wilson et al., 2015). The dosing schedule is dependent on the mother's status as shown below:

- The first dose of 0.5 mL (10 mcg) is given intramuscularly into the anterolateral thigh within 12 hours of birth for babies born to HBsAg-positive mothers. The second dose of vaccine is given at least 1 month after the first dose and followed by a final dose at least 4 months after the first dose and at least 3 months after the second dose, but not before 6 months of age (CDC, 2015b).

- Babies born to HBsAg-negative mothers receive their first dose of vaccine at birth, the second dose at 1 to 2 months, and the third dose at 6 to 18 months (AAP & ACOG, 2012).

- Newborns whose mother's HBsAg status is unknown should receive the same doses of vaccine as babies born to HBsAg-positive mothers.

The only common side effect is soreness at the injection site. Occasionally, there is erythema, swelling, warmth, and induration at the injection site, irritability, or a low-grade fever (37.7°C [99.8°F]). Nursing considerations include:

- The vaccine should be used as supplied. Do not dilute. Shake well.

- Do not inject intravenously or intradermally.

- Monitor for adverse reactions. Monitor temperature closely.

- Have epinephrine available to treat possible allergic reactions.

- Responsiveness to the vaccine is age dependent. Preterm newborns weighing less than 1000 g have lower seroconversion rates. Consider delaying the first dose until the baby is term postconceptual age (PCA) or use a 4-dose schedule.

Teach the family all necessary caregiving methods before discharge. A checklist may be helpful to determine whether the teaching has been completed and to verify the parents' knowledge on leaving the birthing unit (Figure 25–38). Review all areas for understanding or answer outstanding questions with the parents, without rushing, and take time to resolve all queries. Any concerns of yours or the parents should be noted.

COMMUNITY-BASED NURSING CARE

Discuss with parents ways to meet their newborn's needs, ensure safety, and appreciate the newborn's unique characteristics and behaviors. By assisting parents in establishing links with their community-based healthcare provider, you can get the new family off to a good start.

Community-based support for breastfeeding mothers often focuses on breastfeeding support groups. **La Leche League International (LLLI)** is the first (not-for-profit international educational and service organization) mother-to-mother breastfeeding support group formally recognized in the United States. It also has expanded to provide educational breastfeeding conferences for professionals, and it is one of the few organizations to have a peer counselor breastfeeding training program, among other things. Encourage mothers to visit the International Lactation Consultant Association (ILCA) website to find lactation consultants in their geographic areas. Another professional organization, the Academy of Breastfeeding Medicine (ABM), provides many research-based breastfeeding protocols. To access the protocols, visit the ABM website. Many hospitals around the country have lactation programs and may provide lactation services for a fee to anyone seeking services.

Parents need to know the signs of illness, how to reach the pediatrician or after-hours clinic, and the importance of follow-up after discharge. Parents should also check with their healthcare provider for advice about over-the-counter medications to be kept on hand. See *Key Facts to Remember: When Parents Should Call Their Healthcare Provider*.

The family should have the healthcare provider's phone number and address, and any specific instructions. Having the birthing unit or nursery phone number is also reassuring to a newborn's family. Encourage them to call with questions. Follow-up calls lend added support by providing another opportunity for parents to have their questions answered.

KEY FACTS TO REMEMBER
When Parents Should Call Their Healthcare Provider

- Temperature above 38.0°C (100.4°F) axillary or below 36.6°C (97.8°F) axillary
- Continuous rise in temperature
- More than one episode of forceful vomiting or frequent vomiting over a 6-hour period
- Refusal of two feedings in a row
- Lethargy (listlessness), difficulty in awakening baby
- Cyanosis (bluish discoloration of skin) with or without a feeding
- Absence of breathing longer than 20 seconds
- Inconsolable baby (quieting techniques are not effective) or continuous high-pitched cry
- Discharge or bleeding from umbilical cord, circumcision, or any opening (except vaginal mucus or pseudomenstruation)
- Two consecutive green, watery stools or black stools or increased frequency of stools
- No wet diapers for 18 to 24 hours or fewer than six to eight wet diapers per day after 4 days of age
- Development of eye drainage
- Yellowing of skin (jaundice)

The follow-up newborn examination should be within 48 hours of discharge. When the family is unable to visit their primary care healthcare provider within that time period, a home visit should be made. The home visit focuses on normal newborn care, assessment for hyperbilirubinemia (jaundice), extreme weight loss, feeding problems, and knowledge related to newborn care and feeding within the family unit. (For a detailed discussion of home care and the home visit, see Chapter 29.)

Routine well-baby visits should be scheduled with the clinic, pediatric nurse practitioner, or healthcare provider. Regardless of the type of follow-up services available in the community, you must contribute to the newborn's health by stressing the importance of routine care and by helping families who have no follow-up plans to connect to local resources for care.

Evaluation

When evaluating the nursing care provided in preparation for discharge, the following outcomes may be anticipated:

- The parents demonstrate safe techniques in caring for their newborn.
- Parents verbalize developmentally appropriate behavioral expectations of their newborn and knowledge of community-based newborn follow-up care.

NEWBORN CARE TEACHING CHECKLIST

Please read the *New Baby* booklet and view the film before completing this checklist. In the **Need Teaching** column, check off the areas in which you would like further instruction, advice, or demonstration.

	Need Teaching	Teaching Done	Nurse's Initials/Date
Breastfeeding			
Positioning			
Latching on			
Removing baby from nipple			
Let-down reflex			
Supply and demand concept			
How often and for how long			
Knowing if baby is getting enough			
Supplementing			
Expressing milk by hand			
Going back to work while breastfeeding			
Formula Feeding			
Feeding baby a bottle			
Cleaning bottles and nipples			
Choosing a formula			
Preparing formula			
Demand feeding			
Baby Care			
Positioning baby after feeding			
Burping			
Bathing			
Caring for circumcision/genital/umbilical area			
Taking baby's temperature—when to call the doctor			
Using a bulb syringe			
Elimination—what to expect			
Checking for signs of jaundice			
Caring for skin, rashes, milia			
Comforting crying baby			
Signs that baby is sick			
Positioning in crib (Safe to Sleep)			
Safety			
Baby is choking or gagging—what to do			
Shaken baby syndrome			
Newborn screening tests and immunizations			
Using infant car seat			

Other Concerns:	
	Language spoken by mother:
	_____
	Was an interpreter used?
	_____
I understand the teaching instructions given on the specified topics and have no further questions.	Nurse's signature(s):
	_____
Mother's Signature	_____
Date:_____	Date:_____

Figure 25–38 A newborn care teaching checklist is completed before discharge.

SOURCE: Adapted from Presbyterian/St. Luke's medical Center, Denver, CO.

Focus Your Study

- The overall goal of newborn nursing care is to provide comprehensive care while promoting the establishment of a well-functioning family unit.

- The period immediately following birth, during which adaptation to extrauterine life occurs, requires close monitoring to identify any deviations from normal.

- Nursing goals during the first hours after birth (admission and transitional period) are to maintain a clear airway and stable vital signs, maintain a neutral thermal environment, prevent hemorrhage and infection, perform early assessment of neonatal distress, initiate oral feedings, and facilitate attachment.

- The newborn is routinely given prophylactic vitamin K to prevent possible hemorrhagic disease of the newborn.

- Prophylactic eye treatment for *Neisseria gonorrhoeae* is legally required on all newborns.

- Nursing goals in daily newborn care include maintaining cardiopulmonary function, maintaining a neutral thermal environment, promoting adequate hydration and nutrition, preventing complications, promoting safety, and enhancing attachment and family knowledge of child care.

- Following a circumcision, the newborn must be observed closely for signs of bleeding, inability to void, and signs of infection.

- A weight loss of more than 10% is excessive and requires an evaluation and follow-up. Newborns should be back to their birth weight by 10 to 14 days of age. Generally, babies double their birth weight by 5 months, triple their birth weight by 1 year of age, and quadruple their birth weight by 2 years.

- Increases in body length and head circumference for breastfed versus formula-fed babies are the same. A baby gains 1.0 inch per month in the first 6 months, and then 0.5 in. each month for the following 6 months. Length is a better indicator of growth than is weight.

- The American Academy of Pediatrics (AAP) recommends exclusive breastfeeding for the first 6 months and continued breastfeeding until the infant is 1 year old or older.

- Human milk has immunologic and nutritional properties that make it the optimal food for the first year of life.

- Mature breast milk and standard commercially prepared formulas provide 20 kcal/oz.

- Neither cow's milk nor soy milk should be given to babies before 1 year of age. The use of skim milk or low-fat cow's milk is not recommended for children under 2 years old.

- The formula-feeding mother may need help learning about the types of formulas and how to prepare and store formula. Like the breastfeeding mother, she will benefit from understanding feeding cues and proper technique for feeding her baby.

- Most maternal medications are transmitted through human milk to some degree, but few are actually contraindicated. The bioavailability of transmitted drugs to the baby depends on a variety of factors, including route of administration, protein binding, degree of ionization, molecular weight, timing of the dose with respect to feeding time, and absorption across the baby's intestinal tract.

- Signs indicating a newborn's readiness to feed include hand-to-mouth movements, rooting, smacking, fussing, and crying (a late-feeding cue).

- Breastfeeding mothers should be taught to use proper positioning and latch-on techniques and advised to alternate feeding positions periodically to promote efficient drainage of all the ducts in the breast.

- The nurse must be sensitive to cultural beliefs and values of the family and be aware of cultural variation regarding newborn/infant feeding practices.

- During the first few days after birth, the minimum output expectations for an exclusively breastfeeding newborn are the following: one wet/one stool on day 1; two wets/two stools on day 2; three wets/three to four stools on day 3; four wets/three to four stools on day 4; five wets/three to four stools on day 5. Thereafter, an exclusively breastfeeding newborn has a minimum of six to eight wet diapers and three to four yellow stools each day, generally during the first month of life.

- Newborn's stools start as black and sticky at birth and transition to yellow, curdy, or seedy by day 5, or sooner.

- Essential daily care includes assessing vital signs, weight, overall color, intake, output, umbilical cord and circumcision, newborn nutrition, parent education, and attachment.

- Individual birthing units should practice safety measures to prevent newborn abduction and provide information to parents regarding their role in this area and in general newborn safety measures.

- Signs of illness in newborns include temperature above 38°C (100.4°F) axillary or below 36.6°C (97.8°F) axillary, more than one episode of forceful vomiting, refusal of two feedings in a row, lethargy, cyanosis with or without a feeding, and absence of breathing for longer than 20 seconds.

- Newborn blood spot screening may be done on all newborns in the first 1 to 3 days. Hearing screening and critical congenital heart disease screening may be completed before discharge.

Clinical Reasoning in Action

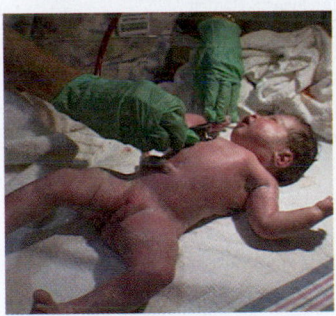

Alice Fine, age 32, G1, now P1001, spontaneously delivers a 7.25–lb baby girl over a median episiotomy. The baby's Apgars are 7 and 9 at 1 and 5 minutes. The baby is suctioned, stimulated, and given free-flow oxygen at birth. As the nurse on duty, you admit baby Fine to the newborn nursery, place her under a radiant heater, and perform a newborn assessment. You obtain the vital signs of temperature 97°F, heart rate 128, respirations 55. A physical examination demonstrates no abnormalities, and you note that there were no significant problems with the pregnancy, the mother's blood type is A+, and she plans to bottle-feed. You monitor the baby until her vital signs are stable and then take her to the mother's room for her first bottle-feeding at 60 minutes old.

1. How would you review measures to promote the safety of the newborn from abduction?
2. How would you explain the technique to suction the newborn with a bulb syringe?
3. Describe the care of the newborn's cord.
4. How would you review breastfeeding and/or bottle-feeding with the mother as appropriate?

References

American Academy of Pediatrics (AAP). (2011). Strategies for implementing screening for critical congenital heart disease. *Pediatrics, 2011*(128), e1259. doi:10.1542/peds.2011-1317

American Academy of Pediatrics (AAP). (2012a). Circumcision policy statement. *Pediatrics, 130,* 585. doi:10.1542/peds.2012-1989

American Academy of Pediatrics (AAP). (2012b). Policy statement: Breastfeeding and the use of human milk. *Pediatrics, 129*(3), e827–841.

American Academy of Pediatrics (AAP). (2014). *Reduce the risk of SIDS.* Retrieved from http://www.healthychildren.org/English/ages-stages/baby/sleep/Pages/Preventing-SIDS.aspx

American Academy of Pediatrics (AAP) Committee on Fetus and Newborn & American College of Obstetricians and Gynecologists (ACOG) Committee on Obstetrics (AAP & ACOG). (2012). *Guidelines for perinatal care* (7th ed.). Evanston, IL: Author.

Association of Women's Health, Obstetrics and Neonatal Nurses (AWHONN). (2013). *Neonatal skin care: Evidence based clinical practice guideline* (3rd ed.). Washington, DC: AWHONN.

Baby-Friendly Hospital Initiative USA. (2016). *Implementing the UNICEF/WHO baby-friendly hospital initiative in the U.S.* Retrieved from https://www.babyfriendlyusa.org/find-facilities

Baker, H. (2016). Child health. In K. Wambach and J. Riordan (Eds.), *Breastfeeding and human lactation* (5th ed. pp. 667-713). Boston, MA: Jones & Bartlett.

Blackburn, S. T. (2013). *Maternal, fetal, & neonatal physiology: A clinical perspective* (4th ed.). St. Louis, MO: Saunders.

Briggs, G. G., & Freeman, R. K. (2015). *Drugs in pregnancy and lactation: A reference guide to fetal and neonatal risk* (10th ed.). Philadelphia, PA: Wolters Kluwer Health

Callister, L. C. (2014). Integrating cultural beliefs and practices when caring for childbearing women and families. In K. R. Simpson & P. A. Creehan (Eds.), *Perinatal nursing* (3rd ed., pp. 29–57). Philadelphia, PA: Lippincott Williams & Wilkins.

Centers for Disease Control and Prevention (CDC). (2015a). *Hearing loss in newborn: Screening and diagnosis.* Retrieved from http://www.cdc.gov/ncbddd/hearingloss/screening.html

Centers for Disease Control and Prevention (CDC) Advisory Committee on Immunization Practices. (2015b).

Recommended childhood and adolescent immunization schedule, United States 2015. Retrieved from http://www.cdc.gov/vaccines/schedules/hcp/child-adolescent.html

Cloherty, J. P., Eichenwald, E. C., Hansen, A. R., & Stark, A. R. (2012). *Manual for neonatal care* (7th ed.). Philadelphia, PA: Lippincott Williams & Wilkins.

Flannery, V. (2014). Increasing breastfeeding rates: Evidence-based strategies. *International Journal of Childbirth Education, 29*(4), 59–62.

Fraser, D. (2014). Newborn adaptation to extrauterine life. In K. R. Simpson & P. A. Creehan (Eds.). *Perinatal nursing* (4th ed., pp. 581–596). Philadelphia, PA: Lippincott Williams & Wilkins.

Genetics Home Reference. (2015). *Newborn screening.* Retrieved from http://www.ghr.nlm.nih.gov/nbs

Hale, T. W. (2014). *Medications and mothers' milk* (16th ed.). Amarillo, TX: Pharmasoft.

Healthy Children. (2015a). *Benefits of breastfeeding for mom.* Retrieved from http://www.healthychildren.org/English/ages-stages/baby/breastfeeding/Pages/Benefits-of-Breastfeeding-for-Mom.aspx

Healthy Children. (2015b). *Breastfeeding benefits your baby's immune system.* Retrieved from http://www.healthychildren.org/English/ages-stages/baby/breastfeeding/Pages/Breastfeeding-Benefits-Your-Baby%27s-Immune-System.aspx

Healthy Children. (2015c). *Car seats: Information for families for 2014.* Retrieved from http://www.healthychildren.org/English/news/Pages/AAP-Updates-Recommendations-on-Car-Seats.aspx http://www.healthychildren.org/English/news/Pages/AAP-Updates-Recommendations-on-Car-Seats.aspx

Healthy Children. (2015d). *Purpose of newborn hearing screening.* Retrieved from http://www.healthychildren.org/English/ages-stages/baby/Pages/Purpose-of-Newborn-Hearing-Screening.aspx

Healthy Children. (2015e). *Reduce the risk of SIDS.* Retrieved from http://www.healthychildren.org/English/ages-stages/baby/sleep/Pages/Preventing-SIDS.aspx

Healthy Children (2015f). *Sleep position: Why back is best.* Retrieved from http://www.healthychildren.org/English/ages-stages/baby/sleep/Pages/Sleep-Position-Why-Back-is-Best.aspx

Healthy Children. (2015g). *Where we stand: Circumcision.* Retrieved from http://www.healthychildren.org/

English/ages-stages/prenatal/decisions-to-make/Pages/Where-We-Stand-Circumcision.aspx

Human Milk Banking Association of North America (HMBANA). (2011). *Best practice for expressing, storing and handling human milk in hospitals, homes and child care settings* (3rd ed.). Raleigh, NC: Author.

Janke, J. (2014). Newborn nutrition. In K. R. Simpson & P. A. Creehan (Eds.), *Perinatal nursing* (4th ed., pp. 626–661). Philadelphia, PA: Lippincott Williams & Wilkins.

Jones, F. (2016). Donor milk banking. In K. Wambach and J. Riordan (Eds.), *Breastfeeding and human lactation* (5th ed., pp. 523–548). Boston, MA: Jones & Bartlett.

Klaus, M., & Klaus, P. (1985). *The amazing newborn.* Menlo Park, CA: Addison-Wesley.

La Leche League International. (2013). *How do I position my baby to breastfeed?* Retrieved from http://www.lll.org/faq/positioning.html

Lipson, J. G., & Dibble, S. L. (2008). *Culture & clinical care* (7th ed.). San Francisco, CA: The Regents, University of California.

Marcewicz, L. (2014). *Late vitamin K deficiency bleeding in infants: Are we seeing a re-emergence?* Medscape. Jan. 27, 2014.

Mercer, A. M., Teasley, S. L., Hopkinson, J., McPherson, D. M., Simon, S. D., & Hall, R. T. (2010). Evaluation of a breastfeeding assessment score in a diverse population. *Journal of Human Lactation, 26*(1), 42–48.

Morrison, B., & Wambach, K. (2016). Women's health and breastfeeding. In K. Wambach and J. Riordan (Eds.), *Breastfeeding and human lactation* (5th ed. pp. 594-634). Boston, MA: Jones & Bartlett

National Conference of State Legislatures. (2015). *Breastfeeding laws.* Retrieved from http://www.ncsl.org/GoogleResults.aspx?q=breastfeeding%20law

Ott, B. B., Al-Khadhuri, J., & Al-Junaibi, S. (2003). Preventing ethical dilemmas: Understanding Islamic health care practices. *Pediatric Nursing, 29*(3), 227–230.

Purnell, L. P. (2013). *Transcultural health care: A culturally competent approach* (4th ed.). Philadelphia, PA: F. A. Davis

Riordan, J. (2016). The biological specificity of breastmilk. In K. Wambach and J. Riordan (Eds.), *Breastfeeding and human lactation* (5th ed. pp. 121–169). Boston, MA: Jones & Bartlett.

Sachs, H. C., & American Academy of Pediatrics (AAP) Committee on Drugs. (2013). Transfer of drugs and therapeutics into human breast milk: An update on selected topics. *Pediatrics, 132*(3), e796–809.

Smith, C. K. (2009). *Some traditional umbilical cord care practices in developing countries.* Retrieved from www.midwiferytoday.com

Spong, C. Y. (2013). Defining "term" pregnancy: Recommendations from the defining "term" pregnancy workgroup. *Journal of the American Medical Association, 309,* 2445–2446.

U.S. Breastfeeding Committee. (2011). *Healthy People 2020: Breastfeeding objectives.* Retrieved from http://www.usbreastfeeding.org/LegislationPolicy/FederalPolicies/HealthyPeople2020BreastfeedingObjectives/tabid/120/Default.aspx

U.S. Department of Labor. (2011). *Section 7(r) of the Fair Labor Standards Act—Break Time for Nursing Mothers Provision.* Retrieved from http://www.dol.gov/whd/nursingmothers/Sec7rFLSA_btnm.htm

U.S. Food and Drug Administration (FDA). (2016). *Bisphenol A (BPA).* Retrieved from https://www.niehs.nih.gov/health/topics/agents/sya-bpa

Walker, M. (2016). Breast pumps and other technologies. In K. Wambach and J. Riordan (Eds.), *Breastfeeding and human lactation* (5th ed. pp. 419–466). Boston, MA: Jones & Bartlett.

Wambach, K. (2016). The cultural context of breastfeeding. In K. Wambach and J. Riordan (Eds.), *Breastfeeding and human lactation* (5th ed., pp. 895–913). Boston, MA: Jones & Bartlett.

Wilson, B. A., Shannon, M. T., & Shields, K. M. (2015). *Prentice Hall nurse's drug guide 2016.* Upper Saddle River, NJ: Pearson Education.

Woodring, B. C., & Andrews, M. M. (2012). Transcultural perspectives in the nursing care of children and adolescents. In M. M. Andrews & J. S. Boyle (Eds.), *Transcultural concepts in nursing care* (6th ed., pp. 123–156). Philadelphia, PA: Lippincott.

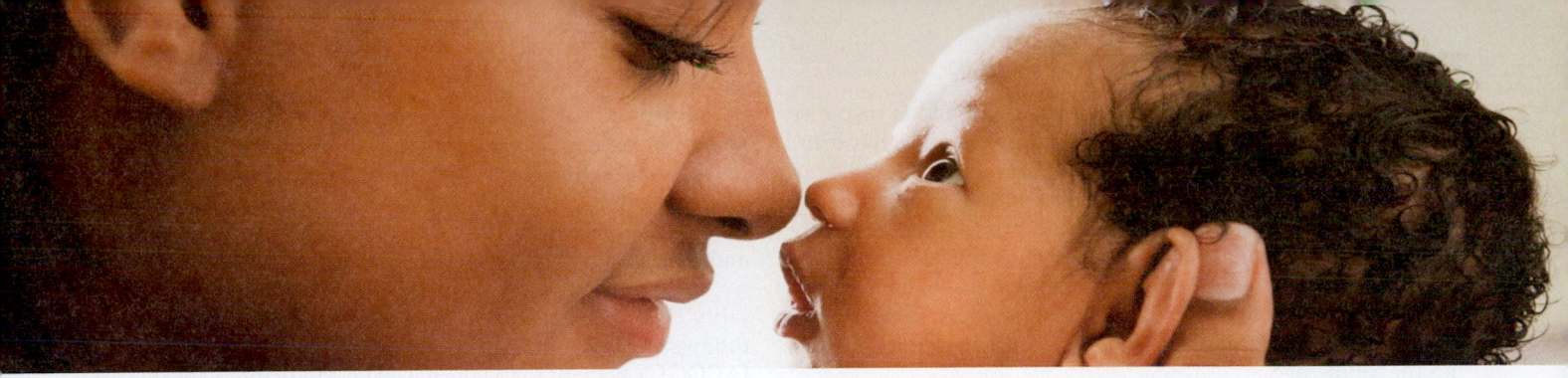

Chapter 26

The Newborn at Risk: Conditions Present at Birth

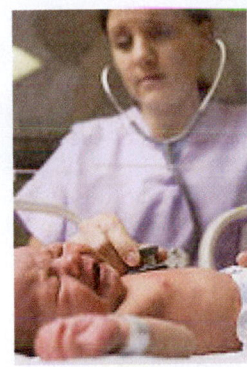

When a newborn is admitted into my unit, and into my care, there is an initial flurry of activity where my entire universe, everything that I am, constricts down to focus on this one little being. Gradually, as the situation stabilizes, I become aware again of the other team members working in concert around me. And I am reassured that this new life is getting the very best care available.

—Neonatal Nurse Practitioner

© RubberBall / SuperStock

⌄ Learning Outcomes

26.1 Explain the factors present at birth that indicate an at-risk newborn.

26.2 Compare the underlying etiologies of the physiologic complications of small-for-gestational-age (SGA) newborns and preterm appropriate-for-gestational-age (Pr AGA) newborns and the nursing management for each.

26.3 Explain the impact of maternal diabetes mellitus on the newborn.

26.4 Compare the characteristics and potential complications that influence nursing management of the postterm newborn and the newborn with postmaturity syndrome.

26.5 Compare the physiologic and behavioral characteristics of the preterm newborn that predispose each body system to various complications and are used in the

development of a plan of care that includes nutritional management.

26.6 Summarize the nursing assessments and initial interventions for a newborn born with selected congenital anomalies.

26.7 Explain the special care needed by an alcohol- or drug-exposed newborn.

26.8 Relate the consequence of maternal HIV/AIDS to the management of and issues for caregivers of newborns at risk for HIV/AIDS in the neonatal period.

26.9 Identify physical examination findings during the early newborn period that would make the nurse suspect a congenital cardiac defect or congestive heart failure.

26.10 Explain the special care needed by a newborn with an inborn error of metabolism.

Many levels of neonatal care have evolved in response to increasing knowledge about at-risk newborns. Along with the newborn's parents, the nurse is an important caregiver in all these settings. As a member of the multidisciplinary healthcare team, the nurse is a technically competent professional who contributes the high-touch human care necessary in the high-tech perinatal environment. In addition to the availability of a high level of newborn care, various other factors influence the outcome of at-risk newborns, including the following:

- Birth weight
- Gestational age
- Type and length of newborn illness
- Environmental factors
- Maternal factors
- Maternal–newborn separation

Identification of At-Risk Newborns

An at-risk newborn is one susceptible to illness (morbidity) or even death (mortality) because of dysmaturity, immaturity, physical disorders, or complications during or after birth. In most cases, the baby is the product of a pregnancy involving one or more predictable risk factors, including the following:

- Low socioeconomic level of the mother
- Limited access to health care or no prenatal care
- Exposure to environmental dangers, such as toxic chemicals and illicit drugs
- Preexisting maternal conditions such as heart disease, diabetes, hypertension, hyperthyroidism, and renal disease
- Maternal factors such as age and parity
- Medical conditions related to pregnancy and their associated complications
- Pregnancy complications such as abruptio placentae, placenta previa, oligohydramnios, preterm labor, premature rupture of membranes, preeclampsia, and uterine rupture

Various risk factors and their specific effects on pregnancy outcomes are listed in Table 9-1. Because these factors and the perinatal risks associated with them are known, the birth of an at-risk newborn can often be anticipated. The pregnancy can be closely monitored, treatment can be started as necessary, and arrangements can be made for birth to occur at a facility with appropriate resources to care for both mother and baby.

Whether or not prenatal assessment indicates that the fetus is at risk, the course of labor and birth and the baby's ability to withstand the stress of labor cannot be predicted. Thus, the nurse's use of electronic fetal heart monitoring or fetal heart auscultation by Doppler plays a significant role in detecting stress or distress in the fetus. Immediately after birth the Apgar score (review Table 18-6) is a helpful tool for identifying the at-risk newborn, but it is not the only indicator of possible long-term outcomes.

The newborn classification and neonatal mortality risk chart is another useful tool for identifying newborns at risk. Before this classification tool was developed, a birth weight of less than 2500 g (5.5 lb) was the sole criterion for determining immaturity. Clinicians then recognized that a newborn could weigh more than 2500 g and still be immature. Conversely, a newborn weighing less than 2500 g might be functionally at term or beyond. Thus birth weight and gestational age together are now the criteria used to assess neonatal maturity, morbidity, and mortality risk.

According to the newborn classification and neonatal mortality risk chart, gestation (postmenstrual age) is divided as follows (American College of Obstetricians and Gynecologists [ACOG] & Society for Maternal-Fetal Medicine [SMFM], 2013; Spong, 2013):

- Preterm: less than or equal to 36 weeks, 6 days
- Late preterm: 34 to 36 weeks, 6 days
- Early Term: 37 weeks, 0 days through 38 weeks, 6 days
- Full Term: 39 weeks, 0 days through 40 weeks, 6 days
- Late Term: 41 weeks, 0 through 6 days
- Postterm: 42 weeks, 0 days and beyond

Late preterm is a new classification. These newborns have demonstrated increased incidences of morbidity and length of stay when compared to full-term newborns (Cloherty, Eichenwald, Hansen, et al., 2012). Morbidities associated with prematurity continue into early-term gestations and are compounded by socioeconomic status (Ruth, Roos, Hildes-Ripstein, et al., 2013).

Large-for-gestational-age (LGA) newborns are those who plot above the 90th percentile curve on intrauterine growth curves. Appropriate-for-gestational-age (AGA) newborns are those who plot between the 10th and the 90th percentile growth curves. **Small-for-gestational-age (SGA)** newborns are those who plot below the 10th percentile growth curve. A newborn is assigned to a category depending on birth weight, length, occipital-frontal head circumference, and gestational age. For example, a newborn classified as Pr SGA is preterm and small for gestational age. The full-term newborn whose weight is appropriate for gestational age is classified F AGA. It is important to note that intrauterine growth charts are influenced by altitude and the ethnicity of the newborn population used to create the chart. Also, the assigned newborn classification may vary according to the intrauterine growth curve chart used; therefore, the chart used should correlate with the characteristics of the patient population.

Neonatal mortality risk is the neonate's chance of death within the newborn period—that is, within the first 28 days of life. Seventy-five percent of all neonatal deaths occur within the first week, with the highest rates occurring during the first day of life. The neonatal mortality risk decreases as both gestational age and birth weight increase. Newborns who are Pr SGA have the highest neonatal mortality risk. The previously high mortality rates for LGA newborns have decreased at most perinatal centers because of improved management of diabetes in pregnancy and recognition of potential complications of LGA newborns.

Neonatal morbidity can be anticipated based on birth weight and gestational age. The neonatal morbidity by birth weight and gestational age tool assists in determining the needs of particular newborns for special observation and care. For example, a baby of 2000 g (4.4 lb) at 40 weeks' gestation should be carefully assessed for evidence of neonatal distress, hypoglycemia, congenital anomalies, congenital infection, and polycythemia.

Identifying the nursing care needs of the at-risk newborn depends on minute-to-minute observations of changes in the newborn's physiologic status. The organization of nursing care must be directed toward the following:

- Decreasing physiologically stressful situations
- Observing constantly for subtle signs of change in clinical condition
- Interpreting laboratory data and coordinating interventions
- Conserving the newborn's energy for healing and growth
- Providing for developmental stimulation and maintenance of sleep cycles
- Assisting the family in developing attachment behaviors
- Involving the family in planning and providing care

Care of the Small-for-Gestational-Age/Intrauterine Growth Restriction Newborn

Currently newborns are considered **small for gestational age (SGA)** when they are less than the 10th percentile for birth weight; very small for gestational age is when they are two standard deviations below the population norm or less than the third percentile (Rozance & Rosenberg, 2012) (Figure 26–1). When possible, the birth weight charts used to assign the SGA classification to a newborn should be based on the local population into which the newborn is born. A SGA newborn may be preterm, term, or postterm. An undergrown newborn may also be said to have **intrauterine growth restriction (IUGR)**, which describes pregnancy circumstances of advanced gestation and limited fetal growth. This classification of abnormal growth is also enhanced by looking at growth potential by adjusting birth weight reference limits for first-trimester maternal height, birth order, and newborn gender.

SGA newborns are commonly seen with mothers who smoke or have high blood pressure, causing these babies to have an increased incidence of perinatal asphyxia and perinatal mortality when compared with appropriate-for-gestational-age (AGA) newborns (ACOG, 2013). The incidence of polycythemia and hypoglycemia is also higher in this group.

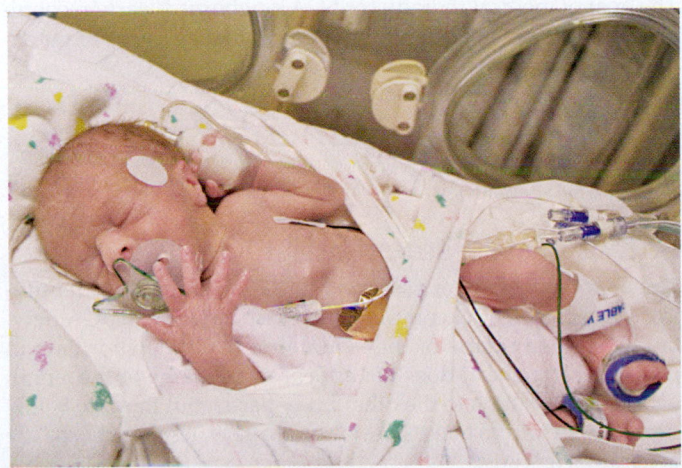

Figure 26–1 **Thirty-one-week gestational age, SGA 2-day-old baby girl.**

SOURCE: Carol Harrigan, RN, MSN, NNP-BC.

Factors Contributing to IUGR

Intrauterine growth restriction may be caused by maternal, placental, or fetal factors and may not be apparent antenatally. Intrauterine growth is linear (follows expected growth line) in the normal pregnancy from approximately 28 to 38 weeks' gestation. After 38 weeks, growth is variable, depending on the growth potential of the fetus and placental function. The most common causes of growth restriction are as follows:

- *Maternal factors.* Primiparity, grand multiparity, multiple-gestation pregnancy (twins and higher-order multiples), lack of prenatal care, age extremes (less than 16 years or more than 40 years), and low socioeconomic status (which can result in inadequate health care, inadequate education, and inadequate living conditions) affect IUGR (Cloherty et al., 2012). Before the third trimester, the nutritional supply to the fetus far exceeds its needs. Only in the third trimester are maternal malnutrition and drug abuse limiting factors in fetal growth.

- *Maternal disease.* Maternal heart disease, substance abuse (drugs, tobacco, alcohol), sickle cell anemia, phenylketonuria (PKU), lupus erythematosus, and asymptomatic pyelonephritis are associated with SGA. Complications associated with preeclampsia, chronic hypertensive vascular disease, and advanced diabetes mellitus can diminish blood flow to the uterus, thereby decreasing oxygen delivery to the fetus and minimizing organ growth.

- *Environmental factors.* High altitude, exposure to X-rays, excessive exercise, work-related exposure to toxins, hyperthermia, and maternal use of drugs that have teratogenic effects, such as nicotine, alcohol, antimetabolites, anticonvulsants, narcotics, and cocaine, affect fetal growth (Cloherty et al., 2012; Mari & Tate, 2013; Resnik & Creasy, 2014).

- *Placental factors.* Placental conditions such as small placenta, infarcted areas, abnormal cord insertions, placenta previa, and thrombosis may affect circulation to the fetus, which becomes more deficient with increasing gestational age (Geary, 2013).

- *Fetal factors.* Congenital infections such as TORCH infections (*t*oxoplasmosis, *o*ther, *r*ubella, *c*ytomegalovirus, *h*erpes simplex virus), syphilis, congenital malformations, discordant twins, gender of the fetus (females tend to be smaller), chromosomal syndromes (trisomies 13, 18, 21), two-vessel umbilical cord, and inborn errors of metabolism can predispose a fetus to fetal growth disturbances.

Identifying fetuses with IUGR is the first step in detecting common disorders associated with affected newborns. The perinatal history of maternal conditions, early dating of pregnancy by first-trimester ultrasound measurements, antepartum testing (non-stress test, contraction stress test, biophysical profile [see Chapter 13 for discussion of antepartum testing]), Doppler velocimetry of placenta, gestational age assessment, and the physical and neurologic assessment of the newborn are also important (Cloherty et al., 2012; Mari & Tate, 2013).

Clinical Tip

In assessing a growth-restricted newborn resulting from unexplained maternal etiology (e.g., hypertension, placental insufficiency), an in utero viral infection may be the answer.

Patterns of IUGR

Intrauterine growth occurs by an increase in both cell number and cell size. If insult occurs early during the critical period of organ development in the fetus, fewer new cells are formed, organs are small, and organ weight is subnormal. In contrast, growth failure that begins later in pregnancy does not affect the total number of cells, only their size. The organs are normal, but their size is diminished. There are two clinical pictures of IUGR newborns:

- *Symmetric (proportional) IUGR* is caused by long-term maternal conditions (such as chronic hypertension, severe malnutrition, chronic intrauterine viral infection, substance abuse [drugs, alcohol, tobacco], anemia) or fetal genetic abnormalities (Resnik & Creasy, 2014). Symmetric IUGR can be noted by ultrasound in the first half of the second trimester. In symmetric IUGR there is chronic, prolonged restriction of growth in the size of organs, weight, length, and, especially, head circumference.

- *Asymmetric (disproportional) IUGR* is associated with an acute compromise of uteroplacental blood flow. Some associated causes are placental infarcts, preeclampsia, and poor weight gain in pregnancy. The growth restriction is usually not evident before the third trimester because, although weight is decreased, length and head circumference (used as a growth indicator) remain appropriate for that gestational age. After 36 weeks' gestation, the abdominal circumference of a normal fetus becomes larger than the head circumference. In asymmetric IUGR, the head circumference remains larger than the abdominal circumference. Thus measuring only the biparietal diameter on ultrasound will not reveal asymmetric IUGR. An early indicator of asymmetric IUGR is a decrease in the growth rate of the abdominal circumference, reflecting subnormal liver growth, a reduction in glycogen stores, and a scarcity of subcutaneous fat (Gleason & Devaskar, 2012). Birth weight is below the 10th percentile, whereas head circumference and/or length may be between the 10th and the 90th percentiles. Asymmetric SGA newborns related to IUGR are particularly at risk for asphyxia, pulmonary hemorrhage, hypocalcemia, and hypoglycemia.

Despite growth restriction, physiologic maturity develops according to gestational age. The SGA newborn's chances for survival are better than those of the preterm AGA newborn because of organ maturity, although this newborn still faces many potential difficulties.

Common Complications of the SGA Newborn

The complications occurring most frequently in the SGA newborn include the following:

- *Fetal hypoxia.* The SGA newborn suffers from chronically lower-than-normal oxygen levels in utero, which leaves little reserve to withstand the demands of normal labor and birth. Thus, intrauterine asphyxia, and its potential systemic problems, can occur. Cesarean birth may be necessary because of worsening fetal compromise and intolerance to labor.

- *Aspiration syndrome.* In utero hypoxia can cause the fetus to gasp during birth, resulting in aspiration of amniotic fluid into the lower airways. It can also lead to relaxation of the anal sphincter and passage of meconium. This may result in aspiration of the meconium in utero or with the first breaths after birth.

- *Hypothermia.* Diminished subcutaneous fat (used for survival in utero), depletion of brown fat in utero, and a large surface area decrease the IUGR newborn's ability to conserve heat. The flexed position assumed by the term SGA newborn diminishes the effect of surface area.

- *Hypoglycemia.* An increase in metabolic rate in response to heat loss and poor hepatic glycogen stores causes hypoglycemia. In addition, the newborn is compromised by inadequate supplies of enzymes to activate gluconeogenesis (conversion of nonglucogen sources such as fatty acids and proteins to glucose).

- *Polycythemia.* The number of red blood cells is increased (central hematocrit greater than 65%) in the SGA newborn. This finding is considered a physiologic response to in utero chronic hypoxic stress. Polycythemia may contribute to hypoglycemia.

Newborns who have significant IUGR tend to have a poor prognosis, especially when born before 37 weeks' gestation. Factors contributing to poor outcome include the following:

- *Congenital malformations.* Congenital malformations occur in 5% of SGA newborns (Cloherty et al., 2012). The more severe the IUGR, the greater the chance for malformation as a result of impaired mitotic activity and cellular hypoplasia.

- *Intrauterine infections.* When fetuses are exposed to intrauterine infections such as rubella and cytomegalovirus, they are profoundly affected by direct invasion of the brain and other vital organs by the offending virus.

- *Continued growth difficulties.* SGA newborns tend to be shorter than newborns of the same gestational age. Asymmetric IUGR newborns can be expected to catch up in weight and approach their inherited growth potential when given an optimal environment.

- *Cognitive difficulties.* Often SGA newborns can exhibit subsequent learning disabilities. The disabilities are characterized by hyperactivity, short attention span, and poor fine motor coordination (writing and drawing). Some hearing loss and speech defects also occur (Gomella, 2013).

Clinical Therapy

The goal of medical therapy for SGA newborns is early recognition and implementation of the medical management of potential problems.

Nursing Management
For the SGA/IUGR Newborn

Nursing Assessment and Diagnosis

You are responsible for assessing gestational age and identifying signs of potential complications associated with SGA newborns. All body parts of the symmetric IUGR newborn are in proportion (the head does not appear overly large or the length excessive in relation to the other body parts), but they are below normal size for the baby's gestational age. These newborns are generally vigorous.

The asymmetric IUGR newborn appears long, thin, and emaciated, with loss of subcutaneous fat tissue and muscle mass. The baby may have loose skin folds; dry, desquamating skin; and a thin and often meconium-stained cord. The head appears relatively large (although it approaches normal size) because the chest size and abdominal girth are decreased. The baby may have a vigorous cry and appear alert and wide eyed.

Nursing diagnoses that may apply to the SGA newborn include those listed in the accompanying *Nursing Care Plan: For the Small-for-Gestational-Age Newborn* and the following (NANDA-I © 2014):

- *Gas Exchange, Impaired,* related to aspiration of amniotic fluid or meconium-stained fluid
- *Injury, Risk for,* related to decreased glycogen stores and impaired gluconeogenesis
- *Tissue Perfusion: Peripheral, Ineffective,* related to polycythemia and increased blood viscosity
- *Parenting, Risk for Impaired,* related to prolonged separation of newborn from parents secondary to illness

Nursing Plan and Implementation

HOSPITAL-BASED NURSING CARE

Hypoglycemia, the most common metabolic complication of IUGR, produces such sequelae as central nervous system (CNS) abnormalities and mental retardation. Conditions such as asphyxia, hyperviscosity, and cold stress may also affect the baby's outcome. Meticulous attention to physiologic parameters is essential for immediate nursing management and reduction of long-term disorders.

COMMUNITY-BASED NURSING CARE

The long-term needs of the SGA newborn include careful follow-up evaluation of patterns of growth and possible disabilities that may later interfere with learning or motor functioning. Long-term follow-up care is essential for newborns with congenital malformations, congenital infections, and obvious sequelae from physiologic problems. Parents of the IUGR newborn need support, because a positive atmosphere can enhance the baby's growth potential and the child's ultimate outcome.

Evaluation

Expected outcomes of nursing care include the following:

- The SGA newborn is free from respiratory compromise.
- The SGA newborn maintains a stable temperature.
- The SGA newborn is free from hypoglycemic episodes and maintains glucose homeostasis.
- The SGA newborn gains weight and takes breast or formula feedings without developing physiologic distress or fatigue.
- The parents verbalize their concerns about their baby's health problems and understand the rationale behind management of their newborn.

Care of the Large-for-Gestational-Age (LGA) Newborn

A newborn whose birth weight is at or above the 90th percentile on the intrauterine growth curve (at any week of gestation) is considered large for gestational age (LGA). Some appropriate-for-gestational-age (AGA) newborns have been incorrectly categorized as LGA because of miscalculation of the date of conception caused by postconceptual bleeding. Careful gestational age assessment is essential to identify the potential needs and problems of these newborns.

The most well-known condition associated with excessive fetal growth is maternal diabetes; however, only a small fraction of large newborns are born to mothers who have diabetes. The cause of the majority of cases of LGA newborns is unclear, but certain factors or situations have been found to correlate with their birth (Cloherty et al., 2012; Hay, 2012):

- Diabetes complications affect 3% to 10% of all pregnancies, it is estimated, with 60% of these women having gestational diabetes and 33% having insulin-dependent (type 1) diabetes.
- Macrosomia (increased size) affecting a LGA infant of a diabetic mother (IDM) is directly proportional to high, unstable maternal glucose concentrations.
- Multiparous women have 2 to 3 times the number of LGA newborns as primigravidas.
- Male newborns are typically larger than female newborns.
- Babies with erythroblastosis fetalis, Beckwith-Wiedemann syndrome (a genetic condition associated with omphalocele, neonatal hypoglycemia, and hyperinsulinemia), or transposition of the great vessels are usually large.

The increase in the LGA newborn's body size is characteristically proportional, although head circumference and body length are in the upper limits of intrauterine growth. The exception to this rule is the baby of the mother with diabetes; such a newborn's body weight is higher, usually greater than 4 kg (8.8 lb), but the baby's length and head circumference may remain in the normal range. Macrosomic newborns have poor motor skills, feeding difficulties, and difficulty regulating behavioral states. LGA newborns tend to be more difficult to arouse to a quiet alert state.

Common Complications of the LGA Newborn

Complications of the LGA newborn can include the following:

- *Birth trauma caused by cephalopelvic disproportion (CPD).* Often LGA newborns have a biparietal diameter greater than 10 cm (4 in.) or are associated with a maternal fundal height measurement greater than 42 cm (16 in.) without the presence of polyhydramnios. Because of their excessive size, there are more breech presentations and shoulder dystocias. These complications may result in asphyxia, fractured clavicles, brachial palsy, facial paralysis, phrenic nerve palsy, depressed skull fractures, cephalohematoma, and intracranial hemorrhage caused by birth trauma.
- *Complications of hypoglycemia, polycythemia, and/or hyperviscosity.* These disorders are most often seen in IDMs, newborns with erythroblastosis fetalis, or newborns with Beckwith-Wiedemann syndrome.

Nursing Management

The perinatal history, in conjunction with ultrasonic measurement of the fetal skull (biparietal diameter) and gestational age testing, is important in identifying an at-risk LGA newborn. Essential components of the nursing assessment are monitoring vital signs, screening for hypoglycemia and polycythemia, and observing for signs and symptoms related to birth trauma.

Nursing Care Plan: For The Small-For-Gestational-Age Newborn

1. Nursing Diagnosis: *Gas Exchange, Impaired,* related to amniotic fluid or meconium aspiration (NANDA-I © 2014)

GOAL: The newborn's respiratory rate and effort will be within normal limits, with no periods of apnea or evidence of worsening distress.

INTERVENTION	RATIONALE
• Obtain maternal prenatal, labor, and delivery records.	• Provides information and clues of potential fetal stress that may have occurred during the antepartum and intrapartum period. In addition, the delivery record will provide information concerning the newborn's respiratory status at birth, such as the Apgar score.
• Maintain airway patency through judicious airway suctioning.	• Respiratory distress in small-for-gestational-age (SGA) newborns is due to in utero hypoxia and aspiration of amniotic fluid or meconium-stained fluid.
• Observe for worsening signs of respiratory distress such as generalized cyanosis, increasing retractions, grunting, and nasal flaring (as evidenced by Silverman respiratory index), sustained tachypnea, apnea episodes, inequality of breath sounds, presence of rales and rhonchi.	
• Monitor and maintain adequate axillary body temperature (36.4°–37.2°C [97.5°–99.0°F]) to avoid increased oxygen consumption.	• Temperature elevation may cause metabolic rate and oxygen needs to increase when associated with meconium aspiration.
• Administer supplemental oxygen or other interventions (e.g., high-flow nasal cannula, nasal continuous positive airway pressure [CPAP], intubation with mechanical ventilation) per order for management of symptoms related to respiratory distress. (See Chapter 27 for nursing care and treatment of meconium aspiration and newborn resuscitation.)	• Provides healthcare personnel with information on cardiac and pulmonary status.
• Implement treatment plan for respiratory distress.	
• Monitor glucose levels.	• Respiratory distress increases consumption of glucose.
• **Collaborative:** Obtain blood gas (ABG or CBG) and pulse oximetry parameters, chest x-ray per healthcare provider orders.	
• Monitor newborn's cardiopulmonary status, pulse oximetry readings, and blood gas values.	• Oxygen demands increase with meconium aspiration. Obtaining serial blood gases and chest x-ray will provide medical personnel with baseline information of newborn's respiratory status, and effective medical interventions can be initiated.

EXPECTED OUTCOMES: The newborn will maintain adequate respiratory gas exchange as evidenced by respirations of 30–60/min with pulse oximetry and blood gases within normal limits and will show no signs and symptoms of respiratory distress.

2. Nursing Diagnosis: *Thermoregulation, Ineffective,* secondary to decreased subcutaneous fat (NANDA-I © 2014)

GOAL: The newborn's temperature will be stable and maintained within normal limits.

INTERVENTION	RATIONALE
• Provide neutral thermal environment (NTE) range for newborn based on postnatal weight.	• Neutral thermal environment charts used for preterm newborn are not reliable for weight of SGA newborn.
• Place a skin probe to maintain newborn's temperature at 36.0°–36.5°C (96.8°–97.8°F).	• A neutral thermal environment requires minimal oxygen consumption to maintain a normal core temperature.

- Obtain axillary temperatures and compare with registered skin probe temperature. If discrepancy exists, evaluate potential cause.

- Adjust and monitor incubator or radiant warmer to maintain set skin temperature, using the servo-control mode.

- Minimize heat losses and prevent cold stress by:

  1. Warming and humidifying oxygen without blowing over face to avoid increasing oxygen consumption

  2. Keeping skin dry, especially immediately following delivery

  3. Keeping incubators, radiant warmers, and open cribs away from windows and cold external walls and out of drafts

  4. Avoiding placing newborn on cold surrounding objects such as metal treatment tables, cold x-ray plates, and scales

  5. Using radiant warmers during procedures

  6. Wrapping the newborn in blankets and covering the head with a hat

- Observe for consequences of cold stress: hypoglycemia, hypoxia, lethargy, pallor, metabolic acidosis (for further discussion see Chapter 27).

- Discrepancies between axillary and skin probe monitor temperatures may be due to mechanical causes or the burning of brown fat.

- Physical principles of heat loss effects include:

  1. Evaporation—loss of heat from newborn by water evaporation from the skin, especially seen immediately after birth

  2. Convection—loss of heat from newborn to the surrounding air

  3. Conduction—loss of heat from newborn to the surface with which the baby is in direct contact

  4. Radiation—loss of heat from newborn to cooler, surrounding surfaces (not in direct contact)

- Hypothermia is a potential problem for an SGA newborn because:

  1. SGA newborn has decreased brown fat stores available for thermogenesis, because they have been used in utero for survival.

  2. SGA newborn has poor insulation due to minimal subcutaneous tissues, because they have been used in utero for survival.

EXPECTED OUTCOMES: The newborn will not exhibit consequences of hypothermia as evidenced by skin temperature maintenance of 36.0°–36.5°C (96.8°–97.8°F) and axillary temperature maintenance of 36.4°–37.2°C (97.5°–99.0°F).

3. **Nursing Diagnosis:** *Injury, Risk for,* **related to decreased glycogen stores and impaired gluconeogenesis (NANDA-I © 2014)**

GOAL: Newborn will have a normal blood glucose level.

INTERVENTION	RATIONALE
• Monitor blood glucose levels per SGA protocol and report values less than 40 mg/dL. (The exact definition of hypoglycemia varies in the literature; it is best to follow your hospital's guidelines.)	• Combined with depletion of glycogen stores, impaired gluconeogenesis predisposes SGA newborns to profound hypoglycemia within first few hours of life.
• Observe, record, and report symptoms of hypoglycemia: irritability, cyanosis, lethargy, hypotonia, poor feeding, temperature instability, tremors, jitteriness, seizure activity, and apnea.	• Target glucose screen >40 mg/dL prior to routine feedings (Armentrout, 2015).
• Initiate feeding schedule for SGA newborns after screening for blood glucose level and symptoms of hypoglycemia per hospital protocol.	• Frequent monitoring of heel stick glucose assists in identifying decreased glucose levels.
• Provide glucose intake either through early enteral feeding (before 1 hr) and/or by intravenous (IV) per healthcare provider order.	• Provision of glucose through early feedings (begin within first hour of age) assists in maintaining glucose levels within the defined parameters. Always treat symptomatic hypoglycemia with IV glucose.

(See further discussion of hypoglycemia in Chapter 27.)

EXPECTED OUTCOME: The newborn will not exhibit signs and symptoms of hypoglycemia as evidenced by a euglycemic state and blood glucose greater than 45 mg/dL.

(continued)

Nursing Care Plan: For the Small-for-Gestational-Age Newborn *(continued)*

4. Nursing Diagnosis: *Nutrition, Imbalanced: Less than Body Requirements,* related to increased metabolic needs in the newborn (NANDA-I © 2014)

GOAL: Newborn will show positive growth as evidenced by increased serial measurements of weight, length, and occipital–fontal circumference (OFC).

INTERVENTION	RATIONALE
• Assess suck, swallow, and breathe reflexes.	• Sterile water or breast milk may be used to test gag and swallow reflex because it causes fewer pulmonary complications in the presence of gastrointestinal tract abnormalities and/or aspiration of feeding.
• Assess for a nondistended, soft abdomen with active bowel sounds.	• Prevents feeding problems and assists in determining the best method of feeding for baby and feeding readiness (Jones, 2012).
• Initiate oral feeding per protocol at 1 hr of age; use expressed breast milk, if available, or commercially prepared formula based on hospital protocol.	• SGA newborns require more calories/kg for growth than appropriate-for-gestational-age (AGA) newborns because of increased metabolic activity and oxygen consumption secondary to increased percentage of body weight made up by visceral organs.
	• Human milk is preferred for feeding term, preterm, and sick babies.
• Supplement oral feedings with IV intake per orders.	• Small, frequent feedings of high-calorie formula are used because of limited gastric capacity and decreased gastric emptying.
• Advance to concentrated formulas that supply more calories in less volume, such as 22 or 24 cal/oz.	
• Promote growth by providing caloric intake of 110–140 cal/kg/day in small amounts.	• Growth is evaluated by increase in weight (about 15–30 g/day), length, and OFC.
• Observe, record, and report signs of feeding intolerance or fatigue occurring during breast-feeding or bottle-feedings.	• Decrease in exhaustion is an important consideration in feeding SGA newborn; gavage tube feeding may need to be initiated.
	• SGA newborns with in utero reversed or absent end-diastolic blood flow are at high risk for developing necrotizing enterocolitis (NEC) (Geary, 2013).
	• Adequate nutritional intake promotes growth and prevents such complications as metabolic catabolism and hypoglycemia.
• Supplement gavage or nipple feedings with IV therapy per healthcare provider order until oral intake is sufficient to support growth.	• Gavage feedings require less energy expenditure on the part of the newborn.
• Establish a nipple-feeding program that is begun slowly and progresses slowly, such as this: nipple-feed once per day, nipple-feed once per shift, progressing to nipple-feed every other feeding.	• Cue-based feedings (based on engagement and hunger cues) allow the baby to become an active participant in the feeding process (Newland, L'Huillier, & Petrey, 2013).
• Initiate breastfeeding attempts when baby shows readiness.	
• Monitor daily weight with anticipation of small amount of weight loss when nipple feedings start.	• Nipple feeding, an active rather than passive intake of nutrition, requires energy expenditure and burning of calories by newborn.
• Weekly OFC and length measurements plotted on growth charts.	• Head circumference is an indicator for brain growth, at the rate of 0.5 cm/week.

EXPECTED OUTCOMES: The newborn will maintain consistent weight gain pattern as evidenced by less than 2%/day weight loss and tolerate enteral feedings.

5. Nursing Diagnosis: *Parenting, Impaired,* **related to lack of knowledge of newborn/infant care and prolonged separation of newborn and parents secondary to illness and prolonged hospitalization (NANDA-I © 2014)**

GOAL: Parents will bond with their newborn and have realistic expectations about their baby. Parents are comfortable taking baby home. They are able to demonstrate normal newborn/infant care and assessments of possible complications and know when to return for follow-up.

INTERVENTION	RATIONALE
• Support emotionally the psychologic well-being of family, including positive parent–newborn attachment and sensory stimulation of baby.	• Parent–newborn attachment begins in first few hours or days following birth. SGA newborns may experience prolonged periods of separation from their parents, which necessitates intervention to ensure parent–newborn attachment.
• Include parents in determining newborn's plan of care and encourage their participation. Encourage parents to visit frequently. Provide opportunities for parents to touch, hold, talk to, and care for baby. Determine the type and amount of appropriate sensory stimulation and implement sensory stimulation program.	• Facilitating kangaroo care allows the newborn to be placed skin-to-skin with a parent, which contributes to the overall health and growth of the baby as well as providing crucial involvement by the parents (Ludington-Hoe, 2013).
• Prepare for discharge by instructing parents in such areas as feeding techniques, formula preparation, and breastfeeding; bathing, diapering, and hygiene; temperature monitoring; administration of vitamins; care of complications and preventing exposure to infections; normal elimination patterns, normal reflexes and activity, and how to promote normal growth and development without being overprotective; returning for continued medical care; and availability of community resources if indicated.	• Parents should receive the same postpartum teaching as any parent taking a newborn home. • Parents need to understand the changes to expect in color of the baby's stool and number of bowel movements plus odor from formula-feeding or breastfeeding to avoid unnecessary concern. SGA newborns usually do not require referral to community agencies such as visiting nurse associations unless there is a specific problem requiring assistance.

EXPECTED OUTCOMES: The parent will demonstrate ability to perform basic newborn/infant care tasks as evidenced by exhibiting appropriate attachment behaviors (e.g., talking to and holding baby), feeding and bathing baby.

Address parental concerns about the visual signs of birth trauma and the potential for continuation of the overweight pattern. Help parents learn to arouse and console their newborn and facilitate attachment behaviors. Mothers of LGA newborns with facial or head bruising may be reluctant to interact with their newborns because they fear hurting their babies. The nursing care involved in the complications associated with LGA newborns is similar to the care needed by the baby whose mother has diabetes and is discussed in the next section.

Care of the Infant of a Diabetic Mother

The **infant of a diabetic mother (IDM)** is considered at risk and requires close observation during the first few hours to the first few days of life. Mothers with severe diabetes or diabetes of long duration associated with vascular complications may give birth to small-for-gestational-age (SGA) newborns. The typical IDM, when the diabetes is poorly controlled or is gestational, is large for gestational age (LGA). The newborn is macrosomic, is ruddy in color, and has excessive adipose (fat) tissue (Figure 26–2). The umbilical cord is thick and the placenta is large. There is a higher incidence of macrosomic newborns born to certain ethnic groups in the United States (Native Americans, Mexican Americans, African Americans, Pacific Islanders).

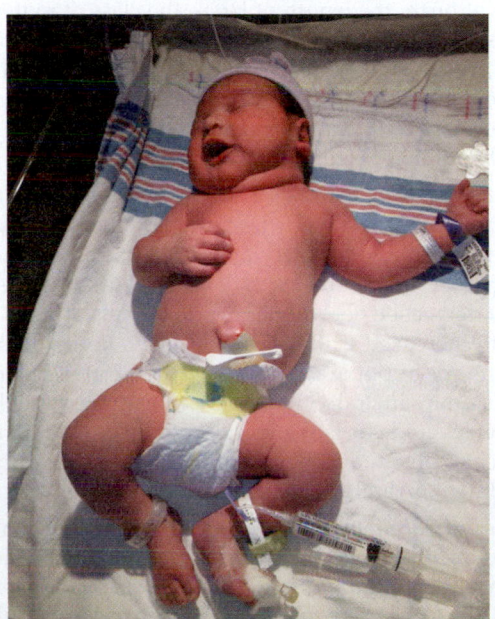

Figure 26–2 Macrosomic newborn of an undiagnosed mother with gestational diabetes born at 35 weeks' gestation weighing 3775 g (8.3 lb). Note the peripheral IV in his foot placed to give a D10W bolus.

SOURCE: Carol Harrigan, RN, MSN, NNP-BC.

IDMs have decreased total body water, particularly in the extracellular spaces, and are therefore not edematous. Their excessive weight is a result of the increased weight of the visceral organs, cardiomegaly (hypertrophy), and increased body fat. The only organ not affected is the brain.

The excessive fetal growth of the IDM is caused by exposure to high levels of maternal glucose, which readily crosses the placenta. The fetus responds to these high glucose levels with increased insulin production and hyperplasia of the pancreatic beta cells. The main action of the insulin is to facilitate the entry of glucose into muscle and fat cells. Once in the cells, glucose is converted to glycogen and stored. Insulin also inhibits the breakdown of fat to free fatty acids, thereby maintaining lipid synthesis; increases the uptake of amino acids; and promotes protein synthesis. Insulin is an important regulator of fetal metabolism and has a "growth hormone" effect that results in increased linear growth. IDMs may be obese as children (Moore, Hauguel-DeMouzon, & Catalano, 2014).

Common Complications of the IDM

Although IDMs are usually large, they have immature physiologic functions and exhibit many of the problems of the preterm (premature) newborn. The complications most often seen in an IDM are as follows:

- *Hypoglycemia.* Hypoglycemia is defined as a blood sugar less than 40 mg/dl. It occurs transiently in the immediate neonatal period for all newborns, but occurs sooner, with increased frequency, and to lower levels in IDMs (Moore et al., 2014). Once the fetus is delivered and the maternal glucose supply is severed, the IDM continues to produce high levels of insulin, which deplete the newborn's blood glucose within hours after birth. IDMs also have less ability to release glucagon and catecholamines, which normally stimulate glucagon breakdown and glucose release. The incidence of hypoglycemia in IDMs varies according to the degree of success in controlling the maternal diabetes, the maternal blood sugar level at the time of birth, the length of labor, the class of maternal diabetes, and early versus late feedings of the newborn (Daley, 2014). Signs and symptoms of hypoglycemia, which usually present within 1 to 2 hours following delivery, include tremors, cyanosis, apnea, temperature instability, poor feeding, and hypotonia. Seizures may occur in severe cases.

- *Hypocalcemia.* Tremors are the obvious clinical sign of hypocalcemia. They may be caused by the IDM's increased incidence of prematurity and by the stresses of difficult pregnancy, labor, and birth. Women with diabetes tend to have decreased serum magnesium levels at term secondary to increased urinary calcium excretion, which causes secondary hypoparathyroidism in their newborns. Other factors may include vitamin D antagonism, which results from elevated cortisol levels, hypophosphatemia from tissue catabolism, and decreased serum magnesium levels. Treatment is rarely necessary.

- *Hyperbilirubinemia.* This condition may be seen at 48 to 72 hours after birth. It may be caused by slightly decreased extracellular fluid volume, which increases the hematocrit level. This elevation facilitates an increase in red blood cell breakdown, thereby increasing bilirubin levels. The presence of hepatic immaturity may impair bilirubin conjugation. Enclosed hemorrhages resulting from complicated vaginal birth may also cause hyperbilirubinemia.

- *Birth trauma.* Because most IDMs are macrosomic, trauma may occur during labor and birth from shoulder dystocia.

- *Polycythemia.* Fetal hyperglycemia and hyperinsulinism result in increased oxygen consumption, which can lead to fetal hypoxia (Raab & Kelly, 2013). Glycohemoglobin (HbA_{1c}) binds to oxygen, decreasing the oxygen available to the fetal tissues. This tissue hypoxia stimulates increased erythropoietin production, which increases both the hematocrit level and the potential for hyperbilirubinemia. See Chapter 14 for a discussion of HbA1c.

- *Respiratory distress syndrome (RDS).* This complication occurs especially in newborns of diabetic mothers in White classifications A to C whose diabetes is not well controlled (Moore et al., 2014). Insulin antagonizes the cortisol-induced stimulation of lecithin synthesis that is necessary for lung maturation. Therefore, IDMs may have less mature lungs than expected for their gestational age. There is also a decrease in the phospholipid phosphatidylglycerol (PG), which stabilizes surfactant. The insufficiency of PG increases the incidence of RDS. Therefore, it is important to test for the presence of PG in the amniotic fluid before birth.

- RDS does not appear to be a problem for babies born of diabetic mothers in White classifications D to F; instead, the stresses of poor uterine blood supply may lead to increased production of steroids, which accelerates lung maturation. IDMs may also have a delay in closure of the ductus arteriosus and decreases in postnatal pulmonary artery pressure (Hay, 2012).

- *Congenital birth defects.* These may include congenital heart defects (transposition of the great vessels, ventricular septal defect, patent ductus arteriosus), small left colon syndrome, renal anomalies, neural tube defects, and sacral agenesis (caudal regression) (Cloherty et al., 2012). Early close control of maternal glucose levels before and during pregnancy decreases the risk of birth defects. See Chapter 14 for more information.

Clinical Therapy

Prenatal management is directed toward controlling maternal glucose levels, which minimizes the common complications of IDMs. Because the onset of hypoglycemia occurs between 1 and 3 hours after birth in IDMs (with a spontaneous rise to normal levels by 4 to 6 hours), blood glucose determinations should be done on cord blood or by heel stick hourly during the first 4 hours after birth and then at 4-hour intervals until the risk period (about 48 hours) has passed or per agency protocol (Figure 26–3).

IDMs whose serum glucose level falls below 40 mg/dL should have early feedings with formula or breast milk (colostrum). If normal glucose levels cannot be maintained with oral feedings, an intravenous (IV) infusion of glucose will be necessary (see Chapter 27 for detailed discussion of hypoglycemia in the newborn).

Clinical Tip

When beginning fluids on an infant of a diabetic mother (IDM), it is sometimes best to start at a higher concentration of dextrose to avoid hypoglycemia episodes.

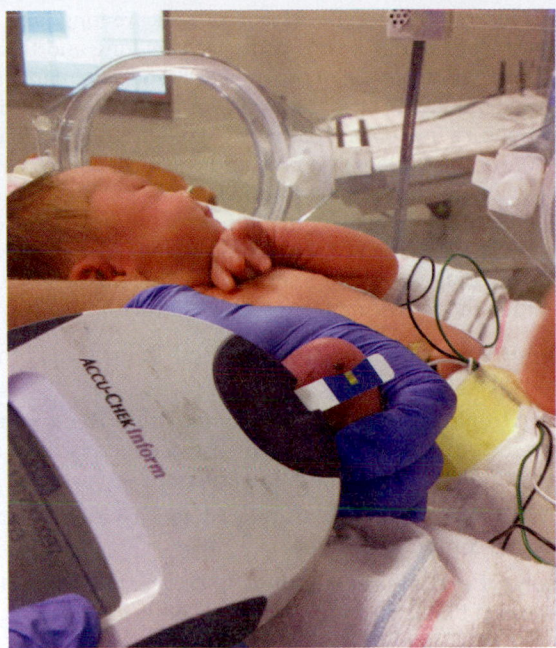

Figure 26–3 Nurse obtaining a bedside blood glucose.

SOURCE: Carol Harrigan, RN, MSN, NNP-BC.

Nursing Management

For the Infant of a Diabetic Mother (IDM)

Nursing Assessment and Diagnosis

Do not be lulled into thinking that a big baby is a mature baby. In almost every case, because of the newborn's large size, the IDM will appear older than gestational age scoring indicates. Consider both the gestational age and whether the baby is AGA or LGA in planning and providing safe care. In caring for the IDM, assess for signs of respiratory distress, hyperbilirubinemia, hypocalcemia, birth trauma, and congenital anomalies.

SAFETY ALERT!

When infusing either a D₁₀W bolus or a constant infusion, be careful not to administer too much glucose too fast in order to prevent hyperglycemic-induced insulin secretion. When beginning IV fluids on a symptomatic IDM, it is best to start an IV glucose infusion at 4 to 6 mg/kg/min to avoid rebound hypoglycemia (Armentrout, 2015).

Nursing diagnoses that may apply to IDMs include the following (NANDA-I © 2014):

- *Nutrition, Imbalanced: Less than Body Requirements,* related to increased glucose metabolism secondary to hyperinsulinemia
- *Gas Exchange, Impaired,* related to respiratory distress secondary to impaired production of surfactant
- *Tissue Perfusion: Peripheral, Ineffective,* secondary to polycythemia related to increased synthesis of erythropoietin, chronic intrauterine hypoxia, and increased metabolic rate

- *Tissue Integrity, Impaired,* related to poor maternal metabolic control
- *Family Processes, Interrupted,* related to the illness of the baby

Nursing Plan and Implementation

Nursing care of the IDM is directed toward early detection and ongoing monitoring of hypoglycemia (by performing glucose tests) and polycythemia (by obtaining central hematocrits), RDS, and hyperbilirubinemia. (These conditions are discussed in Chapter 27.) The nurse also assesses for signs of birth trauma and congenital anomalies.

Parent teaching is directed toward preventing macrosomia and the resulting fetal/neonatal problems by instituting early and ongoing diabetic control. Parents are advised that with early identification and care, most IDMs' complications have no significant sequelae.

Evaluation

Expected outcomes of nursing care include the following:

- The IDM's respiratory distress and metabolic problems are minimized.
- The parents understand the effects of maternal diabetes on the baby's health and preventive steps they can initiate to decrease its impact on subsequent pregnancies.
- The parents verbalize their concerns about their baby's health problems and understand the rationale behind management of their newborn.

Care of the Postterm Newborn

The **postterm newborn** is any newborn born after 42 completed weeks of gestation. Posterm or prolonged pregnancy occurs in approximately 7% of all pregnancies (Bowers, 2014). The cause of posterm pregnancy is not completely understood, but several factors are known to be associated with it. (See Chapter 21 for a discussion of maternal factors.) Many pregnancies classified as prolonged are thought to be a result of inaccurate estimates of date of birth (EDB). Posterm pregnancy is more common in Australian, Greek, and Italian ethnic groups.

Most babies born as a result of prolonged pregnancy are of normal size and health; some continue growing and are over 4000 g (8.8 lb) at birth, which supports the contention that the posterm fetus can remain well nourished. Potential intrapartum problems for these healthy but large fetuses are cephalopelvic disproportion (CPD) and shoulder dystocia (see Chapter 21 for discussion of the necessary assessments and interventions).

Common Complications of the Newborn With Postmaturity Syndrome

The term **postmaturity** applies only to the newborn who is born after 42 completed weeks of gestation and also demonstrates characteristics of *postmaturity syndrome.* Postterm newborns have begun to lose weight but usually have normal length and head circumference (Cloherty et al., 2012).

The characteristics of postmature newborns are primarily caused by a combination of advanced gestational age, placental aging and decreased placental function, and continued exposure to amniotic fluid. The truly postmature newborn is at high risk for morbidity and has a mortality rate 2 to 3 times greater than that of term newborns. Although today the percentages are extremely low, the majority of postmature fetal deaths occur during labor, because the fetus uses up necessary body reserves.

The following are common disorders of the postmature newborn:

- *Hypoglycemia*, from nutritional deprivation and depleted glycogen stores
- *Meconium aspiration* in response to in utero hypoxia as the stress of labor begins. The presence of oligohydramnios increases the danger of aspirating thick meconium. Severe meconium aspiration syndrome increases the baby's chance of developing persistent pulmonary hypertension, pneumothorax, and chemical pneumonitis.
- *Polycythemia* caused by increased production of red blood cells (RBCs) in response to hypoxia (impaired oxygenation)
- *Congenital anomalies* of unknown cause
- *Seizure* activity because of hypoxic insult
- *Cold stress* because of loss or poor development of subcutaneous fat.

Clinical Therapy

The aim of antenatal management is to differentiate the fetus with postmaturity syndrome from the fetus who at birth is large, well nourished, alert, and tolerating the prolonged (postterm) pregnancy. Antenatal tests that are done to evaluate fetal status and determine obstetric management and their use in postterm pregnancy are discussed in more depth in Chapters 14 and 20. If the amniotic fluid is meconium stained, an amnioinfusion may be done during labor. This procedure dilutes the meconium by directly infusing either normal saline or Ringer lactate into the uterus, decreasing the risk of meconium aspiration syndrome. (For detailed discussion of clinical management and care of the newborn at risk for meconium aspiration, see Chapter 27.)

Hypoglycemia is monitored by serial glucose determinations per agency protocols. The baby may be placed on glucose infusions or given early feedings if respiratory distress is not present, but these measures must be instituted with caution because of the frequency of asphyxia in the first 24 hours. Postmature newborns are often voracious eaters.

For the small-for-gestational-age (SGA) newborn who is postmature, peripheral and central hematocrits are tested to determine the presence of polycythemia. Fluid resuscitation can be initiated. In extreme cases a partial exchange transfusion may be necessary to prevent polycythemia and adverse sequelae such as hyperviscosity. Oxygen is provided for respiratory distress. In addition, temperature instability and excessive loss of heat can result from decreased liver glycogen stores. (See Chapter 27 for thermoregulation techniques.)

Nursing Management

For the Newborn With Postmaturity Syndrome

Nursing Assessment and Diagnosis

The newborn with postmaturity syndrome appears alert. This wide-eyed, alert appearance is not necessarily a positive sign because it may indicate chronic intrauterine hypoxia. The newborn typically has dry, cracking, parchmentlike skin without vernix or lanugo (Figure 26–4). Fingernails are long, and scalp hair is profuse. The newborn's body appears long and thin. The wasting involves depletion of previously stored subcutaneous tissue, causing the skin to be loose. Fat layers are almost nonexistent.

Postmature newborns frequently have meconium staining, which colors the nails, skin, and umbilical cord. The varying shades (yellow to green) of meconium staining can give some clue as to whether the expulsion of meconium in utero was a recent or a chronic problem. Green coloring indicates a more recent event.

Nursing diagnoses that may apply to the postmature newborn include the following (NANDA-I © 2014):

- *Hypothermia* related to decreased liver glycogen and brown fat stores
- *Nutrition, Imbalanced: Less Than Body Requirements*, related to increased use of glucose secondary to in utero stress and decreased placenta perfusion
- *Gas Exchange, Impaired*, related to airway obstruction from meconium aspiration
- *Tissue Perfusion: Peripheral, Ineffective*, related to increased blood viscosity caused by polycythemia

Nursing Plan and Implementation

Nursing care of the postmature newborn is directed toward early detection and ongoing monitoring of hypothermia (by regulating thermoregulation), hypoglycemia (by performing glucose tests), polycythemia (by obtaining central hematocrits), and meconium aspiration and respiratory distress syndrome (RDS) (by monitoring cardiopulmonary status). (These conditions are discussed in Chapter 27.)

Encourage parents to express their feelings and fears about the newborn's condition and potential long-term problems. Give careful explanations of procedures, include the parents in the development of care plans for their baby, and encourage follow-up care as needed.

Evaluation

Expected outcomes of nursing care include the following:

- The postterm newborn establishes effective respiratory function.
- The postmature baby is free of metabolic alterations (hypoglycemia) and maintains a stable temperature.

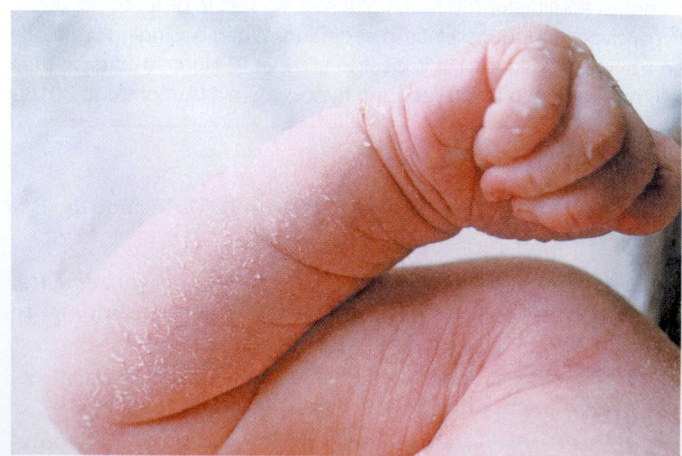

Figure 26–4 The skin of the postterm newborn exhibits deep cracking and peeling of skin.

SOURCE: Pablo Koch/Science Source.

Care of the Preterm (Premature) Newborn

A **preterm newborn** is any baby born at 37 or fewer weeks' gestation (Figure 26–5) (ACOG & Society for Maternal-Fetal Medicine (SMFM), 2013; Spong, 2013). With the help of modern technology, babies are surviving at younger gestational ages, but not without significant morbidity. The incidence of all preterm births in the United States in 2012 was approximately 11.7%, dropping for the fifth consecutive year, with the largest decline seen among babies born at 34 to 36 weeks' gestation (Brooks, 2013; Lynch, Dezen, & Brown, 2013). The United States still has the highest rate of preterm birth of any industrialized country, which costs businesses about 12 times as much as uncomplicated healthy births (Brooks, 2013).

The major problem of the preterm newborn is the variable immaturity of all systems. The degree of immaturity depends on the length of gestation. Because of immaturity, the premature newborn is ill equipped to smoothly traverse the same complex, interconnected pathways from intrauterine to extrauterine life.

Alteration in Respiratory and Cardiac Physiology

The preterm newborn is at risk for respiratory problems because of these critical factors in the development of respiratory distress:

1. The preterm newborn is unable to produce adequate amounts of surfactant. (See Chapter 23 for discussion of respiratory adaptation and development.) Inadequate surfactant lessens compliance (ability of the lung to fill with air easily), thereby increasing the inspiratory pressure needed to expand the lungs with air. This progressive atelectasis leads to an inability to develop a functional residual capacity (FRC), causing an ineffective exchange of oxygen and carbon dioxide. As a result, the baby becomes hypoxic, pulmonary blood flow is inefficient, and the preterm newborn's available energy is depleted.

2. The muscular coat of pulmonary blood vessels is incompletely developed. Consequently, the pulmonary arterioles do not constrict as well in response to decreased oxygen

levels. This lowered pulmonary vascular resistance leads to left-to-right shunting of blood through the ductus arteriosus, which increases the blood flow back into the lungs.

3. Normally the ductus arteriosus responds to increasing oxygen levels and prostaglandin E levels by vasoconstriction; in the preterm newborn, who is more susceptible to hypoxia, the ductus may remain open. A patent ductus increases the blood volume to the lungs, causing pulmonary congestion, increased respiratory effort, carbon dioxide retention, and bounding femoral pulses.

The common complications of the cardiopulmonary system in preterm newborns are discussed later in this chapter and in Chapter 27.

Alteration in Thermoregulation

Heat loss is a major problem in preterm newborns. Two factors limiting heat production, however, are the decreased availability of glycogen in the liver and the limited amount of brown fat available for heat production, which appear in the third trimester. Because the muscle mass is small in preterm babies, and muscular activity is diminished (they are unable to shiver), heat production is further limited.

Five physiologic and anatomic factors increase heat loss in the preterm newborn:

1. The preterm baby has a higher ratio of body surface to body weight. This means that the baby's ability to produce heat (based on body weight) is much less than the potential for losing heat (based on surface area). The loss of heat in a preterm newborn weighing 1500 g (3.3 lb) is five times greater per unit of body weight than in an adult.

2. The preterm baby has very little subcutaneous fat, which is the human body's insulation. Without adequate insulation, heat is easily conducted from the core of the body (warmer temperature) to the surface of the body (cooler temperature). Heat is lost from the body as the blood vessels, which lie close to the skin surface in the preterm newborn, transport blood from the body core to the subcutaneous tissues.

3. The preterm newborn has thinner, more permeable skin than the term baby. This increased permeability contributes to a greater insensible water loss as well as to heat loss.

4. Flexion of the extremities decreases the amount of surface area exposed to the environment. Extension increases the surface area exposed to the environment and thus increases heat loss. The gestational age of the newborn influences the amount of flexion, from completely hypotonic and extended at 28 weeks to strong flexion displayed by 36 weeks.

5. The preterm baby has a decreased ability to vasoconstrict superficial blood vessels and conserve heat in the body core.

In summary, gestational age is directly proportional to the ability to maintain thermoregulation; thus the more preterm the newborn, the less able the baby is to maintain heat balance. Preventing heat loss by providing a neutral thermal environment using a servocontrol skin probe is one of the most important considerations in nursing management of the preterm baby. Other nursing interventions assisting in the thermoregulation of the preterm newborn include increasing the delivery room temperature, loosely covering the baby with polyethylene wrap, placing the baby in a plastic bag from feet to shoulders, and

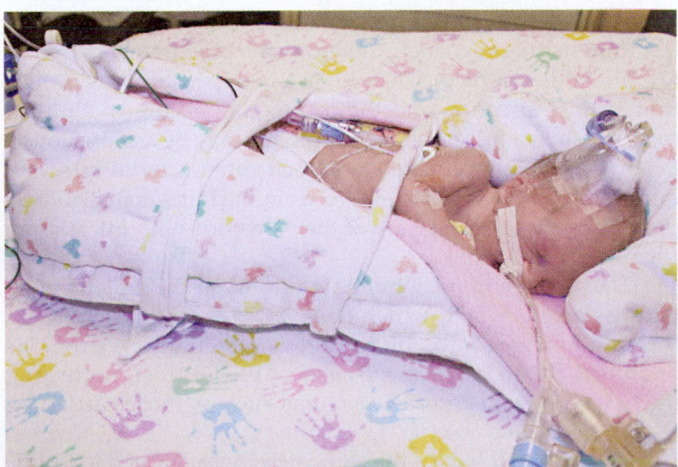

Figure 26–5 A 6-day-old, 26–week gestational age, 960-g preterm newborn.

SOURCE: Carol Harrigan, RN, MSN, NNP-BC.

placing the baby on a chemical mattress. Cold stress, with its accompanying severe complications, can be prevented (see the section Care of the Newborn with Cold Stress in Chapter 27).

Alteration in Gastrointestinal Physiology

Maturation of the digestive and absorptive process is more variable, however, and occurs later in gestation. As a result of GI immaturity, the preterm newborn has the following ingestion, digestive, and absorption problems (Ditzenberger, 2015):

- A marked danger of aspiration and its associated complications because of the baby's poorly developed gag reflex, incompetent esophageal cardiac sphincter, and poor sucking and swallowing reflexes.
- Difficulty in meeting high caloric and fluid needs for growth because of small stomach capacity.
- Limited ability to convert certain essential amino acids to nonessential amino acids. Certain amino acids, such as histidine, taurine, and cysteine, are essential to the preterm newborn but not to the term newborn.
- Inability to handle the increased osmolarity of formula protein because of kidney immaturity. The preterm newborn requires a higher concentration of whey protein than of casein.
- Difficulty absorbing saturated fats because of decreased bile salts and pancreatic lipase. Severe illness of the newborn may also prevent intake of adequate nutrients.
- Difficulty with lactose digestion initially because processes may not be fully functional during the first few days of a preterm newborn's life. The preterm newborn can digest and absorb most simple sugars.
- Deficiency of calcium and phosphorus may exist because two thirds of these minerals are deposited in the last trimester. Rickets and significant bone demineralization caused by deficiency of calcium and phosphorus, which are deposited primarily in the last trimester, are also problems.
- Increased basal metabolic rate and increased oxygen requirements caused by fatigue associated with sucking.
- Feeding intolerance and necrotizing enterocolitis (NEC) as a result of diminished blood flow and tissue perfusion to the intestinal tract because of a combination of contributing factors including prematurity, formula feeding, bacterial colonization, and hypoemia/ischemia events (Bradshaw, 2015).

Alteration in Renal Physiology

Specific characteristics of the preterm newborn that pose clinical problems in the management of fluid and electrolyte balance include the following:

- The glomerular filtration rate (GFR) is directly related to lower gestational age and increases steadily after 34 weeks postconceptual age (PCA). The GFR is also decreased in the presence of diseases or conditions that decrease the renal blood flow and perfusion, such as severe respiratory distress, hypotension, and asphyxia. Preterm newborns usually have some urine output during the first 24 hours of life. By day 3, urine output should be approximately 1 to 3 mL/kg/hr. A low systolic blood pressure can reflect any diseases that decrease cardiac output and affect renal blood flow. Systolic blood pressure (BP) varies with gestational age and PCA.

Clinical Tip

A gradual decline in urine may be associated with a drop in the newborn's blood pressure.

- The preterm newborn's kidneys are limited in their ability to concentrate urine or to excrete excess amounts of fluid, because of a blunted response to antidiuretic hormone (ADH). This means that if excess fluid is administered, the baby is at risk for fluid retention and overhydration. If too little is administered, the baby will become dehydrated because of the inability to retain adequate fluid.
- The preterm newborn's kidneys begin excreting glucose (glycosuria) at a lower serum glucose level than that of the term newborn. Therefore, glycosuria with hyperglycemia can lead to osmotic diuresis and polyuria.
- The kidneys' buffering capacity is reduced, predisposing the newborn to metabolic acidosis. Bicarbonate is excreted at a lower serum level, and acid is excreted more slowly. Therefore, after periods of hypoxia or insult, the preterm baby's kidneys require a longer time to excrete the lactic acid that accumulates.
- The immaturity of the renal system affects the preterm newborn's ability to excrete drugs. Because excretion time is longer, many drugs are given over longer intervals (i.e., every 24 hours instead of every 12 hours). Urine output must be carefully monitored when the baby is receiving nephrotoxic drugs such as gentamicin and vancomycin. In the event that urine output is poor, drugs can become toxic in the baby much more quickly than in the adult.

Alteration in Immunologic Physiology

The preterm newborn has an increased susceptibility to infections acquired in utero that may have precipitated preterm labor and birth. However, all preterm newborns have immature specific and nonspecific immunity.

In utero the fetus receives passive immunity against a variety of infections from maternal IgG immunoglobulins, which cross the placenta. Most passive immunity is acquired in the last trimester of pregnancy; therefore, the preterm newborn has few antibodies at birth. The preterm newborn has less protection against infection and that protection becomes depleted earlier than in a full-term newborn. This may be a contributing factor in the higher incidence of recurrent bacterial infection during the first year of life as well as in the immediate neonatal period. (See the section Care of the Newborn With Infection in Chapter 27.)

The other immunoglobulin significant for the preterm newborn is secretory IgA, which does not cross the placenta but is found in breast milk. Breast milk's secretory IgA provides immunity to the mucosal surfaces of the GI tract, protecting the newborn from enteric infections such as those caused by *Escherichia coli* and *Shigella*.

In very small babies the skin is easily excoriated, and this factor, coupled with many invasive procedures, places the newborn at great risk for nosocomial infections. It is vital to use good hand hygiene techniques in the care of these babies to prevent unnecessary infection.

Alteration in Neurologic Physiology

Because the period of most rapid brain growth and development occurs during the third trimester of pregnancy, the closer
to term a baby is born, the better the neurologic prognosis. A
common interruption of neurologic development in the preterm
newborn is caused by intraventricular hemorrhage (IVH) and
intracranial hemorrhage (ICH). Hydrocephalus may develop as
a consequence of an IVH caused by the obstruction at the cerebral aqueduct (Scher, 2013).

Alteration in Reactivity Periods and Behavioral States

The newborn's response to extrauterine life is characterized by
two periods of reactivity (see Chapter 23). However, the preterm newborn's periods of reactivity are delayed. In the very ill
newborn, these periods of reactivity may not be observed at all
because the baby may be hypotonic and unreactive for several
days after birth.

In general, stable preterm newborns do not demonstrate
the same behavioral states as term newborns. Preterm babies
tend to be more disorganized in their sleep–wake cycles and
are unable to attend as well to the human face and objects in
the environment. Neurologically, their responses (sucking,
muscle tone, states of arousal) are weaker than full-term babies'
responses.

Clinical Tip
After observing a newborn's pattern of behavior and responses,
especially the sleep–wake states, use the time when the baby is
alert and best able to attend to help parents learn about and provide newborn care and form a positive attachment with their child.

Management of Nutrition and Fluid Requirements

Early feedings are extremely valuable for the premature newborn in maintaining normal metabolism and lowering the
possibility of such complications as hypoglycemia, hyperbilirubinemia, hyperkalemia, and osteopenia of prematurity and
other digestive system problems.

NUTRITIONAL REQUIREMENTS

Oral (enteral) caloric intake necessary for growth in a healthy
preterm newborn is 95 to 130 kcal/kg/day (Blackburn, 2013).
Early feedings are associated with improved glucose homeostasis, immune functions, and weight gain patterns, ultimately
resulting in early discharge home. Human milk is preferred

EVIDENCE-BASED PRACTICE | Improving Outcomes for Late Preterm Newborns

Clinical Question
What interventions support the best outcomes for late preterm babies (neonates born between 34 weeks 0 days and
36 weeks 6 days gestation)?

The Evidence
In 2006, the National Institutes of Health recommended using
the term *late preterm* to describe those babies born between
34 0/7 and 36 6/7 weeks of gestation. While these neonates
are often considered *near term*, this reference underestimates
the risks to this population. Nearly 10% of all births fall into this
classification, and the newborns have a higher rate of hypothermia, respiratory complications, feeding difficulty, extended
lengths of stay, and infant mortality. It is now recognized that
this group of babies requires careful perinatal monitoring, cus-
tomized feeding plans, consideration of neurological development, and close follow up after they go home (Baker, 2015a).
An interprofessional team of nurses from labor and delivery,
neonatal ICU, and postpartum care collaborated on a systematic review of the literature to develop an evidence-based
practice guideline for this group of at-risk babies. This type of
structured review based on randomized trials and culminating
in a practice guideline forms the strongest level of evidence.

Best practice focuses on appropriate monitoring and
prevention of complications. Late preterm newborns—or
babies weighing less than 2000 grams (4.4 lb)—should be
admitted to a neonatal ICU for at least 24 hours of observation and monitoring. Babies born between 35 and 36 weeks of
gestation should be monitored for signs of respiratory distress,
particularly those with a birth Apgar of 4 or less. Newborns of
greater than 36 weeks' gestation can be moved to the mother/
baby unit unless clinically unstable. These babies should be
admitted to a specialty care unit if they have persistent oxygen
requirements, any evidence of apnea, inability to take adequate feeding, respiratory distress, or inability to regulate body
temperature (Baker, 2015b). If admitted to a specialty care
unit, these babies should have frequent measurement of vital
signs, an external heat source until body temperature stabilizes, blood glucose on admission and then every 8 hours, and
routine feeding when the respiratory rate is below 60. Transfer
to the mother/baby unit should occur only when all criteria are
met to facilitate mother/baby interaction, achieve adequate
nutritional intake, and breathe without distress.

Best Practice
Late preterm newborns have an elevated risk of complications,
and should be treated as at-risk neonates. Close monitoring
of respiratory condition, feeding behavior, neurological status,
and blood glucose is needed to recognize signs of distress and
other complications. Babies can be transferred to routine care
when they are stable and able to feed adequately.

Clinical Reasoning
What assessments should the nurse include to be sure that the
baby is stable and can be cared for by the mother? What will
be included in the discharge teaching plan for these mothers?

for feeding the preterm newborn with significant benefits for the mother, baby, family, and society (O'Hare, Wood, & Fiske, 2013). Human donor milk is an available option for the high-risk newborn whose mother in unable to produce sufficient amounts of milk. To meet the high caloric needs of the growing premature baby, breast milk may be fortified or special preterm formulas may be used.

Whether breast milk or formula is used, feeding protocols are established based on the baby's weight and estimated stomach capacity. Initial formula-feedings are gradually increased as the baby tolerates them.

In addition to a higher calorie and protein formula, preterm newborns should receive supplemental multivitamins, including vitamins A, D, and E, iron, and trace minerals. A diet high in polyunsaturated fats (which preterm babies tolerate best) increases the requirement for vitamin E. Preterm newborns fed iron-fortified formulas have higher red cell hemolysis and lower vitamin E concentrations and thus require additional vitamin E. Preterm formulas also need to contain medium-chain triglycerides (MCT) and additional amino acids such as cysteine, as well as calcium, phosphorus, and vitamin D supplements to increase mineralization of bones. Rickets and significant bone demineralization have been documented in very-low-birth-weight newborns and otherwise healthy preterm babies.

Nutritional intake is considered adequate when there is consistent weight gain of 20 to 30 g/day. Initially, no weight gain may be noted for several days, but total weight loss should not exceed 15% of the total birth weight or more than 1% to 2% per day. Some institutions add the criteria of head circumference growth and increase in body length of 1 cm (0.4 in.) per week, once the newborn is stable.

METHODS OF FEEDING

The preterm newborn is fed by various methods depending on the baby's gestational age, health and physical condition, and neurologic status. The three most common oral feeding methods are bottle, breast, and gavage.

Bottle-Feeding. Preterm newborns who have a coordinated as well as rhythmic suck–swallow–breathing pattern are usually between 35 and 36 weeks' postconceptual age and may be fed by bottle. Oral readiness to feed is best described by the following engagement and hunger cues (Newland et al., 2013):

- Bringing hands to the mouth
- Being alert
- Exhibiting fussiness
- Sucking on fingers or pacifier
- Exhibiting rooting behavior
- Showing relaxed facial expression and good tone

To avoid excessive expenditure of energy, a soft, yellow, single-hole nipple is usually used (milk flow is less rapid). The baby is fed in a semisitting position and burped gently after each 0.5 to 1 oz. The feeding should take no longer than 15 to 20 minutes (nippling requires more energy than other methods). Premature newborns who are progressing from gavage feedings to bottle-feeding should be assessed for feeding readiness and started with one session of bottle-feeding a day. The number of times a day a bottle is offered should be increased slowly until the baby tolerates all feedings from a bottle (Figure 26–6).

Sucking may be affected by age, asphyxia, sepsis, intraventricular hemorrhage, or other neurologic insult. Before initiating nipple feeding, the nurse observes for signs of stress, such

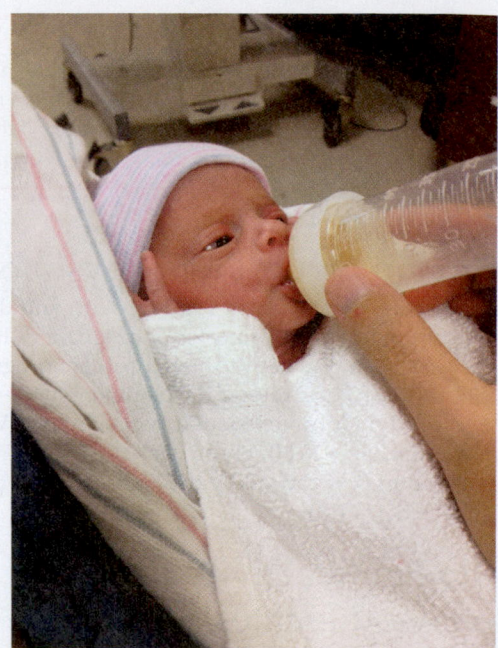

Figure 26–6 Mother bottle-feeding her premature newborn with expressed breast milk.

SOURCE: Carol Harrigan, RN, MSN, NNP-BC.

as tachypnea (more than 60 respirations per minute), respiratory distress, or hypothermia, which may increase the risk of aspiration. During the feeding the nurse observes the newborn for signs of feeding difficulty (tachypnea, decrease in oxygen saturation levels, bradycardia, lethargy, uncoordinated suck and swallow). Difficulty in bottle-feeding is often associated with a milk bolus that is too large for the baby's oral cavity, which can lead to aspiration. Demand feeding protocols, based on the baby's hunger cues, should be considered for a growing premature newborn only when there is sufficient caloric intake to promote consistent weight gain (Newland et al., 2013). See Table 26–1.

Clinical Tip

The more preterm the newborn is at birth, the longer it will take to reach the maturational state required to be successful at oral feedings.

Breastfeeding. Mothers who wish to breastfeed their preterm newborns are given the opportunity to put the baby to the breast as soon as the baby has demonstrated a coordinated suck and swallow reflex, is showing consistent weight gain, and can control body temperature outside of the incubator, regardless of weight. Preterm newborns tolerate breastfeeding with higher transcutaneous oxygen pressures and better maintenance of body temperature than during bottle-feeding. Besides breast milk's many benefits for the newborn, it allows the mother to contribute actively to the baby's well-being (Figure 26–7). The nurse should encourage mothers to breastfeed if they choose to do so. It is important for the nurse to be aware of the advantages of breastfeeding, as well as the possible disadvantages of breast milk as the sole source of food for the preterm newborn (see Chapter 25).

By initiating skin-to-skin holding of premature newborns in the early intensive care phase, mothers can significantly

TABLE 26–1 Cue-Based Feeding Readiness Scales

FEEDING								
Readiness								
Quality								
Caregiver								
Time								
Quantity								
Nipple (circle breast or write nipple color)	Breast Nipple color	Breast Nipple color	Breast Nipple color	Breast Nipple color	Breast Nipple color	Breast Nipple color	Breast Nipple color	Breast Nipple color
Initial								

Readiness

Breastfeed (Bottle)

SCORE	DESCRIPTION
1	Drowsy, alert, or fussy prior to care. Rooting and/or hands to mouth / takes pacifier. Good tone.
2	Drowsy or alert once handled. Some rooting or takes pacifier. Adequate tone.

Breastfeed (No bottle)

SCORE	DESCRIPTION
3	Briefly alert with care. No hunger behaviors. No change in tone.
4	Sleeping throughout care. No hunger cues. No change in tone.

Gavage only

SCORE	DESCRIPTION
5	Needs increased O_2 with care. Apnea/bradycardia (A/B) with care. Tachypnea over baseline with care.

Caregiver Techniques

SCORE	DESCRIPTION
A	Side-lying position
B	External pacing
C	Adding or increasing O_2 during feed
D	Imposed breaks
E	Stimulation for/recovery from A/B
F	Frequent burping
G	Nipple change
H	Other (specify)

Quality Breastfeeding

SCORE	DESCRIPTION
1	Latched well with a strong coordinated suck for >15 min.
2	Latched well with a strong coordinated suck initially, but fatigues with progression. Active suck for 8–15 min.
3	Difficulty maintaining a strong, consistent latch. May be able to nurse intermittently but active for only <15 min.
4	Latch is weak/inconsistent, with a frequent need to relatch. Limited effort with inconsistent pattern. May be considered nonnutritional breastfeeding (NNBF).
5	Unable to latch to breast and achieve suck–swallow-breathe pattern. May have difficulty arousing to a state conducive to breastfeeding. Could result in frequent or significant A/B's and/or tachypnea significantly above baseline with feeding.

Quality Bottle

SCORE	DESCRIPTION
1	Nipples with a strong coordinated suck throughout feed.
2	Nipples with a strong coordinated suck initially, but fatigues with progression.
3	Nipples with consistent suck, but difficulty coordinating swallow; some loss of liquid or difficulty pacing. Benefits from external pacing.
4	Nipples with a weak/inconsistent suck. Little to no rhythm. May require some rest breaks.
5	Disorganized; unable to coordinate suck–swallow–breathe pattern. May result in frequent or significant A/Bs or large amounts of liquid loss and or tachypnea significantly above baseline with feeding.
6	Dysfunctional; abnormal or deviant oral motor patterns evidenced by inability to extract fluid from nipple.

Sources: Data from Baylor University Medical Center, Dallas, Texas; Ludwig, S. M., & Weitzman, K. A. (2007). Changing feeding documentation to reflect infant-driven feeding practice. *Newborn and Infant Nursing Reviews, 7,* 155–160.

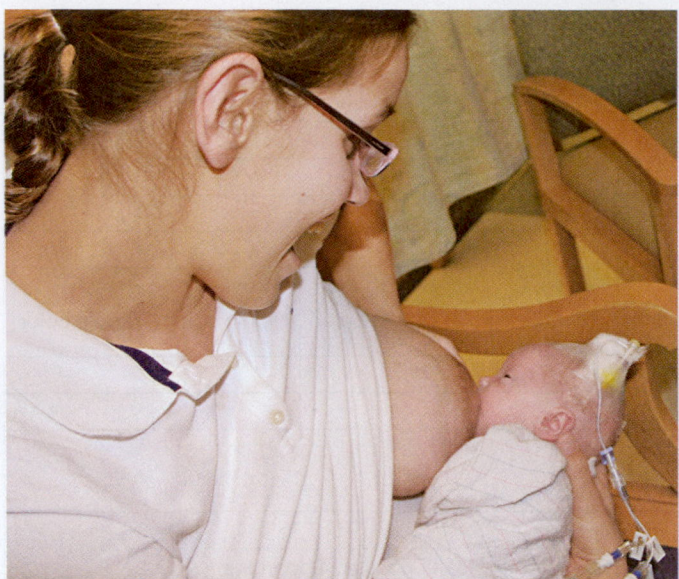

Figure 26–7 This mother is breastfeeding her premature newborn.

SOURCE: Carol Harrigan, RN, MSN, NNP-BC.

increase milk volume, thereby overcoming lactation problems. Many mothers of preterm newborns seem to find that the football hold (refer to Figure 25-16) is a convenient position for breastfeeding preterm babies. Feeding may take up to 45 minutes, and babies should be burped as they alternate breasts. Length of feeding time must be monitored so that the preterm newborn does not expend too many calories.

The nurse should coordinate a flexible feeding schedule so that babies can nurse during alert times and be allowed to set their own pace. Feedings should be on demand, but a maximum number of hours between feedings should be set. A similar regimen should be used for the baby who is progressing from gavage feeding to breastfeeding. The mother begins with one feeding at the breast and then gradually increases the number of times during the day that the baby breastfeeds. Even if the baby cannot be put to the breast, mothers can pump their breasts, and the breast milk can be given via gavage. A double-pumping system produces higher levels of prolactin than sequential pumping of the breasts. When breastfeeding is not possible because the baby is too small or too weak to suck at the breast, an option for the mother may be to express her breast milk into a cup. The milk touches the baby's lips and is lapped by the protruding motions of the tongue.

Gavage Feeding. The gavage feeding method is used with preterm newborns (less than 34 weeks' gestation) who lack or have a poorly coordinated suck and swallow reflex or are ill and ventilator dependent. Gavage feeding may be used as an adjunct to nipple feeding if the newborn tires easily or as an alternative if the baby is losing weight because of the energy expenditure required for nippling (see *Clinical Skill: Performing Gavage Feeding*). Gavage feedings are administered by the intermittent bolus or continuous drip method. In common practice, bolus gavage feedings are usually initiated, but if intolerance occurs, then the feedings are changed to infuse on a pump over a set amount of time (i.e., over an hour) or continuously. Gavage feeding is not without its consequences, including gastroesophageal reflux (GER), which can lead to significant emesis, food refusal, dysphagia, oral eversion, and aspiration (Jones, 2012).

Clinical Skill 26–1
Performing Gavage Feeding

NURSING ACTION

Preparation

- When choosing the catheter size, consider the size of the baby, the area of insertion (oral or nasal), and the desired rate of flow.

Rationale: The size of the catheter will influence the rate of flow.

- Explain the procedure to the parents.

- Elevate the head of the bed and position the newborn on the back or side to allow easy passage of the tube.

- Measure the distance from the tip of the ear to the nose to the xiphoid process, and mark the point with a small piece of paper tape (Figure 26–8) to ensure enough tubing to enter the stomach.

Equipment and Supplies

- No. 5 or No. 8 Fr. feeding tube
- 3- to 5-ml syringe, for aspirating stomach contents

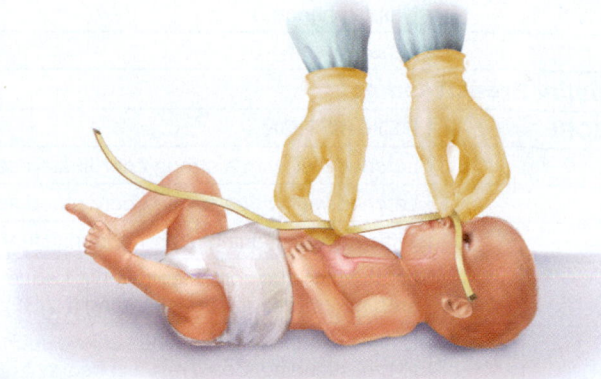

Figure 26–8 Measuring gavage tube length.

- 1/4-in. paper tape, to mark the tube for insertion depth and to secure the catheter during feeding
- Stethoscope, for auscultating the rush of air into the stomach when testing the tube placement
- Appropriate formula
- Small cup of sterile water to act as lubricant
- Clean gloves

Procedure: Clean Gloves

Inserting and Checking Placement of Tube

1. If inserting the tube nasally, lubricate the tip in a cup of sterile water. Use water instead of an oil-based lubricant, in case the tube is inadvertently passed into a lung. Shake any excess drops to prevent aspiration.

2. If inserting the tube orally, the oral secretions are enough to lubricate the tube adequately.

3. Stabilize the baby's head with one hand and pass the tube via the mouth (or nose) into the stomach to the point previously marked. If the baby begins coughing or choking or becomes cyanotic or phonic, remove the tube immediately as the tube has probably entered the trachea.

4. If respiratory distress is not apparent, lightly tape the tube in position, draw up 0.5 to 1.0 ml of air in the syringe, and connect the syringe to the tubing. Place the stethoscope over the epigastrium and briskly inject the air (Figure 26–9). You will hear a sudden rush as the air enters the stomach.

5. Aspirate the stomach contents with the syringe, and note the amount, color, and consistency to evaluate the newborn's feeding tolerance. Return the residual to the stomach unless you are requested to discard it. It is usually not discarded because of the potential for electrolyte imbalance.

Administering the Feeding

1. Hold the baby for feeding, or position the baby on the right side.

Rationale: This position decreases the risk of aspiration in case of emesis during feeding.

2. Separate the syringe from the tube, remove the plunger from the barrel, reconnect the barrel to the tube, and pour the formula into the syringe.

3. Elevate the syringe 6 to 8 inches over the baby's head, and allow the formula to flow by gravity at a slow, even rate. You may need to initiate the flow of formula by inserting the plunger of the syringe into the barrel just until you see formula enter the feeding tube. Do not use pressure.

4. Regulate the rate to prevent sudden stomach distention leading to vomiting and aspiration. Continue adding formula to the syringe until the baby has absorbed the desired volume.

Clearing and Removing the Tube

1. Clear the tubing with 2 to 3 ml of air.

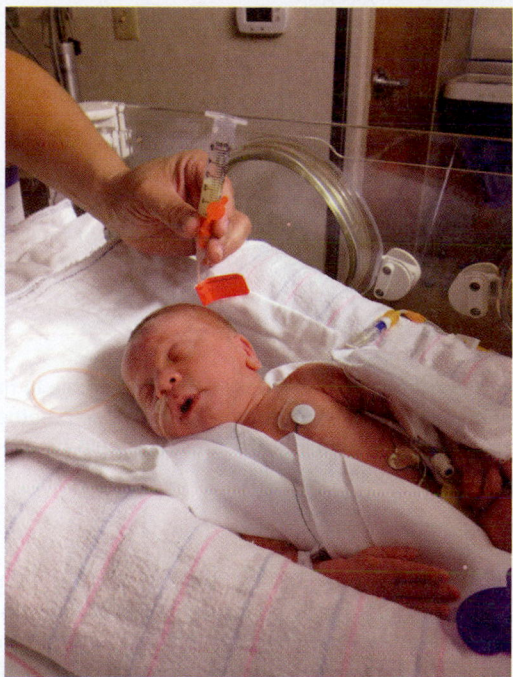

Figure 26–9 Gavage feeding a preterm newborn, flowing in by gravity.

SOURCE: Carol Harrigan, RN, MSN, NNP-BC.

Rationale: This ensures that the baby has received all of the formula. If the tube is going to be left in place, clearing it will decrease the risk of occlusion and bacterial growth in the tube.

2. To remove the tube, loosen the tape, fold the tube over on itself, and quickly withdraw the tube in one smooth motion to minimize the potential for fluid aspiration as the tube passes the epiglottis. If the tube is to be left in, position it so that the baby is unable to remove it. Replace the tube per hospital policy.

Maximize the Feeding Pleasure of the Baby

1. Whenever possible, hold the baby during gavage feeding. If it is too awkward to hold the baby during feeding, be sure to take time for holding after the feeding.

Rationale: Feeding time is important to the newborn's tactile sensory input.

2. Offer a pacifier to the baby during the feeding.

Rationale: Sucking during feeding comforts and relaxes the newborn, making the formula flow more easily. Babies can lose their sucking reflexes when fed by gavage for long periods.

3. Document procedure, including untoward complications, in the baby's medical record.

Early initiation of minimal enteral nutrition (MEN) via gavage is now advocated as a supplement to parenteral nutrition. MEN refers to small-volume feedings of formula or human milk (usually less than 24 ml/kg/day) which are designed to "prime" the intestinal tract, thereby stimulating many of its hormonal and enzymatic functions (Cloherty et al., 2012). Benefits of early feeding (as early as 24 to 72 hours of life) include the following:

- No increase in the incidence of necrotizing enterocolitis
- Fewer days on total parenteral nutrition (TPN), thereby decreasing the incidence of cholestatic jaundice

- Increased weight gain
- Increased muscle maturation of the gut as well as muscle growth
- Increased gut peristalsis and gut hormone levels, which can lead to improved feeding tolerance
- Shorter time required to reach full-volume enteral feedings
- Lower risk of osteopenia
- Possible decrease in the total number of hospital days in the NICU

SAFETY ALERT!

Orogastric gavage catheter placement is preferable to nasogastric because most newborns are obligatory nose breathers. If nasogastric is used, a #5 French catheter should be used to minimize airway obstruction.

Fluid Requirements. The calculation of fluid requirements must take into account the newborn's weight and postnatal age. Recommendations for fluid therapy in the preterm newborn weighing 1500 g are approximately 60 to 80 ml/kg/day for day 1; 80 to 120 ml/kg/day for day 2; and 120 to 160 ml/kg/day by day 3 of life. These amounts may be increased up to 190 ml/kg/day if the newborn is very small, receiving phototherapy, or under a radiant warmer because of the increased insensible water losses. Fluid losses can be minimized through the use of heat shields and added humidification in the incubator. Daily weights, and sometimes weights every 6 to 8 hours, are the best indicator of fluid status in the less than 1000-g preterm newborn. The expected weight loss during the first 5 to 6 days of life in a preterm newborn is 15% to 20% of birth weight (Cloherty et al., 2012).

Common Complications of Preterm Newborns and Their Clinical Management

The goals of medical and nursing care are to meet the preterm newborn's growth and development needs and to anticipate and manage the complications associated with prematurity. The most common complications associated with prematurity are as follows:

- *Apnea of prematurity.* Apnea of prematurity refers to cessation of breathing for 20 seconds or longer or for less than 20 seconds when associated with cyanosis, pallor, and bradycardia. Apnea is a common problem in the preterm newborn less than 36 weeks, presenting between day 2 and day 7 of life. The etiology of apnea is multifactorial but is thought to be primarily a result of neuronal immaturity, a factor that contributes to the preterm newborn's irregular breathing patterns (central apnea). Obstructive apnea can occur when there is cessation of airflow associated with blockage of the upper airway (small airway diameter, increased pharyngeal secretions, altered body alignment and positioning). Gastroesophageal reflux (GER) is defined as a movement of gastric contents into the lower esophagus caused by poor esophageal sphincter tone, causing laryngospasm, which leads to bradycardia and apnea. Apnea of prematurity is then a diagnosis of exclusion.

Clinical Tip

For an otherwise healthy, growing premature newborn who is receiving total enteral intake and has started to experience apnea and bradycardia, one differential diagnosis to think about is reflux rather than sepsis, although sepsis may need to be ruled out.

- *Patent ductus arteriosus (PDA).* The ductus arteriosus fails to close because of decreased pulmonary arteriole musculature and hypoxemia. Symptomatic PDA is often seen around the time when premature newborns are recovering from respiratory distress syndrome (RDS). Patent ductus arteriosus often prolongs the course of illness in a preterm newborn and leads to chronic pulmonary dysfunction.

CLINICAL TIP

A growing premature newborn showing clinical signs of worsening respiratory status (i.e., increased oxygen needs, increased ventilatory settings), acidosis, and hypotension may be exhibiting signs and symptoms of a patent ductus arteriosus (PDA).

- *Respiratory distress syndrome (RDS).* Respiratory distress results from inadequate surfactant production (see Chapter 27).
- *Intraventricular hemorrhage (IVH).* Intraventricular hemorrhage is the most common type of intracranial hemorrhage in small preterm newborns, especially those weighing less than 1500 g or of less than 34 weeks' gestation. Up to 34 weeks' gestation, the preterm newborn's brain ventricles are lined by the germinal matrix, which is highly susceptible to hypoxic events such as respiratory distress, birth trauma, and birth asphyxia. The germinal matrix is highly vascular, and these blood vessels rupture in the presence of hypoxia (Scher, 2013).

SAFETY ALERT!

An extremely premature, low-birth-weight newborn who presents with a sudden drop in hemoglobin along with the onset of severe metabolic acidosis, a "waxy" color, and hypotension may have experienced an intracranial hemorrhage.

Other common problems of preterm newborns such as NEC are briefly discussed earlier in the physiologic sections. (For in-depth discussions of RDS, hyperbilirubinemia, hypoglycemia, anemia of prematurity, and sepsis, see Chapter 27.)

Long-Term Needs and Outcome

The care of preterm newborns and their families does not stop on discharge from the nursery. Within the first year of life, low-birth-weight preterm babies face higher mortality rates than term babies. Causes of death include sudden infant death syndrome (SIDS)—which occurs about five times more frequently in the preterm baby—respiratory infections, and neurologic defects. Morbidity is also much higher among preterm babies, with those weighing less than 1500 g (3.3 lb) at highest risk for long-term complications.

The most common long-term needs observed in preterm newborns include the following:

- *Retinopathy of prematurity (ROP).* Premature newborns are particularly susceptible to characteristic retinal changes, known as ROP, which can result in visual impairment. The disease is now viewed as multifactorial in origin. Increased survival of very-low-birth-weight (VLBW) newborns may be the most important factor in the increased incidence of ROP.

SAFETY ALERT!

According to AAP (2013), all newborns with a birth weight of less than or equal to 1500 g (3.3 lb) or gestational age of 30 weeks or less and selected newborns with a birth weight between 1500 and 2000 g (3.3 and 4.4 lb) or gestational age of more than 30 weeks with an unstable clinical course should have a retinal screening examination (see Figure 26–10).

- *Bronchopulmonary dysplasia (BPD).* Long-term lung disease is a result of damage to the alveolar epithelium secondary to positive pressure respiratory therapy and high oxygen concentration. These babies have long-term dependence on oxygen therapy and an increased incidence of respiratory infection during their first few years of life.
- *Speech defects.* The most frequently observed speech defects involve delayed development of receptive and expressive ability that may persist into the school-age years.
- *Neurologic defects.* The most common neurologic defects include cerebral palsy, hydrocephalus, seizure disorders, lower IQ, and learning disabilities. However, the socioeconomic climate and family support systems are extremely important influences on the child's ultimate school

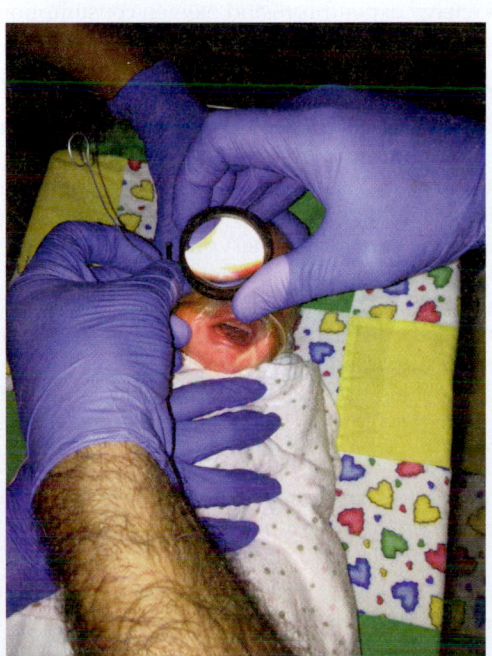

Figure 26–10 A pediatric ophthalmologist performing an eye examination on a preterm newborn screening for ROP.

SOURCE: Carol Harrigan, RN, MSN, NNP-BC.

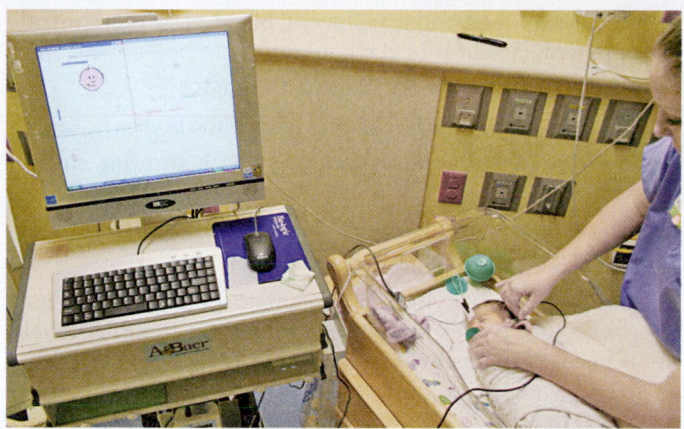

Figure 26–11 Preterm newborns should have a formal hearing test prior to discharge.

SOURCE: Carol Harrigan, RN, MSN, NNP-BC.

performance in the absence of major neurologic defects. Families can be reminded that risk does not equal injury, injury does not equal damage, and description of damage does not allow a precise prediction about recovery or outcome.

- *Auditory defects.* Preterm newborns have a 1% to 4% incidence of moderate to profound hearing loss and should have a formal audiologic examination before discharge and at 3 to 6 months (corrected age). Tests currently used to measure hearing functions of the newborn are the evoked otoacoustic emissions (EOAE) or the automated auditory brain response (AABR) test (Figure 26–11). Any baby with repeated abnormal results should be referred to speech/language specialists.

Healthy People 2020

(ENT-VSL-1.1) Increase the proportion of newborns who are screened for hearing loss no later than age 1 month

---

When evaluating the newborn's abilities and disabilities, parents must understand that developmental progress must be evaluated based on chronologic age from the expected date of birth, not from the actual date of birth (corrected age). In addition, the parents need the consistent support of healthcare professionals in the long-term management of their babies. Many new and ongoing concerns arise as the high-risk infant grows and develops; the goal is to promote the highest quality of life possible.

Nursing Management

For the Preterm Newborn

Nursing Assessment and Diagnosis

Assess the physical characteristics and gestational age of the preterm newborn accurately to anticipate the special needs and problems of the baby. Physical characteristics vary greatly depending on gestational age, but the following characteristics are frequently present:

- *Color.* Usually pink or ruddy but may be acrocyanotic (cyanosis, jaundice, and pallor are abnormal and should be noted)

- *Skin.* Reddened and translucent, blood vessels are readily apparent, lack of subcutaneous fat
- *Lanugo.* Plentiful and widely distributed
- *Head size.* Appears large in relation to the body
- *Skull.* Bones pliable, fontanelle smooth and flat, sutures approximated or overriding
- *Ears.* Minimal cartilage, pliable, folded over
- *Nails.* Soft, short
- *Genitals.* Male: Nonrugated, small scrotum; testes may or may not be descended, or found in the inguinal canals. Female: Prominent clitoris and labia minora.
- *Posture.* Flaccid, froglike position
- *Cry.* Weak, feeble
- *Reflexes.* Poor suck, swallow, and gag; incomplete Moro
- *Activity.* Jerky, generalized movements (not seizure related), decreased tone

Determining gestational age in preterm newborns requires knowledge and experience in administering gestational assessment tools. The tool used should be specific, reliable, and valid. (For a discussion of gestational age assessment tools, see Chapter 24.)

Nursing diagnoses that may apply to the preterm newborn include the following (NANDA-I © 2014):

- *Gas Exchange, Impaired,* related to immature pulmonary vasculature and inadequate surfactant production
- *Breathing Pattern, Ineffective,* related to immature central nervous system
- *Tissue Perfusion: Cardiac, Risk for Decreased,* related to hypotension related to decreased tissue perfusion secondary to PDA
- *Tissue Perfusion: Peripheral, Ineffective,* related to anemia of prematurity
- *Nutrition, Imbalanced: Less Than Body Requirements,* related to weak suck and swallow reflexes and decreased ability to absorb nutrients
- *Thermoregulation, Ineffective,* related to hypothermia secondary to decreased glycogen and brown fat stores
- *Fluid Volume, Deficient,* related to high insensible water losses and inability of kidneys to concentrate urine
- *Family Processes, Dysfunctional,* related to anger or guilt at having given birth to a premature baby

Nursing Plan and Implementation

MAINTENANCE OF RESPIRATORY FUNCTION

There is increased danger of respiratory obstruction in preterm newborns because their bronchi and trachea are so narrow that mucus can obstruct the airway. Maintain patency through judicious suctioning, but only on an as-needed basis.

Positioning can also affect respiratory function. If the baby is in the supine position, slightly elevate the baby's head to maintain the airway, being careful to avoid hyperextension of the neck because the trachea will collapse. Also, because the newborn has weak neck muscles and cannot control head movement, ensure that this head position is maintained by placing a small roll under the shoulders. Because the prone position splints the chest wall and decreases the amount of respiratory effort used to move the chest wall, it facilitates chest expansion and improves air entry and oxygenation. Weak or absent cough or gag reflexes increase the chance of aspiration in the premature newborn. Ensure that the newborn's position facilitates drainage of mucus or regurgitated formula.

Healthy People 2020

(MICU-20) Increase the proportion of infants who are put to sleep on their back

Monitor heart and respiratory rates with cardiorespiratory monitors and observe the newborn to identify alterations in cardiopulmonary status. Signs of respiratory distress include the following:

- Cyanosis (serious sign when generalized)
- Tachypnea (sustained respiratory rate greater than 60/minute after first 4 hours of life)
- Retractions
- Expiratory grunting
- Nasal flaring
- Apneic episodes
- Presence of rales or rhonchi on auscultation
- Diminished air entry

If respiratory distress occurs, administer oxygen per healthcare provider in order to relieve hypoxemia. If hypoxemia is not treated immediately, it may result in patent ductus arteriosus or metabolic acidosis. If oxygen is administered to the newborn, monitor the oxygen concentration with devices such as the transcutaneous oxygen monitor ($tcPO_2$) or the pulse oximeter. Periodic arterial blood gas sampling to monitor oxygen concentration in the baby's blood is essential because hyperoxemia may lead to ROP.

Consider respiratory function before initiation of feedings as well as during feeding to prevent aspiration as well as increased energy expenditure and oxygen consumption.

MAINTENANCE OF NEUTRAL THERMAL ENVIRONMENT

Providing a neutral thermal environment minimizes the oxygen consumption required to maintain a normal core temperature; it also prevents cold stress and facilitates growth by decreasing the calories needed to maintain body temperature. The preterm newborn's immature central nervous system, as well as small brown fat stores, provides poor temperature control. A small newborn (>1200 g [2.6 lb]) can lose 80 kcal/kg/day through radiation of body heat. Implement all the usual thermoregulation measures discussed in Chapter 25.

In addition, to minimize heat loss and temperature instability for preterm and low-birth-weight (LBW) newborns, do the following:

1. Allow skin-to-skin contact (SSC) between mother and newborn to maintain warmth and faster security (see *kangaroo care*, described later).
2. Warm and humidify oxygen to minimize evaporative heat loss and decrease oxygen consumption.
3. Place the baby in a double-walled incubator or use a Plexiglas heat shield over small preterm babies in single-walled incubators to avoid radiative heat losses. Some institutions use radiant warmers and plastic wrap over the baby and pipe in humidity (swamping). Do not use Plexiglas shields on radiant warmer beds because they block the infrared heat.

4. Avoid placing the baby on cold surfaces such as metal treatment tables and cold x-ray plates (conductive heat loss). Pad cold surfaces with diapers and use radiant warmers during procedures, place the preterm newborn on prewarmed mattresses, and warm hands before handling the baby to prevent heat transfer via conduction.

5. Use warmed ambient humidity. Humidity can decrease insensible and transdermal water loss but the optimal level and duration is yet to be determined (Lund, Brandon, Holden, et al., 2013). Humidity, however, should be started only once the baby's temperature is within normal limits.

6. Keep the skin dry (evaporative heat loss) and place a cap on the baby's head. The head makes up 25% of the total body size.

7. Keep radiant warmers, incubators, and cribs away from windows and cold external walls (radiative heat loss) and out of drafts (conductive heat loss).

8. Open incubator portholes and doors only when necessary, and use plastic sleeves on portholes to decrease convective heat loss.

9. Use a skin probe to monitor the baby's skin temperature. Correlate ambient temperatures with the skin probe in the incubator using the servocontrol rather than the manual mode. The temperature should be 36° to 37°C (96.8° to 98.6°F). Temperature fluctuations indicate hypothermia or hyperthermia. Be careful not to place skin temperature probes over bony prominences, areas of brown fat, poorly vasoreactive areas such as extremities, or excoriated areas.

10. Warm formula or stored breast milk before feeding.

11. Use a reflector patch over the skin temperature probe when using a radiant warmer bed so that the probe does not sense the higher infrared temperature as the baby's skin temperature and therefore decrease the heater output.

Once preterm newborns are medically stable, they can be clothed with a double-thickness cap, cotton shirt, and diaper and, if possible, swaddled in a blanket. See *Concept Map: Hypothermia of Prematurity.*

Be familiar with your individual institution's protocol for weaning a preterm newborn from an incubator to a crib.

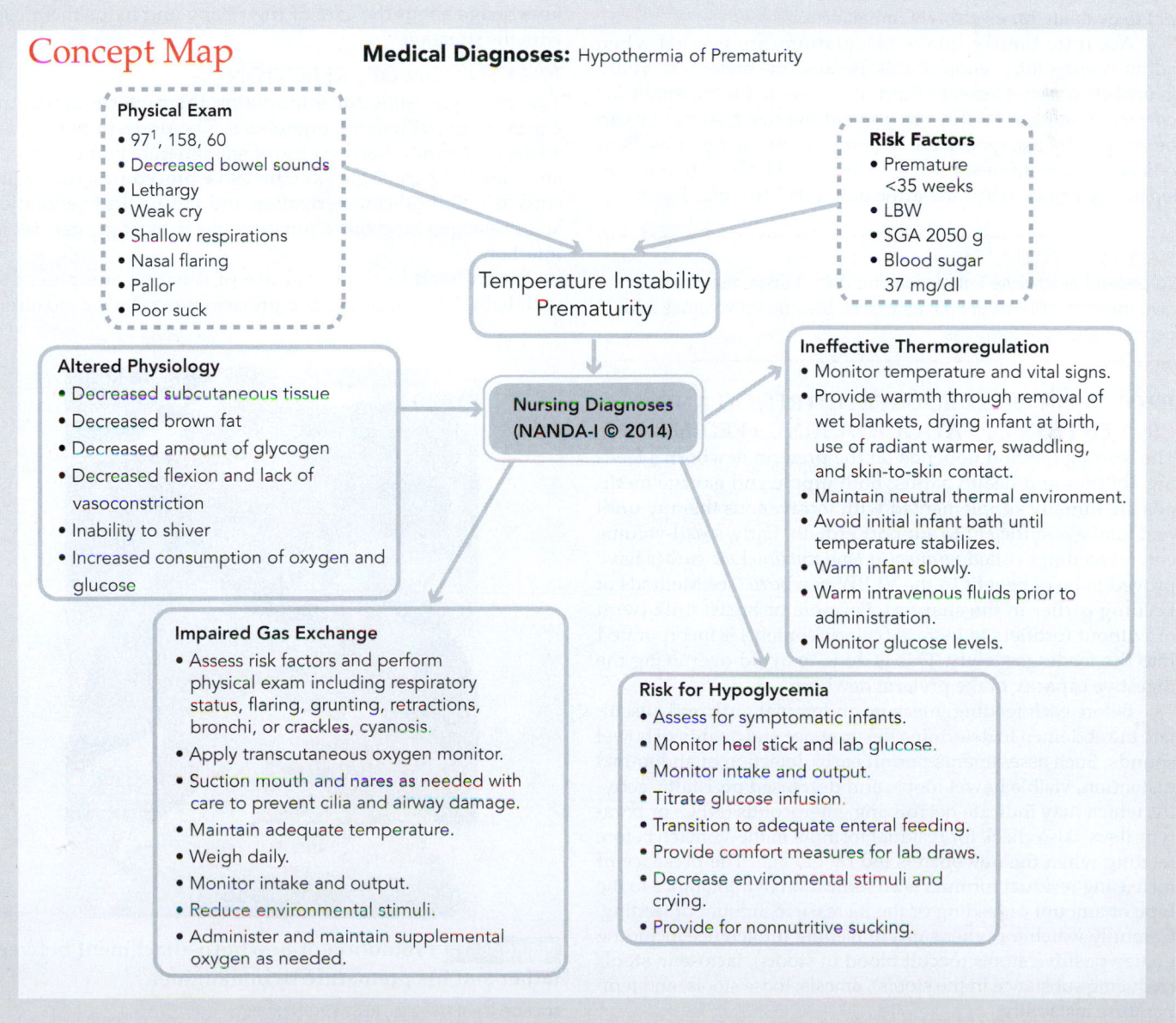

Concept Map

Medical Diagnoses: Hypothermia of Prematurity

Physical Exam
- 97¹, 158, 60
- Decreased bowel sounds
- Lethargy
- Weak cry
- Shallow respirations
- Nasal flaring
- Pallor
- Poor suck

Risk Factors
- Premature <35 weeks
- LBW
- SGA 2050 g
- Blood sugar 37 mg/dl

Temperature Instability Prematurity

Nursing Diagnoses (NANDA-I © 2014)

Altered Physiology
- Decreased subcutaneous tissue
- Decreased brown fat
- Decreased amount of glycogen
- Decreased flexion and lack of vasoconstriction
- Inability to shiver
- Increased consumption of oxygen and glucose

Ineffective Thermoregulation
- Monitor temperature and vital signs.
- Provide warmth through removal of wet blankets, drying infant at birth, use of radiant warmer, swaddling, and skin-to-skin contact.
- Maintain neutral thermal environment.
- Avoid initial infant bath until temperature stabilizes.
- Warm infant slowly.
- Warm intravenous fluids prior to administration.
- Monitor glucose levels.

Impaired Gas Exchange
- Assess risk factors and perform physical exam including respiratory status, flaring, grunting, retractions, bronchi, or crackles, cyanosis.
- Apply transcutaneous oxygen monitor.
- Suction mouth and nares as needed with care to prevent cilia and airway damage.
- Maintain adequate temperature.
- Weigh daily.
- Monitor intake and output.
- Reduce environmental stimuli.
- Administer and maintain supplemental oxygen as needed.

Risk for Hypoglycemia
- Assess for symptomatic infants.
- Monitor heel stick and lab glucose.
- Monitor intake and output.
- Titrate glucose infusion.
- Transition to adequate enteral feeding.
- Provide comfort measures for lab draws.
- Decrease environmental stimuli and crying.
- Provide for nonnutritive sucking.

MAINTENANCE OF FLUID AND ELECTROLYTE STATUS

Maintain hydration by providing adequate intake based on the newborn's weight, gestational age, chronologic age, and volume of sensible and insensible water losses. Adequate fluid intake should compensate for increased insensible losses and the amount needed for renal excretion of metabolic products. Insensible water losses can be minimized by providing high ambient humidity, humidifying oxygen, using heat shields, covering the skin with plastic wrap, and placing the baby in a double-walled incubator.

Evaluate the hydration status of the baby by assessing and recording signs of dehydration. Be sure to identify signs of over-hydration by observing the newborn for edema or excessive weight gain and by comparing urine output with fluid intake.

Weigh the preterm newborn at least once daily at the same time each day. Weight change is one of the most sensitive indicators of fluid balance. Weighing diapers is also important for accurate input and output measurement (1 ml = 1 g). A comparison of intake and output measurements over an 8- or 24-hour period provides important information about renal function and fluid balance. Assessment of patterns and whether they show a net gain or loss over several days is also essential to fluid management. In addition, monitor blood serum levels and pH to evaluate for electrolyte imbalances.

Accurate hourly intake calculations are needed when administering intravenous fluids. Because the preterm newborn is unable to excrete excess fluid, it is essential to maintain the correct amount of IV fluid to prevent overload. Accuracy can be ensured by using neonatal or pediatric infusion pumps. Periodically obtain urine-specific gravity and pH. Hydration is considered adequate when the urine output is 1 to 3 mL/kg/hr.

SAFETY ALERT!

To prevent electrolyte imbalance and dehydration, take care to give the correct IV solutions, as well as the correct volumes and concentrations of formulas.

PROVISION OF ADEQUATE NUTRITION AND PREVENTION OF FATIGUE DURING FEEDING

The feeding method depends on the preterm newborn's feeding abilities and health status. Both nipple and gavage methods are initially supplemented with intravenous therapy until oral intake is sufficient to support growth. Early, small-volume enteral feedings called *minimal enteral nutrition via gavage* have proved to be of benefit to the VLBW newborn (see Methods of Feeding earlier in the chapter). Formula or breast milk (with or without fortifiers to increase caloric content) is incorporated into the feedings slowly. This is done to avoid overtaxing the digestive capacity of the preterm newborn.

Before each feeding, measure abdominal girth and auscultate the abdomen to determine the presence and quality of bowel sounds. Such assessments permit early detection of abdominal distention, visible bowel loops, and decreased peristaltic activity, which may indicate necrotizing enterocolitis (NEC) or paralytic ileus. Also check for residual formula in the stomach before feeding when the newborn is fed by gavage. The presence of increasing residual formula is an indication of intolerance to the type or amount of feeding or the increase in amount of feeding. Carefully watch for other signs of feeding intolerance including guaiac-positive stools (occult blood in stools), lactose in stools (reducing substance in the stools), emesis, loose stools, and temperature instability.

Preterm newborns who are ill or who fatigue easily with nipple feedings are usually fed by gavage. The baby is essentially passive with these methods, thus conserving energy and calories. As the baby matures, gavage feedings are replaced with nipple (breast or formula) feedings to assist in strengthening the sucking reflex and in meeting oral and emotional needs. Signs that indicate readiness for oral feedings are a strong gag reflex, presence of nonnutritive sucking, and rooting behavior. Both low-birth-weight and preterm newborns nipple-feed more effectively in a quiet state. Establish a gradual nipple-feeding program, such as one nipple feeding per day, then one nipple feeding per shift, and then a nipple feeding every other feeding. Daily weights are monitored because often there is a small weight loss when nipple feedings are started. After feedings, place the baby on the right side (with support to maintain this position) or on the abdomen. These positions facilitate gastric emptying and decrease the chance of aspiration if regurgitation occurs. Gastroesophageal reflux is not uncommon in preterm newborns. Long-term gavage feeding may create nipple aversion that will require developmental occupational therapy interventions.

Involve the parents in feeding their preterm baby. This is essential to the development of attachment between parents and newborn (Figure 26–12). In addition, it increases parental knowledge about the care of their baby and helps them cope with the situation.

PREVENTION OF INFECTION

You are responsible for minimizing the preterm newborn's exposure to pathogenic organisms. The preterm newborn is susceptible to infection because of an immature immune system and thin and permeable skin. Invasive procedures, techniques such as umbilical catheterization and mechanical ventilation, and prolonged hospitalization place the baby at greater risk for infection.

Strict hand hygiene and use of separate equipment for each baby help minimize the preterm newborn's exposure to

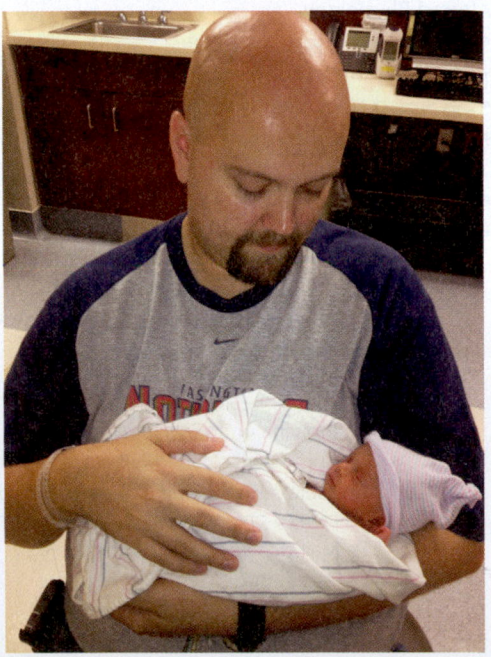

Figure 26–12 Promotion of newborn attachment between father and his premature twin daughter.

SOURCE: Carol Harrigan, RN, MSN, NNP-BC.

infectious agents. Most nurseries have adopted the Centers for Disease Control and Prevention (CDC) (2014) standard precautions of isolating every baby and the Joint Commission requirement that staff members have short-trimmed nails and no artificial nails. Staff members are required to complete a 2- to 3-minute scrub using iodine-containing antibacterial solutions, which inhibit growth of gram-positive cocci and gram-negative rod organisms. Other specific nursing interventions include limiting visitors, requiring visitors to wash their hands, maintaining strict aseptic practices when changing IV tubing and solutions (IV solutions and tubing should be changed every 24 hours or per agency protocols), administering parenteral fluids, and assisting with sterile procedures. Incubators and radiant warmers should be changed weekly. Prevent pressure-area breakdown by changing the baby's position regularly, doing range-of-motion exercises, and using water-bed pillows or an air mattress. To avoid skin tears, a protective transparent covering can be applied over vulnerable joints; however, this method is used sparingly (Blackburn, 2013). Chemical skin preps and tape may cause skin trauma and should be avoided as much as possible.

If infection (sepsis) occurs in the preterm newborn, you may be the first to identify its subtle clinical signs, such as lethargy and increased episodes of apnea and bradycardia. Inform the clinician of the findings immediately and implement the treatment plan per clinician orders in the presence of infection. (For specific nursing care required for the newborn with an infection, see Chapter 27.)

Clinical Tip

By 10 to 14 days of life, the skin integrity of the preterm newborn becomes mature and similar to that of a full-term baby.

PROMOTION OF PARENT–NEWBORN ATTACHMENT

Preterm newborns can be separated from their parents for prolonged periods after illness or complications that are detected in the first few hours or days following birth. The resultant interruption in parent–newborn bonding necessitates intervention to ensure successful attachment.

Measures need to be taken to promote positive parental feelings toward the preterm newborn. You can give photographs of the baby to parents to take home. These can also be given to the mother if she is in a different hospital or too ill to come to the nursery and visit. The newborn's first name is placed on the incubator as soon as it is known to help the parents feel that their baby is a unique and special person. Parents are given a weekly card with the baby's footprint, weight, and length, which helps to promote bonding. They are also given the telephone number of the nursery or intensive care unit and the names of staff members so that they have access to information about their baby at any time of the day or night. Encourage visits from siblings and grandparents to foster attachment.

Early involvement in the care of and decisions about their baby provides the parents with realistic expectations for their baby. The individual personality characteristics of the newborn and the parents influence the bonding and contribute to the interactive process for the family. By observing a baby's patterns of behavior and responses, especially sleep–wake states, you can teach parents optimal times for interacting with their baby. Parents need education to develop caregiving skills and to understand the premature newborn's behavioral characteristics.

Their daily participation (if possible) is encouraged, as are early and frequent visits.

Skin-to-skin care (also called *kangaroo care*) is defined as the practice of holding babies skin to skin next to a parent (Figure 26–13). The baby is usually naked, except for a diaper, and placed on the bare chest of the mother or father/partner. They are then both covered with a blanket. Benefits of skin-to-skin care as a developmental intervention include the following (Ludington-Hoe, 2013):

- Improved oxygenation as evidenced by an increase in transcutaneous oxygen levels
- Enhanced temperature regulation
- Decline in the episodes of apnea and bradycardia
- Increased periods of quiet sleep
- Stabilization of vital signs
- Positive interaction between parent and baby, which enhances attachment and bonding
- Increased growth parameters
- Early discharge

Limitations to skin-to-skin care may be because of staff uneasiness and the lack of protocols or guidelines to safely maneuver, position, and hold the newborn.

You and the parents can plan nursing care around the times when the baby is alert and best able to attend. The more knowledge parents have about the meaning of their baby's responses, behaviors, and cues for interaction, the better prepared they will be able to meet their newborn's needs and form a positive attachment with their child. Parental involvement in difficult care decisions is essential and discussed in greater detail in Chapter 27.

Some parents may progress easily to touching and cuddling their newborn; however, others will not. Parents need to

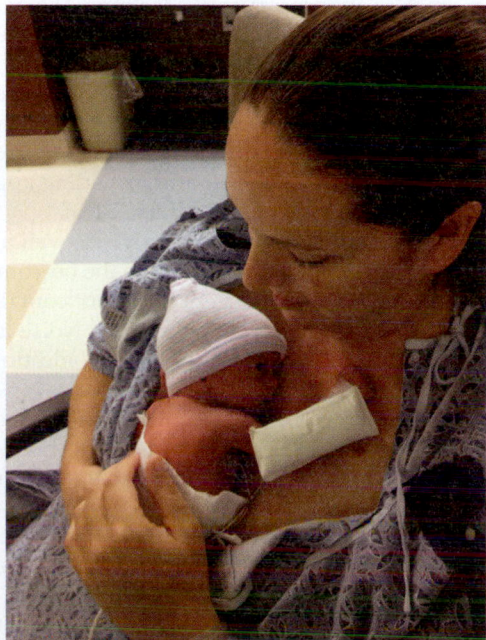

Figure 26–13 Kangaroo (skin-to-skin) care facilitates a closeness and attachment between mother and her premature newborn.

SOURCE: Carol Harrigan, RN, MSN, NNP-BC.

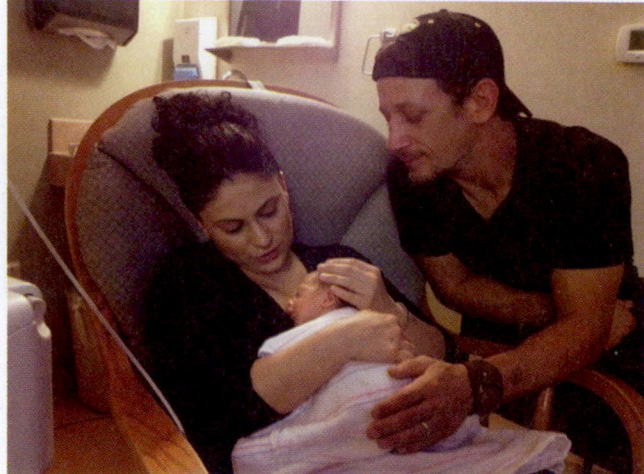

Figure 26–14 Family bonding occurs when parents have opportunities to spend time with their newborn.

SOURCE: Carol Harrigan, RN, MSN, NNP-BC.

know that their feelings are normal and that the progression of acquaintanceship is slow. Rooming-in can provide another opportunity for the stable preterm newborn and family to get acquainted; it offers both privacy and readily available help (Figure 26–14).

PROMOTION OF DEVELOPMENTALLY SUPPORTIVE CARE

Prolonged separation and the NICU environment necessitate individualized baby sensory stimulation programs. You can play a key role in determining the appropriate type and amount of visual, tactile, and auditory stimulation.

Some preterm newborns are not developmentally able to deal with more than one sensory input at a time. The Assessment of Preterm Infant Behavior (APIB) scale identifies individual preterm newborn behaviors according to five areas of development (Als, Butler, & Costa, 2005). The preterm baby's behavioral reactions to stimulation are observed, and developmental interventions are then based on reducing detrimental environmental stimuli to the lowest possible level and providing appropriate opportunities for development (Blackburn, 2013).

Providing developmentally supportive, as well as family-centered, care has been proven to improve the outcomes of the critically ill newborn. The NICU environment contains many detrimental stimuli that you can help reduce. Noise levels can be lowered by replacing alarms with lights. In addition, silencing alarms quickly and keeping conversations away from the baby's bedside can help. Dimmer switches should be used to shield the baby's eyes from bright lights, and blankets may be placed over the top portion of the incubator. Dimming the lights may encourage babies to open their eyes and be more responsive to their parents. Nursing care should be planned to decrease the number of times the baby is disturbed. Signs (e.g., "Quiet Please") can be placed near the bedside to allow the baby some periods of uninterrupted sleep (Blackburn, 2013). Some other suggested developmentally supportive interventions include the following:

- Facilitate handling by using containment measures when turning or moving the newborn or doing procedures such as suctioning. Use your hands to hold the baby's arms and legs flexed close to the midline of the body. This helps

stabilize the baby's motor and physiologic subsystems during stressful activities.

- Touch the newborn gently and avoid sudden postural changes.
- Promote soothing activities, such as placing blanket rolls or approved manufactured devices next to the baby's sides and against the feet to provide "nesting." Swaddle the baby to maintain extremities in a flexed position while ensuring that the hands can reach the face (Figure 26–15). This permits the newborn to do hand-to-mouth activities. Also provide self-consoling objects for the baby to grasp (e.g., a piece of blanket, oxygen tubing, a finger) during caregiving.
- Simulate the kinesthetic advantages of the intrauterine environment by using sheepskin and approved water beds. Water bed and pillow use has been reported to improve sleep and decrease motor activity as well as lead to more mature motor behavior, fewer state changes, and a decreased heart rate.
- Provide opportunities for nonnutritive sucking with a pacifier. This improves transcutaneous oxygen saturation; decreases body movements; improves sleep, especially after feedings; and increases weight gain.

As NICUs become more and more developmentally supportive, complementary care has become an adjunct to that nurturing environment. This holistic approach in caring for the low-birth-weight newborn attempts not only to mimic the intrauterine environment, but also to foster parent–newborn bonding by simultaneously caring for the body, spirit, and mind. See Box 26–1.

PREPARATION FOR HOME CARE

Parents are often anxious when their premature newborn is transferred out of the NICU or is discharged home. Parents of preterm babies should receive the same postpartum teaching as

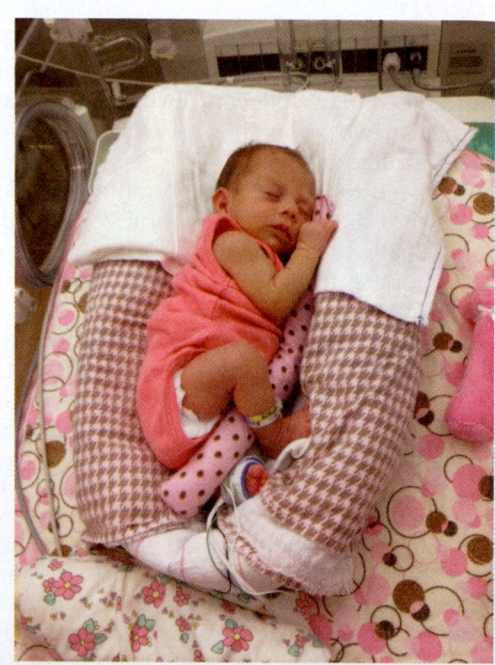

Figure 26–15 A 3-week-old, 31 weeks' gestational age newborn is nested and developmentally positioned. Hand-to-mouth behavior facilitates self-consoling and soothing activities.

SOURCE: Carol Harrigan, RN, MSN, NNP-BC.

Box 26–1 **Complementary Care in the NICU**

- *Aromatherapy* is the use of scent to alter mood or behavior to produce a calming and sedating effect. There is an enhanced bonding process between mothers and newborns associated with the natural body odor emitted from the mother (Kassity-Krich & Jones, 2014). Aromatherapy is utilized in the NICU by placing an article of clothing belonging to the mother next to the newborn to produce a soothing and consoling effect on the baby in her absence. Researchers are also investigating other aromatherapies, including peppermint as a respiratory stimulant, chamomile as a method to regulate sleep–wake cycles, Brazilian guava for its analgesic effects, and lavender sitz baths for management of diaper rash.

- *Music therapy* as a noninvasive auditory stimulus has been shown to be advantageous in the premature newborn. The music used in NICUs includes primarily lullabies and soft acoustical pieces that are pleasant, soothing, and calming. Such music has been shown to effect newborn physiologic responses, such as improving oxygenation and increasing weight gain. It also has behavioral effects, leading to enhanced parental bonding and increased intervals of nonnutritive sucking periods. Language development is also enhanced if the music is live and sung by the mother or another female, which is preferential to the newborn. However, the overall noise level in the NICU needs to be considered before including any extra auditory stimulation, including music therapy (Kassity-Krich & Jones, 2014).

- Infant massage and gentle human touch (GHT) have been practiced for many centuries. The types of stimulation include massage with stroking, gentle touch without stroking, and therapeutic touch or "hands-on" containment. Practitioners report such physiologic benefits as stimulating blood and lymphatic flow, promoting weight gain in premature newborns, regulating sleep patterns, and many emotional and behavioral benefits. Massage demonstrates compassion while increasing parents' empathy and understanding of the baby. It helps parents learn to interpret their baby's behavioral cues such as facial expression, various crying patterns, and other body language. At the same time, it helps babies learn about their various body parts and boundaries and feel how they integrate into the whole. Therapeutic touch reduces motor activity and energy expenditure by the baby and also promotes comfort.

any parent taking a newborn home. In preparing for discharge, encourage the parents to spend time caring directly for their baby. This familiarizes them with their baby's behavior patterns and helps them establish realistic expectations. Some hospitals have a special room near the nursery where parents can spend the night with their baby before discharge.

Discharge instruction includes breastfeeding and formula-feeding techniques, formula preparation, and vitamin administration. If the mother wishes to breastfeed, teach her to pump her breasts to keep the milk flowing and provide milk even before discharge. Provide information on bathing, diapering, hygiene, and normal elimination patterns. Prepare the parents to expect changes in the color of the baby's stool, number of bowel movements, and timing of elimination when the baby is switched from formula-feeding to breastfeeding. This information can prevent unnecessary concern by the parents.

Discuss normal growth and development patterns, reflexes, and activity for preterm babies, especially signs and symptoms of overstimulation. In these discussions, emphasize ways to promote bonding behaviors and deal with newborn crying. Care of the preterm newborn with complications, preventing infections, recognizing signs of a sick baby, and the need for continued medical follow-up are other key issues. Family-care conferences with all the various disciplines involved in the care of the preterm newborn are often helpful just prior to discharge.

Families with preterm newborns usually do not need to be referred to community agencies, such as visiting nurse assistance. However, referral may be necessary if the baby has severe congenital abnormalities, feeding problems, or complications with infections or respiratory problems or if the parents seem unable to cope with an at-risk baby. Parents of preterm newborns can benefit from meeting with others in a similar situation to share common experiences and concerns. Refer parents to support groups sponsored by the hospital or by others in the community and make connections for parents with early education intervention centers.

Preterm and LBW newborns are at greater risk of increased morbidity from vaccine-preventable diseases. Stable preterm newborns show consistently high rates of seroconversion following the first dose of hepatitis B vaccine even when the first dose is given as early as 1 month after birth (American Academy of Pediatrics [AAP] Committee on Fetus and Newborn & American College of Obstetricians and Gynecologists [ACOG] Committee on Obstetrics, 2012). The medically stable preterm newborn and the LBW newborn should receive full doses of diphtheria, tetanus, acellular pertussis, *Haemophilus influenzae* type b (Hib), hepatitis B, inactivated poliovirus, rotavirus, and pneumococcal conjugate vaccines (PCV) at a chronologic age consistent with the schedule recommended for full-term newborns. The influenza vaccine should be administered at 6 months of age before the beginning of and during the influenza season. The vaccine for immunoprophylaxis against respiratory syncytial virus (RSV) is given to those high-risk newborns prior to discharge from the NICU and monthly thereafter during local RSV season.

Evaluation

Expected outcomes of nursing care include the following:

- The preterm newborn is free of respiratory distress and establishes effective respiratory function.

- The preterm newborn gains weight and shows no signs of fatigue or aspiration during feedings.

- The preterm newborn demonstrates a serial head circumference growth rate of 1 cm (0.4 in.) per week.

- The parents are able to verbalize their anger and guilt feelings about the birth of a preterm baby and show attachment behavior such as frequent visits and growing confidence in their participatory care activities.

Care of the Newborn With Congenital Anomalies

The birth of a baby with a congenital defect places both newborn and family at risk. Many congenital anomalies can be life threatening if not corrected within hours after birth; others are very visible and cause the families emotional distress. When one congenital anomaly is found, healthcare providers should look for others, particularly in body systems that develop at the same time during gestation. Table 26–2 identifies common anomalies and their early management and nursing care in the newborn period.

TABLE 26–2 Congenital Anomalies: Identification and Care in the Newborn Period

CONGENITAL ANOMALY	NURSING ASSESSMENTS	NURSING GOALS AND INTERVENTIONS
CONGENITAL HYDROCEPHALUS (progressive ventricular enlargement due to a malformation and obstruction in the flow of the cerebrospinal fluid [CSF] pathways)	Enlarged or full fontanelles Split or widened sutures "Setting sun" eyes Head circumference greater than 90% on growth chart Visibly distended scalp veins Behavioral state changes; may become increasingly irritable or lethargic	Assess presence of hydrocephalus: Measure and plot initial occipital–frontal circumference (OFC) measurement; then measure daily. Check fontanelle for bulging and sutures for widening. Obtain neurosurgery consult. Assist with imaging studies, to include cranial ultrasound, CT scan, and MRI. Maintain skin integrity: Change position frequently. Use gel pillow under head. Postoperatively, position head off operative site, watch for signs of infection.
CHOANAL ATRESIA (unilateral or bilateral bony occlusion of posterior nares)	Respiratory distress (cyanosis and retractions at rest) Noisy respirations Difficulty breathing during feeding (obligatory nose breathers) Obstruction by thick mucus	Assess patency of nares: Listen for breath sounds while holding baby's mouth closed and alternately compressing each nostril. Assist with passing a catheter through each naris to confirm diagnosis. Obtain ENT consult. Maintain respiratory function: Assist with taping airway in mouth to prevent respiratory distress. Position with head elevated to improve air exchange.
CLEFT LIP (unilateral or bilateral visible defect) 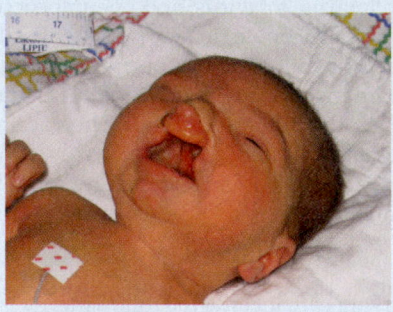 Bilateral cleft lip with cleft abnormality involving both hard and soft palates. SOURCE: Carol Harrigan, RN, MSN, NNP-BC.	May involve upper lip only or may involve external nares, nasal cartilage, nasal septum, and alveolar process Flattening or depression of midfacial contour	Provide nutrition: Feed with special nipple and bottle. Burp frequently (increased tendency to swallow air and reflex vomiting). Obtain craniofacial/ENT consult. Clean cleft with sterile water (to prevent crusting on cleft before repair). Support parental coping: Assist parents with grief over loss of idealized baby. Encourage verbalization of their feelings about visible defect.
CLEFT PALATE (fissure connecting oral and nasal cavity)	May involve uvula and soft palate May extend forward to nostril involving hard palate and maxillary alveolar ridge Difficulty in sucking Expulsion of formula through nose	Prevent aspiration/infection: Place in side-lying position to facilitate drainage. Obtain craniofacial/ENT consult. Feed in upright position (to prevent formula from flowing back into nasal passages, to aid swallowing and discourage aspiration). Provide nutrition: Feed with special nipple and bottle. Formula may escape through the nose, which is common (nasal regurgitation). Burp after each ounce (tend to swallow large amounts of air). Plot weight gain patterns to assess adequacy of diet. Provide parental support: Refer parents to community agencies, support groups, and speech pathologists. Encourage verbalization of frustrations because feeding process is long and frustrating. Praise all parental efforts. Encourage parents to seek prompt treatment for upper respiratory infection (URI) and teach them ways to decrease URI.

CONGENITAL ANOMALY	NURSING ASSESSMENTS	NURSING GOALS AND INTERVENTIONS
Tracheoesophageal Fistula (lower esophageal segment connects to the lower trachea with upper esophageal segment ending blindly [atresia])	History of maternal polyhydramnios Excessive oral secretions Constant drooling Abdominal distention beginning soon after birth Periodic choking and cyanotic episodes Immediate regurgitation when feeding Aspiration of pharyngeal contents into trachea. Signs/symptoms: tachypnea, retractions, rhonchi, decreased breath sounds, cyanotic spells Reflux of gastric contents into trachea leading to aspiration pneumonia Inability to pass nasogastric tube (will not pass beyond 10–15 cm from nares)	Maintain respiratory status and prevent aspiration. Withhold feeding until esophageal patency is determined by chest radiograph Obtain a surgical consult. Place an indwelling Replogle tube attached to low intermittent suction to control saliva and mucus (to prevent aspiration pneumonia) in esophageal pouch. Elevate head of bed 20–40 degrees (to prevent reflux of gastric contents). Keep baby calm (crying causes air to pass through fistula and to distend intestines, causing compression of the diaphragm and respiratory embarrassment). Maintain fluid and electrolyte balance. Begin broad-spectrum antibiotics secondary to risk of aspiration pneumonia. Give fluids to replace esophageal drainage and maintain hydration. Provide parent education: Explain staged repair—primary or staged—provision of gastrostomy, ligation of fistula, repair of atresia. Keep parents informed; clarify and reinforce healthcare provider's explanations regarding malformation, surgical repair, preoperative and postoperative care, and prognosis.

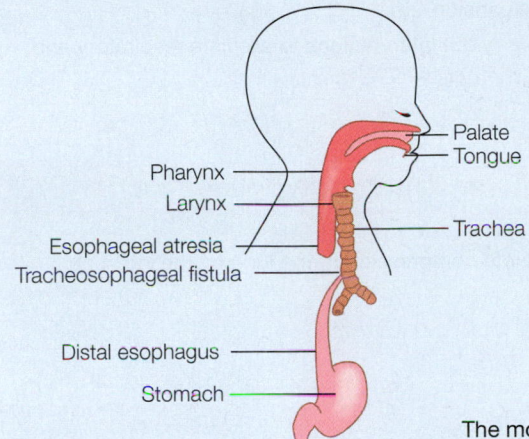

Palate
Tongue
Pharynx
Larynx
Trachea
Esophageal atresia
Tracheoesophageal fistula
Distal esophagus
Stomach

The most frequently seen type of congenital tracheoesophageal fistula with esophageal atresia.

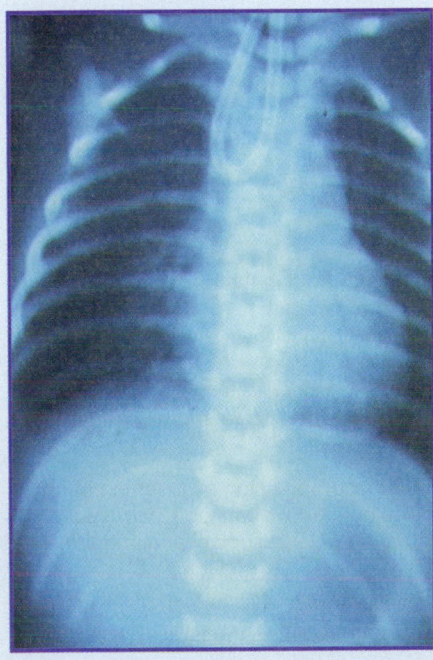

TEF with esophageal atresia. Note coiled NG tube and large stomach bubble.
SOURCE: Carol Harrigan, RN, MSN, NNP-BC.

(continued)

TABLE 26–2 Congenital Anomalies: Identification and Care in the Newborn Period (*continued*)

CONGENITAL ANOMALY	NURSING ASSESSMENTS	NURSING GOALS AND INTERVENTIONS
DIAPHRAGMATIC HERNIA (portion of intestines in the thoracic cavity through abnormal opening in diaphragm, occurring commonly on the left side)	Difficulty initiating respirations secondary to hypoplastic lung on affected side, compression of lung on contralateral side Gasping respirations with nasal flaring and chest retractions Barrel chest and scaphoid abdomen Asymmetric chest expansion Breath sounds may be diminished or absent, usually on affected side Heart sounds displaced to contralateral side Bowel sounds may be heard in thoracic cavity	Do not ventilate with bag and mask O_2 because the stomach and intestines will become air-filled and distended, further compressing the lungs. Obtain chest radiograph to confirm diagnosis. Obtain a surgical consult. Maintain respiratory status: Administer oxygen, prepare for intubation and ventilation (considered a respiratory emergency). Initiate gastric decompression by placing an indwelling Replogle tube attached to low intermittent suction. Place in high semi-Fowler position (to use gravity to keep abdominal organs' pressure off diaphragm). Turn onto affected side to allow unaffected lung expansion. Carry out interventions to alleviate respiratory and metabolic acidosis.

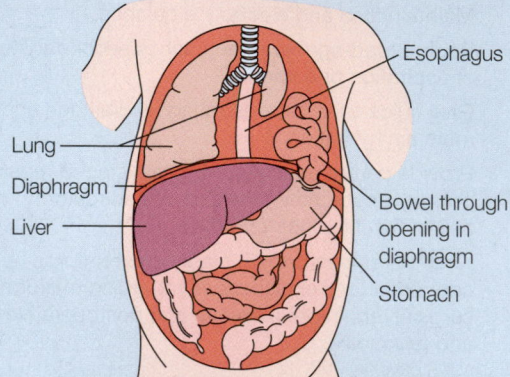

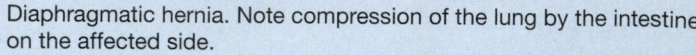

Diaphragmatic hernia. Note compression of the lung by the intestine on the affected side.
SOURCE: Nancy Houck, RN, BSN, NNP-BC.

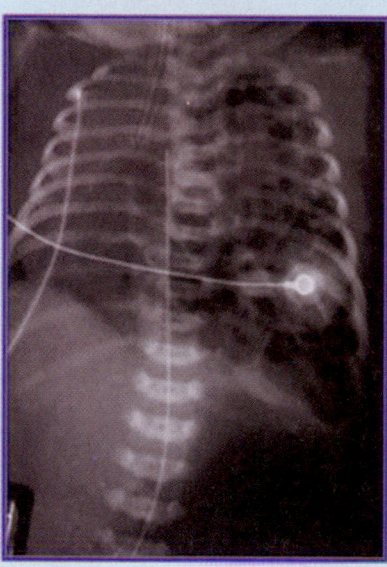

Diaphragmatic hernia. Note bowel gas pattern in the upper left chest with a shift in the mediastinum to the right.
SOURCE: Carol Harrigan, RN, MSN, NNP-BC.

OMPHALOCELE (herniation of abdominal contents into base of umbilical cord)	Abdominal contents encased in a protective, transparent membrane	Maintain hydration and temperature. Place baby in sterile bag up to and covering defect. Obtain surgical consult. Initiate gastric decompression by insertion of an indwelling Replogle tube attached to low suction (to prevent distention of lower bowel and impairment of blood flow). Position to prevent trauma to defect. Administer broad-spectrum antibiotics to prevent infection.

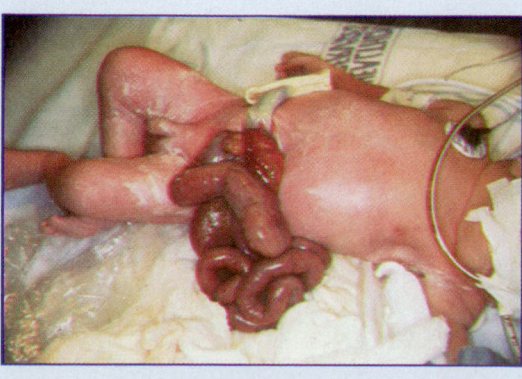

Newborn with omphalocele.
SOURCE: Carol Harrigan, RN, MSN, NNP-BC.

CONGENITAL ANOMALY	NURSING ASSESSMENTS	NURSING GOALS AND INTERVENTIONS
GASTROSCHISIS (full-thickness defect in abdominal wall allowing viscera outside the body to the right of an intact umbilical cord)	No protective covering Intestines exposed to the caustic amniotic fluid Associated with intestinal atresia, malrotation Large amount of evaporative fluid losses from exposed bowel	Maintain hydration and temperature. Provide normal saline for hypovolemia/fluid resuscitation. Place baby in sterile bag up to axilla in a side-lying position to prevent trauma of the bowel. *Do not cover defect with wet saline gauze.* Obtain surgical consult. Initiate gastric decompression by insertion of an indwelling Replogle tube attached to low suction; measure and replace gastric output. Administer broad-spectrum antibiotics to prevent infection of exposed bowel.

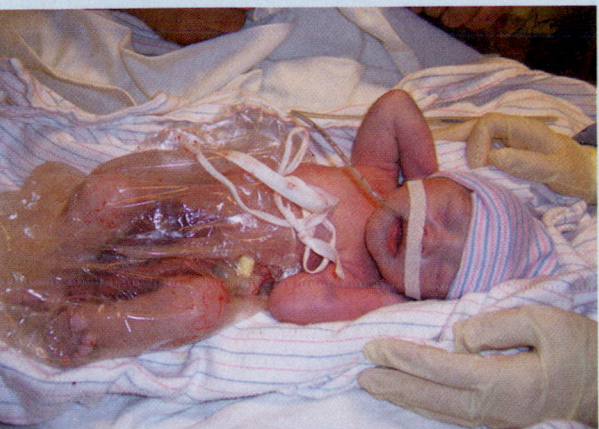

Term newborn with gastroschisis. Note the externalized loops of bowel visible through the bag.
SOURCE: Carol Harrigan, RN, MSN, NNP-BC.

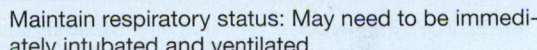

PRUNE BELLY SYNDROME (congenital absence of one or more layers of abdominal muscles)	Oligohydramnios leading to pulmonary hypoplasia common Deficiency of the abdominal wall musculature causing the abdomen to be shapeless Skin hangs loosely and is wrinkled in appearance Associated with urinary abnormalities (urethral obstruction, renal dysplasia) In boys, cryptorchidism is common; rarely occurs in girls	Maintain respiratory status: May need to be immediately intubated and ventilated. Obtain surgical and urology consult. Prevent trauma and infection. Administer broad-spectrum antibiotics. Place a urinary catheter and monitor urinary output. Carry out interventions to alleviate respiratory and metabolic acidosis. Keep parents updated and informed about prognosis.

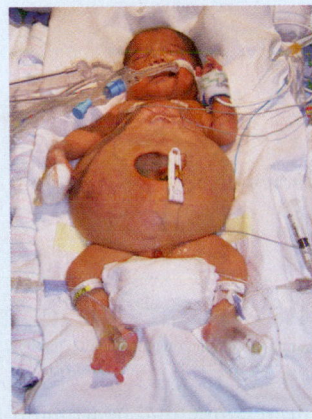

Prune belly syndrome.
SOURCE: Carol Harrigan, RN, MSN, NNP-BC.

(continued)

TABLE 26–2 Congenital Anomalies: Identification and Care in the Newborn Period (*continued*)

CONGENITAL ANOMALY	NURSING ASSESSMENTS	NURSING GOALS AND INTERVENTIONS
MYELOMENINGOCELE (saclike cyst containing meninges, spinal cord, and nerve roots in thoracic and/or lumbar area)	Myelomeningocele directly connects to subarachnoid space so hydrocephalus often associated No response or varying response to sensation below level of defect May have constant dribbling of urine Incontinence or retention of stool Anal wink may or may not be present	Prevent trauma and infection. Position on abdomen or on side and restrain (to prevent pressure and trauma to sac). Obtain neurosurgery and urology consult. Meticulously clean buttocks and genitals after each void and stool (to prevent contamination and infection of sac). Cover with protective plastic wrap over sac (to prevent trauma, rupture and drying). *Do not cover defect with wet saline gauze.* Administer broad-spectrum antibiotics to prevent infection. Observe sac for oozing of fluid. Credé bladder (apply downward pressure on bladder with thumbs, moving urine toward the urethra) as ordered to prevent urinary stasis. Assess amount of sensation and movement below defect. Obtain baseline occipital–frontal circumference (OFC) measurements; then measure head circumference daily (to detect hydrocephalus). Check fontanelle for fullness and bulging.
IMPERFORATE ANUS (absence of anal opening, may or may not have a fistula connection) Boy: fistula between rectum and urinary tract, scrotum, penis, perineum Girl: fistula between rectum and vagina or perineum)	Inability to visualize rectal opening No meconium is passed Meconium passed through fistula or malpositioned anus Gradual abdominal distension if no fistula present	Inspect perineal area for presence of fistula. Initiate gastric decompression by insertion of an indwelling Replogle tube attached to low suction if no fistula present; measure and replace gastric output. Maintain fluid balance. Obtain surgical consult.
CONGENITAL DISLOCATED HIP AND CLUBFOOT	See discussion in Chapter 24	

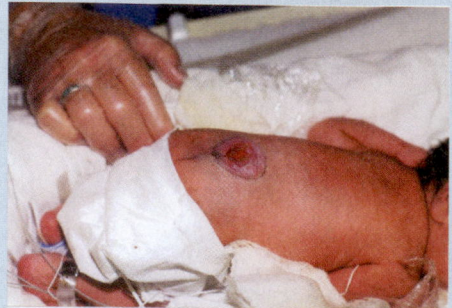

Newborn with lumbar myelomeningocele.
SOURCE: Carol Harrigan, RN, MSN, NNP-BC.

Care of the Newborn With Congenital Heart Defect

Congenital heart defects (CHD), the most common congenital defect, occur in approximately 8 to 12 per 1000 live births (depending on severity of the structural defects). Of those, 7.4% of all infant deaths are related to CHD, with a small percentage being undiagnosed until autopsy (Frank, Bradshaw, Beekman, et al., 2013). Of the cardiac lesions associated with death during the first 2 weeks of life, the most common are coarctation of the aorta, aortic valve stenosis, interrupted aortic arch, hypoplastic left heart syndrome, truncus arteriosus, and critical pulmonary stenosis. Only 25% of all cardiac lesions are identified on a prenatal ultrasound. Some newborns go home with their parents before their heart defect is detected. These babies with *critical congenital heart disease (CCHD)* are at risk for serious complications within the first few days or weeks of life and often require emergency care. It is crucial for the nurse to have comprehensive knowledge of congenital heart disease and perform a thorough cardiac assessment to detect deviations from normal and to initiate interventions prior to hospital discharge following birth.

Healthy People 2020

(MICH-1.7) Reduce the rate of infant deaths related to birth defects (congenital heart defects)

Overview of Congenital Heart Defects

In the majority of cases of congenital heart malformations, the cause is multifactorial with no specific trigger. Other factors that might influence development of congenital heart malformation can be classified as environmental or genetic. Infections of the pregnant woman, such as rubella, cytomegalovirus, coxsackie B, and influenza, have been implicated. Steroids, alcohol, lithium, and some anticonvulsants have been shown to cause malformations of the heart. Seasonal spraying of pesticides has also been linked to an increase in congenital heart defects. Clinicians are also beginning to see cardiac defects in babies of mothers with phenylketonuria (PKU) who do not follow their diets. Babies with Down syndrome, Turner syndrome, Holt-Oram syndrome, trisomy 13, and trisomy 18 frequently have heart lesions. Increased incidence and risk of recurrence of specific defects occur in families.

The most common cardiac defects seen in the first 6 days of life are left ventricular outflow obstructions, such as mitral stenosis and aortic stenosis or atresia; hypoplastic left heart; coarctation of the aorta; patent ductus arteriosus (PDA), which is the most common defect in premature newborns; transposition of the great vessels; tetralogy of Fallot; and large ventricular septal defect or atrial septal defects. Many cardiac defects may not manifest themselves until after discharge from the birthing unit.

Clinical Tip

When cyanosis occurs in an otherwise healthy 12- to-24-hour-old newborn displaying no respiratory distress, and it is not resolved with oxygen, think about cardiac issues, especially a ductal-dependent lesion.

Nursing Management

Your primary goal as a neonatal nurse is to identify cardiac defects early and initiate referral to the physician. The three most common manifestations of cardiac defect are cyanosis, detectable heart murmur, and congestive heart failure signs (tachycardia, tachypnea, diaphoresis, hepatomegaly, cardiomegaly). Table 26–3 presents the clinical manifestations and medical–surgical management of these specific cardiac defects. Initial repair of heart defects in the newborn period is becoming more commonplace. The NICU staff is now involved in both preoperative and postoperative care of newborns. The benefits for the baby being cared for by NICU staff include the staff's knowledge of neonatal anatomy and physiology, experience in supporting the family, and an awareness of the newborn's developmental needs.

After the baby has been stabilized, decisions are made about ongoing care. The parents need careful and complete explanations and the opportunity to take part in decision making. They also require ongoing emotional support. Families with a baby born with any congenital anomaly also need genetic counseling about future conception. Parents need opportunities to verbalize their concerns about their baby's health maintenance and their understanding of the rationale for follow-up care.

Care of the Newborn of a Substance-Abusing Mother

Substance abuse during pregnancy is often undiagnosed and underestimated, putting the pregnant woman at high risk for maternal and fetal morbidity as well as significant neonatal withdrawal. Tetratogenicity, poor maternal nutrition, poor placental perfusion, and placental insufficiency leading to growth restriction in the fetus are common obstetric concerns for the substance-abusing mother. The drug use of the substance-abusing mother may vary from infrequent, recreational use to daily use due to psychologic and physiologic addiction. An **infant of a substance-abusing mother (ISAM)** may be exposed to a number of licit and illicit drugs singularly or in combination (see Table 26–4). Identification of these intrauterine-drug-exposed newborns becomes essential not only to anticipate problems in the delivery room and in the nursery but also to recognize those babies at risk for long-term neurodevelopmental sequelae following discharge.

Alcohol Dependence

Fetal alcohol syndrome (FAS), a leading cause of preventable, nongenetic intellectual disability, includes a group of physical, behavioral, and cognitive abnormalities frequently found in babies exposed to alcohol in utero. It is estimated that complete FAS occurs in up to 1 to 4 per 1000 live births annually in some United States and Western European populations (Chambers & Scialli, 2014). FAS rates are higher among Native Americans, Alaska natives, African Americans, and women of low socioeconomic status.

New guidelines for diagnosis and referral of newborns/infants and children with FAS have been developed. Currently, the term **fetal alcohol spectrum disorder (FASD)** has been used to include all categories of prenatal alcohol exposure, including FAS. The diagnostic categories for FASD take into consideration the various clinical manifestations of FAS, the social and family environment, and, if available, the maternal alcohol history. Five diagnostic categories are used to describe effects of alcohol exposure:

1. FAS with a confirmed history of maternal alcohol intake.
2. FAS with phenotypic features but no confirmed history of maternal alcohol intake.
3. Partial FAS with confirmed history of maternal alcohol intake, some facial abnormalities, and one of the following: central nervous system (CNS) abnormalities, growth restriction, or behavioral or cognitive disabilities.
4. Alcohol-related birth defects (ARBD). These are usually determined only by a positive maternal drinking history. They present with one or more birth defects including malformations and dysplasias of the heart, bone, kidney, vision, or hearing systems and do not exhibit the classic facial dysmorphology of the baby with FAS (Chambers & Scialli, 2014).
5. Alcohol-related neurodevelopmental disorder (ARND). Children with ARND have CNS neurodevelopmental abnormalities and complex behavior and cognitive abnormalities. ARBD and ARND can occur together.

Although it has been known that ethanol freely crosses the placenta to the fetus, it is now known that its by-products are equally responsible for the damage. There is also strong evidence that the amount of alcohol ingested is directly responsible for the neurodevelopmental outcomes of these babies; heavy alcohol use is defined as binge drinking 1 or 2 times per week and consumption of six standard drinks per occasion (Chambers & Scialli, 2014). Often, the consumption of alcohol occurs during conception, when critical fetal organogenesis is most adversely affected. (Chapter 14 discusses alcohol abuse in pregnancy.) The effects of other substances often combined with alcohol, such as nicotine, diazepam (Valium), marijuana, and caffeine, as well as poor diet, enhance the likelihood of FAS.

LONG-TERM COMPLICATIONS FOR THE NEWBORN WITH FASD

Because of the failure-to-thrive appearance, many newborns with FASD are often evaluated for deficiencies in organic and inorganic amino acids. These babies have a delay in oral feeding

TABLE 26–3 Cardiac Defects of the Early Newborn Period

CONGENITAL HEART DEFECT	CLINICAL FINDINGS	MEDICAL/SURGICAL MANAGEMENT
INCREASED PULMONARY BLOOD FLOW		
Patent Ductus Arteriosus (PDA) ↑ in females, maternal rubella, respiratory distress syndrome (RDS), less than 1500 g preterm newborns, high-altitude births 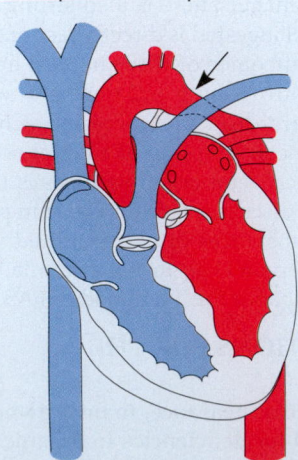	Harsh grade 2–3/6 machinery-type murmur heard at upper left sternal border (LSB) just beneath clavicle ↑ difference between systolic and diastolic pulse pressure Bounding peripheral pulses Hyperactive precordium Can lead to right-sided heart failure and pulmonary congestion ↑ left atrial (LA) and left ventricular (LV) enlargement, dilated ascending aorta ↑ pulmonary vascularity on x-ray Can be evident on day 2 or 3 of life	Indomethacin—0.2 mg/kg IV Q12 hr × 3 doses Neoprofen—10 mg/kg IV × 1 dose then 5 mg/kg IV @ 24 & 48 hr from first dose (both prostaglandin inhibitors) Surgical ligation, occlusion coil Use of O_2 therapy and blood transfusion to improve tissue oxygenation and perfusion Fluid restriction, digoxin, and diuretics to manage symptoms of CHF
	The patent ductus arteriosus is a vascular connection that, during fetal life, bypasses the pulmonary vascular bed and directs blood from the pulmonary artery to the aorta. Postnatally, blood shunts through the ductus from the aorta to the pulmonary artery (left-to-right shunting).	
Atrial Septal Defect (ASD) ↑ in females and Down syndrome	Initially frequently asymptomatic in the newborn period Systolic murmur Grade 2–3/6 second heard at left sternal border left intercostal space (LICS) with splitting second heart sound (S2) With large ASD, diastolic rumbling murmur lower left sternal (LLS) border Failure to thrive, upper respiratory infection (URI), poor exercise tolerance	Surgical closure with patch or suture Umbrella occlude
Ventricular Septal Defect (VSD) ↑ in males Most common heart defect	Initially asymptomatic until end of first month or large enough to cause pulmonary edema Loud, blowing systolic murmur between the third and fourth intercostal space (ICS); pulmonary blood flow heard at lower left sternal border Right ventricular hypertrophy Rapid respirations, growth failure, feeding difficulties Congestive right heart failure at 6 weeks–2 months of age Typically closes spontaneously during first 2 years of life	Follow medically—some spontaneously close Use of digoxin and diuretics to manage congestive heart failure (CHF) Surgical closure with Dacron patch or umbrella occluder
OBSTRUCTION TO SYSTEMIC BLOOD FLOW		
Coarctation of Aorta Can be preductal or postductal	Blood pressure higher above the area of coarctation than below Absent or diminished femoral pulses Increased brachial pulses Late systolic ejection murmur Grade 1–2/6 heard at left intrascapular area, loudest in the back Systolic BP in lower extremities Enlarged left ventricle Can present in CHF at 7–21 days of life Progressive cyanosis as PDA closes	Four-point blood pressure measurements Surgical resection of narrowed portion of aorta Prostaglandin E_1 to maintain patency of PDA to ensure systemic blood flow No afterload reducer drugs
	Coarctation of the aorta is characterized by a narrowed aortic lumen. The lesion produces an obstruction to the flow of blood through the aorta, causing an increased left ventricular pressure and workload, minimizing systemic circulation of blood.	

CONGENITAL HEART DEFECT	CLINICAL FINDINGS	MEDICAL/SURGICAL MANAGEMENT
Hypoplastic Left Heart Syndrome	Normal at birth—cyanosis and shocklike congestive heart failure develop within a few hours to days	Prostaglandin E$_1$ (PGE$_1$) until treatment decision made
	Soft systolic murmur heard just left of the sternum	Norwood procedure
	Diminished pulses	Fontan procedure
	Aortic and/or mitral atresia	Transplant
	Tiny, thick-walled left ventricle	Compassionate care
	Large, dilated, hypertrophied right ventricle	
	X-ray examination: cardiac enlargement: enlarged right atrium and ventricle and pulmonary venous congestion	
	Hypoplastic left heart syndrome is the underdevelopment of the left side of the heart including aortic valve atresia, severe mitral valve stenosis, and small left ventricle.	

DECREASED PULMONARY BLOOD FLOW

CONGENITAL HEART DEFECT	CLINICAL FINDINGS	MEDICAL/SURGICAL MANAGEMENT
Tetralogy of Fallot (TOF) Pulmonary stenosis Ventricular septal defect (VSD) Overriding aorta Right ventricular hypertrophy 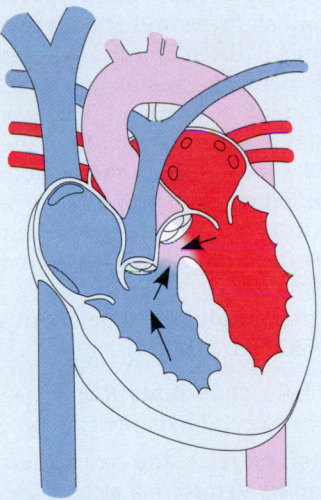	May be cyanotic at birth or within first few months of life	Prevention of dehydration, intercurrent infections
	Harsh systolic murmur LSB	Alleviation of paroxysmal dyspneic attacks
	Crying or feeding increases cyanosis and respiratory distress	Palliative surgery to increase blood flow to the lungs
	X-ray: "boot-shaped" appearance secondary to small pulmonary artery	Corrective surgery—resection of pulmonic stenosis, closure of VSD with Dacron patch
	Right ventricular enlargement	

In tetralogy of Fallot, the severity of symptoms depends on the degree of pulmonary stenosis, the size of the ventricular septal defect, and the degree to which the aorta overrides the septal defect.

MIXED DEFECTS*

CONGENITAL HEART DEFECT	CLINICAL FINDINGS	MEDICAL/SURGICAL MANAGEMENT
Transposition of Great Vessels (TGA) (Most common cyanotic heart defect) ↑ females, infants of diabetic mothers (IDMs), LGAs 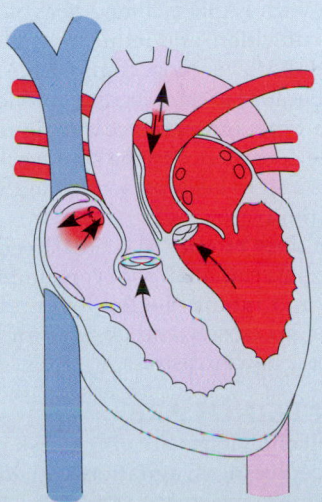	Significant cyanosis at birth or within 3 days as PDA closes	Prostaglandin E to maintain patency of the PDA
	Possible pulmonic stenosis murmur	Initial surgery to create opening between right and left side of heart if none exists
	Right ventricular hypertrophy	Total surgical repair—usually the arterial switch procedure—done within first few days of life
	Polycythemia	
	X-ray: "egg on its side" x-ray appearance	

Complete transposition of great vessels is an embryologic defect caused by a straight division of the bulbar trunk without normal spiraling. As a result, the aorta originates from the right ventricle, and the pulmonary artery from the left ventricle, resulting in a parallel circulatory system. An abnormal communication between the two circulations must be present to sustain life.

*MIXED defects: Postnatal survival is dependent upon mixing of systemic and pulmonary blood flow.

TABLE 26–4 Common Drugs of Abuse

OPIOIDS/OPIATES	CNS STIMULANTS	CNS DEPRESSANTS/SEDATIVES	HALLUCINOGENS
Codeine	Amphetamines	Alcohol	Inhalants
Darvon	Cocaine	Barbiturates	LSD
Demerol	Methamphetamines	Benzodiazepines	Solvents and aerosols (glue, gasoline, paint, cleaning solutions)
Fentanyl	Nicotine	Chloral Hydrate	
Heroin	Phencyclidines	Cannabinoids (marijuana)	
Hydrocodone (Lortab, Vicodin)	Ritalin		
Hydromorphone (Dilaudid)			
Methadone			
Morphine			
Oxycodone (Percocet, OxyContin)			

development but have a normal progression of oral–motor function. Many babies with FASD nurse poorly and have persistent vomiting until 6 to 7 months of age. They have difficulty adjusting to solid foods and show little spontaneous interest in food.

CNS dysfunctions are the most common and serious problem associated with FASD. Hypotonicity and increased placidity are seen in these babies. They also have a decreased ability to block out repetitive stimuli. Children exhibiting FASD can have either severe intellectual disabilities or normal intelligence. These children show impulsivity, cognitive impairment, and speech and language abnormalities indicative of CNS involvement. As they progress through the adolescent years, they change from very thin and underweight children to those who are overweight and often obese. Short stature and microcephaly persist.

Nursing Management

For the Newborn With Fetal Alcohol Spectrum Disorder (FASD)

Nursing Assessment and Diagnosis

Newborns with FASD show the following characteristics:

- *Abnormal structural development and CNS dysfunction.* These include irritability, hypotonia, microcephaly, and hyperactivity and cognitive disability in childhood.
- *Growth deficiencies.* The growth of babies with FAS is often restricted in regard to weight, length, and head circumference. These infants continue to show a persistent postnatal growth deficiency, with head circumference and linear growth most affected.
- *Distinctive facial abnormalities.* These include short palpebral fissures; epicanthal folds; broad nasal bridge; flattened midfaces; short, upturned, or beaklike nose; micrognathia (abnormally small lower jaw); hypoplastic maxilla; thin upper lip or vermilion border; and smooth philtrum (groove on upper lip) (Cloherty et al., 2012).
- *Associated anomalies.* Abnormalities affecting the heart (primarily septal and valvular defects), eyes (optic nerve hypoplasia), ears (conductive and sensorineural hearing loss), kidneys, and skeleton (especially involving joints, such as congenital dislocated hips) systems are often noted.

An alcohol-exposed newborn in the first week of life may show symptoms that include sleeplessness, excessive arousal states, inconsolable crying, abnormal reflexes, hyperactivity with little ability to maintain alertness and attentiveness to environment, jitteriness, abdominal distention, and exaggerated mouthing behaviors such as hyperactive rooting and increased nonnutritive sucking. Seizures may be common. These symptoms commonly persist throughout the first month of life but may continue longer. Alcohol dependence in the newborn is physiologic, not psychologic. Signs and symptoms of withdrawal often appear within 3 to 12 hours and can last up to 18 months (Wang, 2014). Seizures after the neonatal period are rare.

Nursing diagnoses that may apply to the newborn with FASD include the following (NANDA-I © 2014):

- *Nutrition, Imbalanced: Less Than Body Requirements,* related to decreased food intake and hyperirritability
- *Infant Behavior: Disorganized,* related to central nervous system involvement secondary to maternal alcohol use
- *Coping, Ineffective,* related to dysfunctional family dynamics and substance-dependent mother

Nursing Plan and Implementation

HOSPITAL-BASED NURSING CARE

Nursing care of the newborn with FASD is aimed at avoiding heat loss, providing adequate nutrition, and reducing environmental stimuli. The baby with FASD is most comfortable in a quiet, dimly lit environment. Because of their feeding problems, these newborns require extra time and patience during feedings. It is important to provide consistency in the staff working with the baby and the parents and to keep personnel and visitors to a minimum at any one time.

Inform the alcohol-dependent mother that breastfeeding is not contraindicated but that excessive alcohol consumption may intoxicate the newborn and inhibit the let-down reflex. Monitor the newborn's vital signs closely and observe for evidence of seizure activity and respiratory distress.

COMMUNITY-BASED NURSING CARE

Babies affected by maternal alcohol abuse are also at risk psychologically. Restlessness, sleeplessness, agitation, resistance to cuddling or holding, and frequent crying can be frustrating to parents because their efforts to relieve the distress are unrewarded. Feeding difficulties can also result in frustrations for the caregiver and digestive upsets for the baby. Frustration may cause the parents to punish the baby or result in the unconscious desire to stay away from the baby. Either outcome may create an unstable family environment and result in failure to thrive.

Focus on providing support for the parents and reinforcing positive parenting activity. Before discharge, give parents opportunities to provide baby care so that they can feel confident in their interpretations of their baby's cues and ability to meet the baby's needs. Referring the family to social services and visiting nurse or public health nurse associations is essential for the well-being of the child. Follow-up care and teaching can strengthen the parents' skill and coping abilities and help them create a stable, healthy environment for their family. The baby with FASD should be involved in intervention programs that monitor the child's developmental progress, health, and home environment.

Evaluation

Expected outcomes of nursing care include the following:

- The newborn with FASD is able to tolerate feedings and gain weight.
- The hyperirritability or seizures of the newborn with FASD are controlled, and the baby has suffered no physical injuries.
- The parents are able to identify the special needs of their newborn and accept outside assistance as needed.

Opiate Dependency

Patterns of abuse of opiates, including heroin, morphine, codeine, and prescription narcotics, in childbearing women have increased in the last several years (Prasad, 2014). (See section Substances Commonly Abused During Pregnancy in Chapter 14 for more discussion of maternal substance abuse.)

Twenty-one to 94% of newborns with intrauterine opiate exposure are predisposed to a number of physical and neurodevelopmental complications associated with withdrawal (Pritham, Paul, & Hayes, 2012). Of those babies, 46% to 78% will likely go on to require pharmacologic intervention for neonatal withdrawal requiring extended hospital stay (Pritham et al., 2012). Almost all opioid drugs readily cross the placenta and enter the fetal circulation, resulting in problems in the fetus in utero or in the newborn following delivery. Because opioid receptors are primarily in the CNS and GI tract, the signs and symptoms reflect CNS irritability, autonomic irritability, and GI dysfunction (Wang, 2014). The effects of polydrug use on the newborn must always be taken into consideration.

The greatest risks to the fetus of the drug-abusing mother are as follows:

- *Intrauterine asphyxia.* Asphyxia is often a direct result of fetal withdrawal secondary to maternal withdrawal. Fetal withdrawal is accompanied by hyperactivity, with increased oxygen consumption. Insufficiency of oxygen can lead to fetal asphyxia. Moreover, women addicted to narcotics tend to have a higher incidence of preeclampsia, abruptio placentae, and placenta previa, resulting in placental insufficiency and fetal asphyxia.
- *Intrauterine infection.* Sexually transmitted infection, HIV infection, and hepatitis are often connected with the pregnant addict's lifestyle. In addition, intravenous drug abuse

can predispose the mother to many infections including cellulitis, endocarditis, and chorioamnionitis (Cunningham et al., 2014). Such infections can involve the fetus.

- *Intrauterine growth restriction (IUGR).* There is a high correlation between substance abuse and poor maternal nutrition. In addition, diminished placental function has been evident as an additional cause for compromised fetal growth including weight and occipital–frontal circumference (OFC). This in turn contributes to the increase risk for stillbirths (Cunningham et al., 2014). Surveillance during the antenatal period, to include serial fetal ultrasounds, fundal height measurements, Doppler velometry readings, biophysical profiles, and non-stress tests (NSTs), will assist in diagnosing IUGR in the substance-abusing mother.
- *Low Apgar scores.* Low scores may be related to the intrauterine asphyxia or the medication the woman received during labor. The use of a narcotic antagonist (nalorphine or naloxone) to reverse respiratory depression is contraindicated because it may precipitate acute withdrawal in the newborn.

Common Complications of the Drug-Exposed Newborn

The newborn of a woman who abused drugs during her pregnancy is predisposed to the following problems:

- *Respiratory distress.* The heroin-addicted newborn frequently suffers respiratory stress, mainly meconium-aspiration pneumonia and transient tachypnea. Meconium aspiration is usually secondary to increased oxygen consumption and activity experienced by the fetus during intrauterine withdrawal. Transient tachypnea may develop secondary to the inhibitory effects of narcotics on the reflex responsible for clearing the lungs. Respiratory distress syndrome (RDS), however, occurs less often in heroin-addicted newborns, even in those who are premature, because they have tissue-oxygen-unloading capabilities comparable to those of a 6-week-old term infant. In addition, heroin stimulates production of glucocorticoids via the anterior pituitary gland.
- *Jaundice.* Newborns of methadone-addicted women may develop jaundice because of prematurity. By contrast, babies of mothers addicted to heroin or cocaine have a lower incidence of hyperbilirubinemia because these substances contribute to early maturity of the liver.
- *Congenital anomalies and growth restriction.* Babies of cocaine-addicted mothers exhibit congenital malformations involving bony skull defects, such as microcephaly, and symmetric intrauterine growth restriction (IUGR), cardiac defects, and genitourinary defects. In addition, the incidence of sudden infant death syndrome (SIDS) is higher. Congenital anomalies, however, are rare. Newborns exposed to methamphetamines during gestation may show a higher incidence of cardiac anomalies, cleft lip and palate, microencephaly, and low birth weight (LBW) (Blackburn, 2013). However, congenital anomalies are rare.
- *Behavioral abnormalities.* Babies exposed to cocaine have poor state organization. They exhibit decreased interactive behaviors when tested with the Brazelton Neonatal Behavioral Assessment Scale. These newborns also have difficulty moving through the various sleep and wake states and have problems attending to and actively engaging in auditory and visual stimuli.

- *Withdrawal.* The most significant postnatal problem of the drug-exposed newborn is opiate withdrawal (usually from heroin or methadone). The onset of withdrawal manifestations often begins within the first 24 to 48 hours of life; effects can be seen for as long as 21 days (Wang, 2014). See Table 26–5 for the clinical manifestations of newborn withdrawal.

During the first 2 years of life, many cocaine-exposed infants demonstrate susceptibility to behavior lability and the inability to express strong feelings such as pleasure, anger, or distress, or even a strong reaction to being separated from their parents. As a result, these infants have poor social interaction skills; cannot habituate to external stimuli; and become easily overstimulated, having difficulty sleeping. Cocaine-exposed newborns are at higher risk for motor development problems, delays in expressive language skills, and feeding difficulties because of swallowing problems (Cunningham et al., 2014). Behavioral state control is poorly developed in drug-exposed babies, who tend to rapidly progress from sleep to the awake state of crying without a smooth transition from one state to the next. Babies of drug-addicted mothers often demonstrate a higher incidence of gastrointestinal and respiratory illnesses related to the mother's lack of education regarding proper newborn/infant care, feeding, and hygiene. After birth the newborn born to a drug-dependent mother may also be subject to neglect or abuse, or both.

CLINICAL THERAPY

For optimal fetal and neonatal outcome, the heroin-addicted woman should receive complete prenatal care as early as possible to reduce maternal morbidity and mortality rates and to promote fetal stability and growth (Prasad, 2014). Methadone maintenance programs have been the standard treatment for the heroin-addicted mother to combat the cravings and to prevent withdrawal. For those women dependent on narcotics, it is not recommended that they be withdrawn completely while pregnant because this induces fetal withdrawal with poor newborn outcomes.

Newborn treatment may include management of complications; serologic tests for syphilis, HIV, and hepatitis B; urine drug screen and meconium analysis; and social service referral. Screening of meconium provides a more comprehensive and accurate indication of exposure over a longer gestational period than does screening of neonatal urine and is comparable to umbilical cord tissue samples (Wang, 2014).

Pharmacologic management for opiate withdrawal may include oral morphine sulfate solution, paregoric, tincture of opium, oral methadone, phenobarbital (adjunct therapy) clonidine (adjunct therapy), and diazepam. In addition, the use of the mother's expressed breast milk or breastfeeding by women who are in methadone-maintenance programs has been beneficial for substance-exposed babies in decreasing the need for lengthy neonatal abstinence syndrome (NAS) treatment (Wang, 2014). Nutritional support is important in light of the increase in energy expenditure that withdrawal may entail.

Nursing Management
For the Substance-Exposed Newborn

Nursing Assessment and Diagnosis

Early identification of the newborn needing clinical or pharmacologic interventions decreases the incidence of neonatal mortality and morbidity. The identification of substance-exposed newborns is determined primarily by clinical indicators in the prenatal period including maternal presentation, history of substance use or abuse, medical history, or toxicology results. During the newborn period, nursing assessment focuses on the following:

- Discovering the mother's last drug intake and dosage level. Women may be reluctant to disclose this information; therefore, a nonjudgmental interview technique is essential (AAP & ACOG, 2012).

- Assessing for congenital malformations and the complications related to intrauterine withdrawal such as SGA, asphyxia, meconium aspiration, and prematurity.

- Identifying the signs and symptoms of newborn withdrawal or neonatal abstinence syndrome (see Table 26–6).

TABLE 26–5 Clinical Manifestations of Newborn Withdrawal

Central Nervous System Signs
- High-pitched cry
- Hyperirritability, difficult to console, restlessness
- Increased muscle tone
- Exaggerated reflexes
- Tremors, myoclonic jerks
- Seizures
- Sneezing, hiccups, yawning
- Short, unquiet sleep

Gastrointestinal Signs
- Disorganized, vigorous suck
- Excessive sucking
- Vomiting
- Poor weight gain
- Sensitive gag reflex
- Diarrhea
- Poor feeding (less than 15 mL on first day of life; takes longer than 30 minutes per feeding)

Autonomic Signs
- Stuffy nose, sneezing
- Yawning
- Mottled
- Tachypnea (greater than 60 breaths/minute when quiet)
- Sweating
- Hyperthermia

Cutaneous Signs
- Excoriated buttocks, knees, elbows
- Facial scratches
- Pressure-point abrasions

TABLE 26–6 Neonatal Abstinence Syndrome Signs and Symptoms

Central Nervous System Disturbances

Cry	• Continuous high-pitched cry
	• Excessive high-pitched cry
Sleep	• Sleeps less than 3 hours after feeding
	• Sleeps less than 2 hours after feeding
	• Sleeps less than 1 hour after feeding
Moro reflex	• Markedly hyperactive Moro reflex
	• Hyperactive Moro reflex
Tremors	• Moderate–severe tremors undisturbed
	• Mild tremors undisturbed
	• Moderate–severe tremors disturbed
	• Mild tremors disturbed
Convulsions	• Generalized convulsions
	• Myoclonic jerks
	• Increased muscle tone
	• Excoriation (specific area)

Metabolic Disturbances

Thermoregulation	• Sweating
	• Fever over 101°F (38.4°C and higher)
	• Fever, under 101°F (99°–100.8°F/ 37.2°–38.2°C)

Vasomotor Disturbances

	• Frequent yawning (more than 3–4 times/interval)
	• Mottling of the skin
	• Nasal stuffiness
	• Sneezing (more than 3–4 times/interval)

Respiratory Disturbances

Respiration	• Nasal flaring
	• Respiratory rate more than 60 per minute with retractions
	• Respiratory rate more than 60 per minute

Gastrointestinal Disturbances

Feeding	• Poor feeding
	• Excessive sucking
Vomiting	• Projectile vomiting
	• Regurgitation
Stooling	• Watery stools
	• Loose stools

NOTE:
• Signs and symptoms are listed in descending order of severity for each subgroup.
• Signs/symptoms are scored 1–5, with 5 being the most severe using a neonatal abstinence score sheet.
• The newborn should be evaluated every 4 hours and a daily weight noted.

Source: Data from Neonatal Abstinence Syndrome by L. P. Finnegan, in N. Nelson (ed.), *Current Therapy in Neonatal-Perinatal Medicine* (2nd ed.), 1990, Ontario, CA: B. C. Decker; Zahorodny, W., Rom, C., Whitney, W., Giddens, S., Samuel, M., Maichuk, G., & Marshall, R. (1998). The neonatal withdrawal inventory: A simplified score of newborn withdrawal. *Developmental and Behavioral Pediatrics, 19*(2), 89–93. doi:10.1097/00004703-199804000

Although many of the signs and symptoms of drug withdrawal are similar to those seen with hypoglycemia and hypocalcemia, glucose and calcium values are reported to be within normal limits.

Neonatal abstinence syndrome includes both physiologic and behavioral responses. The severity of withdrawal can be assessed by a scoring system based on observations and measurement of the responses to neonatal abstinence such as the Finnegan scale. It evaluates the newborn every 4 hours on 31 potentially life-threatening signs, which are given a score from 1 to 5. A newer option, the Neonatal Withdrawal Inventory (NWI), is another tool that evaluates and scores seven prominent signs of withdrawal; each sign is given a predetermined weight of 1 to 4, with the highest total score of 19 (Zahorodny et al., 1998). Both NAS scoring tools help to guide the need for pharmacologic intervention; pharmacologic treatment is warranted for three consecutive Finnegan or NWI scores greater than 8. Many hospitals have modified existing scales and have created a scoring system of their own.

Nursing diagnoses that may apply to drug-dependent newborns include those in *Nursing Care Plan: For the Newborn of a Substance-Abusing Mother* and the following (NANDA-I © 2014):

• *Infant Behavior: Disorganized,* related to perinatal substance abuse
• *Breathing Pattern, Ineffective,* related to meconium aspiration syndrome due to fetal stress and hypoxia
• *Skin Integrity, Impaired,* related to constant activity, diarrhea
• *Parenting, Impaired,* related to hyperirritable behavior of the newborn and lack of knowledge of newborn care

Nursing Plan and Implementation

HOSPITAL-BASED NURSING CARE

Care of the drug-dependent newborn is based on reducing withdrawal symptoms and promoting adequate respiration, temperature, and nutrition. See *Nursing Care Plan: For the Newborn of a Substance-Abusing Mother* for specific nursing measures. Some general nursery care measures include the following:

• Perform neonatal abstinence scoring per hospital protocol.
• Monitor temperature for hypothermia.
• Monitor pulse and respirations carefully every 15 minutes and pulse oximetry until stable.
• Provide small, frequent feedings, especially in the presence of vomiting, regurgitation, and diarrhea.
• Position on the right side-lying or semi-Fowler position to avoid possible aspiration of vomitus or secretions.
• Monitor weight-gain pattern daily to assess the need for increased calorie content of formula.
• Administer medications as ordered, such as oral morphine elixir, methadone, and deodorized tincture of opium (DTO). A sedative, such as phenobarbital, is usually used in combination with an opioid, as it does not control any of the GI symptoms associated with NAS (Wang, 2014).
• Monitor frequency of diarrhea and vomiting and weigh newborn every 8 hours during withdrawal.
• Swaddle with hands near mouth to minimize injury and achieve more organized behavioral state. Offer a pacifier for nonnutritive, excessive sucking (Figure 26–16). Gentle, vertical rocking can be successful in calming a baby who is out of control.
• Protect newborn's face and extremities from excoriation by using mittens, as well as soft sheets or sheepskin. Apply protective skin emollient to the groin area with each diaper change.
• Place the newborn in a quiet, dimly lit area of the nursery.

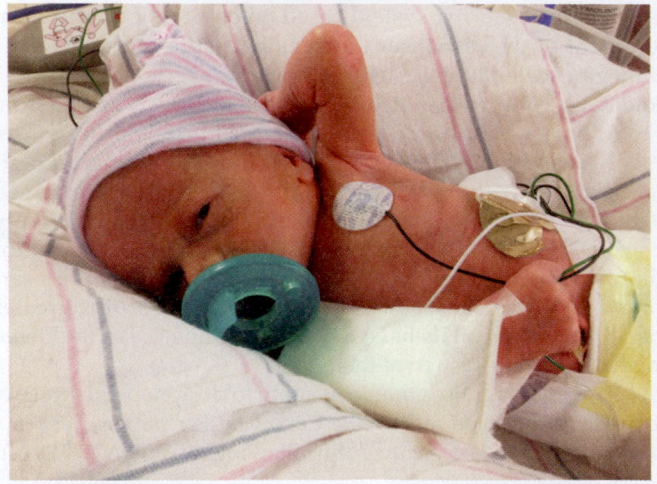

Figure 26–16 Nonnutritive sucking on a pacifier has a calming effect on the preterm newborn and also facilitates readiness to bottle-feed.

SOURCE: Carol Harrigan, RN, MSN, NNP-BC.

COMMUNITY-BASED NURSING CARE

Parents need assistance to prepare for what they can expect for the first few months at home. At the time of discharge, the mother should be instructed to anticipate mild jitteriness and irritability in the newborn, which may persist from 6 days to 8 weeks, depending on the initial severity of the withdrawal (Blackburn, 2013). Babies with neonatal abstinence syndrome are at significantly higher risk for SIDS when the mother used heroin or cocaine. The baby should sleep supine and home apnea monitoring should be implemented. Help the mother learn feeding techniques, comforting measures, how to recognize newborn cues, and appropriate parenting responses. Counsel parents regarding available resources, such as support groups, as well as signs and symptoms that indicate the need for further care. Ongoing evaluation is necessary because of the potential for long-term problems. Follow-up on missed appointments can bring parents back into the healthcare system, thereby improving parent and baby outcomes and promoting a positive, interactive environment after birth (AAP & ACOG, 2012).

Evaluation

Expected outcomes of nursing care include the following:

- The newborn tolerates feedings, gains weight, and has a decreased incidence of diarrhea.
- The parents learn innovative ways to comfort their newborn.
- The parents are able to cope with their frustrations and begin to use outside resources as needed.

Newborns of Mothers Who Are Tobacco Dependent

Despite increased knowledge about the dangers to the fetus and newborn of smoking mothers, 22% of women continue to smoke during pregnancy (Barron, 2014). The common consequence of tobacco use is addiction to nicotine.

RISKS OF TOBACCO TO THE FETUS AND NEWBORN

Preconceptual cigarette smoking has been found to increase infertility. Fortunately, the reduction in fertility is reversible if the woman stops smoking. Smoking during pregnancy has been associated with spontaneous abortion, placenta previa, and abruptio placentae.

The most studied compound found in cigarette smoking that can adversely affect the intrauterine environment is carbon monoxide. Carbon monoxide binds hemoglobin to form carboxyhemoglobin, which reduces the oxygen-carrying capacity of the blood. It also increases the binding of hemoglobin to oxygen, which impairs the release of oxygen to the tissues. Therefore the fetus can experience intrauterine hypoxia and ischemia. This chronic hypoxia causes the fetus to produce more red blood cells to increase available oxygen-carrying sites, resulting in polycythemia/hyperviscosity, which can further impair placental blood flow. Mothers who smoke during pregnancy are more likely to have IUGR and premature babies. These newborns typically weigh 150 to 250 g (0.3 to 0.5 lb) less than babies of nonsmokers (Cloherty et al., 2012). The nicotine in cigarettes acts as a neuroteratogen that interferes with fetal development, specifically the developing nervous system. Additional risks to the fetus and newborn of the mother who smokes include the following (Barron, 2014):

- *Intrauterine distress* presenting as meconium staining and low Apgar scores
- *Neonatal neurobehavioral abnormalities* such as impaired habituation, orientation, consolability, orientation to sound
- *Hypertonia* or *hypotonia, increase in tremors, increased Moro reflex*
- *Signs of nicotine toxicity* (tachycardia, irritability, poor feeding)
- *Sudden infant death syndrome (SIDS)*

CLINICAL THERAPY

Inquiry into tobacco and smoke exposure should be a routine part of the prenatal history. Preconception and prenatal counseling about the effects of cigarette smoking on pregnancy and the fetus should occur. An estimated 5% reduction in perinatal mortality would occur if smoking during pregnancy were eliminated (AAP & ACOG, 2012). Mothers should be counseled that eliminating or reducing smoking even late in pregnancy can improve fetal growth. The use of nicotine patches (instead of smoking) reduces the absorption of nicotine and thereby may increase the birth weight of the fetus. See the section Tobacco in Chapter 10 for further discussion of prenatal smoking cessation and other intervention programs.

Cotinine, a metabolite of nicotine, has been found in fetal body fluids. There is also a positive correlation between the number of cigarettes smoked per day and the concentration of cotinine in maternal urine. Other factors that influence fetal and maternal serum cotinine concentrations are nicotine content of the cigarette and the time elapsed between the last cigarette smoked and the sampling. These findings indicate that cotinine may be used as a marker of maternal–fetal tobacco exposure during pregnancy (Prasad & Jones, 2014).

Nursing Management

Newborns of mothers who are tobacco dependent may be screened with the NICU Network Neurobehavioral Scale (NNNS) to assess their neurologic, behavioral, and stress/abstinence neurobehavioral function.

Nursing Care Plan: For the Newborn of a Substance-Abusing Mother

1. Nursing Diagnosis: *Infant Behavior: Disorganized, Risk for,* **related to perinatal substance abuse** (NANDA-I © 2014)

GOAL: The newborn will be free of signs and symptoms of central nervous system (CNS) effects from maternal substance abuse.

INTERVENTION	RATIONALE
• Obtain prenatal records and question the mother about history of drug use. Include type of drug or drugs used, duration, time and amount of last dose taken during pregnancy and during labor and delivery.	• Confirms what drugs, if any, were abused during pregnancy. If enrolled in a methadone-maintenance program, neonatal abstinence syndrome (NAS) withdrawal will be more significant and predictable. • Noting the mother's last drug ingestion will provide the medical staff with an approximate time frame to expect the newborn to exhibit withdrawal symptoms.
• Obtain meconium drug screen using newborn's first stool.	• Confirms what drugs, if any, were abused during pregnancy. Indications to test a newborn: history of drug abuse, no prenatal care, unexplained placental abruption, changes in behavioral state of newborn.
• Assess newborn for signs and symptoms of withdrawal (e.g., high-pitched shrill cry, sneezing, vomiting, diarrhea, hypertonicity, restlessness, and wakefulness) using neonatal abstinence scoring tool per hospital guidelines.	• The average symptoms of withdrawal occur 72 hr after birth; however, symptoms may appear as early as 6–24 hr after birth.
• Provide a quiet, calm, darkened environment. Swaddle baby tightly and place in a side-lying or prone position.	• Providing a quiet environment decreases stimuli, therefore reducing CNS symptoms.
• Carefully plan tests and/or treatments to avoid excessive stimuli.	• Planning care promotes rest and reduces external stimuli.
• Use soothing techniques such as rocking, cuddling, soft music, and soft tones when speaking.	• These activities promote comfort, security, and newborn bonding.
• Administer appropriate medications as ordered by healthcare provider. Monitor efficacy of these medications as evidenced by a decrease in NAS scores.	• These medications aid the baby in minimizing symptoms related to withdrawal.

EXPECTED OUTCOME: Newborn will have no signs and symptoms of CNS effects of maternal substance abuse as evidenced by reduced hyperactivity and irritability, normal sleep–wake pattern, no jitteriness, and no seizure activity.

2. Nursing Diagnosis: *Airway Clearance, Ineffective,* **related to suppression of respiratory system** (NANDA-I © 2014)

GOAL: Newborn will be free of signs and symptoms of respiratory distress after birth.

INTERVENTION	RATIONALE
• Obtain maternal prenatal, labor, and birth records.	• Provides information about fetal stress that may have occurred during the prenatal or intrapartum period. In addition, the birth record will provide information concerning the newborn's respiratory status at birth, for example, the Apgar score.
• Assess newborn's respiratory rate and effort, skin color, heart rate, presence or absence of cough reflex, and symptoms of respiratory distress.	• Maternal narcotic consumption may depress the cough reflex and respiratory center of the newborn after birth. Symptoms such as cyanosis, tachycardia, grunting, retractions, and nasal flaring may indicate hypoxia.
• Position baby in a side-lying or semi-Fowler position.	• Prevents aspiration.

(continued)

Nursing Care Plan: For the Newborn of a Substance-Abusing Mother (continued)

INTERVENTION	RATIONALE
• Monitor baby for temperature elevation.	• Temperature elevation may cause metabolic rate and oxygen needs to increase when associated with CNS stimulation.
• *Collaborative:* Obtain arterial blood gas (ABG) and chest radiograph as ordered by healthcare provider.	• Oxygen demands increase with drug withdrawal. Obtaining an ABG and chest radiograph will provide healthcare personnel baseline information on newborn's respiratory status, and effective medical interventions can be initiated.
• Monitor newborn's cardiac status and pulmonary status using electrocardiogram (ECG) and pulse oximetry.	• Provides healthcare personnel with cardiac and pulmonary status.

EXPECTED OUTCOME: The newborn will maintain adequate respiratory effort as evidenced by respirations of 30–60/min; no signs of retractions, grunting, or cyanosis; arterial blood gas values within normal range; and normal pulse oximetry saturations for gestational age.

3. **Nursing Diagnosis:** *Nutrition, Imbalanced: Less than Body Requirements,* **related to vomiting and diarrhea, uncoordinated suck and swallow reflex, and hypertonia secondary to withdrawal (NANDA-I © 2014)**

GOAL: The newborn will maintain a consistent weight gain pattern.

INTERVENTION	RATIONALE
• Review gestational age assessment.	
• Assess newborn's sucking and swallowing reflexes.	
• Monitor regurgitation, vomiting, diarrhea.	• Gastrointestinal (GI) hypermobility, irritation, and CNS stimulation can increase nutritional needs.
• Use bulb syringe judiciously before feedings if newborn is having problems with nasal stuffiness and congestion.	• Allows newborn to breathe easier by ridding the nasal passages of excessive mucus.
• Initiate appropriate feedings per healthcare provider orders (e.g., nipple and/or gavage); may need supplemental IV fluids.	• Oral feeding may be difficult because of CNS hyperactivity and GI hypermobility.
• Provide small, frequent feedings of a high-calorie formula.	• Facilitates nutritional intake because small-for-gestational-age (SGA) newborns require 110–140 kcal/kg/day for adequate nutrition.
• Position baby on right side after feedings.	• Prevents regurgitation and promotes gastric emptying.
• Monitor newborn's weight and document on graph.	• Identifies abnormalities in weight gain/loss and allows for early intervention when necessary.
• Offer pacifier between feedings for nonnutritive sucking.	• Nonnutritive sucking allows for sucking practice, management of pain, and self-consoling behaviors.

EXPECTED OUTCOMES: The newborn will tolerate feedings and maintain consistent weight gain pattern evidenced by no regurgitation or aspiration of feedings and adequate weight gain according to weight graph.

4. **Nursing Diagnosis:** *Parenting, Risk for Impaired,* **related to lack of knowledge of newborn/infant care (NANDA-I © 2014)**

GOAL: The parent will demonstrate ability to independently provide newborn/infant care.

INTERVENTION	RATIONALE
• Assess mother's desire to learn newborn/infant care tasks as well as evaluate her present physical and emotional stability.	• Provides knowledge of mother's ability to care for newborn.
• Instruct mother on coping strategies (e.g., exercise, listening to music, and discussing concerns openly) to manage stressful situations.	• Gives mother the tools to handle stress, thereby decreasing the chances of exhibiting abusive behavior.

- Assess mother's insight into her own chemical dependency.

- Instruct mother on signs and symptoms of withdrawal and treatment interventions.

- Offer a night of "nesting in" with baby before discharge.

- Encourage mother and family members to perform basic newborn/infant care tasks.

- Initiate social service consult.

- Assistance in enrollment into a chemical dependency program may be necessary before mother can independently care for baby.

- Assists the mother in understanding newborn's behaviors and gives her the tools to intervene without feeling anxious.

- Assists parents to care for baby by themselves, but with nursing support nearby.

- Facilitates attachment and increases parenting competence.

EXPECTED OUTCOME: The parent will demonstrate the ability to perform basic newborn care tasks as evidenced by exhibiting appropriate attachment behaviors (e.g., talking to and holding baby), and feeding and bathing baby.

The potential for long-term respiratory problems such as asthma, as well as cognitive and receptive language delays that may persist into school age, should be evaluated.

Care of the Newborn Exposed to HIV/AIDS

Approximately 33.3 million people around the world live with HIV (Greenfield, 2013). In the United States, the CDC estimates that each year 215 to 370 babies with HIV infections are born (Gomella, 2013). Preventative strategies, including prenatal testing, antiretroviral therapy, viral load measurements, and scheduled cesarean sections, have reduced the risk of maternal–child transmission of HIV to approximately 1% to 2% (Centers for Disease Control [CDC], 2014). Most HIV transmissions during the perinatal and newborn periods occur across the placenta, across the amniotic membranes, or through breast milk or contaminated blood (Greenfield, 2013). The risk of vertical transmission in mothers not receiving an antiretroviral (ARV) drug regimen such as oral zidovudine (ZDV) during gestation is 25% to 40% in the United States (Greenfield, 2013). Pregnant women should be universally tested (with client notification) for HIV infection as part of the routine battery of prenatal blood tests unless they decline the test (i.e., opt-out approach) as permitted by local and state regulations. Refusal of testing should be documented. (For discussion of maternal and fetal HIV/AIDS, see Chapter 14.) Some infants infected by maternal–fetal transmission suffer from severe immunodeficiency, with HIV disease progressing more rapidly during the first year of life.

Early identification of babies with or at risk for HIV/AIDS is essential during the newborn period in addition to a consultation with a pediatric HIV specialist. Currently available HIV serologic tests (enzyme-linked immunosorbent assay [ELISA] and Western blot test) cannot distinguish between maternal and infant antibodies; therefore, they are inappropriate for babies up to 18 months of age. It may take up to 18 months for infected infants to form their own antibodies to HIV (Greenfield, 2013). The preferred test for diagnosis of HIV infection in newborns is the bDNA polymerase chain reaction (PCR) assay and HIV RNA assays (Smith & Carley, 2014). A positive result by 48 hours of age suggests in utero transmission, thus allowing early identification and treatment. If testing is performed at birth, umbilical cord blood should not be used, as it may be contaminated with maternal blood, leading to a false positive result. A repeat, confirmatory HIV DNA PCR is done at 14 to 21 days, 1 to 2 months, and 4 to 6 months postnatally (Smith & Carley, 2014).

For newborns, AZT is started prophylactically 2 mg/kg/dose PO every 6 hours beginning as soon after birth as possible and continuing for 6 weeks; dosing for preterm newborns is 2 mg/kg/dose PO every 12 hours for the first 2 weeks, then three times a day for the next 4 weeks. If the HIV DNA PCR is positive, the National Institutes of Health (NIH) recommends changing to combination antiretroviral therapy; this has been shown to decrease the rate of servoconversion of babies born to mothers infected with HIV (Davis & Yawetz, 2012). Breastfeeding in developed countries, where there are accessible alternative feeding methods, should be avoided with an HIV-positive mother as transmission of the HIV virus to the newborn in breast milk is well documented (Davis & Yawetz, 2012). A baseline complete blood count (CBC) with differential and platelets is obtained because anemia is one of the side effects of AZT therapy (Smith & Carley, 2014).

NURSING MANAGEMENT
For the Newborn Exposed to HIV/AIDS

Nursing Assessment and Diagnosis

Many newborns exposed to HIV/AIDS are premature or small for gestational age (SGA), or both, and show evidence of failure to thrive during neonatal and infant periods. They can show signs and symptoms of disease within days of birth. Signs that may be seen in the early infancy period include enlarged spleen and liver, swollen glands, recurrent respiratory infections, rhinorrhea, interstitial pneumonia (rarely seen in adults), recurrent GI (diarrhea and weight loss) and urinary system infections, persistent or recurrent oral candidiasis infections, and loss of achieved developmental milestones (McLean, 2014). There is also a high risk of acquiring *Pneumocystis jirovecii* pneumonia. Opportunistic diseases such as gram-negative sepsis and problems associated with prematurity are the primary causes of mortality in babies with HIV infection.

Nursing diagnoses that may apply to a newborn exposed to HIV/AIDS include the following (NANDA-I © 2014):

- *Nutrition, Imbalanced: Less than Body Requirements,* related to formula intolerance and inadequate intake

- *Skin Integrity, Impaired,* related to chronic diarrhea

- *Infection, Risk for* related to perinatal exposure and immunoregulation suppression secondary to HIV/AIDS

- *Mobility: Physical, Impaired,* related to decreased neuromuscular development

- *Development: Delayed, Risk for,* related to lack of attachment and stimulation

- *Parenting, Impaired,* related to diagnosis of HIV/AIDS and fear of future outcome

Nursing Plan and Implementation

HOSPITAL-BASED NURSING CARE

Nursing care of the newborn exposed to HIV/AIDS includes all the care normally given to any newborn in a nursery. In addition, you must include care for a newborn suspected of having a bloodborne infection, as with hepatitis B.

SAFETY ALERT!

Standard precautions should be used when caring for the newborn immediately after birth and when obtaining blood samples via vein puncture or heel stick. The blood of all newborns must be considered potentially infectious because the status of the baby's blood is often not known until after the baby is discharged.

Health Promotion Preventing Infection

Most institutions recommend that their healthcare provider wear gloves during all diaper changes, especially in the presence of diarrhea because blood may be in the stool, and during examination of the newborn. There is a window of time before seroconversion occurs when the baby is still considered infectious. See Table 26–7 for some general issues for all nurses and healthcare providers of the newborn at risk for HIV/AIDS. In addition, provide for comfort; keep the newborn properly nourished and protected from opportunistic infections; provide good skin care to prevent skin rashes; and facilitate growth, development, and attachment.

TABLE 26–7 Issues for Caregivers of Newborns at Risk for HIV/AIDS

Resuscitation	For suctioning use a bulb syringe, mucus extractor, or meconium aspirator with wall suction on low setting. Use masks, goggles, and gloves.
Admission Care	To remove blood from baby's skin, give warm water/mild soap bath using gloves as soon as possible after admission.
Hand Hygiene	Thorough hand washing is indicated before and after caring for baby. Hands must be washed immediately if contaminated with blood or body fluids. Wash hands after removal of gloves.
Gloves	Gloves are indicated with touching blood or other high-risk fluids. Gloves should also be worn when handling newborns before and during their initial baths, cord care, eye prophylactics, and vitamin K administration.
Mask, Goggle, and Gown	Not routinely needed unless coming in contact with placenta or the blood and amniotic fluid on the skin of the newborn.
Needles and Syringes	Used needles should not be recapped or bent; they should be disposed of in a puncture-resistant plastic container belonging specifically to that baby. After the newborn is discharged the container is discarded.
Specimens	Blood and other specimens should be double-bagged and/or sealed in an impervious container and labeled according to agency protocol.
Equipment and Linen	Articles contaminated with blood or body fluids should be discarded or bagged according to isolation or institution protocol.
Body Fluid Spills	Blood and body fluids should be cleaned promptly with a solution of 5.25% sodium hypochlorite (household bleach) diluted 1:10 with water. Apply for at least 30 seconds then wipe after the minimum contact time.
Education and Support	Provide education and psychologic support for family and staff. Nurses and healthcare providers who avoid contact with a baby at risk or who overdress in unnecessary isolation garb subtly exacerbate an already difficult family situation. Information resources include the National AIDS Hotline (1-800-342-2437) and the AIDS Clinical Trials Information Service (1-800-TRIALS-A).
Exempted Personnel	Immunologically compromised staff (pregnant women may be included in this group) and possibly infectious staff members should not care for these newborns.

Sources: Data from Krist, A. H., & Crawford-Faucher, A. (2002). Management of newborns exposed to maternal HIV infection. *American Family Physician, 65*(10), 2049–2056; Smith, J. R., & Carley, A. (2014). Common neonatal complications. In K. R. Simpson & P. A. Creehan (Eds.), *AWHONN's perinatal nursing* (4th ed., pp. 662–698). Philadelphia, PA: Lippincott Williams & Wilkins.

COMMUNITY-BASED NURSING CARE

Hand hygiene is crucial when caring for newborns at risk for AIDS. Parents should be taught proper hand washing technique. Nutrition is essential because failure to thrive and weight loss are common. Small, frequent feedings and food supplementation are helpful. Discuss with parents sanitary techniques for preparing formula. Inform the parents that the baby should not be put to bed with juice or formula because of potential bacterial growth. Parents need to be alert to the signs of feeding intolerance, such as increasing regurgitation, abdominal distention, and loose stools. The newborn should be weighed 3 times a week.

Clinical Reasoning Newborn with Possible HIV

Mrs. Jean Corrigan, a 23-year-old GIPI positive for HIV, has just given birth to a 7 lb, 1 oz baby girl. As she watches you assessing her daughter in the birthing room, she asks why you are wearing gloves and whether her daughter will have to be in isolation.

What will your response be to the new mother?

The baby should have his or her own skin care items, towels, and washcloths. Most clothing and linens can be washed with other household laundry. Linen that is visibly soiled with blood or body fluids should be kept and washed separately in hot, sudsy water with household bleach. Prompt diaper changing and perineal care can prevent or minimize diaper rash and promote comfort.

The diaper-changing area in the home should be separate from the food preparation and serving areas. Soiled diapers should be placed in plastic bags, sealed, and disposed of daily. Diaper-changing areas should be cleaned with a 1:10 dilution of household bleach after each diaper change. Toys should be kept as clean as possible, not shared with other children, and checked for sharp edges to prevent scratches.

Instruct the parents about signs of infection to be alert to and when to call their healthcare provider. The inability to feed without pain may indicate esophageal yeast infection and may require administration of nystatin (Mycostatin) for the oral thrush. Topical Mycostatin or Desitin ointment is used for diaper rashes. If diarrhea occurs, the baby needs frequent perineal care as well as fluid replacement. Antidiarrheal medications are often ineffective. Irritability may be the first sign of fever. Fluids, antipyretics, and sponging with tepid water are of use in managing fever. Preventive care for exposed newborns includes routine immunizations, except the combined measles-mumps-rubella-varicella (MMRV). HIV-1 exposed and infected infants should receive the rotavirus vaccine at 2, 4, and 6 months of age.

Parents and family members need to be reassured that there are no documented cases of people contracting HIV/AIDS from routine care of infected babies. Emotional support for family members is essential because of the stress and social isolation they may face. Because of these stresses, parents may not bond with the baby or they may fail to provide the baby with enough sensory and tactile stimulation. Encourage the parents to hold the baby during feedings because the baby benefits from frequent, gentle touch. Auditory stimulation may also be provided by using music or tapes of parents' voices. Offer families information about support groups, available counseling, and information resources.

All newborns born to HIV-positive mothers require regular clinical, immunologic, and virologic monitoring. At 1 month of age the baby's physical examination should include a developmental assessment and complete blood count, including differential blood count, CD4+ count, and platelet count. Prophylaxis for *Pneumocystis jirovecii* pneumonia for all babies born to women who are HIV infected should be begun after completion of the ZDV prophylaxis regimen (McLean, 2014). Pediatric HIV disease raises many healthcare issues for the family. The parents, depending on their health status, may or may not be able to care for their baby, and they must deal with many psychosocial and economic issues.

Evaluation

Expected outcomes of nursing care include the following:

- The parents are able to bond with their newborn and have realistic expectations about the baby.
- Potential opportunistic infections are identified early and treated promptly.
- The parents verbalize their concerns about their baby's existing and potential health problems and long-term care needs and accept outside assistance as needed.

Care of the Newborn With an Inborn Error of Metabolism

Inborn errors of metabolism (IEM) are a group of hereditary disorders transmitted by mutant genes. Each causes an enzyme defect that blocks a metabolic pathway and leads to an accumulation of toxic metabolites. Most of the disorders are transmitted by an autosomal recessive gene, requiring two heterozygous parents to produce a homozygous child with the disorder. Heterozygous parents carrying some inborn errors of metabolism disorders can be identified by special tests, and some inborn errors of metabolism can be detected and treated in utero. Some of the inborn errors of metabolism (especially those associated with intellectual disability) are now detected neonatally through newborn screening programs. All states require screening of newborns for phenylketonuria (PKU) and congenital hypothyroidism (CH) (Matthews & Robin, 2011). Mandatory newborn screening for other inborn errors of metabolism varies among states and often includes maple syrup urine disease (MSUD), homocystinuria, cystic fibrosis (CF), sickle cell anemia, and congenital adrenal hypoplasia. In several states, newborn screening includes an enzyme assay for galactose 1-phosphate uridyltransferase; however, this test does not detect galactosemia if it is caused by a deficiency of the enzyme galactokinase. With new laboratory technology and the introduction of tandem mass spectrometry (MS/MS), a spot of blood from a newborn can be used to detect more than 50 inborn errors of metabolism (Matthews & Robin, 2011).

Selected Inborn Errors of Metabolism

Phenylketonuria (PKU) is the most common of the amino acid disorders. Newborn screenings have set its incidence at about 1 in 12,000 live births in the United States; however, the incidence varies considerably among ethnic groups (Gleason & Devaskar, 2012). The highest incidence is noted in White populations from northern Europe and the United States. It is rarely observed in people of African, Hispanic, Chinese, or Japanese descent (Kaye & Committee on Genetics, 2006, reaffirmed 2011).

Phenylalanine is an essential amino acid (found in dietary protein) used by the body for growth. In the normal individual any excess is converted to tyrosine. The newborn with PKU lacks this converting ability, which results in an accumulation of phenylalanine in the blood. Phenylalanine produces two abnormal metabolites, phenylpyruvic acid and phenylacetic acid. These are eliminated in the urine, producing a musty odor. Excessive accumulation of phenylalanine and its abnormal metabolites in the brain tissue leads to progressive mental retardation.

The Guthrie blood test for PKU, required for all newborns before discharge, uses a drop of blood collected from a heel stick and placed on filter paper (Figure 26–17). Because phenylalanine metabolites begin to build up in the PKU baby once milk feedings have been initiated, the test is done at least 24 hours after the initiation of feedings containing the usual amounts of breast milk or formula. At-risk newborns should receive a 60% milk intake, with no more than 40% of their total intake from nonprotein intravenous fluids. The PKU testing of at-risk newborns should be deferred for at least 48 hours after hyperalimentation is initiated. It is vital that the parents understand the need for the screening procedure; a follow-up check is necessary to confirm that the test was done.

Another disorder frequently included in mandatory newborn screening blood tests is *congenital hypothyroidism (CH)*. An inborn enzymatic defect, lack of maternal dietary iodine, or maternal ingestion of drugs that depress or destroy thyroid tissue can cause CH. An elevated thyroid-stimulating hormone (TSH) and low T_4 level are commonly seen in the premature newborn following birth; it may be necessary to repeat levels at 2 to 6 weeks of age. Congenital hypothyroidism occurs more often in Hispanic and American Indian/Alaska Native people. Babies with Down syndrome are also at increased risk of having CH (Kaye & Committee on Genetics, 2006, reaffirmed 2011).

The incidence of metabolic errors is relatively low, but for affected newborns and their families these disorders pose a threat to the baby's survival. If they survive, these children frequently require lifelong treatment.

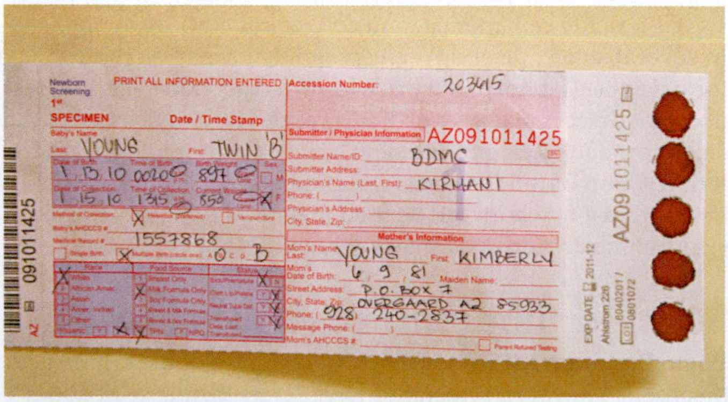

Figure 26–17 Guthrie card for newborn testing.

SOURCE: Carol Harrigan, RN, MSN, NNP-BC.

Clinical Therapy

Identification via newborn screening and early clinical intervention for some inborn errors of metabolism has become more difficult with the advent of early discharge of newborns. If the initial specimen is obtained before the newborn is 24 hours of age, then a second specimen should be obtained before 5 days of age, although few states currently require the second test (Kaye & Committee on Genetics, 2006, reaffirmed 2011). Early collection of specimens may yield false-positive results for certain metabolic disorders. Conversely, certain metabolic disorders may go undetected. Newborns in the NICU who require interhospital transfers as well as early-discharge healthy newborns are at risk for nonscreening. Newborn screen specimens are always collected before a blood transfusion.

Nursing Management

For the Newborn With an Inborn Error of Metabolism

Assess the newborn for signs of inborn errors of metabolism and carry out state-mandated newborn screening tests. Refer parents of affected newborns to support groups. Ensure that parents are informed about centers that can provide information about biochemical genetics and dietary management.

Nursing Plan and Implementation

NEWBORN WITH PHENYLKETONURIA

Typically, a baby with phenylketonuria (PKU) is a normal-appearing newborn, most often with blond hair, blue eyes, and fair complexion. Decreased pigmentation may be related to the competition between phenylalanine and tyrosine for the available enzyme tyrosinase. Tyrosine is needed for the formation of melanin pigment and the hormones epinephrine and thyroxine. Without treatment, the baby fails to thrive and develops vomiting and eczematous rashes. By about 6 months of age, the infant exhibits behaviors indicative of intellectual disability and other central nervous system (CNS) involvement, including seizures and abnormal electroencephalogram (EEG) patterns.

Advise parents that once identified, a baby with PKU can be treated with a special diet that limits ingestion of phenylalanine. Special formulas low in phenylalanine, such as Lofenalac, Minafen, and Albumaid XP, are available. Special food lists are helpful for parents of a child with PKU. If treatment is begun before 1 month of age, CNS damage can be minimized. There is an increased risk of producing a child with intellectual disability if the mother with PKU is not on a low-phenylalanine diet during pregnancy. It is recommended that the woman reinstate her low-phenylalanine diet before becoming pregnant again (Blackburn, 2013).

NEWBORN WITH CONGENITAL HYPOTHYROIDISM

Approximately 5% of newborns with congenital hypothyroidism (CH), generally those who are more severely affected, have recognizable features at birth, including a large tongue, umbilical hernia, cool and mottled skin, low hairline, hypotonia, and large fontanelles (especially the posterior fontanelle in term newborns) (Kaye & Committee on Genetics, 2006, reaffirmed 2011). Early symptoms include prolonged neonatal jaundice, poor feeding, constipation, low-pitched cry, poor weight gain, inactivity, early sleeping through the night, and delayed motor development. In addition, premature newborns of less than 30 weeks' gestation frequently have lower T_4 and TSH values than those of term babies. This difference may reflect the premature newborn's inability to bind thyroid and a risk for hypothyroidism.

Babies with CH need frequent follow-up laboratory monitoring and adjustment of thyroid medication to accommodate the child's growth and development. With adequate treatment, children remain free of symptoms, but if the condition is left untreated, stunted growth (slowed linear growth) and intellectual disability occur.

Evaluation

Expected outcomes of nursing care include the following:

- Newborns at risk for inborn errors of metabolism are promptly identified and receive early intervention.

- The parents verbalize their concerns about their baby's nutritional status, health problems, long-term care needs, and potential outcomes.

- The parents are aware of available community health resources and use them as indicated.

Focus Your STUDY

- Early identification of potential high-risk fetuses through assessment of preconception, prenatal, and intrapartum factors facilitates strategically timed nursing observations and interventions.

- High-risk newborns, whether they are premature, small for gestational age (SGA), large for gestational age (LGA), post-term, infant of a diabetic mother (IDM), or infant of a substance-abusing mother (ISAM), have many similar problems, although their problems are based on different physiologic processes.

- SGA newborns are at risk for perinatal asphyxia and resulting aspiration syndrome, hypothermia, hypoglycemia, hypocalcemia, polycythemia, congenital anomalies, and intrauterine infections. Long-term problems include continued growth and learning difficulties.

- LGA newborns are at risk for birth trauma as a result of cephalopelvic disproportion, hypoglycemia, polycythemia, and hyperviscosity.

- IDMs are at risk for hypoglycemia, hypocalcemia, hyperbilirubinemia, polycythemia, and respiratory distress caused by delayed maturation of their lungs.

- Postterm newborns often encounter intrapartum problems such as cephalopelvic disproportion (CPD) (shoulder dystocia) and birth traumas, hypoglycemia, polycythemia, meconium aspiration, cold stress, and possible seizure activity. Long-term complications may involve poor weight gain and low IQ scores.

- The common problems of the preterm newborn are a result of the baby's immature body systems. Potential problems include respiratory distress syndrome (RDS), patent ductus arteriosus (PDA), hypothermia and cold stress, feeding difficulties and necrotizing enterocolitis (NEC), marked insensible water loss and loss of buffering agents through the kidneys, infection, anemia of prematurity, apnea, intraventricular hemorrhage, retinopathy of prematurity, and behavioral state disorganization. Long-term needs and problems include bronchopulmonary dysplasia, speech defects, sensorineural hearing loss, and neurologic sequelae.

- Cardiac defects are a significant cause of morbidity and mortality in the newborn period. Early identification and nursing and medical care of newborns with cardiac defects are essential to improve the outcomes for these babies. Care is directed toward lessening the workload of the heart and decreasing oxygen and energy consumption.

- Newborns of alcohol-dependent mothers are at risk for physical characteristic alterations and the long-term complications of feeding problems; CNS dysfunction, including low IQ, hyperactivity, and language abnormalities; and congenital anomalies.

- Newborns of drug-dependent mothers experience drug withdrawal as well as respiratory distress, jaundice, congenital anomalies, and behavioral abnormalities. With early recognition and intervention, the potential long-term physiologic and emotional consequences of these difficulties can be avoided or at least lessened in severity.

- Newborns of mothers with HIV/AIDS require early recognition and treatment so that the physiologic and emotional consequences may be lessened in severity and CDC guidelines implemented.

- Inborn errors of metabolism such as phenylketonuria (PKU) and congenital hypothyroidism (CH) are usually included in a newborn screening program designed to prevent intellectual disability through dietary management and medication.

- The nursing care of the newborn with special problems involves the understanding of normal physiology, the pathophysiology of the disease process, clinical manifestations, and supportive or corrective therapies. Only with this theoretical background can the nurse make appropriate observations about responses to therapy and development of complications.

- The nurse facilitates interprofessional communication with the parents. Parents of at-risk newborns need support from nurses and healthcare providers to understand the special needs of their babies and feel confident in their ability to care for them at home.

Clinical Reasoning in Action

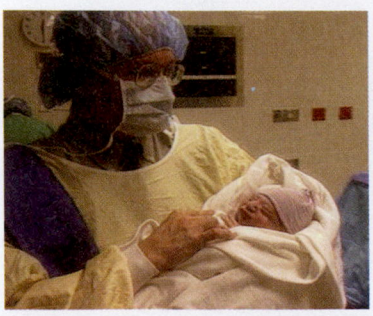

As the nurse on duty, you are caring for baby boy Jonathan, a 38-week infant of a diabetic mother (IDM) born by repeat cesarean birth to a 32-year-old G3 now P3 mother. Jonathan's Apgar scores are 7 and 9 at 1 and 5 minutes. At 2 hours of age, the baby has an elevated respiratory rate of 100 to 110, heart rate of 165 with Grade II/VI intermittent machinery murmur, and mild cyanosis. He is now receiving 30% oxygen and has a respiratory rate of 70 to 80. The baby's clinical course, chest x-ray, and laboratory results are all consistent with transient tachypnea of the newborn and patent ductus arteriosus.

The mother calls you to ask about how her baby is doing. She tells you that her last child was born at 30 weeks and had to be hospitalized for 6 weeks. She says, "I really tried to do it right this time," and asks you if this baby will have the same respiratory problem.

1. What should you tell the mother?
2. What can you do to facilitate mother–newborn attachment?
3. Discuss the emotional response of parents to the birth of an ill or at-risk newborn.
4. Discuss the four psychologic tasks essential for coping with the stress of an at-risk newborn and providing a basis for the maternal–newborn relationship.
5. Baby Jonathan is being discharged tomorrow. Review the elements of discharge and home care instructions.

References

Als, H., Butler, S., & Kosta, S. (2005). The assessment of preterm infant's behavior (APIB): Furthering the understanding and measurement of neurodevelopmental competence in preterm and full-term infants. *Mental Retardation and Developmental Disabilities Research Reviews, 11*(1), 94–102. doi:10.1002/mrdd.20053

American Academy of Pediatrics (AAP). (2013). Policy statement: Screening examination of premature infants for retinopathy of prematurity. *Pediatrics, 131*(1), 189–195. doi: 10.1542/peds.2012-2996

American Academy of Pediatrics (AAP) & American College of Obstetricians and Gynecologists (ACOG). (2012). *Guidelines for perinatal care* (7th ed.). Elk Grove Village, IL: Author.

American College of Obstetricians and Gynecologists (ACOG). (2013). Practice bulletin Number 134: Fetal growth restriction. *Obstetrics & Gynecology, 121,* 1122–1133.

American College of Obstetricians and Gynecologists (ACOG) & Society for Maternal-Fetal Medicine. (2013). Committee opinion No. 579: Definition of term pregnancy. *Obstetrics & Gynecology, 122,* 1139–1140.

Armentrout, D. (2015). Glucose management. In M. Terese Verklan & M. Walden (Eds.), *Core curriculum for neonatal intensive care nursing* (5th ed., pp. 162–171). St. Louis, MO: Saunders.

Baker, B. (2015a). Evidence-based practice to improve outcomes for late preterm infants. *Journal of Obstetric, Gynecological and Neonatal Nursing (JOGNN), 44*(1), 127–134.

Baker, B. (2015b). Improving outcomes for late preterm infants and their mothers. *Journal of Obstetric, Gynecological and Neonatal Nursing (JOGNN), 44*(1), 100–101.

Barron, M. L. (2014). Antenatal care. In K. R. Simpson & P. A. Creehan (Eds.), *AWHONN's perinatal nursing* (4th ed., pp. 89–121). Philadelphia, PA: Lippincott Williams & Wilkins.

Blackburn, S. (2013). *Maternal, fetal, neonatal physiology: A clinical perspective* (4th ed.). Philadelphia, PA: Saunders.

Bowers, B. (2014). Prenatal, intrapartal, and postnatal risk factors. In C. Kenner & J. W. Lott (Eds.), *Comprehensive neonatal nursing care* (5th ed., pp. 28–54). New York, NY: Springer.

Bradshaw, W. T. (2015). Gastrointestinal disorders. In M. T. Verklan & M. Walden (Eds.), *Core curriculum for neonatal intensive care nursing* (5th ed., pp. 583–631). St. Louis, MO: Saunders.

Brooks, M. (2013). *US preterm birth rate drops to 15-year low, but more to go.* Retrieved from http://www.medscape.com/viewarticle/813632

Centers for Disease Control and Prevention (CDC). (2014). *HIV among pregnant women, infants, and children.* Retrieved from http://www.cdc.gov/hiv/risk/gender/pregnantwomen/facts/

Chambers, C., & Scialli, A. R. (2014). Teratogenesis and environmental exposure. In R. K. Creasy & R. Resnik (Eds.), *Maternal-fetal medicine: Principles and practice* (7th ed., pp. 465–472). Philadelphia, PA: Saunders.

Cloherty, J. R., Eichenwald, E. C., Hansen, A. R., & Stark, A. R. (2012). *Manual of neonatal care.* Philadelphia, PA: Lippincott Williams & Wilkins.

Cunningham, F. G., Leveno, K. J., Bloom, S. L., Spong, C. Y., Dashe, J. S., Hoffman, B. L., . . . & Sheffield, J. S. (2014). *Williams obstetrics* (24th ed.). New York, NY: McGraw-Hill.

Daley, J. M. (2014). Diabetes in pregnancy. In K. R. Simpson & P. A. Creehan (Eds.), *AWHONN's perinatal nursing* (4th ed., pp. 203–223). Philadelphia, PA: Lippincott Williams & Wilkins.

Davis, J. A., & Yawetz, S. (2012). Management of HIV in the pregnant woman. *Clinical Obstetrics and Gynecology, 55*(2), 531–540. doi:10.1097/GRF.0b013e31824f3ae1

Ditzenberger, G. R. (2015). Nutritional management. In M. T. Verklan & M. Walden (Eds.), *Core curriculum for neonatal intensive care nursing* (5th ed., pp. 172–196). St. Louis, MO: Saunders.

Frank, L. H., Bradshaw, E., Beekman, R., Mahle, W. T., & Martin, G. R. (2013). Critical congenital heart disease screening using pulse oximetry. *Journal of Pediatrics 162*(3), 445–453.

Geary, E. (2013). Risk of necrotizing enterocolitis and feeding interventions for preterm infants with abnormal umbilical artery doppler. *Neonatal Network, 32*(1), 5–14.

Gleason, C. A., & Devaskar, S. U. (2012). *Avery's diseases of the newborn* (9th ed.) St. Louis, MO: Elsevier Saunders.

Gomella, T. L. (Ed.) (2013). *Neonatology: Management, procedures, on-call problems, diseases, and drugs* (7th ed.). New York, NY: McGraw-Hill Education.

Greenfield, R. A. (2013). *Pediatric HIV infection.* Retrieved from http://emedicine.medscape.com/article/965086-overview?src=wnl_ref_prc_peds&uac

Hay, W. W. (2012). Care of the infant of the diabetic mother. *Current Diabetes Report, 12*(1), 4–15. doi:10.1007/s11892-011-0243-6

Jones, L. R. (2012). Oral feeding readiness in the neonatal intensive care unit. *Neonatal Network, 31*(3), 148–155.

Kassity-Kritch, N. A., & Jones, J. E. (2014). Complementary and integrative therapies. In C. Kenner & J. W. Lott (Eds.), *Comprehensive neonatal nursing care* (5th ed., pp. 773–782). New York, NY: Springer.

Kaye, C. I., & Committee on Genetics. (2006, reaffirmed 2011). Newborn screening fact sheets. *Pediatrics, 118*(3), 934–963. doi:10.1542/peds.2006-1782

Ludington-Hoe, S. M. (2013). Kangaroo care as a neonatal therapy. *NAINR, 13*(2), 73–75.

Lund, C. H., Brandon, D., Holden, A. C., Kuller, J., & Hill, C. M. (2013). Neonatal skin care: Evidence-based clinical practice guidelines (3rd ed.). Washington, DC, AWHONN.

Lynch, E., Dezen, T., & Brown, N. (2013). *U. S. preterm birth rate shows five-year improvement.* Retrieved from http://www.marchofdimes.com/news/united-states-preterm-birth-rate-shows-five-year-improvement.aspx

Mari, G., & Tate, D. L. (2013). *Detection and surveillance of IUGR.* Retrieved from http://contemporaryobgyn.modernmedicine.com/print/374473

Matthews, A., & Robin, N. H. (2011). Genetic disorders, malformation, and inborn errors of metabolism. In S. L. Gardner (Ed.), *Merenstein & Gardner's handbook of neonatal intensive care* (7th ed., pp. 78–112). St. Louis, MO: Mosby.

McLean, K. R. (2014). Emerging infections. In C. Kenner & J. W. Lott (Eds.), *Comprehensive neonatal nursing care* (5th ed., pp. 619–639). New York, NY: Springer.

Moore, T. R., Hauguel-de Mouzon, S., & Catalano, P. (2014). Diabetes in pregnancy. In R. K. Creasy & R. Resnik (Eds.), *Maternal-fetal medicine: Principles and practice* (7th ed., pp. 988–1021). Philadelphia, PA: Saunders.

Newland, L., L'Huillier, M. W., & Petrey, B. (2013). Implementation of cue-based feeding in a level III NICU. *Neonatal Network, 32*(2), 132–137.

O'Hare, E. M., Wood, A., & Fiske, E. (2013). Human milk banking. *Neonatal Network, 32*(3), 175–183.

Prasad, M. (2014). *When opiate abuse complicates pregnancy.* Retrieved from http://contemporaryobgyn.modernmedicine.com/contemporary-obgyn/content/tags/drug-abuse/when-opiate-abuse-complicates-pregnancy

Prasad, M. R., & Jones, H. E. (2014). Substance abuse in pregnancy. In R. K. Creasy & R. Resnik (Eds.), *Maternal-fetal medicine: Principles and practice*

(7th ed., pp. 1132–1145). Philadelphia, PA: Saunders.

Pritham, U. A., Paul, J. A., & Hayes, M. J. (2012). Opioid dependency in pregnancy and length of stay for neonatal abstinence syndrome. *JOGNN: Journal of Obstetric, Gynecologic, and Neonatal Nursing, 41*(2), 180–189.

Raab, E. L., & Kelly, L. K. (2013). Neonatal resuscitation. In A. H. Decheney, L. Nathan, N. Laufer, & A. S. Roman (Eds.), *Current diagnosis & treatment: Obstetrics & gynecology* (11th ed., pp. 369–388). New York, NY: McGraw-Hill/Lange.

Resnik, R., & Creasy, R. K. (2014). Intrauterine growth restriction. In R. K. Creasy & R. Resnik (Eds.), *Maternal-fetal medicine: Principles and practice* (7th ed., pp. 743–755). Philadelphia, PA: Saunders.

Rozance, P. J., & Rosenberg, A. A. (2012). The neonate. In S. G. Gabbe, J. R. Niebyl, J. L. Simpson, M. B. Landon, H. L. Galan, E. R. M. Jauniaux, & D. A. Driscoll (Eds.), *Obstetrics: Normal and problem pregnancies* (6th ed., pp. 481–516). St. Louis, MO: Elsevier.

Ruth, C. A., Roos, N., Hildes-Ripstein, E., & Brownell, M. (2013). The influence of gestational age and

socioeconomic status on neonatal outcomes in late preterm and early term gestation: A population based study. *BioMed Central Pregnancy & Childbirth. 12*(1), 62. doi: 10.1186/1471-2393-12-62

Scher, M. S. (2013). Brain disorders of the fetus and neonate. In A. A. Fanaroff & J. M. Fanaroff (Eds.), *Klaus & Fanaroff's care of the high-risk neonate* (6th ed., pp. 476–524). Philadelphia, PA: Elsevier.

Smith, J. R., & Carley, A. (2014). Common neonatal complications. In K. R. Simpson & P. A. Creehan (Eds.), *AWHONN's perinatal nursing* (4th ed., pp. 662–698). Philadelphia, PA: Lippincott Williams & Wilkins.

Spong, C. Y. (2013). Defining "term" pregnancy: Recommendations from the defining " term" pregnancy workgroup. *JAMA, 309,* 2445–2446.

Wang, M. (2014). *Perinatal drug abuse and neonatal drug withdrawal.* Retrieved from http://emedicine.medscape.com/article/978492

Zahorodny, W., Rom, C., Whitney, W., Giddens, S., Samuel, M., Maichuk, G., & Marshall, R. (1998). The neonatal withdrawal inventory: A simplified score of newborn withdrawal. *Developmental and Behavioral Pediatrics, 19*(2), 89–93. doi:10.1097/00004703-199804000-00004

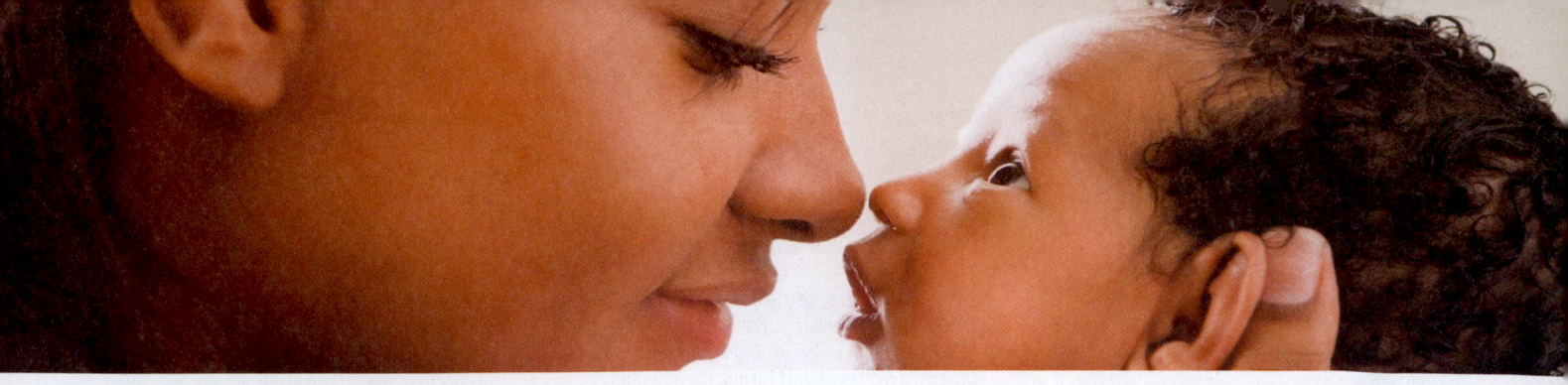

Chapter 27

The Newborn at Risk: Birth-Related Stressors

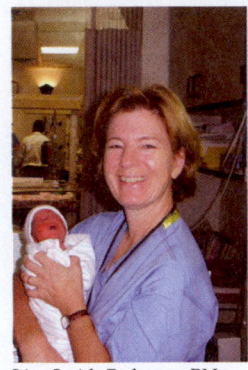

I work primarily in what our system calls the "high-risk transition nursery." When I am called to attend a birth it is usually because the labor and delivery team has detected a potential problem and they think the newborn will need some additional care at birth. The neonatal nurse practitioner (NNP) and I work together to anticipate and respond to whatever is needed at the time. Each situation is unique and deserves our complete attention. But it is also essential that the parents be kept informed and comforted as much as possible. With each newborn that I care for, I ask myself, "If this were my baby, how would I be feeling right now, and what would I want to know?"

—**High-Risk Nursery Nurse**

Lisa Smith-Pedersen, RN, MSN, NNP-BC.

⌄ Learning Outcomes

27.1 Describe how to identify newborns in need of resuscitation and the appropriate method of resuscitation based on the antepartum/labor record and physiologic indicators.

27.2 Differentiate, based on clinical manifestations, among the various types of respiratory distress (respiratory distress syndrome, transient tachypnea of the newborn, and meconium aspiration syndrome) in the newborn and the nursing care related to each type.

27.3 Discuss the types of metabolic abnormalities (cold stress and hypoglycemia), their effects on the newborn, and their nursing implications.

27.4 Differentiate between physiologic and pathologic jaundice according to timing of onset (in hours), cause, possible sequelae, and specific management.

27.5 Explain how Rh incompatibility or ABO incompatibility can lead to the development of hyperbilirubinemia.

27.6 Identify nursing responsibilities and rationales in caring for the newborn receiving phototherapy.

27.7 Describe the causes and nursing management of newborns with anemia.

27.8 Describe the nursing assessments that would lead the nurse to suspect newborn sepsis and the nursing care of the newborn with an infection.

27.9 Relate the expected assessment findings of selected maternally transmitted infections, such as maternal syphilis, gonorrhea, Herpesviridae family (HSV or CMV), and chlamydia, to the nursing management for each of the affected newborns in the neonatal period.

27.10 Describe interventions to facilitate parental attachment and meet the special initial and long-term needs of parents of at-risk newborns.

Marked homeostatic changes occur during the newborn's transition from fetal to neonatal life. Because the most rapid anatomic and physiologic changes occur in the cardiopulmonary system, most major problems of the newborn are usually related to this system. These problems include asphyxia, respiratory distress syndrome (RDS), cold stress, jaundice, hemolytic disease, and anemia. Ideally, most problems are anticipated and identified prenatally. Some treatment may be initiated in the prenatal period, whereas other intervention measures are begun at or immediately after birth.

Care of the Newborn at Risk of Asphyxia

Perinatal asphyxia occurs in 1% to 1.5% of live births, and the incidence increases as the gestational age decreases (Cloherty, Eichenwald, Hansen, et al., 2012; Pappas & Robey, 2015). Neonatal asphyxia results in circulatory, respiratory, and biochemical changes. Circulatory patterns that accompany asphyxia indicate an inability of the newborn to make the transition to extrauterine circulation—in effect, a return to fetal circulatory patterns. Failure of lung expansion and establishment of respiration rapidly produce serious biochemical changes, including hypoxemia (decreased oxygen in the blood), metabolic acidosis (increased acidity of blood reflected by low pH), and hypercarbia (excess levels of carbon dioxide in the blood) (Cloherty et al., 2012).

These biochemical changes produce the following results:

- Pulmonary vasoconstriction and high pulmonary vascular resistance in relation to the lower systemic vascular resistance (following birth the pulmonary vascular resistance should be markedly lower than the systemic vascular resistance)
- Hypoperfusion of the lungs
- A large right-to-left shunt (from the right side of the heart to the left side of the heart) through the ductus arteriosus, bypassing the lungs and impeding oxygenation of the blood

As right atrial pressure exceeds left atrial pressure, the foramen ovale reopens, and blood flows from right to left (Cloherty et al., 2012). See Chapter 23 for a review of normal newborn cardiopulmonary adaptation.

However, the most serious biochemical abnormality is a change from aerobic to anaerobic metabolism in the presence of hypoxia. This change results in the buildup of lactate, which combines with hydrogen to form lactic acid, and the development of metabolic acidosis. Lactic acidosis can develop after prolonged tissue hypoxia (oxygen starvation) as active cells rely on anaerobic metabolism.

The newborn is supplied with several protective mechanisms against hypoxic insult:

- Relatively immature brain
- Resting metabolic rate lower than that of adults
- Ability to mobilize substances within the body for anaerobic metabolism and to use energy more efficiently
- Intact circulatory system able to redistribute lactate and hydrogen ions in tissues still being perfused

Severe prolonged hypoxia overcomes these protective mechanisms, resulting in brain damage or death of the newborn. The newborn suffering apnea requires immediate resuscitative efforts.

The need for resuscitation can be anticipated if specific risk factors are present during the pregnancy or labor and birth period.

Risk Factors Predisposing to Asphyxia

The need for resuscitation may be anticipated if the mother demonstrates the antepartum and intrapartum risk factors described in Table 9–1 and Table 17–2).

Fetal/neonatal risk factors for resuscitation are as follows (Cloherty et al., 2012; Gomella, 2013):

- Nonreassuring fetal heart rate (FHR) pattern/sustained bradycardia
- Impairment of maternal oxygenation (maternal asthma/cardiac disease)
- Anything affecting blood flow through the placenta
- Significant intrapartum bleeding
- Difficult birth, prolonged labor
- Fetal scalp/capillary blood sample acidosis pH less than 7.2
- Narcotic use in labor
- History of meconium in amniotic fluid
- Prematurity
- Male baby
- Small-for-gestational age (SGA) or macrosomia
- Infant of a diabetic mother (IDM)
- Multiple births
- Structural lung abnormality/oligohydramnios (congenital diaphragmatic hernia, lung hypoplasia)
- Congenital heart disease
- Anemia: isoimmunization, fetal–maternal hemorrhage, parvovirus

Clinical Therapy

The initial goal of clinical management is to identify the fetus at risk for asphyxia, so that resuscitative efforts can begin at birth.

Fetal biophysical assessment (see Chapter 13 for discussion), combined with monitoring of fetal pH, FHRs, and fetal oximeter if available during the intrapartum period, may help identify the presence of nonreassuring fetal status. If nonreassuring fetal status is present, appropriate measures can be taken to deliver the fetus immediately, before major damage occurs, and to treat the asphyxiated newborn.

The stress of labor causes an intermittent decrease in exchange of gases in the placental intervillous space, which causes the fall in pH and fetal metabolic acidosis. During labor, a fetal pH of 7.25 or higher is considered normal (nonacidemia). A pH value of 7.20 or less is considered an ominous sign of intrauterine asphyxia (acidemia), whereas a pH of less than 7 is considered pathologic acidemia (Cloherty et al., 2012). However, low fetal pH without associated hypoxia can be caused by maternal acidosis secondary to prolonged labor, dehydration, and maternal lactate production.

Assessment of the newborn's need for resuscitation begins at the time of birth by assessing skin color, heart rate, and respirations/respiratory effort of the newborn. The nurse should note the time of the first gasp, first cry, and onset of sustained respirations in order of occurrence. The Apgar score (see Chapter 18 and Table 18–6 for discussion of the Apgar score) may be helpful in describing the status of the newborn at birth and subsequent adaptation to the extrauterine environment, but should not be used to determine whether certain steps need to be taken during resuscitation. The Apgar can serve as a measure of the neonate's response to effective resuscitation and clinical status (Pappas & Robey, 2015). If indicated, resuscitation should be started before the 1-minute Apgar score is calculated. An assisted Apgar scoring system is recommended by the AAP Committee on the Fetus and Newborn, which documents the assistance the newborn is receiving at the time the score is assigned (American Academy of Pediatrics [AAP] & American College of Obstetricians and Gynecologists [ACOG], 2012). The Apgar score at 1 minute tends to relate to intrapartum depression, an ischemic or hypoxic event in utero, and subsequent scores relate to adequacy of resuscitative efforts (Rubarth, 2012). Retrospective Apgar scores are likely to be assigned when stabilizing critically ill newborns. A score of less than 7 at 5 minutes following birth requires that additional scores be assigned every 5 minutes up to 20 minutes (American Academy of Pediatrics [AAP] & American Heart Association [AHA], 2011).

Resuscitative efforts are required by 10% of all newborns to begin breathing, 3% require positive pressure ventilation, and 1% of all newborns require more extensive resuscitative efforts (AAP & AHA, 2011; Sawyer, Laubach, Hudak, et al., 2013; Trevisanuto et al., 2013). Identification of newborns who may require resuscitation is accomplished by carrying out a rapid assessment of four characteristics by asking the following questions:

1. What is the gestational age?
2. Is the amniotic fluid clear of meconium and evidence of infection?
3. How many babies are expected?
4. Are there any other risk factors?

Following birth, these three questions need to be posed:

1. Is the baby full term?
2. Is the baby breathing or crying?
3. Does the baby have good muscle tone?

If the answers to these questions are "yes" then the baby does not need resuscitation and should not be separated from the mother. If the answer to *any* of the previous questions is "no," the newborn should receive resuscitative assistance (AAP & AHA, 2011). The newborn should receive one or more of the following categories of action:

- Initial steps in stabilization (warming, positioning, clearing the airway as necessary, drying, stimulating, and repositioning)
- Oxygen administration with continuous monitoring of the pulse oximeter, preferably on the right hand or wrist because it will be measuring the amount of oxygen available to the brain (Bagwell, 2014b)
- Positive pressure ventilation
- Chest compressions
- Administration of epinephrine, volume expansion, or both (AAP & AHA, 2011; AAP & ACOG, 2012)

SAFETY ALERT!

In the birthing room exposure to blood or other body fluids is inevitable. Standard precautions must be practiced by wearing caps, goggles or glasses, gloves, and impervious gowns until the cord is cut and the newborn is dried and wrapped (Cloherty et al., 2012).

Resuscitation Management

After the first few breaths, the nurse places the newborn in a level (sniff) position (the head is tilted just far enough back so that the baby appears to be sniffing the air with the nose pointed upward) under a radiant heat source and dries the baby quickly with warm blankets to maintain abdominal skin temperature at about 36.5° to 37.0°C (97.7° to 98.6°F). The stable newborn may be placed on the mother's chest or abdomen "skin-to-skin" as another heat source. If assessment indicates that further assistance and formal resuscitation are necessary, the baby continues in the radiant warmer in a position that facilitates easy access by healthcare providers (Gleason & Devaskar, 2012).

Breathing is established by employing the simplest form of resuscitative measures initially, with progression to more complicated methods as required; for example:

1. Position and clear the airway only as necessary. Simple stimulation is provided by rubbing the newborn's back with a blanket or towel, while simultaneously drying the baby.

2. If respirations have not been initiated or are inadequate (gasping or occasional respirations), the lungs must be inflated with positive pressure (Niermeyer, Clarke, & Hernandez, 2016). The proper size mask is positioned securely on the face (over the nose and mouth, avoiding the eyes) with the baby's head in a *sniffing* or neutral position (Figure 27–1). Hyperextension of the baby's neck will obstruct the trachea and must be avoided. An airtight connection is made between the baby's face and the mask (thus allowing the flow inflating bag to inflate). The lungs are inflated rhythmically by squeezing the bag.

All devices utilized for ventilation of newborns during resuscitation should have a pressure gauge/manometer in place. These devices include the following:

- Self-inflating bag
- Flow inflating/anesthesia bag
- T-Piece resuscitator (AAP & AHA, 2011; Bagwell, 2014b)

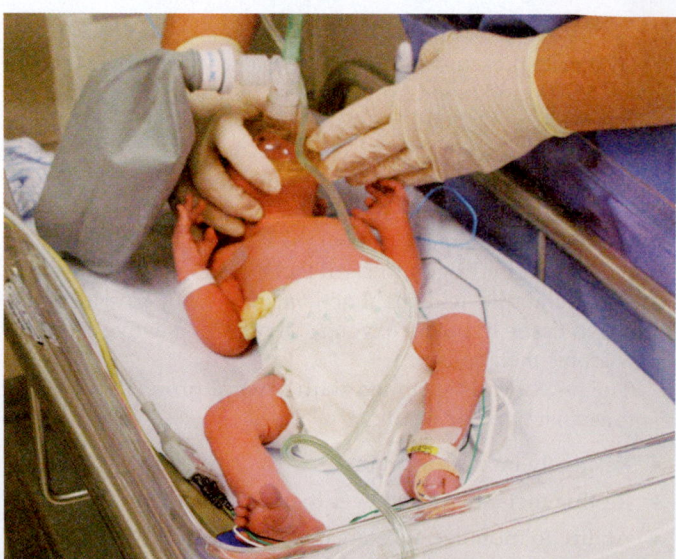

Figure 27–1 Demonstration of resuscitation of a newborn with bag and mask. Note that the mask covers the nose and mouth, and the head is in a neutral position. The resuscitation bag is placed to the side of the baby so that chest movement can be seen.

Supplemental oxygen is not utilized when initiating resuscitation on a term newborn. The amount of oxygen administered is titrated from 21% (room air) to 100% based on clinical assessment of the preterm newborn (Saugstad, Aune, Aguar, et al., 2014; Trevisanuto et al., 2013). Oxygen is a medication, and it is only administered in the presence of central cyanosis or when the pulse oximeter readings are less than expected for the age of the newborn. Too much oxygen can actually cause long-term detrimental outcomes (Sabir, Jary, Tooley, et al., 2012). Oxygen saturation of the neonate in utero is approximately 60%, and it typically increases to greater than 90% during the first 10 minutes following birth. An anesthesia bag with an attached manometer or modified self-inflating bag and adequate liter flow of 5 to 10 L/min is utilized for neonatal resuscitation (AAP & AHA, 2011).

3. Chest movement is observed for proper ventilation. Air entry and heart rate (HR) are checked by auscultation; HR may be quickly checked by palpating the base of the umbilical cord stump and counting the pulsations for 6 seconds and then multiplying by 10. Manual resuscitation is coordinated with any voluntary efforts. During positive pressure ventilation, squeeze the resuscitation bag just enough to improve HR, color, and muscle tone, at a rate of 40 to 60 breaths per minute. Pressure should be adequate to move the chest wall. The pressure gauge (manometer) must be in place to avoid overdistention of the newborn's lungs and other problems such as pneumothorax or abdominal distention. An inspiratory pressure of approximately 20 cmH_2O should be adequate to start. Increasing the pressure to 30 cmH_2O or greater is occasionally necessary if there is no improvement in heart rate, color, and muscle tone; however, the amount of pressure should never exceed 40 cmH_2O (Bagwell, 2014b; AAP & AHA, 2011). If ventilation is adequate, the chest moves symmetrically with each inspiration, bilateral breath sounds are audible, and the lips and mucous membranes become pink. Distention of the stomach is controlled by inserting a nasogastric tube for decompression.

4. Endotracheal intubation is strongly recommended when chest compressions start in order to coordinate ventilation and chest compressions. However, most newborns, except for very-low-birth-weight (VLBW) (<1500 g [3.3 lb]) babies, can be resuscitated by bag and mask ventilation. An increasing heart rate (HR) and CO_2 detection are the primary methods for confirming endotracheal tube placement.

Once breathing has been established, the HR should increase to over 100 beats per minute. If the HR is absent or the HR remains less than 60 beats per minute after 30 seconds of effective positive pressure with oxygen concentration of 21% to 100% to elicit an oxygen saturation of 60% to 65% at 1 minute and 85% to 95% at 10 minutes of age, external cardiac massage (chest compression) is begun (AAP & AHA, 2011).

SAFETY ALERT!

Establishing effective ventilation is the highest priority in neonatal resuscitation. Do not start chest compressions without first establishing effective ventilation (as evidenced by audible bilateral breath sounds and chest movement) (AAP & AHA, 2011).

Chest compressions are started immediately if there is no detectable heartbeat. The following procedure is used for performing chest compressions:

1. The newborn is positioned properly on a firm surface.

2. The resuscitator stands at the foot or head of the newborn and places both thumbs over the lower third of the sternum (just below an imaginary line drawn between the nipples), with the fingers wrapped around and supporting the back (Figure 27–2A). Alternatively, the resuscitator can use two fingers instead of thumbs (Figure 27–2B). The two-thumb method is preferred because it may provide better coronary perfusion pressure and a more consistent and controlled depth of compression; however, it makes access to the umbilical cord for medication administration more difficult (AAP & AHA, 2011).

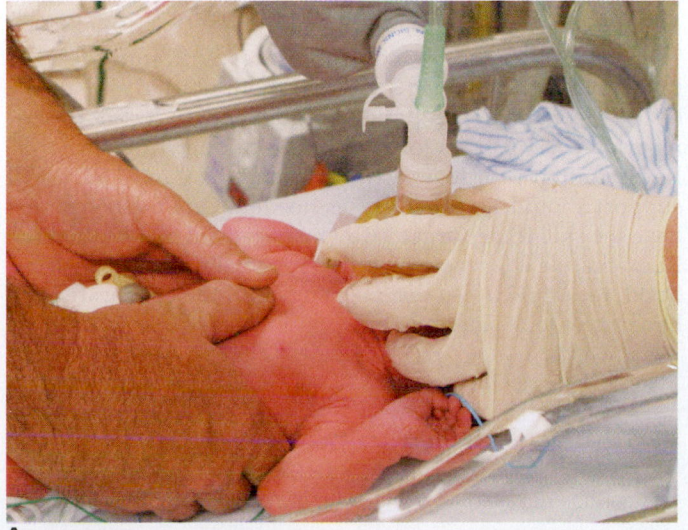

A

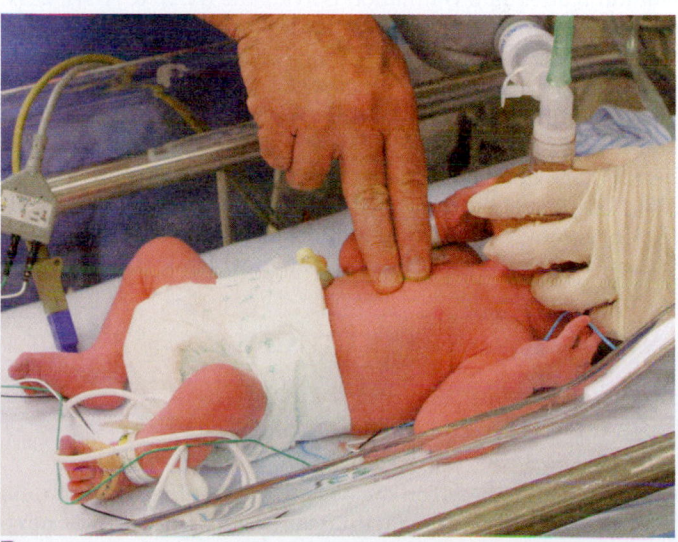

B

Figure 27–2 External cardiac massage. The lower third of the sternum is compressed with two fingertips or thumbs at a rate of 90 beats per minute. A. In the thumb method, the fingers support the baby's back and both thumbs compress the sternum. B. In the two-finger method, the tips of two fingers of one hand compress the sternum, and the other hand or a firm surface supports the baby's back.

3. The sternum is depressed to sufficient depth to generate a palpable pulse or approximately one third of the anterior–posterior depth of the chest at a rate of 90 beats per minute (AAP & AHA, 2011). Use a 3:1 ratio of heartbeat to assisted ventilation, 90 chest compressions: 30 breaths per minute (AAP & AHA, 2011; Hemway, Christman, & Perlman, 2013).

SAFETY ALERT!

Remember to say, "One and two and three and breathe, and one and two and three and breathe" out loud and demonstrate with finger movements so all members of the resuscitation team are aware of where they are in the cycle. There are 5 cycles in 10 seconds.

Drugs that should be available in the birthing area include those needed in the treatment of shock, cardiac arrest, and narcosis. Oxygen, because of its effective use in ventilation, is the drug most often used. After 30 seconds of ventilation and coordinated cardiac compression, the newborn's cardiopulmonary status is reassessed by palpating the umbilical cord for a pulse. If the newborn has not responded with spontaneous respirations and an HR above 60 beats/min, resuscitative medications are necessary (AAP & AHA, 2011; Cloherty et al., 2012; Gomella, 2013).

The most accessible route for administering medications is the umbilical vein (given intravenously [IV]). When the heart rate remains below 60 beats/min despite 45 to 60 seconds of chest compressions and ventilation, then epinephrine, a cardiac stimulant, is indicated. If persistent bradycardia is present, an intravenous dose of epinephrine (0.1 to 0.3 mL/kg [up to 1.0 mL] of a 1:10,000 solution [0.1 mg/mL]) is given through the umbilical vein catheter as rapidly as possible, followed by 0.5 to 1 mL of normal saline. When epinephrine is administered by endotracheal tube, consider a higher dose (0.5 to .01 mL/kg) (AAP & AHA, 2011; Bagwell, 2014b; Gomella, 2013; Sawyer et al., 2013). Naloxone hydrochloride (0.1 mg/kg), a narcotic antagonist, is used to reverse known iatrogenic narcotic depression; however, it is not currently recommended to be given during initial resuscitation if adequate ventilation is available (AAP & AHA, 2011; Gomella, 2013).

If shock develops (low blood pressure, pallor, or poor peripheral perfusion), the baby may be given a volume expander such as normal saline or lactated Ringer solution in a dose of 10 mL/kg via umbilical vein route. If there is a known fetal hemorrhage or fetal anemia, whole blood (O Rh-negative crossmatched against the mother's blood) and packed red blood cells (RBCs) given over a 5- to 10-minute period can also be used for volume expansion and treatment of hypovolemic shock.

Nursing Management

For the Newborn Needing Resuscitation

Nursing Assessment and Diagnosis

Communication between the obstetric (OB) office or clinic and the birthing area nurse facilitates the identification of newborns who may need resuscitation. When the woman arrives in the birthing area, you should have the prenatal/antepartum record and should note any contributory prenatal history factors and assess present fetal status. As labor progresses, nursing assessments include ongoing monitoring of fetal heartbeat and its response to contractions, assisting with fetal scalp blood

sampling (if available), and observing for the presence of meconium in the amniotic fluid, when ruptured, to help identify possible fetal asphyxia. In addition, alert the interprofessional resuscitation team and the practitioner responsible for the care of the newborn of any potential high-risk laboring women.

Nursing diagnoses that may apply to the newborn with asphyxia and the newborn's parents include (NANDA-I © 2014):

- *Breathing Pattern, Ineffective,* related to lack of spontaneous respirations at birth secondary to in utero asphyxia
- *Cardiac Output, Decreased,* related to impaired oxygenation
- *Coping: Family, Compromised,* related to baby's lack of spontaneous respirations at birth and fear of losing their newborn

Plan and Implementation

HOSPITAL-BASED NURSING CARE

Following identification of possible high-risk situations, the next step in effective resuscitation is assembling the necessary equipment and ensuring proper functioning.

Check and maintain equipment to ensure its reliability before an emergency arises. The equipment must be restocked immediately after use and rechecked before every birth. Inspect all equipment—radiant warmer, bag and mask, oxygen, flow meter and blender, pulse oximeter, laryngoscope, and suction machine—for damaged or nonfunctioning parts before a birth or when setting up an admission bed. A systematic check of the emergency cart and equipment is a routine responsibility of each shift. It is desirable to assemble equipment for pH and blood gas determination as well.

During resuscitation, keep the newborn warm. Dry the newborn quickly with warmed towels or blankets and position a hat to prevent evaporative heat loss, then place the baby under a prewarmed radiant warmer with servocontrol set at 36.5°C (97.7°F). This device provides an overhead radiant heat source. (A thermostatic mechanism that is secured to the newborn's abdomen, over a solid organ like the liver, triggers the radiant warmer to turn on or off to maintain a constant temperature.) An open bed is necessary for easy access to the newborn.

Training and knowledge about resuscitation are vital to personnel in the birth setting for both normal and at-risk births. Neonatal Resuscitation Program (NRP) certification is renewed every 2 years for personnel working with newborns. Resuscitation is at least a two-person effort and additional support should be called for as needed. One member must have the skill to perform airway management and ventilation. Resuscitative efforts are recorded in the newborn's electronic health record (EHR) so that all members of the healthcare team have access to the information.

Healthy People 2020

(MICH-1.2) Decrease fetal and infant deaths during perinatal period (28 weeks of gestation to 7 days after birth)

(MICH-1.4) Decrease neonatal deaths (within the first 28 days of life)

(MICH-33) Increase the proportion of very-low-birth-weight (VLBW) infants born at Level III hospitals or subspecialty perinatal centers

---

PARENT TEACHING

The new cardiopulmonary resuscitation (CPR) guidelines favor family members being present during resuscitation in the birthing room and in the neonatal ICU (NICU), but be aware that the procedure is particularly distressing for parents. If the need for resuscitation is anticipated, the parents should be assured that an interprofessional health team will be present at the birth to care specifically for their newborn. Advise parents that a support person will be available for them as well. As soon as the newborn's condition has stabilized, a member of the team needs to discuss the baby's condition with the parents. The parents may have many fears about the reasons for resuscitation and the condition of their baby following resuscitation (White, 2012).

Evaluation

Expected outcomes of nursing care include the following:

- The newborn requiring resuscitation is promptly identified, and intervention is started early.
- The newborn's metabolic and physiologic processes are stabilized, and recovery is proceeding without complications.
- The parents can verbalize the reason for resuscitation and what was done to resuscitate their newborn.
- The parents can verbalize their fears about the resuscitation process and potential implications for their baby's future.

Care of the Newborn With Respiratory Distress

One of the severest conditions to which the newborn may fall victim is respiratory distress—an inappropriate respiratory adaptation to extrauterine life. Only with knowledge of normal pulmonary and circulatory physiology (discussed in Chapter 23), the pathophysiology of the disease process, clinical manifestations, and supportive and corrective therapies can the nurse make appropriate observations about responses to therapy and development of complications. Unlike the verbalizing adult client, the newborn communicates needs only by behavior or physiologic parameters that must be interpreted by the NICU nurse. The neonatal nurse interprets this behavior as clues about the individual baby's condition. This section discusses respiratory distress syndrome, transient tachypnea of the newborn, and meconium aspiration syndrome.

Respiratory Distress Syndrome

Respiratory distress syndrome (RDS), also referred to as *hyaline membrane disease (HMD)*, is characterized by inadequate production of pulmonary surfactant, a substance produced in the lungs that keeps lungs from collapsing on expiration (Smith & Carley, 2014). The syndrome occurs more frequently in premature White newborns than in newborns of African or Hispanic descent and almost twice as often in boys as in girls (Cloherty et al., 2012).

All the factors precipitating the pathologic changes of RDS have not been determined, but the main factors associated with its development include:

- **Prematurity.** All preterm newborns—no matter their size—and especially infants of diabetic mothers (IDM) are at risk for RDS. The incidence of RDS increases with the degree of prematurity, and most deaths occur in newborns weighing less than 1500 g (3.3 lb). The maternal and fetal factors resulting in preterm labor and birth, complications of pregnancy, cesarean birth (and its indications), and familial tendency are all associated with RDS.

- **Surfactant deficiency disease.** Normal pulmonary adaptation requires adequate surfactant, a lipoprotein that coats the inner surfaces of the alveoli. Surfactant provides alveolar stability by decreasing the alveoli's surface tension and tendency to collapse. Surfactant is produced by type II alveolar cells starting at about 24 weeks' gestation. In the normal or mature newborn lung, it is continuously synthesized, oxidized during breathing, and replenished. Adequate surfactant levels lead to better lung compliance and permit breathing with less work. RDS is caused by alterations in surfactant quantity, composition, function, or production (Van Woudenberg, Wills, & Rubarth, 2012).

Development of RDS indicates a failure to synthesize surfactant, which is required to maintain alveolar stability. Upon expiration this instability increases atelectasis, which causes hypoxia and acidosis because of the lack of gas exchange (Smith & Carley, 2014; Van Woudenberg et al., 2012). These conditions further inhibit surfactant production and cause pulmonary vasoconstriction. The resulting lung instability causes the biochemical problems of hypoxemia (decreased Po_2), hypercarbia (increased Pco_2), and acidemia (decreased pH), primarily metabolic, which further increase pulmonary vasoconstriction and hypoperfusion, alveolar endothelial and epithelial damage, and subsequent protein-rich interstitial and alveolar edema. The cycle of events of RDS leading to eventual respiratory failure is diagrammed in Figure 27–3.

Because of these pathophysiologic conditions, the newborn must expend increasing amounts of energy to reopen the collapsed alveoli with every breath, so that each breath becomes more difficult than the last. The progressive expiratory atelectasis upsets the physiologic homeostasis of the pulmonary and cardiovascular systems and prevents adequate gas exchange. Breathing becomes progressively harder as lung compliance decreases, which makes it more difficult to inflate the lungs and breathe.

The physiologic alterations of RDS produce the following complications:

- **Hypoxia.** As a result of hypoxia, the pulmonary vasculature constricts, pulmonary vascular resistance increases, and pulmonary blood flow is reduced. Increased

| TEACHING HIGHLIGHTS | Understanding Respiratory Distress |

You can help parents understand their baby's respiratory distress by having them think of the air sacs (alveoli) of the lungs as tiny balloons filled with water and no air. When the tiny balloon (alveoli) is emptied (as in expiration), water droplets can remain inside the balloon and the sides of the balloons stick together (increasing the surface tension between the sides of the balloon). This increased surface tension makes the next reinflation very difficult and requires an increased amount of energy.

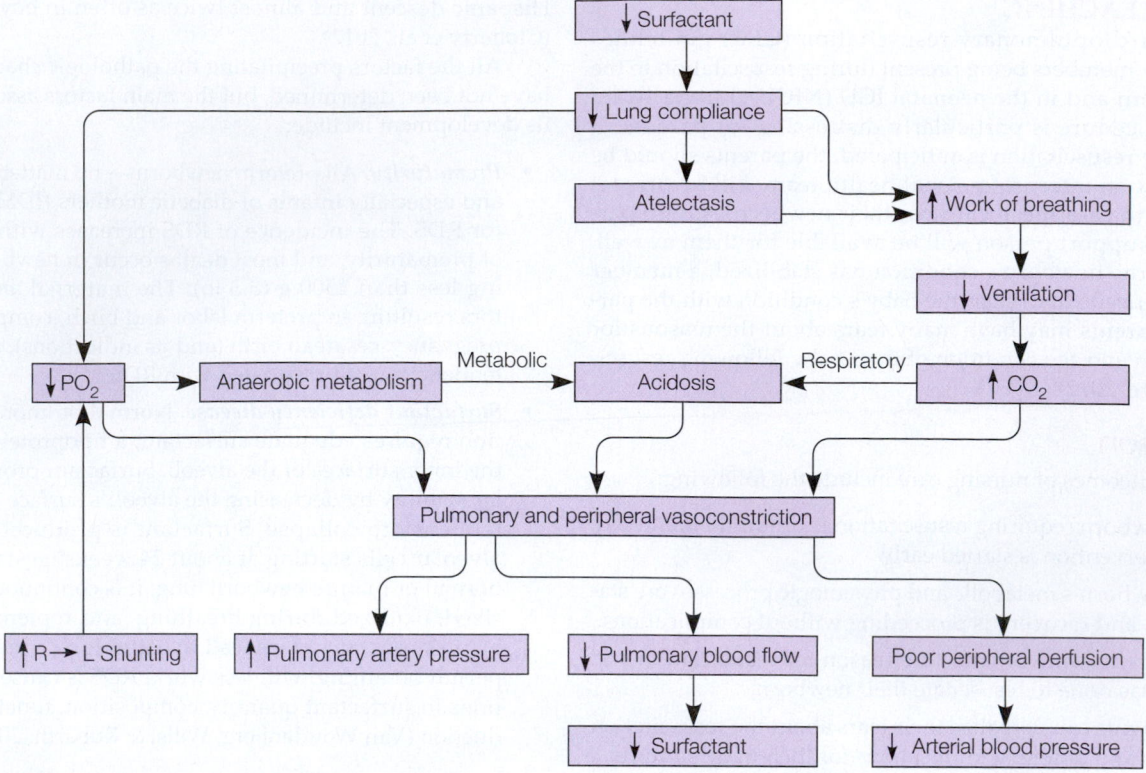

Figure 27–3 Cycle of events of RDS leading to eventual respiratory failure.

SOURCE: Modified from Gluck, L., & Kulovich, M. V. (1973). Fetal lung development. *Pediatric Clinics of North America, 20,* 375.

pulmonary vascular resistance may precipitate a return to fetal circulation as the ductus opens and blood flow is shunted around the lungs in a right-to-left blood flow. This shunting increases the hypoxia and further decreases pulmonary perfusion. Hypoxia also causes impairment or absence of metabolic response to cold; reversion to anaerobic metabolism, resulting in lactate accumulation (acidosis); and impaired cardiac output, which decreases perfusion to vital organs.

- *Respiratory acidosis.* Increased PCO_2 and decreased pH are results of alveolar hypoventilation. A persistent rise in PCO_2 is a poor prognostic sign of pulmonary function and adequacy because the increased PCO_2 and decreased pH are results of alveolar hypoventilation.

- *Metabolic acidosis.* Because of the cells' lack of oxygen, the newborn begins anaerobic metabolism, with an increase in lactate levels and a resulting base deficit (loss of bicarbonate). As the lactate levels increase, the pH decreases in an attempt to maintain acid–base homeostasis.

The classic radiologic picture of RDS is diffuse bilateral reticulogranular (ground glass appearance) density, with portions of the air-filled tracheobronchial tree (air bronchogram) outlined by the opaque ("white-out") lungs with widespread atelectasis, potentially obliterating the heart borders (Figure 27–4) (Cloherty et al., 2012). The progression of x-ray findings parallels the pattern of resolution, which usually occurs in 7 to 10 days, and the time of surfactant reappearance, unless surfactant replacement therapy has been used (Blackburn, 2013). Echocardiography is a valuable tool in diagnosing vascular shunts that move blood either away from or toward the lungs.

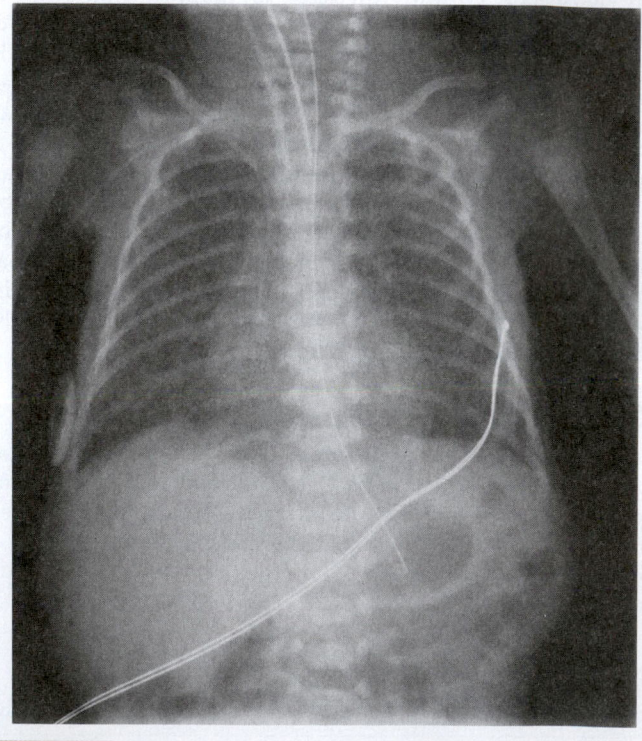

Figure 27–4 RDS chest x-ray. Chest radiograph of respiratory distress syndrome characterized by a reticulogranular pattern with areas of microatelectasis of uniform opacity and air bronchograms.

SOURCE: Carol Harrigan, RN, MSN, NNP-BC.

CLINICAL THERAPY

The primary goal of prenatal management is to prevent preterm birth through early assessment of fetal lung maturity, aggressive treatment of preterm labor, and administration of glucocorticoids to enhance fetal lung development (see discussions in Chapter 15). Antenatal steroids reduce the incidence and severity of RDS and improve survivability of the 24 to 34 weeks' gestation and extremely low-birth-weight (LBW) newborn (less than 1250 g) (Cloherty et al., 2012).

Postnatal surfactant replacement therapy is available for newborns to decrease the severity of RDS in LBW babies (Polin, Carlo, & Committee on the Fetus and Newborn, 2014). Babies born at less than 30 weeks' gestation who receive prophylactic surfactant show increased chronic lung disease (Polin et al., 2014). Surfactant replacement therapy is delivered through an endotracheal tube and may be given in either the birthing room or the nursery as indicated by the severity of RDS. Repeat doses are often required. The most frequently reported response to treatment is rapidly improved oxygenation and decreased need for ventilatory support, sometimes occurring soon after the dose is administered.

Supportive medical management consists of ventilation therapy, blood gas monitoring, pulse oximetry monitoring, correction of acid–base imbalance, environmental temperature regulation, adequate nutrition, and protection from infection. Ventilation therapy is directed toward preventing hypoventilation and hypoxia. Mild cases of RDS may require only increased humidified oxygen concentrations. Use of continuous positive airway pressure (CPAP) may be required in moderately afflicted newborns. Babies with severe RDS require mechanical ventilatory assistance from a respirator (Figure 27–5) (Fanaroff & Fanaroff, 2013).

High-frequency ventilation (HFV) can be tried when conventional ventilator therapy has not been successful, and it sometimes can be the primary mode of ventilation to minimize lung injury in very small and/or sick newborns (Gomella, 2013). In some institutions, morphine or fentanyl is used for its analgesic and sedative effects.

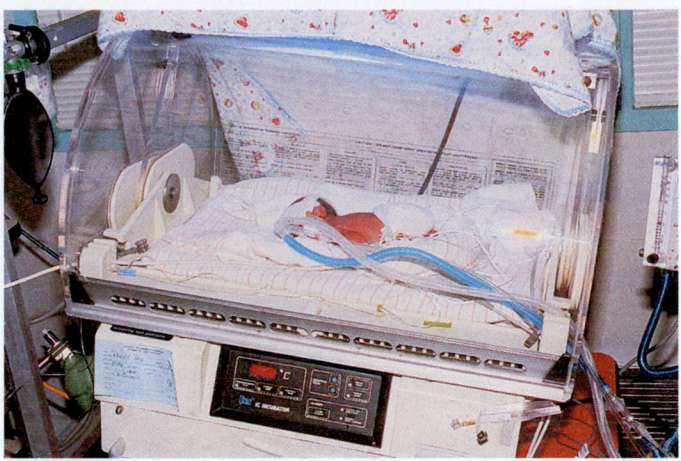

Figure 27–5 **Mechanical ventilator assistance. One-day-old, 29 weeks' gestational age, 1450 g baby on respirator and in isolette.**

SOURCE: Carol Harrigan, RN, MSN, NNP-BC.

helpful in evaluating the signs of respiratory distress observed in the birthing area.

Nursing interventions and criteria for instituting mechanical ventilation depend on institutional protocol. Noninvasive oxygen monitoring provides real-time trend information that is particularly useful in newborns showing frequent swings in PaO_2 and oxygen saturation. These methods (pulse oximetry, transcutaneous oxygen monitor) can also reduce the frequency of blood gas sampling. Methods of noninvasive oxygen monitoring and nursing interventions are included in Table 27–2.

Based on clinical parameters, implement therapeutic approaches to provide the baby with respiratory distress with a very supportive environment (Figure 27–6) that includes maintaining thermoregulation to decrease respiratory effort and decrease infection secondary to invasive procedures and using standard precautions. (See *Nursing Care Plan: For the Newborn With Respiratory Distress Syndrome.*) Newborns with severe respiratory distress are cared for in neonatal intensive care units by nurses with advanced knowledge and training.

Transient Tachypnea of the Newborn

Some newborns, term and late preterm babies, may develop progressive respiratory distress that clinically can resemble RDS and is called *transient tachypnea of the newborn (TTN)*. Other risk factors include maternal diabetes and asthma, male sex of the fetus, macrosomia (possibly related to maternal diabetes), and cesarean section delivery, especially elective cesarean sections without spontaneous labor. Some term babies with progressively worsening respiratory distress may benefit from exogenous surfactant (Gardner, Enzman-Himes, & Nyp, 2016). Typically, supplemental oxygen of less than 40% will alleviate the hypoxia (Cloherty et al., 2012; Fanaroff & Fanaroff, 2013). Newborns with transient tachypnea may have had intrauterine or intrapartum asphyxia because of maternal oversedation or poor uterine perfusion, maternal bleeding, prolapsed cord, or breech presentation. The baby then fails to clear the airway of lung fluid, mucus, and other debris, or the excess of fluid in the lungs due to aspiration of amniotic or tracheal fluid (Gomella, 2013). TTN is also more prevalent in

Clinical Tip

In babies with RDS who are on ventilators, increased diuresis or urination (determined by weighing diapers) may be an early clue that the baby's condition is improving. As fluid moves out of the lungs into the bloodstream, alveoli open and kidney perfusion increases; this results in increased voiding. At this point, the nurse must monitor chest expansion closely. If chest expansion is increasing, pulmonary compliance is improving and ventilator settings may have to be decreased, sometimes quite soon after surfactant dosing. Too high a ventilator setting may "blow the lung," resulting in pneumothorax. If diuresis does not occur, it is a sign that bronchopulmonary dysplasia (BPD), also called *chronic lung disease (CLD) of prematurity*, may be developing (Cloherty et al., 2012).

Nursing Management

Look for characteristics of RDS such as increasing cyanosis, tachypnea (greater than 60 respirations per minute), grunting respirations, nasal flaring, significant retractions, and apnea. Table 27–1 reviews clinical findings associated with respiratory distress in general. The Silverman-Andersen index may be

TABLE 27–1 Clinical Assessments Associated with Respiratory Distress

CLINICAL PICTURE	SIGNIFICANCE
SKIN COLOR	
Pallor or mottling	These represent poor peripheral circulation caused by systemic hypotension and vasoconstriction and pooling of independent areas (usually in conjunction with severe hypoxia).
Cyanosis (bluish tint)	Depending on hemoglobin concentration, peripheral circulation, intensity and quality of viewing light, and acuity of observer's color vision, this is frankly visible in advanced hypoxia. Central cyanosis is most easily detected by examination of mucous membranes and tongue.
Jaundice (yellow discoloration of skin and mucous membranes caused by presence of unconjugated [indirect] bilirubin)	Metabolic alterations (acidosis, hypercarbia, asphyxia) of respiratory distress predispose a newborn to dissociation of bilirubin from albumin-binding sites and deposition in the skin and central nervous system.
Edema (presents as slick, shiny taut skin)	This is characteristic of preterm newborns because their total protein concentration is low, with a decrease in colloidal osmotic pressure and transudation of fluid. Edema of hands and feet is frequently seen within first 24 hours and resolved by fifth day in newborns with severe RDS.
RESPIRATORY SYSTEM	
Tachypnea (normal respiratory rate [RR] 30 to 60/minute, sustained, elevated respiratory rate 60+/minute)	Increased respiratory rate is the easiest detectable sign of respiratory distress after birth. Because of the premature newborn's very compliant chest wall, it is more energy efficient to increase the respiratory rate than to increase the depth of respirations. This compensatory mechanism attempts to increase respiratory dead space to maintain alveolar ventilation and gas exchange in the face of an increase in mechanical resistance. As a decompensatory mechanism it increases workload and energy output by increasing respiratory rate, which causes increased metabolic demand for oxygen and thus increases alveolar ventilation on an already overstressed system. During shallow, rapid respirations, there is an increase in dead space ventilation, thus decreasing alveolar ventilation.
Apnea (episode of nonbreathing for more than 20 seconds); periodic breathing, a common "normal" occurrence in preterm newborns, is defined as apnea of 5–10 seconds alternating with 10–15 seconds of ventilation that is sometimes quite rapid	This poor prognostic sign indicates cardiorespiratory disease, central nervous system (CNS) disease, metabolic alterations, intracranial hemorrhage, sepsis, or immaturity. Physiologic alterations include decreased oxygen saturation, respiratory acidosis, and bradycardia.
CHEST	
Chest movement	Inspection of the thoracic cage includes shape, size, and symmetry of movement. Respiratory movements should be symmetric and diaphragmatic; asymmetry reflects pathology (pneumothorax, diaphragmatic hernia). Increased anteroposterior diameter indicates air trapping (meconium aspiration syndrome).
Labored respirations (Silverman-Andersen index indicates severity of retractions, grunting, and nasal flaring, which are signs of labored respirations)	Indicates marked increase in the work of breathing.
Retractions (inward pulling of soft parts of the chest cage—suprasternal, substernal, intercostals [between the ribs]—at inspiration)	These reflect the significant increase in negative intrathoracic pressure necessary to inflate stiff, noncompliant lungs. Newborns attempt to increase lung compliance by using accessory muscles. Lung expansion markedly decreases. Seesaw respirations are seen when the chest flattens with inspiration and the abdomen bulges. Retractions increase the work of breathing and O_2 need. As a result, assisted ventilation may be necessary because of exhaustion.
Nasal flaring (inspiratory dilation of nostrils)	This compensatory mechanism attempts to lessen the resistance of the narrow nasal passage.
Expiratory grunt (Valsalva maneuver in which the baby exhales against a partially closed glottis, thus producing an audible moan)	This increases intrapulmonary pressure, which decreases or prevents atelectasis, thus improving oxygenation and alveolar ventilation. It allows more time for the passage of oxygen into the circulatory system. Intubation should not be attempted unless the newborn's condition is rapidly deteriorating, because it prevents this maneuver and allows the alveoli to collapse.
Rhythmic body movement with labored respirations (chin tug, head bobbing, retractions of anal area)	This is a result of using abdominal and other respiratory accessory muscles during prolonged forced respirations.
Auscultation of chest reveals decreased air exchange, with harsh breath sounds or fine inspiratory rales; rhonchi may be present	Decrease in breath sounds and distant quality may indicate interstitial or intrapleural air or fluid.

CLINICAL PICTURE	SIGNIFICANCE
CARDIOVASCULAR SYSTEM	
Continuous systolic murmur may be audible	Patent ductus arteriosus is a common occurrence with hypoxia, pulmonary vasoconstriction, right-to-left shunting, and congestive heart failure.
Heart rate usually within normal limits (fixed heart rate may occur with a rate of 110 to 120 beats/min)	A fixed heart rate indicates a decrease in vagal control.
Point of maximal impulse usually located at fourth to fifth intercostal space, left sternal border	Displacement may reflect dextrocardia, pneumothorax, or diaphragmatic hernia.
HYPOTHERMIA	
	This is inadequate functioning of metabolic processes that require oxygen to produce necessary body heat.
MUSCLE TONE	
Flaccid, hypotonic, unresponsive to stimuli; hypertonia and/or seizure activity	These may indicate deterioration in the newborn's condition and possible CNS damage caused by hypoxia, acidemia, or hemorrhage.

TABLE 27–2 Oxygen Monitors

TYPE	FUNCTION AND RATIONALE	NURSING INTERVENTIONS
PULSE OXIMETRY—SPO$_2$		
Estimates beat-to-beat arterial oxygen saturation.	Calibration is automatic.	Understand and use oxyhemoglobin dissociation curve.
Microprocessor measures saturation by the absorption of red and infrared light as it passes through tissue.	Less dependent on perfusion than TcPO$_2$ and TcPCO$_2$, however, functions poorly if peripheral perfusion is decreased because of low cardiac output.	Monitor trends over time and correlate with arterial blood gases. Check disposable sensor at least every 8 hr.
Changes in absorption related to blood pulsation through vessel determine saturation and pulse rate.	Much more rapid response time than TcPO$_2$—offers real-time readings. Can be located on extremity, digit, or palm of hand, leaving chest free; not affected by skin characteristics. Requires understanding of oxyhemoglobin dissociation curve. Pulse oximeter reading of 88% to 93% reflects a PaO$_2$ of 50–80 mm Hg Extreme sensitivity to movement; decreases if average of 7th or 14th beat is selected rather than beat to beat. Poor correlation with extreme hyperoxia.	Use disposable cuffs (reusable cuffs allow too much ambient light to enter, and readings may be inaccurate).
TRANSCUTANEOUS OXYGEN MONITOR—TcPO$_2$		
Measures oxygen diffusion across the skin. Clark electrode is heated to 43°C [109.4°F] (preterm) or 44°C [111.2°F] (term) to warm the skin beneath the electrode and promote diffusion of oxygen across the skin surface. PO$_2$ is measured when oxygen diffuses across the capillary membrane, skin, and electrode membrane.	When transcutaneous monitors are properly calibrated and electrodes are appropriately positioned, they will provide reliable, continuous, noninvasive measurements of PO$_2$, PCO$_2$, and oxygen saturation. Readings vary when skin perfusion is decreased. Reliable as trend monitor. Frequent calibration necessary to overcome mechanical drift. Following membrane change, machine must "warm up" 1 hour prior to initial calibration; otherwise, after turning it on, it must equilibrate for 30 minutes prior to calibration. When placed on newborn, values will be low until skin is heated; approximately 15 minutes required to stabilize. Second-degree burns are rare but can occur if electrodes remain in place too long. Decreased correlations noted with older babies (related to skin thickness), with babies with low cardiac output (decreased skin perfusion), and with hyperoxic babies. The adhesive that attaches the electrode may abrade the fragile skin of the preterm newborn. May be used for both preductal and postductal monitoring of oxygenation for observations of shunting.	Use TcPO$_2$ to monitor trends of oxygenation with routine nursing care procedures. Clean electrode surface to remove electrolyte deposits; change solution and membrane once a week. Allow machine to stabilize before drawing arterial gases; note reading when gases are drawn and use values to correlate. Ensure airtight seal between skin surface and electrode; place electrodes on clean, dry skin on upper chest, abdomen, or inner aspect of thigh; avoid bony prominences. Change skin site and recalibrate at least every 4 hours; inspect skin for burns; if burns occur, use lowest temperature setting and change position of electrode more frequently. Adhesive disks may be cut to a smaller size, or skin prep may be used under the adhesive circle only; allow membrane to touch skin surface at center.

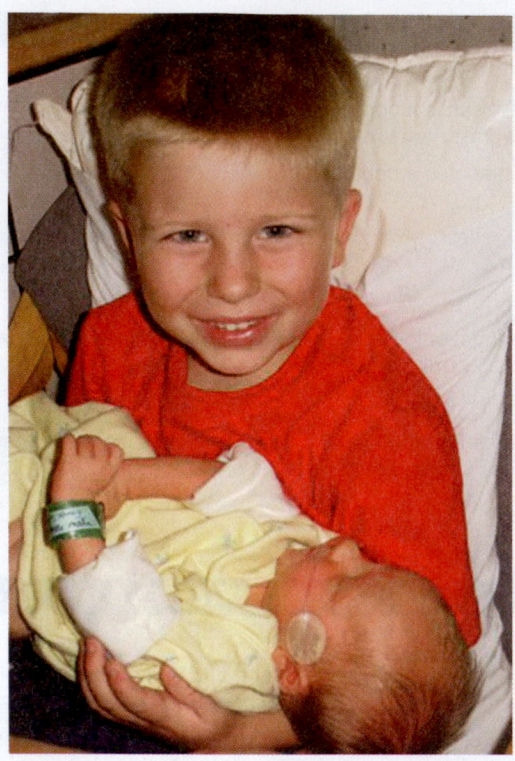

Figure 27–6 This baby born at 36 weeks' gestational age had severe RDS. He has on-going oxygen needs provided by a nasal cannula but still can be held by his proud big brother.

SOURCE: Lisa Smith-Pedersen, RN, MSN, NNP-BC.

cesarean birth newborns who have not had the *thoracic squeeze* that occurs during vaginal birth and removes some of the lung fluid.

Usually the newborn experiences little or no difficulty at the onset of breathing. However, shortly after birth, expiratory grunting, flaring of the nares, and mild cyanosis may be noted in the newborn breathing room air (Gardner et al., 2016). Air will become trapped and an increase in the anterior–posterior diameter of the chest will be observed (Blackburn, 2013). Tachypnea is usually present by 6 hours of age, with respiratory rates consistently greater than 60 breaths per minute, and possibly reaching 80 to 110 breaths/min with a requirement of oxygen. Mild respiratory and metabolic acidosis may be present within the first 6 hours. These clinical signs usually persist for 12 to 24 hours. In mild TTN, the signs can improve within 24 hours but may continue for up to 72 hours when more severe and possibly last up to 1 week (Cloherty et al., 2012).

CLINICAL THERAPY

Initial x-ray findings may be identical to those showing RDS within the first 3 hours. However, radiographs of newborns with transient tachypnea usually reveal a generalized overexpansion of the lungs (hyperaeration of alveoli), which is identified principally by flattened contours of the diaphragm. Dense streaks (increased vascularity) radiate from the hilar region and represent engorgement of the lymphatic vessels, which clear alveolar fluid on initiation of air breathing. Within 48 to 72 hours, the chest x-ray examination is normal with the exception of perihilar markings, which may remain visible for 3 to 7 days because of remaining fluid in the periarterial tissue (Fanaroff & Fanaroff, 2013).

Nursing Care Plan: For the Newborn With Respiratory Distress Syndrome

1. Nursing Diagnosis: *Breathing Pattern, Ineffective,* **related to immature lung development or inadequate lung surfactant (NANDA-I © 2014)**

GOAL: The newborn will maintain an effective breathing pattern.

INTERVENTION	RATIONALE
• Review maternal birth records, noting medications given to mother before birth and the baby's condition at birth such as Apgar scores and resuscitative measures.	• Several drugs suppress respiratory function in the newborn.
• Administer surfactant replacement therapy as ordered. • Surfactant replacement therapy may be administered via endotracheal tube either in the birthing room or in the nursery.	• Surfactant improves lung compliance; therefore the need for ventilatory support may be decreased. Surfactant provides alveolar stability by decreasing the alveoli's surface tension and tendency to collapse. Alterations in surfactant quantity, composition, function, or production result in respiratory distress syndrome.
• Initiate cardiac and respiratory monitoring and calibrate these monitors every 8 hours or per unit protocol.	• Close monitoring detects periodic apneic spells and allows for medical intervention if necessary.
• Monitor newborn's respiratory rate and rhythm, pulse, blood pressure, chest movement, color, and activity.	• Increases in respiratory rate and pulse and alteration in rhythm and blood pressure may indicate respiratory distress.
• Administer warmed, humidified oxygen to the newborn and monitor the oxygen concentrations every 30 minutes or per agency protocol.	• Prevents mucosal dryness and maintains an even level of oxygen administration.
• Oxygen may be administered to the newborn experiencing mild respiratory distress via nasal cannula or oxygen hood. With severe respiratory distress mechanical ventilatory assistance from a respirator may be necessary.	• Oxygenation and ventilatory therapy may prevent hypoventilation and hypoxia. Mild cases of respiratory distress may require only increased humidified oxygen concentrations, whereas more severe cases may require continuous positive airway pressure.

- **Collaborative:** Obtain arterial blood gases (ABGs) per primary care provider order and agency protocol.

- Obtaining ABGs is essential in managing a newborn receiving oxygen.

- Failure to synthesize surfactant increases atelectasis, which causes hypoxia and acidosis caused by lack of gas exchange. Lung compliance will deteriorate and result in difficulty of inflation, labored respirations, and increased work of breathing. Progressive hypoxia may be seen when ABG levels are compared and evaluated.

- Attach pulse oximeter to newborn's extremity to measure tissue oxygenation.

- Monitor transcutaneous pulse oximeter continuously or hourly and record. Rotate sensor site every 3–4 hours.

- Oxygen saturation should be kept at approximately 88% to 92% (Cloherty, 2012). Avoid excessive oxygenation, which can increase the risk of developing chronic lung disease and retinopathy of prematurity.

- Assess newborn's need for mechanical ventilation: apnea present, hypoxia (PaO_2 less than 50 mmHg), hypercapnia ($PaCO_2$ greater than 60 mmHg), respiratory acidosis (pH less than 7.2).

- Administer mechanical ventilation per hospital protocol.

- Mechanical ventilation improves oxygenation and ventilation, resulting in rise in PaO_2 and decrease in $PaCO_2$.

- Continuous positive airway pressure (CPAP) or positive end-expiratory pressure (PEEP) can be administered by nasal prongs, nasopharyngeal or oral intubation.

EXPECTED OUTCOME: The newborn will maintain an effective breathing pattern as evidenced by respirations of 30–60 breaths/min, arterial blood gases are within normal range, baby is free of signs of retractions or nasal flaring, and blood pH is 7.35–7.45.

2. **Nursing Diagnosis:** *Thermoregulation, Ineffective,* related to increased respiratory effort (NANDA-I © 2014)

GOAL: The newborn will exhibit no signs of hypothermia.

INTERVENTION	RATIONALE

- Review maternal prenatal and intrapartum records. Note any medications mother received during these times.

- Medications such as Demerol and magnesium sulfate used by the mother during the prenatal or intrapartum periods significantly interfere with the newborn's ability to retain heat.

- Assess newborn's temperature frequently. Place servoprobe on baby's skin over a solid organ.

- Hypothermia leads to pulmonary vasoconstriction because of the increase in oxygen consumption. Cold stress leads to increased oxygen needs; consequently, brown fat is used to maintain body temperature.

- Observe for signs of increased oxygen consumption and metabolic acidosis.

- Warm and humidify all inspired gases and record temperature of delivered gases

- Hypoxia and acidosis further depress surfactant production.

- Cold air/oxygen blown in face of newborn is stimulus for consumption of oxygen and glucose and increased metabolic rate.

- Use radiant warmers or incubators with servocontrols and open cribs with appropriate clothing.

- Maintains neutral thermal environment.

- Note signs and symptoms of respiratory distress, including tachypnea, apnea, cyanosis, acrocyanosis, bradycardia, lethargy, weak cry, and hypotonia.

- These signs can predispose the newborn to metabolic acidosis.

EXPECTED OUTCOME: The newborn will not exhibit signs and symptoms of hypothermia as evidenced by temperature maintenance of 97.7°F (36.5°C) to 99.1°F (37.3°C) and no signs and symptoms of respiratory distress.

3. **Nursing Diagnosis:** *Nutrition, Imbalanced: Less Than Body Requirements,* related to increased metabolic needs in the newborn (NANDA-I © 2014)

GOAL: The newborn will gain weight in a normal curve.

INTERVENTION	RATIONALE

- Assess suck, swallow, gag, and cough reflexes.

- Prevents feeding problems and assists in determining the best individualized method of feeding for newborn.

- Assess respiratory status of newborn. If any problems are noted, notify physician.

- In the presence of respiratory distress, avoid oral fluids and initiate parenteral nutrition per physician's orders.

(continued)

Nursing Care Plan: For the Newborn With Respiratory Distress Syndrome (*continued*)

- Monitor IV rates per infusion pump (starting at 80 mL/kg/day) as ordered by physician.

- Record hourly intake and output (I&O) and daily weights.

- Provide total parenteral nutrition (TPN) when indicated.

- Advance, based on tolerance, from IV to gastrointestinal (GI) feedings. Gavage or nipple feedings are used, and IV is used as supplement (discontinued when oral intake is sufficient).

- Provide adequate caloric intake: Consider amount of intake, type of formula, route of administration, and need for supplementation of intake by other routes.

- Assess infusion site for signs and symptoms of infection including erythema, edema, and drainage with a foul odor.

- Allows for close monitoring of fluid intake.

- IV fluids are administered to replace sensible and insensible water loss, as well as evaporative water loss secondary to respiratory distress. Monitoring I&O will prevent circulatory system overload that can lead to pulmonary edema and cardiac problems.

- TPN is used as nutritional alternative if bowel sounds are not present and/or baby remains in acute distress.

- If IV is discontinued before oral intake is established, baby will not receive adequate calories.

- Formula or breast milk stimulates GI hormones necessary for a functional absorptive GI tract.

- Avoid complications associated with nutrition by IV route only.

- Calories are essential to prevent catabolism of body proteins and metabolic acidosis because of starvation or inadequate caloric intake.

- Appropriate intervention can be initiated when signs and symptoms of infection are detected early. Treatment may avoid infection and sepsis in the newborn.

EXPECTED OUTCOME: The newborn maintains steady weight gain as evidenced by no more than 2%/day weight loss, tolerates oral feedings, and has a urine output of 1–3 mL/kg/hour.

Clinical Reasoning Transient Tachypnea of the Newborn

You are caring for baby girl Linn, who is a 39-week, AGA female born by repeat cesarean birth to a 34-year-old G3, now P3 mother. Baby Linn's Apgar scores were 7 at 1 minute and 9 at 5 minutes. At 2 hours of age, you note an elevated respiratory rate of 70 to 80 and mild cyanosis. The newborn is now receiving 30% oxygen and has a respiratory rate of 100 to 120. The baby's clinical course, chest x-ray examination, and lab work are all consistent with transient tachypnea of the newborn. Linn's mother calls you to ask about her baby. She tells you that her last child was born at 30 weeks' gestation, had respiratory distress syndrome requiring ventilator support, and was hospitalized for 6 weeks. She asks you, "Is this the same respiratory distress?"

What will you tell Linn's mother?

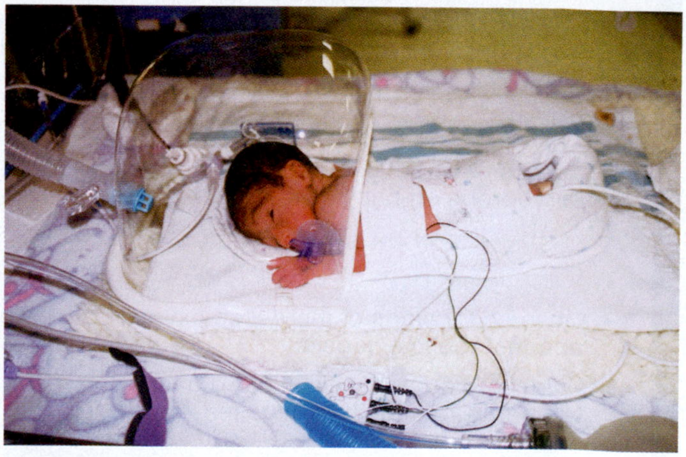

Figure 27–7 Premature newborn under oxygen hood. Baby is nested and has a nonnutritive sucking pacifier.

SOURCE: Lisa Smith-Pedersen, RN, MSN, NNP-BC.

Supplemental oxygen, usually under an oxygen hood, may be required to correct the hypoxemia (Figure 27–7). Fluid and electrolyte requirements should be met with IV during the acute phase of the disease. Oral feedings are contraindicated because of rapid respiratory rates and the subsequent risk of aspiration.

When hypoxemia is severe and tachypnea continues, persistent pulmonary hypertension must be considered and treatment measures initiated. If pneumonia or sepsis is suspected initially, antibiotics may be administered prophylactically.

Nursing Management

For nursing actions, see *Nursing Care Plan: For the Newborn With Respiratory Distress Syndrome.*

The Newborn With Meconium Aspiration Syndrome

Because the body's physiologic response to asphyxia is increased intestinal peristalsis, relaxation of the anal sphincter and the presence of meconium in the amniotic fluid indicate that the fetus may be suffering from asphyxia, either in the immediate period during labor or perhaps some time in the recent past (Marks, 2012). However, if the fetus is in a breech position, the presence of meconium in the amniotic fluid *does not necessarily* indicate asphyxia.

Approximately 8% to 20% of all live-born late-preterm, early-term, or term babies are born through meconium-stained amniotic fluid (MSAF) (Swarnam, Soraisham, & Sivanandan, 2012). Of the newborns born through MSAF, one third develop meconium aspiration syndrome (MAS) (Marks, 2012; Swarnam et al., 2012). The amniotic fluid may be aspirated into the tracheobronchial tree in utero or during the first few breaths taken by the newborn.

Presence of meconium in the lungs produces the following:

- Mechanical obstruction of airways: ball-valve action (air is allowed in but not exhaled), so that alveoli overdistend, with oxygen and carbon dioxide trapping and hyperinflation; air leaks such as pneumothorax are common
- Chemical pneumonitis leading to the possible development of secondary bacterial pneumonia
- Inactivation of natural surfactant (Fanaroff & Fanaroff, 2013; Gomella, 2013).

CLINICAL MANIFESTATIONS OF MAS

Clinical manifestations of MAS include:

- Fetal hypoxia in utero a few days or a few minutes before birth, indicated by a sudden increase in fetal activity followed by diminished activity, slowing of fetal heart rate (FHR) or weak and irregular heartbeat, loss of beat-to-beat variability, and meconium staining of amniotic fluid or particulate meconium.
- Presence of signs of distress or depression at birth, such as pallor, cyanosis, apnea, slow heartbeat, and low Apgar scores (below 6) at 1 and 5 minutes.

After the initial assessment and stabilization, the severity of the ongoing clinical symptoms correlates with the extent of aspiration. Many newborns require mechanical ventilation at birth because of immediate signs of distress (generalized cyanosis, tachypnea, and severe retractions). An overdistended, barrel-shaped chest with increased anteroposterior diameter is common. Auscultation reveals diminished air movement, with prominent rales and rhonchi. Abdominal palpation may reveal a displaced liver caused by diaphragmatic depression resulting from the overexpansion of the lungs. Yellowish/pale green staining of the skin, nails, and umbilical cord is usually present, especially if the incident occurred a good length of time before birth (Fanaroff & Fanaroff, 2013).

The MAS chest X-ray film reveals asymmetric, coarse, patchy densities and possible hyperinflation (9 to 11 rib expansion), which may predispose the newborn to air leak syndrome such as pneumothorax or pneumomediastinum (Fanaroff & Fanaroff, 2013).

CLINICAL THERAPY

The combined efforts of the maternity and the pediatric team are needed to prevent MAS. Previously, the most effective form of preventive management was intrapartum suctioning after the head of the newborn was delivered but when the shoulders and chest were still in the birth canal. Current evidence does not support this practice, as routine intrapartum oropharyngeal and nasopharyngeal suctioning does not prevent or alter the course of MAS (AAP & ACOG, 2012; Fanaroff & Fanaroff, 2013).

If the newborn is vigorous, even if there is meconium-stained amniotic fluid, no subsequent special resuscitation such as tracheal suctioning is indicated. Injury to the vocal cords is also more likely to occur during attempts to intubate a vigorous newborn.

If the newborn has absent or depressed respirations, heart rate less than 100 beats/min, or poor muscle tone, direct tracheal suctioning with a DeLee device attached to low-pressure wall suction by a specially trained healthcare provider is recommended. The glottis is visualized and the trachea suctioned to remove meconium or other aspirated material from beneath the glottis to decrease the possibility of human immunodeficiency virus (HIV) transmission.

Further resuscitative efforts are undertaken as indicated, following the same principles of clinical therapy used for asphyxia (discussed earlier in this chapter). Resuscitated newborns should be transferred immediately to the nursery for closer observation. The newborn should be maintained in a neutral thermal environment and tactile stimulation should be minimized. An umbilical arterial line may be used for direct monitoring of arterial blood pressures, as well as blood sampling for pH and blood gases. An umbilical venous catheter may be placed for infusion of IV fluids, blood, or medications.

Treatment usually involves delivery of high levels of oxygen and high-pressure ventilation. High pressures may be needed to cause sufficient expiratory expansion of obstructed terminal airways or to stabilize airways that are weakened by inflammation so that the most distal atelectatic (collapsed) alveoli are ventilated. Naturally occurring surfactant may be inactivated by the presence of meconium and the subsequent inflammatory response that occurs. Surfactant replacement therapy is most effective when given as a prophylactic measure. Providing exogenous surfactant possibly decreases mortality (Swarnam et al., 2012; Walsh, Daigle, DiBlasi, et al., 2013). Systemic blood pressure and pulmonary blood flow must be maintained. Dopamine or dobutamine, or both, may be used to maintain systemic blood pressure.

Newborns with respiratory failure who are not responding to conventional ventilator therapy may require treatment with high-frequency ventilation and/or nitric oxide therapy or extracorporeal membrane oxygenation (ECMO) if baby is greater than 1.8 kg (4.0 lb) and 34 weeks estimated gestational age (EGA) (Fanaroff & Fanaroff, 2013; Gomella, 2013). Inhaled nitric oxide has proven successful for newborns with meconium aspiration, pneumonia, and persistent pulmonary hypertension of the newborn (PPHN) (failure of the normal circulatory transition that occurs after birth) and it avoids the need for ECMO.

Prophylactic intravenous antibiotics are frequently given. Continuous infusion of bicarbonate to correct metabolic acidosis may be necessary for several days for severely ill newborns. Mortality in term or postterm newborns is very high because the cycle of hypoxemia and acidemia is difficult to break.

Nursing Management
For the Newborn With Meconium Aspiration Syndrome

Nursing Assessment and Diagnosis

During the intrapartum period, observe for signs of fetal hypoxia and meconium staining of amniotic fluid. At birth, assess the newborn for signs of distress. During the ongoing assessment of the newborn, carefully observe for complications such as pulmonary air leaks, PPHN, hypotension and poor cardiac output, renal function, cerebral and pulmonary edema, sepsis secondary to bacterial pneumonia, and any signs of intestinal necrosis from ischemia.

EVIDENCE-BASED PRACTICE | Antibiotics for Meconium-Stained Amniotic Fluid in Labor

Clinical Question

Are antibiotics effective for preventing maternal and neonatal infections when amniotic fluid is meconium stained?

The Evidence

Meconium-stained amniotic fluid (MSAF) increases the risk of maternal and neonatal infections. Pregnant women with MSAF are more likely to develop inflammation of the fetal membranes caused by bacteria (chorioamnionitis). These mothers are also at higher risk of postpartum endometritis, and their babies are at higher risk of neonatal sepsis. Fetal stress may trigger gasping in the fetus, which results in aspiration of the meconium-stained fluid and can cause a host of respiratory difficulties. These investigators conducted a systematic review to determine if the administration of antibiotics could reduce the incidence of maternal infections and neonatal sepsis and other consequences of respiratory compromise. The review, published in the rigorous *Cochrane Database of Systematic Reviews*, is a highly structured review of randomized trials and forms the strongest evidence for practice.

The only antibiotic tested was ampicillin-sulbactam, and it appeared to have no effect on the rate of neonatal sepsis and subsequent neonatal intensive care admission. There was also no measurable effect on maternal endometritis rates. However, there was a significant decrease in the rate of chorioamnionitis,

reducing the mothers' risk of this condition by about a third (Siriwachirachai, Sangkomkamhang, Lumbiganon, et al., 2014). The investigators noted that the evidence that the antibiotic had no effect was weaker for the neonates, as there was a relatively small sample, and a large effect would have been needed to draw a conclusion that it was completely ineffective. In addition, only one antibiotic was tested. However, the effect on maternal infection was so strong that its use is recommended, and no adverse effects were observed in either mother or baby when this antibiotic was used. Additional research with a range of antibiotics is warranted to discover if other antibiotics may be effective in preventing neonatal complications of MSAF.

Best Practice

Antibiotics should be administered to mothers with meconium-stained amniotic fluid to reduce the risk of chorioamnionitis. The drug has no measurable adverse effects and has been shown to be safe for both mother and baby.

Clinical Reasoning

Why might an antibiotic be effective for prevention of maternal infections and not for the neonate? What client teaching is needed for the mother with meconium-stained amniotic fluid in terms of her self-care and care of the neonate?

Nursing diagnoses that may apply to the newborn with MAS and the baby's parents include the following (NANDA-I © 2014):

- *Gas Exchange, Impaired,* related to aspiration of meconium and amniotic fluid during birth
- *Nutrition, Imbalanced: Less Than Body Requirements,* related to respiratory distress and increased energy requirements
- *Coping: Family, Compromised,* related to life-threatening illness in term newborn

Nursing Plan and Implementation

HOSPITAL-BASED NURSING CARE

Initial interventions are aimed at early identification of meconium aspiration. When significant aspiration occurs, therapy is supportive with the primary goals of maintaining appropriate gas exchange and minimizing complications. Nursing interventions after resuscitation should include maintaining adequate oxygenation and ventilation, regulating temperature, performing glucose testing by glucometer to check for hypoglycemia and monitoring calcium levels, observing IV fluid administration, calculating necessary fluids (which may be restricted in the first 48 to 72 hours because of cerebral edema), providing caloric requirements with total parenteral nutrition (TPN), and monitoring IV antibiotic therapy.

Evaluation

Expected outcomes of nursing care include the following:

- The newborn at risk for MAS is promptly identified and early intervention is initiated.

- The newborn is free of respiratory distress and metabolic alterations.
- The parents verbalize their concerns about their baby's health problem and survival and understand the rationale behind the management of their newborn.

Care of the Newborn With Cold Stress

Cold stress is excessive heat loss resulting in the use of compensatory mechanisms (such as increased respirations and nonshivering thermogenesis/use of brown fat stores) to maintain core body temperature close to 37.0°C (98.6°F) (Cloherty et al., 2012). Heat loss that results in cold stress occurs in the newborn through the mechanisms of evaporation, convection, conduction, and radiation. (See Chapter 23 for types of thermoregulation.) Heat loss at birth that leads to cold stress can play a significant role in the severity of respiratory distress syndrome (RDS) and the ultimate outcome for the newborn. Both preterm and small-for-gestational-age (SGA) newborns are at risk for cold stress because they have decreased adipose tissue, brown fat stores, and glycogen available for metabolism (Fanaroff & Fanaroff, 2013).

As discussed in Chapter 23, the newborn's major source of heat production in nonshivering thermogenesis (NST) is brown fat metabolism. The ability of a baby to respond to cold stress by NST is impaired in the presence of several conditions:

- Hypoxemia (PO$_2$ less than 50 torr)
- Intracranial hemorrhage or any central nervous system (CNS) abnormality
- Hypoglycemia (blood glucose level less than 40 mg/dL)

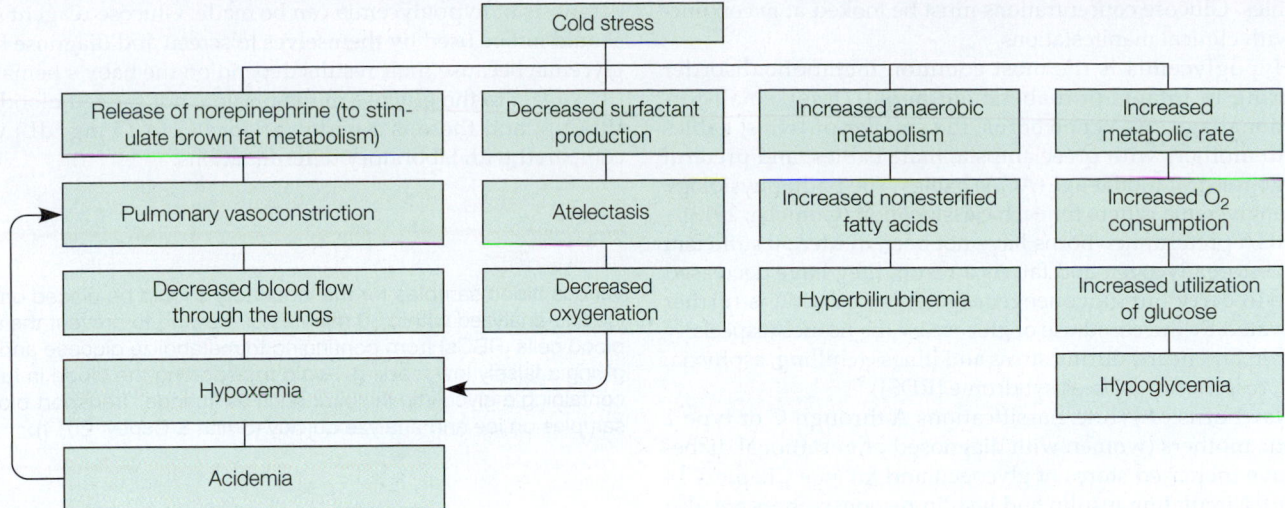

Figure 27–8 **Cold stress chain of events. The hypothermic, or cold-stressed, newborn attempts to compensate by conserving heat and increasing heat production.**

The metabolic consequences of cold stress can be devastating and potentially fatal to a newborn. Oxygen requirements rise; even before a change in temperature is noted, glucose use increases, acids are released into the bloodstream, and surfactant production decreases (Fanaroff & Fanaroff, 2013). The effects are graphically depicted in Figure 27–8.

Nursing Management

The amount of heat a newborn loses depends to a large extent on the actions of the nurse or caregiver. Prevention of heat loss is especially critical in the very-low-birth-weight (VLBW) baby. Use prewarmed blankets and prewarm all contact surfaces. Placing the VLBW newborn in a polyethylene wrapping immediately following birth can decrease the postnatal fall in temperature that normally occurs (Gardner & Hernandez, 2016). Using head coverings made of insulated fabrics, wool, or polyolefin can significantly decrease heat loss after childbirth (Blackburn, 2013). Convective, radiant, and evaporative heat loss can all be reduced. Swaddling and nesting maintain flexion, which reduces exposed surface area and thus convective and radiant losses.

Observe the baby for signs of cold stress. These include increased movements and respirations, decreased skin temperature and peripheral perfusion, development of hypoglycemia, and, possibly, development of metabolic acidosis.

Vasoconstriction is the initial response to cold stress; because it initially decreases skin temperature, the nurse should monitor and assess skin temperature instead of rectal temperature. A decrease in rectal temperature means that the baby has long-standing cold stress. Through monitoring of skin temperature, a possible decrease will become apparent before the baby's core temperature is affected. If a decrease in skin temperature is noted, determine whether hypoglycemia is present. Hypoglycemia is a result of the metabolic effects of cold stress and is suggested by glucometer values below 40 to 50 mg/dL, tremors, irritability or lethargy, apnea, or seizure activity.

If hypothermia occurs, the following nursing interventions should be initiated (Gomella, 2013):

- Maintain a neutral thermal environment (NTE); adjust based on the gestational age and postnatal age.
- Warm the newborn slowly because rapid temperature elevation may cause hypotension and apnea.

- Increase the air temperature in hourly increments of 1°C (33.8°F) until the newborn's temperature is stable.
- Monitor skin temperature every 15 to 30 minutes to determine if the newborn's temperature is increasing, assessing the temperature with the use of skin, axillary (most commonly utilized method), or infrared (IR) thermometers (Smith, Alcock, & Usher, 2013).
- Remove plastic wrap, caps, and heat shields while rewarming the baby so that cool air as well as warm air is not trapped.
- Warm IV fluids before infusion.
- Initiate efforts to block heat loss by evaporation, radiation, convection, and conduction (review ways to prevent heat loss in Chapter 23).
- Maintain the newborn in NTE.

If a decrease in skin temperature is noted, determine whether hypoglycemia is present. Attempts to burn brown fat increase oxygen consumption, lactic acid levels, and metabolic acidosis. Hypoglycemia may be reversed by adequate glucose intake, as described in the following section.

Care of the Newborn With Hypoglycemia

Hypoglycemia, low blood sugar, can affect 1 to 3 newborns per 1000 live births, and up to 15% of them are born growth restricted (Harris, Weston, & Harding, 2012; Smith & Carley, 2014). An operational threshold for intervention in newborn hypoglycemia is a plasma glucose concentration of less than 40 to 45 mg/dL at any time in any newborn. It requires a follow-up glucose measurement to document normal values (AAP & ACOG, 2012; Cloherty et al., 2012; Fanaroff & Fanaroff, 2013; Riley, Spencer, & Prater, 2014). Within the first hours of life, normal asymptomatic newborns may have a transient glucose level in the 30s (mg/dL) that will increase either spontaneously or with feedings. Plasma glucose values of less than 20 to 25 mg/dL should be treated with parenteral glucose D$_{10}$W, regardless of the age or gestation, to raise plasma glucose to greater than 45 mg/dL. There is no absolute threshold that can be applied to all babies. Glucose concentrations must be looked at in conjunction with clinical manifestations.

Hypoglycemia is the most common metabolic disorder occurring in infants of diabetic mothers (IDMs), small-for-gestational-age (SGA) newborns, the smaller of twins, babies born to mothers with preeclampsia, male babies, and preterm average-for-gestational-age (AGA) babies. The pathophysiology of hypoglycemia differs for each classification (Gomella, 2013).

AGA preterm newborns have not been in utero a sufficient time to store glycogen and fat. As a result, they have decreased ability to carry out gluconeogenesis. This situation is further aggravated by increased use of glucose by the tissues (especially the brain and heart) during stress and illness (chilling, asphyxia, sepsis, respiratory distress syndrome [RDS]).

Newborns of White classifications A through C or type 1 diabetic mothers (women with diagnosed or gestational diabetes) have increased stores of glycogen and fat (see Chapters 14 and 26). Circulating insulin and insulin responsiveness are also higher when compared with other newborns. Because the high glucose loads present in utero stop at birth, the newborn experiences rapid and profound hypoglycemia (Blackburn, 2013). Newborns with recurrent episodes of hypoglycemia may have long-term neurologic deficits (Harris et al., 2012).

The SGA newborn has used up glycogen and fat stores because of intrauterine malnutrition and has a blunted hepatic enzymatic response with which to produce and use glucose. Any newborn stressed at birth from asphyxia or cold also quickly uses up available glucose stores and becomes hypoglycemic. In addition, epidural anesthesia may alter maternal–fetal glucose homeostasis, resulting in hypoglycemia.

Clinical Therapy

The goal of management includes early identification of hypoglycemia through observation and screening of newborns at risk (Fanaroff & Fanaroff, 2013; Gomella, 2013; Harris et al., 2012). The newborn may be asymptomatic, or any of the following may occur:

- Lethargy, apathy, and limpness
- Poor feeding, poor sucking reflex, vomiting
- Pallor, cyanosis
- Hypothermia or temperature instability
- Apnea, irregular respirations, respiratory distress
- Tremors, jerkiness, jitteriness, seizure activity
- High-pitched cry (Cloherty et al., 2012)
- Exaggerated Moro reflex
- Temperature instability

Universal blood glucose screening before clinical signs develop is not recommended by the AAP (Committee on the Fetus and Newborn & Adamkin, 2011). Aggressive treatment is recommended after a single low blood glucose value if the baby shows any of these symptoms. In at-risk newborns, routine screening should be done frequently during the first hours of life and then whenever any of the noted clinical manifestations appear or at 1- to 4-hour intervals until the risk period has passed.

Hypoglycemia may also be defined as a *glucose oxidase reagent strip with reflectance meter* below 40 mg/dL, but only when corroborated with laboratory plasma glucose testing. Point-of-care testing (POCT) methods use whole blood, an enzymatic reagent strip, and a reflectance meter or color chart. Bedside glucose oxidase strip tests can screen for hypoglycemia, but laboratory determinations *must confirm* the results before a

diagnosis of hypoglycemia can be made. Glucose reagent strips should not be used by themselves to screen and diagnose hypoglycemia because their results depend on the baby's hematocrit (they react to the glucose in the plasma, not the red blood cells [RBCs]), and there is a wide variance (5 to 15 mg/dL) when compared with laboratory determinations.

Clinical Tip

Venous blood samples for the laboratory should be placed on ice and analyzed within 30 minutes of drawing to prevent the red blood cells (RBCs) from continuing to metabolize glucose and giving a falsely low reading. Avoid transporting the blood in tubes containing a glycolytic inhibitor such as fluoride. Transport blood samples on ice and analyze quickly (Smith & Carley, 2014).

Blood glucose sampling techniques can significantly affect the accuracy of the blood glucose value. It is important to note that whole blood glucose concentrations are 10% to 15% lower than plasma glucose concentrations (Cloherty et al., 2012). The higher the hematocrit, the greater the difference between whole blood and plasma values. Also, venous blood glucose concentrations are approximately 15% to 19% lower than arterial blood glucose concentrations because the tissues extract some glucose before the blood enters the venous system. Newer point-of-care techniques, such as using a glucose oxidase analyzer or an optical bedside glucose analyzer, are more reliable for bedside screening but must also be validated with laboratory chemical analysis.

Adequate caloric intake is important. Early formula-feeding or breastfeeding is one of the major approaches for preventing hypoglycemia. If early feeding or IV glucose is started to meet the recommended fluid and caloric needs, the blood glucose concentration is likely to remain above the hypoglycemic level. During the first hours after birth, asymptomatic newborns may also be given oral glucose contained in formula or breast milk (glucose water should not be used because it causes a rapid increase in glucose followed by an abrupt decrease), and then another plasma glucose measurement is obtained within 30 to 60 minutes after feeding.

IV infusions of a dextrose solution D_5W to $D_{10}W$ (5% to 10%) begun immediately after birth should prevent hypoglycemia. Plasma glucose levels are obtained when the parenteral infusion is started. However, in the very small AGA newborn, infusions of 10% dextrose solution may cause hyperglycemia to develop, requiring an alteration in the glucose concentration. An IV glucose solution should be calculated based on the baby's body weight and fluid requirements and correlated with blood glucose tests to determine adequacy of the infusion treatment.

In more severe cases of hypoglycemia, corticosteroids may be administered. It is thought that steroids enhance gluconeogenesis from noncarbohydrate protein sources (Gomella, 2013; Smith & Carley, 2014).

Nursing Management

For the Newborn With Hypoglycemia

Nursing Assessment and Diagnosis

The objectives of nursing assessment are to identify newborns at risk and to screen symptomatic babies. For newborns diagnosed with hypoglycemia, assessment is ongoing and includes careful monitoring of glucose values. Glucose strips, urine dipstick, and urine volume tests (monitor only if above 1 to 3 mL/kg/hr) may be evaluated frequently for osmotic diuresis and glycosuria.

Nursing diagnoses that may apply to the newborn with hypoglycemia include the following (NANDA-I © 2014):

- *Nutrition, Imbalanced: Less than Body Requirements,* related to increased glucose use secondary to physiologic stress
- *Breathing Pattern, Ineffective,* related to tachypnea and apnea
- *Pain, Acute,* related to frequent heel sticks secondary to glucose monitoring

Nursing Plan and Implementation

Monitor all at-risk groups within 30 to 60 minutes after birth and before feedings or whenever abnormal clinical manifestations appear. Monitor the IDM within 30 minutes of birth. Once an at-risk newborn's blood sugar level is stable, glucose testing every 2 to 4 hours (or per agency protocol), or before feedings,

adequately monitors glucose levels. See *Clinical Skill: Performing a Heel Stick on a Newborn.*

The method of feeding greatly influences glucose and energy requirements; thus careful attention to glucose monitoring is again required during the transition from IV to oral feedings. Titration of IV glucose may be required until the newborn is able to take adequate amounts of formula or breast milk to maintain a normal blood sugar level. Titrate by decreasing the concentration of parenteral glucose gradually to 5% (D$_5$W), then reducing the rate of infusion (mg/kg/min) and slowly discontinuing it over 4 to 6 hours. Enteral feedings are increased to maintain an adequate glucose and caloric intake and maintain normal blood glucose levels.

Evaluation

Expected outcomes of nursing care include the following:

- The newborn at risk for hypoglycemia is identified, and prompt intervention is started.
- The newborn's glucose level is stabilized, and recovery is proceeding without sequelae.

Clinical Skill 27–1
Performing a Heel Stick on a Newborn

NURSING ACTION

Preparation

- Explain to parents what will be done.
- Select a clear, previously unpunctured site.

Rationale: The selection of a previously unpunctured site minimizes the risk of infection and excessive scar formation.

- The newborn's lateral heel is the site of choice because it precludes damaging the posterior tibial nerve and artery, the plantar artery, and the important longitudinally oriented fat pad of the heel, which in later years could impede walking (Figure 27–9). This is especially important for babies undergoing multiple heel-stick procedures. Toes are acceptable sites if necessary.

Equipment and Supplies

- Microlancet (do not use a needle)
- Alcohol swabs or other skin prep per agency protocol
- 2 × 2 sterile gauze squares
- Small bandage (may not use on premature newborn with extremely sensitive skin; instead, hold pressure until bleeding ceases)
- Transfer pipette or capillary tubes
- Glucose reagent strips or reflectance meters
- Gloves

Procedure: Clean Gloves

1. Apply gloves.

Rationale: A needle may nick the periosteum. Gloves are used to implement standard precautions and prevent nosocomial infections.

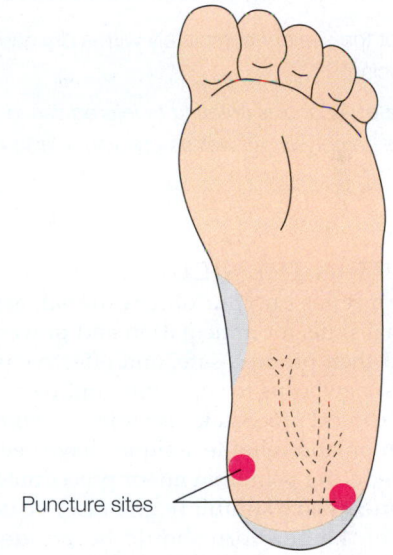

Puncture sites

Figure 27–9 Potential sites for heel sticks. Avoid shaded areas to prevent injury to arteries and nerves in the foot and the important longitudinally oriented fat pad of the heel, which in later years could impede walking.

2. Warming the baby's heel for 5 to 10 seconds to facilitate blood flow is controversial. Check agency policy.

Performing the Heel Stick

1. Grasp the newborn's foot in your nondominant hand so as to impede venous return slightly. Support the dorsum of the foot with your thumb and the ankle with your other fingers. This will facilitate extraction of the blood sample (Figure 27–10).

2. Clean the site by rubbing vigorously with 70% isopropyl alcohol swab or skin prep per agency.

Rationale: Friction produces local heat, which aids vasodilation.

(continued)

Clinical Skill 27–1 (*continued*)

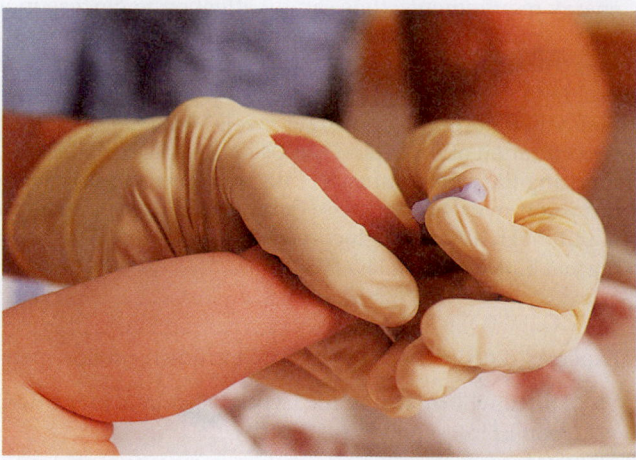

Figure 27–10 **Heel stick. With a quick, piercing motion, puncture the lateral heel with a microlancet. Be careful not to puncture too deeply.**

3. Blot the site dry completely with a dry gauze square before lancing.

Rationale: *Alcohol is irritating to injured tissue and it may also produce hemolysis, as well as causing a false low reading.*

4. With a quick, piercing motion, puncture the lateral heel with a microlancet. Be careful not to puncture too deeply. Optimal penetration is 4 mm.

5. Wipe the first drop of blood away with the gauze.

Rationale: *The first drop may be contaminated by skin contact and the blood cells may have been traumatized during the stick. Blood glucose may be lowered by residual alcohol.*

Collecting the Blood Sample

1. Use a transfer pipette to place a drop of blood on glucose reflectance meter or directly onto the Glucometer test strip.

2. Use capillary tube for hematocrit testing.

Preventing Excessive Bleeding

1. Apply a folded gauze square to the puncture site and secure it firmly with a bandage, or hold pressure until bleeding stops.

2. Check the puncture site frequently for the first hour after sampling.

Documentation: Record the findings in the newborn's electronic health record.

PAIN RELIEF IN THE NICU

The newborn relies on your observational, assessment, and interventional skills for anticipation and prevention of pain if possible and then prompt, safe, and effective pain relief. It is vital to assist newborns to cope with and recover from necessary painful clinical procedures. A variety of nonpharmacologic pain prevention and relief techniques have been shown to be effective in reducing pain from minor procedures in newborns.

Any unnecessary stimuli (e.g., noise, visual, tactile, and vestibular) of the newborn should be avoided, if possible. Developmental care, which includes limiting environmental stimuli, lateral positioning, the use of supportive bedding, and attention to behavioral cues, assists the newborn to cope with painful procedures (Gomella, 2013; Walden, 2014).

Containment with swaddling or facilitated tucking (holding the arms and legs in a flexed position) is effective in reducing excessive immature motor responses. Swaddling also may provide comfort through other senses, such as thermal, tactile, and proprioceptive senses. Breastfeeding and skin-to-skin contact with the mother during the painful procedure may help to relieve pain (Gomella, 2013; Walden, 2014).

Nonnutritive sucking (NNS) refers to the provision of a pacifier into the newborn's mouth to promote sucking without the provision of breast milk or formula for nutrition. NNS is thought to produce analgesia through stimulation of orotactile and mechanoreceptors when the pacifier is placed into the baby's mouth. Allowing nonnutritive sucking with a pacifier aids in the reduction of procedural pain and stress (Gomella, 2013; Walden, 2014).

A wide range of oral sucrose doses have been used for procedural pain relief (heel sticks, venipuncture, IM injections) but while no optimal dose has been established, a solution of 24% sucrose solution is agreed upon (Walden, 2014).

The sweetness of the sucrose, a disaccharide, elevates the pain threshold through endogenous opioid release in the CNS and produces a calming effect (Gomella, 2013; Walden, 2014).

Evaluation

Expected outcomes of nursing care include the following:

- The newborn at risk for hypoglycemia is identified, and prompt intervention is started.

- The newborn's glucose level is stabilized, and recovery is proceeding without sequelae.

Care of the Newborn With Jaundice

The most common abnormal physical finding in newborns is jaundice (*icterus neonatorum*). Some degree of jaundice, resulting from elevated unconjugated bilirubinemia, with total serum bilirubin levels greater than 5mg/dL, occurs in up to 80% of healthy newborns in the first 7 days following birth (Bhutani, Stark, Lazzeroni, et al., 2013; Gomella, 2013; Turnbull & Petty, 2012). **Jaundice** is a yellowish coloration of the skin and sclera of the eyes that develops from deposit of the yellow pigment bilirubin in lipid/fat-containing tissues. Fetal unconjugated (indirect) bilirubin is normally cleared by the placenta in utero, so total bilirubin at birth is usually less than 3 mg/dL unless an abnormal hemolytic process has been present. Postnatally, the newborn must conjugate bilirubin (convert a lipid-soluble pigment into a water-soluble pigment) in the liver.

The rate and amount of conjugation of bilirubin depend on the rate of hemolysis, the bilirubin load, the maturity of the liver, and the presence of albumin-binding sites. (See Chapter

23 for discussion of conjugation of bilirubin.) A normal, healthy, full-term newborn's liver is usually mature enough and produces enough glucuronyl transferase that the total serum bilirubin concentration does not reach a pathologic level. The diagnosis of pathologic jaundice is given to newborns who exhibit jaundice within the first 24 hours of life, have a total serum bilirubin concentration increase of greater than 0.2 mg/dL/hr, surpass the 95th percentile on the nomogram for age in hours, or have persistent visible jaundice after 1 week of age in term newborns or after 2 weeks in preterm newborns (Casey, 2013; Turnbull & Petty, 2012).

Pathophysiology of Hyperbilirubinemia

Serum albumin-binding sites are usually sufficient to conjugate enough bilirubin to meet the normal demands of the newborn. However, certain conditions such as fetal or neonatal asphyxia and neonatal drugs such as indomethacin can decrease the binding affinity of bilirubin to albumin, because acidosis impairs the capacity of albumin to hold bilirubin. Hypothermia and hypoglycemia release free fatty acids that dislocate bilirubin from albumin. Maternal medications such as sulfa drugs and salicylates compete with bilirubin for these sites. Finally, premature newborns have less albumin available for binding with bilirubin. Neurotoxicity is possible because unconjugated bilirubin has a high affinity for extravascular tissue, such as fatty tissue (subcutaneous tissue) and cerebral tissue.

Bilirubin not bound to albumin can cross the blood–brain barrier, damage cells of the CNS, and produce kernicterus or **acute bilirubin encephalopathy (ABE)**. **Kernicterus** (meaning "yellow nucleus") refers to the deposition of indirect or unconjugated bilirubin in the basal ganglia of the brain and to the permanent neurologic sequelae of untreated **hyperbilirubinemia** (elevation of bilirubin level) (Cloherty et al., 2012). The incidence is 0.5 to 2 per 100,000 live births (Maisels, 2012).

The classic acute bilirubin encephalopathy of kernicterus most commonly found with Rh and ABO blood group incompatibility is less common today because of aggressive treatment with phototherapy and exchange transfusions. Kernicterus cases are reappearing as a result of early discharge and the increased incidence of dehydration (as a result of discharge before the mother's milk is established). Unfortunately, current therapy cannot distinguish all newborns who are at risk. It is recommended that *all* newborns be screened for bilirubin level prior to leaving the hospital using total serum bilirubin (TSB) or transcutaneous bilirubin (TcB). It is also advised to record information on gestation, birth weight, bilirubin/albumin ratios, and risk factors (Maisels & Watchko, 2012).

Causes of Hyperbilirubinemia

A primary cause of hyperbilirubinemia is **hemolytic disease of the newborn**. All pregnant women who are Rh negative or who have blood type O (possible ABO blood incompatibility) should be asked about outcomes of any previous pregnancies and history of blood transfusion. Prenatal amniocentesis with spectrophotographic examination may be indicated in some cases. Cord blood from newborns is evaluated for bilirubin level, which normally does not exceed 5 mg/dL. Newborns of Rh-negative and O blood type mothers are carefully assessed for appearance of jaundice and levels of serum bilirubin.

Alloimmune hemolytic disease, also known as **erythroblastosis fetalis**, occurs when an Rh-negative mother is pregnant with an Rh-positive fetus and maternal antibodies cross the placenta.

Maternal antibodies enter the fetal circulation, then attach to and destroy the fetal red blood cells (RBCs). The fetal system responds by increasing RBC production. Jaundice, anemia, and compensatory erythropoiesis result. Because of the widespread use of Rh immune globulin (RhoGAM), the incidence of erythroblastosis fetalis has dropped dramatically (Turnbull & Petty, 2012).

Hydrops fetalis, the most severe form of erythroblastosis fetalis, occurs when maternal antibodies attach to the Rh site on the fetal RBCs, making them susceptible to destruction; severe anemia and multiorgan system failure result. Cardiomegaly with severe cardiac decompensation and hepatosplenomegaly occurs. Severe generalized massive edema (anasarca) and generalized fluid effusion into the pleural cavity (hydrothorax), pericardial sac, and peritoneal cavity (ascites) develops. Jaundice is not present until the newborn period because the bilirubin pigments are excreted through the placenta into the maternal circulation. The hydropic hemolytic disease process is also characterized by hyperplasia of the pancreatic islets, which predisposes the newborn to neonatal hypoglycemia similar to that of infants of diabetic mothers (IDMs). These babies have increased bleeding tendencies because of associated thrombocytopenia and hypoxic damage to the capillaries. Hydrops is a frequent cause of intrauterine death among fetuses with Rh disease.

ABO incompatibility (the mother is blood type O and the baby is blood type A or B) may result in jaundice, although it rarely results in hemolytic disease severe enough to be clinically diagnosed and treated. Hepatosplenomegaly may be found occasionally in newborns with ABO incompatibility, but hydrops fetalis and stillbirth are rare.

Developing Cultural Competence Ethnic Variations and Jaundice

East Asian newborns (Japanese, Chinese, and Filipino ethnic groups) have a higher occurrence of hyperbilirubinemia than White newborns. In addition, newborns with Asian fathers and Caucasian mothers have a higher incidence of jaundice than if both parents are White. Other ethnic groups at risk for increased bilirubinemia are Navajo, Eskimo, and Sioux Native American newborns; Greek newborns; Sephardic-Jewish newborns; and some Hispanic newborns. The incidence is lower in African Americans (Gomella, 2013).

During pregnancy, predisposing maternal conditions include hereditary spherocytosis, diabetes, intrauterine infections, gram-negative bacilli infections that stimulate production of maternal alloimmune antibodies, drug ingestion (such as sulfas, salicylates, novobiocin, and diazepam), and oxytocin administration. Early prenatal identification of the fetus at risk for Rh or ABO incompatibility allows prompt treatment. (See Chapter 15 for discussion of in utero management of this condition.)

The prognosis for a newborn with hyperbilirubinemia depends on the extent of the hemolytic process and the underlying cause. Severe hemolytic disease may result in fetal or early neonatal death from the effects of anemia—cardiac decompensation, edema, ascites, and hydrothorax. Hyperbilirubinemia may lead to kernicterus if not aggressively treated. The initial symptoms requiring acute intervention of an exchange transfusion are poor tone, lethargy, and/or feeding/sucking issues (Kamath-Rayne, Thio, Deacon, et al., 2016). Continuing worsening progression includes neurologic damage, which may cause death, cerebral palsy, cognitive impairment, or hearing loss/nerve deafness, or, to a lesser degree, perceptual impairment, delayed speech development, hyperactivity, muscle incoordination, or learning difficulties (Kamath-Rayne et al., 2016). Intravenous gamma globulin (IVIG) may be used with newborns suffering from isoimmune hemolytic disease, 1 g/kg over 4 hours and repeated in 12 hours if required (Gomella, 2013).

Clinical Therapy

LABORATORY AND DIAGNOSTIC ASSESSMENTS

The best treatment for hemolytic disease is prevention by early recognition of prenatal risk factors such as Rh and ABO incompatibility (see Chapter 15 for discussion of in utero management of these conditions), and attention to certain neonatal clinical conditions. Neonatal hyperbilirubinemia must be considered pathologic and requires further investigation if any of the following criteria are met (Bhutani, Johnson, & Keren, 2004; Gomella, 2013):

1. Clinically evident jaundice appears before 24 hours of life or jaundice seems excessive for the newborn's age in hours.

2. Serum bilirubin concentration rises by more than 0.2 mg/dL per hour.

3. Total serum bilirubin concentration exceeds the 95th percentile on the nomogram.

4. Conjugated bilirubin concentrations are greater than 2 mg/dL or more than 20% of the total serum bilirubin concentration.

5. Clinical jaundice persists for more than 8 days in a term newborn and 14 days in a preterm newborn (Cloherty et al., 2012).

Initial diagnostic procedures are aimed at differentiating jaundice resulting from increased bilirubin production, impaired conjugation or excretion, increased intestinal reabsorption, or a combination of these factors.

Transcutaneous bilirubin (TcB) measurements are a noninvasive method of assessing bilirubin levels and may be used for predischarge risk assessment (Figure 27–11). A TcB can be performed quickly and painlessly, and repeated measures are easily obtained. A TcB can quantify the amount of bilirubin pigment in the newborn's skin. Nurses need to measure bilirubin levels to confirm the presence, absence, or suspicion of jaundice. However, it is important to remember that total serum bilirubin (TSB) levels remain the standard of care for confirmation or diagnosis of hyperbilirubinemia (Maisels & Watchko, 2012).

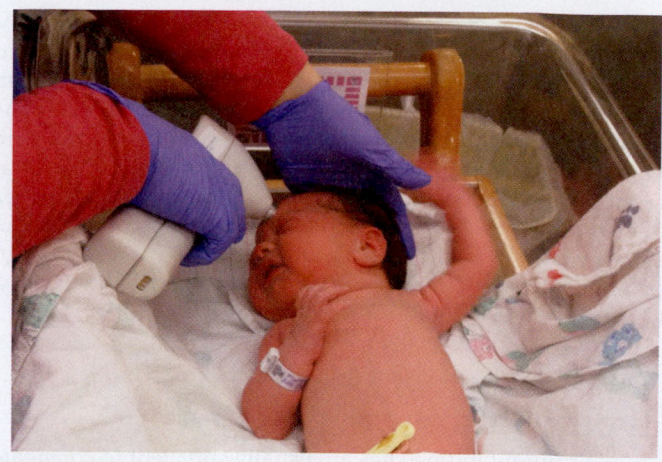

Figure 27–11 A newborn being screened with a transcutaneous bilirubinometer.

SOURCE: Lisa Smith-Pedersen, RN, MSN, NNP-BC.

Because of the shorter lifespan of RBCs in the newborn, a significant bilirubin load is produced. When bilirubin breaks down, carbon monoxide (CO) is released. This production of carbon monoxide is being investigated as a marker in the study of bilirubin production. Measuring end-tidal CO (ETCO) has been shown to provide results similar to laboratory bilirubin; however, devices to measure CO are not widely available (Cloherty et al., 2012).

Essential laboratory evaluations are Coombs test, serum bilirubin levels (direct and total), hemoglobin, reticulocyte percentage, white cell count, and positive smear for cellular morphology.

The Coombs test (DAT-direct antiglobulin) is performed to determine whether jaundice is because of Rh or ABO incompatibility. The indirect Coombs test measures the amount of Rh-positive antibodies in the mother's blood. Rh-positive red blood cells are added to the maternal blood sample. If the mother's serum contains antibodies, the Rh-positive red blood cells will agglutinate (clump) when rabbit immune antiglobulin is added, which is a positive test result. The direct Coombs test reveals the presence of antibody-coated (sensitized) Rh-positive red blood cells in the newborn. Rabbit immune antiglobulin is added to the specimen of neonatal blood cells. If the neonatal red blood cells agglutinate, they have been coated with maternal antibodies, a positive result.

If the hemolytic process is caused by Rh sensitization, laboratory findings reveal the following: (1) an Rh-positive newborn with a positive Coombs test; (2) increased erythropoiesis with many immature circulating red blood cells (nucleated blastocysts); (3) anemia, in most cases; (4) elevated levels (5 mg/dL or more) of bilirubin in cord blood; and (5) a reduction in albumin-binding capacity. Maternal data may include an elevated anti-Rh titer and spectrophotometric evidence of a fetal hemolytic process.

If the hemolytic process is caused by ABO incompatibility, laboratory findings reveal an increase in reticulocytes. The resulting anemia is usually not significant during the newborn period and is rare later on. The direct Coombs test may be negative or mildly positive, whereas the indirect Coombs test may be strongly positive. Newborns with a positive direct Coombs test have increased incidence of jaundice, with bilirubin levels in excess of 10 mg/dL. Increased numbers of spherocytes

Clinical Tip

The transcutaneous bilirubinometer (TcB) is a noninvasive screening tool that can be utilized on all newborns (except those receiving phototherapy) prior to discharge, at any time during hospitalization, or at a follow-up visit at the pediatrician's office. Any elevated results need to be verified with a total serum bilirubin level (TsB). Results are found to be within 2 to 3 mg/dL of the TsB. Depending on the manufacturer, the recommendation is to test on the forehead or the sternum of the neonate (Bosschaart, Kok, Newsum, et al., 2012; Maisels, 2012; Mantagou, Fouzas, Skylogianni, et al., 2012; Wolff, Schinasi, Lavelle, et al., 2012).

(spherical, plump, mature erythrocytes) are seen on a peripheral blood smear. Increased numbers of spherocytes are not seen on blood smears from Rh disease babies.

THERAPEUTIC MANAGEMENT

Whatever the cause of hyperbilirubinemia, management of these newborns is directed toward alleviating anemia, removing maternal antibodies and sensitized erythrocytes, increasing serum albumin levels, reducing serum bilirubin levels, and minimizing the consequences of hyperbilirubinemia. Early discharge of newborns from birthing centers has significantly influenced the diagnosis and management of neonatal jaundice, increasing the emphasis on outpatient and home care management.

If hemolytic disease is present, it may be treated with phototherapy, exchange transfusion, and drug therapy. When determining the appropriate management of hyperbilirubinemia caused by hemolytic disease, the three relevant variables are the newborn's (1) serum bilirubin level, (2) birth weight, and (3) age in hours. If a newborn has hemolysis with an unconjugated bilirubin level of 14 mg/dL, weighs less than 2500 g (5.5 lb) (birth weight), and is 24 hours old or less, an exchange transfusion may be the best management. However, if that same newborn is over 24 hours of age, which is past the time during which an increase in bilirubin would occur because of pathologic causes, phototherapy may be the treatment of choice to prevent the possible complication of kernicterus.

PHOTOTHERAPY

Phototherapy is the exposure of the newborn to high-intensity light. It may be used alone or in conjunction with an exchange transfusion to reduce serum bilirubin levels. Exposure of the newborn to high-intensity light (a bank of fluorescent light bulbs, LEDs [light-emitting diodes], or bulbs in the blue-light spectrum) decreases serum bilirubin levels in the skin by facilitating biliary excretion of unconjugated bilirubin. Phototherapy decreases serum bilirubin levels by changing bilirubin from the non–water-soluble (lipophilic) form to water-soluble by-products that can then be excreted via urine and bile. Photoisomerization occurs when the natural form of bilirubin is exposed to light at a certain wavelength and the bilirubin is converted to a less toxic form. The new isomer, photobilirubin, is created rapidly but is quite unstable. The photobilirubin is bound to albumin, transported to the liver, and incorporated into bile. If it is not quickly eliminated from the bowel, it can convert back to its original form and return to the bloodstream. In addition, the photodegradation products formed when light oxidizes bilirubin can be excreted in the urine.

Phototherapy is an intervention that is used to prevent hyperbilirubinemia in order to halt bilirubin levels from climbing dangerously high. The decision to start phototherapy is based on two factors: gestational age and age in hours. Phototherapy does not alter the underlying cause of jaundice, and hemolysis may continue to produce anemia. Many authors have recommended initiating phototherapy "prophylactically" in the first 24 hours of life in high-risk, very-low-birth-weight (VLBW), or severely bruised, newborns. The risk category of newborns requiring follow-up/intervention for their hyperbilirubinemia is evaluated by plotting their serum bilirubin level and age in hours on a nomogram. Phototherapy is not benign; especially in the preterm neonate, it has been attributed to destruction of platelets, hemolysis, and prolonged patency of the fetal ductus arteriosus (Hintz, Stevenson, Yao, et al., 2011).

Clinical Tip

When excreted, the newborn's urine will be much darker in color/appearance because of the excreted higher conjugated bilirubin content.

Phototherapy can be provided by conventional banks of fluorescent tube phototherapy lights, by a fiberoptic blanket attached to a halogen light source around the trunk of the newborn, by a fiberoptic mattress placed under the baby, or by a combination of these delivery methods. Levels should continue to decline when phototherapy covers a wider surface area. If a drop in bilirubin levels is not reached, then an exchange transfusion should be considered. Most phototherapy units will provide this level of irradiance 45 to 50 cm below the lamps. The nurse can use a photometer to measure and maintain desired irradiance levels. The nurse keeps track of the number of hours each lamp is used so that each can be replaced before its effectiveness is lost (Bhutani & Committee on the Fetus and Newborn, 2011). Disadvantages of lights are that they create a difficult work environment and can distort a baby's color. See *Clinical Skill: Newborn Receiving Phototherapy*).

EXCHANGE TRANSFUSION

Exchange transfusion is the withdrawal and replacement of the newborn's blood with donor blood. It is used to treat anemia with red blood cells that are susceptible to maternal antibodies, to remove sensitized red blood cells that would soon be lysed, to remove serum bilirubin, to provide bilirubin-free albumin, and to increase the binding sites for bilirubin. Concerns about exchange transfusion are related to the use of blood products and the associated potential for HIV infection and hepatitis. If the TSB is at or approaching the exchange level, blood should be sent for immediate type and crossmatch. Blood for exchange transfusion is modified whole blood (red cells and plasma) crossmatched against the mother and compatible with the newborn.

Nursing Management
For the Newborn With Jaundice

Nursing Assessment and Diagnosis

Assessment is aimed at identifying prenatal and perinatal factors that predispose the newborn to the development of jaundice and at recognizing the jaundice as soon as it is apparent. Significant hyperbilirubinemia in the neonatal population is often due to a multitude of causes including a genetic basis. Clinically, ABO incompatibility presents as jaundice and occasionally as hepatosplenomegaly. Fetal hydrops or erythroblastosis is rare (see Chapter 15). Hemolytic disease of the newborn is suspected if one or more of the following are evident:

- The placenta is enlarged.
- The newborn is edematous, with pleural and pericardial effusion plus ascites.
- Pallor or jaundice is noted during the first 24 to 36 hours.
- Hemolytic anemia is diagnosed.
- The spleen and liver are enlarged.

Note changes in behavior and observe for evidence of bleeding. If laboratory tests indicate elevated bilirubin levels, check

Clinical Skill 27–2
Newborn Receiving Phototherapy

NURSING ACTION

Preparation

- Explain the purpose of phototherapy, the procedure itself (including the need to use eye patches), and possible side effects such as dehydration and skin breakdown from more frequent stooling.

- Note evidence of jaundice in the skin, sclera, and mucous membranes (in newborns with darkly pigmented skin). Be sure that recent serum bilirubin levels are available.

Rationale: The decision to use phototherapy is based on a careful assessment of the newborn's condition over a period of time. The most recent results before starting therapy serve as a baseline to evaluate the effectiveness of therapy.

Equipment and Supplies

- Bank of phototherapy lights
- Eye patches
- Small scale to weigh diapers

Procedure

1. Obtain vital signs including axillary temperature.

Rationale: Provides baseline data.

2. Remove all of the baby's clothing except the diaper (keep genitals covered).

Rationale: Exposure of the newborn to high-intensity light (a bank of fluorescent light bulbs or bulbs in the blue-white spectrum) decreases serum bilirubin levels in the skin by aiding biliary excretion of unconjugated bilirubin. Because the tissue absorbs the light, best results are obtained when there is maximum skin surface exposure.

3. Apply eye coverings (eye patches or a Bili mask) to the baby according to agency policy (Figure 27–12).

Rationale: Eye coverings are used because it is not known if phototherapy injures delicate eye structures, particularly the retina.

4. Place the newborn in an open crib or isolette (more commonly used in preterm babies and babies who are sicker) about 45 to 50 cm below the bank of phototherapy lights. Reposition every 2 hours (Gomella, 2013).

Rationale: The isolette helps the newborn maintain body temperature while undressed. Repositioning exposes different areas of skin to the lights, prevents the development of pressure areas on the skin, and varies the stimulation the baby receives.

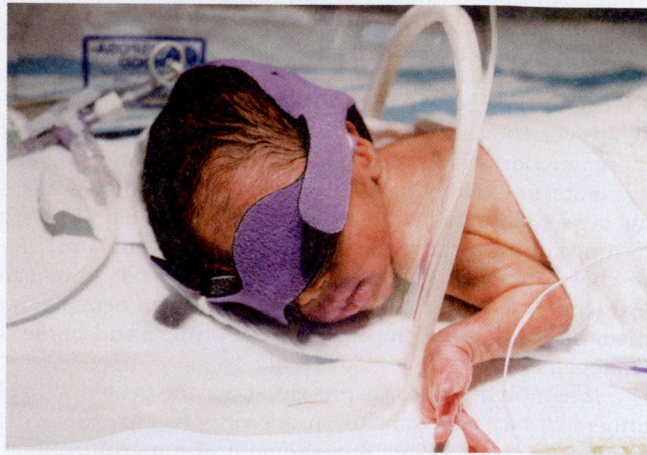

Figure 27–12 Newborn receiving phototherapy. The phototherapy light is positioned over the incubator. Bilateral eye patches are always used during phototherapy to protect the baby's eyes.
SOURCE: Lisa Smith-Pedersen, RN, MSN, NNP-BC.

5. Monitor vital signs every 4 hours with axillary temperatures.

Rationale: Temperature assessment is indicated to detect hypothermia or hyperthermia. Deviation in pulse and respirations may indicate developing complications.

6. Check the lights using a bilimeter to ensure safe, effective treatment.

7. Cluster care activities.

8. Discontinue phototherapy and remove eye patches at least every 2 to 3 hours when feeding the baby and when the parents visit.

Rationale: Care activities are clustered to help ensure that the newborn has maximum time under the lights. Eye patches are removed to assess for signs of complications such as excessive pressure, discharge, or conjunctivitis. Patches are also removed to provide some social stimulation and to promote parental attachment.

9. Maintain adequate fluid intake. Evaluate need for IV fluids.

10. Monitor intake and output (I&O) carefully. Weigh diapers before discarding. Record quantity and characteristics of each stool.

Rationale: Newborns undergoing phototherapy treatment have increased water loss and loose stools as a result of bilirubin excretion. This increases their risk of dehydration.

11. Assess specific gravity with each voiding. Weigh newborn daily.

Rationale: Specific gravity provides one measure of urine concentration. Highly concentrated urine is associated with a dehydrated state. Weight loss is also a sign of developing dehydration in the newborn.

12. Observe the baby for signs of perianal excoriation and institute therapy if it develops.

Rationale: Perianal excoriation may develop because of the irritating effect of diarrhea stools.

13. Ensure that serum bilirubin levels are drawn regularly according to orders or agency policy. Turn the phototherapy lights off while the blood is drawn.

Rationale: Serum bilirubin levels provide the most accurate indication of the effectiveness of phototherapy. They are generally drawn every 12 hours but at least once daily. The phototherapy lights are turned off to ensure accurate serum bilirubin levels.

14. Examine the newborn's skin regularly for signs of developing pressure areas, bronzing, maculopapular rash, and changes in degree of jaundice.

Rationale: Pressure areas may develop if the baby lies in one position for an extended period. A benign, transient bronze discoloration of the skin may occur with phototherapy when the newborn has elevated direct serum bilirubin levels or liver disease. A maculopapular rash is another transient side effect of phototherapy that develops occasionally.

15. Avoid using lotion or ointment on the exposed skin.

Rationale: Lotions and ointments on a newborn receiving phototherapy may cause skin burns.

16. Provide parents with opportunities to hold the newborn and assist in the baby's care. Answer their questions accurately and keep them informed of developments or changes.

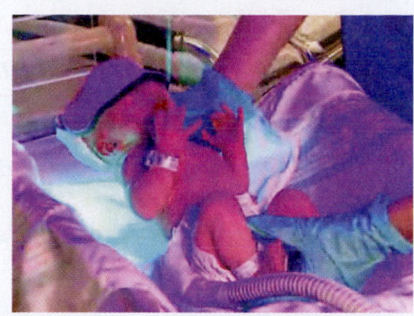

Figure 27–13 Newborn on fiberoptic "bili" mattress and under phototherapy lights. A combination of fiberoptic light source mattress and standard phototherapy light source may also be used.

NOTE: The color is distorted because of the reflection of the bililight mattress.

Rationale: A sick newborn is a source of great anxiety for parents. Information helps them deal with their anxiety. Moreover, they have a right to be kept well informed of their baby's status so that they are able to make informed decisions as needed.

17. May also provide phototherapy using lightweight, fiberoptic blankets ("bili blankets"). The baby is wrapped in the blanket, which is plugged into an outlet (Figure 27–13).

Rationale: With fiberoptic blankets the newborn is readily accessible for care, feedings, and diaper changes. The baby does not get overheated, and fluid and weight loss are not complications of this system. The baby is accessible to the parents and the procedure seems less alarming to parents than standard phototherapy.

the newborn for jaundice about every 2 hours and record observations.

To check for jaundice in lighter-skinned babies, blanch the skin over a bony prominence (forehead, nose, sternum) by pressing firmly with the thumb. After pressure is released, if jaundice is present, the area appears yellow before normal color returns. Check oral mucosa and the posterior portion of the hard palate and conjunctival sacs for yellow pigmentation in darker-skinned babies. Jaundice progresses in a cephalocaudal direction from the face to the trunk and then to the lower extremities. The overall progression of jaundice should be noted. Assessment in daylight gives the best results, because pink walls and surroundings may mask yellowish tints and yellow light makes differentiation of jaundice difficult. The time at onset of jaundice is recorded and reported. If jaundice appears, careful observation of the increase in depth of color and of the newborn's behavior is mandatory.

Assess the newborn's behavior for neurologic signs associated with hyperbilirubinemia, which are rare but may include hypotonia, diminished reflexes, lethargy, or seizures.

Nursing diagnoses that may apply to care of a newborn with jaundice include those discussed in *Nursing Care Plan:*

For the Newborn With Hyperbilirubinemia and the following (NANDA-I © 2014):

- *Injury, Risk for,* related to use of phototherapy
- *Neurovascular Dysfunction: Peripheral, Risk for,* related to neurologic damage secondary to kernicterus

Nursing Plan and Implementation

HOSPITAL-BASED NURSING CARE

Hospital-based care is described in *Nursing Care Plan: For the Newborn with Hyperbilirubinemia.*

Phototherapy success is measured every 12 hours or daily by serum bilirubin levels (more frequently if there is hemolysis or a higher level before initiation of phototherapy). The phototherapy lights must be turned off while drawing blood for serum bilirubin levels. Because it is not known whether phototherapy injures the delicate eye structures, particularly the retina, apply eye patches over the newborn's closed eyes during exposure to banks of phototherapy lights (see Figure 27–12). Discontinue conventional phototherapy and remove the eye

Nursing Care Plan: For the Newborn With Hyperbilirubinemia

1. Nursing Diagnosis: *Tissue Integrity, Impaired,* related to predisposing factors associated with hyperbilirubinemia (NANDA-I © 2014)

GOAL: Newborns at risk for jaundice and early signs of jaundice will be identified.

INTERVENTION	RATIONALE
• Evaluate newborn's history for predisposing factors for hyperbilirubinemia.	• Early identification of risk factors enables the nurse to monitor newborns for early signs of hyperbilirubinemia. Acidosis, hypoxia, and hypothermia increase the risk of hyperbilirubinemia at lower bilirubin levels.
• Observe color of amniotic fluid at time of rupture of membranes.	• Amber-colored amniotic fluid indicates hyperbilirubinemia.
• Assess baby for developing jaundice in daylight if possible.	• Early detection is affected by nursery environment. Artificial lights (with pink tint) may mask beginning of jaundice.
1. Observe sclera.	1. Most visible sign of hyperbilirubinemia is jaundice noted in skin, sclera, or oral mucosa. Onset is first seen on face and then progresses down the trunk.
2. Observe skin color and assess by blanching.	2. Blanching the skin leaves a yellow color to the skin immediately after pressure is released.
3. Check oral mucosa, posterior portion of hard palate, and conjunctival sacs for yellow pigmentation in dark-skinned newborns.	3. Underlying pigment of dark-skinned babies may normally appear yellow.
• Report jaundice occurring within 24 hours of birth.	

EXPECTED OUTCOME: Newborn's jaundice is identified early.

2. Nursing Diagnosis: *Fluid Volume: Imbalanced, Risk for,* related to phototherapy (NANDA-I © 2014)

GOAL: The newborn will not exhibit signs of dehydration and will display appropriate weight gain.

INTERVENTION	RATIONALE
• Offer feedings every 2–3 hr.	• Adequate hydration increases peristalsis and excretion of bilirubin.
• Breastfeed on demand with no supplementation unless excessive weight loss or increasing total serum bilirubin (TSB) with adequate feeding.	
• Provide 25% extra fluid intake.	• Replace fluid losses due to watery stools, if under phototherapy.
• Assess for dehydration:	• Phototherapy treatment may cause liquid stools and increased insensible water loss, which increases risk of dehydration.
1. Poor skin turgor	
2. Depressed fontanelles	
3. Sunken eyes	
4. Decreased urine output	
5. Weight loss	
6. Changes in electrolytes	
• Monitor intake and output (I&O).	
• Weigh daily.	
• Report signs of dehydration.	
• Administer IV fluids:	

INTERVENTION	RATIONALE
1. Monitor flow rates.	• Prevents fluid overload.
2. Assess insertion sites for signs of infection.	• IV fluids may be used if baby is dehydrated or in presence of other complications. IV may be started if exchange transfusion is to be done.

EXPECTED OUTCOMES: Newborn will have good skin turgor, clear amber urine output of 1–3 mL/kg/hr, and six to eight wet diapers/day, and will maintain weight.

---

3. Nursing Diagnosis: *Injury, Risk for,* **related to use of phototherapy (NANDA-I © 2014)**

GOAL: Newborn will not have any corneal irritation/drainage, skin breakdown, or major fluctuations in temperature.

INTERVENTION	RATIONALE
• Cover baby's eyes with eye patches while under phototherapy lights. Cover testes/penis in boys.	• Protects retina from damage due to high intensity light and testes from damage from heat.
• Make certain that eyelids are closed before applying eye patches.	• Prevents corneal abrasions.
• Remove baby from under phototherapy and remove eye patches during feedings.	• Provides visual stimulation and facilitates attachment behaviors.
• Inspect eyes each shift for conjunctivitis, drainage, and corneal abrasions due to irritation from eye patches.	• Prevents or facilitates prompt treatment of purulent conjunctivitis.
• Administer thorough perianal cleansing with each stool or change of perianal protective covering.	• Frequent stooling increases risk of skin breakdown. Prevents infection.
• Provide minimal coverage—only of diaper area.	• Provides maximal exposure. Shielded areas become more jaundiced, so maximum exposure is essential.
• Avoid the use of oily applications on the skin.	• Prevents superficial burns to skin.
• Reposition baby every 2 hr.	• Provides equal exposure of all skin areas and prevents pressure areas.
• Observe for bronzing of skin.	• Bronzing is related to use of phototherapy with increased direct bilirubin levels or liver damage; may last for 2–4 months.
• Place Plexiglas shield between baby and light.	• Hypothermia and hyperthermia are common complications of phototherapy.
• Monitor baby's skin and core temperature frequently until temperature is stable.	• Hypothermia results from exposure to lights, subsequent radiation, and convection losses.
• Check axillary temperature with readings on servo-controlled unit on incubator.	• Hyperthermia may result from the increased environmental heat.
• Regulate incubator temperature as needed.	• Additional heat from phototherapy lights frequently causes a rise in the baby's and incubator's temperatures.
	• Fluctuations in temperature may occur in response to radiation and convection.

EXPECTED OUTCOMES: Newborn's eyes are protected, skin is intact, and baby maintains a stable temperature.

---

4. Nursing Diagnosis: *Parenting, Risk for Impaired,* **related to deficient knowledge of infant care and prolonged separation of newborn and parents secondary to illness (NANDA-I © 2014)**

GOALS: Parents will bond with newborn and have realistic expectations about their baby. Parents are comfortable taking their baby home. They are able to demonstrate normal newborn/infant care and assessments of possible complications, and they know when to return for follow-up.

(continued)

Nursing Care Plan: For the Newborn With Hyperbilirubinemia (continued)

INTERVENTION	RATIONALE
• Encourage parents to provide tactile stimulation during feeding and diaper changes.	• Newborn has normal needs for tactile stimulation.
	• Presence of equipment may discourage parents from interacting with baby.
• Encourage cuddling and eye contact during feedings.	• Provides opportunity for parents to bond with their baby.
• Offer suggestions to comfort restless newborn:	• Provides comfort and decreases sensory deprivation.
• Nesting when beneath bili lights	
• Talking softly and singing quietly to baby	
• Taped music or tape recording of evening activities from home	
• Rhythmic patting of buttocks	
• Firm, nonstroking touch, assisting with control of extremities	
• Pacifier for nonnutritive sucking	
• Encourage family/friend support of mother/parents (e.g., meals, rest, child care for siblings; allow expressions of concerns/feelings).	• Decreases strain on mother/parents by assisting with other responsibilities and allows for additional time with newborn for, e.g., bonding, care.
• Evaluate additional psychosocial needs.	• Parents may not understand what is happening or why.
• Discuss rationale for treatment and possible side effects of phototherapy with family (stool changes, increased fluid loss, possible temp instability, slight lethargy, rash, altered sleep–wake patterns).	• Healthcare provider preference of treatment modalities may vary. Parents may not understand why their newborn is not receiving a treatment that another with the same condition is receiving.
• Instruct family on baby's care while undergoing phototherapy:	
• Safety precautions—bili mask (to protect eyes), incubator door closed and latched, covering genitalia per policy.	
• Skin care, cord care, circumcision care as appropriate.	
• Lab draws, rationale I&O.	
• Encourage parent/significant other/sibling involvement in newborn care as possible.	
• Give explanation of equipment being used and changes in bilirubin levels. Allow parents an opportunity to ask questions; reinforce or clarify information as needed.	
• Evaluate family's understanding of information.	
• As necessary, review role of pumping breasts and offering formula for limited time.	• The etiology of breast milk jaundice remains uncertain. The serum bilirubin levels begin to fall within 48 hr after discontinuation of breastfeeding. Opinion of healthcare providers varies regarding the need for discontinuing breastfeeding.
• Assist mother to pump her breasts to maintain milk supply.	• If breastfeeding is temporarily discontinued, assess mother's knowledge of pumping her breasts in regular increments (q 2–3 hr), and provide information and support as needed.

EXPECTED OUTCOMES: The parent will demonstrate ability to perform basic newborn care tasks as evidenced by exhibiting appropriate attachment behaviors (e.g., talking to and holding baby, feeding baby, and caring for baby under home bili therapy).

Parents verbalize understanding of rationale and possible side effects from phototherapy; parents/family demonstrate safety precautions when caring for baby; parents are getting meals and rest and verbalize support given.

patches at least once per shift to assess the eyes for the presence of conjunctivitis. Also remove eye patches to allow eye contact during feeding (for social stimulation) or when parents are visiting (to promote parental attachment).

Most phototherapy units will provide this level of irradiance: 6 to 12 $\mu W/cm^2/nm$ below the lamps for conventional phototherapy and greater than 25 to 30 $\mu W/cm^2/nm$ for intensive phototherapy (Gomella, 2013; Vandborg, Hansen, Greisen, et al., 2012). A photometer can be used to measure and maintain desired irradiance levels. Disadvantages of lights are that they create a difficult work environment and can distort a baby's color. Be careful about using ointments under bilirubin lights because they may cause burns.

Clinical Tip

If the area of jaundice about the eyes begins to disappear, it is probable that the eye patches are allowing light to enter and better eye protection is needed.

Some parents may feel guilty about their baby's condition and think they have caused the problem. Under stress, parents may not be able to understand the healthcare provider's first explanations. Expect that the parents will need explanations repeated and clarified and that they may need help in voicing their questions and fears. Coach parents when they visit with the baby. Encourage eye and tactile contact with the newborn. After the mother's discharge, keep parents informed of their baby's condition and encourage them to return to the hospital or telephone at any time so that they can be fully involved in the care of their newborn. Advise parents that after discontinuation of phototherapy, a rebound of 1 to 2 mg/dL can be expected and a follow-up bilirubin test may be done (Cloherty et al., 2012).

While the mother is still hospitalized, phototherapy can also be carried out in the parents' room if the only problem is hyperbilirubinemia and the parents agree to do the following:

- Keep the baby in the room for 24 hours a day.
- Take emergency action (e.g., for choking) if necessary.
- Complete instruction checklists.
- Sign a consent form per agency protocol.

Instruct the parents and also continue to monitor the baby's temperature, activity, intake and output, and positioning of eye patches (if conventional light banks are used) at regular intervals.

COMMUNITY-BASED NURSING CARE

Some studies have shown that the early discharge of newborns and their mothers comes with an increase in hospital readmission and elevated risk of pathologic hyperbilirubinemia. Home phototherapy use is recommended only if the bilirubin level is plotted on the nomogram and found to be in the "optional phototherapy" range. Any newborn with a level in the higher range should be hospitalized for continual phototherapy and serum bilirubin levels closely monitored on a regular schedule.

Jaundice and its treatment can be disturbing to parents and may generate feelings of guilt and fear. The parent's perception of and/or misconceptions about jaundice can affect parent–newborn interactions. Explain the causes of jaundice and emphasize that it is usually a transient problem and one to which all babies must adapt after birth. Reassurance and support are vital, especially for the breastfeeding mother, who may question her ability to adequately nourish her newborn.

It is essential that the impact of cultural beliefs be considered. Some Latina women believe that showing strong maternal emotions during pregnancy and breastfeeding can be detrimental. *Bilis* associated with anger may be blamed by some Latina women for jaundice.

If the baby is to receive phototherapy at home, teach the parents to record the baby's temperature, weight, fluid intake and output (I&O), stools, and feedings and how to use the phototherapy equipment. In addition, if conventional phototherapy lights are being used, parents must agree that the baby will be exposed to the lights for long periods of time; that they will hold the baby for only short periods for feeding, comforting, and cleansing of the perineal area; and that the room temperature will be regulated to minimize heat loss. Fiberoptic phototherapy blankets eliminate the need for eye patches, decrease heat loss because the baby is clothed, and provide more opportunities for interaction between the baby and the parents (see Figure 27–13). The best method of home phototherapy depends on the cause of the hyperbilirubinemia and the rate of progression of the jaundice. A combination of phototherapy lights and fiberoptic mattress may be used. Ongoing monitoring of bilirubin levels is essential with home phototherapy and can be carried out in the home, in the follow-up clinic, or in the clinician's office.

Clinical Reasoning Suspected Hyperbilirubinemia

Baby boy Martin is a term baby born by vaginal delivery with vacuum assist. His mother has blood type O positive, and baby Martin has blood type A positive. The baby has a normal complete blood count (CBC) with a hematocrit of 60%. While performing a physical examination on baby Martin on day 2 of life, the nurse notes that he has a large cephalohematoma, has an enlarged liver on palpation (hepatomegaly), and is clinically jaundiced. The nurse suspects that the baby has hyperbilirubinemia and discusses her findings with the healthcare provider, who orders a total bilirubin level to be drawn. The resulting level is 16 mg/dL. The decision is made to start the newborn on phototherapy treatment.

What risk factors and clinical findings does this baby have that predispose him to hyperbilirubinemia? How would the nurse explain baby Martin's hyperbilirubinemia and subsequent treatment and nursing care to his mother?

Evaluation

Expected outcomes of nursing care include the following:

- The newborn at risk for development of hyperbilirubinemia is identified, and action is taken to minimize the potential impact of hyperbilirubinemia.
- The baby does not have any corneal irritation or drainage, skin breakdown, or major fluctuations in temperature.
- Parents understand the rationale for, goal of, and expected outcome of therapy.
- Parents verbalize concerns about their baby's condition and identify how they can facilitate their baby's improvement.

Care of the Newborn With Anemia

Neonatal anemia is often difficult to recognize by clinical evaluation alone. The hemoglobin concentration in greater than 34 weeks' gestational age and full-term newborns is 14 to 20 g/dL (Gomella, 2013). Newborns with central hemoglobin values of less than 11 mg/dL (term) and 7 to 9 g/dL (preterm), at their lowest point at 8 to 12 weeks of age for term-born newborns, and 4 to 8 weeks of age for preterm newborns, are usually considered anemic (Arcara & Tschudy, 2012; Gomella, 2013).

Blood loss (hypovolemia) occurs in utero from placental bleeding (placenta previa or abruptio placentae). Intrapartum blood loss may be fetomaternal, fetofetal, or the result of umbilical cord bleeding. Birth trauma to abdominal organs (adrenal hemorrhage) or the cranium (subgaleal bleed) may produce significant blood loss, and cerebral bleeding may occur because of hypoxia, hypercapnia, or reperfusion injury (Gomella, 2013).

Excessive hemolysis of red blood cells is usually a result of blood group incompatibilities but may be caused by infections. The most common cause of impaired RBC production is a genetically transmitted deficiency in glucose-6-phosphate dehydrogenase (G6PD). Anemia and jaundice are the presenting signs (Gomella, 2013).

A condition known as **physiologic anemia of infancy** is a result of the normal gradual drop in hemoglobin; theoretically, the bone marrow stops production of RBCs in response to higher oxygen levels resulting from initiation of breathing, reaching the lowest point, or nadir, by 2 to 3 months of age for term-born and 3 to 6 or 4 to 8 weeks of age for preterm-born babies. At that point, the bone marrow begins production of RBCs again, and the anemia disappears (Arcara & Tschudy, 2012; Taylor & Kennedy, 2013).

The preterm newborn's hemoglobin reaches a nadir sooner than does the term newborn's because a preterm baby's red blood cell survival time is shorter than that of a term newborn. This difference is because of several factors: the preterm baby's rapid growth rate, decreased iron stores, shortened red blood cell survival time, and inadequate production of erythropoietin (EPO). Iatrogenic causes occur more often in preterm newborns as their condition requires more laboratory assessment (Taylor & Kennedy, 2013).

Clinical Therapy

Hematologic problems can be anticipated based on the pregnancy history and clinical manifestations. The age at which anemia is first noted is also of diagnostic value. Clinically, light-skinned anemic newborns are very pale in the absence of other symptoms of shock and usually have abnormally low red blood cell counts. In acute blood loss, symptoms of shock such as pallor, low arterial blood pressure, and a decreasing hematocrit value may be present.

The initial laboratory workup should include determinations of hemoglobin, hematocrit, bilirubin levels (in hemolytic disease), reticulocyte count, examination of peripheral blood smear, direct Coombs test of newborn's blood, and examination of maternal blood smear for fetal erythrocytes (Kleihauer-Betke test). Mild or chronic anemia in a baby may be treated adequately with iron supplements alone or with iron-fortified formulas. Folate and vitamin E may have to be supplemented depending on the type of formula ingested (Bagwell, 2014a). In severe cases of anemia, transfusions with O-negative or typed and crossmatched packed red cells are the preferred method of treatment.

Management of anemia of prematurity includes treating the causative factor (e.g., antibiotics/antivirals used for infection, steroid therapy for disorders of erythrocyte production) and supplemental iron. Blood transfusions (dedicated units of blood ideally from a single donor source) are kept to a minimum.

Use of recombinant human erythropoietin (rEPO) in preterm neonates can be beneficial in decreasing blood transfusions by stimulating the baby's own red blood cell production (Gomella, 2013; Ohls, Roohi, Peceny, et al., 2012).

Nursing Management

Assess the newborn for symptoms of anemia (pallor). If the blood loss is acute, the baby may exhibit the following signs of shock:

- Capillary filling time greater than 3 seconds
- Decreased pulse
- Tachycardia
- Low blood pressure

Signs of compromise include the following:

- Poor weight gain
- Tachycardia
- Tachypnea
- Apneic episodes

The baby should be placed on constant cardiac and respiratory monitoring. Promptly report any symptoms indicating anemia or shock. Continued observations will be necessary to identify physiologic anemia as the preterm newborn grows. Try to prevent iron deficiency by limiting phlebotomy losses and recording the amount of blood removed in tenths of a milliliter. The total blood removed is assessed and replaced by transfusion when necessary or by starting iron therapy at 2 weeks postnatal age.

Care of the Newborn With Infection

Newborns in the first month of life are particularly susceptible to infection, referred to as **sepsis neonatorum**, caused by organisms that do not typically cause significant disease in older children. Once any infection occurs in the newborn, it can spread rapidly through the bloodstream, regardless of its primary site. The incidence of *early-onset neonatal sepsis (EONS)* is 2.2 per 1000 live births (Gomella, 2013). EONS, seen in the first 7 days of life, is caused primarily by vertical transmission of maternal organisms, commonly group B streptococcus (Polin, Denson, Brady, & the Committee on the Fetus and Newborn & Committee on Infectious Diseases, 2012). *Escherichia coli* was found to be the most common causative agent; however, there is no standard prophylactic treatment (Bondi, Evans, Mischler, et al., 2013; Johnson, 2012). Late-onset sepsis occurs between the second week and the third month of age.

Nosocomial infections are infections acquired while a baby is in the neonatal intensive care unit (NICU) that usually are caused by organisms introduced during procedures or on equipment required to save the life of the neonate (Polin, Denson, Brady, et al., 2012). Methicillin-resistant *Staphylococcus aureus* (MRSA) and *Candida*, which cause 10% of late-onset sepsis, are two of the most common pathogens causing hospital-acquired infections in the NICU population (Johnson, 2012). The general debilitation and underlying illness often associated with prematurity necessitate invasive procedures such as umbilical catheterization, intubation, resuscitation, ventilatory support, monitoring, parenteral alimentation (especially lipid emulsions), and prior broad-spectrum antibiotic therapy.

However, even full-term newborns are susceptible, because their immunologic systems are immature (Figure 27–14). They lack the complex factors involved in effective phagocytosis and the ability to localize infection or to respond with a well-defined, recognizable inflammatory response. In addition, all newborns lack IgM immunoglobin, which is necessary to protect against bacteria, because it does not cross the placenta (see Chapter 23 for immunologic adaptations in the newborn period).

Most nosocomial infections in the NICU present as bacteremia/sepsis, urinary tract infections, meningitis, or pneumonia. Maternal antepartum infections may cause congenital infections and resulting disorders in the newborn. Intrapartum maternal infections, such as amnionitis, are sources of neonatal infection (see Chapter 15 for more detailed information on perinatal infection). Passage through the birth canal and contact with the vaginal flora (β-hemolytic streptococci, herpes, *Listeria*, gonococci) expose the newborn to infection (Table 27–3). With infection anywhere in the fetus or newborn, the adjacent tissues or organs are easily penetrated, and the blood–brain barrier is ineffective. Septicemia is more common in males, except for infections caused by group B β-hemolytic streptococcus.

Gram-negative organisms (especially *Escherichia coli, Enterobacter cloace, Serratia marcesceus,* and *Klebsiella pneumoniae*) account for 15% to 20% of late-onset sepsis and, along with the gram-positive organism β-hemolytic streptococcus, are the most common causative agents. *Pseudomonas* is a common fomite contaminant of ventilator support and oxygen therapy equipment. Gram-positive bacteria, especially coagulase-negative (CoNS) *Staphylococcus epidermidis* and *Staphylococcus aureus,* which combined cause 60% to 70% of infections, are common pathogens in nosocomial bacteremias, pneumonias, and urinary tract infections (Gomella, 2013; Johnson, 2012).

Protection of the newborn from infections starts prenatally and continues throughout pregnancy and birth. Prenatal prevention should include maternal screening for sexually transmitted infections and monitoring of rubella titers in women who test negative. Intrapartally, sterile technique is essential. Visual exam of the lesions is often reported on the labor and birth record to identify a woman with herpes. Placenta and amniotic fluid cultures are obtained if amnionitis is suspected. Local eye treatment with an antibiotic ophthalmic ointment is given to all newborns to prevent damage from gonococcal (occurring 3 days following birth) and possibly chlamydial (occurring 7 to 10 days after birth) infections. Prophylactic antibiotic therapy, for asymptomatic women who test positive for group B streptococcus (GBS) during the intrapartum period, helps prevent EOS sepsis. There has been a decrease in clinical neonatal sepsis rates because of the use of prenatal prophylactic antibiotic therapy (Lukacs & Schrag, 2012; Smith & Carley, 2014).

Health Promotion Preventing Newborn Infections

The following measures will help to prevent newborn infections.

During the prenatal period:

- Conduct maternal screening for sexually transmitted infections.
- Monitor rubella titers in women who test negative.

During the intrapartum period:

- Sterile technique is essential.
- Visual examination of any lesions should be reported on the labor and birth record to identify a woman with herpes.
- Placenta and amniotic fluid cultures are obtained if amnionitis is suspected.
- Prenatal prophylactic antibiotic therapy for asymptomatic women who test positive for GBS helps prevent early-onset sepsis and has shown a decrease in clinical neonatal sepsis rates (Lukacs & Schrag, 2012; Smith & Carley, 2014).

During the postpartum period:

- Local eye treatment with an antibiotic ophthalmic ointment is given to all newborns to prevent damage from gonococcal infections (occurring 3 days following birth) and the possibility of chlamydial infection (occurring 7 to 10 days after birth).

Clinical Therapy

Cultures should be taken as soon after birth as possible for newborns with a history of possible exposure to infection in utero (e.g., premature rupture of membranes [PROM] more than 24 hours before birth, questionable maternal history of infection, maternal fever/chorioamnionitis, or high-risk behavior such as multiple sexual partners or illicit drug use). Cultures are obtained before antibiotic therapy is begun (Bennett, 2013; Polin & Committee on Fetus and Newborn, 2012).

1. Anaerobic and aerobic blood cultures are taken from a peripheral site rather than an umbilical vessel, because catheters have yielded false-positive results caused by contamination. The skin is prepared by cleaning with a unit antiseptic solution and allowed to dry; the specimen is obtained with a sterile needle and syringe to lessen the

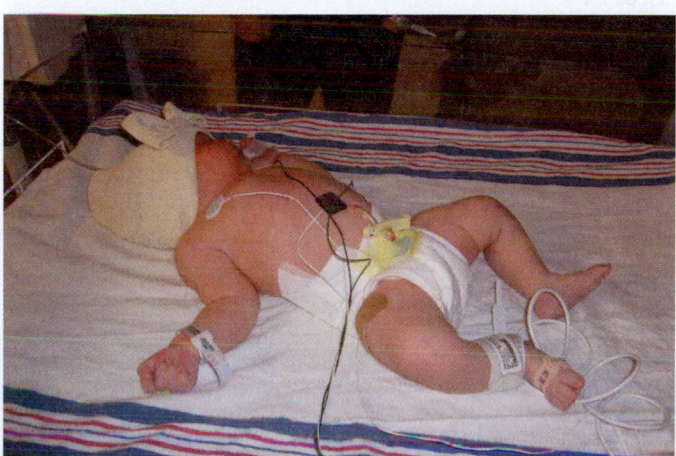

Figure 27–14 Term newborn with suspected sepsis.
SOURCE: Valentina Mescolotto.

TABLE 27–3 Maternally Transmitted Newborn Infections

INFECTION	NURSING ASSESSMENT OF THE NEWBORN	NURSING PLAN AND IMPLEMENTATION
GROUP B STREPTOCOCCUS 1%–2% colonized, with 1 in 10 developing disease. Early onset—usually within hours of birth or within first week. Late onset—1 week to 3 months (Cloherty et al., 2012).	Severe respiratory distress (grunting and cyanosis). May become apneic or demonstrate symptoms of shock. Meconium-stained amniotic fluid seen at birth.	Early assessment of clinical signs necessary. Assist with x-ray examination—shows aspiration pneumonia or respiratory distress syndrome. Immediately obtain blood, gastric aspirate, external ear canal, and nasopharynx cultures. Administer antibiotics, usually aqueous penicillin or ampicillin combined with gentamicin, as soon as cultures are obtained. Early assessment and intervention are essential to survival.

CONGENITAL SYPHILIS
 	
Spirochetes cross placenta after 16th–18th week of gestation.
 	
The more recent the maternal infection, the higher the likelihood of transmission.
 	
Most are asymptomatic at birth but develop symptoms within first 3 months of life.
	Assess newborn for:
	  Elevated cord serum IgM and FTA-ABS (fluorescent treponemal antibody absorbed) IgM
	  Rhinitis (snuffles)
	  Fissures on mouth corners and excoriated upper lip
	  Red rash around mouth and anus
	  Copper-colored rash over face, palms, and soles
	  Irritability, generalized edema, particularly over joints; bone lesions; painful extremities, hepatosplenomegaly, jaundice, congenital cataracts, small for gestational age (SGA), and failure to thrive
		Refer to evaluate for blindness, deafness, learning or behavioral problems.
		
		Initiate standard precautions until newborns have been on antibiotics for at least 24 hours.
		
		Administer penicillin.
		
		Provide emotional support for parents because of their feelings about mode of transmission and potential long-term sequelae.

GONORRHEA
 	
Approximately 30%–35% of newborns born vaginally to infected mothers acquire the infection.
	Assess for:
	  Ophthalmia neonatorum (conjunctivitis)
	  Purulent discharge and corneal ulcerations
	  Neonatal sepsis with temperature instability, poor feeding response, and/or hypotonia, jaundice
		Administer ophthalmic antibiotic ointment or penicillin.
		
		If positive maternal test, single dose systemic antibiotic therapy.
		
		Make a follow-up referral to evaluate any loss of vision.

HERPES TYPE 2 Usually transmitted during vaginal birth; a few cases of in utero transmission have been reported.	Check perinatal history for active herpes genital lesions. Small cluster vesicular skin lesions over all the body about 6 to 9 days of life. Disseminated form—disseminated intravascular coagulation (DIC), pneumonia, hepatitis with jaundice, hepatosplenomegaly, and neurologic abnormalities. Without skin lesions, assess for fever or subnormal temperature, respiratory congestion, tachypnea, and tachycardia	Carry out careful hand washing and contact precautions (gown and glove isolation with linen precautions). Obtain skin, eye, and mucocutaneous membrane lesion and cerebrospinal fluid (CSF) cultures to identify herpes virus type 2 antigen-specific antibodies in serum. Cultures positive in 24–48 hours. Administer intravenous acyclovir. Make a follow-up referral to evaluate potential sequelae of microcephaly, spasticity, seizures, deafness, or blindness. Encourage parental rooming-in and touching of their newborn. Show parents appropriate hand-washing procedures and precautions to be used at home if mother's lesions are active.
CYTOMEGALOVIRUS (CMV) Most common cause of congenital infection in the United States—approximately 1% of all newborns (Cloherty et al., 2012) Transmission occurs in utero or during labor, or may happen postnatally through breast milk.	Congenital CMV disease, including intrauterine growth retardation, jaundice, hepatosplenomegaly, petechiae or purpura (blueberry muffin spots), thrombocytopenia, and pneumonia. Central nervous system (CNS) manifestations are very common and include lethargy and poor feeding, hypertonia or hypotonia, microcephaly, intracranial calcifications, chorioretinitis, and sensorineural deafness.	Diagnosis of congenital CMV infection is established by isolating virus from urine, saliva, or tissue obtained during the first 3 weeks of life. All newborns in whom the diagnosis is suspected should have a viral culture performed; a CT scan of the brain is particularly important to document the extent of CNS involvement; perform eye examination and hearing test; close long-term follow-up evaluation is needed for developmental effects.

INFECTION	NURSING ASSESSMENT OF THE NEWBORN	NURSING PLAN AND IMPLEMENTATION
ORAL CANDIDAL INFECTION (THRUSH)		
Acquired during passage through birth canal	Assess newborn's buccal mucosa, tongue, gums, and inside the cheeks for white plaques (seen 5 to 7 days of age). Check diaper area for bright-red, well-demarcated eruptions. Assess for thrush periodically when newborn is on long-term antibiotic therapy.	Differentiate white plaque areas from milk curds by using cotton-tipped applicator (if it is thrush, removal of white areas causes raw, bleeding areas). Maintain cleanliness of hands, linen, clothing, diapers, and feeding apparatus. Instruct breastfeeding mothers on treating their nipples with nystatin. Administer nystatin swabbed on oral lesions 1 hour after feeding or nystatin instilled in baby's oral cavity and on mucosa. Swab skin lesions with topical nystatin.
CHLAMYDIA TRACHOMATIS		
Acquired during passage through birth canal.	Assess for perinatal history of preterm birth. Symptomatic newborns present with pneumonia. Chlamydial conjunctivitis presents with inflammation, yellow discharge, and eyelid swelling 5 to 14 days after birth. Assess for chronic follicular conjunctivitis (corneal neovascularization and conjunctival scarring).	Treat chlamydial conjunctivitis or pneumonia with oral erythromycin for 14 days (Cloherty et al., 2012). Monitor for hypertrophic pyloric stenosis. Initiate follow-up referral for eye complications and late development of pneumonia at 4 to 11 weeks postnatally.

likelihood of contamination. One mL of blood is recommended for each culture; they should not be divided between anaerobic and aerobic bottles.

2. Spinal fluid culture is done following a spinal tap/lumbar puncture if there are concerns about late-onset sepsis (LOS) or CNS symptoms/pathology. The fluid can be analyzed for culture and Gram stain as well as for glucose, protein, and white blood cell (WBC) count as well as for viral presence.

3. The specimen for urine culture is best obtained by a suprapubic bladder aspiration or sterile catheterization but should not be used in sepsis workup in early-onset sepsis (EOS) (Gomella, 2013).

4. Skin cultures are taken of any lesions or drainage from lesions or reddened areas.

5. Tracheal aspirate cultures may be obtained immediately after intubation.

Other laboratory investigations include a complete blood count, C-reactive protein (CRP), procalcitonin (PCT), chest x-ray examination, serology, and Gram stains of umbilicus. WBC count with differential may indicate the presence or absence of sepsis. A level of 30,000 to 40,000 mm^3 WBCs may be normal in the first 24 hours of life, whereas low WBC (less than 5000 to 7500/mm^3) may be indicative of sepsis. A low neutrophil count and a high band (immature white blood cells) count indicate that an infection is present. Stomach aspirate should be sent for culture and smear if a gonococcal infection or amnionitis is suspected. CRP, an acute-phase reactant protein synthesized in response to inflammation, may or may not be elevated initially. Other inflammatory responses may cause an elevation in the CRP, so it should not be used as the only indicator of infection (Smith & Carley, 2014). The CRP may be helpful in watching for improvement once antibiotic therapy is initiated. PCT is most diagnostic in late-onset septicemia (LOS) as it rises in the first 48 hours (Bennett, 2013; Gomella, 2013).

Serum IgM levels are elevated (normal level less than 20 mg/dL) in response to transplacental infections. If available,

counterimmunoelectrophoresis tests for specific bacterial antigens are performed. In the future repetitive sequence-based polymerase chain reactions (rep-PCR) tests will be used to identify specific infectious organisms within hours instead of days (Cloherty et al., 2012). Evidence of congenital infections may be seen on skull x-ray films for cerebral calcifications (cytomegalovirus, toxoplasmosis), on bone x-ray films (syphilis, cytomegalovirus), and in serum-specific IgM levels (rubella). Cytomegalovirus infection is best diagnosed by urine culture.

Because neonatal infection causes high mortality, therapy is instituted before results of the septic workup are obtained. A combination of two broad-spectrum antibiotics, such as ampicillin and gentamicin, is given in large doses but only until a culture with sensitivities is obtained.

After the pathogen and its sensitivities are determined, appropriate specific antibiotic therapy is begun. Rotating aminoglycosides has been suggested to prevent development of resistance. Use of cephalosporins and, in particular, cefotaxime has emerged as an alternative to aminoglycoside therapy in the treatment of neonatal infections for infants 1 to 3 months of age (Bennett, 2013). For newborns, third-generation cephalosporins are not currently recommended as single-agent therapy (Bennett, 2013).

Duration of therapy varies from 7 to 14 days (Table 27–4). If cultures are negative and symptoms subside, antibiotics may be discontinued after 2 days/ 48 hours of negative blood cultures. A normal CRP at 48 hours also supports discontinuing antibiotics if blood cultures are negative. Supportive physiologic care may be required to maintain respiratory, hemodynamic, nutritional, and metabolic homeostasis.

Nursing Management
For the Newborn With Infection

Nursing Assessment and Diagnosis

Symptoms of infection are most often noticed by the nurse during daily care of the newborn. The baby may deteriorate rapidly in the first 12 to 24 hours after birth if β-hemolytic streptococcal

TABLE 27–4 Neonatal Sepsis Antibiotic/Antiviral Therapy

DRUG	DOSE (MG/KG) TOTAL DAILY DOSE	SCHEDULE FOR DIVIDED DOSES	ROUTE	COMMENTS
Acyclovir (Zovirax)	20 mg/kg	q 8 hr	IV	Length of treatment is 14 days for skin/eye/mouth (SEM) or 21 days for CNS and disseminated disease: *Herpes*
Ampicillin	25–50 mg/kg/dose (100 mg/kg/dose if treating meningitis and severe group B streptococcal sepsis)	q 12 hr* q 8 hr† q 6 hr**	IM or IV	Effective against gram-positive microorganisms, *Listeria*, and most *Escherichia coli* strains. Higher doses indicated for meningitis. Used with aminoglycoside for synergy.
Cefotaxime	50 mg/kg/dose (25 mg/kg/dose gonococcal infection)	q 12 hr* q 8 hr q 6 hr**	IM or IV	Active against most major pathogens in babies; effective against aminoglycoside-resistant organisms; achieves cerebrospinal fluid (CSF) bactericidal activity; lack of ototoxicity and nephrotoxicity; wide therapeutic index (levels not required); resistant organisms can develop rapidly if used extensively; ineffective against *Pseudomonas*, *Listeria*.
Gentamicin	4–5 mg/kg/dose 4–5 mg/kg/dose (first week of life)	q 24–48 hr‡*** q 24–48 hr	IM or IV	Effective against gram-negative rods and staphylococci; may be used instead of kanamycin against penicillin-resistant staphylococci and *E. coli* strains and *Pseudomonas aeruginosa*. May cause neurotoxicity, ototoxicity, and nephrotoxicity. Need to follow serum levels. Must never be given as IV push. Must be given over at least 30–60 minutes. In presence of oliguria or anuria, dose must be decreased or discontinued. In newborns less than 1000 g or 29 weeks, lower dosage to 2.5–3 mg/kg/day. Monitor serum levels before administration of second dose. Peak 5–10 mcg/mL Trough 1–2 mcg/mL
Vancomycin	10–20 mg/kg 30 mg/kg/day	q 12–24 hr*‡ q 8 hr†	IV	Effective for methicillin-resistant strains (*Staphylococcus epidermidis*); must be administered by slow intravenous infusion to avoid prolonged cutaneous eruption. For smaller newborns (less than 1200 g, less than 29 weeks), smaller dosages and longer intervals between doses. Nephrotoxic, especially in combination with aminoglycosides. Slow IV infusion over at least 60 minutes. Peak 25–40 mcg/mL Trough 5–10 mcg/mL

*Up to 7 days of age.

**>45 weeks postmenstrual age.

†Greater than 7 days of age.

‡Dependent on gestational age.

***Dependent on postnatal age.

infection is present, with signs and symptoms mimicking respiratory distress syndrome (RDS). In other cases, the onset of sepsis may be gradual, with more subtle signs and symptoms. The most common signs observed include the following:

- Subtle behavioral changes; the newborn "is not doing well" and is often lethargic or irritable (especially after the first 24 hours) and hypotonic; color changes may include pallor, duskiness, cyanosis, or a "shocky" appearance; skin is cool and clammy.

- Temperature instability, manifested by either hypothermia (recognized by a decrease in skin temperature) or, rarely in newborns, hyperthermia (elevation of skin temperature) necessitating a corresponding increase or decrease in incubator temperature to maintain a neutral thermal environment.

- Feeding intolerance, as evidenced by a decrease in total intake, abdominal distention, vomiting, poor sucking, lack of interest in feeding, and diarrhea.

- Hyperbilirubinemia, hepatosplenomegaly.

- Tachycardia initially, followed by spells of apnea/ bradycardia.

Signs and symptoms may suggest central nervous system (CNS) disease (jitteriness, tremors, seizure activity). A differential diagnosis is necessary because of the similarity of symptoms to other more specific conditions.

Nursing diagnoses that may apply to the newborn with sepsis neonatorum and the family include the following (NANDA-I © 2014):

- *Infection, Risk for,* related to newborn's immature immunologic system

- *Fluid Volume, Deficient,* related to feeding intolerance

- *Coping: Family, Compromised,* related to present illness resulting in prolonged hospital stay for the newborn

Nursing Plan and Implementation

In the nursery, environmental control and prevention of acquired infection are the responsibilities of the neonatal nurse. An infected newborn can be isolated effectively in an isolette and receive close observation. Promote strict hand hygiene technique for all healthcare providers who enter the nursery and for parents. Visits to the nursery area by unnecessary personnel should be discouraged. Be prepared to assist in the aseptic collection of specimens for laboratory investigations. Scrupulous care of equipment—changing and cleaning of incubators at least every 7 days, removing and sterilizing wet equipment every 24 hours, preventing cross use of linen and equipment, cleaning sink-side equipment such as soap containers periodically, and taking special care with the open radiant warmers (access without prior hand washing is much more likely than with the closed incubator)—will prevent contamination.

PROVISION OF ANTIBIOTIC THERAPY

Administer antibiotics as ordered by the healthcare provider/nurse practitioner. It is your responsibility to be knowledgeable about the following:

- The proper dose to be administered, based on the weight of the newborn and desired peak and trough levels
- The appropriate route of administration, because some antibiotics cannot be given intravenously
- Admixture incompatibilities, because some antibiotics are precipitated by intravenous solutions or by other antibiotics
- Side effects and toxicity

For term newborns being treated for infections, neonatal home infusion of antibiotics should be considered as a viable alternative to continued hospitalization. The infusion of antibiotics at home by skilled registered nurses (RNs) facilitates parent–newborn bonding while meeting the baby's ongoing healthcare needs.

PROVISION OF SUPPORTIVE CARE

In addition to antibiotic therapy, physiologic supportive care is essential in caring for a septic baby. Carry out the following:

- Observe for resolution of symptoms or development of other symptoms of sepsis.
- Maintain neutral thermal environment with accurate regulation of humidity and oxygen administration.
- Provide respiratory support: administer oxygen, use pulse oximetry, observe and monitor respiratory effort.
- Provide cardiovascular support: observe and monitor pulse and blood pressure; observe for hyperbilirubinemia, anemia, and hemorrhagic symptoms.
- Provide adequate calories, because oral feedings may be discontinued because of increased mucus, abdominal distention, vomiting, and aspiration.
- Provide fluids and electrolytes to maintain homeostasis; monitor weight changes, urine output, and urine specific gravity.
- Observe for the development of hypoglycemia, hyperglycemia, acidosis, hyponatremia, and hypocalcemia.

Restricting parental visits has not been shown to have any effect on the rate of infection and may be harmful for the newborn's psychologic development. With your instruction and guidance both parents should be allowed to handle the baby and participate in daily care. Support of the parents is crucial.

They need to be informed of the newborn's prognosis as treatment continues and to be involved in care as much as possible. They also need to understand how infection is transmitted.

Evaluation

Expected outcomes of nursing care include the following:

- The risks for development of sepsis are identified early, and immediate action is taken to minimize the development of the illness.
- Appropriate use of aseptic technique protects the newborn from further exposure to illness.
- The baby's symptoms are relieved, and the infection is treated.
- The parents verbalize concerns about their baby's illness and understand the rationale behind the management of their newborn.

Care of the Family With Birth of an At-Risk Newborn

The birth of a preterm or ill baby or a baby with a congenital anomaly is a serious crisis for a family (Sweet & Mannix, 2012). Throughout the pregnancy, both parents, together and separately, have felt excitement, experienced thoughts of acceptance, and pictured what their baby would look like. Both parents have wished for a perfect baby and feared an unhealthy one. Each parent and family member must accept and adjust when the fantasized fears become reality (Zimmerman & Bauersachs, 2012).

Parental Responses

Family members have acute grief reactions to the loss of the idealized baby they have envisioned. In a preterm birth, the mother is denied the last few weeks of pregnancy that seem to prepare her psychologically for the stress of birth and the attachment process. Attachment at this time is fragile, and interruption of the process by separation can affect the future mother–child relationship (Discenza, 2012b; Sweet & Mannix, 2012). Parents express grief as shock and disbelief, denial of reality, anger toward self and others, guilt, blame, and concern for the future. Self-esteem and feelings of self-worth are jeopardized (Walker, 2013).

Feelings of guilt and failure often plague mothers of preterm newborns. Guilt fantasies may lead her to wonder what she might have done to cause the early labor. She may ask herself questions such as: "Why did labor start?" or "What did I do (or not do)?" A woman may have guilt fantasies and wonder what she may have done to cause the early labor: "Was it because I had sexual intercourse with my husband (a week, 3 days, a day) ago?" "Was it because I carried three loads of wash up from the basement?" or "Am I being punished for something done in the past—even in childhood?"

The period of waiting between suspicion and confirmation of abnormality or dysfunction is a very anxious one for parents because it is difficult, if not impossible, to begin attachment to the baby if the newborn's future is questionable. During the waiting period, parents need support and acknowledgment that this is an anxious time. They must be kept informed about tests and efforts to gather additional data, as well as efforts to improve their baby's outcome (Sweet & Mannix, 2012). It is helpful to tell both parents about the problem at the same time, with the baby present. An honest discussion of the problem and anticipatory management at the earliest possible time by health professionals help the parents (1) maintain trust in the healthcare provider and nurse, (2) appreciate the reality of the situation by dispelling fantasy and misconception, (3) begin the grieving process, and (4) mobilize internal and external support.

Nurses need to be aware that anger is a universal response by parents to a preterm birth. It is best that the parents direct it outward because holding it in check requires great energy, which is then diverted away from grieving and physical recovery from pregnancy and giving birth. Anger may be directed at the healthcare provider and/or nurse, at the food, at nursing care, or at hospital regulations and routines (Discenza, 2012b). Perceived maternal stress may be lessened and the mother empowered if information is provided regarding preterm behavioral cues. This empowers the mother and allows her to better care for her child. The mother of a preterm baby who has to spend time in a neonatal intensive care unit (NICU) suffers from psychologic distress similar to posttraumatic stress disorder (PTSD). The nurse working with a mother in the NICU setting has the opportunity to encourage maternal competence and confidence, both during and after hospitalization, by teaching interpretation of her baby's behavioral cues, prompting maternal care of the baby while in the NICU, and facilitating expression of her feelings (for more detailed discussion of PTSD see Chapter 30). The father also may suffer from depression both before and after the birth of the child, adding to the discord in the family unit and compounding the perceived stress experienced by the mother.

A variety of behavioral patterns may occur. For example, one or more members of the family may make a scapegoat of the child. Another may become the youngster's champion to the exclusion of others. One or the other spouse may feel pushed aside or denied attention, and thus may withdraw or leave the family unit. Parents or siblings may feel that their own needs (schooling, material goods, freedom of movement) are being set aside whereas all assets (financial and other) go to support the one child's needs. There may also be an increase in child abuse.

Solnit and Stark (1961) postulate that grief and mourning over the loss of the loved object—the idealized child—mark parental reactions to a child with abnormalities. *Grief work*, the emotional reaction to a significant loss, must occur before adequate attachment to the actual child is possible. Parental detachment precedes parental attachment. The parents must first grieve the loss of the wished-for perfect child, and then must adopt the imperfect child as the new love object.

Some degree of postpartum depression occurs in new mothers up to 15% of the time, and rates can be as high as 32% to 63% in mothers with babies in the NICU. Maternal depression can have a negative impact on attachment with the newborn (Bicking & Moore, 2012). Other members of the family also may suffer from depressive symptoms (Sweet & Mannix, 2012). Although reactions and steps of attachment are altered by the birth of these babies, a healthy parent–child relationship can occur.

Developmental Consequences

The baby who is born prematurely, is ill, or has a malformation or disorder is at risk for emotional, intellectual, and cognitive development delays. The risk is directly proportional to the seriousness of the problem and the length of treatment. The necessary physical separation of family and newborn and the tremendous emotional and financial burdens may adversely affect the parent–child relationship. The recent trends to involve the parents with their newborn early, repeatedly, and over protracted periods of time has done much to facilitate positive parent–child relationships (Bicking & Moore, 2012).

Parents must have a clear picture of the reality of the handicap and the types of developmental hurdles ahead. Unexpected behaviors and responses from the baby because of the defect or disorder can be upsetting and frightening. The demands of care for the child and disputes regarding management or behavior stress family relationships. The entire interprofessional healthcare team may need to pool its resources and expertise to help parents of children born with problems or disorders so that both parents and children can thrive. Involving the parents in rounds can be a valuable tool to enhance their feelings of inclusion in the care and decision-making process of their NICU baby (Graci, 2013).

Nursing Management
For the Family of an At-Risk Newborn

Nursing Assessment and Diagnosis

A concurrent illness of the mother or other family members or other concurrent stress (lack of hospitalization insurance, loss of job, age of parents) may alter the family response to the baby. Feelings of apprehension, guilt, failure, and grief expressed verbally or nonverbally are important aspects of the nursing history. These observations enable all professionals to be aware of the parental state, coping behaviors, and readiness for attachment, bonding, and caretaking. Appropriate nursing assessments during interviewing and relating to the family include the following:

- *Level of understanding.* Observations concerning the family's ability to assimilate information given and to ask appropriate questions; the need for constant repetition of information
- *Behavioral responses.* Appropriateness of behavior in relation to information given; lack of response; flat affect
- *Difficulties with communication.* Deafness (reads lips only); blindness; dysphasia; understanding only a non-English language
- *Paternal and maternal education level.* Parents who are unable to read or write; parents with eighth-grade–level education or lower; parents with a graduate-level degree or healthcare background

Documentation of such information, gathered through continuing contact and development of a therapeutic family relationship, allows all professionals to understand and use the nursing history to provide continuous individualized care.

A record of visits, caretaking procedures, affect (in relating to the newborn), and telephone calls indicates the level or lack of parental attachment. Serial observations, rather than just isolated observations that cause concern, must be obtained. Grant (1978) developed a conceptual framework depicting adaptive and maladaptive responses to parenting of a preterm or less-than-perfect baby (Table 27–5).

If a pattern of distancing behaviors evolves, institute appropriate interventions. Follow-up studies have found that a statistically significant number of preterm, sick, and congenitally defective babies suffer from failure to thrive, battering, or other parenting disorders. Early detection and intervention will prevent these aberrations in parenting behaviors from leading to irreparable damage or death.

Nursing diagnoses that may apply to the family of a newborn at risk include the following (NANDA-I © 2014):

- *Grieving, Complicated,* related to loss of idealized newborn
- *Fear* related to emotional involvement with an at-risk newborn
- *Parenting, Impaired,* related to impaired bonding secondary to feelings of inadequacy about caretaking activities

TABLE 27–5 Adaptive and Nonadaptive Parental Responses to a Newborn's Health Crisis

PARENTAL TASKS AT THIS TIME INCLUDE THE FOLLOWING:

- Understanding the newborn's medical condition and needs
- Adapting to the NICU environment
- Assuming the main caretaking role
- Taking responsibility for the baby after discharge
- Coping with the death of the baby

ADAPTIVE RESPONSES	NONADAPTIVE RESPONSES
• Frequent visits to baby and calls to the unit	• Failure to visit baby or communicate with unit
• Emotional involvement with baby	• Emotional withdrawal from baby
• Positive interaction with baby during hospitalization	• Lack of interaction with baby during hospitalization
• Eagerness to assume caretaking during baby's hospitalization	• Resistance to providing care of the baby during hospitalization
• Increasing sense of parental competence	• Lack of a sense of parental competence
• Growing attachment to baby	• Failure to achieve attachment to baby
• Realistic interpretation of medical information	• Inability to understand or accept medical information
• Acceptance of baby's condition	• Unhealthy preoccupation with baby's condition
• Understanding of the causes of baby's condition	• Blaming others for baby's condition
• Eagerness to assume total responsibility for baby	• Fear of going home with baby
• Realistic understanding of baby's needs at discharge	• Negative view of baby and baby's needs at discharge
• Open discussion of concerns and needs to staff and family	• Inability to discuss needs and concerns with staff and family
• Fair and realistic expectations of staff	• Distrustful and hostile attitude toward staff

POSITIVE OUTCOME	NEGATIVE OUTCOME
• Healthy parent–child relationship	• Poor parent–child relationship
• Marital and family equilibrium is maintained	• Failure to thrive
	• Vulnerable child syndrome
	• Marital and family equilibrium is compromised

Source: Data from Grant, P. (1978). *Family & community health*. Philadelphia, PA: Lippincott Williams & Wilkins.

Nursing Plan and Implementation

HOSPITAL-BASED NURSING CARE

In their sensitive and vulnerable state, parents are acutely perceptive of others' responses and reactions (particularly nonverbal) to the child. Parents can be expected to identify with the responses of others. Therefore, it is imperative that medical and nursing staff be fully aware of the parents' feelings and come to terms with their own feelings so that they are comfortable and at ease with the baby and the grieving family.

Nurses may feel uncomfortable, may not know what to say to parents, or may fear confronting their own feelings as well as those of the parents. Each nurse must work out personal reactions with instructors, peers, clergy, parents, or significant others. It is helpful to have a stockpile of therapeutic questions and statements to initiate meaningful dialogue with parents. Opening statements might include the following:

"You must be wondering what could have caused this."

"Are you thinking that you (or someone else) may have done something?"

"How can I help?"

"Are you wondering how you are going to manage?"

Avoid statements such as:

"It could have been worse."

"It's God's will."

"You have other children."

"You are still young and can have more."

"I understand how you feel."

Always remember that this child and this situation are important now.

Support of Parents for Initial Viewing of the Newborn

Before parents see their newborn, prepare them for the visit. It is important to maintain a positive, realistic attitude regarding the baby. An overly negative, fatalistic attitude further alienates the parents from their baby and retards attachment behaviors. Instead of beginning to bond with their baby, the parents will anticipate their loss and the process of grieving. Once started, this process is very difficult to reverse.

All babies exhibit strengths as well as deficiencies; prepare the parents to see both the deviations and the normal aspects of their newborn. You might say, "Your baby is small, about the length of my two hands. She weighs 2 lb, 3 oz, but is very active and cries when we disturb her. She is having some difficulty breathing but is breathing without assistance. She is breathing 35% oxygen and room air is 21%." Many NICUs have booklets for parents to read before entering the units. Through explanations and pictures, the parents are better prepared to deal with the feelings they may experience when they see their baby for the first time (Figure 27–15). Describe the equipment being used for the at-risk newborn and its purpose before the parents enter the intensive care unit.

Upon entering the unit, parents may be overwhelmed by the sounds of monitors, alarms, and respirators, as well as by

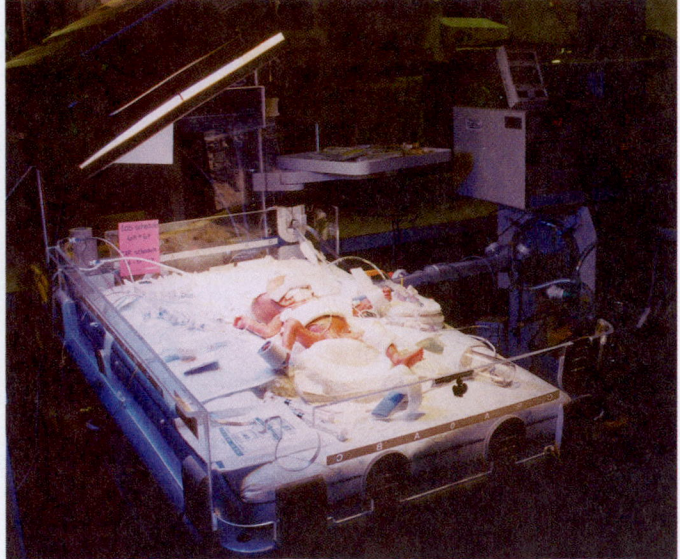

Figure 27–15 This 25 weeks' gestational age newborn with respiratory distress syndrome may be frightening for her parents to see for the first time because of the technology that is attached to her.

SOURCE: Lisa Smith-Pedersen, RNC, MSN, NNP-BC.

the unfamiliar language and "foreign" atmosphere. Preparing the parents by having familiar healthcare providers accompany them to the unit can be reassuring. The primary nurse and healthcare provider caring for the newborn need to be with the parents when they first visit their baby. Parental reactions vary, but initially there is usually an element of shock. Providing chairs and time to regain composure assists the parents. Slow, complete, and simple explanations—first about the baby and then about the equipment—allay fear and anxiety.

Concern about the baby's physical appearance is common yet may remain unvoiced. Parents may express concerns such as "He looks so small and red—like a drowned rat," "Why do her genitals look so abnormal?" and "Will that awful-looking mouth [cleft lip and palate] ever be normal?" Anticipate and address such questions. Use of pictures, such as of a baby after cleft lip repair, may be reassuring to doubting parents. Knowledge of the development of a "normal" preterm baby allows you to make reassuring statements such as "The baby's skin may look very red and transparent with lots of visible veins, but it is normal for her maturity. As she grows, subcutaneous fat will be laid down, and these superficial veins will begin to disappear."

The nursing staff sets the tone of the NICU. Nurses foster the development of a safe, trusting environment by viewing the parents as essential caregivers, not as visitors or nuisances in the unit. It is important to provide parents privacy when needed and easy access to staff and facilities. An uncrowded and welcoming atmosphere lets parents know "You are welcome here." However, even in crowded physical surroundings, you can convey an attitude of openness and trust.

A trusting relationship is essential for collaborative efforts in caring for the newborn. Work toward therapeutically using your own responses to relate to the parents on a one-to-one basis. Each individual has different needs, different ways of adapting to crisis, and different means of support. Use techniques that are real and spontaneous to them and avoid words

or actions that are foreign to them. Gauge your interventions so that they match the parents' pace and needs.

Implementation of family-centered care, a team approach with healthcare professionals and the family, in which the parents, grandparents, and older siblings are vital members of the team, is important to bonding and the development of the family unit (Chinchilla, 2012). Show concern and support by planning time to spend with the parents, by being psychologically as well as physically present, by encouraging open discussion and grieving, by repetitious explanations (as necessary), by providing privacy as needed, and by encouraging contact with the newborn. Identifying and clarifying feelings and fears decrease distortions in perception, thinking, and feeling. Invest the baby with value in the eyes of the parents by providing meticulous care to the newborn, talk and coo (especially in the face-to-face position) while holding or providing care to the baby, refer to the child by gender or name, and relate the baby's activities ("He took a whole ounce of formula," "She took hold of the blanket and just wouldn't let go"). Also note the "normal" characteristics and capabilities of each newborn as well as the baby's needs. When the baby is physiologically stable and of an appropriate weight, allowing the baby to be dressed in clothes has been determined to aid the mother in perceiving the baby as a "person" or "actual baby."

Facilitation of Attachment If Neonatal Transport Occurs

Transport to a regional referral center some distance from the parents may be necessary. It is essential that the mother see and touch her newborn before the baby is transported. Bring the mother to the nursery or take the baby in a warmed transport incubator to the mother's bedside to allow her to see the baby before transportation to the center. When the baby reaches the referral center, a staff member should call the parents with information about the baby's condition during transport, safe arrival at the center, and present condition.

Support of parents, with explanations from the professional staff, is crucial. Occasionally the mother may be unable to see the baby before transport (e.g., if she is still under general anesthesia or experiencing complications such as shock, hemorrhage, or seizures). In these cases, the baby should be photographed before transport. The picture should be given to the mother, along with an explanation of the baby's condition, present problems, and a detailed description of the baby's characteristics, to facilitate the attachment process until the mother can visit. An additional photograph is also helpful for the father to share with siblings or extended family. If the mother is hospitalized apart from the newborn, the first person to visit the baby should relay information regarding the baby's care and condition to the mother and family. Because the mother has had minimal contact, if any, with her baby she may mistrust all those who provide information (the father, nurse, physician, or extended family) until she sees the baby for herself. This can put tremendous stress on the relationship between spouses.

With the increased attention on improved fetal outcome, prenatal maternal transports, rather than neonatal transports, are occurring more frequently. This practice gives the mother of an at-risk baby the opportunity to visit and care for her baby during the early postpartum period.

Promotion of Touching and Parental Caretaking

Parents visiting a small or sick newborn may need several visits to become comfortable and confident in their ability to touch the baby without injuring the baby. Barriers such as incubators, incisions, monitor electrodes, and tubes may delay the mother's development of comfort in touching the newborn.

Klaus and Kennell (1982) have demonstrated a significant difference in the amount of eye contact and touching behaviors of mothers of normal newborns and mothers of preterm newborns. Whereas mothers of normal newborns progress within minutes to palm contact of the baby's trunk, mothers of preterm newborns are slower to progress from fingertip to palm contact and from the extremities to the trunk. The progression to palm contact with the baby's trunk may take several visits to the nursery.

Through support, reassurance, and encouragement, you can facilitate the mother's positive feelings about her ability and her importance to her baby. Touching facilitates "getting to know" the baby and thus establishes a bond with the baby. Touching and seeing the newborn help the mother realize the "normals" and potential of her baby (Figure 27–16).

Encourage parents to meet their newborn's need for stimulation. Stroking, rocking, cuddling, singing, and talking should be an integral part of the parents' caretaking responsibilities. Bonding can be facilitated by encouraging parents to visit and become involved in their baby's care. Skin-to-skin contact (kangaroo care), usually between the mother, father, or surrogate (another person instead of the parents) and the neonate, was first introduced over 40 years ago. It is now utilized to enhance bonding and impacts positively both the behavior and physiology of the newborn (Figure 27–17) (Discenza, 2012a; Ludington-Hoe, 2011). Something as simple as softly reading a book to the baby can help during this time (Walker, 2013). When visiting is impossible, the parents should feel free to phone when they wish to receive information about their baby. Your warm, receptive attitude provides support. Facilitate parenting by personalizing the baby to the parents, by referring to the baby by name, or relating personal behavioral characteristics. Remarks such as "Jenny loves her pacifier" help make the baby seem individual and unique.

The variety of equipment needed for life support is hardly conducive to anxiety-free caretaking by the parents. However, even the sickest newborn may be cared for, if only in a small way, by the parents. As a facilitator of parental caretaking,

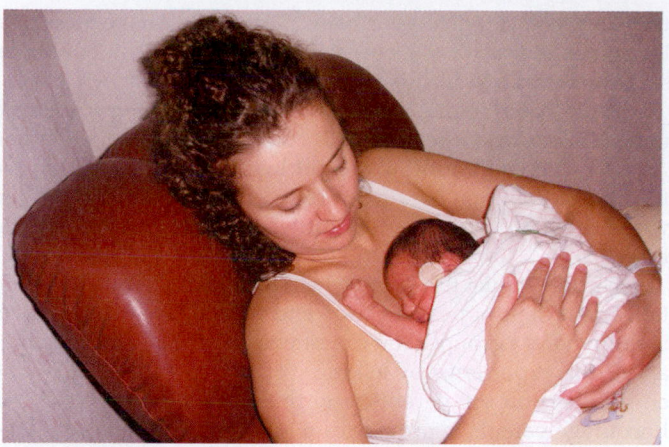

This mother of a 31 weeks' gestational age newborn with respiratory distress syndrome is spending time with her newborn and meeting the baby's need for cuddling.

SOURCE: Lisa Smith-Pedersen, RN, MSN, NNP-BC.

you can help promote the parents' success (Zimmerman & Bauersachs, 2012). Demonstration and explanation, followed by support of the parents in initial caretaking behaviors, positively reinforce this behavior. Changing their newborn's diaper, providing skin or oral care, or helping to turn the baby may at first provoke anxiety, but the parents will become more comfortable and confident in caretaking and feel satisfied by the baby's reactions and their ability "to do something" (Skene, Franck, Curtis, et al., 2012). Complimenting the parents' competence in caretaking also increases their self-esteem, which has received recent "blows" of guilt and failure. *It is vitally important that you never give the parents a task that they might not be able to accomplish.* Cues that the parents are ready to become involved with the child's care include their reference to the baby by name and their questioning as to amount of feeding taken, sleeping patterns, appearance today, and the like. Simple inclusion of the parents in providing comfort care for their baby is an early step in transferring care from the medical staff to the parents (Skene et al., 2012).

Often parents of high-risk newborns have ambivalent feelings toward the nurse. These feelings may take the form of criticism of the care of the baby, manipulation of staff, or personal guilt. Accept this behavior, but continue to remind the parents that it is okay and natural to feel disappointment, a sense of failure, helplessness, or anger. Overprotectiveness and overoptimism are defense mechanisms. To deny the negative feelings only entrenches them further, delays their resolution, and delays realistic planning. Instead of fostering (by silence) these inferiority feelings of parents, recognize that such feelings are needed to intervene appropriately to enhance parent–newborn attachment. Deal with ambivalent feelings that contribute to a competitive atmosphere. For example, avoid making unfavorable comparisons between the baby's responses to parental and nursing caretaking. Verbalizations that improve parental self-esteem are essential and easily shared. You can point out that, in addition to physiologic use, breast milk is important because of the emotional investment of the mother. Pumping, storing, labeling, and delivering quantities of breast milk is a time-consuming "labor of love" for mothers. Positive remarks about breast milk reinforce the maternal behavior of caretaking and providing for her baby: "Breast milk is something

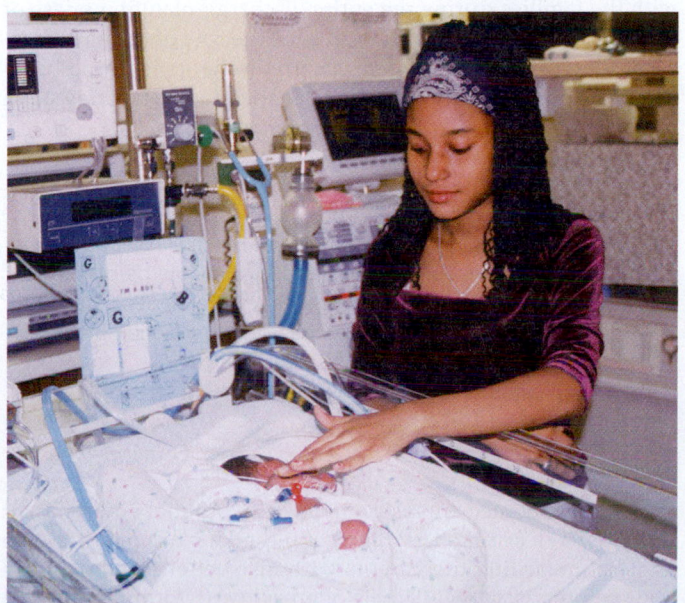

Mother of this 26 weeks' gestational age 600g baby begins attachment through fingertip touch.

SOURCE: Lisa Smith-Pedersen, RN, MSN, NNP-BC.

that only you can give your baby," "You really have brought a lot of milk today," "Look how rich this breast milk is," or "Even small amounts of milk are important, and look how rich it is."

If the baby begins to gain weight while being fed breast milk, it is important to point this correlation out to the mother. Advise parents that initial weight loss with beginning nipple feedings is common because of the increased energy expended when the baby begins active rather than passive nutritional intake.

During a quiet time it may help to encourage the parents to talk about their hopes and fears and to facilitate their involvement in parent groups. You can often elicit the parents' feelings about the experience by asking, "How are you doing?" The emphasis is on the parents, and the interest must be sincere. Encourage parents to provide care for their newborn even if the baby is very sick and likely to die. Detachment is easier after attachment, because the parents are comforted by the knowledge that they did all they could for their child while the baby was alive.

Facilitation of Family Adjustment During Crisis

During crisis, it is difficult to maintain interpersonal relationships. Yet in a newborn intensive care area, the parents are expected to relate to many different care providers. It is important that parents have as few professionals as possible relaying information to them. A primary nurse should coordinate care and provide continuity for parents. Care providers are individuals and thus will use different terms, inflections, and attitudes. These subtle differences are monumental to parents and may confuse, confound, and produce anxiety. The transfer of the baby from the NICU to a step-down unit or transport back to the home hospital provokes parental anxiety because they must now deal with new healthcare providers. You will not only function as a liaison between the parents and the various healthcare professionals interacting with the baby and parents but also offer clarification, explanation, interpretation of information, and support to the parents (Chinchilla, 2012).

Encourage parents to deal with the crisis with help from their support system. Biologic kinship is not the only valid criterion for a support system; an emotional kinship is the most important factor. In our mobile society of isolated nuclear families, the support system may be a next-door neighbor, a best friend, or perhaps a schoolmate. Search out the significant people in the lives of the parents and help them understand the problems so that they can be a constant parental support.

The impact of the crisis on the family is individual and varied. To institute appropriate interventions, you will need to view the birth of the baby, whether it is a healthy term newborn, preterm newborn, or a baby with a congenital anomaly, as experienced by the family. It is important to encourage open intrafamily communication. Discourage the family from keeping secrets from one another, especially between spouses, because secrets undermine the trust of relationships. Well-meaning rationales such as "I want to protect her," "I don't want him to worry about it," and so on can be destructive to open communication and to the basic element of a relationship: trust.

The needs of siblings should not be overlooked. Siblings have been looking forward to the new baby, and they, too, suffer a degree of loss. Young children may react with hostility and older ones with shame at the birth of a baby with an anomaly. Both reactions may make siblings feel guilty. Parents, who may be preoccupied with working through their own feelings, often cannot give the other children the attention and support they need. Sometimes another child becomes the focus of family tension. Anxiety thus directed can take the form of finding fault or

of overconcern. This is a form of denial; the parents cannot face the real worry: the newborn at risk. After carefully assessing the situation, you can work to ensure that another family member or friend steps in to support the siblings of the affected baby.

Parents from minority cultures must deal with language barriers and cultural differences that can make feelings of isolation and uncertainty more acute. Healthcare providers have the professional responsibility to be aware of the cultural needs of all clients and to ensure those needs are met. Feelings of isolation and uncertainty influence not only the parent's emotional responses to the ill newborn, but also the utilization of services and their interaction with health professionals. Hospital cultural interpreter programs can assist families with interactions with staff, as well as provide translation during family meetings, collaborative-care family conferences, and parent support groups.

Families with babies in the NICU may become friends and support one another. To encourage the development of these friendships and to provide support, many units have established parent groups. The core of a group consists of parents whose babies were once in the intensive care unit. Most groups make contact with families within a day or two of the newborn's admission to the unit, through either phone calls or visits to the hospital. Early one-on-one parent contacts are more effective than discussion groups in helping families work through their feelings. This personalized method gives the grieving parents an opportunity to express personal feelings about the pregnancy, labor, and birth and their "different from expected" baby with others who have experienced the same feelings and with whom they can identify.

COMMUNITY-BASED NURSING CARE

Predischarge planning begins once the newborn's condition becomes stable and it seems likely the baby will survive. These medically fragile babies remain vulnerable for several years (Holditch-Davis, Miles, Burchinal, et al., 2011). Discharge preparation and care conferences should involve a collaborative-care team approach. NICU nursing staff members are the fulcrum for aiding in the transition of high-risk newborns from the intensive care unit to the home. Effective open communication with the families during the entire discharge-planning phase of care empowers the families to assume the role of primary caregiver for their children. Adequate predischarge teaching helps parents transform any feelings of inadequacy they may have into feelings of self-assurance and attachment.

SAFETY ALERT!

The high incidence of prematurity and LBW in multiple-birth babies and the corresponding risks for SIDS should be considered. As with all families at discharge, parents of multiples should be taught SIDS risk-reduction practices. SIDS reduction practices include supine positioning, babies sleeping in parents' room, firm bedding surface, no loose coverings/items, and no barriers between babies.

Provide home care instructions in an optimal environment for parental learning. Learning should take place over time, to avoid bombarding the parents with instructions in the day or hour before discharge. Parents often enjoy performing minimal caretaking tasks, with gradual expansion of their role. Many NICUs provide facilities for parents to room in with their babies for a few days before discharge. This allows parents a degree of independence in the care of their baby with the security of nursing help nearby. Families can interact with staff while gradually transitioning to being the sole caretakers of their medically complex high-risk baby. This practice is particularly helpful for anxious parents, parents who have not had the opportunity to spend extended time with their baby, or parents who will be giving complex physical care at home, such as gastrostomy feeding, medication administration, and other care (Lopez, Anderson, & Feutchinger, 2012; Schlittenhart, Smart, Miller, et al., 2012). According to a study by Sneath (2009), parents of NICU graduates do not feel adequately prepared for discharge from the NICU with their babies. Teaching that occurs with daily interaction of the NICU staff is not always perceived by the family as adequate, and the stress levels of the family while in the NICU can be a barrier to a learning environment.

When discharging a medically fragile baby to home, schedule a predischarge home visit by a public health nurse or home health agency. This discharge visit evaluates the home for any possible issues that may complicate the parents' ability to care for their at-risk baby, especially if there are multiple monitoring equipment needs.

The basic elements of discharge and home care instruction are as follows:

1. Teach the parents routine well-baby care, such as bathing, taking a temperature, preparing formula, and breastfeeding.

2. Help parents learn to do special procedures as needed by the newborn, such as gavage or gastrostomy feedings, tracheostomy or enterostomy care, medication administration, cardiopulmonary resuscitation (CPR), and operation of the apnea monitor. Before discharge, the parents should be as comfortable as possible with these tasks and should demonstrate independence. Written tools and instructions are useful for parents to refer to once they are home with the baby, but they should not replace actual participation in the baby's care.

3. Make sure that all applicable screening (metabolic, vision, hearing) tests, immunizations, and respiratory syncytial virus (RSV) prophylaxis are done before discharge and that all records are given to the healthcare provider and parents.

4. Refer parents to community health and support organizations. The Visiting Nurse Association, public health nurses, or social services can assist the parents in the stressful transition from hospital to home by providing the necessary home teaching and support. Some NICUs have their own parent support groups to help bridge the gap between hospital and home care. Parents can also find support from a variety of community organizations, such as mothers-of-twins groups, March of Dimes Birth Defects Foundation, services for children with disabilities, and teen mother and child programs. Each community has numerous agencies capable of assisting the family in adapting emotionally, physically, and financially to the chronically ill baby. The nurse should be familiar with community resources and help the parents identify which agencies may benefit them.

5. Help parents recognize the growth and development needs of their baby. A development program begun in the hospital can be continued at home, or parents may be referred to an infant development program in the community.

6. Arrange medical follow-up care before discharge. The baby will need to be followed up by a family pediatrician, a well-baby clinic, or a specialty clinic. The first appointment should be made before the baby is discharged from the hospital.

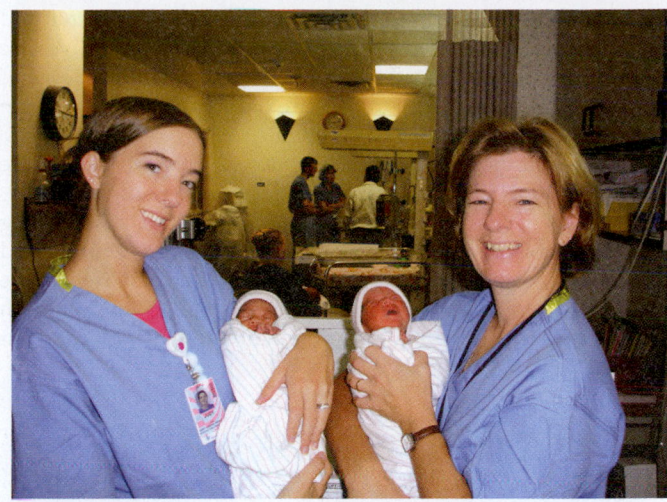

Figure 27–18 Discharge day. These 33 weeks' gestational age twins are being held by staff in the NICU on the happy day of discharge. This is what is so rewarding about working in the NICU: Healthy babies going home to their families.

SOURCE: Lisa Smith-Pedersen, RN, MSN, NNP-BC.

7. Evaluate the need for special equipment for care (such as a respirator, oxygen, an apnea monitor, a feeding pump) in the home. Any equipment or supplies should be placed in the home before the baby's discharge.

8. Ensure that a medical home for continuing medical care for the baby has been identified and a plan for transfer of information and care has been completed as needed.

9. Arrange for neonatal hospice for parents of the medically fragile baby as needed.

Further evaluation after the baby has gone home is useful in determining whether the crisis has been resolved satisfactorily. The parents are usually given the intensive care nursery's telephone number to call for support and advice. The ability to contact the NICU, perhaps even utilizing video conferencing, can be an effective method of support following discharge (Lopez et al., 2012). The staff can follow up with visits or telephone calls at intervals for several weeks to assess and evaluate the baby's (and parents') progress (Figure 27–18).

Evaluation

Expected outcomes of nursing care include the following:

- The parents are able to verbalize their feelings of grief and loss.

- The parents verbalize their concerns about their baby's health problems, care needs, and potential outcome.

- The parents are able to participate in their baby's care and show attachment behaviors.

Considerations for the Nurse Who Works With At-Risk Newborns

The birth of a baby with a problem is a traumatic event with the potential for either disruption or growth of the involved family. The NICU staff nurses may never see the long-term results of the specialized sensitive care they give to parents and their newborns. Their only immediate evidence of effective care may be the beginning resolution of parental grief; discharge of a recovered, thriving baby to the care of happy parents; and the beginning of reintegration of family life.

Nurses cannot provide support unless they themselves are supported. Working in an emotional environment of "lots of living and lots of dying" takes its toll on staff. NICUs are among the most stressful areas in health care for clients, families, and nurses. Nurses bear much of the stress and largely determine the atmosphere of the NICU. The nurse's ability to cope with stress is the key to creating an emotionally healthy environment and a positive working atmosphere. The emotional needs and feelings of the staff must be recognized and dealt with so that staff can support the parents. An environment of openness to feelings and support in dealing with their human needs and emotions is essential for staff.

As caregivers, nurses may be unaware of their need to grieve for their own losses in the NICU. Nurses must also go through the grief work that parents experience. Techniques such as group meetings, individual support, and primary care nursing may assist in maintaining staff mental health. Reunions in some nurseries are beneficial for the families and healthcare providers so they are able to see the children after discharge.

Focus Your Study

- The sick newborn—whether preterm, term, or postterm—must be managed within narrow physiologic parameters. These parameters (respiratory, cardiovascular, and thermal regulation) maintain physiologic homeostasis and prevent introduction of iatrogenic stress to the already stressed baby.

- The nursing care of the newborn with special problems involves the understanding of normal physiology, the pathophysiology of the disease process, clinical manifestations, and supportive or corrective therapies. Only with this knowledge can the nurse caring for newborns make appropriate observations concerning responses to therapy and development of complications.

- Asphyxia results in significant circulatory, respiratory, and biochemical changes in the newborn that make the successful transition to extrauterine life difficult. Asphyxia requires early identification and resuscitative management. Newborns needing resuscitation have a weak cry, poor respiratory effort, and retractions at birth.

- Resuscitation methods include:
  - Stimulation by rubbing the newborn's back. (Done initially to all newborns.)
  - Use of positive pressure to inflate the lungs. (Used if respirations are inadequate or have not been initiated.)
  - Endotracheal intubation. (Used immediately for severely premature newborns, newborns with known congenital anomalies, and newborns who do not respond to stimulation or bag and mask.)
  - Medications: Naloxone (Narcan) may be used to reverse effects of narcotics given to mother prior to birth.

- Newborn conditions that commonly present with respiratory distress and require oxygen and ventilatory assistance are as follows:
  - Respiratory distress syndrome (RDS) is a lack of sufficient surfactant that causes labored respirations and increased work at breathing. It is seen most frequently in premature newborns. Nursing care involves administration of surfactant, close assessment, and supportive care if mechanical ventilation is needed.

- Transient tachypnea of the newborn usually results from excess fluid in the lungs. Baby breathes normally at birth, but develops symptoms of respiratory distress by 4 to 6 hours of age. Nursing care involves initiating oxygen therapy and restricting oral feedings until respiratory status improves.

- Meconium aspiration syndrome (MAS) shows signs and symptoms of respiratory distress beginning at birth. Care depends on the amount of meconium that is aspirated and the activity level of the newborn. If baby is vigorous even in the presence of meconium—no subsequent special resuscitation. If baby has absent or depressed respirations, HR less than 100 beats per minute, or poor muscle tone—direct tracheal suctioning by specially trained personnel.

- After initial suctioning and/or resuscitation efforts, nursing care involves ongoing assessment for signs and symptoms of respiratory distress and supportive care of the newborn requiring mechanical ventilation or ECMO.

- Cold stress sets up the chain of physiologic events of hypoglycemia, pulmonary vasoconstriction, hyperbilirubinemia, respiratory distress, and metabolic acidosis.

- Nurses are responsible for early detection and initiation of treatment for hypoglycemia. Nursing interventions include: keep the baby warm during any transport; observe for any subtle signs of hypoglycemia; have baby go to breast or feed early in neonatal period; and assess blood glucose frequently.

- Physiologic jaundice occurs in 50% of all newborns; appears after 24 hours of age; is not visible after 10 days of age; and may require phototherapy. Pathologic jaundice is usually caused by ABO or Rh incompatibility; may be present within 24 hours of birth; treatment begins with phototherapy, but may progress to exchange transfusions. Untreated hyperbilirubinemia (because of either type of jaundice) may result in neurotoxicity.

- In Rh incompatibility: Maternal antibodies enter the fetal circulation, then attach to and destroy fetal red blood cells; fetal system produces more RBCs and hyperbilirubinemia, anemia, and jaundice result. In ABO incompatibility the mother is type O and newborn is type A or B and it is less severe than Rh incompatibility.

- Nursing responsibilities for the newborn receiving phototherapy include: expose maximum amount of skin surface for optimal therapeutic results; apply eye patches while banks of phototherapy lights are in progress; assess eyes for signs/symptoms of conjunctivitis per agency protocol; frequently monitor temperature; offer baby breast milk or formula frequently to assist in excretion of bilirubin. Additionally, keep parents informed of need for phototherapy and encourage them to hold and care for baby while undergoing phototherapy.

- Anemia (decreased amount of red blood cell volume) in newborns results from prenatal blood loss, birth trauma, infection, or blood group incompatibility. Anemia places the newborn at risk for alterations in blood flow and the oxygen-carrying capacity of the blood.

- Nursing assessment of the septic newborn involves identifying very subtle clinical signs that are also seen in other clinical disease states such as: lethargy or irritability, pallor or duskiness, hypothermia, feeding intolerance, hyperbilirubinemia, and tachycardia, bradycardia, or apneic spells. The nursing care includes: obtain cultures before antibiotic therapy starts; carry out laboratory sepsis workup; and administer antibiotics as prescribed. Also provide supportive care to include NTE, respiratory and cardiovascular support, nutrition, monitoring of fluid and electrolyte homeostasis, and observation for complications.

- All newborns receive eye prophylaxis with ophthalmic antibiotic because of the possibility of transmission of gonorrhea or chlamydia during the birth process. Maternal syphilis requires that the baby be isolated from other newborns and receive antibiotics at birth. Maternal herpes virus infection requires administration of IV antiviral medications in the immediate newborn period as well as multiple cultures (skin, spinal fluid) for presence of herpes virus.

- The nurse is the facilitator for interprofessional communication with the parents, identifying their level of understanding of their baby's care and their need for emotional support. Initially, the parents need to understand the baby's problem, including expected treatments.

- The nurse needs to prepare and facilitate the parents' viewing of the newborn by promoting touching and parental participation in care of the baby. The nurse should ensure parents understand routine well-baby care as well as normal growth and development of newborns/infants, and have referrals for normal newborn/infant screening procedures.

- Parents should have medical follow-up arranged and referral for any special equipment required at home and understand how to perform any special procedures needed to care for the baby.

- Parents of at-risk newborns need support from nurses and healthcare providers to understand the special needs of their baby and to feel comfortable in an overwhelming and often unfamiliar environment.

Clinical Reasoning in Action

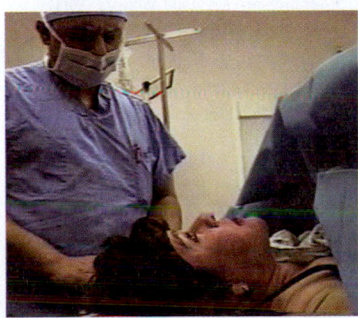

Rebecca Prince, age 21, G2 now P2, gives birth to a 5 lb baby at 38 weeks' gestation by primary cesarean birth for fetal distress. The baby's Apgars are 7 and 9 at 1 and 5 minutes. The newborn is suctioned and given free-flow oxygen at birth, then is admitted to the newborn nursery for transitional care and does well. You are the nurse caring for baby Prince at 36 hours old. You review the newborn's record and note that the baby's blood type is A+ and his mother is O+. Rebecca wants to breastfeed. You are performing a shift assessment on baby Prince when you observe that the baby has a unilateral cephalohematoma and is lethargic. You blanch the skin over the sternum and observe a yellow discoloration of the skin. Laboratory tests reveal a serum bilirubin level of 12 mg/dL, hematocrit 55%, a mildly positive direct Coombs test, and a positive indirect Coombs test. Baby Prince is diagnosed with hyperbilirubinemia secondary to ABO incompatibility and cephalohematoma. You provide phototherapy by fiberoptic blanket around the trunk of the newborn and take the baby to his mother's room.

1. How would you explain the purpose of phototherapy with the mother?

2. Plot the bilirubin on the hour-specific nomogram to assess the zone.

3. Explain the follow-up laboratory testing required and when it will be required.

4. Describe the care the mother can give to the newborn.

5. Discuss the advantage of the fiberoptic blanket phototherapy for the newborn.

References

American Academy of Pediatrics (AAP) & American Heart Association (AHA). (2011). *Textbook of neonatal resuscitation* (6th ed.). Elk Grove Village, IL: American Academy of Pediatrics & American Heart Association.

American Academy of Pediatrics (AAP), Committee on the Fetus and Newborn, & Adamkin, D. H. (2011). Clinical report: Postnatal glucose homoeostasis in late-preterm and term infants. *Pediatrics, 127*(3), 575–579.

American Academy of Pediatrics (AAP), Committee on the Fetus and Newborn, & American College of Obstetricians and Gynecologists (ACOG), Committee on Obstetric Practice. (2012). *Guidelines for perinatal care* (7th ed.). Elk Grove Village, IL: Author.

Arcara, K., & Tschudy, M. (2012). *The Harriet Lane handbook: Mobile medicine series, expert consult: Online* (19th ed.). New York, NY: Elsevier Health Sciences.

Bagwell, G. A. (2014a). Hematologic system. In C. Kenner & J. W. Lott (Eds.), *Comprehensive neonatal nursing care* (5th ed., pp. 334–375). New York, NY: Springer.

Bagwell, G. A. (2014b). Resuscitation and stabilization of the newborn and infant. In C. Kenner & J. W. Lott (Eds.), *Comprehensive neonatal nursing care* (5th ed., pp. 55–70). New York, NY: Springer.

Bennett, N. J. (2013). Bacteremia. *Medscape reference: Drugs, diseases & procedures.* Retrieved from http://emedicine.medscape.com/article/961169-overview

Bhutani, V. K., & Committee on the Fetus and Newborn. (2011). Phototherapy to prevent severe neonatal hyperbilirubinemia in the newborn infant 35 or more weeks of gestation. *Pediatrics 128*, e1046–1052. doi:10.1542/peds.2011-1494

Bhutani, V. K., Johnson, L. H., & Keren, R. (2004). Diagnosis and management of hyperbilirubinemia in the term neonate: For a safer first week. *Pediatric Clinics of North America, 51*(4), 843–861.

Bhutani, V. K., Stark, A. R., Lazzeroni, L. C., Poland, R., Gourley, G. R., Kazmierczak, S., . . . Stevenson, D. K. (2013). Predischarge screening for severe neonatal hyperbilirubinemia identifies infants who need phototherapy. *The Journal of Pediatrics, 162*, 477–482.

Bicking, C., & Moore, G. A. (2012). Maternal perinatal depression in the neonatal intensive care unit: The role of the neonatal nurse. *Neonatal Network, 31*(5), 295–304.

Blackburn, S. T. (2013). *Maternal, fetal, & neonatal physiology: A clinical perspective* (4th ed.). St. Louis, MO: Saunders.

Bondi, E., Evans, R., Mischler, M., Benel-Stenzel, M., Horstmann, S., Lee, V., . . . Gigliotti, F. (2013). Epidemiology of bacteremia in febrile infants in the United States. *Pediatrics, 132*(6), 990–996.

Bosschaart, N., Kok, J. H., Newsum, A. M., Ouweneel, D. M., Mentink, R., van Leeuwen, T. G., & Aalders, M. C. G. (2012). Limitations and opportunities of transcutaneous bilirubin measurements. *Pediatrics, 129*(4), 689–694.

Casey, G. (2013). Jaundice: An excess of bilirubin. *Kai Tiaki Nursing New Zealand, 19*(1), 20–24.

Chinchilla, M. K. (2012). Patient family-centered care: A bedside RN's perspective. *Neonatal Network, 31*(5), 341–344.

Cloherty, J. P., Eichenwald, E. C., Hansen, A. R., & Stark, A. R. (2012). *Manual of neonatal care* (7th ed.). Philadelphia, PA: Lippincott Williams & Wilkins.

Discenza, D. (2012a). Kangaroo care: Worth the time and effort. *Neonatal Network, 31*(3), 189.

Discenza, D. (2012b). Preemie parent frustration: Dealing with insensitive comments. *Neonatal Network, 31*(1), 52–53.

Fanaroff, A. A., & Fanaroff, J. M. (2013). *Klaus and Fanaroff's care of the high-risk neonate* (6th ed.). Philadelphia, PA: Elsevier Saunders.

Gardner, S. L., Enzman-Himes, M., & Nyp, M. (2016). Respiratory diseases. In S. L. Gardner, B. S. Carter, M. Enzman-Hines, & J. A. Hernandez (Eds.), *Merenstein & Gardner's handbook of neonatal intensive care* (8th ed., pp. 565–648). St. Louis. MO: Mosby Elsevier.

Gardner, S. L., & Hernandez, J. (2016). Heat balance. In S. L. Gardner, B. S. Carter, M. Enzman-Hines, & J. A. Hernandez (Eds.), *Merenstein & Gardner's handbook of neonatal intensive care* (8th ed., pp. 105–125). St. Louis. MO: Mosby Elsevier.

Gleason, C. A., & Devaskar, S. U. (2012). *Avery's diseases of the newborn* (9th ed.). St. Louis, MO: Elsevier Saunders.

Gomella, T. L. (2013). *Neonatology: Management, procedures, on-call problems, diseases, and drugs* (7th ed.). New York, NY: Lange McGraw-Hill.

Graci, A. (2013). A rounding system to enhance patient, parent, and neonatal nurse interactions and promote patient safety. *Journal of Obstetric, Gynecological, and Neonatal Nursing (JOGNN), 42*, 239–242.

Grant, P. (1978). Psychological needs of families of high risk infants. *Family and Community Health, 1*(3), 91–102.

Harris, D. L., Weston, P. J., & Harding, J. E. (2012). Incidence of neonatal hypoglycemia in babies identified as at risk. *The Journal of Pediatrics, 161*, 787–791.

Hemway, R. J., Christman, C., & Perlman, J. (2013). The 3:1 is superior to a 15:2 ratio in a newborn manikin model in terms of quality of chest compressions and number of ventilations. *Archives of Disease in Childhood. Fetal and Neonatal Edition, 98*(1), F42–45.

Hintz, S. R., Stevenson, D. K., Yao, Q., Wong, R. J., Das, A., Van Meurs, K. P., . . . Higgins, R. D. (2011). Is phototherapy exposure associated with better or worse outcomes in 501- to 1000-g-birth-weight infants? *Acta Paediatrica, 100*, 960–965. doi:10.1111/j.1651-2227.02175x

Holditch-Davis, D., Miles, M. S., Burchinal, M. R., & Goldman, B. D. (2011). Maternal role attainment with medically fragile infants: Part 2. Relationship to the quality of parenting. *Research in Nursing Health, 34*(1), 35–48. doi:10.1002/nur.20418

Johnson, P. J. (2012). Antibiotic resistance in the NICU. *Neonatal Network, 31*(2), 109–114.

Kamath-Rayne, B. D., Thio, E. H., Deacon, J., & Hernandez J. J. (2016). Neonatal hyperbilirubinemia. In S. L. Gardner, B. S. Carter, M. Enzman-Hines, & J. A. Hernandez (Eds.), *Merenstein & Gardner's handbook of neonatal intensive care* (8th ed., pp. 511–536). St. Louis, MO: Mosby Elsevier.

Klaus, M. H., & Kennell, J. H. (1982). *Maternal-infant bonding* (2nd ed.). St. Louis, MO: Mosby.

Lopez, G. L., Anderson, K. H., & Feutchinger, J. (2012). Transition of premature infants from hospital to home life. *Neonatal Network, 31*(4), 207–214.

Ludington-Hoe, S. M. (2011). Thirty years of kangaroo care science and practice. *Neonatal Network, 30*(5), 357–362.

Lukacs, S. L., & Schrag, S. J. (2012). Clinical sepsis in neonates and young infants, United States, 1988–2006. *The Journal of Pediatrics, 160*, 960–965.

Maisels, M. J. (2012). Noninvasive measurements of bilirubin. *Pediatrics, 129*(4), 779–781.

Maisels, M. J., & Watchko, J. F. (2012). Treatment of hyperbilirubinemia. In G. Buonocore, R. Bracci, & M. Weindling (Eds.), *Neonatology: A practical approach to neonatal management* (pp. 629–640). Milan, Italy: Springer-Verlag.

Mantagou, L., Fouzas, S., Skylogianni, E., Giannakopoulos, I., Karatza, A., & Varvarigou, A. (2012). Trends in transcutaneous bilirubin in neonates who develop significant hyperbilirubinemia. *Pediatrics, 130*, e898–e904.

Marks, M. (2012). Evidence-based midwifery: The case against newborn suctioning. *Midwifery Today (Summer 2012)*, 21–22.

Niermeyer, S., Clarke, S. B., & Hernandez J. J. (2016). Delivery room care. In S. L. Gardner, B. S. Carter, M. Enzman-Hines, & J. A. Hernandez (Eds.), *Merenstein & Gardner's handbook of neonatal intensive care* (8th ed., pp. 47–70). St. Louis, MO: Mosby Elsevier.

Ohls, R. K., Roohi, M., Peceny, H. M., Schrader, R., & Bierer, R. (2012). A randomized, masked study of weekly erythropoietin dosing in preterm infants. *The Journal of Pediatrics, 160*, 790–795.

Pappas, B. E., & Robey, D. L. (2015). Neonatal delivery room resuscitation. In M. T. Verklan & M. Walden (Eds.),

Core curriculum for neonatal intensive care nursing. (5th ed., pp. 77–94). St. Louis, MO: Saunders.

Polin, R. A., Carlo, W. A., & the Committee on the Fetus and Newborn. (2014). Surfactant replacement therapy for preterm and term neonates with respiratory distress. *Pediatrics, 133*(1), 156–163. doi:10.1542/peds.2013-3443

Polin, R. A., & the Committee on the Fetus and Newborn. (2012). Management of neonates with suspected or proven early-onset bacterial sepsis. *Pediatrics, 129*, 1006–1015.

Polin, R. A., Denson, S., Brady, M. T., & the Committee on the Fetus and Newborn and Committee on Infectious Diseases. (2012). Strategies for prevention of health care-associated infections in the NICU. *Pediatrics, 129*(4), e1085–e1093.

Riley, C., Spencer, B., & Prater, L. S. (2014). Normal term newborn. In C. Kenner & J. W. Lott (Eds.), *Comprehensive neonatal nursing care* (5th ed., pp. 113–132). New York, NY: Springer.

Rubarth, L. (2012). The Apgar score: Simple yet complex. *Neonatal Network, 31*(2), 169–176.

Sabir, H., Jary, S., Tooley, J., Liu, X., & Thoresen, M. (2012). Increased inspired oxygen in the first hours of life is associated with adverse outcome in newborns treated for perinatal asphyxia with therapeutic hypothermia. *The Journal of Pediatrics, 161*, 409–416.

Saugstad, O. D., Aune, D., Aguar, M., Kapadia, V., Finer, N., & Vento, M. (2014). Systematic review and meta-analysis of optimal initial fraction of oxygen levels in the delivery room at ≤ weeks. *Acta Paediatrica 103*(7), 744.

Sawyer, T., Laubach, V. A., Hudak, J., Yamamura, K., & Pocrnich, A. (2013). Improvements in teamwork during neonatal resuscitation after interprofessional Team STEPPS training. *Neonatal Network, 32*(1), 26–33. doi:10.1891/0730-0832.32.1.26

Schlittenhart, J. M., Smart, D., Miller, K., & Severtson, B. (2012). Preparing parents for NICU discharge: An evidence-based teaching tool. *Nursing for Women's Health, 15*(6), 486–494.

Siriwachirachai, T., Sangkomkamhang, U., Lumbiganon, P., & Laopaiboon, M. (2014). Antibiotics for meconium-stained amniotic fluid in labour for preventing maternal and neonatal infections. *Cochrane Database of Systematic Reviews, Issue 11*. Art. No. CD007772.

Skene, C., Franck, L., Curtis, P., & Gerrish, K. (2012). Parental involvement in neonatal comfort care. *Journal of Obstetric, Gynecological, and Neonatal Nursing (JOGNN), 41*, 786–797.

Smith, J., Alcock, G., & Usher, K. (2013). Temperature measurement in the preterm and term neonate: A review of the literature. *Neonatal Network, 32*(1), 16–25.

Smith, J. R., & Carley, A. (2014). Common neonatal complications. In K. R. Simpson & P. C. Creehan (Eds.), *AWHONN perinatal nursing* (4th ed., pp. 662–698). Philadelphia, PA: Wolter Kluwer.

Sneath, N. (2009). Discharge teaching in the NICU: Are parents prepared? An integrative review of parents' perceptions. *Neonatal Network, 28*(5), 237–246.

Solnit, A., & Stark, M. (1961). Mourning and the birth of a defective child. *Psychoanalytic Study of the Child, 16*, 505.

Swarnam, K., Soraisham, A. S., & Sivanandan, S. (2012). Advances in the management of meconium aspiration syndrome. *International Journal of Pediatrics* 2012. doi: 10:1155/2012/359571

Sweet, L., & Mannix, T. (2012). Identification of parental stressors in an Australian neonatal intensive care unit. *Neonatal, Paediatric and Child Health Nursing, 15*(2), 8–16.

Taylor, T. A., & Kennedy, K. A. (2013). Randomized trial of iron supplementation versus routine iron intake in VLBW infants. *Pediatrics, 131*(2), e433–e438.

Trevisanuto, D., Cengio, V. D., Doglioni, N., Cavallin, F., Zanardo, V., Parotto, M., & Weiner, G. (2013). Oxygen delivery using a neonatal self-inflating resuscitation bag: Effect of oxygen flow. *Pediatrics, 131,* e1144–e1149.

Turnbull, V., & Petty, J. (2012). Early onset jaundice in the newborn: Understanding the ongoing care of mother and baby. *British Journal of Midwifery, 20*(9), 615–622.

Van Woudenberg, C. D., Wills, C. A., & Rubarth, L. B. (2012). Newborn transition to extrauterine life. *Neonatal Network, 31*(5), 317–322.

Vandborg, P. K., Hansen, B. M., Greisen, G., & Ebbesen, F. (2012). Dose-response relationship of photo-therapy for hyperbilirubinemia. *Pediatrics, 130,* e352–e357.

Walden, M. (2014). Pain in the newborn and infant. In C. Kenner & J. W. Lott (Eds.), *Comprehensive neonatal nursing care* (5th ed., pp. 571–587). New York, NY: Springer.

Walker, L. J. (2013). Bonding with books: The parent-infant connection in the neonatal intensive care unit. *Neonatal Network, 32*(2), 104–109.

Walsh, B. K., Daigle, B., DiBlasi, R. M., & Restrepo, R. D. (2013). AARC clinical practice guideline. Surfactant replacement therapy: 2013. *Respiratory Care, 58*(2), 367–375.

White, A. L. (2012). Parents vs. neonatal resuscitation team: Who should decide? *The Kansas Nurse, 87*(3), 17–19.

Wolff, M., Schinasi, D. A., Lavelle, J., Boorstein, N., & Zorc, J. J. (2012). Management of neonates with hyperbilirubinemia: Improving timelines of care using a clinical pathway. *Pediatrics, 130,* e1688–e1694.

Zimmerman, K., & Bauersachs, C. (2012). Empowering NICU parents. *International Journal of Childbirth Education, 27* (1), 50–53.

Chapter 28
Postpartum Adaptation and Nursing Assessment

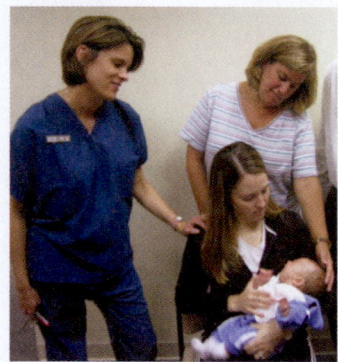

My position as a postpartum nurse involves helping the new family get to know one another. The real challenge is to balance the introduction of new skills and information with the time and space needed for the family to recover, both physically and mentally, from the birth experience. I want the families I care for to regard me as a resource, not an authority.

—Postpartum Nurse

Learning Outcomes

28.1 Describe the basic physiologic changes that occur in the postpartum period as a woman's body returns to its prepregnant state and the related nursing care.

28.2 Describe the psychologic adjustments that normally occur during the postpartum period and the related nursing care and support.

28.3 Explain the impact of cultural influence on providing nursing care during the postpartum period.

28.4 Describe the physiologic and psychologic components of a systematic normal postpartum assessment.

28.5 Describe the common concerns of the mother that are considered in a postpartum assessment.

28.6 Examine the physical and developmental tasks that the mother must accomplish during the postpartum period.

28.7 Relate how the nursing assessment of early attachment incorporates factors that influence the development of positive parent–newborn attachment.

During the **puerperium**, or *postpartum period*, the woman readjusts, physically and psychologically, from pregnancy and birth. The period begins immediately after birth and continues for approximately 6 weeks, or until the body has returned to a near prepregnant state.

This chapter describes the physiologic and psychologic changes that occur postpartum and the basic aspects of a thorough postpartum assessment.

Postpartum Physical Adaptations

Comprehensive nursing assessment is based on a sound understanding of the normal anatomic and physiologic processes of the puerperium. These processes involve the reproductive organs and other major body systems.

Reproductive System

INVOLUTION OF THE UTERUS

The term **involution** is used to describe the rapid reduction in size of the uterus and the return of the uterus to a nonpregnant state. Following separation of the placenta, the decidua of the uterus is irregular, jagged, and varied in thickness. The spongy layer of the decidua is cast off as lochia, and the basal layer of the decidua remains in the uterus to become differentiated into two layers within the first 48 to 72 hours after birth. The outermost layer becomes necrotic and is sloughed off in the lochia. The layer closest to the myometrium contains the fundi of the uterine endometrial glands, and these glands lay the foundation for the new endometrium. Except at the placenta site, this process is completed in approximately 3 weeks. The placenta site can take up to 6 weeks to be completely healed (Cunningham, Leveno, Bloom, et al., 2014; Pessel & Tsai, 2013). Bleeding from the larger uterine vessels of the placenta site is controlled by compression of the retracted uterine muscle fibers. The clotted blood is gradually absorbed by the body. Some of these vessels are eventually obliterated and replaced by new vessels with smaller lumens.

Rather than forming a fibrous scar in the decidua, the placenta site heals by a process of exfoliation and growth of endometrial tissue. This occurs with upward endometrial growth in the decidua basalis under the placenta site, with simultaneous growth of endometrial tissue from the margins of the site. The infarcted superficial tissue then becomes necrotic and is sloughed off (Blackburn, 2013). *Exfoliation* is a very important aspect of involution; if healing of the placenta site leaves a fibrous scar, the area available for future implantation is limited, as is the number of possible pregnancies.

With the dramatic decrease in the levels of circulating estrogen and progesterone following placental separation, the uterine cells atrophy, and the hyperplasia of pregnancy begins to reverse. Proteolytic enzymes are released, and macrophages migrate to the uterus to promote autolysis (self-digestion) (James, 2014). Protein material in the uterine wall is broken down and absorbed. Factors that enhance involution include an uncomplicated labor and birth, complete expulsion of the placenta or membranes, breastfeeding, manual removal of the placenta during a cesarean birth, and early ambulation. Factors that slow uterine involution and the rationale for each factor are listed in Table 28–1.

CHANGES IN FUNDAL POSITION

The **fundus** (top portion of the uterus) is situated in the midline midway between the symphysis pubis and the umbilicus (Figure 28–1). Immediately following the birth of the placenta, the uterus contracts to the size of a large grapefruit. The walls of the contracted uterus are in proximity, and the uterine blood vessels are firmly compressed by the myometrium. Within 6 to 12 hours after birth, the fundus of the uterus rises to the level of the umbilicus because of blood and clots that remain within the uterus and changes in support of the uterus by the ligaments. A fundus that is above the umbilicus and boggy (feels soft and spongy rather than firm and well contracted) is associated with excessive uterine bleeding. As blood collects and forms clots within the uterus, the fundus rises; firm contractions of the uterus are interrupted, causing a **boggy uterus (uterine atony)**.

When the fundus is higher than expected on palpation and is not in the midline (usually deviated to the right), distention of the bladder should be suspected; the bladder should be emptied

TABLE 28–1 Factors that Slow Uterine Involution

FACTOR	RATIONALE
Prolonged labor	Muscles relax because of prolonged time of contraction during labor.
Anesthesia	Muscles relax.
Difficult birth	The uterus is manipulated excessively.
Grand multiparity	Repeated distention of uterus during pregnancy and labor leads to muscle stretching, diminished tone, and muscle relaxation.
Full bladder	As the uterus is pushed up and usually to the right, pressure on it interferes with effective uterine contraction.
Incomplete expulsion of placenta or membranes	The presence of even small amounts of tissue interferes with the ability of the uterus to remain firmly contracted.
Infection	Inflammation interferes with the uterine muscle's ability to contract effectively.
Overdistention of uterus	Overstretching of uterine muscles with conditions such as multiple gestation, hydramnios, or a very large baby may set the stage for slower uterine involution.

immediately and the fundal height remeasured (Figure 28–2). If the woman is unable to void, in-and-out catheterization of the bladder may be required. In the immediate postpartum period, many women may not be aware of a full bladder. Because the uterine ligaments are still stretched, a full bladder can move

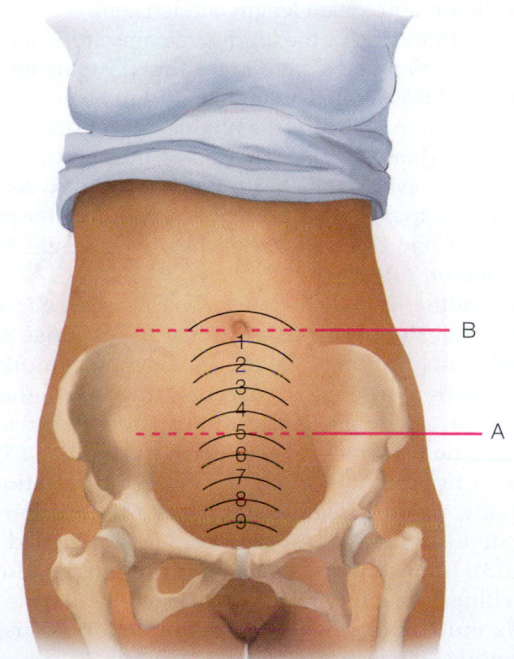

Figure 28–1 Involution of the uterus. A. Immediately after delivery of the placenta, the top of the fundus is in the midline and approximately halfway between the symphysis pubis and the umbilicus. About 6 to 12 hours after birth, the fundus is at the level of the umbilicus. B. The height of the fundus then decreases about one fingerbreadth (approximately 1 cm) each day.

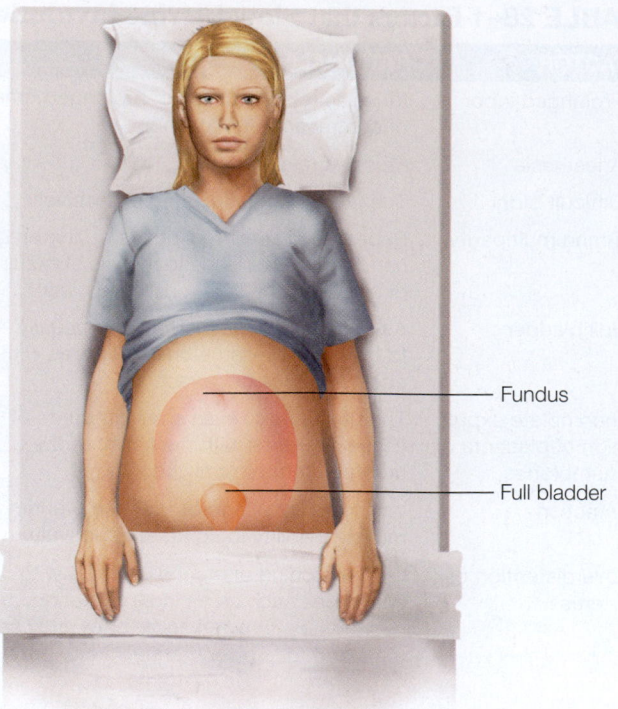

Fundus

Full bladder

Figure 28–2 The uterus becomes displaced and deviated to the right when the bladder is full.

the uterus. By the end of the puerperium, these ligaments have regained their nonpregnant length and tension.

After birth the top of the fundus remains at the level of the umbilicus for about half a day. On the first postpartum day, the top of the fundus is located about 1 cm (0.4 in.) below the umbilicus. On day 3 after delivery, the fundus is 3 cm (1.18 in.) below the umbilicus (James, 2014). The top of the fundus descends approximately one fingerbreadth (width of index, second, or third finger), or 1 cm, per day until it descends into the pelvis on about the 10th day. By 6 to 8 weeks, the uterus weighs 60 grams (2 oz) (Whitmer, 2016).

If the mother is breastfeeding, the release of endogenous oxytocin from the posterior pituitary in response to suckling hastens involution of the uterus. Barring complications, such as infection or retained placental fragments, the uterus approaches its prepregnant size and location by 5 to 6 weeks. In women who had an oversized uterus during the pregnancy (because of hydramnios, birth of a large-for-gestational-age [LGA] baby, or multiple gestation), the time frame for an immediate uterine involution process is lengthened (Blackburn, 2013). If intrauterine infection is present, in addition to foul-smelling lochia or vaginal discharge, the uterine fundus descends much more slowly. When infection is suspected, other clinical signs such as fever and tachycardia in addition to delay in involution must be assessed. Any slowing of descent is called **subinvolution** (for further discussion of subinvolution, see Chapter 30).

LOCHIA

The uterus rids itself of the debris remaining after birth through a discharge called **lochia**, which is classified according to its appearance and contents. **Lochia rubra** is dark red.

It occurs for the first 2 to 3 days and contains epithelial cells, erythrocytes, leukocytes, shreds of decidua, and occasionally fetal meconium, lanugo, and vernix. Clotting is often the result of pooling of blood in the upper portion of the vagina. A few small clots (no larger than a nickel) are common, particularly in the first few days after birth. However, lochia should not contain large (plum-size) clots; if it does the cause should be investigated without delay. **Lochia serosa** is a pinkish color. It follows from about day 3 until day 10. Lochia serosa is composed of serous exudate (hence the name), shreds of degenerating decidua, erythrocytes, leukocytes, cervical mucus, and numerous microorganisms (Blackburn, 2013).

The red blood cell (RBC) component decreases gradually, and a creamy or yellowish discharge persists for an additional week or two. This final discharge, termed **lochia alba** from the Latin word for *white*, is composed primarily of leukocytes, decidual cells, epithelial cells, fat, cervical mucus, cholesterol crystals, and bacteria.

Recent studies examining lochia patterns have found that the lochia rubra phase lasts longer than generally assumed and that it varies according to breastfeeding practice and parity (Blackburn, 2013). Variation in the duration of lochia discharge is not uncommon; however, the trend should be toward a lighter amount of flow and a lighter color of discharge. When the lochia flow stops, the cervix is considered closed, and chances of infection ascending from the vagina to the uterus decrease.

Like menstrual discharge, lochia flow has a musty, stale odor that is not offensive. Microorganisms are always present in the vaginal lochia, and by the second day following birth the uterus is contaminated with the vaginal bacteria. It is thought that an infection does not develop because the organisms involved are relatively nonvirulent. Any foul smell to the lochia or used peripad suggests infection and the need for prompt additional assessment, such as white blood cell count and differential and assessment for uterine tenderness and fever.

The total average volume of lochia is about 225 mL, and the daily volume gradually decreases (Blackburn, 2013). Discharge is greater in the morning because of pooling in the vagina and uterus while the mother lies sleeping. The amount of lochia may also be increased by exertion or breastfeeding. Multiparous women usually have more lochia than first-time mothers. Women who undergo a cesarean birth typically have less lochia than women who give birth vaginally (Blackburn, 2013).

Evaluation of lochia is necessary not only to determine the presence of hemorrhage but also to assess uterine involution. The type, amount, and consistency of lochia determines the stage of healing of the placenta site, and a progressive change from bright red at birth to dark red to pink to white or clear discharge should be observed. Persistent discharge of lochia rubra or a return to lochia rubra indicates subinvolution or late postpartum hemorrhage (see Chapter 30).

The nurse should exercise caution when evaluating bleeding immediately after birth. The continuous seepage of blood is consistent with cervical or vaginal lacerations and may be effectively diagnosed when the bleeding is evaluated in conjunction with the consistency of the uterus. Lacerations should be suspected if there is a continuous trickle of blood present but the uterus is firm and of expected size and if no clots can be expressed.

Clinical Reasoning   **Variations in Fundus Status**

You have completed your assessment of Patty Clark, a 24-year-old, G2P2 woman who is 24 hours past childbirth. The fundus is just above the umbilicus and slightly to the right. Lochia rubra is present, and a pad is soaked every 2 hours.

What would you do?

CERVICAL CHANGES

Following birth the cervix is spongy, flabby, and formless, and may appear bruised. The lateral aspects of the external os are frequently lacerated during the birth process (Cunningham et al., 2014). The external os is markedly irregular and closes slowly. It admits two fingers for a few days following birth, but by the end of the first week it admits only a fingertip.

The shape of the external os is permanently changed by the first childbearing. The characteristic dimple-like os of the nullipara changes to the transverse slit (fish-mouth) os of the multipara (Pessel & Tsai, 2013). After significant cervical laceration or several lacerations, the cervix may appear lopsided. Because of the slight change in the size of the cervix, a diaphragm or cervical cap will need to be refitted if the woman is using one of these methods of contraception.

VAGINAL CHANGES

Following birth the vagina appears edematous and may be bruised. Small superficial lacerations may be evident, and the rugae are obliterated. The apparent bruising is caused by pelvic congestion and trauma and will quickly disappear. The hymen, torn and jagged, heals irregularly, leaving small tags called *carunculae myrtiformes*.

The size of the vagina decreases and rugae return within 3 to 4 weeks (Blackburn, 2013; James, 2014). This facilitates the gradual return to smaller, although not nulliparous, dimensions. By 6 weeks the nonbreastfeeding woman's vagina usually appears normal. The lactating woman is in a hypoestrogenic state because of ovarian suppression, and her vaginal mucosa may be pale and without rugae; the effects of the lowered estrogen level may lead to dyspareunia (painful intercourse), which may be reduced by the addition of a water-soluble personal lubricant. Tone and contractility of the vaginal orifice may be improved by perineal tightening exercises such as Kegel exercises (see Chapter 10), which may begin soon after birth. The labia majora and labia minora are more flaccid in the woman who has borne a child than in the nullipara woman.

PERINEAL CHANGES

During the early postpartum period, the soft tissue in and around the perineum may appear edematous, with some bruising. If an episiotomy or a laceration is present, the edges should be drawn together. Occasionally, ecchymosis occurs, and this may delay healing. Initial healing of the episiotomy or laceration occurs in 2 to 3 weeks after the birth, although complete healing may take up to 4 to 6 months (Blackburn, 2013). Perineal discomfort may be present during this time.

RECURRENCE OF OVULATION AND MENSTRUATION

The return of ovulation and menstruation varies for each postpartum woman. Menstruation generally returns as soon as 7 weeks in 70% and by 12 weeks in all nonlactating mothers or as late as 3 years in 70% of breastfeeding mothers (Pessel & Tsai, 2013). The return of ovulation is directly associated with a rise in the serum progesterone level. In nonlactating mothers the average time to first ovulation can occur within 70 to 75 days, with a mean time of 6 months to first ovulation in lactating women (Pessel & Tsai, 2013).

The return of ovulation and menstruation in breastfeeding mothers is usually prolonged and is associated with the length of time the woman breastfeeds and whether formula supplements are used. If a mother breastfeeds for less than 1 month, the return of menstruation and ovulation is similar to that of the nonbreastfeeding mother. In women who exclusively breastfeed, menstruation is usually delayed for at least 3 months. Suckling by the baby typically results in alterations in gonadotropin releasing hormone (GnRH) production, which is thought to be the cause of amenorrhea (Blackburn, 2013). Although exclusive breastfeeding helps to reduce the risk of pregnancy for the first 6 months after birth, it should be relied on only temporarily and if it meets the observed criteria for the lactational amenorrhea method (LAM). Furthermore, because ovulation precedes menstruation and women often supplement breastfeeding with bottles and pacifiers, breastfeeding is not considered a reliable means of contraception.

Abdomen

The uterine ligaments (notably the round and broad ligaments) are stretched and require the length of the puerperium to recover. Although the stretched abdominal wall appears loose and flabby, it responds to exercise within 2 to 3 months. **Diastasis recti abdominis**, a separation of the abdominal muscle, may occur with pregnancy, especially in women with poor abdominal muscle tone (Figure 28–3). If diastasis occurs, part of the abdominal wall has no muscular support but is formed only by skin, subcutaneous fat, fascia, and peritoneum. This may be especially pronounced in women who have undergone a cesarean section, because the rectus abdominis muscles are manually separated to access the uterine muscle. Improvement depends on the physical condition of the mother, the total number of pregnancies, pregnancy spacing, and the type and amount of physical exercise (Cunningham et al., 2014). This may result in a pendulous abdomen and increased maternal backache. Fortunately, diastasis responds well to exercise, and abdominal muscle tone can improve significantly.

The striae (stretch marks), which occurred as a result of stretching and rupture of the elastic fibers of the skin, take on different colors based on the mother's skin color. The striae of White mothers are red to purple at the time of birth and gradually fade to silver or white. The striae of mothers with darker skin, in contrast, are darker than the surrounding skin and remain darker. These marks gradually fade after a time but remain visible.

Lactation

During pregnancy, breast development in preparation for lactation results from the influence of both estrogen and progesterone. After birth, the interplay of maternal hormones leads to milk production. (For further details, see the section on breastfeeding in Chapter 25.)

Gastrointestinal System

Hunger following birth is common, and the mother may enjoy eating a light meal. Frequently, she is quite thirsty

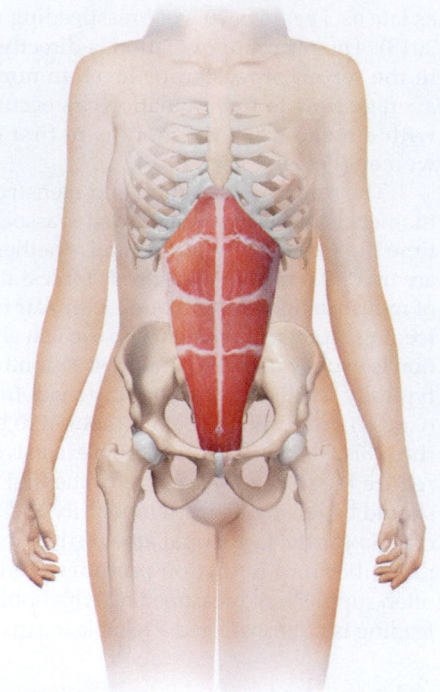

Normal location of rectus
muscles of the abdomen

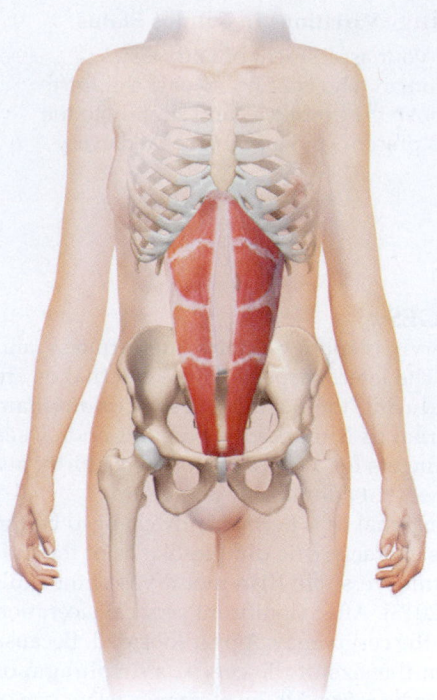

Diastasis recti: separation
of the rectus muscles

Figure 28–3 Diastasis recti abdominis, a separation of the abdominal musculature, commonly occurs after pregnancy.

and will drink large amounts of fluid. Drinking fluids helps replace fluids lost during labor, in the urine, and through perspiration.

The bowels tend to be sluggish following birth because of the lingering effects of progesterone, decreased abdominal muscle tone, and bowel evacuation associated with the labor and birth process (Whitmer, 2016). Pain medications and narcotics also can contribute to constipation and sluggish bowels. Women who have had an episiotomy, lacerations, or hemorrhoids may tend to delay elimination for fear of increasing their pain or because they believe their stitches will be torn if they bear down. In resisting or delaying a bowel movement, the woman may cause increased constipation and more pain when bowel elimination finally occurs.

The woman with a cesarean birth may receive clear liquids shortly after surgery; once bowel sounds are present, her diet is quickly advanced to solid food. In addition, the woman may experience some initial discomfort from flatulence, which is relieved by early ambulation and use of antiflatulent medications. Chamomile tea and peppermint tea may also be helpful in reducing discomfort from flatulence. It may take a few days for the bowel to regain its tone, especially if general anesthesia was used. The woman who has had a cesarean or a difficult birth may benefit from stool softeners.

Urinary Tract

The postpartum woman has an increased bladder capacity, swelling and bruising of the tissue around the urethra, decreased sensitivity to fluid pressure, and a decreased sensation of bladder filling. Consequently, she is at risk for

overdistention, incomplete bladder emptying, and a buildup of residual urine. Women who have had an anesthetic block have inhibited neural functioning of the bladder and are more susceptible to bladder distention, difficulty voiding, and bladder infections. In addition, immediate postpartum use of oxytocin to facilitate uterine contractions following expulsion of the placenta has an antidiuretic effect. Following cessation of the oxytocin, the woman will experience rapid bladder filling.

Urinary output increases during the early postpartum period (first 12 to 24 hours) because of *puerperal diuresis*. The kidneys must eliminate an estimated 2000 to 3000 mL of extracellular fluid with the normal pregnancy, which causes rapid filling of the bladder (Blackburn, 2013). Thus adequate bladder elimination is an immediate concern. Women with preeclampsia, chronic hypertension, and diabetes experience greater fluid retention than other women, and postpartum diuresis is increased accordingly.

If urine stasis exists, chances for urinary tract infection increase because of bacteriuria and the presence of dilated ureters and renal pelves, which persist for about 6 weeks after birth. A full bladder may also increase the tendency of the uterus to relax by displacing the uterus and interfering with its contractility, leading to hemorrhage. In the absence of infection, the dilated ureters and renal pelves return to prepregnant size by the end of the sixth week.

Vital Signs

During the postpartum period, with the exception of the first 24 hours, the woman should be afebrile. A maternal temperature of up to 38°C (100.4°F) may occur after childbirth as a result of the exertion and dehydration of labor. An increase in temperature to between 37.8° and 39°C (100° and 102.2°F) may also occur during the first 24 hours after the mother's milk comes in (Cunningham et al., 2014). However, in women not meeting these criteria, infection must be considered in the presence of an increased temperature (see discussion in Chapter 30).

Immediately following childbirth, many women experience a transient rise in both systolic and diastolic blood pressure, which spontaneously returns to the prepregnancy baseline during the next few days (James, 2014). A decrease may indicate physiologic readjustment to decreased intrapelvic pressure, or it may be related to uterine hemorrhage. Orthostatic hypotension, as indicated by feelings of faintness or dizziness immediately after standing up, can develop in the first 48 hours as a result of abdominal engorgement that may occur after birth. A low or decreasing blood pressure may reflect hypovolemia secondary to hemorrhage, but it is a late sign. Blood pressure elevations may result from excessive use of oxytocin or vasopressor medications. Because preeclampsia can persist into or occur first in the postpartum period, routine evaluation of blood pressure is needed. If a woman complains of headache, hypertension must be ruled out before analgesics are administered.

Puerperal bradycardia with rates of 50 to 70 beats per minute (beats/min) commonly occurs during the first 6 to 10 days of the postpartum period. It may be related to decreased cardiac effort, the decreased blood volume following placental separation and contraction of the uterus, and increased stroke volume. A pulse rate greater than 100 beats/min may be indicative of hypovolemia, infection, fear, or pain and requires further assessment (Whitmer, 2016).

Blood Values

Blood values should return to the prepregnant state by the end of the postpartum period. Pregnancy-associated activation of coagulation factors may continue for variable amounts of time after birth. This condition, in conjunction with trauma, immobility, or sepsis, predisposes the woman to the development of thromboembolism. The incidence of thromboembolism is reduced by early mobilization.

Nonpathologic leukocytosis often occurs during labor and in the immediate postpartum period, with white blood cell (WBC) counts of 25,000 to 30,000/mm³. WBC values typically return to normal levels by the end of the first postpartum week. Leukocytosis combined with the normal increase in erythrocyte sedimentation rate (ESR) may obscure the diagnosis of acute infection at this time (James, 2014).

Hemoglobin and hematocrit levels may be difficult to interpret in the first 2 days after birth because of the changing blood volume. This loss in blood in the first 24 hours accounts for half of the RBC volume gained during the course of the pregnancy. Blood loss averages 200 to 500 mL with a vaginal birth and nearly 1000 mL or more with a cesarean birth (Pessel & Tsai, 2013). Lochia constitutes less than 25% of this blood loss. As extracellular fluid is excreted, hemoconcentration occurs, with a concomitant rise in hematocrit. A drop in values indicates an abnormal blood loss. The following is a convenient rule to remember: A 2- to 3- percentage point drop in hematocrit equals a blood loss of 500 mL (James, 2014). After 3 to 4 days, mobilization of interstitial fluid leads to a slight increase in plasma volume. This hemodilution leads to a decrease in hemoglobin, hematocrit, and plasma protein

by the end of the first postpartum week. Decreases in plasma volume reach nonpregnant levels by 4 to 6 weeks postpartum (Blackburn, 2013).

Platelet levels typically fall as a result of placental separation. They then begin to increase by the third to fourth postpartum day, gradually returning to normal by the sixth postpartum week. Fibrinolytic activity typically returns to normal during the hours following birth. The hemostatic system as a whole reaches its normal prepregnant status by 3 to 4 weeks postpartum; however, the diameter of deep veins can take up to 6 weeks to return to prepregnant levels (Blackburn, 2013). This is why there is a prolonged risk of thromboembolism in the first 6 weeks following birth.

Cardiovascular Changes

The cardiovascular system undergoes dramatic changes during the birth that can result in cardiovascular instability because of an increase in the cardiac output. The cardiac output typically stabilizes and returns to pregnancy levels within an hour following birth (Blackburn, 2013). Maternal hypervolemia acts to protect the mother from excessive blood loss. Cardiac output declines by 30% in the first 2 weeks following birth and reaches normal levels by 6 to 12 weeks (Blackburn, 2013). Diuresis in the first 2 to 5 days assists to decrease the extracellular fluid and results in a weight loss of 3 kg (6.6 lb) (James, 2014). The failure of diuresis to occur in the immediate postpartum period can lead to pulmonary edema and subsequent cardiac problems. This is seen more commonly in women with a history of preeclampsia or preexisting cardiac problems (James, 2014).

Neurologic and Immunologic Changes

Neurologic problems and disorders can predispose women to higher rates of morbidity and mortality during pregnancy and in the postpartum period. Headaches are the most common neurologic symptoms encountered by postpartum women. Headaches may result from fluid shifts in the first week after birth, leakage of cerebrospinal fluid into the extradural space during spinal anesthesia, pregnancy-induced hypertension, or stress (James, 2014). It is estimated that up to 40% of postpartum women develop headaches within the first week following birth when estrogen drops precipitously (James, 2014; Lim, Evangelou, & Jurgens, 2014). There may be an increased incidence of headache if the woman had spinal or epidural anesthesia. Migraine headaches, although less frequent during pregnancy, tend to resume in the postpartum period, usually in the first week following birth (Nicholson, 2014).

Women with epilepsy are 9 times more likely to have a seizure during labor or in the first 24 hours after birth than during pregnancy (Samuels & Niebyl, 2012). The postpartum woman with epilepsy is more likely to be diagnosed with depression and referral to a therapist or support group should be made (Klein, 2012). The physiologic changes of pregnancy that may have required increasing antiepileptic drug (AED) dosage are now removed, and retitration of the AEDs is required to prevent toxicity. Women with multiple sclerosis (MS) and Guillain-Barré syndrome are more likely to have symptoms in the postpartum period than during pregnancy (Nicholson, 2014; Samuels & Niebyl, 2012). Myasthenia gravis (autoimmune disease) affects the neuromuscular junctions. The increase in symptoms during pregnancy is variable; however, the first month of pregnancy and the first month of the postpartum period are the most critical (Kalayjian, Goodwin, & Lee, 2013).

Weight Loss

An initial weight loss of about 10 to 12 lb (4.5 to 5.4 kg) occurs as a result of the birth of the baby, delivery of the placenta, and loss of amniotic fluid. Diuresis accounts for the loss of an additional 5 lb (2.3 kg) during the early puerperium. By the sixth to eighth week after birth, many women have returned to their approximate prepregnant weight if they gained the average 25 to 30 lb (11.3 to 13.6 kg). Women often express concern about the slow pace of their postpartum weight loss. Multiparas tend to be more positive than primiparas, probably because the multipara's previous experience has prepared her for the fact that the body does not immediately return to a prepregnant state.

Postpartum Chill

Frequently the mother experiences intense tremors that resemble shivering from a chill immediately after birth. Several theories have been offered to explain this shivering: It is the result of the sudden release of pressure on the pelvic nerves after birth, a response to a fetus-to-mother transfusion that occurred during placental separation, a reaction to maternal epinephrine production during labor and birth, or a reaction to epidural anesthesia. If not followed by fever, this chill is of no clinical concern, but it is uncomfortable for the woman. The nurse can increase the woman's comfort by covering her with a warmed blanket and reassuring her that the shivering is a common, self-limiting situation. If she allows herself to go with the shaking, the shivering will last only a short time. Some women may also find a warm beverage helpful. Later in the puerperium, chill and fever indicate infection and require further evaluation.

Postpartum Diaphoresis

The elimination of excess fluid and waste products via the skin during the puerperium produces increased perspiration. Diaphoretic (sweating) episodes frequently occur at night, and the woman may awaken drenched with perspiration. This perspiration is not significant clinically, but the mother should be protected from chilling.

Afterpains

Afterpains are more common in multiparas than in primiparas and are caused by intermittent uterine contractions. Although the uterus of the primipara usually remains consistently contracted, the lost tone of the multiparous uterus results in alternate contraction and relaxation. This phenomenon also occurs if the uterus has been markedly distended, as with a multiple-gestation pregnancy or hydramnios, or if clots or placental fragments were retained. These afterpains may cause the mother severe discomfort for 2 to 3 days after birth. The administration of oxytocic agents stimulates uterine contraction and increases the discomfort of the afterpains. Because endogenous oxytocin is released when the baby suckles, breastfeeding also increases the frequency and severity of the afterpains.

A warm water bottle placed against the lower abdomen may reduce the discomfort of afterpains. In addition, the breast-feeding mother may find it helpful to take a mild analgesic agent approximately 1 hour before feeding her baby. The nurse can assure the nursing mother that the prescribed analgesics are not harmful to the newborn and help improve the quality of the breastfeeding experience. An analgesic is also helpful at bedtime if the afterpains interfere with the mother's rest.

Postpartum Psychologic Adaptations

The postpartum period is a time of readjustment and adaptation for the entire childbearing family, but especially for the mother. The woman experiences a variety of responses as she adjusts to a new family member, postpartum discomforts, changes in her body image, and the reality that she is no longer pregnant.

Taking-In and Taking-Hold

Soon after birth, the woman tends to be passive and somewhat dependent. The new mother follows suggestions, is hesitant about making decisions, and is still rather preoccupied with her needs (Rubin, 1984). She may have a great need to talk about her perceptions of her labor and birth. This *taking-in* period helps her work through the process, sort out the reality from her fantasized experience, and clarify anything that she did not understand. Food and sleep are major needs.

By the second or third day after birth, the new mother is often ready to resume control of her body, her mothering, and her life in general. Rubin (1984) labeled this the *taking-hold* period. If she is breastfeeding, she may worry about her technique or the quality of her milk. If her baby spits up after a feeding, she may view it as a personal failure. She may also feel demoralized by the fact that the nurse or an older family member handles her baby proficiently while she feels unsure and tentative. She requires assurance that she is doing well as a mother. Today's mothers seem to be more independent and adjust more rapidly, exhibiting behaviors of "taking-in" and "taking-hold" in shorter time periods than those previously identified.

Becoming a Mother

Maternal role attainment (MRA) is the process by which a woman learns mothering behaviors and becomes comfortable with her identity as a mother. As the mother grows to know her baby and forms a relationship, the mother's maternal identity gradually and systematically evolves and she "binds in" to the infant (Rubin, 1984). In most cases maternal role attainment occurs within 3 to 10 months following birth.

Mercer proposed replacing the term *maternal role attainment (MRA)* with the term **becoming a mother (BAM)**. She stated that BAM "more accurately encompasses the dynamic transformation and evolution of a woman's persona than does MRA, and the term MRA should be discontinued" (Mercer, 2004, p. 226). BAM more accurately reflects the transitional process of becoming a mother that changes throughout the maternal–child relationship.

Postpartum nurses need to be aware of the long-term adjustments and stresses that the childbearing family faces as its members adjust to new and different roles. Nursing interventions that foster the process of becoming a mother include the following categories:

- Instructing for newborn/infant caregiving
- Building awareness of and responsiveness to newborn interactive capabilities
- Promoting maternal–newborn attachment
- Preparing the woman for the maternal social role
- Encouraging interactive therapeutic nurse–client relationships

Maternal/social role preparation and interactive therapeutic nurse–client relationships have a greater impact on the progress of becoming a mother than formal teaching.

depression (Ding, Wang, Qu, et al., 2014). Managing acute postpartum pain supports the new mother's ability to emotionally attach and care for her baby.

Professionalism in Practice Enhancing Patient-Centered Care

Mercer (2006) emphasized the importance of individualized dialogue between the mother and the nurse, which involves "a mutual identification by the mother and the nurse of the mother's needs and the available resources among the mother's family and friends, her community, and the larger society. With the mother's input about her preferences for available assistance. . . . Appropriate referrals may be made" (p. 650). Professional nurses who follow Mercer's recommendations enhance the process of becoming a mother and engage in patient-centered care.

Developing Cultural Competence Postpartum Depression

Nurses should take cultural and ethnic influences into account when assessing for the signs of postpartum depression (PPD). In a Pregnancy Risk Assessment Monitoring System survey, women of Asian/Pacific Islander descent had more than 3 times the rate of PPD that their White counterparts had and were more likely to be diagnosed with PPD after the birth of a female baby (Liu & Tronick, 2013). Gestational diabetes was a risk factor for PPD among African American women. Some characteristics, such as the baby's gender, are not commonly thought of as predictors for depression, but are predictive in specific ethnic groups. Across all the ethnic groups, prenatal depression is a strong predictor of PPD and assessment for signs of depression both before and after the birth is best practice.

Postpartum Blues

The **postpartum blues** consist of a transient period of depression that occurs during the first few days of the puerperium. It may be manifested by mood swings, anger, weepiness, anorexia, difficulty sleeping, and a feeling of being let down. This mood change frequently occurs while the woman is still hospitalized, but it may occur at home as well. Changing hormone levels are certainly a factor; psychologic adjustments, an unsupportive environment, and insecurity also have been identified as potential causes. In addition, fatigue, discomfort, and overstimulation may play a role. Postpartum pain after both vaginal and cesarean births has been shown to be associated with postpartum

Postpartum blues usually resolve naturally within 10 to 14 days, but if they persist or symptoms worsen, the woman may need evaluation for postpartum depression. Ideally a depression assessment should be completed each trimester to update a pregnant woman's risk status. If this is not done previously, the nurse assesses the woman for predisposing factors during labor and the postpartum stay. Several depression scales are available for assessing postpartum depression (see Chapter 30 for further discussion).

EVIDENCE-BASED PRACTICE | Psychosocial and Psychologic Interventions for Preventing Postpartum Depression

Clinical Question
What kinds of psychosocial and psychologic interventions may be helpful in the prevention of postpartum depression?

The Evidence
There is substantial evidence identifying the risk factors for the development of postpartum depression. It has been theorized that these risk factors could serve as the basis for designing psychosocial and psychologic interventions that could be offered during pregnancy and the immediate postpartum period to prevent the occurrence of this serious condition. Two researchers conducted a systematic review to first discover if these types of interventions are effective preventive measures. A secondary goal of the review was to determine the specific aspects of these interventions that were effective, such as professionally versus lay-based interventions; individually based versus group-based interventions; effects of interventions on onset and duration of depression; and relationship of treatment and specific risk factors. This review was structured and peer reviewed and published in the rigorous *Cochrane Database of Systematic Reviews*, which forms the strongest level of evidence. Twenty-eight studies with samples totaling almost 17,000 women were represented in this review.

Women who received psychosocial and/or psychologic interventions were considerably less likely to experience postpartum depression (Dennis & Dowswell, 2014). The most promising interventions were the provision of intensive, individualized postpartum home visits provided by nurses or nurse-midwives. These women had nearly half the rate of postpartum depression as women without this support. Peer-provided telephone support by lay women was also successful, as was interpersonal psychotherapy provided by professional counselors. Using risk factors to identify mothers who were most likely to develop postpartum depression aided in its prevention.

Best Practice
Psychosocial and psychologic interventions are clearly effective in preventing postpartum depression. Mothers should be assessed for risk factors and interventions should be applied accordingly. These interventions can be provided through professionally based home visits or psychotherapy, or by lay peers via telephone consultation.

Clinical Reasoning
What are some of the prenatal risk factors that might help identify women who should receive interventions for prevention of postpartum depression? What might be the major components of a psychosocial or psychologic intervention?

Importance of Social Support

After the birth of a baby, women and their partners may find that family relationships become increasingly important. The attention that their baby receives from family members is a source of satisfaction to the new parents. In many cases, the ties to the woman's family become especially good. Fathers may report that their relationships with their in-laws become far more positive and supportive. However, the increased family interaction can be a source of stress, especially for the new mother, who tends to have more contact with the families.

The new parents may also have increasing contact with other parents of small children while contact with coworkers declines. Of great concern are women and their partners who have no family or friends with whom to form a social network. Isolation at a time when the woman feels an increased need for support can result in tremendous stress and is often a contributing factor in situations of postpartum depression, child neglect, or abuse. New mother support groups are helpful for women who lack a social support system. Postpartum doulas are professionals trained to help the new mother be as rested and well nourished as possible, and to take responsibility for keeping the household in good order so that she can focus her energy on her new baby.

Developing Cultural Competence Middle Eastern Initial Postpartum Experience

In many countries in the Middle East that follow a patriarchal system, the new mother and her baby stay with the husband's family following the birth. Frequent visits from the woman's family are discouraged and may even be viewed as burdensome by the husband's family. Typically, only women visit the new mother during the postpartum period. For the birth of the first baby, the wife's parents are expected to purchase all of the baby's supplies and clothing.

Development of Family Attachment

Some parents may lack any experience with babies and may feel overwhelmed by the newborn. Bonding is a series of steps in which the mother, father, and baby develop relationships.

Maternal–Newborn Attachment Behavior

A mother's first interaction with her newborn is influenced by many factors, including her involvement with her family of origin, her relationships, the stability of her home environment, the communication patterns she has developed, and the degree of nurturing she received as a child. These factors have shaped the person she has become. The following personal characteristics are also important:

- *Level of trust.* What level of trust has this mother developed in response to her life experiences? What is her philosophy of childrearing? Will she be able to treat her baby as a unique individual with changing needs that should be met as much as possible?

- *Level of self-esteem.* How much does she value herself as a woman and as a mother? Does she feel generally able to cope with the adjustments of life?

- *Capacity for enjoying herself.* Is the mother able to find pleasure in everyday activities and human relationships?

- *Adequacy of knowledge about childbearing and childrearing.* What beliefs about the course of pregnancy, the capabilities of newborns, previous experiences with babies/children, and the nature of her emotions may influence her behavior at first contact with her newborn and later?

- *Prevailing mood or usual feeling tone.* Is the woman predominantly contented, angry, depressed, or anxious? Is she sensitive to her own feelings and those of others? Will she be able to accept her own needs and to obtain support in meeting them?

- *Reactions to the present pregnancy.* Was the pregnancy planned? Did it go smoothly? Were there ongoing life events that enhanced her pregnancy or depleted her reserves of energy? How have other life roles changed because of her pregnancy and motherhood?

By the time of birth, each mother has developed an emotional orientation of some kind to the baby based on these factors.

INITIAL MATERNAL ATTACHMENT BEHAVIOR

After labor and birth, a new mother will demonstrate a fairly regular pattern of maternal behaviors as she continues to familiarize herself with her newborn. In a progression of touching activities, the mother proceeds from fingertip exploration of the newborn's extremities toward palmar contact with larger body areas and finally to enfolding the baby with the whole hand and arm. The time taken to accomplish these steps varies from minutes to days. The mother increases the proportion of time spent in the *en face* position (Figure 28–4). She arranges herself or the newborn so that she has direct face-to-face and eye-to-eye contact. There is an intense interest in having the baby's eyes open. When the baby's eyes are open, the mother characteristically greets and talks in high-pitched tones to her baby.

In most instances the mother relies heavily on her senses of sight, touch, and hearing in getting to know what her baby is really like. She tends also to respond verbally to any sounds emitted by the newborn, such as cries, coughs, sneezes, and grunts. The sense of smell may be involved as well.

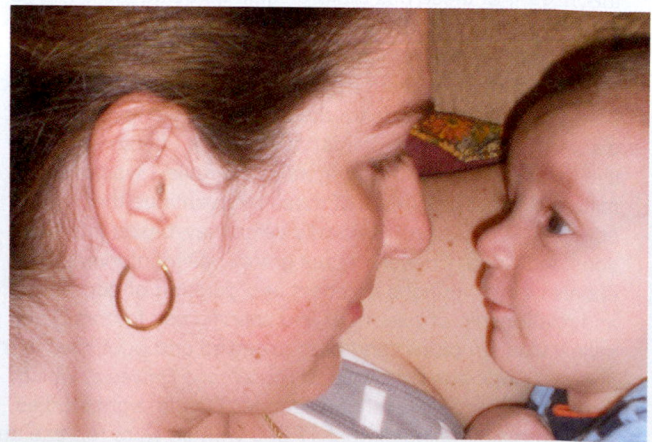

Figure 28–4 The mother has direct face-to-face and eye-to-eye contact in the *en face* position.

SOURCE: Joanna Allen.

While interacting with her newborn, the mother may be experiencing shock, disbelief, or denial. She may state, "I can't believe she's finally here" or "I feel like he is a stranger." On the other hand, feelings of connectedness between the newborn and the rest of the family can be expressed in positive or negative terms: "She's got your cute nose, Daddy" or "Oh, no! He looks just like Matthew, and he was an impossible baby." A mother's facial expressions or the frequency and content of her questions may demonstrate concerns about the newborn's general condition or normality, especially if her pregnancy was complicated or if a previous baby was not healthy.

During the first few days after her baby's birth, the new mother applies herself to the task of getting to know her baby. This is termed the *acquaintance phase*. If the newborn gives clear behavioral cues about needs, his or her responses to mothering efforts will be predictable, which will make the mother feel effective and competent. Other behaviors that make a baby more attractive to caretakers are smiling, grasping a finger, nursing eagerly, and being easy to console.

During this time the newborn is also becoming acquainted. Within a few days after birth, the baby shows signs of recognizing recurrent situations and responding to changes in routine. To the extent that the newborn's mother is his or her world, it can be said that the baby is actively becoming acquainted with her.

During the *phase of mutual regulation*, mother and newborn seek to determine the degree of control each partner in their relationship will exert. A balance is sought between the needs of the mother and the needs of the baby. The most important consideration is that each should obtain a good measure of enjoyment from the interaction. During this phase, negative maternal feelings are likely to surface or intensify. Because "everyone knows that mothers love their babies," these negative feelings often go unexpressed and are allowed to build up. If they are expressed, the response of friends, relatives, or healthcare personnel is often to deny the feelings to the mother: "You don't mean that." Some negative feelings are normal in the first few days after birth, and the nurse should be supportive when the mother vocalizes these feelings.

When mutual regulation arrives at the point where both mother and newborn primarily enjoy each other's company, reciprocity has been achieved. **Reciprocity** is an interactional cycle that occurs simultaneously between mother and baby. It involves mutual cuing behaviors, expectancy, rhythmicity, and synchrony. The mother develops a new relationship with an individual who has a unique character and evokes a response entirely different from the fantasy response of pregnancy. When reciprocity is synchronous, the interaction between mother and baby is mutually gratifying and is sought and initiated by both partners (Feldman, 2012).

FAMILY–NEWBORN INTERACTIONS

In Western cultures, commitment to family-centered maternity care has fostered interest in understanding the feelings and experiences of the new father. Evidence suggests that the father has a strong attraction to his newborn and that the feelings he experiences are similar to the mother's feelings of attachment. The characteristic sense of absorption, preoccupation, and interest in the newborn demonstrated by fathers during early contact is termed **engrossment** (Figure 28–5). Differences in involvement still exist among fathers in Western culture and may be influenced by factors other than culture (e.g., previous experience with paternal role or exposure to male/father role models).

Siblings and Others

Babies are capable of maintaining a number of strong attachments without loss of quality. These attachments may include siblings, grandparents, aunts, and uncles. The social setting and personality of the individual seem to be significant factors in the development of multiple attachments. Birth centers are especially geared toward the inclusion of the family in the

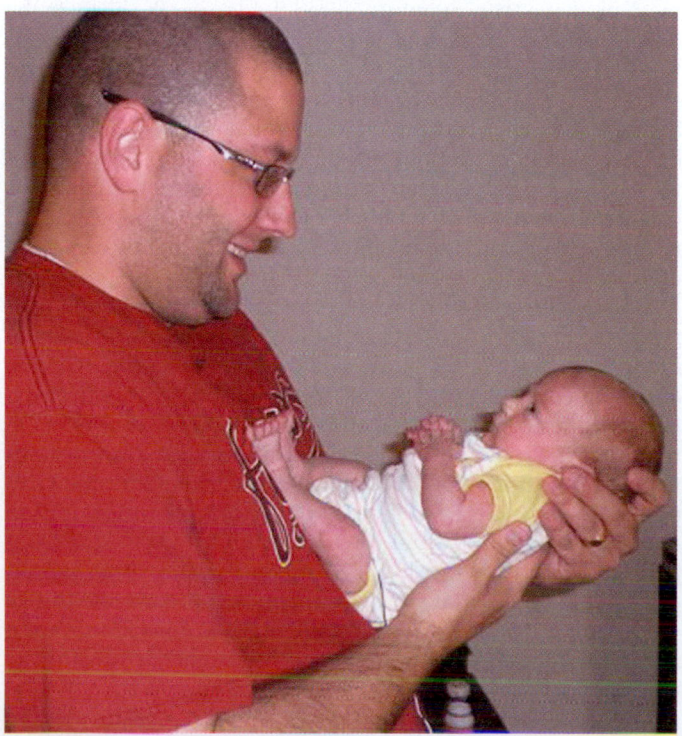

Figure 28–5 The father experiences strong feelings of attraction during engrossment.

SOURCE: Christopher Allen.

birth process. In the hospital setting, the advent of open visiting hours and rooming-in permits siblings and others to participate in the attachment process.

Cultural Influences in the Postpartum Period

Whereas Western culture places primary emphasis on the events of birth, many other cultures place greater emphasis on the postpartum period. For women not of the dominant American culture, the new mother's culture and personal values influence her beliefs about her postpartum care. Her expectations about food, fluids, rest, hygiene, medications and relief measures, support, and counsel—as well as other aspects of her life—will be influenced by the beliefs and values of her family and cultural group. Sometimes, a new mother's wishes will differ from the expectations of the healthcare provider/CNM or nurse.

All nurses belong to their particular ethnoculture and also share in the culture of health care. As a part of the healthcare cultural group, nurses implement practices that support their general beliefs, such as offering food in the recovery period following birth, providing iced fluids, expecting the woman to ambulate as soon as possible, and assuming the woman will want to shower and perhaps wash her hair soon after birth. It is important for nurses to recognize that they are approaching their clients' care from their own perspectives and that, to individualize care for each mother, they need to assess each woman's preferences, her level of acculturation and assimilation to Western culture, her linguistic abilities, and her educational level (Callister, 2014; Lauderdale, 2012). In addition, the nurse should have the mother exercise her choices when possible and support those choices, with the help of cultural awareness and a sound knowledge base.

The woman of European heritage may expect to eat a full meal and have large amounts of iced fluids after the birth, in the belief that the food restores energy and the fluids help replace fluid lost during the labor. She may want to ambulate shortly after the birth, shower, wash her hair, and put on a fresh gown. She may expect a short stay in the hospital and may or may not be interested in educational classes. Women of the Islamic faith may have specific modesty requirements; the woman must be completely covered, with only her feet and hands exposed, and no man, other than the husband or a family member, may be alone with her (Lauderdale, 2012).

Some cultures emphasize certain postpartum routines or rituals for mother and baby that are designed to restore the hot–cold balance of the body. Some women of Latino, African, and Asian cultures may avoid cold after birth. This prohibition includes cold air, wind, and all water (even if heated). On the other hand, some women of traditional Mexican descent may avoid eating "hot" foods such as pork just after the birth of a baby (considered a "hot" experience). It is important to note that each individual or cultural group may define hot and cold conditions and foods differently. The nurse should ask each woman what she can eat and what foods she thinks would be helpful for healing. The nurse may encourage family members to bring preferred foods and drinks for the mother.

In many cultures, the extended family plays an essential role during the puerperium. The grandmother is often the primary helper to the mother and newborn. She brings wisdom and experience, allowing the new mother time to rest and giving her ready access to someone who can help with problems and concerns as they arise. African American mothers often model their mothering skills after their older female relatives. In addition, these same older female relatives frequently provide child care as needed (Purnell, 2013).

It is important to ensure access of all family members to the mother and newborn. Visiting hours may be waived to allow family members or authority figures access to the mother and newborn. These practices show respect and foster a blending of old and new behaviors to meet the goals of all concerned (Purnell, 2013).

Developing Cultural Competence Caring for the Orthodox Jewish Couple

The orthodox Jewish couple's beliefs and practices are strictly adhered to in their dress, communication, dietary practices, and activities of daily living in the postpartum time. Jewish mothers may request a kosher diet. The nurse should assist the woman in maintaining her modesty in her dress and keeping her hair covered at all times. For the first 7 days after delivery, the woman will be given special treatment and will be cared for by family members. Some traditional Jewish couples avoid physical contact while the woman is experiencing any vaginal discharge; unfortunately the man following this custom may be viewed as unsupportive by the staff during the postpartum period. Resting after childbirth is considered crucial for the first 6 weeks. The woman will breastfeed her newborn. The baby will not be named nor will the newborn male be circumcised until a later date after discharge from the hospital. The Sabbath is sacred and begins at sundown on Friday evening and ends after dark on Saturday. During this time neither the man nor the woman will use electricity, travel, or write. They will not tear or cut anything. So if the woman is in the hospital during the Sabbath, the nurse should be sensitive to the fact that any forms that need to be signed will have to be signed before or after the Sabbath. The woman will need the nurse to adjust an electric bed, turn off/on lights, tear pieces of toilet paper for her to use, etc. The woman will not leave the hospital and travel home until after the Sabbath (Lauderdale, 2012).

Postpartum Nursing Assessment

Comprehensive care is based on a thorough assessment that identifies individual needs or potential problems.

Risk Factors

Ongoing assessment and patient education during the puerperium is designed to meet the needs of the childbearing family and to detect and treat possible complications. Table 28–2 identifies factors that may place the new mother at risk during the postpartum period. The nurse uses this knowledge during the assessment and is particularly alert for possible complications associated with identified risk factors.

Physical Assessment

The nurse should remember several principles when preparing for and completing the assessment of the postpartum woman:

TABLE 28–2 Postpartum High-Risk Factors

Preeclampsia	↑ Blood pressure ↑ CNS irritability ↑ Need for bed rest → ↑ risk thrombophlebitis
Diabetes	Need for insulin regulation Episodes of hypoglycemia or hyperglycemia ↓ Healing
Cardiac disease	↑ Maternal exhaustion
Cesarean birth	↑ Healing needs ↑ Pain from incision ↑ Risk of infection ↑ Length of hospitalization
Overdistention of uterus (multiple gestation, hydramnios)	↑ Risk of hemorrhage ↑ Risk of thrombophlebitis (cesarean section [C/S] risk) ↑ Risk of anemia ↑ Risk of breastfeeding problems (C/S risk) ↑ Stretching of abdominal muscles ↑ Incidence and severity of afterpains
Abruptio placentae, placenta previa	Hemorrhage → anemia ↓ Uterine contractility after birth → ↑ infection risk
Precipitous labor (less than 3 hours)	↑ Risk of lacerations to birth canal → hemorrhage
Prolonged labor (greater than 24 hours)	Exhaustion ↑ Risk of hemorrhage Nutritional and fluid depletion ↑ Bladder atony and/or trauma
Difficult birth	Exhaustion ↑ Risk of perineal lacerations ↑ Risk of hematomas ↑ Risk of hemorrhage → anemia
Extended period of time in stirrups at birth	↑ Risk of thrombophlebitis
Retained placenta	↑ Risk of hemorrhage ↑ Risk of infection

- Select a time that will provide the most accurate data. Palpating the fundus when the woman has a full bladder, for example, may give false information about the progress of involution. Ask the woman to void before assessment.
- Consider the woman's need for possible premedication before any painful assessment such as fundal massage.
- Explain the purpose of regular assessment to the woman.
- Ensure that the woman is relaxed before starting; perform the procedures as gently as possible to avoid unnecessary discomfort.
- Document and report the results as clearly as possible.
- Take appropriate precautions to prevent exposure to body fluids.

The physical assessment is an excellent opportunity for patient teaching. For example, when assessing the breasts of a lactating woman, the nurse can discuss breast care, breast milk production, the let-down reflex, and breast self-examination. A new mother may be very receptive to instruction on postpartum abdominal tightening exercises when the nurse assesses the woman's fundal height and diastasis. The assessment is also an excellent time to provide information about the body's postpartum physical and anatomic changes as well as danger signs to report. See *Teaching Highlights: Common Postpartum Concerns*. Because the time new mothers spend in the postpartum unit is limited, nurses need to use every available opportunity for patient education about self-care. To assist nurses in recognizing these opportunities, examples of patient teaching during the assessment are provided throughout the following discussion.

VITAL SIGNS

Many nurses begin by assessing vital signs because the findings are more accurate when they are obtained with the woman at rest. In addition, establishing whether the vital signs are within the expected normal range will assist the nurse in determining if other assessments are needed. For instance, if the temperature is elevated, the nurse considers the time since birth and gathers information to determine whether the woman is dehydrated or whether an infection is developing.

Temperature elevations (less than 38°C [100.4°F]) caused by normal processes should last for only 24 hours. The nurse evaluates any elevation of temperature in light of associated signs and symptoms and carefully reviews the woman's history to

TEACHING HIGHLIGHTS	Common Postpartum Concerns

Source of Concern	Explanation
Gush of blood that sometimes occurs when she first arises	Because of normal pooling of blood in the vagina when the woman lies down to rest or sleep. Gravity causes blood to flow out when she stands.
Passing clots	Blood pools at the top of the vagina and forms clots that are passed upon rising or sitting on the toilet.
Night sweats	Normal physiologic occurrence that results as the body attempts to eliminate excess fluids that were present during pregnancy. May be aggravated by a plastic mattress pad.
Afterpains	More common in multiparas. Caused by contractions and relaxation of uterus. Increased by oxytocin, breastfeeding. Relieved with mild analgesics and time.
"Large stomach" after birth and failure to lose all weight gained during pregnancy	The baby, amniotic fluid, and placenta account for only a portion of the weight gained during pregnancy. The remainder takes approximately 6 weeks to lose. Abdomen also appears large because of decreased muscle tone. Postpartum exercises will help.

identify other factors, such as premature rupture of membranes (PROM) or prolonged labor, that might increase the incidence of infection in the genital tract.

Alterations in vital signs may indicate complications, so the nurse assesses them at regular intervals. After an immediate, transient rise after birth, blood pressure (BP) should remain stable. The pulse often shows a characteristic slowness that is no cause for alarm. Pulse rates return to prepregnant norms very quickly unless complications arise.

SAFETY ALERT!

During the first few hours after birth, the woman may have some orthostatic hypotension. This will cause her to have a lower blood pressure reading in a sitting position. For the most accurate reading, use manual BP cuffs and measure the woman's BP with her in the same position each time, preferably lying on her back with her arm at her side. Because of the propensity for hypotension, assist the mother the first few times she attempts to ambulate after childbirth.

The nurse informs the woman of her vital signs and provides information about the normal changes in BP and pulse. This may be an opportunity to determine whether the mother knows how to assess her own and her baby's temperature, how to read a thermometer, and how to select a thermometer from the wide variety available.

AUSCULTATION OF LUNGS

The breath sounds should be clear. Women who have been treated for preterm labor or preeclampsia are at higher risk for pulmonary edema (see section Care of the Woman with a Hypertensive Disorder in Chapter 15 for further discussion).

BREASTS

Before examining the breasts, the nurse dons gloves and then assesses the fit and support provided by the woman's bra and, if appropriate, offers information about how to select a supportive bra. A properly fitting bra supports the breasts and helps maintain breast shape by limiting stretching of supporting ligaments and connective tissue. If the mother is breastfeeding, the straps of the bra should be cloth, not elastic (because cloth has less stretch and provides more support), and easily adjustable. The back should be wide and have at least three rows of hooks to adjust for fit. Traditional nursing bras have a fixed inner cup and a separate half cup that can be unhooked for breastfeeding while the inner cup continues to support the breast. Purchasing a nursing bra one size larger than the prepregnant size will usually result in a good fit because the breasts increase in size with milk production.

Clinical Tip

An easy way to remember the components specific to the postpartum examination is to remember the term BUBBLEHE: **B** – breast, **U** – uterus, **B** – bladder, **B** – bowel, **L** – lochia, **E** – episiotomy/laceration/edema, **H** – Homans/hemorrhoids, **E** – emotional. Some agencies include a final **R** (BUBBLEHER) to represent RhoGAM and rubella immunizations. (See Chapter 29 for further discussion.)

The nurse can then ask the woman to remove her bra so the breasts can be examined. The nurse notes the size and shape of the breasts and any abnormalities, reddened or hot areas,

or engorgement. The breasts are also lightly palpated for softness, slight firmness associated with filling, firmness associated with engorgement, warmth, and tenderness. The nipples are assessed for fissures, cracks, soreness, and inversion. The nurse teaches the woman the characteristics of the breast and explains how to recognize problems such as fissures and cracks in the nipples.

The nonbreastfeeding mother is assessed for evidence of breast discomfort, and relief measures are instituted if necessary. (See discussion of lactation suppression in the nonbreastfeeding mother in Chapter 29.) Breast assessment findings for a nonbreastfeeding woman may be recorded as follows: "Breasts soft, filling, no evidence of nipple tenderness or cracking, nipples everted."

ABDOMEN AND FUNDUS

Before examination of the abdomen, the woman should void. This practice ensures that a full bladder is not displacing the uterus or causing any uterine atony; if atony is present, other causes (such as uterine relaxation associated with a regional block, overstretched uterus, or distended bladder) must be investigated.

Clinical Tip

Gloves may be put on before assessing the abdomen and fundus and must be worn when you are ready to assess the perineum and lochia.

The nurse determines the relationship of the fundus to the umbilicus and also assesses the firmness of the fundus. The top of the fundus is measured in fingerbreadths above, below, or at the umbilicus (Figure 28–6). See *Clinical Skill: Assessing the Status of the Uterine Fundus After Vaginal or Cesarean Birth*. The nurse notes whether the fundus is in the midline or displaced to either side of the abdomen. If not midline, the uterus position should be located. The most common cause of displacement is a full bladder; this finding requires further assessment. If the fundus is in midline but higher than expected, it is usually associated with clots within the uterus. The nurse should then record the results of the assessment.

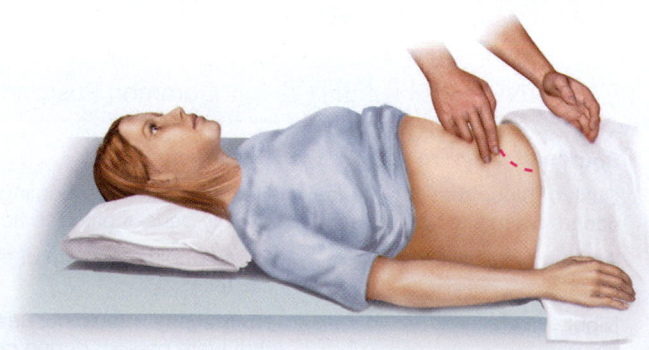

Figure 28–6 Measurement of descent of the fundus for the woman with vaginal birth. The fundus is located two fingerbreadths below the umbilicus. Always support the bottom of the uterus during any assessment of the fundus.

Clinical Skill 28–1

Assessing the Status of the Uterine Fundus After Vaginal or Cesarean Birth

NURSING ACTION

Preparation

- Consider offering to premedicate 30 to 45 minutes before assessing the fundus, especially if the woman has had a cesarean section.

Rationale: The postoperative area will be very tender, and she may be very fearful of the potential pain.

- Explain the procedure, the information it provides, and what it might feel like.
- Ask the woman to void.

Rationale: A full bladder can cause uterine atony.

- Have the woman lie flat in bed with her head on a pillow. If the procedure is uncomfortable, she may find that it helps to flex her legs. Flexing the legs and providing support under them with folded pillows is especially helpful with women who have had a cesarean.

Rationale: The supine position prevents a falsely high assessment of fundal height. Flexing the legs relaxes the abdominal muscles.

Equipment and Supplies

- Clean perineal pad
- Clean gloves

Procedure

1. Gently place one hand on the lower segment of the uterus. Using the side of the other hand, palpate the abdomen until you locate the top of the fundus.

Rationale: One hand stabilizes the uterus while the other hand locates the top of the fundus. (Support of the uterus prevents stretching of the ligaments that support the uterus.)

2. Determine whether the fundus is firm. If it is, it will feel like a hard round object (similar to a grapefruit) in the abdomen. If it is not firm, massage the abdomen lightly until the fundus is firm, then check for bleeding.

Rationale: A firm fundus indicates that the uterine muscles are contracted and bleeding will not occur.

3. Measure the top of the fundus in fingerbreadths above, below, or at the fundus (Figure 28–6).

Rationale: Fundal height gives information about the progress of involution.

4. Determine the position of the fundus in relation to the midline of the body. If it is not in the midline, locate it and then evaluate the bladder for distention.

Rationale: The fundus may deviate from the midline when the bladder is full because the enlarged bladder pushes the uterus aside.

5. If the bladder is distended, use nursing measures to help the woman void. If she is not able to void after a specified period of time, catheterization may be necessary.

6. Measure urine output for the next few hours until normal elimination is established.

Rationale: During the postpartum period as diuresis occurs, the bladder may fill far more rapidly than normal, putting the woman at risk for uterine atony and hemorrhage. (Diminished tone of the uterus may cause loss of the urge to void.)

7. Assess the lochia (see *Clinical Skill: Evaluating Lochia*).

8. During the first few hours postpartum, if the fundus becomes boggy frequently or is located high above the umbilicus and the woman's bladder is empty, the uterine cavity may be filled with clots of blood. In this case, do the following:

   - Release the front of the perineal pad and lay it back so that you can see the perineum and the pad laying between the woman's legs.
   - Massage the uterine fundus until it is firm.
   - Keep one hand in position, stabilizing the lower portion of the uterus. With the hand you used to massage the fundus, put steady pressure on the top of the now-firm fundus and see if you are able to express any clots. (Watch the pad between her legs for clots to pass from the vagina.)

Rationale: If the woman's uterus is filled with blood, it acts as an irritant and the uterus will not remain contracted. When the muscle fibers relax, bleeding results, further aggravating the problem. Pushing on a uterus that is not firm is dangerous because it is possible to cause the uterus to invert, a true emergency.

9. If measurement of the blood loss is needed, the perineal pads and absorbent pad can be weighed.

10. Provide the woman with a clean perineal pad.

11. Record findings. Fundal height is recorded in fingerbreadths (e.g., "2 FB ↓ U" or "1 FB ↑ U"). If fundal massage was necessary, note that fact: "Uterus boggy → firm with light massage."

12. Communicate bogginess or heavy flow to healthcare provider.

13. If the woman is post–cesarean section, inspect the abdominal incision for signs of healing, such as approximation or bleeding, and for any signs of infection, including drainage, edema, foul odor, or redness. Observe whether internal sutures, Steri-Strips, or staples are intact. If dressing is in place over the incision, observe for the dressing to be clean, dry, and intact.

Rationale: If drainage is present on the dressing, mark the outline of the drainage and reevaluate 30 minutes later for further bleeding or drainage.

14. Document findings according to hospital or unit policy.

15. Communicate active bleeding, increasing drainage, redness, foul odor, or incision edges not approximated to healthcare provider.

Assessing the status of the uterine fundus may be uncomfortable. In addition to explaining the importance of the assessment to the mother, you can show her how to perform frequent light massage of the fundus herself to promote uterine involution. She may be delighted to be able to feel the difference between where the fundus is now and where "the top of the uterus" was just prior to delivery. Involving her in her own care encourages her participation. In addition, having her massage her own uterus may lessen bleeding and reduce the need for more thorough massage.

In the woman who has had a cesarean birth, the abdominal incision is extremely tender. The nurse should palpate the fundus with extreme care and inspect the abdominal incision for signs of healing, such as approximation (edges of incision appear "glued" together), bleeding, and any signs of infection, including drainage, foul odor, or redness. The nurse should document whether internal sutures, Steri-Strips, or staples are intact. The nurse can also review characteristics of normal healing and incision care, and discuss signs of infection.

LOCHIA

Lochia is then assessed for character, amount, odor, and the presence of clots. Nurses must wear disposable gloves when assessing the perineum and lochia. Nurses may put on the gloves before beginning the assessment, just before assessing the abdomen and fundus, or when they are ready to assess the perineum and lochia. During the first 1 to 3 days, the lochia should be rubra. A few small clots are normal and occur as a result of blood pooling in the vagina. However, the passage of numerous or large clots is abnormal, and the cause should be investigated immediately.

Lochia should never exceed a moderate amount, such as that needed to partially saturate perineal pads daily, with an average of six. However, because this number is influenced by an individual woman's pad-changing practices, as well as the absorbency of the pad, the nurse needs to question her about the length of time the current pad has been in use, whether the amount is normal compared with her typical menstrual period, and whether any clots were passed before this examination, such as during voiding. If heavy bleeding is reported but not seen, the nurse asks the woman to put on a clean perineal pad and then reassess the woman's pad in 1 hour (see Figure 28–7 in *Clinical Skill: Evaluating Lochia*).

If blood loss exceeds the guidelines given in this chapter, weigh the perineal pads and the absorbent pads to estimate the blood loss more accurately. Typically, 1 g = 1 mL blood. Because blood can pool below the woman on the absorbent pad, the pads are included in your assessment.

Clots and heavy bleeding may be caused by uterine relaxation (atony), retained placental fragments, or, rarely, an unknown cervical laceration, seen as heavy bleeding but with firm fundus, that may require further assessment (Table 28–3). Because of the evacuation of the uterine cavity during cesarean birth, women with such surgery usually have less lochia after the first 24 hours than mothers who give birth vaginally. If the woman is at increased risk for bleeding, or is actually experiencing heavy flow of lochia rubra, her blood pressure, pulse, and uterus need to be assessed frequently, and the healthcare provider/CNM may prescribe oxytocin (Pitocin), methylergonovine maleate (Methergine) or misoprostol (Cytotec).

Teaching during assessment of the lochia may center on normal changes, the effect of position changes, or what can be expected in the amount and color of the flow. Hygienic measures, such as wiping the perineum from front to back and washing her hands after toileting and changing pads, may be reviewed if appropriate. The nurse should approach the timing of teaching hygienic practices delicately, along with the content to be included. By establishing positive goals for the teaching—promoting comfort, enhancing tissue healing, and preventing infection—the nurse can avoid value-laden statements regarding personal beliefs about the need for cleanliness or control of body odor. The nurse should review with the mother the need to notify a healthcare professional if there is regression in the lochia flow pattern (i.e., color or amount).

The parity, length of time since delivery, method of delivery, size of baby/gestation (and other factors that could cause hyperextension of the uterus such as multiple gestation, polyhydramnios, and large-for-gestational age) must be considered when deciding whether the amount and color of the lochia is appropriate.

PERINEUM

The perineum is inspected with the woman lying in a Sims position. The nurse lifts the buttock to expose the perineum and anus.

If an episiotomy was done or a laceration required suturing, the nurse assesses the wound. To evaluate the state of healing, the nurse inspects the wound according to the REEDA scale and responds appropriately to findings. After

TABLE 28–3 Changes in Lochia That Cause Concern

CHANGE	POSSIBLE PROBLEM	NURSING ACTION
Presence of clots	Inadequate uterine contractions that allow bleeding from vessels at the placental site	Assess location and firmness of fundus. Assess voiding pattern. Record and report findings.
Persistent lochia rubra	Inadequate uterine contractions; retained placental fragments; infection; undetected cervical laceration	Assess location and firmness of fundus. Assess activity pattern. Assess for signs of infection. Record and report findings.

Clinical Skill 28–2

Evaluating Lochia

NURSING ACTION

Preparation

- Explain why lochia occurs, why it is assessed, how it is assessed, and how it changes during the postpartum period.

- Ask the woman to void.

Rationale: A full bladder can cause uterine atony and increase the amount of lochia.

- Complete the assessment of uterine fundal height and firmness.

Rationale: In almost all cases, fundal height and firmness are evaluated with an assessment of lochia. This practice provides a more thorough assessment.

- If she has not already done so for the fundal assessment, ask the woman to flex her legs. Then ask her to spread her legs apart. Use the bed sheet as a drape to preserve her modesty.

Rationale: This position allows you to see the perineum and the perineal pad more effectively.

Equipment and Supplies

- Clean gloves
- Clean perineal pad

Procedure

1. Don gloves before assessing the perineum and lochia.

2. Lower the perineal pad and observe the amount of lochia on the pad. Because women's pad-changing practices vary, ask her about the length of time the current pad has been in use, whether the amount is normal, and whether any clots were passed before this examination, such as during voiding.

Rationale: During the first 1 to 3 days, the woman's lochia should be rubra, which is dark red in color. A few small clots are normal and occur as a result of pooling of blood in the vagina when the woman is lying down. The passage of large clots is abnormal and the cause should be investigated immediately.

3. If the woman reports heavy bleeding or clots, ask her to put on a clean perineal pad and then reassess the pad in 1 hour. Also ask her to call you before flushing any clots she passes into the toilet during voiding.

4. When the uterine fundus is firm and stabilized with the non-dominant hand, press down on it with the dominant hand while watching to see if any clots are expelled.

(see *Clinical Skill: Assessing the Status of the Uterine Fundus After Vaginal or Cesarean Birth*, Step 8).

5. Determine the amount of lochia, using the following guide (Figure 28–7):

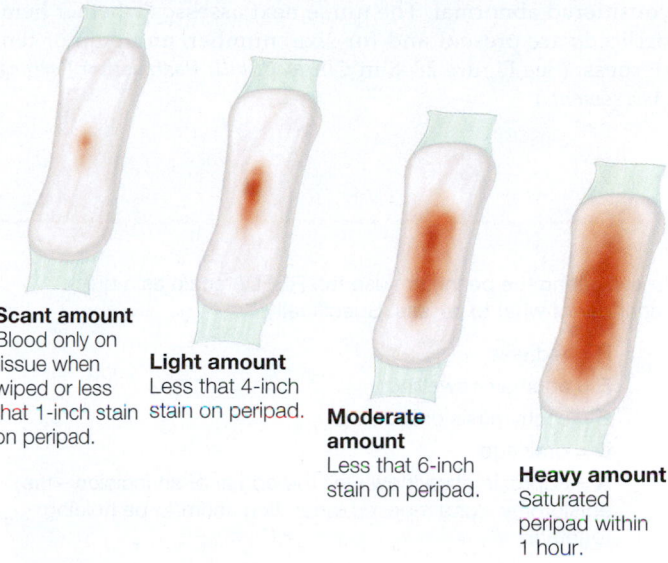

Scant amount
Blood only on tissue when wiped or less that 1-inch stain on peripad.

Light amount
Less that 4-inch stain on peripad.

Moderate amount
Less that 6-inch stain on peripad.

Heavy amount
Saturated peripad within 1 hour.

Figure 28–7 Suggested guideline for assessing lochia volume.

- Heavy amount—Perineal pad has a stain larger than 6 inches in length within 1 hour; 30 to 80 mL lochia.

- Moderate amount—Perineal pad has a stain less than 6 inches in length within 1 hour; 25 to 50 mL lochia.

- Light amount—Perineal pad has a stain less than 4 inches in length after 1 hour; 10 to 25 mL lochia.

- Scant amount—Perineal pad has a stain less than 1 inch in length after 1 hour or lochia is only on tissue when the woman wipes.

Rationale: Lochia should never exceed a moderate amount such as four to eight partially saturated perineal pads daily. Using a consistent standard for measuring lochia improves the accuracy of the information charted and conveyed to others.

6. In most cases, a woman is discharged while her lochia is still rubra. Provide her with information about lochia serosa and lochia alba.

Rationale: Accurate discharge information enables the woman to assess herself more accurately and enables her to judge better when to contact her caregiver.

7. Document the findings according to hospital/unit policy. For example, "Uterus firm, 1 FB ↓ U. Lochia: moderate rubra, no clots passed."

24 hours some edema may still be present, but the skin edges should be well approximated so that gentle pressure does not separate them. Gentle palpation should elicit minimal tenderness, and there should be no hardened areas suggesting infection. Ecchymosis interferes with normal healing, as does infection. Foul odors associated with drainage indicate infection. Hematomas sometimes occur, although these are considered abnormal. The nurse next assesses whether hemorrhoids are present and for size, number, and pain or tenderness. (See Figure 28–8 in *Clinical Skill: Postpartum Perineal Assessment*.)

Clinical Tip

In evaluating the perineum, use the REEDA scale as a quick reminder of what to assess. Specifically:

R = redness

E = edema or swelling

E = ecchymosis or bruising

D = drainage

A = approximation (how well the edges of an incision — the episiotomy — or a repaired laceration seem to be holding together)

During the assessment, the nurse talks with the woman to determine the effectiveness of comfort measures that have been used. The nurse provides teaching about the episiotomy or perineal laceration. Some women do not thoroughly understand what and where an episiotomy is, and they may believe that the stitches must be removed as with other types of surgery. Frequently, when women fear that the stitches must be removed manually, they are afraid to ask about them. While explaining the findings of the assessment, the nurse provides information about the episiotomy, its location, and the signs that are being assessed. In addition, the nurse can casually add that the sutures are special and will dissolve slowly over the next few weeks as the tissues heal. By the time the sutures are dissolved the tissues are strong and the incision edges will not separate. This is also an opportunity to teach comfort measures that may be used and reinforce the need to consult with the healthcare provider/CNM before using over-the-counter (OTC) medications/supplements if breastfeeding (see the section Relief of Perineal Discomfort in Chapter 29).

Clinical Tip

Lysine, an essential amino acid, has been identified as a supplement that decreases the incidence of pain following an episiotomy. The recommended adult dosage is 12 mg/kg of body weight per day. It is also present in dietary sources including meat, cheese, fish, eggs, soybeans, and nuts.

Clinical Skill 28–3

Postpartum Perineal Assessment

NURSING ACTION

Preparation

- Explain the purpose of and the procedure for assessing the perineum during the postpartum period.

- Complete the assessment of fundal height and lochia as described in *Clinical Skill: Assessing the Status of the Uterine Fundus After Vaginal or Cesarean Birth* and *Clinical Skill: Evaluating Lochia*.

Rationale: Typically, perineal assessment follows the fundal and lochial assessments.

- At this point in a postpartum assessment, the woman is lying on her back with her knees flexed. Her perineal pad has already been lifted away from her perineum to permit inspection of the lochia. If an episiotomy was performed or if the birth was difficult, the woman may be using an ice pack on her perineum to reduce swelling. The ice pack would also have been removed for inspection of the lochia.

- Ask her to turn onto her side with her upper knee drawn forward and resting on the bed (Sims position).

Rationale: When the woman is supine, even with her knees flexed, it is very difficult to expose the posterior portion of the perineum. Thus, Sims position makes it easiest to inspect the perineum and anal area.

Equipment and Supplies

- Clean perineal pad, clean ice pack if desired or needed

- Small light source such as a penlight may be necessary

Procedure: Clean Gloves

1. Use a systematic approach to assessment.

Rationale: A systematic approach helps ensure that you do not overlook a significant finding.

2. In evaluating the perineum, begin by asking about the woman's perceptions. How does she describe her discomfort? Does it seem excessive to her? Has it become worse since the birth? Does it seem more severe than you would expect?

Rationale: Information from the woman herself often helps identify developing problems.

Note: Pain that seems disproportionately severe may indicate that the woman is developing a vulvar hematoma.

3. After talking with the woman, assess the condition of the tissue. To allow for full visualization, it may be helpful to ask the woman to lift the knee of her upper leg to expose her perineum more fully. In some cases it may help to use the nondominant gloved hand to lift the buttocks and tissue. Note any swelling (edema) and bruising (ecchymosis). (Use the REEDA scale to recall what to assess.)

Rationale: The tissue is often traumatized by the birth and mild bruising is not unusual. However, excessive bruising may indicate that a hematoma is developing.

4. Evaluate the episiotomy, if there is one, or any repaired laceration for its state of healing. Is it reddened? Note the edges of the incision. Are they well approximated? Tell the woman that you are going to palpate the incision gently, then do so. Note any areas of hardness. Note whether the incision is warmer to the touch than the surrounding tissue.

Rationale: Gentle palpation should elicit minimal tenderness and there should be no redness, warmth, or areas of hardness, which suggest infection. Both bruising and infection interfere with normal healing. Typically, within 24 hours the edges of the incision should be "glued" together (well approximated).

5. During the assessment be alert for odors. Typically the lochia has an earthy, but not unpleasant, smell that is easily identifiable.

Rationale: A foul odor associated with drainage often indicates infection.

6. Finally, assess for hemorrhoids. To visualize the anal area, lift the upper buttocks to fully expose the anal area (Figure 28–8).

   If hemorrhoids are present, note the size, number, and pain or tenderness.

Rationale: Hemorrhoids often develop during pregnancy or labor and can cause considerable discomfort. If hemorrhoids are present, the woman may benefit from available comfort measures.

7. During the assessment, talk to the woman about the effectiveness of comfort measures being used. Provide teaching about care of the episiotomy, hemorrhoids, and the like.

Rationale: Health teaching is an important part of nursing care. Many women have concerns about the episiotomy and may not know, for example, that the suture used is dissolvable. This is an excellent time to provide information about good healthcare practices in both the short and the long term.

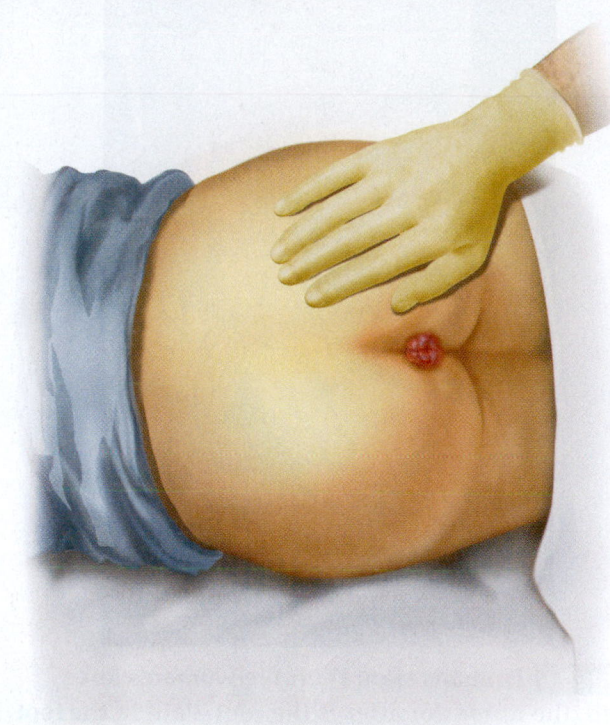

Figure 28–8 Intact perineum with hemorrhoids.

8. Provide the woman with a clean perineal pad. Replenish the ice pack if necessary.

9. Document findings according to hospital or unit policy. For example: "Midline episiotomy; no edema, ecchymosis, or tenderness. Skin edges well approximated. Woman reports pain relief measures are controlling discomfort" or "Perineal repair is approximated, minimal edema, no ecchymosis or tenderness; ice pack to perineum relieves pain."

LOWER EXTREMITIES

Postpartum women are at increased risk for *thrombophlebitis,* thrombus formation, and inflammation involving the leg veins (see the section Care of the Woman with Postpartum Thromboembolic Disease in Chapter 30). To assess for thrombophlebitis, the nurse should have the woman stretch her legs out with the knees slightly flexed and the legs relaxed. The nurse then grasps the woman's foot and sharply dorsiflexes it. The second leg is assessed in the same way. No discomfort or pain should be present. If pain is elicited, the nurse notifies the healthcare provider/CNM that the woman has a positive Homans sign (Figure 28–9). The pain is caused by inflammation of the vessel. The nurse also evaluates the legs for edema by comparing both legs, because usually only one leg is involved. Any areas of redness, tenderness, and increased skin temperature are also noted.

Some facilities have discontinued performing a Homans sign in the nursing assessment, stating it is not diagnostic and could lead to emboli if the clot is dislodged during assessment. Supporters advocate its use as a screening tool, and there are no published reports of an embolus occurring as a result of performing a Homans sign. In the event of a positive Homans sign, diagnosis is made by compression or duplex ultrasonography. Low-dose heparin therapy is used in postpartum women who do develop a deep venous thrombosis (Cunningham et al., 2014; James, 2014).

Early ambulation is an important aspect in the prevention of thrombophlebitis. Most women are able to be up shortly after birth or once they have fully recovered from the effects of regional anesthetic agents, if they have been used. The mother's legs should be assessed for return of sensation following regional anesthesia. The cesarean birth mother requires range-of-motion exercises until she is ambulating more freely. If the mother is unable to get up soon after delivery, sequential compression devices may be used.

Client teaching associated with assessment of the lower extremities focuses on the signs and symptoms of thrombophlebitis. In addition, the nurse may review self-care measures to promote circulation and measures to prevent thrombophlebitis, such as leg exercises that may be performed in bed, dorsiflexion on an hourly basis while on bed rest, ambulation, and avoiding pressure behind the knees and crossing the legs.

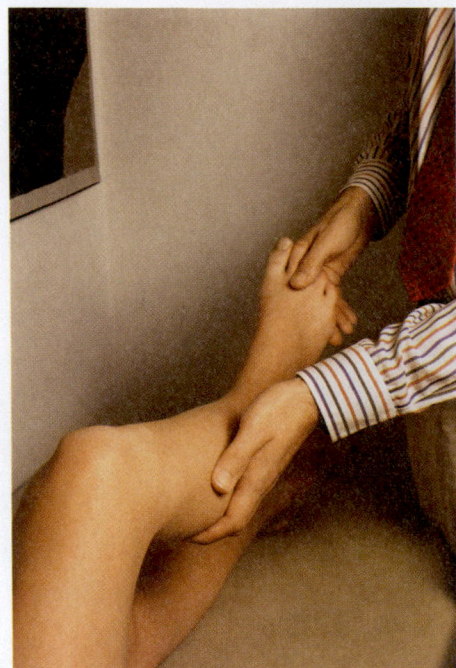

Figure 28–9 Homans sign: With the woman's knee flexed, the nurse dorsiflexes the foot. Pain in the foot or leg is a positive Homans sign.

SOURCE: © Image Source / Getty Images.

The nurse documents the results of the assessment in the medical record. If tenderness and warmth have been noted, they might be recorded as follows: "Tenderness, warmth, slight edema, and slight redness noted on posterior aspect of left calf—positive Homans sign. Woman advised to avoid pressure to this area; lower leg elevated and moist heat applied per agency protocol. Call placed to Dr. Garcia to report findings."

ELIMINATION

During the hours after birth, the nurse carefully monitors the new mother's bladder status. A boggy uterus, a displaced uterus, or a palpable bladder are signs of bladder distention and require nursing intervention.

The postpartum woman can quickly show signs of bladder distention, possibly as soon as 1 to 2 hours after childbirth. This distention results because of normal postpartum diuresis. The nurse should assess the bladder for distention until the woman demonstrates complete emptying of the bladder with each voiding. The nurse may employ techniques to facilitate voiding, such as helping the woman out of bed to void or pouring warm water on the vulva, running water in the sink, and encouraging the woman to relax and take deep breaths. The healthcare provider/CNM will order catheterization when the bladder is distended and the woman cannot void, when she is voiding small amounts (less than 100 mL) frequently, or when no voiding has occurred in 8 hours. The nurse needs to assess the bladder and any voiding pattern frequently before the end of the 8-hour period. Some women require catheterization sooner. The mother who has had a cesarean birth may have an indwelling catheter inserted prophylactically. The same assessments should be made in evaluating bladder emptying once the catheter has been removed.

The nurse should elicit information from the woman about the adequacy of her fluid intake, whether she feels she is emptying her bladder completely when she voids, and any signs of urinary tract infection (UTI) she may be experiencing.

In the same way, the nurse obtains information about the new mother's intestinal elimination and any concerns she may have about it. Many mothers fear that the first bowel movement will be painful and possibly even damaging if an episiotomy has been done. Often, women have defecated during labor or childbirth; therefore, bowel movements normally return within 2 to 3 days after a vaginal childbirth. Stool softeners may be ordered to increase bulk and moisture in the fecal material and to allow more comfortable and complete evacuation. Constipation should be prevented to prevent pressure on sutures and increased discomfort. To enhance bowel elimination and help the woman re-establish her normal bowel pattern, the nurse can encourage ambulation, increased fluid intake (up to 2000 mL/day or more), and additional fresh fruits and roughage in her diet.

During the assessment, the nurse may provide information about postpartum diuresis and explain why the woman may be emptying her bladder so frequently. Information about the need for additional fluid intake, with suggestions of specific amounts, may be helpful. The woman should drink at least eight 8-oz glasses of water or juice in addition to other fluids each day. Breastfeeding mothers will have a higher requirement. The nurse discusses signs of urinary retention and overflow voiding and may review symptoms of UTI if it seems an appropriate moment for teaching. The nurse can also review methods of assisting bowel elimination and provide opportunities for the woman to ask questions.

REST AND SLEEP STATUS

Physical fatigue often affects other adjustments and functions of the new mother. The mother requires energy to make the psychologic adjustments to a newborn and to assume new roles. Fatigue is often a highly significant factor in a new mother's apparent disinterest in her newborn. Frequently the woman is so tired from a long labor and birth that everything seems to be an effort. To avoid inadvertently classifying a very tired mother as one with a potential attachment problem, the nurse should do a psychologic assessment on more than one occasion. After a nap the new mother is often far more receptive to her baby and her surroundings. During the postpartum assessment, the nurse evaluates the amount of rest a new mother is getting. If the woman reports difficulty sleeping at night, the nurse should try to determine the cause. If it is simply the strange environment, a warm drink, back rub, or mild sedative may prove helpful. Appropriate nursing measures are indicated if the woman is bothered by normal postpartum discomforts such as afterpains, diaphoresis, or episiotomy or hemorrhoidal pain. The impact of rooming-in on the mother's ability to rest should be assessed. See Chapter 29 for more detailed discussion of comfort/pain relief measures.

The nurse should encourage a daily rest period and schedule hospital activities to allow time for napping. The nurse can also provide information about the fatigue a new mother experiences, strategies to promote rest/sleep at home, and the impact fatigue can have on a woman's emotions and sense of control.

NUTRITIONAL STATUS

As a part of the nutritional assessment, the nurse can provide teaching about the nutritional needs of the woman during the postpartum period. See the nutrition discussion in Chapter 11. Visiting the mother during mealtime provides an opportunity for unobtrusive nutritional assessment and counseling.

During pregnancy the daily recommended dietary allowances call for increased amounts of calories, protein, and most vitamins and minerals. After birth, the nonbreastfeeding mother should be advised about the need to reduce her caloric intake by about 300 kcal and to return to prepregnancy levels for other nutrients. The breastfeeding mother should increase her caloric intake by about 200 kcal over the pregnancy requirements, or a total of 500 kcal over the prepregnant requirement. New mothers are advised that it is common practice to prescribe iron supplements for 3 months after birth. The hemoglobin and hematocrit values are then checked at the postpartum visit to detect any anemia.

Basic discussion often proves helpful, followed by referral as needed. In all cases, literature on nutrition should be provided, so that the woman will have a source of information after discharge. The nurse should inform the dietitian of any mother who is a vegetarian, who has food allergies or lactose intolerance, or whose cultural or religious beliefs require specific foods. Appropriate meals can then be prepared for her. Many women, especially those who gained more than the recommended number of pounds, are interested in losing weight after birth. The dietitian can design weight-reduction diets to meet nutritional needs and food preferences. The nurse may also refer women with unusual eating habits or numerous questions about good nutrition to the dietitian.

Psychologic Assessment

During the first several postpartum weeks, the woman must accomplish certain physical, psychologic, and developmental tasks:

- Restoring physical condition
- Developing competence in caring for and meeting the needs of her baby
- Establishing a relationship with her new baby
- Adapting to altered lifestyles and family structure resulting from the addition of a new member

Adequate assessment of the mother's psychologic adjustment is an integral part of postpartum evaluation. Some new mothers have little or no experience with newborns and may feel totally overwhelmed. They may show these feelings by asking questions and reading all available material or by becoming passive and quiet because they simply cannot deal with their feelings of inadequacy. Unless a nurse questions the woman about her plans and previous experience in a supportive, nonjudgmental way, the nurse might conclude that the woman is disinterested, withdrawn, or depressed. Clues indicating adjustment difficulties include excessive continued fatigue, marked depression, excessive preoccupation with physical status or discomfort, evidence of low self-esteem, lack of support systems, marital problems, inability to care for or nurture the newborn, and current family crises (illness or unemployment). These characteristics frequently indicate a potential for maladaptive parenting, which may lead to child abuse or neglect (physical, emotional, intellectual) and cannot be ignored. Referrals to public health nurses or other available community resources may provide greatly needed assistance and alleviate potentially dangerous situations.

Assessment of Early Attachment

The beginnings of parent–newborn attachment may be observed in the first few hours after birth. Continued assessments may occur during the postpartum stay and during home visits after discharge. A nurse in any of the postpartum settings should note progress toward attachment. The assessment should include both parents when possible; as discussed previously, research shows that fathers experience similar attachment feelings to those experienced by mothers. The following behaviors focus primarily on the mother's attachment process and can be addressed in the course of nurse–client interactions:

- Is the mother attracted to her newborn? To what extent does she seek face-to-face contact and eye contact? Has she progressed from fingertip touch, to palmar contact, to enfolding the baby close to her own body? Is attraction increasing or decreasing? If the mother does not exhibit increasing attraction, why not? Do the reasons lie primarily within her, in the baby, or in the environment?

- Is the mother inclined to nurture her baby? Is she progressing in her interactions with her baby?

- Does the mother act consistently? If not, is the source of unpredictability within her or her baby?

- Is her mothering consistently carried out? Does she seek information and evaluate it objectively? Does she develop solutions based on adequate knowledge of valid data? Does she evaluate the effectiveness of her maternal care and adjust appropriately?

- Is she sensitive to the newborn's needs as they arise? How quickly does she interpret her baby's behavior and react to cues? Does she seem happy and satisfied with the baby's responses to her efforts? Is she pleased with feeding behaviors? How much of this ability and willingness to respond is related to the baby's nature and how much to her own?

- Does she seem pleased with her baby's appearance and sex? Is she experiencing pleasure when interacting with her baby? What interferes with the enjoyment? Does she speak to the baby frequently and affectionately? Does she call him or her by name? Does she point out family traits or characteristics she sees in the newborn?

- Are there any cultural factors that might modify the mother's response? For instance, is it customary for the grandmother to assume most of the child care responsibilities while the mother recovers from childbirth?

When the nurse has addressed these questions and assembled the facts, the nurse's intuition and knowledge should combine to answer three more questions: Is there a problem in attachment? What is the problem? What is its source? The nurse can then devise a creative approach to the problem as it presents itself in the context of a unique, developing mother–newborn relationship. See *Assessment Guide: Postpartum—First 24 Hours After Birth.*

Discharge Assessment and Follow-Up

The final discharge assessment should include a physical examination and appropriate discharge teaching that includes both maternal and newborn care guidelines. A home visit or follow-up phone call provides opportunities for further assessment of mothers and their newborns and teaching. (See *Assessment Guide: Postpartum—First Home Visit and Anticipated Progress at 6 Weeks* in Chapter 29.)

Women With Special Needs Modifications for Mobility Disorders

For the woman with a mobility disorder, specialized equipment will be needed in order for her to care for the baby. Modifications should include a lower crib and changing table height, arrangement of care supplies in an area she can adequately reach, and space in the nursery or a designated sleep location for the baby in which a wheelchair or walker can move easily, if used.

During this time period, infections, poor feeding, excessive weight loss, jaundice, and other problems in the newborn become apparent (James, 2014). The follow-up phone call is often initiated by a nurse from the postpartum unit of the agency where the mother gave birth. It is made soon after discharge and is designed to provide assessment and, if necessary, care; to reinforce knowledge and provide additional teaching; and to make referrals if indicated. Alternatively, a follow-up phone call from a nurse from the healthcare provider/CNM's office can provide new mothers with a source of support and an opportunity to ask questions. Women who appear to be having adjustment problems should be scheduled for an appointment for further evaluation.

In ideal situations, a family approach involving the father/partner, newborn, and other siblings permits a total evaluation and provides an opportunity for all family members to ask questions and express concerns. In addition, a family approach can sometimes enable the nurse to identify disturbed family patterns more readily and suggest, or even institute, therapeutic measures to prevent potential future problems of neglect or abuse.

ASSESSMENT GUIDE	Postpartum—First 24 Hours After Birth	
Physical Assessment/ Normal Findings	**Alterations and Possible Causes***	**Nursing Responses to Data†**
Vital Signs		
Blood pressure (BP): Should remain consistent with baseline BP during pregnancy.	High BP (preeclampsia, essential hypertension, renal disease, anxiety). Drop in BP (may be normal; uterine hemorrhage).	Evaluate history of preexisting disorders and check for other signs of preeclampsia (edema, proteinuria). Assess for other signs of hemorrhage (↑ pulse, cool clammy skin).
Pulse: 50–90 beats/min. May be bradycardia of 50–70 beats/min.	Tachycardia (difficult labor and birth, hemorrhage).	Evaluate for other signs of hemorrhage (↓ BP, cool clammy skin).
Respirations: 16–24/min.	Marked tachypnea (respiratory disease).	Assess for other signs of respiratory disease.
Temperature: 36.6°–38.0°C (98.0°–100.4°F).	After first 24 hr temperature of 38.0°C (100.4°F) or above suggests infection.	Assess for other signs of infection; notify healthcare provider/CNM.
Breasts		
General appearance: Smooth, even pigmentation, changes of pregnancy still apparent; one may appear larger.	Reddened area (mastitis).	Assess further for signs of infection.
Palpation: Depending on postpartum day, may be soft, filling, full, or engorged.	Palpable mass (caked breast, mastitis). Engorgement (venous stasis). Tenderness, heat, edema (engorgement, caked breast, mastitis).	Assess for other signs of infection: If blocked duct, consider heat, massage, position change for breastfeeding. Assess for further signs. Report mastitis to healthcare provider/CNM.

Physical Assessment/ Normal Findings	Alterations and Possible Causes*	Nursing Responses to Data†
Nipples: Supple, pigmented, intact; become erect when stimulated.	Fissures, cracks, soreness (problems with breastfeeding), not erectile with stimulation (inverted nipples).	Reassess technique; recommend appropriate interventions.
Lungs		
Sounds: clear to bases bilaterally.	Diminished (fluid overload, asthma, pulmonary embolus, pulmonary edema).	Assess for other signs of respiratory distress.
Abdomen		
Musculature: Abdomen may be soft, have a "doughy" texture; rectus muscle intact.	Separation in musculature (diastasis recti abdominis).	Evaluate size of diastasis; teach appropriate exercises for decreasing the separation.
Fundus: Firm, midline; following expected process of involution.	Boggy (full bladder, uterine bleeding).	Massage until firm; assess bladder and have woman void if needed; attempt to express clots when firm.
		If bogginess remains or recurs, report to healthcare provider/CNM.
May be tender when palpated.	Constant tenderness (infection).	Assess for evidence of endometritis.
Cesarean section incision dressing: dry and intact.	Moderate to large amount of blood or serosanguineous drainage on dressing.	Assess for hemorrhage. Reinforce dressing and notify healthcare provider/CNM.
Lochia		
Scant to moderate amount, earthy odor; no clots.	Large amount, clots (hemorrhage).	Assess for firmness, express additional clots; begin peripad count.
	Foul-smelling lochia (infection).	Assess for other signs of infection; report to healthcare provider/CNM.
Normal progression: First 1–3 days: rubra.	Failure to progress normally or return to rubra from serosa (subinvolution).	Report to healthcare provider/CNM.
Following rubra: Days 3–10: serosa (alba seldom seen in hospital).		
Perineum		
Slight edema and bruising in intact perineum.	Marked fullness, bruising, pain (vulvar hematoma).	Assess size; apply ice glove or ice pack; report to healthcare provider/CNM.
Episiotomy: No redness, edema, ecchymosis, or discharge; edges well approximated.	Redness, edema, ecchymosis, discharge, or gaping stitches (infection).	Encourage sitz baths; review perineal care, appropriate wiping techniques.
Hemorrhoids: None present; if present, should be small and nontender.	Full, tender, inflamed hemorrhoids.	Encourage sitz baths, side-lying position; Tucks pads, anesthetic ointments, manual replacement of hemorrhoids, stool softeners, increased fluid intake.
Costovertebral Angle (CVA) Tenderness		
None.	Present (kidney infection).	Assess for other symptoms of urinary tract infection (UTI); obtain clean-catch urine; report to healthcare provider/CNM.
Lower Extremities		
No pain with palpation; negative Homans sign.	Positive findings (thrombophlebitis).	Report to healthcare provider/CNM.
Elimination		
Urinary output: Voiding in sufficient quantities at least every 4–6 hr; bladder not palpable.	Inability to void (urinary retention). Symptoms of urgency, frequency, dysuria (UTI).	Employ nursing interventions to promote voiding; if not successful, obtain order for catheterization.
		Report symptoms of UTI to healthcare provider/CNM.
Bowel elimination: Should have normal bowel movement by second or third day after birth.	Inability to pass feces (constipation caused by fear of pain from episiotomy, hemorrhoids, perineal trauma).	Encourage fluids, ambulation, roughage in diet; sitz baths to promote healing of perineum; obtain order for stool softener.

(continued)

ASSESSMENT GUIDE | Postpartum—First 24 Hours After Birth (*continued*)

Cultural Assessment‡	Variations to Consider*	Nursing Responses to Data†
Determine customs and practices regarding postpartum care.	Individual preference may include room-temperature or warmed fluids rather than iced drinks.	Provide for specific request if possible. If woman is unable to provide specific information, the nurse may draw from general information regarding cultural variation.
Ask the mother whether she would like fluids, and ask what temperature she prefers.		
Ask the mother what foods or fluids she would like.	Special foods or fluids to hasten healing after childbirth.	Mexican women may want food and fluids that restore hot–cold balance to the body.
		Women of European background may ask for iced fluids.
Ask the mother whether she would prefer to be alone during breastfeeding.	Some women may be hesitant to have someone with them when their breast is exposed.	Provide privacy as desired by mother.

Psychologic Adaptation

During first 24 hr: Passive; preoccupied with own needs; may talk about her labor and birth experience; may be talkative, elated, or very quiet.	Very quiet and passive; sleeps frequently (fatigue from long labor; feelings of disappointment about some aspect of the experience; may be following cultural expectation).	Provide opportunities for adequate rest; provide nutritious meals and snacks that are consistent with what the woman desires to eat and drink; provide opportunities to discuss birth experience in nonjudgmental atmosphere if the woman desires to do so.
Usually by 12 hr: Beginning to assume responsibility; some women eager to learn; others easily feel overwhelmed.	Excessive weepiness, mood swings, pronounced irritability (postpartum blues; feelings of inadequacy; culturally proscribed behavior).	Explain postpartum blues; provide supportive atmosphere; determine support available for mother; consider referral for evidence of profound depression.

Attachment

En face position; holds baby close; cuddles and soothes; calls by name; identifies characteristics of family members in baby; may be awkward in providing care.	Continued expressions of disappointment in sex, appearance of baby; refusal to care for baby; derogatory comments; lack of bonding behaviors (difficulty in attachment, following expectations of cultural/ethnic group).	Provide reinforcement and support for newborn/infant caretaking behaviors; maintain nonjudgmental approach and gather more information if caretaking behaviors are not evident.
Initially may express disappointment over sex or appearance of baby but within 1–2 days demonstrates attachment behaviors.		

Patient Education

Demonstrates basic understanding of self-care activities and newborn/infant care needs; can identify signs of complications that should be reported.	Unable to demonstrate basic self-care and newborn/infant care activities (knowledge deficit; postpartum blues; following prescribed cultural behavior and baby will be cared for by grandmother or other family member).	Identify dominant learning style. Determine whether woman understands English and provide interpreter if needed; provide reinforcement of information through conversation and through written material (remember that some women and their families may not be able to understand written materials because of language difficulties or inability to read); provide information regarding newborn/infant care skills that are culturally consistent; give woman opportunity to express her feelings; consider social service home referral for women who have no family or other support, are unable to take in information about self-care and newborn/infant care, and demonstrate no caretaking activities.

*Possible causes of alterations are identified in parentheses.
†This column provides guidelines for further assessment and initial nursing actions.
‡These are only a few suggestions. It is not our intent to imply this is a comprehensive cultural assessment.

Focus Your Study

- The uterus involutes rapidly, primarily through a reduction in cell size.

- Involution is assessed by measuring fundal height. The fundus is at the level of the umbilicus within a few hours after childbirth and should decrease by approximately one fingerbreadth per day.

- The placental site heals by a process of exfoliation, so no scar formation occurs.

- Lochia progresses from rubra to serosa to alba and is assessed in terms of type, quantity, and characteristics.

- The abdomen may have decreased muscle tone (flabby consistency) initially. The nurse should assess for diastasis recti abdominis, separation of the rectus abdominis muscles.

- Constipation may develop in the postpartum period because of decreased tone, limited diet, and denial of the urge to defecate because of fear of pain.

- Decreased bladder sensitivity, increased capacity, and postpartum diuresis may lead to problems with bladder elimination. Frequent assessment and prompt intervention are indicated. A fundus that is boggy but does not respond to massage, is higher than expected, or deviates to the side usually indicates a full bladder.

- Postpartum a healthy woman should be normotensive and afebrile. Bradycardia is common.

- The white blood cell count is often elevated. Activation of clotting factors predisposes the woman to thrombus formation.

- Psychologic adaptations of the postpartum woman are traditionally described as "taking-in" and "taking-hold."

- Postpartum "blues" is a common occurrence and ways to prevent and cope with it should be discussed with not only the mother but also her significant other(s). Signs of postpartum depression should be discussed as well.

- In consideration of the woman's background, the nurse should recognize and respect cultural variations and individual preferences.

- Postpartum assessment should be completed in a systematic way, usually from head to toe, and should include assessment of rest and sleep, nutrition, and attachment. The assessment provides opportunities for informal patient teaching.

- In the weeks following birth, the woman's physical condition returns to a nonpregnant state and she gains competence and confidence in herself as a parent.

Clinical Reasoning in Action

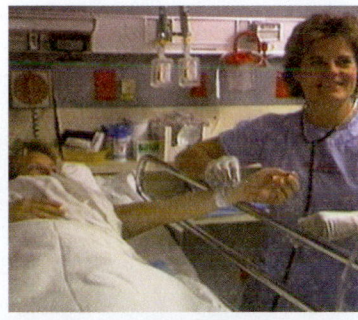

Janet Burns, a 25-year-old G3P3, is 2 hours past a low forceps vaginal birth with a right medial lateral episiotomy of a live 8-pound baby boy. You obtain vital signs of BP 118/70, T 98.8°F, P 76, R 14. You observe the fundus is +1 finger above the umbilicus and slightly to the right. Her episiotomy is slightly ecchymotic and well approximated without edema or discharge. Ice has been applied to the episiotomy for the last 20 minutes. Lochia rubra is present and a pad was saturated in 90 minutes. Janet has an intravenous of Ringer lactate with 10 units of Pitocin infusing at 100 mL/hr in her lower left arm and is complaining of moderate abdominal cramping. Janet's baby is sleeping peacefully in the bassinet next to her bed. She tells you that she is very tired and requests some pain medication so she can sleep for a while.

1. What nursing assessment is of immediate concern?
2. Discuss care of her episiotomy and perineum.
3. What other self-care measures could you advise?
4. Discuss postpartum occurrences that may cause special concern for the mother.
5. Janet expressed concern about her episiotomy healing. What information can you offer?

References

Blackburn, S. T. (2013). *Maternal, fetal, & neonatal physiology: A clinical perspective* (3rd ed.). St. Louis, MO: Saunders.

Callister, L. C. (2014). Integrating cultural beliefs and practices when caring for childbearing women and families. In K. R. Simpson & P. A. Creehan (Eds.), *Perinatal nursing* (4th ed., pp. 41–64). Philadelphia, PA: Lippincott Williams & Wilkins.

Cunningham, F. G., Leveno, K. J., Bloom, S. L., Spong, C. Y., Dashe, J. S., Hoffman, B. L., . . . Sheffield, J. S. (2014). *Williams obstetrics* (24th ed.). New York, NY: McGraw-Hill.

Dennis, C., & Dowswell, T. (2013). Psychosocial and psychological interventions for preventing postpartum depression. *Cochrane Database of Systematic Reviews*, Issue 2. Art. No.:CD001134.

Ding, T., Wang, D., Qu, Y., Chen, Q., & Zhu, S. (2014). Epidural labor analgesia is associated with a decreased risk of postpartum depression: A prospective cohort study. *Anesthesia & Analgesia 119*(2), 383–92.

Feldman, R. (2012). Parent-infant synchrony: A biobehavioral model of mutual influences in the formation of affiliative bonds. *Monographs of the Society for Research in Child Development, 77*(2), 42–51.

James, D. C. (2014). Postpartum care. In K. R. Simpson & P. A. Creehan (Eds.), *Perinatal nursing* (4th ed., p. 530). Philadelphia, PA: Lippincott Williams & Wilkins.

Kalayjian, L., Goodwin, T. M., & Lee, R. H. (2013). Nervous system & autoimmune disorders in pregnancy. In A. H. DeCherney, L. Nathan, T. M. Goodwin, N. Laufer, & A. Roman (Eds.), *Current diagnosis and treatment: Obstetrics & gynecology* (11th ed., pp. 533–542). Boston, MA: McGraw-Hill.

Klein, A. (2012). The postpartum period in women with epilepsy. *Neurologic Clinics, 30*(3), 867–875.

Lauderdale, J. (2012). Transcultural perspectives in childbearing. In M. M. Andrews & J. S. Boyle (Eds.), *Transcultural concepts in nursing care* (6th ed., pp. 91–122). Philadelphia, PA: Lippincott Williams & Wilkins.

Lim, S. Y., Evangelou, N., & Jurgens, S. (2014). Postpartum headache: Diagnostic considerations. *Practical Neurology, 14*(2), 92–99.

Liu, C., & Tronick, E. (2013). Rates and predictors of postpartum depression by race and ethnicity: Results from the 2004 to 2007 New York City PRAMS Survey (Pregnancy Risk Assessment Monitoring System.) *Maternal Child Health, 17*, 1599–1610.

Mercer, R. T. (2004). Becoming a mother versus maternal role attainment. *Journal of Nursing Scholarship, 36*(3), 226–232.

Mercer, R. T. (2006). Nursing support of the process of becoming a mother. *JOGNN: Journal of Obstetric, Gynecologic, & Neonatal Nursing, 35*(5), 649–651. doi:10.1111/J.1552-6909.2006.00086.x

Nicholson, T. B. (2014). Neurological disorders. In R. G. Jordan, J. L. Engstrom, J. A. Marfell, & C. L. Farley (Eds.), *Prenatal and postnatal care: A woman-centered approach* (1st ed., pp. 570–579). Ames, IA: Wiley Blackwell.

Pessel, C., & Tsai, M. C. (2013). The normal puerperium. In A. H. DeCherney, L. Nathan, N., & A. S. Roman (Eds.), *Current diagnosis & treatment: Obstetrics & gynecology* (11th ed., pp. 190–213). New York, NY: McGraw-Hill.

Purnell, L. D. (2013). *Transcultural health care: A culturally competent approach* (4th ed.). Philadelphia, PA: F. A. Davis.

Rubin, R. (1984). *Maternal identity and the maternal experience.* New York, NY: Springer.

Samuels, P. & Niebyl, J. R. (2012). Neurologic disorders. In S. G. Gabbe, J. R. Niebyl, & J. L. Simpson (Eds.), *Obstetrics: Normal and problem pregnancies* (6th ed.). Philadelphia, PA: Churchill Livingstone Elsevier.

Whitmer, T. (2016). Physical and psychologic changes after childbirth. In S. Mattson & J. E. Smith (Eds.). *Core curriculum for maternal-newborn nursing* (6th ed.). Philadelphia, PA: Association of Women's Health, Obstetric and Neonatal Nurses/Elsevier.

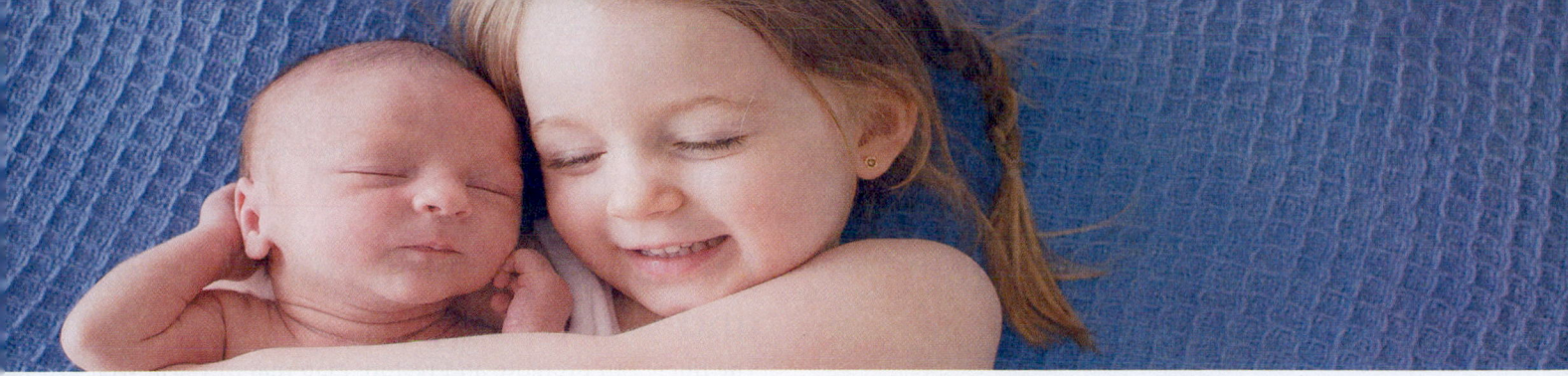

Chapter 29

The Postpartum Family: Early Care Needs and Home Care

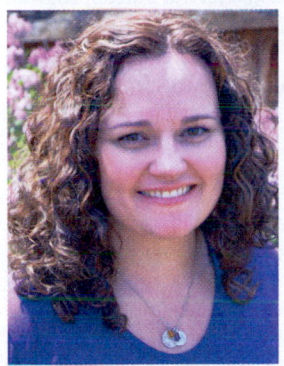

When I first became a nurse I thought I would always practice maternity nursing in a hospital. I loved the pace, the excitement! I began making home visits at the request of my supervisor when our unit partnered with the local midwives and obstetricians to provide postpartum follow-up services. Now I can't imagine doing anything else. Each day is different as I am challenged to improvise and help families deal with issues that arise. I value the independence of this role and the feeling that I am making a difference.

—A Home Care Nurse Working with Postpartum Families

∨ Learning Outcomes

29.1 Formulate nursing diagnoses and nursing care based on the findings of the "normal" postpartum assessment and teaching needs.

29.2 Discuss nursing interventions to promote postpartum maternal comfort, rest, and well-being.

29.3 Explain factors that affect postpartum family wellness in the provision of nursing care and client teaching.

29.4 Compare the postpartum nursing needs of the woman who experienced a cesarean birth with the needs of a woman who gave birth vaginally.

29.5 Examine the nursing needs of the childbearing adolescent during the postpartum period.

29.6 Describe possible approaches to sensitive, holistic nursing care for the woman who relinquishes her newborn.

29.7 Identify teaching topics related to postpartum discharge.

29.8 Identify the main purposes and components of home visits during the postpartum period.

29.9 Summarize actions a nurse should take to ensure personal safety and to foster a caring relationship during a home visit.

29.10 Discuss maternal and family assessment and anticipated progress after birth.

29.11 Delineate interventions to address the common concerns of breastfeeding mothers following discharge.

29.12 Describe the assessment and care of the newborn during postpartum home care.

A thorough discussion of postpartum adaptation and nursing assessment is provided in Chapter 28. This chapter describes how the nurse can use the remaining steps of the nursing process effectively to plan and provide postpartum care. Specific nursing responses to the mother's physical needs and the family's psychosocial needs and the provision of quality postpartum home care are discussed.

Nursing Care During the Early Postpartum Period

For most postpartum women, physical recovery goes smoothly and is considered a healthy process. Because of this perception, caregivers too often assume that the woman and her family have no real needs and that no care plan is needed. Nothing could be further from the truth. Every member of the family has needs, although the needs may not be obvious, especially if they are psychologic or educational.

Nursing Diagnoses

The postpartum family's needs, which should be identified during assessment, are the basis for developing nursing diagnoses. Many nurses have suggested that nursing diagnoses are difficult to make in a wellness setting because of their emphasis on "problems." Nurses involved in the effort to formulate standardized diagnoses recognize this difficulty and continue working to develop nursing diagnoses that are more congruent with wellness settings.

Many agencies that use nursing diagnoses prefer to use only the NANDA list. Consequently, physiologic alterations form the basis of many postpartum diagnoses. Examples of such diagnoses include (NANDA-I © 2014):

- *Breastfeeding, Ineffective,* related to postpartum pain from a cesarean birth or maternal fatigue
- *Constipation* related to fear of tearing stitches or pain
- *Pain, Acute,* related to perineal trauma secondary to episiotomy or birth

Diagnoses related to family coping or instructional needs are also used frequently. Examples of these diagnoses include (NANDA-I © 2014):

- *Knowledge, Readiness for Enhanced,* about infant care related to an expressed desire to improve parenting skills
- *Anxiety* related to self and infant care secondary to lack of knowledge of appropriate care practices
- *Coping: Family, Readiness for Enhanced,* related to successful adjustment to new baby

Nursing Plan and Implementation

An important component of postpartum nursing care is client teaching, which must be individualized to the learning capabilities and readiness of the parent(s). As part of the teaching role, the nurse discusses desired outcomes and goals with the mother and family members as soon as possible following the birth. Interventions can then be designed to achieve optimal health promotion. Strategies for promoting effective parent learning are discussed shortly, and specific teaching content is provided throughout the rest of this chapter. Home care visits and phone contacts help ensure that new parents have the necessary skills and resources to care for their baby.

Promotion of Maternal Comfort and Well-Being

The nurse can promote and restore maternal physical well-being by monitoring uterine status, vital signs, cardiovascular status, elimination patterns, nutritional needs, sleep and rest, and learning needs. Some women also require medication to relieve pain, treat anemia, provide immunity to rubella, and prevent development of antibodies (the latter applies to a nonsensitized Rh-negative woman). Most postpartum women need nursing interventions to promote their comfort and relieve stress. During the postpartum period, ongoing assessments are warranted to assess the physiologic changes that have occurred and ensure that adequate return to a nonpregnant state is occurring. After birth, the examination of the uterine status, lochia, and episiotomy is performed every 15 minutes for 1 hour, then every 30 minutes × 2, then every hour × 2, then every 4 hours × 2, and then every 8 hours until the woman is discharged home (Berens, 2016).

Postpartum Examination

A complete assessment for the postpartum woman should include assessing the breasts, uterus, bowels, bladder, lochia, episiotomy, hemorrhoids, and emotional status. The mnemonic BUBBLEHE provides the nurse with a means to memorize these components of a postpartum assessment. Table 29–1 provides the normal and abnormal findings that can be identified in the postpartum period and interventions for routine care.

Occasionally, medications are needed to promote uterine contractions. These include oxytocin (Pitocin), discussed in Chapter 22, and methylergonovine maleate (Methergine). The nurse also monitors the amount, consistency, color, and odor of the lochia on an ongoing basis. Continued assessment is warranted during the first 24 hours because early postpartum hemorrhage typically occurs in the 24 hours after birth and is most commonly related to uterine atony (the top portion of the uterus is soft and spongy rather than firm and well contracted) (Lowe, 2012). Postpartum hemorrhage remains the primary cause of maternal death globally (Smith, 2014). Table 29–2 describes the position of the uterine fundus following birth. See Chapter 30 for treatment of uterine atony.

Relief of Perineal Discomfort

Before selecting a method to help relieve perineal discomfort, the nurse needs to assess the perineum to determine the degree of edema and other problems. It is also important to ask the woman if she believes any special measures will be particularly effective and to offer her choices when possible. The nurse uses disposable gloves while applying all relief measures and washes hands before and after using the gloves. At all times it is essential for the nurse to remember hygienic practices, such as moving from the front of the perineum (area of the symphysis pubis) to the back (area around the anus). Avoiding contamination between the anal area and the urethral/vaginal area is vital to the prevention of infection.

TABLE 29–1 BUBBLEHE Mnemonic for Postpartum Examination

AREA TO BE ASSESSED	NORMAL FINDINGS	ABNORMAL FINDINGS	INTERVENTIONS FOR ROUTINE CARE
Breasts	Soft or filling No cracking or bleeding from nipples Nipples erect with stimulation Colostrum present	Nipples flat or inverted Unable to obtain erect nipples with feeding or use of breast pump Reddened, tender area warm to touch (possible mastitis or engorgement) Cracked, bleeding nipples (possible trauma from breastfeeding, fissure, infection)	Advise use of a supportive bra. Suggest that breast shells be worn for flat or inverted nipples. Obtain an order for a lactation consult as needed. Note that cracking and bleeding are most commonly related to improper positioning with feeding. Contact healthcare provider immediately if symptoms of infection are present.
Uterus	Fundus firm, midline, position dependent on time since birth but should be at or below umbilicus (see Table 29–2 and Figure 28-1)	Uterus boggy, soft, shifted to the right or not midline, position above umbilicus (possible full bladder, subinvolution) Excessive tenderness with palpation (possible endometritis)	Teach woman to monitor her uterus for firmness. Advise frequent voiding to reduce incidence of bleeding. Suggest use of ibuprofen for any afterbirth pains. Inform woman that breastfeeding aids with involution process. For heavier than expected bleeding, try uterine massage.
Bowels	Abdomen soft, nondistended Normal bowel sounds in all quadrants Passing flatus Bowel movements occur without difficulty	Abdomen distended with discomfort noted No flatus Constipation, reduced bowel sounds	Encourage ambulation, fluids, diet high in fiber, stool softeners. Enema may be needed. Note that women with third- or fourth-degree lacerations need stool softeners.
Bladder	Nondistended, nonpalpable on examination Adequate voiding Urine clear yellow (may contain lochia)	Distended Unable to void or inadequate voiding pattern that does not fully empty bladder	Encourage frequent voiding. Measure first three voids after birth to ensure adequate bladder emptying.
Lochia	Lochia rubra immediately after birth until 3 days Lochia serosa from 3–10 days Lochia alba after that Scant to moderate amount with earthy odor	Heavy amount Clotting Foul smelling Persistent lochia rubra that does not change to serosa	Teach that perineal hygiene includes frequent voiding and cleaning self from front to back. Instruct on consistent use of a "peribottle" while lochia present. Provide sitz bath if ordered.
Episiotomy	Episiotomy or perineum with mild edema Laceration or episiotomy should be intact and well approximated	Excessive edema Bruising Hematoma Discharge Sutures not well approximated or loose	Apply ice to perineum for 20 min on then 20 min off for first 24 hr. Give local perineal medication preparations. Provide sitz baths after first 24 hr. Review perineal hygiene measures.
Hemorrhoids	Rectum intact Hemorrhoids may be present but are small and nontender	Full Tender Inflamed	Teach client about helpful topical agents: witch hazel pads, anesthetic ointments or creams. Try manual replacement of hemorrhoids. Increase fluids and fiber. Encourage sitz baths and side-lying position.
Emotional status	Adequate maternal–newborn attachment is observed Verbalization on proper care of baby Some anxiety is normal	Lack of interest in newborn Lack of expected maternal–newborn attachment behaviors Excessive worrying Depression	Provide education on newborn/infant care practice, postpartum needs. Explore support system availability. Refer to support groups and new mother groups. Encourage frequent rest periods. Review baby blues and signs of postpartum depression.

TABLE 29–2 Position of the Uterine Fundus Following Birth

TIME	POSITION OF FUNDUS
Immediately after birth	Top of fundus is in the midline about midway between the symphysis pubis and the umbilicus.
6–12 hr after birth	Top of fundus is in the midline and at the level of the umbilicus.
1 day after birth	Top of fundus is in the midline and 1 fingerbreadth below the umbilicus.
Second day after birth and thereafter	Top of fundus remains in the midline and descends about 1 fingerbreadth per day.

PERINEAL CARE

Perineal care after each elimination cleanses the perineum, prevents infection, and helps promote comfort. The woman should be instructed to wash her hands before and after changing peripads or performing pericare. The nurse demonstrates how to cleanse the perineum and assists the woman as necessary. Many agencies provide peri-bottles that the woman can use to squirt

Developing Cultural Competence The Orthodox Jewish Woman

It is important to remember that in Orthodox Judaism, women enter a state known as *yoledat*, a period that starts with the birth of the baby and lasts for a period of time before any physical contact between the husband and wife may occur. However, going to the *mikvah* (ritual cleansing bath before sexual relations may occur) is usually delayed for much longer as most doctors today recommend that women wait at least 6 weeks before resuming marital relations. A 30-day convalescent period is considered a cultural norm, and during this time the woman may receive assistance from family members (Jewish Women's Health, 2016).

warm tap water over her perineum following elimination. To cleanse her perineum, the woman should use moist antiseptic towelettes in a blotting (patting) motion and should be taught to start at the front and proceed toward the back to prevent contamination from the anal area.

Many women have never used perineal pads and will need teaching and assistance in using them during the postpartum period. To prevent contamination, the perineal pad should be applied from front to back (place the front portion against the perineum first) and changed when saturation occurs or after each perineal cleansing. The woman is advised to hold the pad on the sides to prevent contamination. The pad needs to be placed snugly against the perineum but should not produce pressure. If the pad is worn too loosely, it may rub back and forth, irritating perineal tissues and causing contamination between the anal and vaginal areas. The pad should be changed after urination and defecation and should be kept dry, which initially will result in frequent pad changes. Women should be advised to cleanse the perineal area with soap and water at least one time per day in addition to using the peri-bottle after each void or pad change. Women should be encouraged to shower daily, preferably after bowel movements to avoid contamination (Women's and Children's Health Network, 2016).

For centuries, lavender oil infusions have been used for relief of perineal pain and as an aromatherapy agent known for its anti-anxiety properties and calming effect. Marzouk and colleagues (2015) examined the use of lavender infusions on the perineum for pain relief in women who had episiotomies. In a randomized double blind study of 60 primigravida women, the women in the experimental group had less discomfort and dyspareunia at 7 weeks postpartum (Marzouk, Barakat, Ragab, et al., 2015). Women should be advised that perineal pain is common and will decrease gradually each day. Most women note complete resolution within 8 weeks of birth (Marzouk et al., 2015). (For information regarding the care of the perineum following an episiotomy, see *Teaching Highlights: Episiotomy Care*.)

ICE PACK

If an episiotomy is done at the time of birth, an ice pack is generally applied to the perineum to reduce edema and provide numbing of the tissues, which promotes comfort. In some agencies, chemical ice bags are used. These are usually

TEACHING HIGHLIGHTS | Episiotomy Care

- Describe the process of wound healing.
- Discuss the risks of contamination of the episiotomy by bacteria from the anal area.
- Describe techniques that are used to keep the episiotomy clean and promote healing:
  - Sitz bath
  - Use of peri-bottle following each voiding or defecation
  - Use of premoistened antiseptic wipes
  - Pad change following each elimination and at regular intervals
  - Ice pack or ice-filled glove to perineum immediately following childbirth
  - Judicious use of analgesics or topical anesthetics
  - Tightening buttocks before sitting
- Identify signs of episiotomy infection (redness, edema, drainage, incomplete approximation of the edges).
- Advise the woman to contact her healthcare provider if signs of infection develop.

activated by folding both ends toward the middle. The nurse can create inexpensive ice bags by filling a disposable glove with ice chips or crushed ice and then taping the top of the glove. Disposable diapers can also be used as an ice bag by placing ice between the diaper layers; this method is less likely to result in chemical burns because of the extra padding. To protect the perineum from burns caused by contact with such an ice pack, the glove needs to be rinsed under running water to remove any powder and then wrapped in an absorbent towel or washcloth before placing it against the perineum. To attain the maximum effect of this cold treatment, a pattern of applying the ice pack for approximately 20 minutes and then removing it for about 10 minutes should be followed during the first 2 hours to reduce edema. Usually ice packs are needed for the first 24 hours to reduce pain (King, Brucker, Kriebs, et al., 2013). The nurse provides information about the purpose of the ice pack, as well as anticipated effects, benefits, and possible problems, and explains how to prepare an ice pack for home use if edema is present and early discharge is planned.

SITZ BATH

The warmth of the water in a sitz bath provides comfort, decreases pain, and promotes circulation to the tissues, which promotes healing and reduces the incidence of infection (Figure 29–1). In some facilities, the use of the sitz bath has declined and is reserved only for women who have third- and fourth-degree lacerations, whereas in other facilities, it is offered to all women who have edema or a laceration following birth. Sitz baths may be ordered three times a day (tid) and as needed (PRN) and usually begin 24 hours after birth. The nurse prepares the sitz bath by cleaning the equipment and adding water at 38.9° to 40.6°C (102° to 105°F). The woman is encouraged to remain in the sitz bath for about 20 minutes. It is important for the woman to have a clean, unused towel to pat dry her perineum after the sitz bath and to have a clean perineal pad to apply. The nurse places a call bell within reach and asks the woman to use it if she feels dizzy or light-headed or develops difficulty hearing. The nurse also checks on the woman at frequent intervals.

Cool sitz baths have been used because they are effective in reducing perineal edema and reducing the response of nerve endings that cause perineal discomfort (Brincat, Crosby, McLeod, et al., 2015). Because women may find the practice uncomfortable, nurses should ask the woman if she would prefer a warm or cool sitz bath based on personal choice. In administering a cool sitz bath, have the woman start with the water at room temperature and add ice according to the woman's comfort.

The nurse provides information about the purpose and use of the sitz bath; anticipated effects, benefits, and possible problems; and safety measures to prevent overheating, scalds, chills, or injury from fainting or slipping while getting into or out of the tub. Home use of sitz baths may be recommended for the woman with an extensive episiotomy. The woman may use a portable sitz bath or her bathtub. It is important for the nurse to emphasize that in using a bathtub, the woman draws only 4 to 6 in. of water, assesses the temperature, and uses the water only for the sitz and not for bathing. If the woman takes a sitz bath, she should release the water, have a helper clean the tub, and draw new water before bathing to prevent infection.

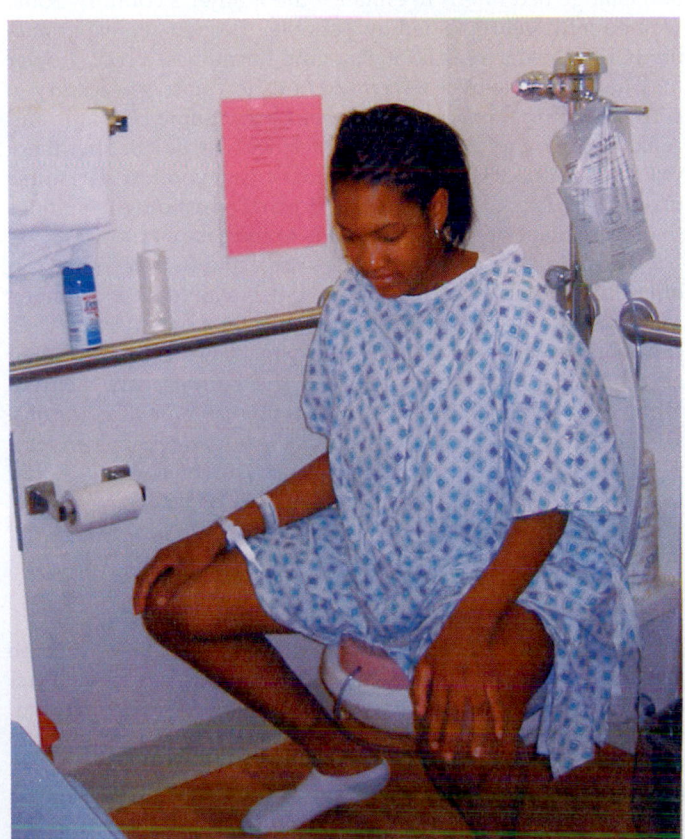

Figure 29–1 A sitz bath promotes healing and provides relief from perineal discomfort during the initial weeks following birth.

SOURCE: Michele Davidson.

Clinical Tip

After the mother completes the sitz bath, show her how to inspect the perineal area for burns (that could be related to using water that is too hot), edema, and approximation by using a handheld mirror. If the mother routinely inspects the area, she will be aware of changes that may indicate an infection, such as redness, poor approximation, drainage, or odor.

Box 29–1 Infrared Heat Lamp Therapy

In the past, heat lamps were widely used in the postpartum period for episiotomy care. Although the use has significantly decreased, Kakade (2015) conducted a double blind controlled clinical trial with primiparous women who had undergone an episiotomy and found that the woman treated with infrared heat lamp therapy to the perineum had reduced redness, edema, ecchymosis, and discharge; increased pain relief and comfort; better approximation of the wound edges; and faster wound healing. Infrared heat lamp use is associated with increased blood circulation to the wound, prevention of growth of micro-organisms, loosening of tight muscles, and increased healing of the damaged tissue (Kakade, 2015).

TOPICAL AGENTS

Topical anesthetics such as benzocaine aerosol spray (e.g., Dermoplast, Americaine) may be used to relieve perineal discomfort. The woman is advised to apply the anesthetic after a sitz bath or perineal care and should hold the spray can 6 to 12 inches from the perineal site. Spray duration should not exceed 1 minute. Women with infection should not use the spray (Berens, 2016). Witch hazel compresses (Tucks pads) may be used to relieve perineal or hemorrhoid discomfort and edema. Pads can also be refrigerated or the liquid can be poured over an ice pad pack for additional relief. The nurse should emphasize the need for the woman to wash her hands before and after using the topical treatments.

The nurse provides information about the anesthetic spray or topical agent. The woman needs to understand the purpose, use, anticipated effects and benefits, and possible problems associated with the product. The nurse can combine a demonstration of application with teaching. A return demonstration is a useful method for evaluating the woman's understanding.

Relief of Hemorrhoidal Discomfort

Some mothers experience hemorrhoidal pain after giving birth. Relief measures include hydrocortisone acetone (Anusol-HC, Tucks); hydrocortisone acetone and pramoxine aerosol spray (Proctofoam-HC), dibucaine 1% ointment (Nupercaine) all applied to the rectal area, and the use of sitz baths. The woman may be taught to digitally replace external hemorrhoids in her rectum. Hand washing to prevent contamination to the vagina is essential. She may also find it helpful to maintain a side-lying position when possible and to avoid prolonged sitting. The mother is encouraged to maintain an adequate fluid intake, and stool softeners are administered to ensure greater comfort with bowel movements. Mothers should be advised to avoid straining with bowel movements because this can increase the severity and discomfort associated with hemorrhoids. The hemorrhoids usually disappear a few weeks after birth if the woman did not have them before her pregnancy.

Relief of Afterpains

Afterpains are the result of intermittent uterine contractions. A primipara may not experience afterpains because her uterus is able to maintain a contracted state. However, multiparous women and those who have had a multiple-gestation pregnancy or hydramnios frequently experience discomfort from afterpains as the uterus contracts intermittently. Breastfeeding women are also more likely to experience afterpains than formula-feeding women because of the release of oxytocin when the baby suckles.

The nurse can suggest that the woman lie prone, with a small pillow under her lower abdomen, and explain that the discomfort may feel intensified for about 5 minutes but then diminishes greatly if not completely. The prone position applies pressure to the uterus and therefore stimulates contractions. When the uterus maintains a constant contraction, the afterpains cease. Additional nursing interventions include a sitz bath (for warmth), positioning, ambulation, or administration of an analgesic agent. For breastfeeding mothers, an analgesic administered 30 minutes to an hour before nursing helps promote comfort and enhances maternal–newborn interaction.

The nurse provides information about the cause of afterpains and methods to decrease discomfort. The nurse explains any medications that are ordered, including their expected effect, benefits, and possible side effects, and any special considerations such as the possibility of dizziness or sleepiness with particular medications.

Relief of Discomfort From Immobility and Muscle Strain

Discomfort may be caused by immobility. The woman who has been in stirrups or has pulled back on her legs for an extended period of time may experience muscular strain from extreme positioning. It is not unusual for women to experience joint pains and muscular pain in both arms and legs, depending on the effort they exerted during the second stage of labor.

Early ambulation is encouraged to help reduce the incidence of complications such as constipation and thrombophlebitis. It also helps promote a feeling of general well-being and aids in the woman's recovery to a prepregnancy state. The nurse provides information about ambulation and the importance of monitoring any signs of dizziness or weakness.

SAFETY ALERT!

Assist the woman the first few times she gets up during the postpartum period. Fatigue, effects of medications, loss of blood, and lack of food intake may cause feelings of dizziness or faintness when the woman stands up.

Because dizziness and light-headedness may be a problem during the woman's first shower, the nurse should remain in the room, check the woman frequently, and have a chair close by in case she becomes faint. During this first shower the nurse instructs the woman in the use of the emergency call button in the bathroom; she is advised that if she becomes faint during a future shower, she should sit down and press the call button for assistance immediately.

Relief of Discomfort From Postpartum Diaphoresis

Postpartum diaphoresis (excessive perspiration) may cause discomfort for new mothers. The nurse can offer a fresh, dry gown and change bed linens to enhance the mother's comfort. Some women may feel refreshed by a shower. For women experiencing hot flashes as a result of changing hormones, a cool shower may be preferable over a warm or hot shower. It is necessary to consider cultural practices and realize that some Hispanic and Asian women prefer to delay showering. Nurses can offer these women a warm or cool washcloth to increase comfort. The nurse provides information about the normal physiologic changes that cause diaphoresis and methods to increase comfort.

Because diaphoresis may also increase thirst, the nurse can offer fluids as the woman desires. Women should be encouraged to hydrate with fluids to prevent dehydration and increase milk production for those who are breastfeeding. Ask the woman about her preferred beverage and the temperature desired. Women of Western European background may prefer iced drinks, whereas Asian women may prefer hot tea or water at room temperature. It is important to ascertain the woman's wishes rather than operate from one's own values or cultural beliefs.

Suppression of Lactation in the Nonbreastfeeding Mother

For the woman who chooses not to breastfeed, lactation may be suppressed by mechanical inhibition (previously used pharmacological agents are no longer used). Although signs of engorgement (excessive breast fullness) do not usually appear until the second or third postpartum day, engorgement is best prevented by beginning mechanical methods of lactation suppression as soon as possible after birth. Ideally, this involves having the woman begin wearing a supportive, well-fitting bra within 6 hours after birth. A tight-fitting sports bra may be preferred by some women. The bra is worn continuously until lactation is suppressed (usually about 5 to 7 days) and is removed only for showers. The bra provides support and eases the discomfort that can occur with tension on the breasts because of fullness.

Ice packs should be applied over the axillary area of each breast for 20 minutes four times daily, beginning soon after birth. In addition, ice is useful in relieving discomfort if engorgement occurs. A gel-filled ice pack can be worn in the bra to increase comfort (Australian Breastfeeding Association, 2016).

The mother is advised to avoid any stimulation of her breasts by her baby, herself, breast pumps, or her sexual partner until the sensation of fullness has passed. Such stimulation increases milk production and delays the suppression process. Heat is avoided for the same reason; therefore, the mother is encouraged to let shower water flow over her back rather than her breasts.

Some mothers may experience excessive engorgement and may find relief by pumping or expressing a small amount of milk. Because stimulation can increase production, care should be given to only express a small amount to relieve significant engorgement. During the acute engorgement period, women can be encouraged to sleep on their backs or to use pillows to support their breasts in a side-lying position.

Women seeking complementary therapies for reducing engorgement or decreasing milk supply when weaning can utilize oral ingestion of common herbs including lemon balm, oregano, parsley, peppermint, menthol, sage, spearmint, and thyme (Sim, Hattingh, Sheriff, et al., 2015).

<hr>

Clinical Tip

To treat severe engorgement that typically occurs on days 3 and 4 postpartum, some mothers find relief by applying raw chilled, green cabbage leaves topically to their breasts. After the veins in the leaves have first been crunched using the fist or a rolling pin, the leaves are applied directly to the bare breasts using a bra to hold the leaves in place. Leaves are changed out every couple of hours when they have become wilted or when the mother awakens during the night until breast swelling resolves (Australian Breastfeeding Association, 2016). Women may also try employing hollyhock leaf compresses to provide relief from engorgement (Khosravan, Mohammadzadeh-Moghadam, Mohammadzadeh, et al., 2015); Sim et al., 2015).

<hr>

Relief of Emotional Stress

The time after birth brings significant physical, emotional, and relationship stressors. For many women, the onset of so many new and changing factors can lead to feelings of being overwhelmed. Hormonal shifts, physical factors, role transition, and sleep disturbances can all impact the new mother's well-being and adjustment process.

During the early postpartum period, the mother may be emotionally labile, and mood swings and tearfulness are common. Discussion and reliving of the birth experience allows the mother to integrate her experiences. Women who feel they did not cope well with labor may have feelings of inadequacy and may benefit from reassurance that they did well. Alterations in time perception and recalling of details of the labor and birth are common. Providing the woman with this information and allowing her to repeat her birth story or ask questions are helpful in her emotional recovery. Women with traumatic birth experiences are at risk for perinatal-related posttraumatic stress disorder. These women have increased risks of postpartum mood and anxiety disorders and will need closer follow-up in the postpartum period.

Attachment is a developmental process that evolves over time and describes a relationship between the baby and a caregiver, usually the mother. During the time after childbirth, the new mother must adjust and accept the actual child she gave birth to, rather than a fantasized child that she envisioned during pregnancy. This initial transition occurs as emotional attachment begins. For some women, unexpected factors may impact this transition, such as birth of a different gender than desired or the presence of birth defects. Reva Rubin first described the psychological process of becoming a mother with three phases: taking in, taking hold, and letting go (Hollway, 2015).

Immediately after the birth, the *taking-in* phase, the mother is focused on bodily concerns and may not be fully ready to learn about personal and newborn care. For most new mothers, the *taking-hold* phase, which can last from 2 days to 2 weeks, is characterized by maternal concerns about her ability to be a successful parent and to provide emotional attachment and physical care to her newborn. The *letting-go* phase typically occurs after 2 weeks and represents the time when mothers strive to be independent with their parenting skills. Because this is usually the period when "baby blues" can occur, advise family members of symptoms of postpartum depression to facilitate early detection and treatment.

Attachment that is consistent builds stability in the maternal–newborn relationship. Most experts believe that stages of attachment occur as the baby develops and experiences new developmental needs. Consistency in the parent–newborn/infant relationship results in children who are happier and more socially skilled, competent, compliant, and empathetic than children who were insecurely attached as infants. Preschoolers with secure attachments also were more popular with their peers, had higher self-esteem, and were less dependent and negative. Positive parent–newborn/infant attachment results in a higher incidence of positive adult relationships and reduced aggression in adolescence and adulthood (Hollway, 2015).

<hr>

SAFETY ALERT!
A woman who voices concerns over hurting herself or her baby is experiencing symptoms that are much more severe than baby blues and requires emergency psychiatric intervention.

<hr>

Promotion of Maternal Rest and Activity

Following childbirth, maternal fatigue often occurs and is typically associated with energy exertion during labor and birth. These women may benefit from prolonged rest periods with limited visitors to promote rest and relaxation. Other women may be euphoric and full of psychic energy, ready to relive and recount the experience of birth repeatedly. The nurse can provide a period for airing of feelings and then encourage a period of rest. Nurses also promote rest by organizing their activities to avoid frequent interruptions for the woman.

Relief of Fatigue

Physical fatigue often affects other adjustments and functions of the new mother. For example, fatigue can reduce milk flow, thereby increasing problems with establishing breastfeeding. Energy is also needed to make the psychologic adjustments to a new baby and to assume new roles. It is helpful for the new mother to know that fatigue may persist for several weeks or even months. Nighttime feedings result in disruption of sleep and can lead to a cycle of fatigue and sleep disturbance. Persistent fatigue is especially common when mothers attempt to perform activities while their babies are napping, instead of resting themselves. Mothers who have other children may feel overwhelmed with trying to meet their needs as well (Hollway, 2015). The nurse teaches women that this practice can lead to chronic fatigue and should be avoided. Severe ongoing fatigue can also be a symptom of a thyroid disorder and should be evaluated by a clinician. Although most new mothers feel tired, if they have perceived the pregnancy and birth as a natural process, they tend to view themselves as healthy and well. Fatigue can also be a symptom of postpartum depression and should be discussed with the healthcare provider if symptoms continue or are accompanied by other signs of depression. Complete inability to sleep may be associated with postpartum mood and anxiety disorders, including postpartum psychosis, and warrant immediate assessment.

Specific groups of mothers are at a higher risk for postpartum fatigue. These include mothers of multiples, mothers with babies who are still hospitalized and who must engage in multiple trips to the hospital to visit their babies, mothers of babies with birth defects or special needs, mothers who lack social support, mothers without additional caretakers in the home, and mothers who return to work before the advised 6-week time period. A mother who has been on extended bed rest during the pregnancy may also be more at risk for fatigue. Because many family members are geographically separated and may be unable to come and spend time with the mother and new baby, the woman may experience fatigue caring for herself and the baby unaided in the early postpartum period.

Developing Cultural Competence Postpartum Recuperation

Most mothers view the postpartum period as a time for recuperation. In many non-Western cultures, the 40 days following the birth are a time of recovery when female relatives or friends assist the new mother in her daily activities (McFarland & Wehbe-Alamah, 2014).

In northern Africa, for example, the 40-day period after birth is considered a time of transition for the mother. The mother and the baby are not separated during this time. This practice is known to prevent postpartum psychosis and facilitate bonding (McFarland & Wehbe-Alamah, 2014). This is also the custom in India, where it is believed that the mother and new baby need protection from evil spirits as well as from exposure to illness, because they are both considered vulnerable during this time period (McFarland & Wehbe-Alamah, 2014).

In Mexico, this period is briefer, lasting only 20 days. During the first 7 days, non–household members are not permitted to visit or enter the home. The mother gradually increases activity after the first week. The end of the postpartum period is marked by a *sobada*, a massage performed by the midwife on the 20th day after birth (McFarland & Wehbe-Alamah, 2014).

Women With Special Needs Mental Illness

Women with a history of mental illness are at an increased risk for postpartum mood and anxiety disorders. Risks increase with lack of sleep. These women should be counseled to take frequent naps and avoid sleep deprivation.

Resumption of Activity

Ambulation and activity should gradually increase after birth. The new mother should avoid heavy lifting, excessive stair climbing, and strenuous activity. One or two daily naps are essential and are most easily achieved if the mother sleeps when her baby does. Women with older children often find it difficult to get adequate rest because they want to spend time with their older children when the baby is napping. The woman should be cautioned that fatigue and exhaustion can become a vicious cycle and should be avoided. Assistance in the household can help prevent this and can enable the mother to spend special time with older children while others take over household tasks.

By the second week at home, the woman may resume light housekeeping. Although it is customary to delay returning to work for 6 weeks, most women are physically able to resume practically all activities by 4 to 5 weeks. In some cases, if bleeding returns, it is often a sign that the mother is overdoing her activities and should decrease some activity. Delaying the return to work until after the final postpartum examination minimizes the possibility of problems.

Postpartum Exercises

The woman should be encouraged to begin simple exercises while in the birthing unit and to continue them at home. Kegel exercises (see Chapter 10 and Figure 10–12) should be reviewed and begun while the woman is still in the hospital. She is advised that increased lochia or pain means she should reevaluate her activity and make necessary alterations. Most agencies provide a booklet describing suggested postpartum exercises. (Exercise routines vary for women undergoing cesarean birth or tubal ligation after childbirth.)

Exercise during the postpartum period has several health benefits for new mothers. Exercise can help maintain insulin and high-density lipoprotein (HDL) cholesterol levels, as well as improve aerobic fitness. The postpartum woman is more likely to have positive views of her well-being, more self-esteem, and less fatigue if she continues to do stretching and her own pattern of exercise after she is home. Walking is an excellent exercise that enables the woman to include her baby in her routine, eliminates the need for child care, and does not require transportation. The addition of pelvic floor exercises can also decrease such problems as urinary leakage or urinary incontinence. Exercise has been shown to have multiple benefits to the new mother. It facilitates postpartum weight loss, reduces stress, increases energy, decreases postpartum depression, promotes sleep and relaxation, and strengthens and tones abdominal muscles. Some women may utilize exercise as a time for being alone (American College of Obstetricians and Gynecologists [ACOG], 2015a).

Sexual Activity and Contraception

Typically, postpartum couples are advised they may resume sexual intercourse after the 6-week postpartum visit. Clinically, sexual relations can resume once any sutures have healed and lochia has ceased. Approximately 64% of postpartum women experience sexual dysfunction in the first year following birth, with 70% experiencing dissatisfaction with sexual relations (Khajehei, Doherty, Tilley, et al., 2015). The resumption of sexual activity is related to multiple factors including maternal fatigue, fear of pain, breastfeeding, time wakening patterns, newborn sleep disturbances, alterations in body image, child care needs of other children, reduction in desire, arousal, and orgasm related to hormonal factors, and perceptions of the sexual partner. Risk factors for sexual dysfunction after childbirth include primiparity, lack of initiation of sexual activity by the postpartum woman, delaying sexual activity beyond 9 weeks after birth, relationship strain during the first 5 months after birth, and postpartum depression (Khajehei et al., 2015).

Education that addresses expectations for resumption of sexual activity should include a brief description of estrogen deficiency and how it reduces lubrication and pliability of vaginal tissue. Lubricants should be used along with slow progression with penetration, and altering positions that allow the woman to control the depth of penetration may help to increase comfort for the woman. Discomfort is common and can persist for 6 months or more. Increased frequency of intercourse can aid in the physiological stretching of the perineum when sutures have been placed (Khajehei et al., 2015). Breastfeeding couples should be forewarned that during orgasm milk may be discharged. This can be reduced by nursing prior to sexual activity or wearing a bra with absorbent pads to absorb milk.

With anticipatory guidance during the prenatal and postpartum periods, the couple can be forewarned of potential temporary problems. Anticipatory guidance is enhanced if the couple can discuss their feelings and reactions as they are experienced. (See *Teaching Highlights: Resumption of Sexual Activity After Childbirth.*)

Information on contraception is often provided as part of discharge teaching if it is permissible within the healthcare agency. The nurse can also be an important resource for the woman and her partner during postpartum follow-up. Couples typically choose to use contraception to control the number of children they will have or to determine the spacing of future children. However, some religious-based hospital facilities prohibit nurses and other healthcare providers from discussing contraception. If the nurse is discussing birth control, it is important to emphasize that in choosing a specific method, consistency of use is essential. The nurse needs to identify the advantages, disadvantages, risks, and contraindications of the various methods to help the couple, or the single mother, make an informed choice about the most practical and compatible method. (For a more detailed discussion of contraceptive methods, see Chapter 5.) Breastfeeding women are commonly concerned that a contraceptive method will interfere with their ability to breastfeed. Breastfeeding women should be given available options and choose the method that best fits their lifestyle, financial situation, and personal preference.

Pharmacologic Interventions

Pharmacologic preparations, including pain medications, vaccinations (rubella and Tdap [reduced diphtheria toxoid and acellular pertussis]), and Rh immune globulin, are frequently administered in the postpartum period (see Table 29–3).

Promotion of Effective Parent Learning

Meeting the educational needs of the new mother and her family is a primary task of the postpartum nurse. Each woman's educational needs vary based on her age, parity, background, availability of primary language instruction, educational level, previous experiences, disabilities, and expectations. Cultural influences can also impact learning and expectations for the postpartum period. Because of brief hospital stays, assessing the learning needs of the new mother through observation, sensitivity to nonverbal cues, and tactfully phrased questions is vital. For example, "What plans have you made for handling things when you get home?" may elicit a response of several words and may provide the opportunity for some information sharing and guidance. Some agencies also use checklists of common concerns for new mothers. The woman can check the concerns that are of interest to her. Effective education provides the family with knowledge of maternal and newborn health needs and how to seek assistance when necessary.

Teaching during the postpartum period is a continuous process in which the nurse takes opportunities throughout interactions with the new parents to identify learning opportunities and offer teaching interventions. The nurse can also plan and implement teaching in a logical, nonthreatening way based on knowledge and respect of the family's cultural values and beliefs. Unless the nurse believes a culturally related activity would be harmful, it can be supported and encouraged.

Nurses need to consider the mother's physical and psychosocial needs when conducting postpartum teaching. Initially, women may be exhausted from the birth experience and their concentration may be impaired. Later, the new mother may be preoccupied with visitors and phone calls. Information should be delivered a little at a time and repeated to make sure that the parents understand what the nurse has discussed with them. Repetition is a valuable tool in the postpartum environment.

TEACHING HIGHLIGHTS	Resumption of Sexual Activity After Childbirth

- Delay intercourse until no lochia is present because lochia indicates that healing is not yet complete.
- Tenderness of the vagina and perineum may cause discomfort. The partner may test the woman's level of comfort by slipping a lubricated finger inside her vagina. The female-superior and side-lying positions may be preferable because they let the woman control the depth of penetration of the penis.
- Vaginal dryness may occur because the vagina is "hormone poor." Discomfort as a result of dryness can be avoided by using a water-soluble lubricant.
- Based on the amount of breast engorgement and tenderness present, the partner may need to avoid breast stimulation during foreplay or use a very gentle approach.
- Escape of milk during sexual activity can be minimized by breastfeeding immediately beforehand.
- Fatigue and the new baby's schedule may have a negative impact on the woman's feelings of desire. Napping when the baby sleeps helps decrease fatigue. However, fatigue may be a reality couples need to accept during the early postpartum months.
- Contraception is important even during the early postpartum period. The woman's body needs adequate time to heal and recover from the stress of pregnancy and childbirth. Couples opposed to contraception may choose abstinence at this time.

TABLE 29–3 Vaccinations for Postpartum Administration

RUBELLA VIRUS VACCINE, LIVE (MERUVAX 2)

Dose/Route:

Single-dose vial, inject subcutaneously in outer aspect of the upper arm.

Indication:

Stimulate active immunity against rubella virus. Rubella titer of less than 1:10 or antibody negative on enzyme-linked immunosorbent assay (ELISA) test.

Adverse Effects:

Burning or stinging at the injection site; about 2– 4 weeks later may have rash, malaise, sore throat, or headache.

Nursing Implications:

Obtain informed consent. Determine whether woman has sensitivity to neomycin (vaccine contains neomycin); is immunosuppressed, or has received blood transfusions (not to be administered within 3 months of blood transfusion, plasma transfusion, or serum immune globulin). To be given at discharge.

Client Teaching:

Name of drug, expected effect, possible adverse effects, possible comfort measures to use if adverse effects occur; rubella titer will be assessed in about 3 months. Instruct woman to AVOID PREGNANCY FOR 30 DAYS following vaccination. Provide information regarding contraceptives and their use.

Nursing Diagnoses (NANDA-I © 2014) Related to Drug Therapy:

Knowledge, Deficient, regarding drug therapy

Self-Health Management, Readiness for Enhanced, related to information about postpartum contraception regarding an expressed desire to avoid pregnancy following rubella vaccination

Pain related to rash and malaise

TDAP (REDUCED DIPHTHERIA TOXOID AND ACELLULAR PERTUSSIS)

Dose/Route:

Single-dose vial, inject subcutaneously in outer aspect of the upper arm.

Indication:

Any woman who is nonimmune and has not received the vaccination during pregnancy should be vaccinated in the postpartum period.

Adverse Effects:

Soreness, redness or swelling at injection site, fever, headache, nausea, vomiting, diarrhea, stomach upset, swelling of the entire arm (rare)

Nursing Implications:

Confirm criteria for administration are present.

Inject entire contents of vial. Advise woman of potential adverse reactions.

Client Teaching:

Name of drug, expected action, possible side effects; report soreness at injection site to nurse; advise primary care provider of any vaccinations received in the postpartum period.

Nursing Diagnoses (NANDA-I © 2014) Related to Drug Therapy:

Self-Health Management, Readiness for Enhanced, related to information about need for updated immunizations to reduce the incidence of contracting and spreading disease

Pain related to soreness at injection site

RHOGAM (RH IMMUNE GLOBULIN SPECIFIC FOR D ANTIGEN)

Dose/Route:

Postpartum: One vial IM within 72 hr of birth. *Antepartum:* One vial microdose RhoGAM IM at 28 weeks in Rh-negative women; after amniocentesis, spontaneous or therapeutic abortion, or ectopic pregnancy.

Indication:

Prevention of sensitization to the Rh factor in Rh-negative women and to prevent hemolytic disease in the newborn in subsequent pregnancies (see Chapter 15). Mother must be Rh negative, not previously sensitized to Rh factor. Newborn must be Rh positive, direct antiglobulin negative.

Adverse Effects:

Soreness at injection site.

Nursing Implications:

Confirm criteria for administration are present. Ensure correct vial is used for the client (each vial is crossmatched to the specific woman and must be carefully checked).

Inject entire contents of vial.

Client Teaching:

Name of drug, expected action, possible side effects; report soreness at injection site to nurse; woman should carry information regarding Rh status and dates of RhoGAM injections with her at all times; explain use of RhoGAM with subsequent pregnancies.

Nursing Diagnoses (NANDA-I © 2014) Related to Drug Therapy:

Self-Health Management, Readiness for Enhanced, related to information about future need for Rh immune globulin regarding an expressed desire to understand the long-term implications of her Rh-negative status

Pain related to soreness at injection site

When performing teaching sessions, the partner should be included if possible. Flexible scheduling that takes into account the partner's schedule with work and home responsibilities can increase participation (Figure 29–2). In some cultures female relatives often assist the new mother and baby. It is important to include any care providers in the teaching session.

Postpartum units use a variety of instructional methods, including printed handouts, formal classes, videos, televised educational programming, and individual interaction. Printed materials are helpful for new mothers to consult if questions arise at home. Some facilities offer a hotline service that new mothers can call with questions or concerns. As the culturally diverse populations in the United States continue to grow, the need for culturally sensitive information is imperative. Along with culturally diverse material, teaching aids should be presented in the woman's native language when possible. Written materials should be available and translators or language (translation) lines should be utilized. Many clients are now accustomed to using the Internet and may prefer to use online support groups and access educational materials found online. As technology expands, the nurse must remain current with the changing technology and the resources it creates. Evaluation of learning may also take several forms: return demonstrations, question-and-answer sessions, and even formal evaluation tools. Follow-up phone calls after discharge provide additional evaluative information and continue the helping process for the family.

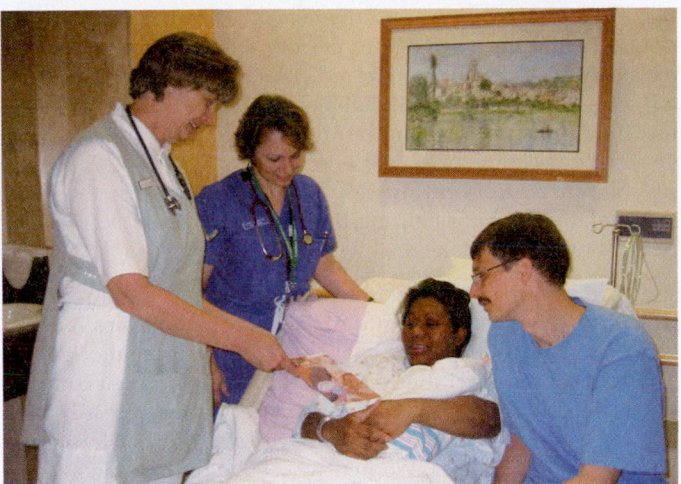

Figure 29–2 The nurse provides educational information to both parents.

SOURCE: Michele Davidson.

Teaching content should include information on role changes and psychologic adjustments as well as skills. Risk factors and signs of postpartum mood and anxiety disorders should be reviewed with all women. Information is also essential for women with specialized educational needs such as the mother who has had a cesarean birth, the parents of twins, the parents of a baby with congenital anomalies, parents with other young children, and parents with a child that will require long-term hospitalization. Because more and more women with disabilities are now having children, they may require additional support and education. Anticipatory guidance can help prepare parents for the many changes they will experience with a new family member.

Promotion of Family Wellness

A positive maternity experience is likely to have a positive effect on the entire family. The family that receives appropriate information and has adequate time to interact with its newest member in a supportive environment will feel more comfortable and secure at home.

Today most facilities support *family-centered care* that is focused on keeping the mother and baby together as much as the mother desires. This type of care is called **mother–baby care**, or **couplet care**, and provides increased opportunities for parent–newborn interactions because the newborn shares the mother's room, allowing the baby and mother to be cared for together. Mother–baby care promotes maternal–newborn attachment while enabling the mother to care for the baby in a supportive environment. It is especially conducive to on-demand feeding schedules for both breast- and formula-feeding babies. This arrangement also allows the father/partner, siblings, grandparents, and others to participate in the care of the new baby. Women who give birth in a facility that offers mother–baby care are often more satisfied with their postpartum experience than women who are cared for under different care models (Brockman, 2015).

Mother–baby unit policies must be flexible enough to permit the mother to return the baby to the nursery if she finds it necessary because of fatigue or physical discomfort. Some mother–baby units also return the newborns to a central nursery at night so the mothers can get more rest.

Reactions of Siblings

Mother–baby care provides excellent opportunities for family bonds to grow when the mother, father/partner, newborn, and siblings begin functioning as a family unit immediately after the birth. When mother–baby care is not available, liberal sibling visitation policies can meet the family's needs. A visit to the mother–baby unit reassures children that their mother is well and still loves them. It also provides an opportunity for the children to become familiar with the new baby. For the mother, the pangs of separation are lessened as she interacts with her children and introduces them to the newest family member (Figure 29–3). Even newborns who require intensive care nursery admissions should be allowed to have sibling visits whenever possible. Although preventing infection in the newborn who requires intensive care services is a valid concern, policies that involve taking the sibling's temperature before each visit and documenting the sibling's health status can provide a safeguard that still promotes family bonding. Some babies may be hospitalized for weeks or months. Sibling visitation allows the early incorporation of the baby into the family unit for siblings.

Clinical Tip

Because siblings may feel left out with the addition of a new family member, provide positive feedback to promote attachment. For example, pointing out to the older child that "Carlos is looking at you" or asking, "Do you think he knows you're his big sister?" can help make siblings feel accepted and valued. Also identify ways in which siblings can help the new mother, for example, by bringing her a cup of water or singing the baby a favorite lullaby.

Teach parents that although they may have prepared their children for the presence of a new brother or sister, the actual arrival of the newborn in the home requires some adjustments. Although it may be more chaotic for the parents, allowing the children to come to the hospital to pick up mom and the new baby can signify their importance in the family process. If small children are waiting at home, it is helpful if the father carries the

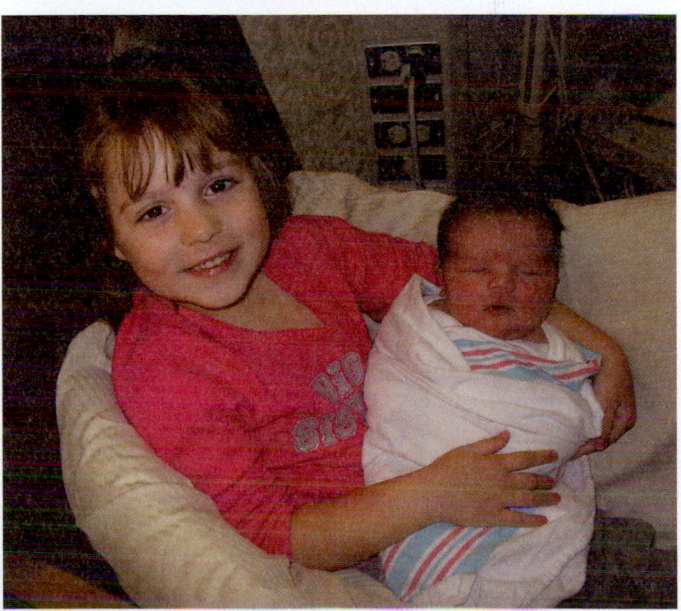

Figure 29–3 The sister of this newborn becomes acquainted with the new family member.

SOURCE: Wilson Garcia.

baby inside. This practice keeps the mother's arms free to hug and touch her older children. Many mothers bring a doll home with them for an older child. Caring for the doll alongside the mother or father helps the child to identify with the parents. This identification helps decrease anger and the need to regress for attention.

Parents may also provide supervised times when older children can hold the new baby and perhaps even help with a feeding or diapering. Many parents may have concerns about the children "hurting" the new baby, but with proper supervision, the children are more likely to develop an attachment to their new sibling. The other children feel a sense of accomplishment and learn tenderness and caring. The nurse also suggests that parents spend one-to-one quality time with each of their older children each day. This may require some careful planning, but it confirms the parents' continuing love for the other children and promotes their acceptance of the newborn.

Parent–Newborn Attachment

Nursing interventions to enhance the quality of parent–newborn attachment should be designed to promote feelings of well-being, comfort, and satisfaction. See Chapter 28 to review parent/maternal–newborn attachment and bonding behaviors.

Nursing Care Following Cesarean Birth

After a cesarean birth the new mother has postpartum needs similar to those of women who have given birth vaginally. Because she has undergone major abdominal surgery, however, the woman's nursing care needs are also similar to those of other surgical patients.

Health Promotion **Reducing Cesarean Births**

Healthy People 2020 objectives (U.S. Department of Health and Human Services [USD-HHS], 2015) include reducing the number of cesarean births in low-risk women. Nurses can explain to women that even though a cesarean birth was performed for this birth, a trial of labor after cesarean (TOLAC) may be a viable option in the future.

Promotion of Maternal Physical Well-Being After Cesarean Birth

The chances of pulmonary infection are increased because of immobility after the use of narcotics and sedatives and because of the altered immune response in postoperative patients. Therefore, the woman is encouraged to cough and deep breathe every 2 to 4 hours while awake until she is ambulating frequently. Leg exercises are also encouraged every 2 hours until the woman is ambulating. These exercises increase circulation, help prevent thrombophlebitis, and also aid intestinal motility by tightening abdominal muscles.

Early ambulation, eating a low roughage diet shortly after birth, and breastfeeding as soon as possible after birth (ideally within the first hour) all enhance the recovery of the mother and decrease complications in the postoperative period. Even though a cesarean birth is an operative procedure, most women giving birth are relatively healthy and therefore are less likely to experience postoperative complications when compared with other surgical patients.

The nurse monitors and manages the woman's pain experience during the postpartum period. Sources of pain include incisional pain, gas pain, referred shoulder pain, periodic uterine contractions (afterbirth pains), discomfort related to breastfeeding, pain from getting in and out of bed, and pain from voiding, defecating, or constipation.

Nursing interventions are oriented toward preventing or alleviating pain or helping the woman cope with pain. The nurse should undertake the following measures:

- Administer analgesics as needed, especially during the first 24 to 72 hours after childbirth. Use of analgesics relieves the woman's pain and enables her to be more mobile and active. Some facilities administer ibuprofen on a continuous basis in the early postpartum period to decrease swelling, reduce pain, and decrease the need for, or frequency of, narcotic agents. Women who have undergone a cesarean birth may receive a morphine sulfate injection (Duramorph) via the epidural or spinal anesthesia catheter, which provides 16 to 24 hours of pain relief.

- Promote comfort through proper positioning, frequent position changes, massage, back rubs, oral care, and the reduction of noxious stimuli such as noise and unpleasant odors.

- Encourage visits by significant others, including the newborn and older children. These visits distract the woman from the painful sensations and help reduce her fear and anxiety.

- Encourage the use of breathing, relaxation, guided imagery, and distraction (e.g., stimulation of cutaneous tissue) techniques taught in childbirth preparation class.

The standard of practice for pain control after cesarean birth is the **continuous epidural infusion (CEI),** which uses a combination of opioid and local anesthesia medication that is continually administered via an electric pump. The device also has a button that the woman can depress if additional pain relief is needed. Fentanyl is the most commonly used drug because it tends to provide good pain relief (ACOG, 2015b). Nursing assessments are hourly for women with a CEI in place and include vital signs, level of pain, amount of drug received, and amount of self-administration. The tubing is inspected to ensure connections are maintained because movement by the woman in bed could disrupt the line. The epidural site should also be assessed to ensure the catheter has not been displaced. Because up to 43% of women experience increased motor weakness, which can lead to impaired mobility, duration of use is typically limited to 24 hours. Removal at 24 hours is associated with a reduction in pruritus, urinary retention, and infection (ACOG, 2015b). *Patient-controlled epidural analgesia (PCEA)* has been introduced in obstetric analgesia during the past decade. Many studies have shown that the consumption of analgesic is reduced when the woman requests her own doses.

Patient-controlled analgesia (PCA) uses intravenous administration of a narcotic agent, such as morphine, hydromorphone hydrochloride, or fentanyl to provide postoperative pain control. The woman is given a bolus of analgesia at the beginning of therapy. A continuous low-dose infusion rate is ordered. Using a special intravenous (IV) pump system, the woman presses a button to self-administer small doses of the medication as needed. For safety, the pump is preset with a time lockout so that the woman cannot deliver another dose until a specified period of time has elapsed. While PCA was once widely used, it has been largely replaced by PCEA and is typically used in facilities where PCEA is unavailable or for women who have had general anesthesia. The advantages of PCA and PCEA include providing the woman with a greater sense of control and reduced dependence on staff. The frequent, smaller doses help the woman experience rapid pain relief without grogginess and avoid the discomfort associated with injections.

The use of general anesthesia in modern practice is rare because of the increased risks and side effects including abdominal distention. Interventions for abdominal distention include low-residue diet and dietary interventions to decrease flatus, early ambulation, and left side lying positioning. If the woman is unable to pass flatus, rectal suppositories and/or enemas to stimulate passage of flatus and stool can be given. Women who receive general anesthesia warrant additional assessments in the immediate postpartum period. Vital signs should be monitored continually until the woman has regained consciousness. Cardiopulmonary equipment should be in close range with cardiac monitoring available as needed.

Many physicians also order a nonsteroidal anti-inflammatory drug (NSAID) in addition to the previously mentioned agents once the woman is tolerating oral fluids well. Nonsteroidal anti-inflammatory drugs (NSAIDs) assist with decreasing inflammation and do not have the negative side effects associated with many narcotics, such as sedation and constipation. NSAIDs are often given in combination with narcotic agents in the immediate postpartum period and often result in a decreased intake of narcotic agents. In 2015, the Food and Drug Administration (FDA) issued a warning that the use of NSAIDs can increase the risk of myocardial infarction and cerebral vascular accident. Consideration should be given for the women with cardiac risk factors or with previous adverse cardiac events. The risk increases with higher dosages, so the lowest effective dose should be administered (Food & Drug Administration [FDA], 2015).

Sometimes women who have had a cesarean birth have other discomforts that can be relieved with pharmacologic interventions. The nurse assesses the woman for other symptoms, such as nausea, itching (which is typically related to the morphine used in the epidural), and headache. If the woman is experiencing nausea, an antiemetic can be administered. Itching can also be relieved with pharmacologic interventions. NSAIDs are effective in managing headaches and other body aches.

Nursing Management

Prior to the first time out of bed (at least 30 minutes prior to ambulation), provide oral pain medication to the woman; elevate the head of the bed to a comfortable position, and ensure side rails are up. Allow the woman to ease herself up without pulling on her to assist her. Use supportive measures instead, letting the woman guide the process. Once in a seated position, have the woman remain at the bedside for approximately 1 minute. Show the woman how to splint her incision with a rolled towel for support. Encourage the woman to stand up straight, ensuring she feels steady before taking her initial steps. Do not leave the woman unattended during the initial ambulation. Other measures that are unique to the woman who has had an operative birth include the following (Davidson, 2013; Santos, Epstein, & Chaudhuri, 2015; Gabbe, Niebyl, Simpson, et al., 2016).

- Facilitate early contact between mother and baby; allow newborn to remain with support person close to mother as surgical procedure is completed.

- Provide skin-to-skin contact to facilitate attachment as soon as possible after birth; encourage early breastfeeding prior to newborn being moved to nursery.
- Perform a head to toe examination of the mother per agency protocol.
- Assess breasts and nipples to determine if lactation consult is necessary.
- Assess abdomen for consistency; a distended abdomen may be caused by an increase in flatus. Frequent position changes and early ambulation can improve discomfort.
- Assess for nausea, vomiting, and abdominal pain. Provide small quantities of oral fluids within 2 hours of surgery and begin light meals within 8 hours.
- Assess for risk factors for DVT (see Chapter 30 for risk factors).
  - Low risk: cesarean birth
  - Moderate risk: cesarean birth and one additional risk factor
  - High risk: cesarean birth and two or more risk factors
- Low-risk woman: Provide compression stockings; encourage early ambulation, dorsiflexing feet, and frequent turning during bedrest; advise to avoid prolonged sitting and ambulate every 2 hours.
- Moderate- or high-risk woman: Apply sequential compression devices; begin anti-coagulation therapy within 12 to 24 hours after birth.
- Assess IV site, flow rate, and patency of the IV tubing.
- Monitor incision site using the REEDA scale (redness, edema, ecchymosis, discharge, approximation of the suture line); assess skin temperature around the incision line.
- Assess for anesthesia and surgical complications (e.g., nausea, vomiting, pruritus, uncontrolled pain, urinary complaints).
- Monitor nutritional status and intake and output.
- Assess for attachment behaviors, psychological adjustment, and symptoms of postpartum depression, mood changes, or anxiety symptoms.
- Assess for symptoms related to adverse outcomes including DVT, pulmonary embolus, postpartum hemorrhage, surgical site infections, urinary tract infection, and endometritis.

The mother who has had a cesarean birth usually does extremely well postoperatively. Most women are ambulating by the day after the surgery. Usually by the second postpartum day the woman can shower, which seems to provide a mental as well as physical lift. Most women are discharged by the third day after birth. Women with maternal risk factors during pregnancy, such as gestational diabetes, obesity, and preeclampsia warrant closer follow-up postoperatively.

Promotion of Parent–Newborn Interaction After Cesarean Birth

Many factors associated with cesarean birth may hinder successful and frequent parent–newborn interaction. These factors include the physical condition of the mother and newborn and maternal reactions to stress, anesthesia, and medications. The father/partner may be concerned about the mother and preoccupied with her condition, resulting in less interaction with the newborn. The mother and her baby may be separated after birth because of birthing unit routines, prematurity, or neonatal complications or a birth defect. A healthy baby born by uncomplicated cesarean is no more fragile than one born vaginally.

In some cases, signs of depression, anger, or withdrawal may indicate a grief response to the loss of the fantasized birth experience. Fathers as well as mothers may experience feelings of "missing out," guilt, or even jealousy toward another couple who had a vaginal birth. The couple who have experienced a cesarean birth may need the opportunity to tell their story repeatedly to work through these feelings. The nurse can provide factual information about their situation and support the couple's effective coping behaviors. The nurse should acknowledge their feelings while emphasizing the importance of a healthy birth outcome.

Fu and colleagues (2015) examined different care models and measured maternal cortisol levels as a measure of maternal stress after birth in three groups that had (a) routine care by the circulating nurse prior to surgery with written psychological resources provided (b) collaborative care by multidisciplinary team care that initiated care prior to surgery and throughout the hospitalization, and (c) routine care following medical orders. Women in the collaborative care group with multidisciplinary teams had the lowest cortisol levels (Fu, Jiang, Wang, et al., 2015).

Enhanced communication during labor and birth, and in the immediate period following birth, along with specific teaching related to issues regarding a cesarean birth, is associated with less maternal distress and improved satisfaction with the birth experience. While some women may have negative feelings about a cesarean birth, others may have chosen an operative birth and have no negative feelings. During the initial taking-in phase, the new parents are processing their new role and may be nurturing themselves and each other. This is normal and expected.

By the second or third day, the mother who has had a cesarean birth moves into the *taking-hold* period and is usually receptive to learning how to care for herself and her newborn. During this period, the focus shifts from the mother and father/partner to the baby. Vulnerability can occur during this period and the parents may feel overwhelmed. The need for nursing intervention to guide the new parents is essential. Special emphasis should be given to home management. The nurse can encourage the mother to let others assume responsibility for housekeeping and cooking. Fatigue not only prolongs recovery but also interferes with breastfeeding and mother–newborn interaction, increases the risk of prolonged postpartum blues and postpartum mood and anxiety disorders, and leads to feelings of being overwhelmed.

The presence of the father/partner during the birth process positively influences the woman's perception of the birth event. The father's/partner's presence reduces the woman's fears, enhances her sense of control, and enables the couple to share feelings and respond to each other with touch and eye contact. Later, they have the opportunity to relive the experience and fill in any gaps or missing pieces. The presence of the father/partner is especially valuable if the mother has had general anesthesia or experienced complications that resulted in maternal–newborn separation. The father/partner can take pictures, hold the baby, and foster the discovery process by directing the mother's attention to the details of the newborn.

Sometimes, during the *taking-hold* phase, the father/partner can feel neglected or excluded. This will soon pass as the *letting-go* stage begins. During this transition, the family incorporates the baby into the family unit and other family members, such as grandparents and siblings, get to know the baby and are included in the new family routine.

Historically, the baby born by cesarean was removed from the operating room after a brief introduction to the parents. It was also common for the father/partner to accompany the baby to the nursery, leaving the mother without support. Separation of the family unit is not medically necessary unless the newborn needs to be stabilized or a complication occurred in the operating room. Family-centered care advocates keeping the family unit together. The nurse can be an advocate in facilitating family attachment by:

- Encouraging the father/partner to stand beside the warmer and interact with the baby
- Giving the baby to the father/partner to hold as soon as medically stable
- Encouraging the father/partner to place the newborn in close contact with the mother
- Allowing the woman to touch her baby
- Allowing the mother to hold the baby skin-to-skin during surgical closure (if approved by the healthcare provider). If not, allowing skin-to-skin contact immediately after the procedure is completed (Frederick, Busen, Engebretson, et al., 2015).
- Advocating for the newborn to stay with the parents in recovery and be transferred to the postpartum unit to enable interaction when the baby is in an alert state.

Nursing Care of the Postpartum Adolescent

The adolescent mother may have special postpartum needs, depending on her level of maturity and support system. The nurse needs to observe maternal–newborn interaction, interactions of support people, knowledge of childrearing, and plans for follow-up care in order to provide a basis to customize education and discharge teaching. Community resources and appointments with pediatric and pregnancy healthcare providers prior to discharge are important.

Because one in five teen births involve a repeat birth, contraception counseling is imperative (National Campaign to Prevent Teen and Unplanned Pregnancy, 2016). Nurses should be aware of the state laws that govern their jurisdiction in order to determine if providing contraception without parental consent is allowed. In states where adolescents can obtain birth control without parental consent, it is often more comfortable for the adolescent to address these issues without others present (Chapter 12 discusses adolescent pregnancy in depth). Adolescents may encounter obstacles when attempting to obtain contraceptives, including embarrassment, concerns about confidentiality, unwillingness to discuss with parents when parental consent is needed, and lack of knowledge regarding the most effective methods (Centers for Disease Control & Prevention [CDC], 2016). Establishing a therapeutic trusting relationship, treating young mothers with respect, and modeling a positive caretaker role often facilitates open communication in which the young mother feels comfortable discussing sensitive topics.

Postpartum teaching for young parents can be achieved through positive role modeling and utilizing a teaching method that is embraced by the young parents. Verbal explanations with hands-on demonstration with an opportunity for the family to ask questions and to provide a return demonstration may be an effective teaching strategy. Repetition is important for all new mothers. Young mothers may not have the confidence and life experiences that older mothers do, so additional support and teaching are important. Inclusion of other family members is also important and should be encouraged (Cherry & Dillon, 2014).

The newborn examination should be done at the bedside to teach the parents information about their baby's health, demonstrate proper handling and holding positions, and inform the parents about newborn/infant behavior. It is important that teen parents have a realistic expectation of the baby's needs, so they can provide the appropriate care and lessen frustration (Cherry & Dillon, 2014).

When working with an adolescent mother, provide positive feedback about her newborn and her developing maternal responses; provide praise and encouragement to increase her confidence and self-esteem.

Young mothers have significant lifetime implications that result from teen pregnancy. Low self-esteem, family conflict, absence of peer relationships, reduced social supports, and risk of postpartum mood and anxiety disorders are common. Academic advancement is the single most significant indicator of teen parenting outcomes. More than half of teen mothers do not graduate from high school; only 2% have graduated from college at the age of 30. Teen fathers also have lower levels of educational achievement. Low educational achievement is directly correlated with low socioeconomic status and inability to obtain well-paying jobs. Seventy-five percent of teen mothers receive public assistance in the first five years after birth. Teen fathers also earn 10% to 15% less than their peers (National Campaign to Prevent Teen and Unplanned Pregnancy, 2016).

Along with the economic consequences, only 20% of teen fathers marry the mother of their first child. Teen mothers also have a reduced chance of being married by age 35. Parent–child relationships are also at risk for adolescent parents. Teen parents experience more stressors and are more likely to neglect or abuse their children. Children of teen parents have more academic difficulties and decreased high school graduation rates. Their daughters have a higher incidence of teen pregnancy and their sons are more likely to enter the criminal justice system (National Campaign to Prevent Teen and Unplanned Pregnancy, 2016).

Young mothers are often eager to meet peers and share experiences with young mothers the same age. Group classes for adolescent mothers provide an environment for peer support, role modeling, and mothering and caregiving skills. Educational content should include: newborn/infant care skills, signs of illness in the baby, clinical resources, parenting tips and strategies, and normal newborn growth and development. Teaching at an age-appropriate level is associated with better outcomes. Group sessions should address the impact of changes on peer relationships, dealing with added responsibilities, and short- and long-term goal setting. Successful strategies to keep young mothers in school include a specialized small setting with other young mothers; use of community-based resources; inclusion of health care, child care, counseling services, and mentoring; academic support; career counseling; and case management services (National Campaign to Prevent Teen and Unplanned Pregnancy, 2016).

Nursing Care of the Woman Who Relinquishes Her Baby

It is estimated that less than 1% of American women place their babies for adoption. Characteristics of women who relinquish their newborns include being academically focused and being less likely to live in poverty or receive public assistance. They often marry later than their peers and have lower divorce rates. When comparing single mothers with women who relinquished their babies, the women who relinquished their babies were more likely to be employed within 12 months of birth. These women have similar rates of psychological issues as women who were single mothers and did not opt for adoption (American Adoptions, 2016).

Adoption has changed dramatically over the last 50 years. It peaked in 1971, when 47.5 per 1000 births resulted in adoption. In 1975, when abortion became legal, adoptions dramatically decreased. During that time, single mother births were not considered acceptable. Today's birth mothers are much different today in that they have the freedom to make better-informed decisions and do not feel cultural pressures that were prominent in the past.

Birth mothers now have the ability to choose the families that will adopt their children, meet them in person if desired, and maintain an open relationship if desired. This may be limited to annual photos and child updates or involve an ongoing relationship with the family. Women who choose to relinquish their babies are typically single, White, and never married. Some cultures do not embrace adoption as evidenced by the low rates of relinquishment among Black and Hispanic women. A small number of mothers are forced to relinquish their babies because of lifestyle choices such as illicit drug use, past history of abusing children, and incarceration. The number of babies placed for adoption because of these circumstances is unknown. Many of these babies may be placed with relatives or in the foster care system. There are several state and federal laws that inadvertently have led to termination of parental rights for women who have committed minor crimes (Child Welfare Information Gateway, 2016).

SAFETY ALERT!

Starting in 1997, Infant Safe Haven Acts were enacted to protect newborns from death caused by abandonment; to enable babies to be placed for adoption anonymously; and to ensure that relinquished babies are left with safe providers who can provide medical services. The relinquishing mother is protected from prosecution for neglect or abandonment under the law (Child Welfare Information Gateway, 2016).

Surrogacy

Surrogacy is becoming more common in the United States, resulting in relinquishment agreements that may not show up in the adoption statistics. Even though the mother has entered a legal agreement to give up the child she is carrying, she still faces grief issues. The mother who chooses to let her child be adopted usually experiences intense ambivalence. Several factors contribute to this ambivalence. First, there are social pressures against giving up one's child. Additionally, the woman has usually made considerable adjustments in her lifestyle to carry and give birth to this child, and may be unaware of the growing bond between her and her child. Birth mothers need to complete a grieving process to work through their loss and its accompanying grief, loneliness, guilt, and other feelings. Mothers who relinquish their babies through open adoptions experience comparable psychological difficulties to those of single mothers who keep their babies (American Adoptions, 2016).

Nursing Interventions

The nurse focuses on assisting the mother with grief, which occurs as part of the relinquishment process. Mothers who relinquish their babies often experience disenfranchised grief, that is, grief that is unrecognized or not socially accepted.

Interventions designed to decrease stress and assist the mother in her grieving process include accommodating special requests for the birth and providing opportunities for her to express her emotions. After the birth, it is the mother's decision to have contact with her baby or not. Seeing the newborn often aids the grieving process and provides an opportunity for the birth mother to say goodbye. When the mother sees her baby, she may feel strong attachment and love. Provide reassurance to the woman that these feelings are natural and do not necessarily reflect that she has changed her mind.

Postpartum nursing care also includes ensuring postpartum follow-up, providing contraceptive teaching, interventions for milk suppression, and facilitating early discharge if requested.

Postpartum Care for Special Populations

Nursing Care of the Obese Postpartum Woman

Obesity is increasing in the United States, and the postpartum nurse will care for a growing number of women who are obese or morbidly obese. The woman with obesity has needs similar to those of all postpartum women, but she needs special attention to prevent injury, respiratory complications, thromboembolic disease, and infection, for which she is at high risk.

The nurse should carefully assess the woman for airway obstruction and hypoxia, particularly if she received opioids. Ambulation should be encouraged as soon as possible to prevent pneumonia. The use of sequential compression devices (SCDs) and early ambulation is essential to the prevention of deep vein thrombosis, especially if the woman had a cesarean birth. If mechanical vacuum devices are used to facilitate drainage from her incision following a cesarean birth, the woman should be educated about them. The mother should demonstrate how to visualize, clean, and completely dry her incision prior to discharge. The use of a mirror may be helpful. She needs to recognize and report signs of infection or dehiscence of her surgical incision or episiotomy repair promptly.

SAFETY ALERT!

The nurse needs to utilize adequate personnel and appropriate assistive devices to maintain safety for both the woman who is obese and staff members during position changes, transport, and ambulation. Additionally, the new mother may need extra supervision and assistance when breastfeeding her baby to ensure newborn safety.

Nursing Care of the Lesbian Mother

Although the literature regarding gay and lesbian families is growing, much of it is focused on options for conception,

---

EVIDENCE-BASED PRACTICE | Experiences of Pregnancy for Lesbian Mothers

Clinical Question

How is the experience of conception, pregnancy, and birth different for lesbian mothers?

The Evidence

Societal definitions of "family" have changed substantially and a larger number of lesbian committed couples are opting for one partner to undergo physiologic birth. The 2000 census revealed more than 300,000 self-reported lesbian families, of which more than a third were raising biologic children. While research has shown that the desire and motivation to have children among lesbian couples is quite similar to those in heterosexual relationships, little is known about the experience of conception, pregnancy, and birth as it applies to this population. These researchers conducted an in-depth qualitative study to understand the reactions of lesbian couples to the normal processes of conception, birth, and parenting. More than 120 hours of interviews and observation were included in this integrative study. While quantitative model-testing will make this evidence stronger for practice, the large sample size and extended contact make this good evidence for practice.

These mothers felt differently about the conception, pregnancy, and birth process than mothers from more traditional families. This sense of "differentness" permeated the entire experience. Several themes illustrated their sense of being different. The woman who elected to be the biologic mother often felt "normal" about the pregnancy, while the nonbiologic mother had strong legal and biologic concerns. This sense of uncertainty about legal rights was an ongoing concern for the woman who elected not to carry the pregnancy. These women also were concerned about losing their relationship, and therefore custody, since the rights of lesbian mothers have not been clearly established. The nonbiologic mother often felt incomplete and inadequate as a parent, and there was little support because the population of lesbian mothers is often hidden and not publicly acknowledged (Wojnar & Katzenmeyer, 2014). A surprising finding was that the condition of postpartum depression affected both biologic and nonbiologic parents in these relationships.

Best Practice

Lesbian couples have unique needs during conception, pregnancy, and birth. Sensitivity to the special conditions surrounding these pregnancies is needed to reassure the mothers of their adequacy as parents and to ease their concerns. Finding support for these women can help them deal with the uncertainty and demands of motherhood.

Clinical Reasoning

How can the nurse provide support to lesbian mothers so that they have an optimal pregnancy and birth experience? How might these mothers find support systems that can ease their concerns?

challenges experienced by gay parents, and legal issues. Lesbian women without partners or spouses represent a small number of lesbian mothers. The care of lesbian families focuses on providing culturally appropriate care that provides holistic care to both of the mothers. Showing respect and acceptance of nontraditional families and conveying a sense of equality between both mothers is essential for the nurse.

Spidsberg and Sørlie (2012) examined lesbian couples and found that lesbian couples have a unique and different bond compared to heterosexual couples. In general, most lesbian partners often feel more at ease in the delivery room than many fathers. The nonpregnant partner often assumes a co-mothering role in the family unit. The main needs of lesbian couples identified in Spidsberg and Sørlie's qualitative study were to have an open relationship with healthcare providers who were accepting of their differences and to be able to build a rapport between the nurse and the couple. Nurses need to examine their own feelings about how they perceive alternative families and be mindful of their nonverbal expressions when interacting with these families (Spidsberg & Sørlie, 2012).

The nurse should maintain an attitude that is respectful, caring, and open to sexual diversity when working with all clients. Providing quality client-centered care for any postpartum woman involves acknowledging and welcoming her intimate partner/spouse and involving her in care and decision making. The nurse should be aware that standardized postpartum instructions, particularly those related to intercourse and contraception, need to be individualized and amended.

Nursing Care of the Postpartum Mother With a Developmental Disability

The postpartum period is one of great growth in the maternal mothering role. New mothers are faced with various challenges and different learning opportunities. Women with developmental or intellectual disabilities are at particular risk during this time period. Material should be presented to them in an easy-to-understand format. Peer mentors are often helpful role models for these women. Teaching should be conducted at a level that is achievable for the individual woman. A needs assessment should be performed to determine what needs the mother and new family may have. Community and private resources should be available to make the transition to the postpartum period as flawless as possible.

Nursing Care of the Mother With a History of Sexual Abuse

Women who have previously been sexually abused tend to have more anxiety and stress related to hospital procedures, interactions with unfamiliar staff, and being touched in general. The postpartum woman who has a history of sexual abuse may have difficulty establishing trust and may feel uncomfortable when private information is being given or demonstrations are being performed. The nurse should treat the woman with respect by providing draping whenever possible. Speaking to the woman in private protects her fragile emotions from being observed by others. Support groups may offer the mother with a history of sexual abuse a safe haven to share her experiences and the impact they have on her mothering.

Preparation for Discharge

In preparation for discharge, the nurse evaluates the mother's and the newborn's progress toward identified outcomes and provides discharge teaching.

Discharge Criteria

Ideally, preparation for discharge begins the moment a woman is admitted to the birthing unit. Before discharge, the nurse assesses the mother's physical and psychologic condition, the newborn's adjustment to extrauterine life, the family's overall adjustment, and the need for outside resources. Nursing efforts should be directed toward assessing the parents' knowledge, expectations, and beliefs and then providing anticipatory guidance and teaching accordingly. Because teaching is one of the primary responsibilities of the postpartum nurse, many agencies have elaborate teaching programs and specialized channels to teach newborn/infant care and maternal postpartum care. The nurse should spend time with the parents to determine if they have any last-minute questions. In general, the following criteria should be assessed and met before discharge:

- Normal vital signs
- Appropriate involution of the uterus
- Appropriate amount of lochia without evidence of infection
- Knowledge of signs of infection
- Episiotomy or laceration well approximated with a decrease in edema or bruising
- Ability to perform pericare and apply medications to perineal or anal area if ordered
- Ability to void and pass flatus
- Ability to take fluids and foods without difficulty
- Ability to care for self and newborn
- Has received rubella vaccine, Tdap, influenza vaccine, and RhoGAM if indicated (see Table 29–2). Women < 26 years of age not previously vaccinated may begin the HPV series. Inactivated vaccines can be provided as needed.

Additional outcomes for the mother who has had a cesarean birth include the following:

- States in own words the reason for the cesarean birth
- Maintains desired pain control
- Maintains moderate mobility level

Ensuring that the woman has met the criteria before discharge decreases the incidence of complications or readmission in the postpartum period.

Discharge Teaching

In general, discharge teaching includes at least the following information and maternal activities:

1. Review of literature and multimedia the woman has received or viewed that explain recommended postpartum exercises, the need for adequate rest, the need to avoid overexertion initially, and the recommendation to abstain from sexual intercourse until lochia has ceased. (If the family desires information about birth control methods, the nurse can provide information at this time.)

2. Information geared to the specific nutritional needs of breastfeeding or formula-feeding mothers. (If the mother has been receiving vitamins and/or iron supplements, the nurse encourages her to continue until the first postpartum examination.) Mother demonstrates proper breastfeeding techniques and breast care or describes formula preparation, formula-feeding techniques, and nonlactating breast care.

3. How to provide basic care for the newborn; when to anticipate that the cord will fall off; when the baby can have a tub bath; when the baby will need her or his first immunizations; and so on. (Parents should also be comfortable feeding and handling the baby, and should practice basic principles of safety, including the need to use a car seat when the baby is in a car.)

4. Procedure for obtaining copies of her newborn's birth certificate.

5. When to schedule the first appointment for her postpartum examination and for her newborn's first well-baby examination.

6. Signs of possible complications and encouragement for the woman to contact her caregiver if she develops any of them (see *Key Facts to Remember: When to Contact the Healthcare Provider*). Signs and symptoms that indicate possible problems in the baby and who the parents should contact about them.

7. Information on local agencies and/or support groups, such as La Leche League, Mothers of Twins, adolescent groups, or new mother support groups that might be of particular assistance to the family. Displays appropriate interaction with baby. Identifies the symptoms of postpartum depression and available resources.

8. Phone number of the mother–baby unit or information hotline and encouragement to call if she has any questions or concerns. Plans for home care visits so that the parents know when to expect the visit and what it entails.

KEY FACTS TO REMEMBER
When to Contact the Healthcare Provider

After discharge, a woman should contact her healthcare provider if any of the following develop:

- Sudden, persistent, or spiking fever
- Change in the character of the lochia—foul smell, return to bright-red bleeding, excessive amount, passage of large clots
- Pain at the site of a laceration, an episiotomy, or an abdominal incision
- Evidence of wound infection including redness, swelling, severe or worsening pain, or foul-smelling discharge
- Evidence of mastitis, such as breast tenderness, reddened areas, malaise
- Evidence of thrombophlebitis, such as calf pain, tenderness, redness
- Evidence of urinary tract infection, such as urgency, frequency, burning on urination
- Continued severe or incapacitating postpartum depression, anxiety, psychosis, or PTSD
- Inability to care for self or baby for any physical or psychologic reason

In addition, the nurse performs a postpartum depression (PPD) screening and educates the parents about the symptoms of postpartum mood and anxiety disorders. The nurse assesses for risk factors and schedules women at risk for screening at 2 weeks.

The nurse can also use this final opportunity to reassure the couple of their ability to be successful parents. The nurse can stress the newborn's need to feel loved and secure and urge parents to talk to each other and work together to solve any problems that arise.

Considerations for Follow-Up Care

In 1998, the Newborns' and Mothers' Health Protection Act went into effect ensuring that insurance companies cover a 48-hour stay for vaginal deliveries and a 96-hour stay for cesarean births (U.S. Department of Labor, 2016). Discharge before 48 hours at the family's request should be considered if no maternal or newborn risk factors are present. Approximately 50% of states have legislation in place ensuring that women discharged before 48 hours will receive a home visit.

The concerns regarding early discharge revolve around complications that may occur in the first 48 hours after birth. These include risks of postpartum hemorrhage, breastfeeding issues, elevated newborn bilirubin levels, and presence of symptoms of postpartum mood or anxiety disorder (PMAD). In addition, early discharge leaves little time for client education, and opportunities for the mother to become comfortable with her new baby may be compromised. The risk of postpartum depression is highest in the first month following the birth. Women who received PPD screening in the perinatal period and education about PMAD are more likely to be screened earlier in the postpartum period if risk factors are present, are diagnosed earlier, and receive prompt treatment with diagnosis. However, in the first 24 hours after childbirth, the mother may be too tired or may not be ready emotionally to participate in learning activities. In addition, family members who have agreed to assist the new family in the first few weeks after birth may not have arrived yet. In all cases of early discharge, a home visit by an experienced postpartum nurse can be invaluable.

Early discharges present a challenge to nurses because many conditions in the newborn, such as jaundice, ductal-dependent cardiac lesions, and gastrointestinal obstructions, may take longer than 2 days to develop, and identification of these problems depends on a skilled, experienced professional (American Academy of Pediatrics [AAP] Committee on Fetus and Newborn, 2014). Medical providers also contend that breastfeeding may not be well established before 48 hours and discharge before this time can lead to increased rates of dehydration and poor breastfeeding outcomes (AAP Committee on Fetus and Newborn, 2014).

Special emphasis has also been placed on the needs of **late-preterm newborns**, born between 34 and 36 6/7 weeks (Barfield & Lee, 2015). These babies are at a greater risk for increases in mortality and morbidity because they are not physically mature and are more prone to have physiologic and metabolic complications (Barfield & Lee, 2015). Readmissions for infection and jaundice are more common in late-preterm newborns than in term newborns (Barfield & Lee, 2015). The American Academy of Pediatrics (AAP) has identified specific risk factors in late-preterm newborns that increase the likelihood of readmission and neonatal mortality. These include being first born, breastfeeding at the time of discharge, having a mother who has had labor and childbirth complications, and having public insurance as the source of payment (Barfield & Lee, 2015). Special attention by the home health nurse is warranted for these babies to ensure a proper home transition and to identify possible early complications (Barfield & Lee, 2015).

Following discharge, various services are available in most communities to meet the needs of the postpartum family. The goal is to help ensure that all family members have the opportunity to meet healthcare needs, regardless of their resources. Types of follow-up care include telephone follow-up and home visits.

TELEPHONE FOLLOW-UP

In the past, and currently in some settings, telephone follow-up for postpartum mothers is a routine practice. Effective telephone assessment requires active listening, asking open-ended questions, and projecting an attitude of caring. When complications are identified, referral to the healthcare provider is indicated.

More commonly, women are given an emergency number to call and these calls must be triaged immediately. Calls with urgent or life-threatening implications should be referred appropriately, either by initiating an immediate call to the healthcare provider or, in rare circumstances, calling 911. Many facilities offer 24-hour help lines for new parents to call when they have questions or need support. Some organizations, such as Postpartum Support International (PSI), offer specialized 24-hour support for women with postpartum mood and anxiety disorders.

HOME VISIT

In some states, if the mother, family, and healthcare provider have chosen discharge earlier than 48 hours after vaginal birth, the mother may request a total of three home visits. The home setting provides an opportunity for the nurse and the family to interact in a more relaxed environment in which the family has control. In some instances, the challenges of assessing and enhancing self-care and newborn care may be unique in the home, and the nurse will have many opportunities to exercise critical thinking to develop creative options with the family. The nurse should explain that, unlike community health visits, only one or two home visits are typically planned and are spaced out over a week and that long-term follow-up by the postpartum nurse is not anticipated. Occasionally the nurse may schedule additional home visits based on the findings of the first home visit and the follow-up phone call.

Evaluation

Anticipated outcomes of comprehensive postpartum nursing care of the family include the following:

- The mother is reasonably comfortable and has learned pain relief measures.
- The mother is rested and understands how to add more activity during the next few days and weeks.
- The mother's physiologic and psychologic well-being have been supported.
- The mother verbalizes her understanding of self-care measures.
- The new parents demonstrate how to care for their baby.
- The new parents have had opportunities to form attachments with their baby.
- Follow-up care contacts have been initiated as needed.

Considerations for the Home Visit

Before the home visit, the nurse (who is experienced in postpartum maternal and newborn care) prepares by identifying the purpose of the home visit and gathering needed materials and equipment. A personal contact while the woman is still in the birth setting or a previsit telephone call is used to arrange the appointment with the woman and her family. During the previsit contact, it is important for the nurse to clearly identify the purpose and goals of the visit and to begin establishing rapport.

Purpose and Timing of the Home Visit

Postpartum home care is focused more on assessment, teaching and facilitating learning, and counseling than on physical care.

- *Assessment of mother and newborn health status.* The established guidelines for discharge of the mother and baby mean the nurse can expect certain levels of health and wellness. However, because the status of the mother and the newborn can change, the nurse should stay alert for deviations from the norm and identify conditions that may warrant further medical evaluation or rehospitalization. The nurse can also complete follow-up blood work if needed.

- *Assessment of family adaptation.* The nurse assesses adaptation of the family to the new baby and adjustment of any siblings. The nurse also assesses the parents' skill in bathing, dressing, handling, and comforting their newborn, and the appropriateness and safety of the home environment.

- *Teaching and facilitating learning.* The nurse ascertains current informational needs and offers requested information. Postpartum home care provides opportunities for enhancing self-care and newborn/infant care techniques, including breastfeeding, initially presented in the birth setting. Many times, questions and concerns arise at home that were not identified in the hospital or birthing center.

- *Counseling.* The nurse provides support and encouragement, and addresses the need for referrals to clinics, classes, or postpartum support groups.

Maintaining Safety

In the past, nurses were perceived as a mainstay of communities and could move in most settings without fear or concern for safety. Today, some communities are not safe for visiting nurses. It is important for the nurse to follow basic safety rules when conducting a home visit, including the following:

- Know the specific address and ask for directions during the previsit contact. If the area is not familiar, trace out the route on a map or use an Internet program to provide directions before leaving for the visit and take a map along. Even with a global positioning system (GPS), some newer areas may not be included or found within the system, so always have a backup plan in place.

- Carry a fully charged cellular phone and a working flashlight, especially for night visits.

- Notify an instructor or supervisor when leaving for a visit and check in as soon as the visit is completed.

Many agencies that provide home care services have established violence prevention programs to help ensure safety. Nurses in the community need to be aware of their environment and alert to environmental cues, whether overt or subtle. In addition, the following recommendations are important:

- Investigate the neighborhood prior to leaving the car.
- Avoid walking in crowded, violent areas.
- Visit the family during the day in high-risk areas. Inform the family of your arrival time and ask them to call a supervisor if you do not arrive after 15 minutes.
- Park in well-lit, populated areas with car windows and doors locked.
- Before leaving for the visit, lock personal belongings in the trunk of the car, out of sight.
- Wear clothing and identification consistent with agency policy. Wear a name tag identifying you as a nurse and carry identification.
- Avoid wearing expensive jewelry or pins of a religious or political nature that might be seen as offensive.
- Use appropriate personal body language that does not exhibit fear, aggression, or anger.
- Observe all family members' body language during the visit and be prepared to terminate the visit quickly if you feel discomfort.
- Be alert for signs that a person is becoming enraged (reddened neck and/or face, clenched fists, pacing). If any family member is violent, or if drug or alcohol abuse is occurring, leave the home and report the incident to your supervisor.
- Leave the home immediately in a nonconfrontational manner if any weapons or illegal substances are visible.
- Terminate the visit immediately if a situation arises that feels unsafe, or a "gut feeling" tells you something is not right.

SAFETY ALERT!

If the visit is in an area that seems unsafe, it may be wise for two nurses to go together. Nurses should avoid entering areas where violence is in progress. In such cases, they should return to the car and contact the police or dial 9-1-1. Most people are more comfortable in familiar neighborhoods and have some hesitation when entering homes in other residential areas. First home visits may feel uncomfortable because they are unfamiliar, but with experience comfort increases.

Fostering a Caring Relationship With the Family

Although the nurse in the birthing center strives to enhance family autonomy and control, the atmosphere of the institutional environment may cause the new mother and family to feel disempowered. It is important for the professional nurse to recognize that the parameters of a home visit are different. In the home, the family members have control of their environment and the nurse is an invited visitor (Figure 29–4). The nurse can rely on the same characteristics of a caring relationship that have been integral to hospital-based practice—regard for clients, genuineness, empathy, and establishment of trust and rapport—when providing care in the home setting. Evidence of these characteristics forms the foundation

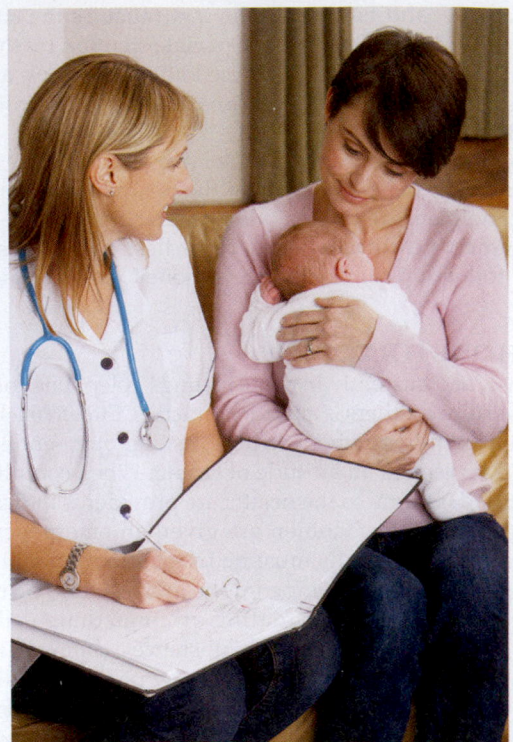

Figure 29–4 Nurse providing care and teaching to a new mother and baby at the home visit.

SOURCE: Monkey Business Images/Shutterstock.

for a caring relationship. See *Key Facts to Remember: Fostering a Caring Relationship*.

In ideal situations a family approach involving the presence of the father/partner and any siblings provides an opportunity to observe family interactions and opportunities for all family members to ask questions and express concerns. In addition, any questionable family interaction pattern such as one suggestive of abuse or neglect may be evident and further referral could be considered if needed.

Professionalism in Practice Reporting Unsanitary Conditions in the Home

As healthcare professionals, nurses are required to report newborn/infant neglect or abuse. When practicing in private homes, the nurse will be exposed to a wide range of home management practices with regard to aesthetics and sanitation. For example, the nurse will need to distinguish a home that is simply messy from a home that is unsanitary. It is important to develop rapport with the parents and to provide education as needed when sanitation issues are present. In certain cases, a follow-up visit is warranted. In cases of extreme filth or severe pest infestations, the nurse will need to use critical thinking skills to determine whether the most vulnerable client—the newborn—is at risk for injury. If that is the case, the nurse should notify the appropriate authorities and follow the home care agency plan for such contingencies. If in doubt, the nurse should call upon resource persons and supervisors for assistance.

KEY FACTS TO REMEMBER
Fostering a Caring Relationship

Use the following approaches to achieve the demonstrated goals that form the foundation of a caring relationship.

Demonstrated Goal: Regard

- Introduce yourself to the family. Call the family members by their surnames until you have been invited to use the given or a less formal name.
- Ask to be introduced to other members of the family who are present. Allow the mother or spokesperson to assume this role. Remember, in some cultures, it may be a male figure or a mother figure who assumes the primary role.
- Ask permission before sitting.
- Accept offered refreshment graciously. Many cultures have strong ties to certain foods and beverages during the postpartum period. Accepting the food or beverage conveys acceptance of cultural norms.
- Use active listening.
- Maintain objectivity.

Demonstrated Goal: Genuineness

- Mean what you say. Make sure that your verbal and nonverbal messages are congruent.
- Be nonjudgmental. Do not make assumptions about individuals or settings.
- Always strive to demonstrate caring behaviors.
- Be prepared for the visit, honestly answer questions and provide information, and be truthful.
- If you do not know the answer to a question, tell the woman you will find the answer and report back.

Demonstrated Goal: Empathy

- Listen to the mother and the family "where they are" without judgment.
- Be attentive to what the birthing experience is for them so that you will understand from their perspective.
- Remember that empathy denotes understanding, not sympathy.

Demonstrated Goal: Trust and Rapport

- Do what you say you will do.
- Be prepared for the visit and be on time.
- Follow up on any areas as needed.

Developing Cultural Competence   Role of Extended Family

In some cultures, extended family members such as grandmothers and aunts play a major role in the care of the postpartum woman and her family. Sometimes, these family members take full responsibility for running the household throughout the postpartum period. In other families, they concentrate entirely on the mother's or the newborn's care. When culturally appropriate, include these extended family members in postpartum education sessions (McFarland & Wehbe-Alamah, 2015).

Home Care: The Mother and Family

During the first home visit, the nurse completes a physical assessment of the mother, a maternal psychologic assessment (attachment, adjustment to the parental role, her perception of her new role, coping skills, educational needs), and a psychosocial assessment of the family (including sibling adjustment). Teaching for self-care is commonly required for new mothers, especially breastfeeding mothers with nipple soreness, engorgement, and other concerns. Family teaching related to resumption of sexual activity and contraception may also be required.

Assessment of the Mother and the Family

Before performing the physical assessment, the nurse should ensure the mother's privacy. The physical assessment focuses on maternal physical adaptation, which is assessed by focusing on vital signs, breasts, abdominal musculature, elimination patterns, reproductive tract, and laboratory values. The nurse also talks with the mother about her diet, fatigue level, ability to rest and sleep, pain management, and signs of postpartum complications. In addition, for breastfeeding mothers, the nurse assesses the woman's feeding technique and presents information about possible problems that may occur. See *Assessment Guide: Postpartum—First Home Visit and Anticipated Progress at 6 Weeks.*

Many new mothers are concerned about weight loss. Women who have gained excess weight during the pregnancy are at risk for obesity in later life. Counseling the mother about proper diet and exercise is an effective strategy for losing weight in the postpartum period. Nursing women should be counseled that extreme weight loss strategies are not advised, but that healthy food choices and exercise can aid in weight reduction. Some weight loss programs are designed specifically for nursing mothers and offer counseling, group support, and monitoring in the postpartum period.

Breastfeeding Concerns Following Discharge

Because mothers are discharged from the birthing unit before breastfeeding is well established, they are frequently alone when they encounter changes in the breastfeeding process. Many women stop nursing if the situations they encounter seem problematic. For this reason, the nurse providing a home visit is in a unique position to positively impact the success of breastfeeding (Newman & Pitman, 2015). Table 29–3 summarizes self-care measures the nurse can suggest to a woman with a breastfeeding problem.

Regardless of feeding method (newborn feeding is discussed in detail in Chapter 25), it is important for the nurse to assess the newborn's fluid and nutritional intake. As part of the physical assessment, the newborn's nude weight is determined. If the weight loss since birth is 10% or more, the nurse assesses the baby for signs of dehydration such as loose skin with decreased skin turgor, dry mucous membranes, sunken anterior fontanelle, and decreased frequency and amount of voiding and stooling. Risk factors for suboptimal breastfeeding include maternal obesity, primiparity, young maternal age, use of formula supplementation, use of pacifiers, cesarean birth, second stage of labor greater than 1 hour, low birth weight, breastfeeding difficulty, and flat or inverted nipples (Newman & Pitman, 2015).

NIPPLE SORENESS

Some discomfort often occurs initially with breastfeeding; it peaks between days 3 and 6 and then recedes. Breastfeeding difficulty and nipple soreness are often causes for women to discontinue breastfeeding. The nurse should counsel the mother not to switch to formula-feeding or delay feedings because these measures cause engorgement and more soreness (Newman & Pitman, 2015). Discomfort that lasts throughout the feeding or past the first week demands attention.

ASSESSMENT GUIDE	Postpartum—First Home Visit and Anticipated Progress at 6 Weeks	
Physical Assessment/Normal Findings	**Alterations and Possible Causes***	**Nursing Responses to Data†**
Vital Signs		
Blood pressure: Return to normal prepregnant level.	Elevated blood pressure (anxiety, essential hypertension, renal disease), preeclampsia (can occur postpartum).	Review history, evaluate normal baseline; refer to healthcare provider if necessary.
Pulse: 60–100 beats/min (or prepregnant normal rate).	Increased pulse rate, tachycardia, chest pain (excitement, anxiety, cardiac disorders).	Count pulse for full minute, note irregularities; marked tachycardia or beat irregularities require additional assessment and possible healthcare provider referral.
Respirations: 12–20/min.	Marked tachypnea or abnormal patterns (respiratory disorders).	Evaluate for respiratory disease; refer to healthcare provider if necessary.
Temperature: 36.6°–37.6°C (98°–99.6°F).	Increased temperature (infection).	Assess for signs and symptoms of infection or disease state.
Weight		
2 days: Possible weight loss of 12–20+ lb.	Minimal weight loss (fluid retention, preeclampsia).	Evaluate for fluid retention, edema, deep tendon reflexes, and blood pressure elevation.
6 weeks: Returning to normal prepregnant weight.	Retained weight (excessive caloric intake).	Determine amount of daily exercise. Provide dietary teaching. Refer to dietitian if necessary for additional dietary counseling.
	Extreme weight loss (excessive dieting, inadequate caloric intake)	Discuss appropriate diets, refer to dietitian for additional counseling if necessary.
Breasts		
Nonbreastfeeding: 2 days: May have mild to moderate tenderness; small amount of milk may be expressed. **6 weeks:** Soft, with no tenderness; return to prepregnant size.	Some engorgement (incomplete suppression of lactation). Redness; marked tenderness (mastitis). Palpable mass (tumor).	Engorgement may be seen in nonbreastfeeding mothers. Advise woman to wear a supportive, well-fitted bra; avoid very warm showers; avoid pumping or any stimulation of breasts; use ice packs for comfort; evaluate for signs and symptoms of mastitis (rare in nonbreastfeeding mothers). Par-cooked or fresh cabbage leaves can be placed against the breasts to relieve engorgement.
Breastfeeding: Full, with prominent nipples; lactation established.	Cracked, fissured nipples (feeding problems). Redness, marked tenderness, or even abscess formation (mastitis). Palpable mass (full milk duct, tumor).	Counsel about nipple care. Observe baby feeding. Evaluate the mother's condition, evidence of fever, redness, or tender area; refer to healthcare provider for initiation of antibiotic therapy if indicated. Opinion varies as to value of breast examination for breastfeeding mothers; some feel a breastfeeding mother should examine her breasts monthly, after feeding, when breasts are empty; if palpable mass is felt, refer to healthcare provider for further evaluation. For breast inflammation instruct the mother to: 1. Keep breast empty by frequent feeding. 2. Rest when possible. 3. Take prescribed pain relief med. 4. Force fluids. 5. Take antibiotics if ordered. If symptoms are accompanied by fever, flulike symptoms, or redness, instruct woman to call her healthcare provider and take an analgesic.

Abdominal Musculature

2 days: Improved firmness, although "bread dough" consistency is not unusual, especially in multipara. Striae pink and obvious.	Marked relaxation of muscles.	Evaluate exercise level; provide information on appropriate exercise program.
Cesarean incision healing.	Use the REEDA scoring system (**r**edness, **e**cchymosis, **e**dema, **d**ischarge from incision site, and **a**pproximation). Assess for tenderness and pain.	Evaluate for infection; refer to healthcare provider if necessary.
6 weeks: Muscle tone continues to improve; striae may be beginning to fade, may not achieve a silvery appearance for several more weeks; linea nigra fading.		

Elimination Pattern

Urinary tract: Return to prepregnant urinary elimination routine.	Urinary incontinence, especially when lifting, coughing, laughing, and so on (urethral trauma, cystocele).	Assess for cystocele; instruct in appropriate muscle-tightening exercises; refer to healthcare provider.
	Pain or burning when voiding, urgency and/or frequency, pus, blood, or white blood cells (WBC) in urine, pathogenic organisms in culture (urinary tract infection).	Evaluate for urinary tract infection; obtain clean-catch urine; refer to healthcare provider for treatment if indicated.
Routine urinalysis within normal limits (proteinuria disappeared).	Sugar or ketone in urine—may be some lactose present in urine of breastfeeding mothers (diabetes).	Evaluate diet; assess for signs and symptoms of diabetes; refer to healthcare provider.
Bowel habits: 2 days: May be some discomfort with defecation, especially if woman had severe hemorrhoids or third- or fourth-degree extension.	Severe constipation or pain when defecating (trauma or hemorrhoids).	Discuss dietary patterns; encourage fluids and high-fiber diet, adequate roughage. Counsel on the effects of medications. Continue use of stool softener if necessary to prevent pain associated with straining; continue sitz baths, periods of rest for severe hemorrhoids; assess healing of episiotomy and/or lacerations; severe constipation may require administration of laxatives, stool softeners, and an enema if not contraindicated (check with healthcare provider).
6 weeks: Return to normal prepregnancy bowel elimination.	Marked constipation (inadequate fluid/fiber intake).	See previous discussed interventions.
	Fecal incontinence or constipation (rectocele).	Assess for evidence of rectocele; instruct in muscle-tightening exercises; refer to healthcare provider.

Reproductive Tract

Lochia: 2 days: Lochia rubra or lochia serosa, scant amounts, fleshy odor.	Excessive amounts and/or large clots (nonfirm uterus), foul odor (infection), passing tissue (possible retained placenta).	Assess for evidence of infection and/or failure of the uterus to decrease in size; refer to healthcare provider.
6 weeks: No lochia, or return to normal menstruation pattern.	See above.	See above.
Fundus and perineum: 2 days: Fundus is at least two fingerbreadths below the umbilicus; uterine muscles still somewhat lax; introitus of vagina lacks tone—gapes when intra-abdominal pressure is increased by coughing or straining.	Uterus not decreasing in size appropriately (infection).	Assess fundus for firmness and/or signs of infection; refer to healthcare provider if indicated.
Episiotomy and/or lacerations healing; no signs of infection; may have some bruising and tenderness.	Evidence of redness, severe pain, poor tissue approximation in episiotomy and/or laceration (wound infection).	Utilize cool or warm sitz baths, topical medications.

(*continued*)

ASSESSMENT GUIDE | Postpartum—First Home Visit and Anticipated Progress at 6 Weeks (*continued*)

6 weeks: Uterus almost returned to prepregnant size with almost completely restored muscle tone.	Continued flow of lochia, failure to decrease appropriately in size (subinvolution).	Assess for evidence of subinvolution and/or infection; refer to healthcare provider for further evaluation and treatment if necessary.
Hemoglobin and Hematocrit Levels		
6 weeks: Hemoglobin (Hb) 12 g/dL; hematocrit (Hct) 37% ± 5%	Hb less than 12 g/dL; Hct 32% (anemia)	Assess nutritional status, assess for signs or symptoms of anemia, begin (or continue) supplemental iron; for marked anemia (Hb less than or equal to 9 g/dL), additional assessment and/or healthcare provider referral may be necessary.
Attachment		
Bonding process demonstrated by soothing, cuddling, and talking to baby; appropriate feeding techniques; eye-to-eye contact; calling baby by name.	Failure to bond demonstrated by lack of behaviors associated with bonding process, calling baby by nickname that promotes ridicule, inadequate weight gain, baby is dirty, hygienic measures are not being maintained, severe diaper rash, failure to obtain adequate supplies to provide newborn/infant care (malattachment).	Provide counseling; talk with the woman about her feelings regarding the baby; provide support for the caretaking activities that are being performed; refer to public health nurse for continued home visits; refer if abuse or neglect is suspected.
Parent interacts with baby and provides soothing, caretaking activities.	Parent is unable to respond to baby's needs (inability to recognize needs, inadequate education and support, fear, family stress).	Provide support for caretaking activities observed; provide information regarding caretaking activities, such as responding to crying by the baby; methods of wrapping the baby; methods of soothing the baby such as swaddling, rocking, increasing stimuli by singing to the baby or decreasing stimuli by putting the baby to rest in quiet room; methods of holding the baby; differences in the cry. Identify support system such as friends, neighbors; provide information regarding community resources and support groups.
Parents express feelings of comfort and success with the parental role.	Evidence of stress and anxiety (difficulty moving into or dealing with the parental role).	Provide support and encouragement; provide information regarding progression into parental role and assist parents in talking through their feelings; refer to community resources and support groups.
Woman is in the informal or personal stage of maternal role attainment.	Woman is still greatly influenced by others, has not developed an image or style of her own (woman remains in the anticipatory stage).	Provide role modeling for the woman in working through problem solving with the baby; provide encouragement as she thinks through decisions and develops her sense of problem solving; encourage her to make decisions regarding newborn/infant care.
Adjustment to Parental Role		
Parents are coping with new roles in terms of division of labor, financial status, communication, readjustment of sexual relations, and adjusting to new daily tasks.	Inability to adjust to new roles (immaturity, inadequate education and preparation, ineffective communication patterns, inadequate support, current family crisis).	Provide counseling, refer to parent groups.
Education		
Mother understands self-care measures.	Inadequate knowledge of self-care (inadequate education).	Provide education and counseling.
Parents are knowledgeable regarding newborn/infant care.	Inadequate knowledge of newborn/infant care (inadequate education).	
Siblings are adjusting to new baby.	Excessive sibling rivalry.	
Parents have a method of contraception.	Birth control method not chosen.	

*Possible causes of alterations are identified in parentheses.

†This column provides guidelines for further assessment and initial nursing intervention.

TABLE 29–3 Common Breastfeeding Problems and Remedies

NIPPLES NOT GRASPABLE	Flat or inverted nipples	• Use Hoffman technique to break adhesions.
		• Wear breast shells to encourage nipples to protrude.
		• Grasp nipples and roll gently between the fingers to increase protractility.
		• Form the nipple before breastfeeding by hand shaping, ice, or wearing nipple shells a half-hour before feeding.
		• Use a breast pump to draw nipples out so that the mother can then put the baby to the breast.
	Engorged breasts	• Treat engorgement by feeding the baby more frequently.
		• A hand or electric pump or manual emptying of the breast can be done if the baby is unable to grasp the nipple.
	Large breasts	• Support breast with opposite hand, or use rolled towel under breast to bring nipple to the level of baby's mouth.
		• Avoid having the nipple pointing downward because this makes latch-on more difficult.
		• Use C-hold to make nipple accessible to baby (see Figure 25–18).
ENGORGEMENT	Missed or infrequent feedings	• Breastfeed frequently (every 1 1/2 hours).
		• Massage and hand express or pump to empty breasts completely when feedings are missed or when a full feeling develops in breasts and baby is not available or willing to feed.
		• Avoid excessive stimulation or pumping between feedings because this will increase milk production.
		• Place warm compresses on breast just before feeding to soften breast.
		• Use cold applications between feedings to slow milk production (frozen bagged vegetables, ice packs, and par-cooked cabbage leaves (Newman & Pitman, 2015).
	Breasts not emptied at feedings	• Massage breasts and use warm cloths before feedings.
		• Breastfeed long enough to empty breasts (10 to 15 minutes on each side at each feeding).
		• If baby will not feed long enough to empty breasts, hand express or pump after feeding.
	Inadequate let-down	• Use relaxation techniques, massage, and warm compresses before breastfeeding.
		• Relax in warm shower with water running from back over shoulders and breasts, hand expressing to relieve fullness.
		• Use hand or electric pump before placing baby on breast to encourage let-down.
		• Listen to soothing music, use visualization or breathing techniques.
		• If caused by anxiety, try to eliminate the source of tension.
	Baby sleepy or not eager to feed	• Use rousing techniques (e.g., hold baby upright, unwrap blanket, change diaper).
		• Pre-express milk onto nipple or baby's lips to entice baby.
		• Avoid use of bottles of water or formula; these will decrease baby's willingness to suckle.
INADEQUATE LET-DOWN	Let-down not well established	• Give the baby ample time at the breast (at least 15 minutes per side) to allow for let-down and complete emptying.
		• Breastfeed in a quiet spot away from distractions.
		• Massage breasts and apply warm compresses before breastfeeding.
		• Drink juice, water, or tea (no caffeine) before and during breastfeeding.
		• Condition let-down by setting up a routine for beginning feedings.
		• Use relaxation, visualization, and breathing techniques.
		• Stimulate the nipple manually before breastfeeding.
		• Concentrate thought on the baby and milk flow; turn on a faucet so that the sound of running water helps stimulate let-down.
		• Take a warm shower before feedings.
		• Use breast pump to stimulate the let-down.
		• Avoid waiting to put baby to breast until the baby is famished because this may increase maternal anxiety.
		• Assess for maternal pain, cold temperature, or anxiety before feeding.

(continued)

TABLE 29–3 Common Breastfeeding Problems and Remedies (*continued*)

	Mother overtired or overextended	• Nap or rest when the baby rests. • Limit distractions, limit visitors, focus on personal needs. • Lie down to breastfeed. • Simplify daily chores; set priorities.
	Mother tense, pressured	• Identify the causes of tensions and eliminate or minimize them. • Decrease fatigue. • Have others assist with other household duties or tasks. • Use relaxation, visualization, and breathing exercises to promote relaxation and comfort.
	Mother caught in cycle of little milk, worry, less milk	• Try all the actions above. • Counsel mother that most women do produce enough milk. • Have baby weighed to ensure adequate weight gain, which is a reflection of milk supply. • Encourage frequent, uninterrupted feedings. • Consult a lactation consultant as needed.
CRACKED NIPPLES	All causes of sore nipples carried to extreme	• Refer to all actions for sore nipples. • Ensure baby is properly positioned. • Feed baby more frequently. • Avoid soaps, perfumes, or other cleaning products that can dry out nipples and predispose them to cracking. • Express milk after feeding and rub into nipple, allowing it to air dry. • Use emollients or lanolin as directed by physician/CNM/lactation consultant. • Consult doctor about using ibuprofen (Motrin), acetaminophen (Tylenol), or other painkiller. • Improve nutritional status, increasing protein, vitamin C, zinc.
	Local infection (baby with staph or other organism may have infected mother's nipples)	• Refer to physician.
PLUGGED DUCTS	Poor positioning	• Try a variety of positions for complete emptying. • Alternate positions so that different areas of the nipple have different compression pressure. • Incomplete emptying of breast. • Breastfeed at least 10 minutes per side after let-down. • Alternate breastfeeding positions. • If baby does not empty breasts, pump or express milk after feedings.
	External pressure on breast	• Use larger-size bra, insert bra extender, or go braless. • Wear a sports bra instead of a traditional bra. • Use nursing bra instead of pulling up conventional bra to breastfeed to avoid pressure on ducts. • Avoid bunching up sweater or nightgown under arm during breastfeeding.
SORE NIPPLES	Poor positioning	• Alternate breastfeeding positions throughout the day. • Bring the baby close to feed so the baby does not pull on the breast. • Place the nipple and some of the areola in the baby's mouth. • Check to ensure the baby is put on and off the breast properly. • Check to ensure the nipple is back far enough in the baby's mouth. • Hold the baby closely during feeding so the nipple is not constantly being pulled. • Ensure that shoulder, hip, and knees are all properly aligned and facing the mother.
	Baby chewing or nuzzling onto nipple	• Form the nipple for the baby. • Set up a pattern of getting the baby onto the breast using the rooting reflex.

Baby sucking on end of nipple	• Ensure the nipple is way back in the baby's mouth by getting the baby properly onto the breast. • Check for an inverted nipple. • Check for engorgement. • If baby is initially placed incorrectly on the end of the nipple, break the suction using a fish hook motion with your index finger and reposition baby on nipple properly. • Do not allow baby to nurse on end of nipple; reposition immediately.
Baby chewing his or her way off the nipple (nipple being pulled out of baby's mouth at end of feeding)	• Remove the baby from the breast by placing a finger between the baby's gums to ensure suction is broken. • End feeding when the baby's suckling slows, before he or she has a chance to chew on the nipple.
Baby overly eager to nurse	• Breastfeed more often. • Pre-express milk to hasten let-down, avoiding vigorous suckling.
Dry colostrum or milk causing nipple to stick to bra or breast pads	• Moisten bra or pads before taking off so as not to remove keratin. • Ensure that nipples are dry before replacing bra or clothing against nipples.
Nipples not allowed to dry	• Remove plastic liners from milk pads. • Air dry breast completely after nursing. • Change nursing pads frequently. • Switch to cotton nursing pads.
Nipple skin not resistant to stress	• Improve diet; in particular, add fresh fruits and vegetables and vitamin supplements. • Eliminate or decrease use of sugary foods, alcohol, caffeine, cigarettes. • Check use of cleansing or drying agents.
Natural oils removed or keratin layers broken down by drying agents (soap, alcohol, shampoo, deodorant)	• Eliminate irritants. • Wash breasts with water only.

The baby's position at the breast is a critical factor in nipple soreness. The mother's hand should be off the areola, and the baby should be facing the mother's chest, with ear, shoulder, and hip aligned (see Figure 25–14). Because the area of greatest stress to the nipple is in line with the newborn's chin and nose, nipple soreness may be decreased by encouraging the mother to rotate positions when feeding the baby. Changing positions alters the focus of greatest stress and promotes more complete breast emptying.

Nipple soreness may also develop if the baby has faulty sucking habits. Nipples may have injured tips that are bruised, scabbed, or blistered from the nipple entering the baby's mouth at an upward angle and rubbing against the roof of the mouth or from poor latch-on (Newman & Pitman, 2015). Soreness may also result from continuous negative pressure if the baby falls asleep with the breast in the mouth.

Chewed nipples, which result from improper positioning, are cracked or tender at or near the base. In these cases, the baby's jaws close only on the nipple instead of on the areola, or the baby's mouth is not opened wide enough or has slipped down to the nipple from the areola as a result of engorgement. Soreness on the underside of the nipple is caused by the baby nursing with the bottom lip tucked in rather than out, causing a friction burn. In such cases, even vigorous sucking produces little milk because the milk sinuses under the areola are not compressed. This situation results in a frustrated baby and marked soreness for the mother. The problem is overcome by manipulating the baby's bottom lip with a fingertip before beginning the feeding, positioning the baby with as much areola as possible in the mouth, and rotating the baby's positions at the breast.

Nipple soreness is especially pronounced during the first few minutes of a feeding. If the mother is not expecting this discomfort, she may become discouraged and quickly stop. The let-down reflex may take a few minutes to activate, and it may not occur if the mother stops nursing too quickly. The baby is unsatisfied, and the possibility of breast engorgement increases.

Clinical Tip

If the mother continually has soreness because of a delay in let-down, encourage her to massage the breast in a circular pattern and apply warm compresses just before each breastfeeding session. These activities encourage let-down, increasing the chance that it will occur at the same time that the baby is placed on the breast.

Nipple soreness can also result from the vigorous feeding of an overeager baby. Thus the mother may find it helpful to nurse more frequently. Again, promoting let-down just before feeding may help. Other self-care measures include applying ice to the nipples and areola for a few minutes before feeding to promote nipple erectness and numb the tissue initially. To promote dryness, the mother may leave her bra flaps down for a few minutes after feeding (Figure 29–5) or expose her nipples to sunlight or ultraviolet light for 30 seconds at first, gradually increasing to 3 minutes. Drying the nipples with a hair dryer on a low heat setting also facilitates drying and promotes healing (Newman & Pitman, 2015). The use of petroleum-based products such as Vaseline, A+D ointment, cocoa butter, and baby oil to lubricate the nipples is discouraged because

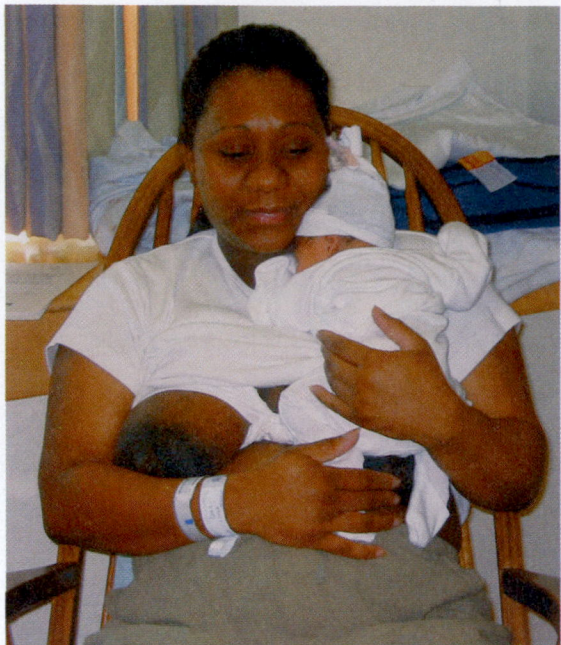

Figure 29–5 Mothers with sore nipples can leave bra flaps down after feedings to promote air drying and prevent chapping.

SOURCE: Michele Davidson.

the petroleum interferes with skin respiration and may prolong soreness. Because of the risk of allergic reactions, Massé cream (risk of peanut allergy) is discouraged. During bathing, mothers should be advised to only rinse their nipples with water and to avoid soap because this can dry the nipple out and lead to soreness.

Current research as to the effectiveness of nipple lubricants is inconclusive. Almost universally, lactation experts recommend that the mother's own milk should be applied to the nipples and allowed to air dry. Breast milk is high in fat, fights infection, and will not irritate the nipples. Moreover, it is readily available at no cost to the mother. For some women with very dry or severely sore nipples, hypoallergenic medical-grade anhydrous lanolin cream or aloe vera peppermint gel may help prevent or aid in healing cracked nipples (Saeidi, Tafazoli, Gholami, et al., 2015). This product poses a low risk of allergy because the alcohols that contribute to the allergic response have been removed.

If the woman finds that her bra or clothing rubs against her nipples and adds to her discomfort, she may insert shells into her bra. Medela shells relieve friction and promote air circulation. If a woman uses breast pads inside her bra to keep milk from leaking onto her clothes, she should change the pads frequently so the nipples remain dry. Some women may be sensitive to the plastic liner within the disposable pad. In such cases, the plastic can be removed or the women can be encouraged to try cotton pads.

If nipple soreness persists, the woman should be advised to consult a certified lactation consultant to determine the etiology of the soreness. Nipple dermatitis, which causes swollen, reddened, burning nipples, is most commonly caused by thrush or by allergic response to breast cream preparations. If the nipple soreness has a sudden onset and is accompanied by burning or itching, shooting pains through the breast, and a deep pink coloration of the nipple, it may be caused by a thrush infection transmitted from the baby to the mother. White patches or streaks in the baby's mouth indicate a need for treatment of the mouth and nipple infection. The infection can be treated

with a variety of antifungal preparations and does not preclude breastfeeding. It is important for both the mother and the baby to receive treatment to prevent cross-transferring of the fungus (*Candida albicans*).

Older remedies for nipple soreness are receiving renewed acceptance. For instance, tea bags may be moistened in warm water and applied to the nipples. The tannic acid seems to help toughen the nipples, and the warmth is soothing and promotes healing. Tannic acid also has anti-inflammatory properties that can help relieve discomfort. Other therapies have included warm compresses and heat applications.

CRACKED NIPPLES

When a breastfeeding mother complains of soreness, the nurse carefully examines the nipples for fissures or cracks and observes the mother during breastfeeding to see whether the baby is correctly positioned at the breast. If the positioning is correct and cracks exist, interventions are necessary. All the interventions described for sore nipples may be used. It may also help the mother to begin nursing on the breast that is less sore. This approach allows the let-down reflex to occur in the affected breast and permits the baby to do more vigorous sucking on the less tender breast, which decreases trauma to the cracked nipple. For the mother's comfort, analgesics may be taken approximately 1 hour before nursing.

BREAST ENGORGEMENT

A distinction exists between breast fullness and engorgement. All lactating women experience a transitional fullness at first, initially caused by venous congestion and later caused by accumulating milk. However, this fullness generally lasts only 24 hours, the breasts remain soft enough for the newborn to suckle, and there is no pain. Engorged breasts are hard, painful, and warm, and appear taut and shiny. The consistency is like gravel.

The newborn should suckle for an average of 15 minutes per feeding and should feed at least 8 to 12 times in 24 hours (Newman & Pitman, 2015). If the baby is unable to nurse more frequently, the mother may express some milk manually or with a pump, taking care to avoid traumatizing the breast tissue. As noted, warm compresses before nursing stimulate let-down and soften the breast so that the baby can grasp the areola more easily. Cool compresses after nursing can help slow refilling of the breasts and provide comfort to the mother. Ice packs may also be used as a comfort measure. The mother should wear a well-fitted nursing bra 24 hours a day to support the breasts and prevent discomfort from tension.

Clinical Reasoning Difficulties With Breastfeeding

Ann Nyembe calls you from home in tears on her third postpartum day. She states breastfeeding was going well in the hospital but now her breasts are swollen, hard, and very painful, and her baby is refusing to suckle. Ann expresses some disappointment that "the breastfeeding didn't work" because she truly believes that breastfeeding is best for babies, and she enjoyed her breastfeeding experience in the hospital, especially breastfeeding the baby immediately after birth. But she also states she has been crying all day and can no longer tolerate her painful breasts. In addition, she says the baby "seems happier" with the bottle.

What actions can the nurse recommend to Ann to increase the likelihood that she will continue breastfeeding and to decrease her discomfort?

PLUGGED DUCTS

Some mothers experience plugging of one or more ducts, especially in conjunction with or following engorgement. When breast milk pools within a duct and then dries, it forms a white, hardened plug that is typically visible at the outlet of the duct at the nipple surface. Because milk accumulates behind a plugged duct, women also experience an area of fullness, tenderness, and/or lumpiness in the associated region of the breast.

Self-care measures include the use of heat and massage. The nurse can encourage the mother to massage her breasts from her chest wall forward to the nipple while standing in a warm shower or following the application of moist heat to the breast. Warm compresses can be used and changed as temperature requires. The mother should then nurse her baby starting on the unaffected breast if the plugged breast is tender. Some lactation consultants advocate starting on the affected side because the more vigorous sucking may help dislodge the plug. A breast pump may also be effective in unplugging the duct.

Prevention of plugged ducts involves frequent nursing and the use of a variety of positions to ensure complete emptying. Some mothers discover that pressure from a shoulder strap on a purse, their baby sling, or a car seat belt causes recurring plugged ducts in the compressed area. Repositioning the device may help prevent plugged ducts in these women. Prevention and prompt correction are important because plugged ducts can lead to *mastitis* (inflammation of the breast). Mastitis is discussed in detail in Chapter 30.

EFFECT OF ALCOHOL AND MEDICATIONS

Mothers may ask the home care nurse about the use of alcohol and medications when breastfeeding. According to the American Academy of Pediatrics (2012), alcohol consumption should be limited to occasional use in breastfeeding mothers. Mothers who do occasionally drink while lactating should be advised to consume the alcohol after breastfeeding and limit intake to less than 0.5 mg/kg, in addition to refraining from nursing until at least 2 hours after alcohol use. Mothers with alcoholism who consume large quantities of alcohol daily may be advised not to breastfeed.

As discussed in Chapter 25, most medications pass into the breast milk. Women should consult their healthcare provider before taking over-the-counter medications, prescription medications, or herbal supplements.

Smoking is not an absolute contraindication to breastfeeding; however, women who smoke should be strongly encouraged to quit. If unable or not desiring to cease smoking, mothers should be advised not to smoke in the presence of the baby because of smoke inhalation, which has been associated with respiratory allergies in babies. Babies of smokers have a higher incidence of poor weight gain and SIDS (AAP, 2012). Although not specifically addressed in guidelines, women with substance abuse issues may be advised to formula-feed.

BREASTFEEDING AND THE WORKING MOTHER

The best preparation for maintaining lactation after returning to work is frequent, unlimited breastfeeding. Even when well planned, the first day back to work may be fraught with emotional and physical distress. Anticipatory guidance from the nurse may facilitate the transition from maternity leave to work. The earlier the breastfeeding mother returns to work, the more often she will need to pump her breasts to express the breast milk. Because milk production follows the principle of supply and demand, if breasts are not pumped, the milk supply will decrease.

Professionalism in Practice Workplace Issues Related to Breastfeeding

"As part of the Affordable Care Act enacted in 2010, the Fair Labor Standards Act was amended to require employers to provide reasonable break time and a private place for nursing mothers to express milk while at work" (USD-HHS, 2013). Many working mothers, particularly lower-income employees, may not be aware of their right to continue breastfeeding after they return to work. The professional nurse can advocate for clients by informing and encouraging them to discuss breastfeeding and the law with their employers.

Electric breast pumps and double collection systems are considered the optimal means of milk expression (see Figures 25–28 and 25–29). However, this is not the only method; mechanical means may not suit some women. Sometimes a mother has a flexible schedule and can return home or have the baby brought to her to nurse at lunch time. If this is not possible, the baby may be fed expressed milk via a bottle or spoon. (For proper storage of breast milk, see section Bottle-Feeding Breast Milk in Chapter 25.) The mother should wait until lactation is well established before introducing the bottle. Most babies adjust to the bottle within 7 to 10 days.

To maintain a milk supply, the working mother must pay special attention to her fluid intake. She can ensure adequate intake by drinking extra fluid at each break and when possible during the day. It is also helpful to nurse more on weekends, nurse during the night, eat a nutritionally sound diet, and continue manual expression or pumping when not nursing.

Night nursing presents a dilemma: It may help a working mother maintain her milk supply, but it may also contribute to fatigue. Some women choose to have the baby sleep nearby so that breastfeeding is more easily accomplished; other women find it difficult to sleep soundly when the baby is in proximity. For the mother who works long hours or has a rigid work schedule, the best alternative may be to limit breastfeeding to morning and evening feedings, with supplemental feedings at other times. This choice allows her to maintain a close relationship with the baby and provides some of the unique benefits of breast milk.

WEANING

The decision to wean the baby from the breast may be made for a variety of reasons, including family or cultural pressures, changes in the home situation, pressure from the woman's partner, or a personal opinion about when weaning should occur. Some babies wean themselves spontaneously, despite the wishes of the mother. For the woman who is comfortable with breastfeeding and well informed about the process, the appropriate time to wean her baby will become evident if she is sensitive to the child's cues. Often weaning falls between periods of great developmental activity for the child. Thus weaning commonly occurs at 8 to 9 months, 12 to 14 months, 18 months, 2 years, and 3 years of age. The baby who is weaned before 12 months should be given iron-fortified infant formula, not cow's milk. The World Health Organization (WHO) (2016) recommends 6 months of exclusive breastfeeding before any solids are introduced and breastfeeding for 2 years (WHO, 2016). The AAP (2012) recommends breastfeeding for at least 12 months or longer if the mother desires.

If weaning is timed to respond to the child's cues, and if the mother is comfortable with the timing, it can be accomplished with less difficulty than if the process begins before mother and child are ready emotionally. Nevertheless, weaning is a time of emotional separation for mother and baby; it may be difficult for them to give up the closeness of their nursing sessions. The nurse who shows understanding about this possibility can help the mother see that her infant is growing up and plan other comforting, consoling, and play activities to replace breastfeeding. A gradual approach is the easiest and most comforting way to wean the child from breastfeedings.

During weaning, the mother should substitute one cup feeding or bottle feeding for one breastfeeding session over a few days to a week so that her breasts gradually produce less milk. Eliminating the breastfeedings associated with meals first facilitates the mother's ability to wean the infant, because satiation with food lessens the desire for milk. Over a period of several weeks she can substitute more cup feedings or bottle feedings for breastfeedings. The slow method of weaning prevents breast engorgement, allows infants to alter their eating methods at their own rates, and provides time for psychologic adjustment.

Clinical Tip

Babies with special needs sometimes benefit from a longer duration of breastfeeding. Preterm babies also benefit from prolonged breastfeeding. Babies who are prone to allergies, gastrointestinal reflux, or impaired motility of the gastrointestinal tract may receive benefits from continued breastfeeding that the mother may be unaware of. These women should be counseled to discuss weaning with their healthcare provider or infant specialist before weaning because the benefits of breastfeeding may influence the woman's choice of timing regarding weaning.

Home Care: The Newborn

In the home, a newborn physical examination is performed as described in Chapter 24. The nurse also assesses and reinforces knowledge related to newborn/infant care as detailed in the following sections.

Handling and Positioning

The nurse demonstrates methods of handling and positioning the newborn as needed. As the family members provide care, the nurse can instill confidence by giving them positive feedback. If a family member encounters problems, the nurse can suggest alternatives and serve as a role model.

When holding the newborn, one of the following positions can be used (Figure 29–6). The *cradle hold* is frequently used during feeding. It provides a sense of warmth and closeness, permits eye contact, frees one of the adult's hands, and provides security because the cradling protects the newborn's body. Extra security is provided by gripping the baby's thigh with the hand while the arm supports the newborn's body. This grip is important to use when the baby is being carried. The *upright position* provides security and a sense of closeness and is ideal for burping the baby. One hand should support the neck and shoulders, while the other hand holds the buttocks or is placed between the newborn's legs. The newborn may also be held upright in a cloth sling carrier that gently holds the baby against the parent's chest and frees the hands for other tasks. The *football hold* frees one of the caregiver's hands and permits eye contact. This hold is ideal for shampooing, carrying, or breastfeeding. It frees the caregiver to talk on the telephone, answer the door, or do the myriad tasks that await attention at this busy time.

The baby's position should be changed periodically throughout the early months of life because skull bones are soft, and permanently flattened areas may develop if the baby consistently lies in one position. The awake newborn is frequently positioned on her or his side with the dependent arm forward to provide support and to prevent rolling. The side-lying position aids

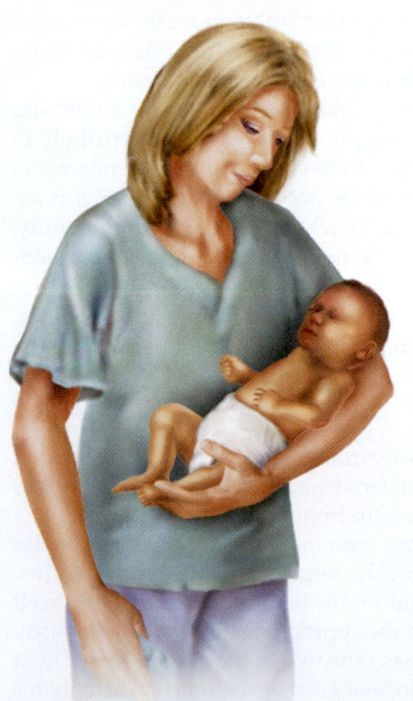
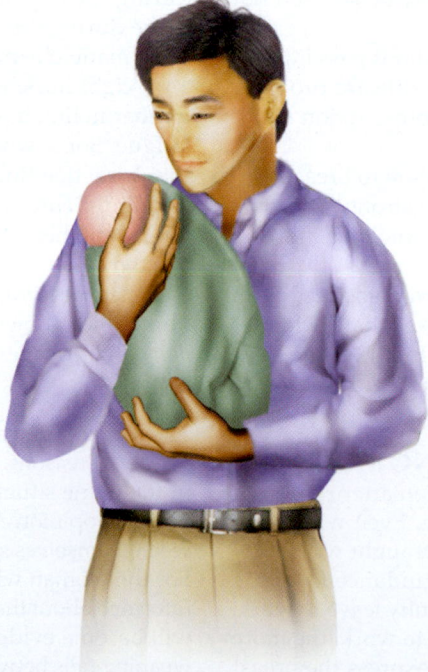
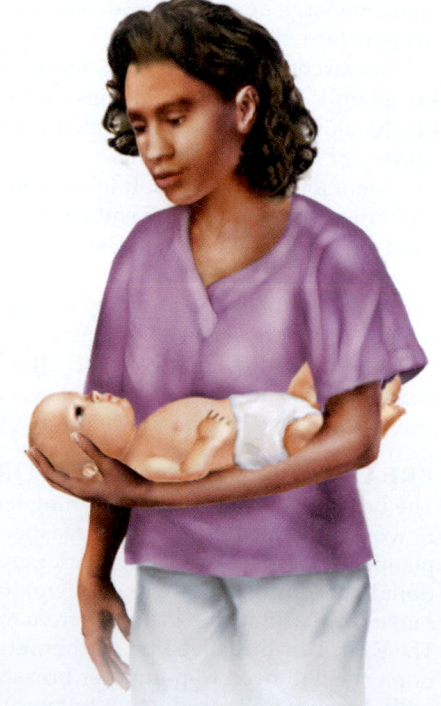

Figure 29–6 Various positions for holding a baby. A. Cradle hold. B. Upright position. C. Football hold.

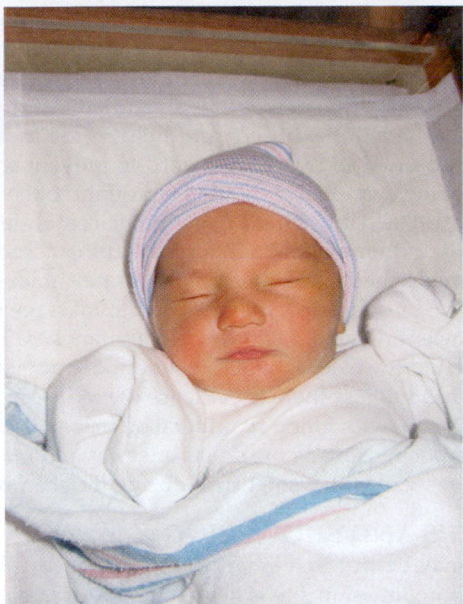

Figure 29–7 Babies should be placed on their backs when sleeping.

SOURCE: Michele Davidson.

drainage of mucus and allows air to circulate around the cord. It is also comfortable for the newly circumcised male. After feeding, the newborn may be placed on the right side to aid digestion and to prevent aspiration of regurgitated feedings; this position also makes it easier to expel air bubbles from the stomach.

Although the side-lying position is appropriate when the baby is awake and under observation, babies should always sleep on their backs (Figure 29–7). The American Academy of Pediatrics has recommended sleeping in nonprone positions since 1992 to reduce the risk of sudden infant death syndrome (SIDS). Since the initiation of the "Safe to Sleep" campaign, there has been an increase in malformation of the skull caused by a decrease in prone positioning. The syndrome is also known as *deformational plagiocephaly*, or positional plagiocephaly. These babies commonly have a flat spot on their skull, usually on the back or side, that is caused by continued placement in the same position. Babies who are not placed on their stomachs while awake at least three times daily are at risk for this skull malformation. If malformations do not resolve by 6 months of age, infants may need to wear a specially fitted helmet to correct the malformation.

Healthy People 2020

(MICH-20) Increase the proportion of infants who are put to sleep on their backs

---

Prone positioning while awake, also known as **tummy time**, is important for all babies because it assists them with learning developmentally appropriate skills; builds muscle strength for their shoulders, neck, and back; and prevents deformational plagiocephaly (National Institute of Child Health & Human Development, 2011). Babies should be placed on their tummies only when they are under the direct supervision of a parent or adult.

SAFETY ALERT!

Never leave a baby unattended on anything with height, such as a bed, sofa, or changing table, because of the risk of falls and subsequent injury. Encourage parents to leave the baby in a crib or on the floor if they are not within immediate sight of the baby.

Bathing

An actual bath demonstration is the best way for the nurse to provide information to parents. Because excess bathing and the use of soap remove natural skin oils and dry out the newborn's sensitive skin, bathing should be done every other day or twice a week. Sponge baths are recommended for the first 2 weeks or until the umbilical cord completely falls off and the umbilicus has healed.

At home, bath supplies can be kept in one convenient place. For the baby's tub, the family may want to use a plastic baby tub, a plastic dishpan, a clean kitchen or bathroom sink, or a large bowl. If using a sink, care should be taken to keep the baby away from faucets via which accidental burns could occur.

Before starting, if no one else is at home, the parent may want to take the phone off the hook and put a sign on the door to prevent being disturbed. Having someone assist the parent during the first few baths will be helpful, because that person can get forgotten items, attend to interruptions, and provide moral support. The room should be warm and free of drafts.

SPONGE BATHS

After the supplies are gathered, the tub (or any of the containers mentioned) is filled with water that is warm to the touch. Even though the newborn will not be placed in the tub, the bath giver carefully tests the water temperature with an elbow or forearm. Families may also choose to purchase a thermometer to help them determine when the bath water is at approximately 37.8°C (100°F) and safe to use. An unperfumed, mild soap such as Castile or Neutrogena should be used and kept on a soap dish or paper towel, not added to the water. Before the bath, the newborn should be wrapped in a blanket, with a T-shirt and diaper on, to keep the baby warm and secure.

To start the bath, the adult wraps a washcloth once around the index finger and wets it with water. *Soap is not used on the face.* Each eye is gently wiped from inner to outer corner. This direction prevents the potential for clogging the tear duct at the inner corner, where the eye naturally drains. A different portion of the washcloth is used for each eye to prevent cross contamination. Cotton balls can also be used for this purpose, a new one for each eye. Some swelling and drainage may be present the first few days after birth because of eye prophylaxis.

The bath giver washes the ears next by wrapping the washcloth once around an index finger and gently cleaning the external ear and behind the ear. Cotton swabs are never used in the ear canal because it is possible to put the swab too far into the ear and damage the ear drum. In addition, the swab may push any discharge farther down into the ear canal. The caregiver then wipes the remainder of the baby's face. Many babies start to cry at this point. The face should be washed every day and the mouth and chin wiped off after each feeding.

The neck is washed carefully but thoroughly with the washcloth. Soap may now be used. Formula or breast milk and lint collect in the skin folds of the neck, so it may be helpful to sit the newborn up, supporting the neck and shoulders with one hand while washing the neck with the other hand.

Next the bath giver unwraps the blanket, removes the T-shirt, and wets the chest, back, and arms with the washcloth. The bath giver may then lather the hands with soap and wash the baby's chest, back, and arms. The umbilical cord should be kept clean and dry. Wetting the cord is avoided, if possible, because it delays drying. The proximity of the umbilical vessels makes the cord a possible entry area for infection. See Chapter 25 for care of the umbilical cord and signs and symptoms of problems. Soap is rinsed off with the wet washcloth, and the upper part of the body is dried with a towel or blanket. The newborn's upper body is then wrapped with a clean, dry blanket to prevent a chill.

The bath giver then unwraps the newborn's legs, wets them with the washcloth, and lathers, rinses, and dries them well. If the newborn has dry skin, a small amount of unscented lotion or ointment (petroleum jelly or A+D ointment) may be used. Ointments are thought to be better than lotions for dry, cracked feet and hands. Baby oil is not recommended, because it clogs skin pores. Powders are not currently recommended. Families should be warned that baby powder can cause serious respiratory problems if inhaled. If parents want to use powder, they should be advised to use one that is talc free. The powder should be shaken into the hand and then placed on the newborn rather than shaken directly onto the baby.

The genital area is cleansed with soap and water daily and with water after each wet or dirty diaper. Girls are washed from the front of the genital area toward the anus to prevent fecal contamination of the urethra and thus the bladder. Newborn girls often have a thick, white mucous discharge or a slight bloody discharge from the vaginal area. This discharge is normal for the first 1 to 2 weeks after birth and should be wiped off with a damp cloth during diaper changes. The labia should be wiped, but the inner labial folds should not be aggressively cleaned.

Parents of uncircumcised boys should cleanse the penis daily. Even minimal retraction of the foreskin is not advised (see in-depth discussion of care of uncircumcised male babies in Chapter 25). Boys who have been circumcised also need daily gentle cleansing. Squeeze warm water over the baby's penis, letting the warm water run over the circumcision site. The area is rinsed off with warm water and lightly patted dry. A small amount of petroleum jelly, A+D ointment, or bactericidal ointment may be put on the circumcised area until the healing is complete, but excessive amounts may block the meatus and should be avoided. It is important to avoid using ointments if a Plastibell is in place because use of ointments may cause the Plastibell ring to slip off the penis too early. The Plastibell usually falls off within 5 to 8 days.

It is important to cleanse the diaper area with each diaper change to prevent diaper rash. Although this cleansing is done on a routine basis, a diaper rash may occasionally occur. Baby powder or cornstarch is not recommended for diaper rash. Baby powder may cake with urine and irritate the perineal area; cornstarch may promote fungal infection. Ointments that provide a barrier, such as zinc oxide, A+D ointment, and petroleum jelly, are more effective for diaper rash. If the ointment does not help the rash, families using single-use (disposable) diapers should try another brand. If they use cloth diapers, a different detergent or fabric softener, more thorough rinsing, and hanging them in the sun to dry may alleviate the problem. If the rash persists, parents should discuss the problem with their nurse practitioner or physician, because it may be caused by a fungal infection.

The last step in bathing is washing the hair (a step some suggest doing first). The newborn is swaddled in a dry blanket, leaving only the head exposed, and held in the football hold with the head tilted slightly downward to prevent water from running into the eyes. Water should be brought to the head by a cupped hand. The baby should never be placed under running water because extreme changes in temperature can lead to burns. The hair is moistened and lathered with a small amount of mild shampoo. A very soft brush may be used to massage the shampoo over the entire head, including the fontanelles. The hair is then rinsed and toweled dry. Oils or lotions are not used on the newborn's head unless there is evidence of cradle cap. Moistening the scaly area with lotion or mineral oil half an hour or more before shampooing softens the crusts or scales and makes it easier to remove them with a soft brush during the shampoo.

TUB BATHS AND SHOWERING

The baby may be put in a small tub after the cord has fallen off and the circumcision site is healed (approximately 2 weeks) (Figure 29–8). Newborns usually enjoy a tub bath more than a sponge bath, although some cry during either type. Only 3 or 4 inches of water is needed in the tub. To prevent slipping, a washcloth can be placed in the bottom of the tub or sink. Some parents choose to bring the newborn into the tub with them.

The baby's face is washed in the same manner as for a sponge bath. The parent then places the newborn in the tub using the cradle hold and grasping the distal thigh. The neck is supported by the parent's elbow in the cradle position. An alternative hold is to support the newborn's head and neck with the forearm while grasping the distal shoulder and arm.

Because wet newborns are slippery, some parents pull a cotton sock (with holes cut out for the fingers) over the supporting arm to provide a "nonskid" surface. The newborn's body may be washed with a soapy washcloth or hand. To wash the back, the bath giver places his or her noncradling hand on the newborn's chest with the thumb under the newborn's arm closest to the adult. Gently tipping the newborn forward onto the

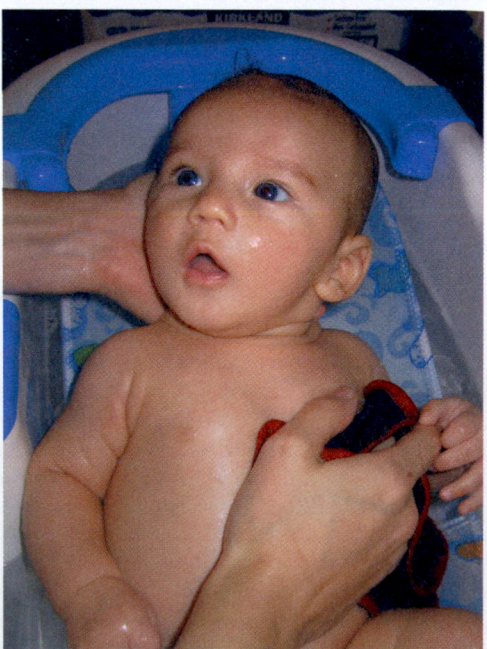

Figure 29–8 When bathing the newborn, the caregiver must support the head. Wet babies are very slippery.

supporting hand frees the cradling arm to wash the back. After the bath, the newborn is lifted out of the tub in the cradle position, dried well, and wrapped in a dry blanket. The hair is then washed in the same way as for a sponge bath.

Some parents prefer to shower their babies during the time of their shower. Parents should be cautioned that babies may become very slippery and are easily dropped so showering should be done with great care. Some parents may wish to place the infant tub on the floor of the shower to ensure adequate safety during a shower.

Nail Care

The nails of the newborn are seldom cut in the birthing center. During the first days of life, the nails may adhere to the skin of the fingers, and cutting is contraindicated. Within a week the nails separate from the skin and frequently break off. If the nails are long or if the newborn is scratching his or her face, the nails may be trimmed. Trimming is most easily done while the baby is asleep. Nails should be cut straight across using adult cuticle scissors or blunt-ended infant cuticle scissors; they may also be filed.

Dressing the Newborn

Newborns need to wear a T-shirt, diaper (and diaper cover or plastic pants if using cloth diapers), and a sleeper. On a fairly cool day, they should be wrapped in a light blanket while being fed. Newborns should be covered with a blanket in air-conditioned buildings. The blanket should be unwrapped or removed when inside a warm building. At home, the amount of clothing the newborn wears is determined by the temperature. Families who maintain their home at 15.5° to 18.3°C (60° to 65°F) should dress the baby more warmly than those who maintain a temperature of 21.1° to 23.9°C (70° to 75°F).

Newborns should wear head coverings outdoors to protect their sensitive ears from drafts. A blanket can be wrapped around the baby, leaving one corner free to place over the head while outdoors or in crowds for added protection. The nurse must advise families about the ease with which a newborn's skin can burn when exposed to the sun. To prevent sunburn, the newborn should remain shaded, wear a light layer of clothing, or be protected with sunscreen specifically formulated for babies.

Diaper shapes vary and are subject to personal preference (Figure 29–9). Prefolded and disposable diapers are usually rectangular. Cloth diapers may also be triangular or kite folded.

Extra material is placed in front for boys and toward the back for girls to increase absorbency. Cloth diapers, some of which now use Velcro and highly absorbent materials, have been used more frequently in recent years because of the environmental concerns related to disposable diapers.

Baby clothing should be laundered separately with a mild soap or detergent. Cloth diapers may be presoaked before washing. All clothing should be rinsed twice to remove soap and residue and to decrease the possibility of rash. Some newborns may not tolerate clothing treated with fabric softeners added to the washer or dryer.

Temperature Assessment

As the nurse prepares to teach parents about taking their baby's temperature, it is important to provide opportunities for discussion and demonstration. Families often need a review of how to take the baby's temperature and when to call their primary healthcare provider.

The nurse discusses the different types of thermometers available for home use. It is important that parents understand the differences and how to select the appropriate one. Tympanic membrane (ear) thermometers use infrared temperature scanning techniques to determine the baby's temperature. Infrared forehead thermometers are also available, but these devices may be less accurate than internal monitoring techniques. Other parents elect to use a digital thermometer. The nurse reviews the correct procedure for using the chosen thermometer. The same digital thermometers should not be used for both oral and rectal temperature taking. Parents should label the thermometer and use it for only one route.

Clinical Tip

Healthcare facilities no longer use glass thermometers because of the risks associated with resulting mercury spillage should one break. Parents should be advised not to use mercury thermometers and should be encouraged to discard them at a hazardous materials site specific to mercury thermometers. Before teaching families about temperature taking, you might find it helpful to visit a local pharmacy and review the types of thermometers available, the costs of the most commonly used methods, and the instructions provided. This will enable you to answer questions accurately when you work with parents or caregivers.

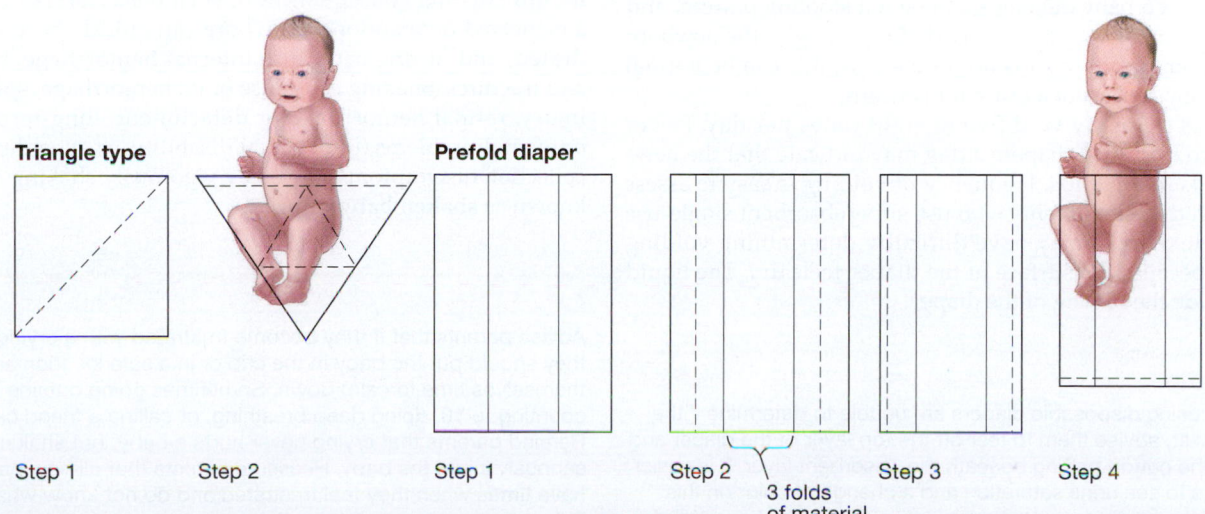

Triangle type		Prefold diaper			
Step 1	Step 2	Step 1	Step 2	Step 3	Step 4

3 folds of material

Figure 29–9 Two basic cloth diaper shapes. Dotted lines indicate folds.

Parents need to take the newborn's temperature only when the signs of illness are present. They should call their healthcare provider immediately if the temperature exceeds 38.4°C (101.0°F) rectally or 38.0°C (100.4°F) axillary. In premature newborns, a low temperature may be a sign of infection; therefore, if the temperature is below 36.1°C (97.0°F) rectally or 36.6°C (97.8°F) axillary, the healthcare provider should be notified.

Parents should discuss management of flu, colds, teething, constipation, diarrhea, gas discomfort, and other common ailments with their clinician before they occur. When analgesic or antipyretic medication is needed, clinicians frequently recommend acetaminophen or ibuprofen drops. Parents should not give any form of aspirin for an illness unless specifically directed to do so by their healthcare provider; use of aspirin in viral illnesses has been linked to Reye syndrome in children.

Stools and Urine

The appearance and frequency of a newborn's stools can cause concern for parents. The nurse prepares them by discussing and showing pictures of meconium stools and transitional stools and by describing the difference between breast milk and formula stools. Although babies develop their own stooling patterns, parents can expect the following (see Figure 25–24).

- Breastfed newborns may have 6 to 10 small, semiliquid, yellow stools per day by the third or fourth day, when milk production is established, unless the mother is having problems with her milk supply. Once breastfeeding is well established, usually by 1 month, the newborn may have only one stool every few days because of the increased digestibility of breast milk. However, they may still have several daily. Constipation is unlikely to occur in newborns receiving only breast milk. Infrequent stooling in the first few weeks may indicate inadequate milk intake.

- Formula-fed babies may have only one or two stools a day; they are more formed and yellow or yellow-brown.

The parents may also be shown pictures of a constipated stool (small, pellet-like) and diarrhea (loose, green, or perhaps blood tinged). Families should understand that a green color is common in transitional stools, so that transitional stools are not confused with diarrhea during the first week of a newborn's life. Constipation may indicate that the newborn needs additional fluid intake. Parents may try offering additional water in an attempt to reverse the constipation. Parents should be counseled that each baby develops a personal stooling pattern, and some babies may not pass a stool daily. As long as the newborn appears comfortable and is not in distress, this can be normal for that baby and is not a cause for concern.

Babies normally void five to eight times per day. Fewer than six to eight wet diapers a day may indicate that the newborn needs more fluids. Frequency of voiding is easy to assess with cloth diapers. Parents who use superabsorbent single-use disposable diapers may have difficulty determining voiding patterns because the surface of the diaper feels dry. The liquid pools inside the batting of the diaper.

Clinical Tip

If parents using disposable diapers are unable to determine if the diaper is wet, advise them to tear off the top layer of the diaper and examine the cotton batting beneath the absorbent layer. It is easier for parents to see urine saturation and a change of color on this portion of the diaper in order to determine if the baby has voided.

Sleep and Activity

The newborn demonstrates several different sleep–wake states after the initial periods of reactivity described in Chapter 23. Six newborn sleep–wake states have been identified (Table 29–4). It is not uncommon for a newborn to sleep almost continuously for the first 2 to 3 days following birth, awakening only for feedings every few hours. Indeed, it is not uncommon to have difficulty feeding the baby during the first 24 to 48 hours because of this deep sleep. Some newborns bypass this stage and require only 12 to 16 hours of sleep. The parents need to know that this pattern is normal.

Babies typically do not sleep through the night until they are at least 3 months of age or weigh 12 to 13 lb (5443 to 5897 g). Some babies sleep through the night as early as 8 weeks, whereas others do not sleep through the night until 6 months of age or beyond. It is estimated that two thirds of infants sleep through the night by the age of 6 months. Although newborns typically sleep up to 16 hours per day, they do so in short time intervals. Some parents may be tempted to try home remedies, such as giving babies cereal in their bottles or other additives that are said to assist their children in sleeping through the night. Parents should be counseled that these remedies are not recommended.

Crying

For the newborn, crying is the only means of expressing needs vocally. Families learn to distinguish different tones and qualities of the newborn's cry. The amount of crying is highly individual. Some cry as little as 15 to 30 minutes in 24 hours, and others cry as long as 2 hours every 24 hours. When crying continues after causes such as discomfort and hunger are eliminated, the newborn may be comforted by swaddling or by rocking and other reassuring activities. There is some indication that newborns who are held more tend to be calmer and cry less when not being held. Some parents are afraid that holding may "spoil" the newborn and need reassurance that this is not the case. Picking babies up when they cry teaches them that adults are responsive to them. This helps build a sense of trust in humankind. Excessive crying should be noted and assessed, taking other factors into consideration. After the first 2 or 3 days, newborns settle into individual patterns.

Coping with prolonged crying may be a challenge for new parents, who may respond by withdrawing their affection from the newborn, providing routine care and feeding, but not becoming emotionally attached. Other parents may respond by neglecting, abandoning, or even hitting or shaking their newborn. Parents need to understand the serious, even life-threatening consequences of such behavior. For example, a neglected or abandoned newborn can quickly become dehydrated, and hitting can cause internal hemorrhage, bruising, and fractures. Shaking can cause brain hemorrhage, spinal cord injury, retinal hemorrhage or detachment, long-term developmental problems, intellectual disability, or even death. This collection of symptoms caused by vigorously shaking a baby is known as **shaken baby injuries**.

Clinical Tip

Advise parents that if they become frustrated with a crying baby, they should put the baby in the crib or in a safe location and allow themselves time to calm down. Sometimes going outside the door, counting to 10, doing deep breathing, or calling a friend can help. Remind parents that crying never hurts a baby, but shaking can seriously injure the baby. Reassure parents that all new parents have times when they feel frustrated and do not know what to do. This is a normal part of parenting a newborn.

To increase parents' coping abilities, suggest that they initially respond to the baby's crying by checking for hunger, a wet or soiled diaper, excessive cold or heat, restrictive or chafing clothing or blankets, or other comfort concerns. If these are not present, suggest holding or rocking the baby as previously discussed. Other calming measures include burping the baby (which provides repetitive tactile stimulation and disperses air bubbles), placing the baby in a mechanized infant swing, or taking the baby for a ride in a stroller or car. Some babies are soothed by white noise such as the sound of a clothes dryer or the static on an untuned radio, whereas others are soothed when bound "papoose style" on the mother's or father's chest, swaddled, bathed, or massaged.

Crying can also be associated with gastrointestinal upset in babies. The parents should discuss concerns with the physician or nurse practitioner to ensure the crying is not associated with a physical cause, such as acid reflux, ear infections, or other physical conditions. In addition, it is not uncommon for babies to cry after feedings because of pain from a buildup of air bubbles in the stomach and an inability to pass flatus. Some practitioners recommend simethicone after each feeding to decrease the incidence of flatus pain. Placing the baby in a prone position across the lap while burping the baby can also aid in passing flatus.

Safety Considerations

Newborns should not have pillows, blankets, or stuffed animals in the crib while they sleep; these items could cause suffocation. Mattresses should fit snugly in a crib to prevent entrapment and suffocation, and the crib should be inspected regularly to determine whether it is in safe working order. Crib slats should be no more than 2⅜ in. apart. Parents can be encouraged to attend infant cardiopulmonary resuscitation (CPR) classes, especially if there is a family history of sudden infant death syndrome (SIDS) or the baby requires special care.

Many families, especially breastfeeding families, practice **cosleeping**, in which the baby sleeps with the mother or both parents during the night. The American Academy of Pediatrics does not recommend cosleeping because it is considered a risk factor for SIDS (Blair, 2015). Some families and cultures, however, may still participate in this practice and thus warrant appropriate teaching measures.

Cosleeping families should be counseled to follow these safety guidelines:

- Place the baby on a firm mattress, never on comforters, pillows, or a waterbed.
- Never sleep with your baby if you have been using drugs or have become intoxicated.
- Ensure that the baby is protected from rolling off the bed or becoming entrapped in bed rails or a space between the frame and the mattress.
- As with crib sleeping, remove all decorative pillows, stuffed animals, toys, or blankets that could impair the baby's breathing. Do not cover the baby with blankets, sheets, or down comforters.
- Make sure the baby is sleeping on his or her back.
- Ensure plenty of ventilation to the baby.
- Avoid overdressing the baby because the parent's body heat will reduce the need for excess clothing.
- Never smoke in bed with the baby. Family members should smoke outdoors and not in the household with the baby.
- If additional children are sleeping in the bed, make sure they are not sleeping directly next to the baby.

The American Academy of Pediatrics recommends that the safest place for the baby to sleep is in the parents' room with the baby in a crib in proximity to the parents for the first 6 months of life. The use of pacifiers has also been associated with a reduction in SIDS deaths (Blair, 2015).

Smoking in the home poses multiple risks to the newborn and any older children. Infants living in a household with a smoker have a higher rate of hospital admissions during the first year of life. They are more prone to ear infections, asthma, allergies, and other respiratory problems. Smoking also creates a fire hazard within the household. Smoking is the primary cause of household fires in the United States. The incidence of such fires increases dramatically when other intoxicating agents are ingested, such as alcohol or drugs. Parents should be counseled to smoke outdoors; use large, heavy ashtrays to avoid tipping; ensure that all cigarette butts are properly extinguished; and never smoke in bed.

Healthy People 2020

(MICH-18) Reduce postpartum relapse of smoking among women who quit smoking during pregnancy

---

Postpartum Classes and Support Groups

These services range from educational, such as classes on nutrition, exercise, newborn/infant care, and parenting, to specific healthcare programs, such as well-baby checks, immunization clinics, family-planning services, new mother support groups, and more.

Postpartum classes are becoming more common as caregivers recognize the continuing needs of the childbearing family. In many instances, classes are prepared to meet the specific needs of a variety of families so that, for example, single mothers and adolescent mothers can attend class with peers. A series of structured classes may focus on topics such as parenting, postpartum exercise, or nutrition, or loosely structured group sessions may address mothers' concerns as they arise. Such classes offer chances for the new mother to socialize, share her concerns, and receive encouragement. Because baby-sitting arrangements may be difficult or expensive, it is desirable to provide child care for newborns and siblings; in some instances babies may remain with mothers in the class.

Many communities offer support groups through birthing centers, hospitals, or other facilities. La Leche League, an excellent support group for breastfeeding mothers, typically meets monthly and is open to all pregnant and breastfeeding mothers of newborns, infants, and toddlers. Women who have children with special needs may need additional support. Referring them to peer counselors or support groups is an effective way to help them find both support and information. Once again, such groups provide an opportunity for parents to share information, advice, and experiences.

Many parents today look to the Internet for information on parenting and newborn care. Nurses have an opportunity to assist parents in evaluating the reliability of the information they find. Criteria that suggest that Internet information is reliable and of high quality include affiliation with a university medical or nursing school or a government agency; inclusion of authors' credentials, education, board certification, and affiliations; referencing of information; currency of information; similarity of information when compared with other sources; and easy accessibility.

TABLE 29–4 Newborn Sleep and Awake States*

NEWBORN STATES	PHYSICAL CHARACTERISTICS	BODY ACTIVITY	EYE MOVEMENTS
Sleep States			
Deep or quiet sleep	Anabolic, restorative sleep, increased cell mitosis and replication, lowered oxygen consumption, release of growth hormone.	Typically still, may occasionally startle or twitch.	None.
Active or light sleep (also known as rapid eye movement [REM] state)	Processing and recording information. Often linked to learning. Is the highest proportion of sleep and precedes awakening.	Some body movements.	REM, eyelids flutter beneath closed eyelids.
Awake States			
Drowsy or semidozing	May return to sleep or awaken further.	Smooth movements with variable activity level. May experience mild startles intermittently.	Eyes may open and close. May appear heavy-lidded, or eyes may appear like slits.
Quiet alert	Attentive to environment, focuses attention on stimuli.	Minimal.	Eyes bright and wide.
Active alert	Baby's eyes are open, not as bright as in quiet alert. More body activity than in a quiet alert state.	Smooth movements may be interspersed with mild startles from time to time.	Eyes open with a glazed, dull appearance.
Crying	Communication tool, response to unpleasant stimuli from environment or internal stimuli. Characterized by intense crying for more than 15 seconds.	Increased motor activity, skin color changes to darkened appearance, red, or ruddy.	Eyes may be tightly closed or open.

FACIAL MOVEMENTS	BREATHING PATTERN	RESPONSES	CAREGIVER IMPLICATIONS
None or may have occasional sucking movements.	Slow and regular.	Only intense or disturbing stimuli will arouse baby; threshold to stimuli is high.	Difficult to arouse for feedings. Teach parents to time feedings when baby is in a more responsive state.

Baby may arouse slightly if an attempt is made to awaken but typically returns to the quiet sleep state. |
| May smile or make fussing or crying noises. | Irregular. | More responsive to internal stimuli (hunger) and external stimuli (such as being picked up by caregiver).

When stimulated may arouse, return to quiet sleep, or remain in active sleep. | Inexperienced care providers may attempt to feed when baby makes normal crying sounds. |
| May have no facial movements and appear still, or may have some facial movements. | Irregular. | Usually reacts to stimuli but may be slowed. May change to other states such as quiet alert, active alert, or crying. | To stimulate baby, provide verbal, sight, or oral stimulation. If left alone, baby may return to a sleep state. |
| Attentive appearance. | Regular. | Most attentive, focuses attention on stimuli. | In the first hours after birth, may experience intense alertness before going into a long sleeping period. This state increases in intensity as the baby becomes older.

Providing stimuli will help maintain an active alert state or a drowsy awake or quiet alert state. Baby provides pleasure and positive feedback to care providers. Good time to feed baby. |
| May be still with or without facial movements. | Irregular. | Reacts to stimuli with delayed responses to stimuli, or may change to quiet alert or crying state. | Baby may be fussy and become sensitive to stimuli, may become more and more active and start crying. If fatigue or caregiver interventions disturb this state, baby may return to a drowsy awake or sleep state. |
| Grimaces. | More irregular than in other states. | Very responsive to internal or external unpleasant stimuli. | Indicates that the baby's limits have been reached. May be able to console self and return to an alert or sleep state, or may need intervention from caregiver. |

*A *state* is a group of characteristic behaviors and physiologic changes that occur together in a regular pattern.

Source: Healthy Children, (2013). Ages & stages. Retrieved from http://www.healthychildren.org/English/ages-stages/baby/Pages/States-of-Consciousness-in-Newborns.aspx

Focus Your Study

- Nursing diagnoses can be used effectively in caring for women during the postpartum period.

- Postpartum discomfort may be caused by a variety of factors, including engorged breasts, an edematous perineum, an episiotomy or laceration, engorged hemorrhoids, or hematoma formation. Various self-care approaches are helpful in promoting comfort.

- Lactation suppression may be accomplished by mechanical techniques.

- The new mother requires opportunities to discuss her childbirth experience with an empathetic listener.

- Mother–baby care provides the childbearing family with opportunities to interact with their new member during the first hours and days of life. It enables the family to develop some confidence and skill in a safe environment.

- Sexual intercourse may resume once the episiotomy/laceration has healed and lochia has ceased.

- After a cesarean birth, the woman has the nursing care needs of an abdominal surgical patient in addition to her needs as a postpartum mother. She may also require assistance in working through her feelings if the cesarean birth was unexpected.

- The nurse evaluates the postpartum adolescent mother in terms of her level of maturity, available support systems, cultural background, and existing knowledge and then plans care accordingly.

- The mother who decides to relinquish her baby needs emotional support. She should be able to decide whether to see and hold her baby, and any special requests regarding the birth should be honored.

- The woman who is obese has needs similar to those of all postpartum women, but she needs special attention to prevent injury, respiratory complications, thromboembolic disease, and infection, for which she is at high risk.

- Providing quality client-centered care for the lesbian mother involves acknowledging and welcoming her intimate partner, and involving her in care and decision making, as well as individualizing standard postpartum instructions, particularly those related to intercourse and contraception.

- Teaching should be conducted at a level that is achievable for the postpartum woman who has a developmental disability; a needs assessment should be performed.

- The postpartum woman who has a history of sexual abuse may have needs that can be addressed by the nurse by providing modesty draping, speaking to the woman in private, and offering information about support groups.

- Before discharge the couple should be given any information necessary for the woman to provide appropriate self-care. Parents should have a beginning skill in caring for their newborn and should be familiar with warning signs of possible complications for mother or baby. Printed information is valuable in helping couples deal with questions that may arise at home.

- Because of the trend toward early discharge, follow-up care is more important than ever. Many approaches are used, especially home visits and telephone follow-up.

- The Newborns' and Mothers' Health Protection Act provides for a guaranteed minimum stay of up to 48 hours following an uncomplicated vaginal birth and 96 hours following an uncomplicated cesarean birth. For women discharged earlier than the mandated time, more than half of all U.S. states require coverage for home care follow-up.

- The overall goal of postpartum home visits is to enhance opportunities for smooth transition of the new family. The home visit provides opportunities for assessment, teaching, and fostering a caring relationship with new families.

- Nurses need to act proactively to maintain their safety when making home visits by exercising reasonable caution and remaining alert to environmental cues.

- The primary focus of the maternal assessment includes a physical and psychologic assessment and identification of teaching needs for the new mother.

- To prevent nipple soreness, cracked nipples, engorgement, and plugged ducts, the nurse can encourage the breastfeeding mother to nurse frequently, to change the baby's position regularly, and to allow her nipples to air dry after breastfeeding.

- Teaching goals during home visits include reinforcement of daily newborn care, discussion of temperature assessment and maintenance of a neutral thermal environment, promotion of adequate hydration and nutrition, prevention of complications, promotion of safe and appropriate newborn sleeping, encouragement of newborn screenings and immunizations, and enhancement of family attachment and confidence in newborn care.

- Parents should be instructed on proper bathing techniques for newborns and safety issues directly related to bathing practices should be addressed.

- The healthcare provider should be notified if there is evidence of redness around the umbilicus, bright-red bleeding, or pus-like drainage near the cord stump, or if the umbilicus remains unhealed.

- Primary risk factors for sudden infant death syndrome (SIDS) are sleeping in the prone position and smoking within the household. Cosleeping is also a risk factor for SIDS.

- Return visits, telephone follow-up, classes, and support groups can provide valuable information and support to new mothers and their families.

Clinical Reasoning In Action

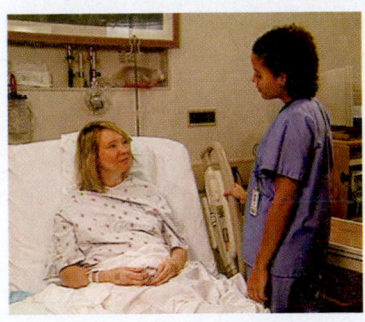

Wendy Callahan, a 31-year-old G3P2, gave birth to an 8.5-pound baby boy by primary cesarean birth for failure to progress. The baby's Apgar scores were 9 and 9 at 1 and 5 minutes. The baby was admitted to the newborn nursery for transitional observation. Wendy was transferred to the postpartum unit, where you assume her care. You introduce yourself and orient her to the room, call bell, and safely measures. You perform an initial assessment, with all findings within normal limits. Wendy tells you she is very tired and would like to rest while her baby is in the nursery. Her husband and family have left the hospital after spending time with her in the recovery room but will return later. She admits she is disappointed that she could not give birth vaginally even though she pushed for 2 hours. She says. "This baby was just too big."

1. How would you discuss with Wendy the need for frequent assessments after birth?

2. Explain "maternity blues" or "baby blues."

3. Explore activities to minimize maternity blues.

4. Discuss concerns of a woman experiencing her second pregnancy.

5. Discuss behaviors that inhibit paternal attachment.

References

American Academy of Pediatrics. (AAP). (2012). Breast-feeding and the use of human milk. AAP Policy Statement. Washington, DC: AAP.

American Academy of Pediatrics (AAP) Committee on Fetus and Newborn. (2011). SIDS and other sleep-related infant deaths: Expansion of recommendations for a safe infant sleeping environment. *Pediatrics, 128*, 1341–1347. doi:10.1542/peds.2011-2285

American Academy of Pediatrics (AAP) Committee on Fetus and Newborn. (2014). Hospital stay for healthy term newborns. Washington, DC: Author.

American Adoptions. (2016). *Adoption statistics.* Retrieved from https://www.americanadoptions.com/pregnant/adoption_stats

American College of Obstetricians and Gynecologists (ACOG). (2015a). Exercise after pregnancy. Patient Education FAQ 131. Washington, DC: Author.

American College of Obstetricians and Gynecologists. (2015b). Obstetric analgesia and anesthesia. ACOG Practice Bulletin No. 36. Washington, DC: Author.

Australian Breastfeeding Association. (2016). *Lactation suppression.* Retrieved from https://www.breastfeeding.asn.au/bfinfo/lactation-suppression

Barfield, W. D., & Lee, K. G. (2015). *Late-preterm infants.* UpToDate. Retrieved from http://www.uptodate.com/contents/late-preterm-infants

Berens, P. (2016). *Overview of postpartum care.* UpToDate. Retrieved from http://www.uptodate.com/contents/overview-of-postpartum-care

Blair, P. S. (2015). Co-sleeping and suffocation. *Forensic Science, Medicine, and Pathology, 11*(2), 1–2.

Brincat, C., Crosby, E., McLeod, A., & Fenner, D. E. (2015). Experiences during the first four years of a postpartum perineal clinic in the USA. *International Journal of Gynecology & Obstetrics, 128*(1), 68–71.

Brockman, V. (2015). Implementing the mother-baby model of nursing care using models and quality improvement tools. *Nursing for Women's Health, 19*: 490–503. doi:10.1111/1751-486X.12245

Centers for Disease Control & Prevention. (CDC). (2016). *Preventing repeat teen births.* Retrieved from http://www.cdc.gov/vitalsigns/teenpregnancy/

Cherry, A., & Dillon, M. (2014). *International handbook of adolescent pregnancy: Medical, psychosocial, and public health responses.* New York, NY: Springer.

Child Welfare Information Gateway. (2016). *Grounds for involuntary termination of parental rights.* Retrieved from http://www.childwelfare.gov/systemwide/laws_policies/statutes/groundtermin.cfm

Davidson, M. R. (2013). *Fast facts for the antepartum and postpartum nurse.* New York, NY: Springer.

Food & Drug Administration. (2015). *Non-aspirin nonsteroidal anti-inflammatory drugs (NSAIDs): Drug safety communication—FDA strengthens warning of increased chance of heart attack or stroke.* Retrieved from http://www.fda.gov/Safety/MedWatch/SafetyInformation/SafetyAlertsforHumanMedicalProduct

Frederick, A. C., Busen, N. H., Engebretson, J. C., Hurst, N. M., & Schneider, K. M. (2015). Exploring the skin-to-skin contact experience during cesarean section. *Journal of the American Association of Nurse Practitioners, 28*(1), 33–38. doi:10.1002/2327-6924.12229

Fu, D. Y., Jiang, J. N., Wang, B. C., & Guo, W. J. (2015). The impact of collaborative care on intraoperative stress in patients undergoing cesarean. *Journal of the Bonoi Academy of Science & Education.* Retrieved from http://www.bonoi.org/sites/default/files/files/Article-30Oct2015.pdf

Gabbe, S. G., Niebyl, J. R., Simpson, J. L., Landon, M. B., Galan, H. L., Jauniaux, E. R. M., ...Grobman, W. A. (2016). *Obstetrics: Normal & problem pregnancies* (7th ed.). Philadelphia, PA: Elsevier.

Hollway, W. H. (2015). *Knowing mothers: Researching maternal identity change.* London, UK: Palgrave Macmillan.

Jewish Women's Health. (2016). *Childbirth in Jewish Law.* Retrieved from http://www.jewishwomenshealth.org/article.php?article=20

Kakade, S. V. (2015). Effectiveness of infrared lamp therapy on healing of episiotomy wound among postnatal mothers. *Health Science Journal.* Retrieved from http://www.hsj.gr/medicine/effectiveness-of-infrared-lamp-therapy-on-healing-of-episiotomy-wound-among-post-natal-mothers.pdf

Khajehei, M., Doherty, M., Tilley, P. J. M., & Sauer, K. (2015). Prevalence and risk factors of sexual dysfunction in postpartum Australian women. *Journal of Sexual Medicine, 12*, 1415–1426. doi:10.1111/jsm.12901

Khosravan, S., Mohammadzadeh-Moghadam, H., Mohammadzadeh, F., Fadafen, S. A. K., &

Gholami, M. (2015). The effect of hollyhock (Althaea officinalis L) leaf compresses combined with warm and cold compress on breast engorgement in lactating women: A randomized clinical trial. *Journal of Evidence-Based Complementary & Alternative Medicine*, published online before print November 23, 2015. doi:10.1177/2156587215617106

King, T. L., Brucker, M. C., Kriebs, J. M., & Fahey, J. O. (2013). *Varney's midwifery* (5th ed.). Burlington, MA; Jones & Bartlett Learning.

Lowe, N. K. (2012). The persistent problem of postpartum hemorrhage. *Journal of Obstetric, Gynecologic, & Neonatal Nursing, 41*(4), 459–460. doi:10.1111/j.1552-6909.2012.01397.x

McFarland, M. R., & Wehbe-Alamah, H. B. (2014). *Leininger's culture care diversity and universality: A worldwide nursing theory* (3rd ed.). Oxford, UK: Jones & Bartlett.

Marzouk, T., Barakat, R., Ragab, A, Badria, F., & Badawy, A. (2015). Lavender-thymol as a new topical aromatherapy preparation for episiotomy: A randomised clinical trial. *Journal of Obstetrics and Gynaecology, 3*(5), 472–475. doi:10.3109/0144361 5.2014.970522

National Campaign to Prevent Teen and Unplanned Pregnancy. (2016). *2016 survey data.* Retrieved from http://thenationalcampaign.org/resource/survey-says-april-2016

National Institute of Child Health & Human Development. (2011). *Back to sleep public education campaign.* Retrieved from http://www.nichd.nih.gov/sids

Newman, J., & Pitman, T. (2015). *Dr. Jack Newman's guide to breastfeeding.* London, UK: Pinton & Martin Ltd.

Saeidi, R., Tafazoli, M., Gholami, M., & Mazloom, R. (2015). New treatment for nipple soreness in breast-feeding mothers: A clinical trial study. *Iranian Journal of Neonatology IJN, 6*(2), 48–51.

Santos, A., Epstein, J., & Chaudhuri, K. (2015). *Obstetric anesthesia.* New York, NY: McGraw-Hill.

Sim, T. F., Hattingh, H. L., Sheriff, J. & Tee, L. B. G. (2015). The use, perceived effectiveness and safety of herbal galactagogues during breastfeeding: A qualitative study. *International Journal of Environmental Research & Public Health, 12*(9): 11050–11071. doi:10.3390/ijerph120911050

Smith, J.R. (2014). Postpartum hemorrhage. Medscape. Retrieved from http://emedicine.medscape.com/article/275038-overview

Spidsberg, B. D., & Sørlie, V. (2012). An expression of love—midwives' experiences in the encounter with lesbian women and their partners. *Journal of Advanced Nursing, 68*(4), 796–805. doi:10.1111/j.1365-2648.2011.05780.x

U.S. Department of Labor. (2016). *Fact sheet: Newborn & mother's health protection act.* Retrieved from http://www.dol.gov/ebsa/newsroom/fsnm-hafs.html

U.S. Department of Health and Human Services (USD-HHS). (2013). *The surgeon general's call to action to support breastfeeding.* Washington, DC: U.S. Department of Health and Human Services, Office of the Surgeon General. Retrieved from http://www.surgeongeneral.gov/library/calls/breastfeeding/callto-actiontosupportbreastfeeding.pdf

U.S. Department of Health and Human Services (USD-HHS). (2015). *Healthy People 2020: Topics and objectives.* Retrieved from http://www.healthypeople.gov/2020/topicsobjectives2020/default.aspx

Wojnar, D., & Katzenmeyer, A. (2014). Experiences of preconception, pregnancy, and new motherhood for lesbian nonbiological mothers. *Journal of Obstetrical, Gynecological, and Neonatal Nursing (JOGNN), 43*(1), 50–60.

Women's and Children's Health Network. (2016). *Care of the perineum after birth.* Retrieved from http://www.cyh.com/HealthTopics/HealthTopicDetails.aspx?p=438&np=464&id=2819

World Health Organization. (WHO). (2016). *Breastfeeding recommendations.* Retrieved from http://www.who.int/topics/breastfeeding/en/

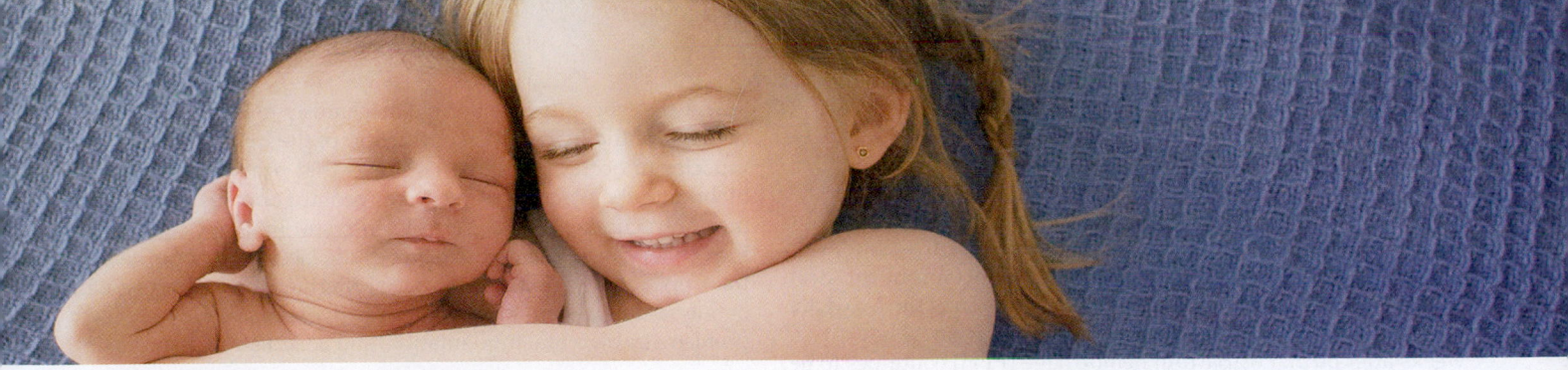

Chapter 30
The Postpartum Family at Risk

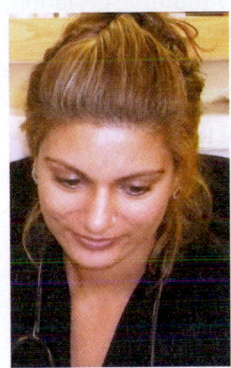

With hospital stays lasting only a couple of days, postpartum problems often develop after the family goes home. Fortunately, in my community, families receive a minimum of two postpartum visits, and more if a specific problem is identified. Whenever I encounter a family needing readmission or referral, I wonder about the new moms, dads, and babies that don't have this type of follow-up care. It is so needed.

—Home Care/Postpartum Nurse

⌄ Learning Outcomes

30.1 Identify the causes, contributing factors, signs and symptoms, clinical therapy, and nursing interventions for early and late postpartum hemorrhage.

30.2 Explain the causes, contributing factors, signs and symptoms, clinical therapy, and nursing interventions for reproductive tract infection.

30.3 Develop a nursing care plan that reflects the etiology, pathophysiology, current clinical therapy, nursing management, and preventive management for the woman with urinary tract infection, lactation mastitis, thromboembolic disease, or a postpartum psychiatric disorder.

30.4 Explain the causes, contributing factors, signs and symptoms, clinical therapy, and nursing interventions for postpartum thromboembolic disease.

30.5 Identify the woman's knowledge of self-care measures, signs of complications to be reported to the healthcare provider, and measures to prevent recurrence of complications.

The postpartum period is typically viewed as a smooth, uneventful transition time—and often it is, even with the challenges of new parenthood and the integration of a new person into the family. However, it is important for the nurse to be aware of physical or emotional complications that may develop in the postpartum period. The nurse should teach the family the signs of postpartum complications, findings to report to the healthcare provider/certified nurse–midwife (CNM), and preventive measures, if available.

Early postpartum discharge challenges the nurse to impart anticipatory information about normal postpartum recovery and self-care for the mother and her newborn, as well as be vigilant about recognizing when things go wrong. Postpartum complications sometimes necessitate readmission of the woman to the hospital, thereby disrupting the family and adding concerns about not only her health but also the way in which care of the newborn will be managed. The most common complications of the postpartum period are hemorrhage, infection, thromboembolic disease, and postpartum psychiatric disorders. This chapter will focus on these issues.

Healthy People 2020

(MICH-5) Reduce the rate of maternal mortality to 11.4 maternal deaths per 100,000 live births

(MICH-6) Reduce maternal illness and complications due to pregnancy (complications during hospitalized labor and delivery) to 28.0%

Care of the Woman With Postpartum Hemorrhage

Hemorrhage in the postpartum period is described as either early (immediate or primary) or late (delayed or secondary). **Early (primary) postpartum hemorrhage** occurs in the first 24 hours after childbirth and is the more common of the two. **Late (secondary) postpartum hemorrhage** occurs from 24 hours to 6 weeks after birth. Postpartum hemorrhage (PPH) continues to be a cause of significant maternal mortality and morbidity, although there has been a decrease in the Western world over recent years. The decrease in mortality and morbidity has been attributed to better management of uterine atony, the primary cause of PPH. However, cases of PPH due to uterine rupture and placenta accreta are on the rise—a direct consequence of the increasing rate of cesarean births (Sosa, 2014). Worldwide, PPH is the leading cause of pregnancy-related deaths, and it is estimated that 140,000 women die from postpartum hemorrhage every year, approximately one sixth of them in the United States (Poggi, 2013).

The traditional definition of postpartum hemorrhage has been a blood loss of greater than 500 mL following childbirth. That definition is currently being questioned, however, because careful quantification indicates that the average blood loss in a vaginal birth is actually greater than 500 mL, and the average blood loss after a cesarean childbirth exceeds 1000 mL (Harvey & Dildy, 2013). Clinically, PPH can be defined as a drop in maternal hematocrit levels of 10% or more from predelivery baseline or excessive bleeding that causes hemodynamic instability or the need for a blood transfusion (Sosa, 2014).

Clinical estimates of blood loss tend to underestimate actual loss by up to 50%. Clinical estimation of blood loss at childbirth is difficult because blood mixes with amniotic fluid and is obscured as it oozes onto sterile drapes or is sponged away. As the amount of blood loss increases, as in the case of hemorrhage, estimates are likely to be even less accurate than with normal childbirth. Moreover, postpartum hemorrhage may occur intra-abdominally, into the broad ligament, or into hematomas arising from genital tract trauma, wherein the blood loss is concealed. Given the increased blood volume of pregnancy, the clinical signs of hemorrhage—increasing pulse, decreased blood pressure, and decreasing urinary output—do not appear until as much as 1000 to 2000 mL or 10% or more of the woman's hematocrit has been lost (Robbins, Martin, & Wilson, 2014).

SAFETY ALERT!

To meet the standard of care in cases of postpartum hemorrhage, rapid response systems are needed in every obstetric setting that enable nurses to respond quickly to implement certain actions independently based on evidence-based protocols, similar to a call for coding someone experiencing a cardiac arrest. This multidisciplinary team approach helps to organize roles and prioritize care to stabilize the woman in a timely manner, thus averting massive hemorrhage.

Early (Primary) Postpartum Hemorrhage

At term, blood volume and cardiac output have increased so that 20% of cardiac output, or 750 to 1000 mL per minute, perfuses the pregnant uterus, supporting the developing fetus (Sosa, 2014). When the placenta separates from the uterine wall, the many uterine vessels that have carried blood to and from the placenta are severed abruptly. The normal mechanism for hemostasis after delivery of the placenta is contraction of the interlacing uterine muscles to occlude the open sinuses that previously brought blood into the placenta. Absence of prompt and sustained uterine contractions (uterine atony) can result in significant blood loss. Other causes of hemorrhage include laceration of the genital tract; episiotomy; retained placental fragments; vulvar, vaginal, or subperitoneal hematomas; uterine inversion; uterine rupture; problems of placental implantation; and coagulation disorders.

UTERINE ATONY

Uterine atony (relaxation of the uterus) is a common cause (as many as 50% of cases) of early postpartum hemorrhage. Although uterine atony can occur after any childbirth, its contributing factors include the following (Cunningham, Leveno, Bloom, et al., 2014; Poggi, 2013; Sosa, 2014):

- Overdistention of the uterus caused by multiple gestation, hydramnios, or a large baby (macrosomia)
- Dysfunctional or prolonged labor, which indicates that the uterus is contracting abnormally
- Oxytocin augmentation or induction of labor
- Grand multiparity, because stretched uterine musculature contracts less vigorously
- Use of anesthesia (especially halothane) or other drugs, such as magnesium sulfate, calcium channel blockers such as nifedipine, or tocolytics like terbutaline (Brethine), any of which causes the uterus to relax
- Prolonged third stage of labor—more than 30 minutes
- Preeclampsia
- Asian or Latino heritage
- Operative birth (includes vacuum extraction or forceps-assisted births)
- Retained placental fragments
- Placenta previa or accreta
- Obesity (Wetta, Szchowski, Seals, et al., 2013)

Hemorrhage from uterine atony may be slow and steady rather than sudden and massive. The blood may escape the vagina or collect in the uterus, where it is evident as large clots. The uterine cavity may distend with up to 1000 mL or more of blood, although the perineal pad and linen protectors remain suspiciously dry. A treacherous feature of postpartum hemorrhage is that maternal vital signs may not change until significant blood loss has occurred because of the increased blood volume associated with pregnancy.

SAFETY ALERT!

It is critical to remember that a woman with no identifiable risk factors may hemorrhage after childbirth as well.

The woman and her partner may wish to have some private time engaging with the newborn when he or she is appropriately warm and ready for an early visit. But postpartum women must be assessed at frequent intervals, especially in the initial hours after delivery of the placenta when most deaths from hemorrhage occur.

Ideally, PPH is prevented, beginning with adequate prenatal care, good nutrition, avoidance of traumatic procedures, risk assessment, early recognition, and management of complications as they arise. Review of maternal records for risk factors will help nurses to plan assessment timelines to maximize early identification and management of excessive bleeding. A prior history of PPH increases the woman's risk by double in a subsequent pregnancy (Oberg, Hernandez-Diaz, Palmsten, et al., 2014).

There is evidence that active management of the third stage of labor through administration of an oxytocic after delivery, controlled traction on the umbilical cord, and uterine massage after birth could prevent half of the cases of postpartum hemorrhage (Poggi, 2013).

Clinical Therapy. The goals of medical management of PPH are to stop the hemorrhage, correct hypovolemia, and treat the underlying cause. After expulsion of the placenta, the fundus is palpated to ensure that it is firmly contracted. If it is not firm, gentle fundal massage is performed until the uterus contracts. Fundal massage is uncomfortable for the woman who has not received regional anesthesia; she will need an explanation for why this procedure is necessary and support as massage is initiated. Clinical guidelines schedule vital signs and assessment of fundal contractility and lochia at regular intervals (see Chapter 28). When excessive bleeding continues despite external uterine massage, the healthcare provider/CNM may elect to do a bimanual massage (Figure 30-1A).

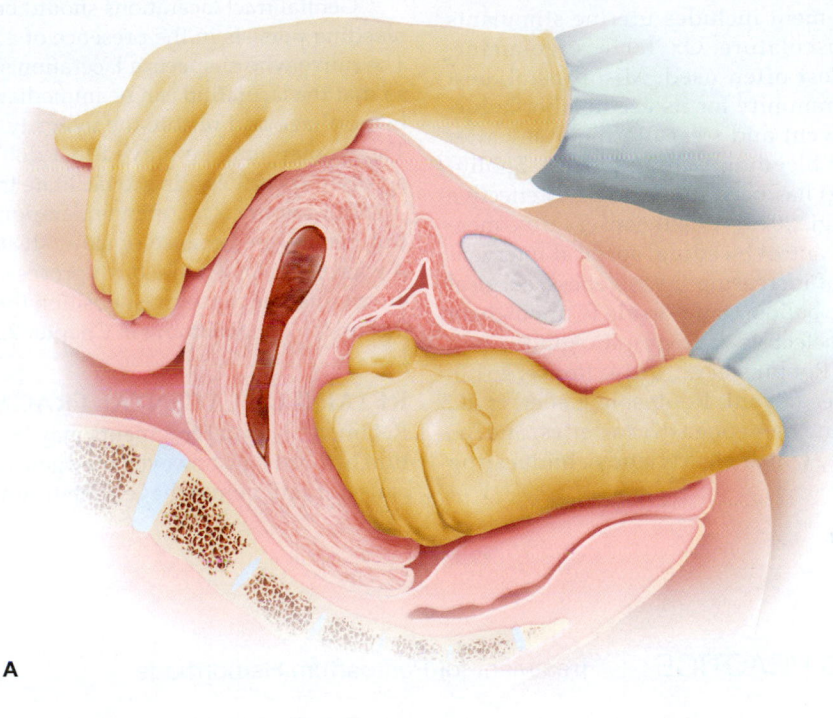

A

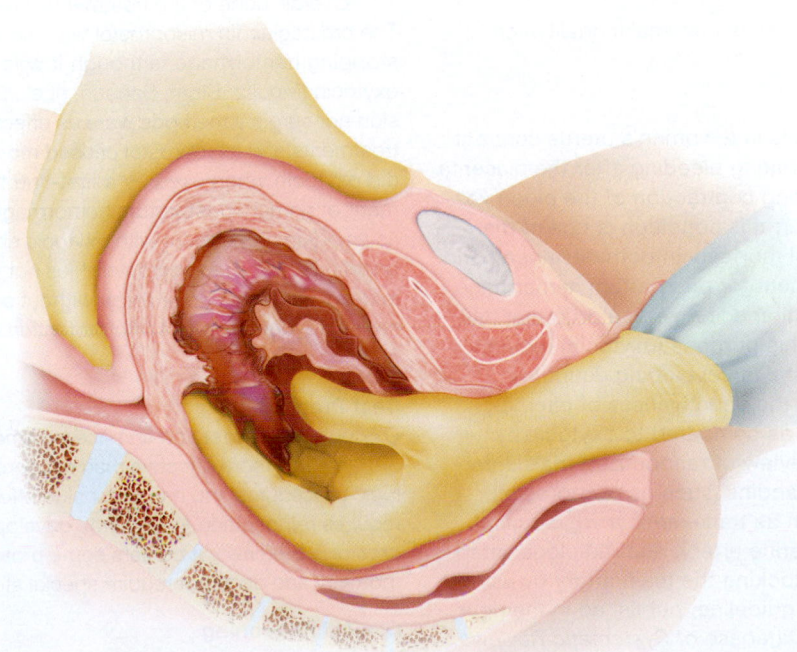

B

Figure 30-1 A. Manual compression of the uterus and massage with the abdominal hand usually will effectively control hemorrhage from uterine atony. B. Manual removal of placenta. The fingers are alternately abducted, adducted, and advanced until the placenta is completely detached. Both procedures are performed only by the healthcare provider.

Bimanual massage compresses the body of the uterus from below while the abdominal hand massages the fundus from above.

If uterine massage is not effective, uterine stimulants (uterotonic agents) will be administered to contract the atonic musculature. Oxytocin, ergotamine, prostaglandin analog, and misoprostol are most often used (Thorp & Laughton, 2014). See *Medications Used to Treat: Uterine Stimulants Used to Prevent and Manage Uterine Atony* for a summary of critical nursing information about the use of uterine stimulants to control bleeding. The need for IV fluid replacement and blood transfusion is determined on the basis of hemoglobin and hematocrit results as well as coagulation studies.

Conservative management includes uterine stimulants to contract the atonic musculature. Oxytocin, ergotamine, and prostaglandin are most often used. Misoprostol, best known to the obstetric community for its use in labor induction, is being used to prevent and treat uterine atony after failed attempts to control bleeding with oxytocics. Sublingual misoprostol (800 mcg) has been found to be as effective as oxytocin (40 U/L) (Poggi, 2013). When conservative measures do not successfully control bleeding, surgical intervention is required. In order of increasing invasiveness, surgical procedures include uterine balloon tamponade (Cunningham et al., 2014; Poggi, 2013), selective radiographic-guided pelvic arterial embolization (Robbins et al., 2014; Rouse, 2013), uterine suturing techniques (Ayadi, Robinson, Geller, et al., 2013), ligation of the uterine or hypogastric arteries, and, as a last resort, hysterectomy, which clearly ends childbearing (Harvey & Dildy, 2013).

LACERATIONS OF THE GENITAL TRACT

Early postpartum hemorrhage is associated with lacerations of the perineum, vagina, or cervix. Several factors predispose women to higher risk of reproductive tract lacerations:

- Nulliparity
- Epidural anesthesia
- Precipitous childbirth (less than 3 hours)
- Forceps- or vacuum-assisted birth
- Macrosomia
- Use of oxytocin

Genital tract lacerations should be suspected when vaginal bleeding persists in the presence of a firmly contracted uterus. The nurse who suspects a laceration should notify the clinician so that the laceration can be immediately sutured to control the hemorrhage and restore the integrity of the reproductive tract. The woman may be moved to a delivery or surgical area for access to special lighting to facilitate treatment.

Episiotomy is an often underappreciated source of postpartum blood loss because of slow, steady bleeding, especially if it was done early in the birth process. To fully assess the episiotomy site, the nurse must position the woman on her side. (See discussion of episiotomy in Chapter 22.)

RETAINED PLACENTAL FRAGMENTS

Retained placental fragments may be a cause of early postpartum hemorrhage; however, they generally are the most common cause of late hemorrhage. Retention of fragments is usually

---

EVIDENCE-BASED PRACTICE | Treatment for Postpartum Hemorrhage

Clinical Question

What treatment reduces the risk of maternal mortality from postpartum hemorrhage?

The Evidence

After birth, the blood vessels in a woman's uterus contract, clamping blood flow and limiting bleeding after the placenta has detached. Without strong contraction of the blood vessels, hemorrhage can occur; this condition is one of the top five causes of maternal mortality in both developed and developing nations. Treatment for postpartum hemorrhage is essential to save the mother's life, yet the drug that has been proven effective for this purpose (oxytocin) requires refrigeration and is not useful in developing countries. These researchers studied the effectiveness of alternative drugs and procedures as compared to oxytocin by conducting a systematic review of randomized trials. Interventions included prostaglandins (such as misoprostol), blood-clotting agents (such as tranexamic acid), surgical techniques to ligate the uterine artery, and radiologic interventions that assisted in blocking the main artery by using gel foams. This structured guideline, published in the rigorously reviewed *Cochrane Database of Systematic Reviews*, forms the strongest level of evidence. This review included 10 randomized controlled trials involving more than 4000 women.

Overall, none of the treatments worked as well as oxytocin. The prostaglandin misoprostol was moderately successful in stopping hemorrhage, although it was not as effective as oxytocin (Mousa, Blum, Senoun, et al., 2014). Neither compression nor surgical methods were as effective as oxytocin. These treatments and misoprostol caused more side effects than did oxytocin when used as a first-line therapy for the treatment of primary postpartum hemorrhage. Using misoprostol as an adjunct treatment with oxytocin showed no additional benefit. However, misoprostol does not need refrigeration, and in developing nations or areas without adequate medication storage, it does confer some protection against mortality from hemorrhage.

Best Practice

Oxytocin is the best and first-line treatment for postpartum hemorrhage. It is more effective than misoprostol or surgical/radiologic procedures and has fewer side effects. However, oxytocin requires refrigeration, so in some developing countries, misoprostol is preferred; it confers some protection against maternal mortality and does not require special storage.

Clinical Reasoning

What are some creative ways for refrigerating oxytocin when standard refrigeration is unavailable? What are ways to estimate blood loss so that interventions can be applied in a timely way?

Medications Used to Treat Uterine Stimulants Used to Prevent and Manage Uterine Atony

DRUG	DOSING INFORMATION	CONTRAINDICATIONS	EXPECTED EFFECTS	SIDE EFFECTS
Oxytocin (Pitocin, Syntocinon)	IV use: 10–40 units in 500–1000 mL crystalloid fluid at 50 milliunits/min administration rate. Onset: immediate. Duration: 1 hr. **IV bolus administration not recommended.** IM use: 10 units. Onset: 3–5 min. Duration: 2–3 hr.	None for use in postpartum hemorrhage. Avoid undiluted rapid IV infusion, which causes hypotension.	Rhythmic uterine contractions that help to prevent or reverse postpartum hemorrhage caused by uterine atony.	Uterine hyperstimulation, mild transient hypertension, water intoxication rare in postpartum use.
Methylergonovine maleate (Methergine)	IM use: 0.2 mg every 2–4 hr. Onset: 2–5 min. Duration: 3 hr (for 5 dose maximum). PO use: 0.2 mg every 4 hr (for 6 doses). Onset: 7 to 15 min. Duration: 3 hr (for 1 week). **IV administration not recommended—can cause dangerous hypertension and stroke.**	Women with labile or high blood pressure or known sensitivity to drug, cardiac disease, and Raynaud disease. Use with caution during lactation.	Sustained uterine contractions that help to prevent or reverse postpartum hemorrhage caused by uterine atony; management of postpartum subinvolution.	Hypertension, dizziness, headache, flushing/hot flashes, tinnitus, nausea and vomiting, palpitations, chest pain. Overdose or hypersensitivity is recognized by seizures; tingling and numbness of fingers and toes.
Prostaglandin (PGF_{2a}, Carboprost tromethamine [Hemabate], Prostin/15M)	IM use: 0.25 mg repeated every 15–90 min, up to 8 doses max. Healthcare provider/CNM may elect to administer by direct intramyometrial injection.	Women with active cardiovascular, renal, liver disease, or asthma or with known hypersensitivity to drug.	Control of refractory cases of postpartum hemorrhage caused by uterine atony; generally used after failed attempts at control of hemorrhage with oxytocic agents.	Nausea, vomiting, diarrhea, headache, flushing, bradycardia, bronchospasm, wheezing, cough, chills, fever.
Dinoprostone (Prostin E_2)	Vaginal or rectal suppository 20 mg every 2 hr. Stored in frozen form—must be thawed to room temperature.	Avoid if woman is hypotensive or has asthma or acute inflammatory disease.	Stimulate uterine contractions	Fever is common and occurs within 15–45 min of insertion; bleeding, abdominal cramps, nausea and vomiting.
Misoprostol (Cytotec)	800–1000 micrograms rectally. Rapid effects, contractions within minutes.	History of allergies to prostaglandins.	Used to prevent and treat uterine atony after failed attempts to control bleeding with oxytocics.	Diarrhea, abdominal pain, headache

NURSING IMPLICATIONS WITH UTERINE STIMULANTS

- Note expected duration of action of drug being administered and take care to recheck fundus at that time for adequate tone.
- When the drug is ineffective and the fundus remains atonic (boggy or uncontracted) and bleeding continues, massage the fundus. If massage fails to cause sustained contraction, consider the status of the urinary bladder. If uterine tone is not restored after the bladder is empty and fundal massage has been performed, notify the healthcare provider/CNM immediately.
- Monitor woman for signs of known side effects of the drug; report to healthcare provider/CNM if side effects occur.
- Remind the woman and her support person that uterine cramping is an expected result of these drugs and that medication is available for discomfort. Administer analgesic medications as needed for pain relief. Provide nonpharmacologic comfort measures. If analgesic medication ordered is insufficient for pain relief, notify the healthcare provider/CNM.
- Provide information to the woman and her family regarding the importance of not smoking during Methergine administration (nicotine from cigarettes leads to constricted vessels and may lead to hypertension) and signs of toxicity.

When Prostaglandin Is Used

- Check temperature every 1–2 hr. Administer antipyretic medication as ordered for prostaglandin-induced fever.
- Auscultate breath sounds frequently for signs of adverse respiratory effects.
- Assess for nausea, vomiting, and diarrhea. Administer antiemetic and antidiarrheal medications as ordered. (In some settings, women are premedicated with these drugs.)

Sources: Data from Robbins, K. S., Martin, S. R., & Wilson, W. C. (2014). Intensive care considerations for the critically ill parturient. In R. K. Creasy & R. Resnik (Eds.), *Maternal–fetal medicine: Principles and practice* (7th ed., pp. 1182–1214). Philadelphia, PA: Saunders; Sosa, M. E. (2014). Bleeding in pregnancy. In K. R. Simpson & P. A. Creehan (Eds.), *AWHONN's perinatal nursing* (4th ed., pp. 143–162). Philadelphia, PA: Lippincott Williams & Wilkins.

attributable to partial separation of the placenta during massage of the fundus before spontaneous placental separation, so this practice should be avoided.

SAFETY ALERT!

Postpartum nurses are wise to appreciate that most deaths from postpartum hemorrhage are not caused by catastrophic bleeding episodes but by ineffective management of slow, steady blood loss.

Following birth, the placenta should always be inspected for intactness and for evidence of missing fragments or cotyledons on the maternal side and for vessels that transverse to the edge of the placenta outward along the membranes of the fetal side, which may indicate succenturiate placenta and a retained lobe. Uterine exploration may be required to remove missing fragments. This cause should be immediately suspected if bleeding persists and no lacerations are noted (Figure 30-1B). Sonography may be used to diagnose retained placental fragments. Curettage, formerly standard treatment, is now thought by some to traumatize the implantation site, thereby increasing bleeding and the potential for uterine adhesions. However, it may be necessitated by the degree of hemorrhage (Poggi, 2013).

VULVAR, VAGINAL, AND PELVIC HEMATOMAS

Hematomas occur as a result of injury to a blood vessel from birth trauma, often without noticeable trauma to the superficial tissue, or from inadequate hemostasis at the site of repair of an incision or laceration. The soft tissue in the area offers no resistance, and hematomas containing 250 to 500 mL of blood may develop rapidly. Signs and symptoms vary somewhat with the type of hematoma. Hematomas may be vulvar (involving branches of the pudendal artery), vaginal (especially in the area of the ischial spines), vulvovaginal, or subperitoneal. The latter are rare; however, they are the most dangerous because of the large amount of blood loss that can occur without clinical symptoms until the woman becomes hemodynamically unstable. Subperitoneal hematomas involve the uterine artery branches or vessels in the broad ligaments and require laparotomy for surgical correction.

Risk factors for hematomas include preeclampsia, use of pudendal anesthesia, first full-term birth, precipitous labor, prolonged second stage of labor, macrosomia, forceps- or vacuum-assisted births, and history of vulvar varicosities (Distefano, Casarella, Amoroso, et al., 2013). Hematomas less than 3 cm (1.2 in.) in size and nonexpanding are managed expectantly with ice packs and analgesia. Small hematomas usually resolve over several days. For larger hematomas and those that expand, surgical management is usually required using incision and drainage (I&D); the hematoma is evacuated, the bleeding vessel ligated, and the wound closed, with or without vaginal packing. A temporary indwelling urinary catheter may be necessary because voiding may be impossible with packing in place (Francois & Foley, 2012).

The hematoma site is an ideal medium for the growth of flora normally present in the genital tract. Consequently, broad-spectrum antibiotics are usually ordered to prevent infection or abscess.

UTERINE INVERSION

Uterine inversion—a prolapse of the fundus to or through the cervix so that the uterus is, in effect, turned inside out after birth—is a rare but life-threatening cause of postpartum hemorrhage. Although not always preventable, uterine inversion is often associated with factors such as fundal implantation or abnormal adherence of the placenta, protracted labor, weakness of the uterine musculature, uterine relaxation secondary to anesthesia or drugs such as magnesium sulfate, and excess traction on the umbilical cord or vigorous manual removal of the placenta. Most cases of uterine inversion are managed by immediate repositioning of the uterus within the pelvis by the healthcare provider under intravenous tocolysis or general anesthesia (Robbins et al., 2014).

Late (Secondary) Postpartum Hemorrhage

Although early postpartum hemorrhage usually occurs within hours after birth, delayed hemorrhage generally occurs within 1 to 2 weeks after childbirth, most frequently as a result of **subinvolution** (failure to return to normal size) of the placental site or retention of placental fragments. Blood loss at this time may be excessive but rarely poses the same risk as that from immediate postpartum hemorrhage. Late postpartum hemorrhage is much less common but can be extremely stressful for the woman and her family who are at home by this time.

The site of placental implantation is always the last area of the uterus to regenerate after childbirth. In the case of subinvolution, adjacent endometrium and the decidua basalis fail to regenerate to cover the placental site. Faulty implantation in the less vascular lower uterine segment, retention of placental tissue, or infection may contribute to subinvolution. With subinvolution, the postpartum fundal height is greater than expected. In addition, lochia flow often fails to progress normally from rubra to serosa to alba. Lochia rubra that persists longer than 2 weeks postpartum is highly suggestive of subinvolution, although studies show there is a great variability in normal lochia patterns (Fletcher, Grotegut, & James, 2012). Some women report scant brown lochia or irregular heavy bleeding. Leukorrhea, backache, and foul lochia may occur if infection is a cause. There may be a history of heavy early postpartum bleeding or difficulty with expulsion of the placenta. When portions of the placenta have been retained in the uterus, bleeding continues because normal uterine contractions that constrict the bleeding site are prohibited. Presence of placental tissue within the uterus can be confirmed by pelvic ultrasound.

Subinvolution is most commonly diagnosed during the routine postpartum examination at 4 to 6 weeks. The woman may relate a history of irregular or excessive bleeding or describe the symptoms listed previously. An enlarged, softer-than-normal uterus palpated bimanually is an objective indication of subinvolution. Treatment includes oral administration of methylergonovine maleate. When uterine infection is present, antibiotics are also administered. The woman is reevaluated in 2 weeks.

Nursing Management

For the Postpartum Woman With Hemorrhage

Nursing Assessment and Diagnosis

Careful and ongoing assessment of the woman during labor and birth and evaluation of her prenatal history will help identify factors that put her at risk for postpartum hemorrhage. Following birth, periodically assess for evidence of vaginal bleeding. Regular and frequent assessment of fundal height and evidence of uterine tone or contractility will alert you to the possible development or recurrence of hemorrhage. Monitoring the bladder for evidence of increasing distention, with immediate intervention, can sometimes help to prevent excessive bleeding that occurs when a full bladder displaces the uterus and interferes with contractility. This assessment can be done visually, by pad counts, or by weighing the perineal pads. In cases of excessive bleeding, be alert for signs of impending hypovolemic shock and the development of coagulation problems, such as disseminated intravascular coagulation (DIC) (see Chapter 15 for an in-depth discussion of DIC).

For all complaints of perineal pain examine the perineal area for signs of hematomas: ecchymosis, edema, tenseness of tissue overlying the hematoma, a fluctuant mass bulging at the introitus, and extreme tenderness to palpation. Estimating the size on first assessment of the perineum enables you to better identify increases in size and the potential blood loss. Notify the physician/CNM if a hematoma is suspected. Help to decrease the risk of vulvar or vaginal hematoma by applying an ice pack to the woman's perineum during the first hour after birth and intermittently thereafter for the next 8 to12 hours. If a small hematoma develops despite preventive measures, a sitz bath after the first 12 hours will aid fluid absorption once bleeding has stopped and will promote comfort, as will the judicious use of analgesic agents. Close monitoring of the woman who has had excessive bleeding is important during sitz baths to ensure safety. In cases of excessive bleeding, be alert for signs of impending hypovolemic shock. Frequent noninvasive monitoring should continue: heart rate, blood pressure, auscultation of heart sounds and breath sounds, oxygen saturation, skin turgor, color, temperature, color and moisture of mucous membranes, capillary refill, level of consciousness, and urinary output, possibly with Foley catheter/urometer, and electrocardiogram (ECG) readings.

Development of a rapid response team is a patient safety initiative. When obstetric postpartum hemorrhage occurs, the interprofessional perinatal rapid response team needs to work collaboratively to treat the underlying cause, manage the blood loss, and lessen the risk to the mother (ACOG Committee on Patient Safety and Quality Improvement, 2014; James, 2014).

Nursing diagnoses that may apply to a woman experiencing postpartum hemorrhage include the following (NANDA-I © 2014):

- *Fluid Volume: Deficient*, related to blood loss secondary to uterine atony, lacerations, retained placental fragments, or coagulopathies
- *Tissue Perfusion: Peripheral, Risk for Ineffective*, related to hypovolemia
- *Bleeding, Risk for*, related to lack of information about signs of delayed postpartum hemorrhage

Nursing Plan and Implementation

HOSPITAL-BASED NURSING CARE

If you detect a soft, boggy uterus, massage it until firm. If the uterus is not contracting well and appears larger than anticipated, you may express clots during fundal massage. Once clots

have been expressed, the uterus tends to contract more effectively. Overly aggressive massage should be avoided so as not to injure the vessels in the broad ligaments or cause reactive relaxation of the musculature.

If the woman seems to have a slow, steady, free flow of blood, do pad counts and if possible begin to weigh the perineal pads (1 mL = 1 g) (Harvey & Dildy, 2013). Monitor the woman's vital signs every 15 minutes, or more frequently if indicated (James, 2014). If the fundus is displaced upward or to one side because of a full bladder, encourage the woman to empty her bladder—or catheterize her if she is unable to void—to allow for efficient uterine contractions. Excessive bleeding or uterine atony despite fundal massage necessitates prompt notification to the healthcare provider/CNM.

When there are risk factors for postpartum hemorrhage or frequent fundal massage has been necessary to sustain uterine contractions, maintain any vascular access (IV) started during labor and anticipate the need for a second IV in case additional fluids, medications, or blood is necessary. If blood has been crossmatched earlier, check that blood is available in the blood bank. Sometimes healthcare providers write orders that specify "discontinue IV after present bottle." The astute postpartum nurse will assess the consistency of the fundus and the presence of normal versus excessive lochia before discontinuing the infusion. If the assessments are not reassuring, continue the IV infusion and notify the healthcare provider/CNM.

Clinical Tip

Bogginess indicates that the uterus is not contracting well, which results in increased uterine bleeding. This blood may remain in the uterus and form clots or may result in increased flow. In assessing the amount of blood loss, first massage the uterus until it is firm and then express clots. Do not be misled by the fact that a woman has a firm uterus. Significant bleeding can occur from causes other than uterine atony. To accurately determine the amount of blood loss, it is not sufficient to assess only the peripads. You should also ask the woman to turn on her side so you can assess underneath her for pooling of blood.

As the woman's blood volume becomes depleted, positioning her with her legs elevated to 30 degrees facilitates venous return and promotes oxygenation. Unlike the Trendelenburg position used in the past for those in shock, this position does not impede breathing or cardiac function and promotes cerebral circulation. Supplemental oxygen may be necessary to keep peripheral tissues oxygenated when blood is shunted to protect vital organs like the brain and kidneys. See *Box 30-1: Nursing Actions During Postpartum Hemorrhage.*

Fluid Replacement and Transfusion

A prominent role of the nurse during PPH is the administration of crystalloid fluids (normal saline and lactated Ringer solution) or of blood and blood products. Typically, lost intravascular volume is replaced initially with rapid administration of warmed crystalloid solutions, in a 3 mL solution per 1 mL of estimated blood lost ratio (Francois & Foley, 2012). With rapid attempts to replace depleted blood volume, you must carefully monitor the woman for evidence of fluid overload.

When blood loss is significant and vital signs become unstable, crystalloid fluid replacement can no longer

BOX 30-1 Nursing Actions During Postpartum Hemorrhage

- Call for help. Initiate response team as per hospital protocol.
- Massage uterus until firm.
- Administer prescribed medications.
- Ensure large-bore (14-, 16-, or 18-gauge) needle IV access (consider starting a second line).
- Replace volume with normal saline or lactated Ringer solution.
- Apply pulse oximeter and administer oxygen according to agency protocol.
- Insert a Foley catheter to empty the bladder and accurately measure output.
- Maintain accurate intake and output measurements.
- Assess blood loss; weigh peri-pads or absorbent dressing for objective estimate of blood loss.
- Monitor pulse and blood pressure every 15 minutes or more often as indicated.
- Assess for shock.
- Elevate the legs to a 20- to 30-degree angle to increase venous return.
- Draw blood for CBC, type and crossmatch, coagulation studies, and blood chemistry.
- Notify blood bank that transfusion may be necessary; administer blood products as ordered.
- Continuous electrocardiogram (ECG) monitoring may be indicated for hypotension, continuous bleeding, tachycardia, or shock.
- Prepare for additional interventions such as uterine tamponade, exploratory laparotomy, or uterine artery embolization.
- Anticipate pain management needs for fundal massage and uterotonic medications.
- Provide emotional support for the woman and her family.

Sources: Data from James, D. C. (2014). Postpartum care. In K. R. Simpson & P. A. Creehan (Eds.), *AWHONN's perinatal nursing* (4th ed., pp. 553–555); American College of Obstetrics & Gynecology. (2006). ACOG Practice Bulletin: Clinical management guidelines for obstetrician-gynecologists #76. *Obstetrics & Gynecology, 108*(4), 1039–1046.

compensate for the loss, and transfusion of blood products becomes necessary. When blood products are transfused, watch for transfusion reactions and respond promptly according to hospital procedures.

Keeping the woman as comfortable as possible with perineal care and frequent changes of disposable pads is important, but her position cannot be allowed to compromise venous return or oxygenation. She will be kept NPO in case surgery is needed, so oral care is important for comfort. There are many interruptions when the woman is experiencing a complication, so you will need to seek opportunities

to promote rest whenever possible. Any intervention to help with maternal–newborn bonding in the interval of separation is of great value to the woman—photographs or videos of the newborn, direct reports from the nursery staff, and brief visits to the room if her condition allows. Encourage the father to visit the newborn and bring information to the mother.

Clearly, the care of the woman experiencing postpartum hemorrhage depends on good nursing assessment and prompt reporting of nonreassuring findings to the healthcare provider. However, direct treatment methods require the collaboration of a healthcare provider and, in some cases, radiographic or surgical staff. You will become an important liaison between these departments, keeping the necessary individuals apprised of the woman's status. For example, if additional transfusions of whole blood or blood products are anticipated, you will need to keep the hospital laboratory informed to facilitate timely response. Care may well include the preprocedural preparation of the woman for surgery or for procedures such as arterial embolization performed by a radiologist.

Evaluate the woman for signs of anemia, such as fatigue, pallor, headache, thirst, and orthostatic changes in pulse or blood pressure (BP), and review the results of all hematocrit determinations. All medical interventions, IV infusions, blood transfusions, oxygen therapy, and medications such as uterine stimulants are monitored as necessary and evaluated for effectiveness. Urinary output should be monitored to determine adequacy of fluid replacement and renal perfusion, with amounts less than 30 mL per hour reported to the physician (Sosa, 2014).

Help the woman plan activities so that adequate rest is possible. The woman who is experiencing anemia and fatigue may need assistance with self-care and progressive ambulation for several days. When she is able to be out of bed to shower, use of a shower chair permits independence while providing a measure of safety should the woman experience weakness or dizziness.

SAFETY ALERT!
The emergency call light should be easily accessible whenever you have left the bedside, even temporarily.

The mother may find it difficult to care for her baby because of the fatigue associated with blood loss. You can often find ways to promote maternal–newborn attachment while accommodating the mother's health needs. The mother may require additional assistance in caring for her baby. If she has intravenous lines in place, even carrying the newborn may be awkward. For the mother who feels compelled to do as much as possible, you may need to give the mother "permission" to return her baby to the nursery so she can have adequate periods of uninterrupted rest.

If the father/partner is involved in the birth experience, including that person in the plan of care is a productive strategy. This person can support the mother's recovery by helping to meet her physical needs while encouraging her to rest. The mother is likely to feel less concern over her limited opportunities for the newborn's care if she can witness the father/partner interacting with and caring for the newborn. The extent to which the father/partner becomes involved with the care of the mother and the baby must be carefully balanced with the need to be rested for the extra responsibilities the support person will assume when the mother and newborn child are discharged from the hospital.

SAFETY ALERT!
Good hand hygiene using standard precautions throughout the hospitalization and emphasizing proper hand washing for home care is important to minimize risk of postpartum infection.

Clinical Reasoning Postpartum Hemorrhage

Betsy Lambert is a primigravida who had a spontaneous vaginal delivery at 09:41 today. An overview of her history reveals the following: 23 years old, married, G1P0 on admission to Labor Unit. Pregnancy normal. Rh positive. No drug allergies. Labs on admission to L&D normal with exception of hemoglobin 11 g and hematocrit 32%. Labor: 13 hours. Estimated blood loss: 450 mL. Delivered female (7 lb 7 oz) spontaneously after epidural anesthesia. APGAR 9/10. Newborn examination was within normal limits and routine newborn orders were implemented. Day shift reports firm fundus; voided 210 mL around 1100; vital signs stable. Baby visited and breastfed briefly with help from lactation nurse. Ate lunch and had Tylenol #3 at 1300 for perineal pain. Has been sleeping for long intervals.

You find Mrs. Lambert still dozing but awaken her for examination and note the following: B/P 112/60, HR 116, R 20, T 100. Breasts—soft, nontender, wearing support bra. Uterus—fundus firm and 2 cm below umbilicus slightly left of midline. Bladder—possibly slightly distended but she feels no urge to void. Lochia—the two perineal pads and blue absorbent underpads are covered with bright red blood. Perineum—covered with blood, as are thighs. Some of the blood has dried on the skin. Slight edema noted—midline episiotomy intact. Ice pack in place but ice melted. Homans sign—negative. Emotional status—reports her husband went home to rest and will be back at dinnertime. Talks with excitement about first attempt to nurse baby. Asks for something cold to drink. The woman cannot remember when she was last checked for bleeding. You don gloves and wash her perineum gently and her thighs and change all her pads so you can better assess her degree of bleeding. An IV is in place with 10 units of oxytocin (Pitocin) (100 mL is left in the IV bag).

You return, as promised, in 15 minutes to reevaluate her lochia and find that her perineal pads are again covered in blood.

Based on your assessments and Mrs. Lambert's laboratory findings, what actions will you take first?

If one of your anticipated actions is to inform the healthcare provider, what specific information will you report and what management should you anticipate initially?

What follow-up care will you anticipate performing during the remainder of your shift?

Health Promotion Preventing Postpartum Bleeding

The woman and her family or other support persons should receive clear, preferably written, explanations of the normal postpartum course, including changes in the lochia and fundus and signs of abnormal bleeding. Instructions for the prevention of bleeding should include fundal massage, ways to assess the fundal height and consistency, and inspection of any episiotomy and lacerations, if present. The woman should receive instruction in perineal care (see discussion of perineal care in Chapter 29). The mother and her family are advised to contact her healthcare provider if any of the signs of postpartum hemorrhage occur (see *Key Facts to Remember: Signs of Postpartum Hemorrhage*.)

If iron supplementation is ordered, instructions for proper dosage should be provided along with client teaching to enhance absorption and avoid constipation and nausea. The Western herb shepherd's purse can be used in tea or tincture form to help control postpartum bleeding. Yarrow is often used with shepherd's purse as a homeostatic agent. Cinnamon and cayenne have also been used. Always report bleeding to a healthcare provider.

KEY FACTS TO REMEMBER
Signs of Postpartum Hemorrhage

- Excessive or bright-red bleeding (saturation of more than one pad per hour)
- A boggy fundus that does not respond to massage
- Abnormal clots
- High temperature
- Any unusual pelvic discomfort or backache
- Persistent bleeding in the presence of a firmly contracted uterus
- Rise in the level of the fundus of the uterus
- Increased pulse or decreased BP
- Hematoma formation or bulging/shiny skin in the perineal area
- Decreased level of consciousness

COMMUNITY-BASED NURSING CARE

For postpartum women, the usual discharge instructions include advice such as "You take care of your baby, and let someone else care for you, the family, and the household." Because of her fatigue and weakened condition, the woman who has experienced postpartum hemorrhage may be unable even to care for her newborn unassisted. The caregivers at home need clear, concise explanations of her condition and needs for recovery. For example, they should understand the woman's need to rest and to be given extra time to rest after any necessary activity. They should also be told that anemia is associated with postpartum depression so that they can be vigilant for and promptly report any change in the woman's affect (Albacar, Sans, Martín-Santos, et al., 2011).

To ensure her safety, advise the woman to rise slowly to minimize the likelihood of orthostatic hypotension. Until she regains strength, she should be seated when holding the newborn.

The person who assumes responsibility for grocery shopping and meal preparation needs advice about the importance of including foods high in iron in the daily menus. Having the woman indicate her preferences from a list of such foods will promote cooperation with the diet. Explain the rationale for continuing medications containing iron and remind the woman that vitamin C–containing fluids maximize absorption of iron, and tea or milk products prevent absorption.

Instruct the woman to continue to count perineal pads for several days so that she can recognize any recurring problems with excessive blood loss (hypovolemia). Invasive procedures, her debilitated condition, and anemia associated with hemorrhage increase the woman's risk of puerperal infection. She and her caregivers should use good hand hygiene technique and minimize exposure to infection in the home. Give the woman's caregivers a list of the signs of infection and ensure that they understand the importance of alerting the healthcare provider immediately if signs occur.

In addition to meeting the woman's physical needs, assess the couple's coping strategies and resources for dealing with the impending crisis. Providing realistic information, offering to call those in their support network, and exploring effective coping strategies can be of immeasurable value as the couple tries to maintain a sense of balance in this difficult situation. A sense of emergency often accompanies late postpartum hemorrhage. Because it commonly occurs 1 to 2 weeks after birth, the couple is generally at home, involved in the day-to-day activities demanded by their new roles, when the unexpected, excessive bleeding begins. Quick decisions about childcare arrangements must often be made so that the mother can return to the hospital. Both mother and father/partner are likely to be alarmed by the excessive bleeding and concerned about her prognosis. There may be additional worries about separation from the newborn, especially when the mother is breastfeeding. The father/partner may be torn between the needs of the mother and those of the newborn. Ideally, arrangements can be made to minimize separation of the family members.

Evaluation

Expected outcomes of nursing care include the following:

- Signs of postpartum hemorrhage are detected quickly and managed effectively.
- Maternal–newborn attachment is maintained successfully.
- The woman is able to identify abnormal changes that might occur following discharge and understands the importance of notifying her caregiver if they develop.

Care of the Woman With a Reproductive Tract Infection or Wound Infection

Puerperal infection is an infection of the reproductive tract associated with childbirth that occurs any time up to 6 weeks postpartum. The most common postpartum infection is endometritis (metritis), which is infection limited to the uterine lining. Indeed, the cause of postpartum fever is presumed to be metritis until proven otherwise. However, infection can be spread by way of the lymphatic and circulatory systems to become a progressive disease resulting in parametrial cellulitis and **peritonitis** (infection involving the peritoneal cavity). Other causes of postpartum fever should be considered, including respiratory complications such as atelectasis or pneumonia,

acute pyelonephritis, thrombophlebitis, or breast engorgement, which rarely lasts more than 24 hours (Duff, 2014).

Maternal death from sepsis is increasing in countries with advanced healthcare systems (Acosta, Kurinczuk, Lucas, et al., 2014). Although the death rate from postpartum infection is low in the United States, infection accounts for 11% of pregnancy-related deaths. Uterine infections are relatively uncommon following uncomplicated vaginal births, but they continue to be a major source of morbidity for women who give birth by cesarean section. Routine antibiotic prophylaxis for cesarean childbirth in conjunction with aseptic technique, fewer traumatic operative births, a better understanding of labor dystocia, improved surgical intervention, and a population that is generally at less risk from malnutrition and chronic debilitative disease have contributed to a reduction in overall postpartum morbidity and mortality.

The standard definition of **puerperal morbidity**, established by the Joint Committee on Maternal Welfare, is a temperature of 38°C (100.4°F) or higher, with the temperature occurring on any 2 of the first 10 postpartum days, exclusive of the first 24 hours, and when taken by mouth by standard technique at least four times a day. During today's short obstetric hospital stays, the temperature is measured every 6 hours in most settings, consistent with the definition for puerperal morbidity. However, serious infections can occur in the first 24 hours or may cause only persistent low-grade temperatures. Therefore, careful assessment of all postpartum women with elevated temperatures is essential.

The vagina and cervix of approximately 70% of all healthy pregnant women contain pathogenic bacteria that, alone or in combination, are sufficiently virulent to cause extensive infections. Although the uterus is considered a sterile cavity before rupture of the fetal membranes, bacterial contamination of amniotic fluid with membranes still intact at term is more common than previously believed and may contribute to premature labor. Following rupture of membranes and during labor, contamination of the uterine cavity by vaginal or cervical bacteria can easily occur. Other factors must also be present for infection to occur such as the change in the postpartum period to an alkaline pH of the vagina that favors growth of aerobes.

Because shortened inpatient stays are the norm in maternity care, women will likely be discharged following childbirth before clinical signs of puerperal infection are evident. According to Bianco, Roccia, Pileggi, et al. (2013), 84% of postpartum infections manifest after hospital discharge. Consequently, perinatal nurses are challenged to analyze the woman's history and clinical course for risk assessment and to recognize the early subtle signs of infection so that discharge may be delayed as needed. Before discharge, the nurse advises the woman about preventive measures, including scrupulous hand hygiene and signs of infection. Nurses should educate the client and her family about the risk of infection and how to recognize and respond appropriately should it occur.

Postpartum Endometritis

Postpartum endometritis (metritis), an inflammation of the endometrium portion of the uterine lining occurring any time up to 6 weeks postpartum, may occur in 30% to 35% of those who give birth by cesarean after an extended period of labor and ruptured membranes (Duff, 2014).

Postpartum infection from vaginal delivery primarily affects the placental implantation site, the decidua, and adjacent myometrium. Bacteria that colonize the cervix and vagina gain access to the amniotic fluid during labor and postpartum and begin to invade devitalized tissue (the lower uterine segment, lacerations, and incisions). The same pathogenesis, polymicrobial proliferation and tissue invasion, is associated with cesarean delivery, but surgical trauma, additional devitalization of tissue, blood and serum accumulation, and foreign bodies (sutures, staples) provide additional favorable anaerobic bacterial conditions. For highly indigent populations, the risk remains high (Poggi, 2013). See Table 30-1 for a list of common causative organisms.

Risk factors for postpartum uterine infection include the following:

- Cesarean deliveries prior to onset of labor—the single most significant risk (5% to 15% increased incidence)

- Preterm premature rupture of the amniotic membranes (PPROM)

- Prolonged labor preceding cesarean birth

- Multiple vaginal examinations during labor

- Compromised health status (low socioeconomic status, obesity, smoking, use of illicit drugs or alcohol, poor nutritional intake, and anemia)

- Use of fetal scalp electrode or intrauterine pressure catheter for internal monitoring during labor

- Obstetric trauma—episiotomy and lacerations of perineum, vagina, or cervix

- Chorioamnionitis—infection of placenta, chorion, and amnion

- Diabetes mellitus

- Preexisting bacterial vaginosis or *Chlamydia trachomatis* infection

- Instrument-assisted childbirth—vacuum or forceps

- Manual removal of the placenta, retained placental fragments, or uterine exploration after delivery

- Lapses in aseptic technique by surgical staff

Assessment findings consistent with endometritis are foul-smelling lochia, sawtooth fever (usually between 38.3°C [101.0°F] and 40°C [104°F]), uterine tenderness on palpation, lower abdominal pain, tachycardia that parallels the temperature increase, and chills (James, 2014).

Prophylactic antibiotics during cesarean section decrease the incidence of endometritis by as much as 60%, particularly after prolonged labor or ruptured membranes. Traditionally, antibiotics are given to the mother during surgery after the umbilical cord

TABLE 30-1 Common Causative Organisms in Metritis

AEROBES	ANAEROBES
• Group A, B, D streptococci	• *Peptostreptococcus*
• *Enterococcus*	• *Clostridium* species
• *Staphylococcus* species	• *Bacteroides* species
• *Escherichia coli*	• *Chlamydia trachomatis*
• *Klebsiella pneumonia*	• Genital mycoplasma
• *Proteus mirabilis*	
• *Gardnerella vaginalis*	
• *Neisseria gonorrhoeae*	

Sources: Data from Duff, P. (2014). Maternal and fetal infectious disorders. In R. K. Creasy & R. Resnik (Eds.), *Maternal–fetal medicine: Principles and practice* (7th ed., pp. 823–851). Philadelphia, PA: Saunders; Poggi, S. B. H. (2013). Postpartum hemorrhage & the abnormal puerperium. In A. H. DeCherney, L. Nathan, & A. S. Roman (Eds.), *Current diagnosis & treatment: Obstetrics & gynecology* (11th ed., pp. 349–368). New York, NY: McGraw-Hill.

is cut, thus avoiding difficulties in evaluating the baby for sepsis should the baby develop symptoms of infection. More recent evidence supports the administration of antibiotics 30 to 60 minutes prior to surgery, with no increase in neonatal infection (Duff, 2014).

PELVIC CELLULITIS (PARAMETRITIS)

Pelvic cellulitis (parametritis) is infection involving the connective tissue of the broad ligament or, in more severe forms, the connective tissue of all pelvic structures. The infection generally ascends upward in the pelvis by way of the lymphatics in the uterine wall but may also occur if pathogenic organisms invade a cervical laceration that extends upward into the connective tissue of the broad ligament—a direct pathway into the pelvis. Infection involving the peritoneal cavity is peritonitis. A pelvic abscess may form in the case of postpartum peritonitis and is most commonly found in the uterine ligaments, the cul-de-sac of Douglas, and the subdiaphragmatic space. Parametritis may be a secondary result of pelvic vein thrombophlebitis. This condition occurs when the clot, usually in the right ovarian vein, becomes infected and the wall of the vein breaks down from necrosis, spilling the infection into the connective tissues of the pelvis.

A woman suffering from parametritis may demonstrate a variety of symptoms, including marked high temperature (38.9° to 40°C [102° to 104°F]), chills, malaise, lethargy, abdominal pain, subinvolution of the uterus, tachycardia, and local and referred rebound tenderness (Poggi, 2013). If peritonitis develops, the woman becomes acutely ill, with severe pain, marked anxiety, high fever, rapid and shallow respirations, pronounced tachycardia, excessive thirst, abdominal distention, nausea, and vomiting.

Perineal Wound Infections

Given the degree of bacterial contamination that occurs with normal vaginal births, it is surprising that more women do not have infections of the episiotomy or repaired lacerations of the perineum, vagina, or vulva. Good aseptic technique is the likely rationale. When perineal wound infection occurs, it is recognized by the classic signs: redness, warmth, edema, purulent drainage, and, later, gaping of the wound that had previously been well approximated. Local pain may be severe.

After cesarean delivery, wound infection is most often associated with concurrent endometritis. The wound is typically red, indurated, tender at the margins, and draining purulent exudate. Some women have cellulitis without actual purulent drainage. Clinical examination is usually sufficient for diagnosis but culture of the exudate should be routinely done because community-acquired methicillin-resistant *Staphylococcus aureus* (CA-MRSA) infections are possible (Cunningham et al., 2014).

Clinical Therapy

The infection site and causative organism(s) are diagnosed by careful history and complete physical examination, blood tests, aerobic and anaerobic endometrial cultures (although this may be of limited value, because multiple organisms are usually present), and urinalysis to rule out urinary tract infection (UTI).

Localized wound infection is treated with broad-spectrum antibiotics, sitz baths, and analgesics as necessary for pain relief. Wounds with evidence of pus or serosanguineous effusion or an infected stitch site are opened and drained completely. Once the incision and drainage (I&D) of the wound is complete, it should be irrigated with warm saline 2 to 3 times daily and a clean dressing should be applied. It is then allowed to heal by secondary intention (Duff, 2014). Alternatively, it may be packed with saline dampened gauze and repacked 2 to 3 times daily and covered with clean gauze using aseptic technique. This allows removal of necrotic debris when packing is removed. Antibiotics with coverage against *Staphyloccus aureus* should be given. Antibiotics are typically continued until the wound base is clean and any signs of cellulitis have resolved.

Endometritis is treated with intravenous antibiotics, such as cephalosporins or penicillins. Women generally improve within 2 days of initiating antibiotics, which are continued until the client has been afebrile and asymptomatic for 24 hours. If fever continues at 48 hours after antibiotic therapy, an additional workup is necessary to check for refractory pelvic infection.

Parametritis and peritonitis are treated with aggressive IV therapy. Broad-spectrum antibiotics effective against the most common causative organisms are chosen initially until the results of culture and sensitivity reports are available. If multiple organisms are present, the approach to antibiotic therapy is continued unless no improvement is observed; then the antibiotic is changed. With appropriate antibiotic coverage, improvement should occur within a few days. Antibiotics are generally continued until the woman is afebrile and asymptomatic for 24 hours (Duff, 2014).

Approximately 90% to 95% of women with postpartum infection respond quickly to antibiotic therapy or drainage of abscesses and are associated with complete recovery and no long-term sequelae (Duff, 2014).

Nursing Management

For the Postpartum Woman With Puerperal Infection

Nursing Assessment and Diagnosis

Inspect the woman's perineum every 8 to 12 hours for signs of early infection. The REEDA scale helps you remember to consider *r*edness, *e*dema, *e*cchymosis, *d*ischarge, and *a*pproximation. Report immediately any degree of induration (hardening) to the clinician.

Document and report the presence of fever, malaise, abdominal pain, foul-smelling lochia, larger-than-expected uterus, tachycardia, and other signs of infection so that treatment can begin. The white blood cell (WBC) count, a usual objective measure of infection, cannot be used reliably because of the normal increase in WBCs during the postpartum period; a WBC count of 14,000 to 16,000 mm³ is not an unusual finding. An increase in WBC level of more than 30% in a 6-hour period, however, is indicative of infection.

Nursing diagnoses that may apply to the women with a puerperal infection include the following (NANDA-I © 2014):

- *Injury, Risk for,* related to the spread of infection
- *Pain* related to the presence of infection
- *Parenting, Risk for Impaired,* related to delayed parent–newborn attachment secondary to malaise and other symptoms of infection as well as possible separation of the newborn from the mother.

Nursing Plan and Implementation

HOSPITAL-BASED NURSING CARE

In caring for a woman during the postpartum period, you are responsible for teaching the woman self-care measures that are helpful in preventing infection. Careful attention to standard precautions and aseptic techniques during labor, birth, and postpartum are essential. If the woman has a draining wound or purulent lochia, it is especially important that those in contact with soiled items and linens practice good hand hygiene. Provide clear, concise instructions about wound care and how to discard soiled dressings appropriately to safeguard the woman and her caregivers.

If the woman is seriously ill, ongoing assessment of urine-specific gravity, as well as intake and output, is necessary. Carefully administer antibiotics as ordered and regulate the intravenous fluid rate. Ongoing assessment of the woman's condition is vital to detect subtle changes in her health status. Also address the woman's comfort needs related to hygiene, positioning, oral hygiene, and pain relief. See *Nursing Care Plan: For the Woman With a Puerperal Infection* for specific nursing care measures.

Promoting maternal–newborn attachment can be difficult with the acutely ill woman. You may provide pictures of the baby and keep the mother informed of the baby's well-being. Mementos, such as a footprint, a note written by the father "from the baby," or a video of the baby can be comforting to the mother during their separation. If she feels up to it, the new mother will also benefit from brief visits with her newborn.

The woman who wishes to breastfeed when her condition allows can maintain lactation by pumping her breasts regularly. Understanding that the opportunity to breastfeed is simply delayed, not eliminated, by the infectious process may improve the woman's morale. The partner of a seriously ill woman will be concerned about her condition and torn about spending time with her and with their newborn. Because maternal–newborn bonding may be compromised, allow for privacy with limited interruptions to facilitate father–newborn bonding.

COMMUNITY-BASED NURSING CARE

The woman with a puerperal infection needs assistance when she is discharged from the hospital. If the family cannot provide this home assistance, a referral to home care services is needed. Home care services should be contacted as soon as puerperal infection is diagnosed so that the home care nurse can meet with the woman for a family and home assessment and development of a home care plan.

Instruct the family in the care of a newborn, including feeding, bathing, cord care, immunizations, and significant observations that should be reported. A well-baby appointment should be scheduled. The woman who wishes to breastfeed when her condition allows can maintain lactation by pumping her breasts regularly. Instruct breastfeeding mothers receiving antibiotics to inspect the baby's mouth for signs of thrush and to report the finding to their healthcare provider.

Instruct the mother regarding activity, rest, medications, diet, and signs and symptoms of complications. Schedule her for a return medical visit. Emphasize the importance of taking the entire course of prescribed antibiotics even though she may begin to feel better before the bottle is empty. Inform her about the importance of pelvic rest; that is, she should not use tampons or douches nor have intercourse until she has been examined by her healthcare provider and told it is safe to resume those activities.

Evaluation

Expected outcomes of nursing care include the following:

- The infection is quickly identified and treated successfully, without further complications.
- The woman understands the infection and the purpose of therapy; she cooperates with ongoing antibiotic therapy after discharge.
- Maternal–newborn attachment is maintained.

Nursing Care Plan: For the Woman With a Puerperal Perineal Wound Infection

1. Nursing Diagnosis: *Infection, Risk for,* related to traumatized tissues (NANDA-I © 2014)

GOAL: The woman will be free of complications associated with infection.

INTERVENTION	RATIONALE
• Encourage the woman, staff, and family members to adhere to a strict hand hygiene policy.	• Hand hygiene kills bacteria and prevents cross-contamination.
• Review the woman's prenatal, intrapartum, and postpartum records for underlying problems that could contribute to poor wound healing or increased risk for spread of infection.	• Identifying underlying problems gives the caregiver an opportunity to initiate preventive measures that will promote healthy wound healing and stop the spread of infection.
• Monitor blood pressure, pulse, respiration, and temperature.	• Obtain baseline data; signs and symptoms of septic shock produce a decrease in blood pressure and an increase in respirations. Temperature increase of 38.0°C (100.4°F) or greater on any 2 days after the first 24 hr indicates infection.
• Instruct the woman on proper perineal care including wiping perineum from front to back after voiding, washing the perineum after voiding and defecating, and changing peri-pads frequently.	• Proper perineal care techniques enhance good hygiene and assist in removing urine and fecal contaminants from perineum. Changing peri-pads frequently decreases skin contact with a moist medium that favors bacterial growth.
• Encourage a well-balanced diet with adequate protein, calories, and vitamin C.	• Protein and vitamin C are essential nutrients for tissue healing and repair.
• Continue prenatal vitamins and iron as ordered.	
• Encourage the woman to consume 2000 mL of fluid a day.	• Maintains hydration and increases circulating volume. Dilutes organisms that are eliminated with voiding.
• Encourage use of the sitz bath, Surgigator, or the perineal light 2 to 4 times a day for at least 10–15 min.	• Moist or dry heat to the perineum increases localized blood flow, promotes healing, and provides comfort.
• Encourage early ambulation.	• Enhances circulation and drainage of lochia.
• Assess and report signs and symptoms of infection in perineum including redness, erythema, edema, discharge, approximation of wound edges (REEDA), and pain.	• Identifying signs and symptoms of infection early allows for prompt treatment and healing.
• **Collaborative:** Obtain lab work as ordered by the healthcare provider including culture and sensitivity, complete blood count (CBC) with differential, and white blood cell (WBC) count.	• Identifies abnormal lab values for early intervention. In addition, identifies infection and its causative organism for appropriate antibiotic treatment.
• Administer antibiotic therapy as ordered by the healthcare provider.	• Fights infection and helps prevent ascension of organisms into further tissue.
• Promote wound drainage by assisting healthcare provider in opening the wound if necessary. Also, if the wound is greater than 2–3 (0.8–1.2 in.) cm, pack with iodoform gauze.	• Iodoform gauze is used to maintain patency of wound opening. This promotes drainage and prevents abscesses from developing.
• Report signs and symptoms of severe infections: foul-smelling lochia, uterine subinvolution, uterine tenderness, severe lower abdominal pain, elevated temperature, elevated WBC count, general malaise, chills, lethargy, tachycardia, nausea and vomiting, and abdominal rigidity.	• Reporting signs and symptoms of severe infections early allows for initiation of appropriate therapy by the healthcare provider and prevents further spread of the invading pathogen.

EXPECTED OUTCOME: The woman will be free of complications associated with infection as evidenced by practicing behaviors that prevent the spread of infection and promote timely wound healing.

(continued)

Nursing Care Plan: For the Woman With a Puerperal Perineal Wound Infection (*continued*)

2. Nursing Diagnosis: *Pain, Acute,* related to the infection process (NANDA-I © 2014)

GOAL: The woman will be free of pain or have a level of relief that is acceptable.

INTERVENTION	RATIONALE
• Assess pain location and intensity; have the woman describe on a scale from 1 (mild) to 10 (severe). Assess nonverbal signs of pain, including facial grimacing and agitation.	• Assesses the need for pain management and evaluates interventions already implemented.
• Encourage the woman to discuss anxiety and fears.	• Reduces anxiety/fear and may decrease the woman's perception of pain.
• Encourage frequent rest periods and decrease disturbing environmental stimuli.	• Frequent rest periods will conserve woman's energy. Excessive environmental stimuli may increase woman's pain perception.
• Promote relaxation by encouraging diversionary activities including radio/television, reading, guided imagery, deep breathing techniques, massage, visualization, and meditation.	• Promotes relaxation and refocuses woman's attention away from the intensity of pain.
• **Collaborative:** Administer analgesics as ordered by the healthcare provider, evaluating the response to the analgesic and any adverse effects in a timely manner.	• Relieves pain and interrupts the pain, fear, tension cycle to facilitate relaxation.

EXPECTED OUTCOME: Woman is free of pain or has an acceptable level of pain as evidenced by verbalization of pain relief and the exhibition of a relaxed demeanor.

3. Nursing Diagnosis: *Parenting, Risk for Impaired,* related to pain secondary to maternal infection and/or separation from newborn to minimize exposure (NANDA-I © 2014)

GOAL: Mother will have no problems bonding with newborn and assuming responsibility for the care of the baby with assistance and later independently.

INTERVENTION	RATIONALE
• Provide quality time for mother and newborn contact.	• Aids in the bonding process.
• Encourage the partner or family members to give the woman videos and pictures of the newborn if the mother's condition requires separation from the baby.	• Promotes bonding and gives the mother reassurance that the newborn is being cared for.
• Encourage the partner and family members to become involved with the care of the baby and verbalize interaction to the mother.	• Allows the mother to feel as though she is involved in the care of the newborn.
• Encourage the mother to feed (breast or bottle) newborn if her condition is stable. If the mother is unable to breastfeed, encourage and assist her in pumping her breasts to maintain milk production.	• Hands-on participation in the newborn's care gives mother a positive outlook.
• Assess maternal support systems.	• As the mother is recovering, she will need assistance in household organization and personal care.
• **Collaborative:** Offer referrals to home health services, doula services, lactation services, and/or support groups.	• Ensures the woman's well-being and identifies problems that may require intervention.

EXPECTED OUTCOME: Mother will bond with the newborn as evidenced by exhibiting appropriate attachment behaviors when interacting with baby, providing care to self and baby, and verbalization of understanding of the parenting role.

Care of the Woman With a Urinary Tract Infection

The postpartum woman is at increased risk of developing urinary tract infection (UTI) caused by the normal postpartum diuresis, increased bladder capacity, decreased bladder sensitivity from stretching or trauma, and possible inhibited neural control of the bladder following the use of general or regional anesthesia and contamination from catheterization. The number of catheterizations performed during labor has increased in the population in recent years. It is essential that the mother empty her bladder completely with each voiding.

Overdistention of the Bladder

Overdistention occurs in the postpartum period when the woman is unable to empty her bladder, usually because of trauma or the effects of anesthesia. Women who have not sufficiently recovered from the effects of anesthesia cannot void spontaneously, and catheterization is necessary. After the effects of regional anesthesia have worn off, if the woman cannot void, postpartum urinary retention is highly indicative of UTI (Poggi, 2013). Other risk factors for urinary retention after childbirth include nulliparity, instrumental childbirth, and prolonged labor (Pessel & Tsai, 2013).

CLINICAL THERAPY

Overdistention in the early postpartum period is often managed by draining the bladder with a straight catheter as a one-time measure. If the overdistention recurs or is diagnosed later in the postpartum period, an indwelling catheter is generally ordered for 24 hours. An alternative urinary retention protocol involves bladder ultrasound scans with intervention based on the amount of urine volume.

Nursing Management

For the Postpartum Woman With a Urinary Tract Infection

Nursing Assessment and Diagnosis

The overdistended bladder appears as a large mass, reaching sometimes to the umbilicus and displacing the uterine fundus upward and to one side. Increased vaginal bleeding occurs, the fundus is boggy, and the woman may complain of cramping as the uterus attempts to contract. Some women also experience backache and restlessness.

Nursing diagnoses that may apply when a woman has difficulties with overdistention of the bladder include the following (NANDA-I © 2014):

- *Infection, Risk for,* related to urinary stasis secondary to overdistention of the bladder
- *Urinary Retention* related to decreased bladder sensitivity and normal postpartum diuresis

---

Clinical Tip

Postpartum urinary retention is often defined as "the absence of spontaneous urination within 6 hours of a vaginal delivery or within 6 hours after removal of an indwelling catheter post–cesarean delivery." The astute nurse will watch the woman's bladder for signs of retention—not the clock! Because urinary retention promotes uterine atony and a subsequent increase in bleeding and also contributes to the possibility of UTI, timely intervention is crucial.

Nursing Plan and Implementation

Diligent monitoring of the bladder during the recovery period and preventive health measures greatly reduce the chances for overdistention of the bladder. Encourage the mother to void spontaneously and help her use the toilet, if possible, or the bedpan, if she has received conductive anesthesia. Assist the woman to a normal position for voiding (i.e., sitting with the legs and feet lower than the trunk) and provide privacy to encourage voiding. The woman should receive medication for whatever pain she may be having before she attempts to void because pain may cause a reflex spasm of the urethra. Applying perineal ice packs after childbirth helps minimize edema, which may interfere with voiding. Pouring warm water over the perineum or having the woman void in the sitz bath may also be effective. Some women note that hearing running water nearby, blowing bubbles through a straw into a glass of water, or voiding onto a bedpan into which a few drops of tincture of peppermint have been added helps stimulate voiding.

If catheterization becomes necessary, employ careful, meticulous aseptic technique during catheter insertion. The vagina and vulva are traumatized to some degree by vaginal birth, and edema is common. This edema may obscure the urinary meatus; therefore, be extremely careful in cleansing the vulva and inserting the catheter. It is imperative to discard a catheter that has inadvertently been introduced into the vagina and thus contaminated. Catheterization is an uncomfortable procedure because of the postpartum trauma and edema of the tissue, so be careful and gentle not only in inserting the catheter but also in handling and cleaning the perineal area.

If the amount of urine drained from the bladder reaches 800 mL, the catheter is clamped and taped firmly to the woman's leg. Take the woman's vital signs before and after the procedure and note the woman's responses. After an hour, the catheter may be unclamped and placed on gravity drainage. This technique protects the bladder and prevents rapid intra-abdominal decompression (James, 2014). When the indwelling catheter is removed, a urine specimen is often sent to the laboratory. The tip of the catheter may also be removed and sent for culture.

Evaluation

Expected outcomes of nursing care include the following:

- The woman voids adequately to meet the demands of the increased fluid shifts during the postpartum period.
- The woman does not develop infection caused by stasis of urine.
- The woman actively incorporates self-care measures to decrease bladder overdistention.

Cystitis (Lower Urinary Tract Infection)

Retention of residual urine, bacteria introduced at the time of catheterization, and a bladder traumatized by birth combine to provide an excellent environment for the development of cystitis (lower UTI). *Escherichia coli* has been demonstrated to be the causative agent in most cases of postpartum cystitis and pyelonephritis (upper UTI). *Klebsiella pneumoniae* and *Proteus* species are significant pathogens, especially in women with histories of recurrent UTIs (Poggi, 2013). Generally, the infection ascends the urinary tract from the urethra to the bladder. If cystitis is not treated, the infection can spread to the kidneys because vesicoureteral reflux (backward flow of urine) forces contaminated urine into the renal pelvis.

CLINICAL THERAPY

When cystitis is suspected, a clean-catch, midstream urine sample is obtained for microscopic examination, culture, and sensitivity tests. The specimen may require collection by the nurse with the woman on a bedpan because few postpartum women can collect a true midstream, clean-catch specimen without contaminating the specimen with lochia. A catheterized specimen is avoided when possible because of the increased risk of infection. When the bacterial concentration is greater than 100,000 colonies of the same organism per milliliter of fresh urine, infection is generally present. Counts between 10,000 and 100,000 suggest infection, particularly if clinical symptoms are noted.

In the clinical setting, antibiotic therapy is often initiated before culture and sensitivity reports are available. Frequently used antibiotics include a preparation of trimethoprim–sulfamethoxazole double strength (Bactrim DS, Septra DS), one of the short-acting sulfonamides, nitrofurantoin (Macrobid), and, in the case of sulfa allergy, ampicillin or amoxicillin–clavulanic acid (Augmentin). The antibiotic is changed later if indicated by the results of the sensitivity report. Antispasmodics or urinary analgesic agents, such as Pyridium, may be given to relieve discomfort.

Nursing Management

For the Postpartum Woman With Cystitis

Nursing Assessment and Diagnosis

Acute cystitis usually causes symptoms of frequency, dysuria, urgency, hesitancy and dribbling, nocturia, and suprapubic pain. Encourage women to void every 2 to 4 hours to prevent urinary stasis and to report any sensations of incomplete emptying of the bladder or dysuria. Symptoms of cystitis often appear 2 to 3 days after childbirth and may include frequency, urgency, dysuria, and nocturia. Gross hematuria may be noted but high fever and systemic symptoms are not expected.

When a UTI progresses to pyelonephritis, systemic symptoms usually occur, and the woman becomes acutely ill. Symptoms include chills, high fever, flank pain (unilateral or bilateral), nausea, and vomiting, in addition to the signs of lower UTI. Costovertebral angle (CVA) tenderness may be noted on examination but is not required for diagnosis. Clean-catch urine specimens show large numbers of white blood cells and are positive for infection (bacterial growth more than 100,000 colony forming/mL of urine) (James, 2014).

Nursing diagnoses that may apply if a woman develops a postpartum UTI include the following (NANDA-I © 2014):

- *Pain, Acute,* with voiding related to dysuria secondary to infection
- *Health Management, Ineffective,* related to need for information about self-care measures to prevent UTI

Nursing Plan and Implementation

Screening for asymptomatic bacteriuria in pregnancy should be routine. Encourage frequent emptying of the bladder during labor and postpartum to prevent overdistention and trauma to the bladder. Catheterization technique and nursing actions to prevent overdistention (previously discussed) also apply. The woman with pyelonephritis must understand the importance of follow-up care after discharge to prevent recurrence or further complications.

Evaluation

Expected outcomes of nursing care include the following:

- The woman identifies the signs of UTI and her condition is treated successfully.
- The woman incorporates self-care measures to prevent the recurrence of UTI as part of her personal hygiene routine.
- The woman continues with any long-term therapy or follow-up as appropriate for the diagnosis.
- Maternal–newborn attachment is maintained and the woman is able to care for her baby effectively.

Care of the Woman With Postpartum Mastitis

Mastitis is an infection of the interlobular connective tissue in the breast that occurs primarily in lactating women. (Chapter 29 discusses the breastfeeding difficulties of the woman with mastitis.) Onset is usually between 2 and 8 weeks postpartum or any time that nursing frequency decreases. It ranges in severity from local inflammation to abscess and septicemia. The incidence of mastitis is estimated to be as high as 33% in breastfeeding mothers and less than 1% in nonlactating mothers (Jahanfar, Ng, & Teng, 2013).

The usual causative organisms are *Staphylococcus aureus, Haemophilus parainfluenzae, H. influenzae, Escherichia coli,* and *Streptococcus* species (Poggi, 2013). Infectious mastitis is a very serious infection, with fever, chills, headache, flulike muscle aches and malaise, and a warm, reddened, painful area of the breast, often wedge shaped because of the connective tissue septal divisions of the breast (James, 2014) (Figure 30-2).

The infection usually begins when bacteria invade the breast tissue after it has been traumatized in some way (see the factors commonly associated with mastitis in Table 30-2). Milk serves as a favorable medium for the invasive bacteria; thus milk stasis is another risk factor. (See *Concept Map: Milk Stasis.*) The most common sources of pathogenic organisms are the baby's nose and throat, although other sources include the hands of the mother or birthing unit personnel and the woman's circulating blood. Babies of women with mastitis generally remain well unless the causative organism is *Candida albicans.*

Concept Map

Medical Diagnoses: Milk stasis

Physical Exam
- Unilateral redness, warmth, tenderness
- Sensation of fullness above area of discomfort

Risk Factors
- Failure to empty all lobes
- Failure to alternate breasts at feeding
- Poor suck
- Poor let-down

Plugged Ducts

Nursing Diagnoses (NANDA-I © 2014)

Risk for infection secondary to milk stasis A&B swollen tender area on breast
- Monitor maternal temperature frequently
- Observe for symptoms of mastitis (fever, chills, hot, red, tender area on breast)
- Apply moist, warm compress—can also apply water directly in warm shower
- Nurse infant frequently on affected side
- Increase fluid intake

Acute pain secondary to milk stasis A&B redness and tenderness
- Apply warm compresses to affected areas
- Utilize circular pattern of massage to entire breast
- Establish frequent feeding patterns
- Change infant feeding position frequently
- Medications prn for pain

Risk for interrupted breastfeeding related to knowledge deficit
- Reinforce need to continue breast-feeding
- Advise frequent feeding
- Promote comfort with warm compresses, massage, medications
- Wear supportive bra

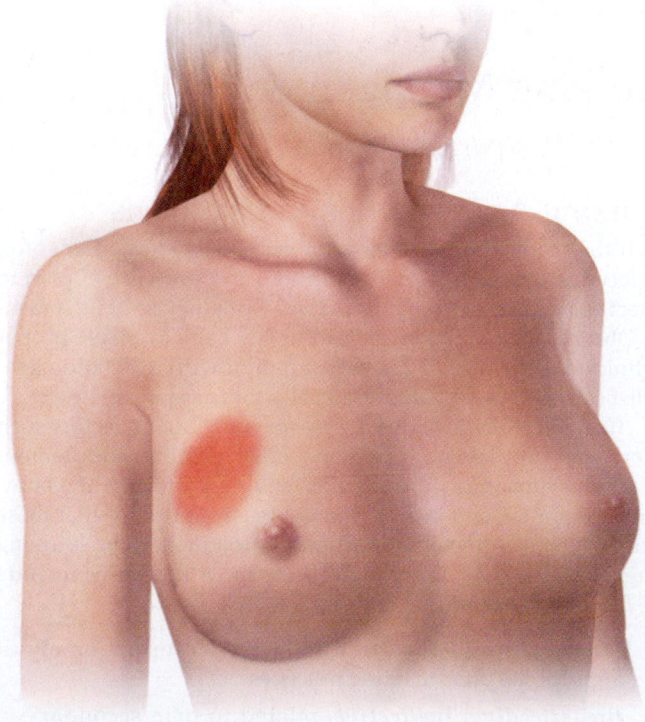

Figure 30–2 **Mastitis. Erythema and swelling are present in the upper outer quadrant of the breast. Axillary lymph nodes are often enlarged and tender. The segmental anatomy of the breast accounts for the demarcated, often V-shaped wedge of inflammation.**

When *Candida albicans* is the causative organism of mastitis, entering the breast through a small fissure or abrasion on the nipple, the baby will often have thrush, a candidal infection of the mouth. There may be a history of a recent course of antibiotics in the woman. Signs include late-onset nipple pain and burning pain of the nipple/areola, followed by stabbing pain of the breast during and between feedings, often radiating to the chest wall (Lawrence & Lawrence, 2014). Eventually, the skin of the affected breast becomes pink, shiny, flaking, and pruritic. Women may notice a yeasty odor to their milk. Unless the mother and her newborn are treated for *Candida*, recolonization will occur when breastfeeding is resumed.

Clinical Therapy

The diagnosis of mastitis is usually made based on clinical signs and symptoms. Culture and sensitivity of the breast milk may be done in some cases where the woman does not respond to antibiotics or has a severe, unusual, or recurring case of mastitis (Wambach, 2016). If a culture of the breast milk is ordered, it is more reliable with a midstream-type collection process. The nipple is washed first; then the first 3 mL of breast milk is manually expressed and discarded, after which the actual specimen is collected.

Treatment of mastitis primarily includes frequent and complete emptying of the breasts, as well as antibiotic coverage. Supportive measures such as rest, increased fluid intake (at least 2.0 to 2.5 L/day), a supportive bra, local application of warm, moist heat or ice packs, and analgesics should also be implemented (James, 2014). Nonsteroidal anti-inflammatory agents are recommended to treat both fever and inflammation. The preferred antibiotics are usually penicillinase-resistant penicillins, such as dicloxacillin 500 mg every 6 hours orally

TABLE 30-2 Factors Associated with Development of Mastitis

MILK STASIS

Failure to change the baby's position to allow emptying of all lobes

Failure to alternate breasts at feedings

Poor suck

Poor let-down

ACTIONS THAT PROMOTE ACCESS/MULTIPLICATION OF BACTERIA

Poor hand hygiene technique

Improper breast hygiene

Failure to air dry breasts after breastfeeding

Use of plastic-lined breast pads that trap moisture against nipple

BREAST/NIPPLE TRAUMA

Incorrect positioning for breastfeeding

Poor latch-on

Failure to rotate position on nipple

Incorrect or aggressive pumping technique

Cracked nipples

Obstruction of Ducts

Restrictive clothing

Constricting bra

Underwire bra

CHANGE IN NUMBER OF FEEDINGS/FAILURE TO EMPTY BREASTS

Attempted weaning

Missed feeding

Prolonged sleeping, including sleeping through night

Favoring side of nipple soreness

LOWERED MATERNAL DEFENSES

Fatigue

Stress

"life" versus *antibiotic*, which literally means "against life"). Probiotics compete with disease-causing microorganisms in the gastrointestinal tract. When antibiotics are taken, they kill many of the beneficial bacteria that exist naturally in the digestive tract. Supplementing with probiotics after a course of antibiotics is frequently prescribed by nutritionists and complementary practitioners. Commonly used probiotics include *Lactobacillus acidophilus* and *Bifidobacterium bifidum*; there are other species of *Lactobacillus* and *Bifidobacterium* that have been shown to be effective in treating such conditions as diarrhea and vaginal infections. Bifidobacterium also competes against *Candida albicans.* Probiotics can be taken in the form of powder, capsules, and suppositories, or in fermented milk products such as yogurt or kefir

Other complementary therapies used for mastitis include belladonna, acupuncture, oxytocin nasal spray to improve milk ejection, a traditional Chinese herb known as extracts of *Fructus gleditsiae*, application of cabbage leaves over the affected area to relieve engorgement, and application of a solution of bacteriocins to nipple and areola to treat staphylococcal mastitis (Wambach, 2016).

Abscess formation is a complication of mastitis, resulting from delayed treatment, treatment failure, or abrupt weaning of the baby. Abscesses are usually in the upper outer quadrants of the breast and will show a localized area of erythema, exquisite tenderness, and induration. Breast abscess may require incision and drainage. Breastfeeding can usually continue on the affected breast, as long as the incision is well away from the areola. The baby can continue to nurse on the unaffected breast (Walker, 2014).

Improved outcome, a decreased duration of symptoms, and decreased incidence of a breast abscess result if the breasts continue to be emptied by either breastfeeding or pumping. Thus continued breastfeeding is recommended in the process of mastitis. The plan of care should include contacting the woman within 24 hours of initiation of treatment to ensure that symptoms are subsiding.

Nursing Management

For the Postpartum Woman With Mastitis

Nursing Assessment and Diagnosis

Each day assess the mother's breast consistency, skin color, surface temperature, nipple condition, and presence of pain to detect early signs of problems that may predispose her to mastitis. Observe the mother breastfeeding her baby to ensure proper technique (see Chapter 25). Consultation with a lactation specialist can be of great value, especially for first-time mothers.

If an infection develops, assess for contributing factors such as cracked nipples, poor hygiene, engorgement, supplemental feedings, change in routine or feeding pattern of the baby, abrupt weaning, and lack of proper breast support so that these factors can be corrected as part of the treatment plan. Nursing diagnoses that may apply to the woman with mastitis include the following (NANDA-I © 2014):

- *Trauma, Risk for,* related to lack of information about appropriate breastfeeding practices
- *Breastfeeding, Ineffective,* related to pain secondary to development of mastitis

Nursing Plan and Implementation

Preventing mastitis is far simpler than treating it. Ideally mothers are instructed in proper breastfeeding technique prenatally. Assist the mother to breastfeed soon after childbirth and review

or, with history of mild milk allergy, a cephalosporin such as cephalexin 500 mg every 6 hours orally (Duff, 2014). The woman should continue to breastfeed; in fact, regular drainage of both breasts actually helps by preventing milk stasis and abscess formation, and there is virtually no risk to the newborn. If there has been no change in symptomatology in 48 hours, modification of the antibiotic therapy will be considered. There have been increasing cases of methicillin-resistant *Staphylococcus aureus (MRSA)* mastitis. When a woman does not respond to first-line antibiotics, MRSA should be considered and a breast milk culture and antibiotic sensitivity should be ordered (Wambach, 2016).

Candidal infections can be especially stubborn. Initial treatment generally involves antifungal creams or ointments once or twice daily, as well as treating the baby with oral nystatin for a full 2 weeks (Lawrence & Lawrence, 2014). Another treatment option is oral fluconazole (Diflucan), which is excreted in breast milk but is not considered to be toxic to the baby and can be used if other agents fail (Lawrence & Lawrence, 2014). Women should be instructed to cleanse their nipples with warm water and allow air drying before application of the antifungal medication (Lawrence & Lawrence, 2014).

Probiotics are a category of dietary supplements consisting of beneficial microorganisms (*pro* means "for" and *biotic* means

TABLE 30-3 Symptoms of Engorgement, Plugged Duct, and Mastitis

ONSET	LOCATION	HEAT/SWELLING	TEMPERATURE	PAIN	GENERAL SYMPTOMS
ENGORGEMENT					
Gradual; postpartum	Entire breast	Breast is hot and swollen	Less than 38.4°C (101.1°F)	Entire breast	None
PLUGGED DUCT					
Gradual; after feedings	One side of breast	Little or no heat; there may be swelling	Less than 38.4°C (101.1°F)	Mild pain on affected side	None
MASTITIS					
Sudden; usually after about 10 days	Generally one side of breast	Swelling on affected side; skin is red and hot	Greater than 38.4°C (101.1°F)	Intense pain on affected side	Similar to flu

Source: Data from Lawrence, R. A., & Lawrence, R. M. (2014). *Breastfeeding: A guide for the medical profession* (8th ed.). Philadelphia, PA: Elsevier Mosby.

correct technique. Comanagement of breastfeeding between the nurse and a certified lactation specialist is often possible. Encourage all women, even those not breastfeeding, to wear a good supportive bra at all times to prevent milk stasis, especially in the lower lobes, and to change breast pads frequently (James, 2014).

Meticulous hand hygiene by the breastfeeding mother and all personnel is the primary measure in preventing epidemic nursery infections and subsequent maternal mastitis. Prompt attention to mothers who have blocked milk ducts eliminates stagnant milk as a growth medium for bacteria. If the mother finds that one area of her breast feels distended, she can rotate the position of her baby for nursing, manually express milk remaining in the breast after feeding (usually necessary only if the baby is not sucking well), or massage the caked area toward the nipple as the baby nurses. Mothers who develop mastitis can apply warm, moist compresses to the affected area before and during breastfeeding. Encourage the mother to breastfeed frequently, starting with the unaffected breast until let-down occurs in the affected breast, then switching to the affected breast until it is emptied completely. After nursing, the mother can leave a small amount of milk on each nipple to prevent cracking, allow nipples to air dry, and apply cold packs to reduce pain and edema (James, 2014). Early identification of and intervention for sore nipples are also essential, as is prompt assessment of the breastfeeding mother's breast when thrush is discovered in her newborn's mouth. For a detailed discussion of breastfeeding problems, see the section Breastfeeding Concerns Following Discharge in Chapter 29.

DISCHARGE PLANNING AND HOME CARE TEACHING

The woman should be aware of the importance of regular, complete emptying of the breasts to prevent engorgement and stasis. She should also understand the role of let-down in successful breastfeeding, correct positioning of the baby on the nipple, proper latch-on, and the principle of supply and demand. If the mother is taking antibiotics, she needs to understand the importance of completing the full course of antibiotics, even if the infection seems to clear quickly. Babies tolerate the small amount of antibiotics in breast milk without difficulty. Breastfeeding mothers who are returning to work outside the home need information on how to do so successfully. Because mastitis tends to develop after discharge, it is important to include information about signs and symptoms in the discharge teaching and printed materials (Table 30-3). All flulike symptoms should be considered a sign of mastitis until proven otherwise. If symptoms develop, the woman should contact her caregiver immediately because prompt treatment helps to prevent abscess formation.

COMMUNITY-BASED NURSING CARE

Because symptoms seldom occur before the second to fourth week postpartum, birthing unit nurses often are not fully aware of how uncomfortable and acutely ill the woman can be. The home care nurse who suspects mastitis on the basis of assessment findings refers the woman to her healthcare provider. As the home care nurse, you may be asked to obtain a sample of breast milk to be cultured for the causative organism.

If the mother feels too ill to breastfeed or develops an abscess that prevents nursing, you can help the mother obtain a breast pump to help her maintain lactation and can provide opportunities for demonstration and return demonstration of pumping. Assist the mother to deal with her feelings about temporarily being unable to breastfeed. Referral to a lactation consultant or to La Leche League can be invaluable to the woman's physical and emotional adjustment to mastitis.

Evaluation

Expected outcomes of nursing care include the following:

- The woman is aware of the signs and symptoms of mastitis.
- The woman reports the mastitis signs and symptoms early and is treated successfully.
- The woman resumes breastfeeding if she chooses.
- The woman understands self-care measures she can employ to prevent the recurrence of mastitis.

Care of the Woman With Postpartum Thromboembolic Disease

Thromboembolic disease may occur antepartum, but it is generally considered a postpartum complication. *Venous thrombosis* refers to blood clot (thrombus formation) at an area of impeded blood flow in a superficial or deep vein, usually in the legs.

When the thrombus is formed in response to inflammation in the vein wall, it is termed **thrombophlebitis**. Pulmonary embolism, a rare, life-threatening condition, occurs when thrombi formed in the deep leg veins are carried to the pulmonary artery, obstructing pulmonary blood flow to one or both lungs.

Three major causes of thromboembolic disease, often referred to as the *Virchow triad*, are hypercoagulability of blood, venous stasis, and injury to the epithelium of the blood vessel. Changes in the woman's coagulation system in pregnancy contribute to hypercoagulability and compression of the common iliac vein by the gravid uterus, which leads to venous stasis (Witcher & Hamner, 2013). These factors increase the risk of thromboembolic disease in pregnant and postpartum women approximately 2 to 6 times. In contrast, deep vein thrombosis (DVT), which is more serious, occurs most commonly in postpartum women between postpartum days 10 to 20.

Risk factors associated with increased risk of thromboembolic disease include the following:

- Cesarean birth
- Immobility (prolonged)
- Obesity
- Cigarette smoking
- Previous thromboembolic disease or strong family history
- Trauma to extremity (can include injury from incorrect positioning or prolonged interval in stirrups during labor)
- Varicose veins
- Diabetes mellitus
- Advanced maternal age
- Multiparity
- Anemia
- Malignancy
- Inherited coagulation pathway deficiency
- Protein C & S deficiency

Factors contributing directly to the development of thromboembolic disease postpartum include (1) increased amounts of certain blood-clotting factors; (2) postpartum thrombocytosis (increased quantity of circulating platelets and their increased adhesiveness); (3) release of thromboplastin substances from the tissue of the decidua, placenta, and fetal membranes; and (4) increased amounts of fibrinolysis inhibitors. Because all women are at risk for thromboembolic disease during the childbearing period, attention should be given to measures that might prevent this complication (see Table 30-4).

Superficial Leg Vein Disease

Superficial thrombophlebitis is far more common in the postpartum period than during pregnancy. Often the clot involves one of the saphenous veins. This disorder is more common in women with preexisting varices (enlarged veins), although it is not limited to these women. They may also occur as a sequelae to IV catheterization. Symptoms—tenderness in a portion of the vein, some local heat and redness, normal temperature or low-grade fever, and occasionally slight elevation of the pulse—usually become apparent about the third or fourth postpartum day. A tender palpable cord may be noted along a portion of the veins. Treatment involves application of local heat, elevation of the affected limb, bed rest, analgesics, and the use of elastic support hose (James, 2014). Anticoagulants are usually not necessary unless complications develop. Pulmonary embolism is extremely rare.

Women With Special Needs Lupus

Women with lupus have a higher incidence of thromboembolic disease and need close observation for the development of deep vein thrombosis (DVT) and pulmonary embolism (PE). Early ambulation and frequent leg exercises should be encouraged. Symptoms of thromboembolic disease should be reviewed. Hormonal contraceptives that contain estrogen are contraindicated in these women.

Deep Vein Thrombosis

Deep vein thrombosis (DVT) is more frequently seen in women with a history of thrombosis. Certain obstetric complications, such as polyhydramnios, preeclampsia, and operative birth, are also associated with an increased incidence. After a clinical diagnosis of DVT, a woman's risk in a subsequent pregnancy increases.

Clinical manifestations may include edema of the ankle and leg and an initial low-grade fever often followed by high temperature and chills. Other findings include tenderness or pain, a palpable cord, changes in limb color, and difference in limb circumference of more than 2 cm (0.8 in.). Depending on the vein involved, the woman may complain of pain in the popliteal and lateral tibial areas (popliteal vein), pain in the entire lower leg and foot (anterior and posterior tibial veins), inguinal tenderness (femoral vein), or pain in the lower abdomen (iliofemoral vein). Homans sign (see Figure 28–9) may or may not be positive. Most DVTs occur in the left leg. Because of reflex arterial spasm, sometimes the limb is pale and cool to the touch and peripheral pulses may be diminished or difficult to palpate. These signs and symptoms have less than 50% specificity, however, and diagnosis of DVT is usually confirmed by compression ultrasound and D-dimer assays (Leung & Lockwood, 2014).

Clinical Reasoning Postpartum Leg Pain

Wanda Sugiyama, G1P1, had a cesarean birth after a prolonged labor and failure to progress. As she is walking in the hallway with her husband, you notice that Wanda is limping slightly, and you comment on that observation. Wanda responds that she is having pain in her right lower leg. She says, "Maybe I pulled a muscle during labor." *What would you do?*

Clinical Therapy

Treatment involves the immediate intravenous (IV) administration of either standard unfractionated heparin or low-molecular-weight heparin (LMWH) using an infusion pump to permit continuous, accurate infusion to stabilize the clot. An example of a possible regimen is a subcutaneous injection of enoxaparin 1 mg/kg twice daily (Witcher & Hamner, 2013). Heparin therapy is continued until the international normalized ratio (INR) with oral warfarin is achieved at 2.0 to 3.0. An advantage of LMWH is a safe profile and dosing not reliant on monitoring the *activated partial thromboplastin time (aPTT)* at a laboratory. Maintenance with warfarin sodium (Coumadin) is started at 1 to 5 days. In some cases thrombolytics (streptokinase or urokinase) or an embolectomy may be used. Strict bed rest and elevation of the affected leg are required, and analgesics are given as necessary to relieve discomfort. In most cases thrombectomy (surgical removal of the clot) is not necessary.

TABLE 30-4 Measures to Decrease Risk of Thromboembolic Disease in Childbearing Women

ANTEPARTUM MEASURES	INTRAPARTUM MEASURES	POSTPARTUM MEASURES
• Advise woman to avoid sedentary lifestyle and to exercise as possible (walking is ideal). • Advise to quit smoking. • Teach to avoid prolonged standing or sitting in one position or sitting with legs crossed. • Encourage elevation of legs when sitting. • Teach to avoid tight knee-high hose or other constrictive garments. • Encourage to take frequent breaks during long car trips to walk around, thereby preventing prolonged venous stasis.	• Encourage ambulation unless contraindicated in early labor; later, encourage leg exercises. • Do not gatch bed or use pillows under knees. • Pad stirrups to prevent pressure on popliteal vessels. • Ensure correct positioning in stirrups to minimize pressure on the popliteal area. • Limit time in stirrups as possible because trauma is a factor. • After cesarean birth, initiate leg/foot exercises as soon as possible (in recovery) to promote venous return. • Use antiembolism stockings for women at risk for DVT.	• Encourage early ambulation. • For women on bed rest, advise or assist with turning and leg exercises every 2 hours (woman may be encouraged to rotate ankles and to "write baby's name in the air with her toes"). • Encourage fluids to avoid dehydration. • Advise no smoking. • Use antiembolism stockings with those at risk, including after cesarean birth. • Advise against prolonged sitting and crossing of legs. • Encourage elevation of legs while sitting.

Once the symptoms have subsided (usually in several days), the woman may begin walking while wearing elastic support stockings. The woman will continue on warfarin sodium (Coumadin) for 4 to 6 weeks postpartum or up to a minimum of 3 months (Witcher & Hamner, 2013). While taking warfarin sodium (Coumadin), prothrombin times are assessed periodically to maintain correct dosage levels. Periodic assessment for signs of bleeding is essential, including those for hematuria and fecal occult blood. In those who cannot be given anticoagulants or have had a venous thromboembolism (VTE) event despite full anticoagulation, a vena cava filtering device may be considered (American College of Obstetrics & Gynecology [ACOG], 2011; Cunningham et al., 2014). To prevent recurrence in subsequent pregnancies, prophylactic treatment will be considered.

Nursing Management
For the Woman With Postpartum Thromboembolic Disease

Nursing Assessment and Diagnosis

Carefully assess the woman's history for factors predisposing her to development of thrombosis or thrombophlebitis. In addition, as part of regular postpartum assessment, be alert to any complaints of pain in the legs, inguinal area, or lower abdomen because such pain may indicate DVT. Also assess the woman's legs for evidence of edema, temperature change, or pain with palpation.

Nursing diagnoses that may apply to a postpartum woman with a thrombotic disease include the following (NANDA-I © 2014):

- *Tissue Perfusion: Peripheral, Ineffective,* related to obstructed venous return
- *Pain, Acute,* related to tissue hypoxia and edema secondary to vascular obstruction
- *Knowledge, Deficient,* related to self-care after discharge on anticoagulant therapy

Nursing Plan and Implementation

HOSPITAL-BASED NURSING CARE

Women are at risk for thromboembolic disease during the childbearing period, especially during labor and the postpartum period. Attention should be given to nursing measures that might prevent or deal with this complication (Table 30-4).

Once DVT is diagnosed, provide appropriate comfort measures, maintain the heparin therapy, monitor the woman during warfarin sodium (Coumadin) therapy, and watch closely for signs of pulmonary embolism. Assess for evidence of bleeding related to heparin and keep the antagonist for heparin, protamine sulfate, readily available. Women discharged on warfarin sodium (Coumadin) should be taught about the drug and safety factors associated with its use. See *Teaching Highlights: What the Postpartum Woman Taking Warfarin Needs to Know.*

Remind the woman to mention her history of thrombosis or thrombophlebitis to her healthcare provider/CNM during subsequent pregnancies so that preventive measures can be instituted early (James, 2014). See *Nursing Care Plan: For the Woman With Thromboembolic Disease.*

COMMUNITY-BASED NURSING CARE

Because the mother with postpartum thromboembolic disease will depend on others for much of her initial home care, it is helpful for the father of the newborn to be involved in preparations for discharge. Provide ample time to answer questions and clarify instructions, verbally and in writing. Evaluate the extent to which both the mother and the father have understood instructions regarding the plan of care. It is especially important to assess the couple's plans to ensure complete bed rest for the mother. They might explore ways for her to maintain bed rest and still spend quality time with her newborn and any other children. For example, young children can sit on the bed for storytelling or play quiet games, and the newborn's crib can be placed next to the mother's bed.

The father/partner may be assuming multiple roles in these circumstances—household manager, parent, worker, and caregiver. Fatigue is inevitable. There may also be financial concerns as a result of prolonged health care or extended time away from work to care for the family. Many concerns will not surface until the couple actually returns home and fully comprehends the reality of their situation. For that reason, it is valuable to provide them with an accessible resource person and to plan telephone or home visit follow-up care.

Signs of postpartum thrombophlebitis may not occur until after discharge from the birthing unit. Consequently all couples must be taught to recognize its signs and symptoms and appreciate the importance of reporting them immediately and not massaging the affected leg. If signs and symptoms occur after discharge, a short readmission may be required. In that case

| TEACHING HIGHLIGHTS | What the Postpartum Woman Taking Warfarin Needs to Know |

- Warfarin is compatible with breastfeeding (Hale & Rowe, 2014).
- Foods high in vitamin K lessen warfarin's effectiveness; thus you will need to strive for consistent daily intake so that accurate dosage of the drug can be achieved. If intake of vitamin K decreases significantly, there is a risk of bleeding.
- Foods high in vitamin K include cauliflower, soybean and canola oil, mayonnaise, broccoli, green and black tea, peppers, spinach, collard, and other leafy greens. Many multivitamins contain vitamin K; you may take them but, again, should do so consistently.
- Cranberry juice increases the effects of warfarin and, if desired, should be consumed in moderation and with consistency.
- Binge alcohol use inhibits warfarin metabolism; an occasional alcoholic beverage does not affect coagulation adversely.
- Several herbals affect the efficacy of warfarin sodium; for example, garlic, ginger, and ginkgo prolong prothrombin time (PT) and should be avoided.
- Vitamin C doses up to 500 mg per day and vitamin E doses up to 400 international units per day are considered safe; higher doses can affect coagulation.
- Certain medications such as aspirin and other nonsteroidal anti-inflammatory drugs increase anticoagulant activity and should be avoided.
- Be alert for signs of bleeding, such as bleeding gums, epistaxis, petechiae or ecchymosis, and evidence of blood in the urine or stool.
- Check for possible medication interaction with warfarin before taking any other medication.
- Be cautious about using sharp objects such as knives or razor blades to avoid injury.
- Avoid risky behaviors that could contribute to falls.
- Wear protective gloves during gardening or heavy housework and always wear shoes to keep hands and feet safe from injury.
- Carry a MedicAlert card or wear a bracelet stating that you are taking warfarin in case of emergency.
- Inform all healthcare providers (including dentists) that you are taking anticoagulants and to have vitamin K available in case of bleeding.
- Bleeding should be reported if it fails to stop within 10 minutes.
- Keep scheduled appointments for PT assessment to guide dosing.
- Consider utilizing point-of-care testing, which decreases the inconvenience of going to the laboratory. Home self-testing involves a single capillary fingerstick (CoaguChek, ProTime, Avocet) to test thromboplastin-mediated clotting expressed as PT or INR. The therapeutic range of INR is 2–3, and the risk of bleeding increases significantly when the INR is 3 or greater (Leung & Lockwood, 2014).

every effort is made to allow mother, father/partner, and newborn to remain together.

After DVT, some women continue to have leg pain, edema, and dermatitis of the affected extremity for prolonged periods caused by a residual venous abnormality. This situation can significantly affect quality of life. Continuing use of compression stockings for a minimum of 1 year after diagnosis will help to prevent this complication of DVT.

Evaluation

Expected outcomes of nursing care include the following:

- The woman seeks treatment for her thrombophlebitis early and it is managed successfully, without further complications.
- At discharge the woman is able to explain the purpose, dosage regimen, and necessary precautions associated with any prescribed medications such as anticoagulants.
- The woman can discuss the self-care measures and ongoing therapies (such as the use of elastic stockings) that are indicated.

- The woman has bonded successfully with her newborn and is able to care for her baby effectively.

Care of the Woman With a Postpartum Psychiatric Disorder

Types of Postpartum Psychiatric Disorders

The classification of postpartum psychiatric disorders is a subject of some controversy. The *Diagnostic and Statistical Manual of Mental Disorders (DSM-5)* (American Psychiatric Association [APA], 2013) contains a peripartum onset specifier to the mood disorder diagnostic category of psychiatric disorders. It is proposed that postpartum psychiatric disorders be considered one diagnosable syndrome with three subclasses: (1) adjustment reaction with depressed mood, (2) postpartum mood episodes with psychotic features, and (3) peripartum major mood episodes (also known as postpartum depression). The incidence, etiology, symptoms, treatment, and prognosis vary with each subclass.

Nursing Care Plan: For the Woman With Thromboembolic Disease

1. Nursing Diagnosis: *Tissue Perfusion: Peripheral, Ineffective,* related to interruption of venous blood flow secondary to complications of labor and birth (NANDA-I © 2014)

GOAL: The woman's presenting signs and symptoms are relieved.

INTERVENTION	RATIONALE
• Assess, record, and report signs of thrombophlebitis.	• Early detection of developing thrombophlebitis permits prompt treatment. As the thrombus increases in size, signs of obstruction also increase.
• Assess leg for edema, peripheral pulse, temperature, color, and tenderness every 8 hours. Initially note presence of palpable cord. Homans sign may be assessed, but is only positive in less than 50% of clients with a DVT (James, 2014).	• Edema/swelling, diminished or absent peripheral pulse, pallor, cool skin temperature, and tenderness are symptoms of deep vein thrombosis (DVT) and indicate dysfunction of peripheral circulation in the lower extremities. Measure circumference of lower leg to monitor for swelling. Peripheral pulses in both legs should be palpated for pulse rate and pulse strength to allow for comparison. A lower extremity cool to the touch may be due to reflex arterial spasm.
• Maintain bed rest during the acute phase.	• Bed rest is ordered to decrease the possibility that a portion of the clot will dislodge and result in pulmonary embolism.
• Provide warm, moist soaks as ordered.	• Warmth promotes blood flow to affected area.
• Maintain limb in elevated position.	• Elevation of affected limb promotes venous return and helps decrease edema.
• Initiate progressive ambulation following the acute phase and provide properly fitting compression stockings before ambulation. These should be properly measured.	• Elastic compression stockings or "TEDs" help prevent pooling of venous blood in lower extremities. Stockings should be carefully measured according to guidelines to ensure proper pressure gradient and avoid "garter-like" roll at top.
	• Woman may begin to ambulate within a few days when symptoms subside.
• **Collaborative:** Administer unfractionated heparin as ordered, by continuous intravenous drip, heparin lock, or subcutaneously, or administer low molecular weight heparin (LMWH) subcutaneously as ordered including:	• Heparin does not dissolve blood clot but is administered to prevent further clotting and improve tissue perfusion. It is safe for breastfeeding mothers because heparin is not excreted in breast milk.
1. Monitor IV or heparin lock site (if in use) for patency, signs of infiltration, or signs of infection.	
2. Obtain international normalized ratio (INR) and partial thromboplastin time (PTT) per healthcare provider order and review before administering heparin.	
3. Observe for signs of anticoagulant overdose with resultant bleeding including:	
a. Hematuria	
b. Epistaxis	
c. Ecchymosis or petechiae	
d. Bleeding gums	
4. Provide protamine sulfate, per healthcare provider order, to combat bleeding problems related to heparin overdose.	• Protamine sulfate is a heparin antagonist, given intravenously, which is almost immediately effective in counteracting bleeding complications caused by heparin overdose.
5. Monitor and report any signs of pulmonary embolism.	• Pulmonary embolism is a major complication of DVT/thrombophlebitis.

(continued)

Nursing Care Plan: For the Woman With Thromboembolic Disease (continued)

6. Initiate or support any emergency treatment.	• Signs and symptoms may occur suddenly and require immediate emergency treatment; prognosis is related to size and location of embolism.
7. Obtain prothrombin time (PT) and review before beginning warfarin. Repeat periodically per healthcare provider order.	• PT is the test most commonly used to monitor the blood of women receiving warfarin.

EXPECTED OUTCOME: Woman will have increased venous return from lower leg as evidenced by decreased edema in lower leg, negative Homans sign, and no pain or tenderness in lower leg.

2. **Nursing Diagnosis:** *Pain, Acute,* related to tissue hypoxia and edema secondary to vascular obstruction (NANDA-I © 2014)

GOAL: Woman will obtain relief of pain or experience level of pain that is acceptable.

INTERVENTION	RATIONALE
• Administer analgesics per healthcare provider order. Notify healthcare provider if pain is not relieved.	• Analgesics act to relieve pain and enable the woman to rest. Aspirin or ibuprofen products are contraindicated because they inhibit platelet adhesiveness. Acetaminophen may be ordered by the healthcare provider.
• Observe or report disruptive effects of pain on emotions and behavior.	• Once pain decreases, woman is more likely to ambulate, which will help increase venous return and decrease edema.
• Provide supportive nursing comfort measures such as backrubs, provision of quiet time for sleep, diversional activities, or imagery.	

EXPECTED OUTCOME: Woman will have reduction in pain as evidenced by a pain level less than 5 at all times.

3. **Nursing Diagnosis:** *Parenting, Risk for Impaired,* related to decreased maternal-newborn interaction secondary to bed rest and IVs (NANDA-I © 2014)

GOAL: Woman will demonstrate evidence of positive physical and social interaction with newborn.

INTERVENTION	RATIONALE
• Maintain mother–newborn attachment when mother is on bed rest:	• Maternal–newborn attachment is enhanced by frequent contact and opportunities to interact.
• Provide frequent contacts for mother and baby; modified rooming-in if possible by having the crib placed close to the mother's bed and nurse checking often to help mother lift or move baby.	
• Encourage mother to continue feeding newborn.	

EXPECTED OUTCOME: Woman will develop attachment bonds as evidenced by physical interactions: good eye contact, touching the baby, holding baby close, attempting to comfort baby, and kissing baby, and social interactions: calling baby by name, making positive comments about baby, asking questions about baby, asking questions about baby care, and talking to baby.

4. **Nursing Diagnosis:** *Family Processes, Interrupted,* related to illness of family member (NANDA-I © 2014)

GOAL: Woman and her family will cope effectively with her illness.

INTERVENTION	RATIONALE
• Encourage woman to express her concerns to her partner. Assist couple in planning ways to manage while woman is hospitalized and after her discharge.	• Illness of any family member impacts the entire family. This is especially true when the family situation is such that the mother is the primary nurturer and she is absent. Family members attempt to continue their own roles while also assuming the tasks of the missing mother. This can result in crisis.
• Encourage partner or support person to bring other children to the hospital to visit mother and meet new sibling.	
• Encourage partner or support person to bring in family pictures and notes from other children. Encourage phone calls.	
• Contact social services if indicated to obtain additional assistance for family if needed.	

EXPECTED OUTCOMES: Woman expresses assurance that her family misses her but is coping effectively as evidenced by:

- Family visits woman frequently.
- Woman and family verbalize plan for division of family tasks while the woman is hospitalized and understanding of potential needs of woman once released from hospital.

5. **Nursing Diagnosis:** *Bleeding, Risk for,* related to lack of information about DVT/thrombophlebitis, its treatment, preventive measures, and the medication warfarin sodium (Coumadin) (NANDA-I © 2014).

GOAL: Woman will understand her condition, its treatment, safety during treatment, and long-term implications.

INTERVENTION	RATIONALE
- Provide information (both verbal and written supplements) about the woman's condition, its treatment regimen, the importance of compliance, and safety factors. Provide contact information that the woman can access 24/7.	- Such discussion is essential to help the woman understand the condition, her medication, and its implications. She must have a clear understanding to be able to provide effective self-care.
- Discuss ways of avoiding circulatory stasis such as avoiding prolonged standing, sitting, crossing legs, and wearing restrictive clothing.	- Prolonged sitting, standing, and crossing legs should be avoided, as these activities decrease venous return.
- Review need to wear support stockings and to plan for rest periods with legs elevated.	
- In the presence of DVT, discuss the following:	- Woman placed on warfarin (Coumadin) therapy for 2–6 months at home.
1. The use of warfarin, its side effects, possible interactions with other medications, and the need to have dosage assessed through periodic checks of the prothrombin time.	
2. Signs of bleeding, which may be associated with warfarin sodium and need to be reported immediately, include the following: hematuria, epistaxis, ecchymosis, bleeding gums, and rectal bleeding.	
3. Monitor menstrual flow: bleeding may be heavier.	
4. Review need for woman to eat a consistent amount of leafy green vegetables (lettuce, cabbage, brussels sprouts, broccoli) every day.	- These foods are high in vitamin K and will affect balance between dose of warfarin and prothrombin.
5. Instruct the woman to report any bleeding that continues more than 10 minutes.	
6. Instruct the woman to do the following:	
a. Routinely inspect the body for bruising.	
b. Carry medical alert card indicating she is on anticoagulant therapy.	
c. Use electric razor to avoid scratching skin.	
d. Use soft-bristle toothbrush.	
e. Avoid binge alcohol intake or keep at minimum.	
f. Avoid taking certain herbs such as ginger, garlic, and ginkgo and any other drugs that can prolong PT without checking with the healthcare provider.	
g. Note that stools may change color to pink, red, or black as a result of anticoagulant use.	
h. Advise all health providers, including dentists, that she is taking anticoagulants.	

EXPECTED OUTCOMES: Woman has health promotion knowledge as evidenced by:

- Woman verbalizes understanding of ways to avoid circulatory stasis; need to wear supportive stockings; medications, dosages, and side effects; and the importance of a balanced diet.
- Woman verbalizes understanding of signs and symptoms of bleeding that need to be reported to healthcare provider.

ADJUSTMENT REACTION WITH DEPRESSED MOOD

Adjustment reaction with depressed mood is also known as **postpartum blues** or as *maternal blues* or *baby blues.* It occurs in as many as 85% of mothers and is characterized by mild depression interspersed with happier feelings (Pessel & Tsai, 2013). The condition is more severe in primiparas than in multiparas and seems related to the rapid alteration of estrogen, progesterone, and prolactin levels after birth, challenges of new motherhood, fatigue, and lifestyle adjustments. New mothers experiencing postpartum blues commonly report feeling overwhelmed, unable to cope, fatigued, anxious, irritable, and oversensitive. A key feature is episodic tearfulness and rapid mood shifts, often without an identifiable reason. Not uncommonly, when asked why she is crying, this woman responds that she does not know. Cunningham et al. (2014) identifies several factors that contribute to the "blues":

- Emotional letdown that follows labor and childbirth
- Physical discomfort typical in the early postpartum
- Fatigue
- Anxiety about caring for the newborn after discharge
- Severe PMS (premenstrual syndrome)
- Depression during pregnancy or previous depression unrelated to pregnancy

Validating the existence of this phenomenon, labeling it as a real but normal adjustment reaction, and providing reassurance can offer a measure of relief. Assistance with self-care and newborn/infant care, rest, good nutrition, information, and family support aid recovery. Helping the new mother anticipate a transient emotional letdown after discharge is important guidance from the nurse, as is talking with her about her view of "the perfect mother." Trying to achieve that image can contribute to fatigue and exacerbate the let-down feeling. The partner should be encouraged to watch for and report signs that the new mother is not returning to a more normal mood but slipping into a deeper depression or that happier times are no longer interspersed with the blues.

POSTPARTUM MAJOR MOOD EPISODES

Peripartum major mood episodes, also known as **postpartum depression (PPD)**, is clinical depression, categorized by the *Diagnostic and Statistical Manual of Mental Disorders* (DSM-5) as Major Depressive Disorder with Peripartum Onset (APA, 2013). Postpartum depression has been shown to occur in 10% to 20% of all postpartum women across several studies (APA, 2013).

Risk factors for postpartum depression include the following:

- History of major depression
- Depression during pregnancy
- History of postpartum depression or bipolar illness (recurrence rates are ≥ 20%)
- Stressful life events
- Primiparity
- Ambivalence about maintaining the pregnancy
- Occurrence of postpartum blues
- Lack of social support
- Lack of a stable and supportive relationship with parents (especially her father, as a child) or partner

- The woman's dissatisfaction with herself, including body image problems and eating disorders
- Complications of delivery
- Loss of newborn
- Age (adolescence increases risk)

Although it may occur at any time during the first postpartum year, the periods of greatest risk occur around the fourth week, just before the initiation of menses, and upon weaning. It is not always associated with depression during pregnancy, although gestational depression is a strong predictor of PPD.

Women with postpartum depression are at risk for suicide, most prominently as they enter or exit the deeply depressed state. In a deep depression, the woman is unlikely to be able to plan and carry out suicide. For that reason, signs of improvement in depression should be celebrated with some caution. Whereas the woman with postpartum psychosis may attempt suicide because of illogical thought processes, the woman with major depression attempts suicide because her suffering is so great that dying seems a more favorable option than continuing to live in such pain. She may also attempt suicide to save her newborn from some perceived or real threat—including the possibility that she herself might harm the baby. The risk of suicide is greater in those who have attempted suicide previously, have a specific plan, and can access the means or weapon identified within the plan. The more specific the plan, the greater is the probability of an attempt.

For women considered to be at high risk, telephone follow-up after delivery or an earlier clinic appointment than 6 weeks may be helpful. Nurses in the pediatrician's office assisting with well-child visits have an excellent opportunity to screen women for PPD (Liberto, 2012). Community health nurses who are seeing other members of the family or parish nurses who know new mothers in their congregation can observe for evidence of depression. The Postpartum Depression Screening Scale (PDSS) and the Edinburgh Postnatal Depression Scale (EPDS) are useful and validated for screening for postpartum depression.

The woman's safety, and that of her child(ren), is a priority. Inquiring about suicidal ideas and assessment for thoughts and feelings toward the baby, hallucinations and delusions, and impulsiveness that might put the newborn and siblings at risk is critical. The woman and her family need information about the illness and its expected course, including the risk of recurrence, as well as comprehensive information about the treatment plan. They need opportunities to clarify misconceptions about mental illness and to have answers to questions. Referral to local or online support groups may be helpful.

Treatment for PPD is most successful with a combination of individual or group psychotherapy and antidepressants (Burt & Stein, 2013). The expected outcomes for mild to moderate depression treated with antidepressants and psychotherapy are good; recurrence rates are increased after each episode of depression. The serotonin reuptake inhibitors (SSRIs) are used most often, as well as tricyclic antidepressants. Monoamine oxidase inhibitors (MAOIs) are rarely used in the treatment of PPD because these drugs have a high profile of interacting with other medications. Women typically continue antidepressants for 1 year after symptoms abate.

All current antidepressant agents are excreted into breast milk. However, most SSRIs and tricyclic antidepressants are considered safe with breastfeeding. Because of its prolonged half-life, fluoxetine (Prozac) is usually not recommended for nursing mothers as a first choice (Hale & Rowe, 2014). Healthcare providers need to educate their breastfeeding postpartum clients who need antidepressants about the different alternatives and help them to balance the risks and benefits with the safety profiles. The final decision about continuing to breastfeed and to take antidepressants is the informed woman's. To help in making the decision, she and her spouse/partner need to be helped to consider how she will respond without pharmacologic therapy and how unmedicated depression will affect the maternal–newborn relationship and the baby's well-being and development. An invaluable online resource for prescribers with current information on drug safety and toxic effects during pregnancy and lactation is the LactMed Database.

Electroconvulsive therapy (ECT) is used as a more rapid treatment for those with severe depression or mania, for those who are unresponsive to other treatment, or for those who are at high risk of suicide. Antidepressants may take 2 to 3 weeks to become effective. ECT results often become noticeable within 1 week (Kellner et al., 2012).

POSTPARTUM MOOD EPISODES WITH PSYCHOTIC FEATURES

The most serious of postpartum psychiatric disorders is **postpartum mood episodes with psychotic features**, also called **postpartum psychosis**. Although relatively rare (1 to 2 in 1000), this disorder gains considerable national attention in the media and is considered an emergency, given the risk of infanticide or suicide. Symptoms usually become evident within the first few days after birth. Clinical features progress rapidly and include the following (Burt & Stein, 2013):

- Sleep disturbances—the woman is unable to sleep, even when her baby is sleeping

- Depersonalization—seeming unaware of or distant from the immediate environment and individuals within it

- Confusion; irrational or disorganized thinking; bizarre behaviors

- Hallucinations; delusions

- Psychomotor disturbances—stupor or agitated state sometimes with rapid and incoherent speech

Significant risk factors include previous postpartum psychosis and/or a history of bipolar disorder. Family history of postpartum psychosis and bipolar disorder have also been found to increase the risk (Burt & Stein, 2013).

Women With Special Needs Bipolar Disorder

Women with a history of bipolar disorder have a 100 times higher risk of developing postpartum psychosis. A complete assessment should include administering a postpartum depression scale and assessing the woman for symptoms that would be considered atypical and may be an indicator of psychosis. The woman and her support persons should be educated about symptoms that warrant immediate medical intervention.

The woman with a psychosis experiences delusions and/or visual, auditory, or tactile hallucinations. In some women, these symptoms support her perceptions that the baby should not be allowed to live or that she should commit suicide. For example, she may believe that her newborn is evil, is some form of "changeling," and will harm her or others or she may believe that her newborn would be "better off dead" than living in such an evil world. She may contemplate suicide because she believes

that her child would be better off without a mother than with her as such a "terrible, crazy mother." Illogical thinking or evidence of bonding difficulties may serve as cues to infanticide and suicide risk; however, this assessment is often challenging because of periods of lucidity seen in some psychotic women. Nurses in various clinical settings who come in contact with this woman may note that the child has been neglected or the woman is practicing unsafe behaviors because of the woman's cognitive impairment. For example, a pediatric nurse noticed that one of her clients placed her newborn across the room at the edge of the narrow examination table while she paced back and forth across the room, muttering to herself, appearing not to notice the baby. This same woman came to her appointment during heavy snow with both her baby and herself underdressed for warmth.

Provisions for safety of the woman and the baby are paramount. This woman needs immediate referral to psychiatric care, usually requiring admission to an inpatient psychiatric hospital. Continued assessment of her symptomatology, safety, and functional capacity is a major nursing role in the setting. An initial history, physical examination, and laboratory work will help to rule out an organic cause of acute psychosis.

POSTTRAUMATIC STRESS DISORDER

Many women envision their own labor and delivery unfolding in a particular way and may experience angst if their labor reality fails to match their expectations. Labor and birth situations that go awry, including those associated with complications, may cause **posttraumatic stress disorder (PTSD)** (also called *posttraumatic stress syndrome [PTSS]*), which the APA's *Diagnostic and Statistical Manual of Mental Disorders* (DSM-5) (2013) describes as "the development of characteristic symptoms following exposure to one or more traumatic events." Traumatic events during childbirth may include emergency cesarean sections, surgery or medical interventions without adequate anesthesia, or the loss of a baby.

Vossbeck-Elsebusch, Freisfeld, and Ehring (2014) found that 1% to 6% of postpartum women meet the diagnostic criteria for PTSD. At particular risk for PTSD are women who have histories of prior trauma and/or prior psychiatric histories and women who undergo emergency cesarean sections (Whitmer, 2016). For this woman, the facts of the labor and birth have become distorted, perhaps because of pain or change in consciousness related to medications she received. Perhaps she underwent an emergency cesarean delivery or her baby had a serious physical anomaly. Perhaps her labor coach could not make the trip to the hospital in time for the birth or she experienced a postpartum hemorrhage. Her perceptions of what occurred and the actions of those involved frequently are far different from the reality, perhaps even seeming delusional.

Clinical features of PTSD include feeling numb, seeming dazed and unaware of her environment, intrusive thoughts and flashbacks to the threatening event, difficulty thinking, difficulty sleeping, irritability, and avoidance of others and reminders of the traumatic event. These signs and symptoms may not be evident until after the woman has left the birth setting. Distress associated with the original traumatic event can recur at anniversaries, and some women are hesitant to consider future pregnancies because of this birth trauma (Beck & Watson, 2010). Based on qualitative research and the work of others related to traumatic birth experiences, Beck and Watson (2010) suggest the following implications for nursing care:

1. Intervene, whenever possible, to prevent traumatic birth experiences.

2. Provide technically competent, concerned care for the woman and the family.

3. Assess for anxiety and fears on admission to labor and provide information to dispel myths.

4. Debrief the woman and family after a stressful traumatic childbirth experience.

5. Visit the woman during her hospitalization to assess for evidence of signs of early trauma.

Women should be asked to tell their birth story, to compare and contrast the actual experience with their birth plan or prior visions of the special day, and to tell what went well for them and what part, if any, of the experience was unexpected, troublesome, disappointing, or distressing.

Nurses who work in childbirth settings should appreciate that a woman they are admitting at any point in time may have previously had a traumatic birth. That woman will need sensitive healthcare providers who provide additional support and information and follow the birth plan to the extent possible. Subsequent childbirth following a traumatic birth experience provides a woman an opportunity to heal, and nurses have the responsibility to help these women to "reclaim their bodies and complete their journey to motherhood" (Beck & Watson, 2010).

Clinical Therapy

Women with a history of postpartum psychosis or depression or other risk factors should be referred to a mental health professional for counseling and biweekly visits between the second and sixth weeks postpartum for evaluation. Medication, individual or group psychotherapy, electroconvulusive therapy in combination with psychotherapy, psychoeducation (family therapy), and practical assistance with child care and other demands of daily life are common treatment measures for both disorders; however, the specific therapies used may vary.

It is important for the nurse to realize that many of the psychotropic drugs used in treating postpartum psychiatric conditions are contraindicated in breastfeeding women. Since newborns have immature hepatic and renal systems and a more permeable blood–brain barrier, they may be vulnerable to side effects, especially when younger than 2 months of age, premature, or exposed to these medications in utero. With the exception of lithium (which is rated a category 5 [use with caution] by the American Academy of Pediatrics), the amount of psychotropic drugs excreted into breast milk appears to be modest and not to compromise growth and development (Rowe, Baker, & Hale, 2016). Parents of a newborn need to be educated to consider these factors in making a decision about the use of psychotropic medications: (1) severity of symptoms and their effect on the newborn if medications are not used; (2) benefits of breastfeeding to the baby; (3) potential risks to the baby if psychotropics are used; and (4) preferences of the woman. If psychotropics are prescribed, the lowest dose possible of monotherapy should be used, and the baby should be monitored carefully by a pediatrician for difficulty being aroused from sleep, rigidity, tremors, irritability, poor hydration, and poor feeding with failure to gain weight (Rowe et al., 2016)

Support groups have proved to be successful adjuncts to previously discussed treatments. Within a support group of postpartum women and their partners, a couple may feel consolation that they are not alone in their experience. Moreover, the group provides a forum for exchanging information about postpartum depression, learning stress reduction measures, and experiencing renewed self-esteem and support. The most effective support groups provide for safe child care

to facilitate attendance. If a support group is not available locally, the woman and her family may be encouraged to contact Depression after Delivery Inc. (DAD), now a national Web-based support network that provides education and volunteers, or Postpartum Support International. The Mills Depression and Anxiety Symptom-Feeling Checklist also is available online.

Nursing Management

For the Postpartum Woman With a Psychiatric Disorder

Nursing Assessment and Diagnosis

Assessment for factors predisposing a woman to postpartum depression or psychosis should begin prenatally and continue during her labor and postpartum stay. Questions designed to detect problems can be included as part of the routine prenatal history interview or questionnaire. Answers to open-ended questions can be telling: What has been your greatest surprise about motherhood? Your greatest disappointment? Biggest concern? Biggest challenge? Or, How does being a mother compare to what you had envisioned? Women with a personal or family history of psychiatric disease, particularly postpartum depression or psychosis, need prenatal instructions on the signs and symptoms of depression and may need additional emotional support.

New mothers and their families expect a challenging adjustment period after bringing home a new baby; they may not realize that their experiences are outside the norm. There is general anticipation that motherhood will be a happy occasion; a woman may not be able to admit her unhappiness out of shame or embarrassment that she is somehow different as a mother. The woman might be concerned that telling someone, even a professional, about her symptoms makes her sound "crazy" and that her baby might be taken away (Logsdon, Tomasulo, Eckert, et al., 2012). One woman reported that she wanted help and sensed she needed it, but did not know which doctor to call. "I had only been home for 3 weeks and my postpartum clinic visit was 3 weeks away when I started feeling so desperate. Should I call my OB? The pediatrician had seen the baby in the hospital nursery but we hadn't visited him yet and, besides, I'm not his patient—I'm an adult. My family doctor doesn't see pregnancy-related problems, so who do I call?"

Several screening tools are available for assessing postpartum depression. The routine use of a screening tool in a matter-of-fact approach significantly increases the diagnosis. The Edinburgh Postnatal Depression Scale is the most widely used screening tool for postpartum depression in large populations of women. The tool has been validated, computerized, and used in telephone screening. Recent studies looked at the use of an interactive voice response system that delivered an automated version of the EPDS via telephone. Results suggested that the use of automated telephone screening may be a useful adjunct to office-based screening for postpartum depression (Kim, Geppert, Quan, et al., 2012). Mothers who score above 12 on the EPDS are likely to be suffering from postpartum depression. Another tool is Beck's (2002) revised Postpartum Depression Predictors Inventory (PDPI–Revised) (Table 30-5). This tool is also a practical and simple screening checklist to use during routine care with all postpartum women to identify those who might be experiencing postpartum depression so that early management might be initiated. The Postpartum

Depression Screening Scale (PDSS) is another widely used and validated tool and has the highest sensitivity. No matter what approach is used to assess for postpartum depression, enabling the woman's voice to be heard about her feelings of maternal role transition and how she is adjusting in this vulnerable time is of inestimable value. Listening to her story provides a critical emic (insider's) view of her circumstances as opposed to an etic (outsider's) view.

In providing daily care, observe the woman for objective signs of depression—anxiety, irritability, poor concentration, forgetfulness, sleep difficulties, appetite change, fatigue, and tearfulness—and listen for statements indicating feelings of failure and self-accusation. Severity and duration of symptoms should be noted. Behavior and verbalizations that are bizarre or seem to indicate a potential for violence against herself or others, including the baby, are reported as soon as possible for further

TABLE 30-5 Postpartum Depression Predictors Inventory (PDPI)—Revised and Guide Questions for Its Use

DURING PREGNANCY		
MARITAL STATUS		**CHECK ONE**
1. Single		❑
2. Married/cohabitating		❑
3. Separated		❑
4. Divorced		❑
5. Widowed		❑
6. Partnered		❑
SOCIOECONOMIC STATUS		
Low		❑
Middle		❑
High		❑
SELF-ESTEEM	Yes	No
Do you feel good about yourself as a person?	❑	❑
Do you feel worthwhile?	❑	❑
Do you feel you have a number of good qualities as a person?	❑	❑
PRENATAL DEPRESSION		
1. Have you felt depressed during your pregnancy?	❑	❑
If yes, when and how long have you been feeling this way?		
If yes, how mild or severe would you consider your depression?		
PRENATAL ANXIETY		
1. Have you been feeling anxious during your pregnancy?	❑	❑
If yes, how long have you been feeling this way?		
UNPLANNED/UNWANTED PREGNANCY		
Was the pregnancy planned?	❑	❑
Is the pregnancy unwanted?	❑	❑
HISTORY OF PREVIOUS DEPRESSION		
1. Before this pregnancy, have you ever been depressed?	❑	❑
If yes, when did you experience this depression?		
If yes, have you been under a healthcare provider's care for this past depression?	❑	❑
If yes, did the healthcare provider prescribe any medication for your depression?	❑	❑
SOCIAL SUPPORT		
1. Do you feel you receive adequate emotional support from your partner?	❑	❑
2. Do you feel you receive adequate instrumental support from your partner (e.g., help with household chores or babysitting)?	❑	❑
3. Do you feel you can rely on your partner when you need help?	❑	❑
4. Do you feel you can confide in your partner? (Repeat same questions for family and again for friends.)	❑	❑
MARITAL SATISFACTION		
1. Are you satisfied with your marriage (or living arrangement)?	❑	❑
2. Are you currently experiencing any marital problems?	❑	❑
3. Are things going well between you and your partner?	❑	❑

(continued)

TABLE 30–5 Postpartum Depression Predictors Inventory (PDPI)—Revised and Guide Questions for Its Use (*continued*)

DURING PREGNANCY		
LIFE STRESS	Yes	No
1. Are you currently experiencing any stressful events in your life such as:		
Financial problems?	❑	❑
Marital problems?	❑	❑
Death in the family?	❑	❑
Serious illness in the family?	❑	❑
Moving?	❑	❑
Unemployment?	❑	❑
Job change?	❑	❑
AFTER DELIVERY, ADD THE FOLLOWING ITEMS		
CHILDCARE STRESS		
1. Is your baby experiencing any health problems?	❑	❑
2. Are you having problems with your baby feeding?	❑	❑
3. Are you having problems with your baby sleeping?	❑	❑
INFANT TEMPERAMENT		
1. Would you consider your baby irritable or fussy?	❑	❑
2. Does your baby cry a lot?	❑	❑
3. Is your baby difficult to console or soothe?	❑	❑
MATERNITY BLUES		
Did you experience a brief period of tearfulness and mood swings during the first week after delivery?	❑	❑
COMMENTS:		

Source: Beck, C. T. (2002). Revision of the Postpartum Predictors Inventory. *Journal of Obstetric, Gynecologic, and Neonatal Nursing*, 30(4), 394–402 (Table 2 on PDPI, pp. 399–400). Washington, DC: AWHONN. © 2002 by the Association of Women's Health, Obstetric and Neonatal Nurses. All rights reserved.

evaluation. Be aware that many normal physiologic changes of the puerperium are similar to symptoms of depression (lack of sexual interest, appetite change, fatigue). It is essential that your observations be as specific and as objective as possible and that they are carefully documented.

Beck (2008) found that anxiety was a prominent feature of illness for some women and suggested that women be assessed for their level of anxiety, particularly regarding newborn/infant care. Because of the strong association between interrupted sleep and postpartum depression and the finding that severe fatigue was an excellent predictor of postpartum depression, assessing fatigue level at 2 weeks postpartum by telephone may be helpful in predicting depression risk early. Restorative sleep improves one's ability to cope and make decisions, thereby producing a sense of better self-control.

A central challenge for nursing is identifying women at risk of suicide. Family members of the depressed woman should also be alert to signals that she may be intent on self-harm; advise them that threats should always be taken seriously. Tell family members to be especially vigilant for suicide when the woman seems to be feeling better.

If a woman admits that she has thought of hurting herself, assessment of the risk that she will follow through is imperative. The mnemonic *SAL* is useful for risk assessment:

- Is there a *Specific* plan with a designated time?
- Is there an *Accessible* weapon or other means?
- How *Lethal* is the method identified in the plan?

A specific plan that identifies a highly lethal method that is immediately accessible is evidence of very high risk of suicide. Immediate intervention is critical; emergency psychiatric hospitalization is likely necessary. Those considered a threat to themselves or others may be admitted to involuntary hospitalization for a minimum of 48 hours until further evaluation is complete.

Family members of the depressed woman should also be alert to signals that she may be intent on self-harm; they must be advised that threats should always be taken seriously. Clues to suicide that might be noted by family are comments such as, "I don't deserve to live," "Life is no longer worth living," or "You won't have to worry about me for long." Someone who is considering suicide may also telephone or write family or friends to say good-bye or give away prized possessions. Family members should be told to be especially vigilant for suicide when the woman seems to be feeling better.

Possible nursing diagnoses that may apply to a woman with a postpartum psychiatric disorder include the following (NANDA-I © 2014):

- *Coping, Ineffective,* related to postpartum depression
- *Parenting, Risk for Impaired,* related to postpartum mental illness
- *Violence, Self-Directed, Risk for,* related to possible suicide
- *Violence, Other-Directed, Risk for,* related to violence directed at newborn and other children related to depression

Nursing Plan and Implementation

Nurses working in antepartum settings or teaching childbirth classes play indispensable roles in helping prospective parents appreciate the lifestyle changes and role demands associated with parenthood. Offering realistic information and anticipatory guidance and debunking myths about the perfect mother or perfect newborn may help prevent postpartum depression. Social support teaching guides are available for nurses to help postpartum women explore their needs for postpartum support.

Alert the mother, spouse/partner, and other family members to the possibility of postpartum blues in the early days after birth and reassure them of the short-term nature of the condition. Symptoms of postpartum depression should be described and the mother encouraged to call her healthcare provider if symptoms become severe, if they fail to subside quickly, or if at any time she feels she is unable to function. Encouraging the mother to plan how she will manage at home and providing concrete suggestions on how to cope will aid in her adjustment to motherhood. *Teaching Highlights: Primary Prevention Strategies for Postpartum Depression* provides suggestions that serve as important prevention measures for postpartum depression.

Information, emotional support, and assistance in providing or obtaining care for the baby may be needed. Assist family members by identifying community resources, making referrals to public health nursing services and social services, and providing a list of telephone numbers as well as emergency services that they may need. Postpartum follow-up is especially important, as well as visits from a psychiatric home health nurse.

COMMUNITY-BASED NURSING CARE

Home visits, especially for early discharge families, are invaluable in fostering positive adjustments for the new family. Telephone follow-up at 2 to 3 weeks postpartum to ask whether the mother is experiencing difficulties is also helpful. Monitoring for signs of depression or performing brief screening at well-child follow-ups also can be valuable for early identification and timely intervention.

Depression does appear to interfere with optimal mothering; it is associated with less interaction between mother and child, more mood and cognitive development problems, and more visits to the doctor in these children. A diagnosis of postpartum depression or other psychiatric disorder will pose major problems for the family, especially the father/partner. The symptoms of these disorders are difficult to witness and may be harder to understand than physical problems such as hemorrhage and infection. The father/partner may feel hurt by the new mother's hostility, worry that she is becoming insane, or be baffled by her mood swings and lack of concern about herself, the newborn, or household responsibilities. Certainly, there is cause for concern about how the newborn and any other children are being affected. Very real practical matters—running the household; managing the children, including the totally dependent newborn; and caring for the mother—may be added to his usual routines and work responsibilities. It is not surprising that, even in the most supportive families, relationships may suffer in

---

TEACHING HIGHLIGHTS | Primary Prevention Strategies for Postpartum Depression

1. Celebrate childbirth but appreciate that it is a life-changing transition that can be stressful—at times it can seem overwhelming. Share your feelings with each other and/or others.

2. Consider keeping a journal in which you write down feelings. Not only is it emotionally cathartic, it provides a great memory book.

3. Appreciate that you do not have to know everything to be a good parent—it is okay to seek advice during this transition.

4. Connect with others who are parents—use them as a support and information network.

5. Set a daily schedule and follow it even if you do not feel like it. Structuring activity helps counteract the inertia that comes with feeling sad or unsettled.

6. Prioritize daily tasks. Decide what must be done and what can wait. Try to get one major thing done every day. Remember, you do not always have to look like a magazine fashion model.

7. Remember that you do not have to entertain or care for everyone who drops by. Doing something for someone else, however, often tends to make you feel better.

8. If people volunteer to help you with tasks or baby care, take them up on it. While your volunteer is in action, do something pleasurable or get some rest.

9. Maintain outside interests. Plan some time every day—even if it's just 15 minutes—to do something exclusively for "you" that is pleasurable.

10. Eat a healthful diet. Limit alcohol. Quit smoking. Get some exercise. (All of these can positively affect the immune system.)

11. Get as much sleep as possible. Rest whenever you can, such as when the baby is napping. If you have other young children, bring them onto your bed to read or play quietly while you lie down.

12. Limit major changes (moves, job changes, etc.) the first year insofar as possible.

13. Spend time with others.

14. If things get overwhelming, and you feel yourself slipping into depression, reach out to someone for help.

15. Attend a local postpartum support group if one is available. Consider also an international program such as Postpartum Support International.

response to these circumstances. It is often the father/partner or another close family member who in desperation makes contact with the healthcare agency. This is especially difficult when the mother is reluctant to admit she is suffering emotional difficulty or is too ill to recognize her own needs.

The integration of the newborn into the family and care of the newborn and other children can be further compromised by concurrent postpartum depression in the father/partner. With both parents having depressive symptoms, the baby and other children are further at risk.

Evaluation

Expected outcomes of nursing care include the following:

- The woman's signs of depression are identified and she receives therapy quickly.
- The newborn is cared for effectively by the father/partner or another support person until the mother is able to provide care.
- The mother and the newborn remain safe.
- The newborn is integrated into the family.

Focus Your Study

- Nursing assessment and intervention play a large role in preventing postpartum complications.
- The main causes of early postpartum hemorrhage and the appropriate nursing interventions include:
  - Uterine atony: perform fundal massage and check for clots.
  - Laceration of vagina and cervix (suspect if mother is bleeding heavily in presence of firmly contracted fundus): contact healthcare provider to suture the laceration.
  - Retained placental fragments (suspect if woman is bleeding, fundus is firm and no lacerations are present): thoroughly inspect placenta.
  - General assessment includes fundus for signs of bogginess, perineal pads for excessive vaginal bleeding and for normal changes in lochia progression.
- Late postpartum hemorrhage most often originates from retained placental fragments, and usually occurs 1 to 2 weeks after birth; although not usually as catastrophic as early hemorrhage, it may require readmission. The appropriate nursing interventions include: provide mother with discharge instructions, including information about possible complications.
- Document a thorough nursing history for causes and contributing factors for reproductive tract infection such as: C-section, prolonged labor preceding C-section, prolonged premature rupture of the amniotic membranes, oxytocin induction of labor, chorioamnionitis, obstetric trauma: episiotomy laceration of perineum, vagina, or cervix and multiple vaginal examinations. The most common postpartum infection is metritis, which is limited to the uterine cavity.
- To prevent postpartum reproductive tract infections, the nurse will:
  - Assess woman in general and incisions for signs of infection such as: temperature of 38.0°C (100.4°F) or higher, with temperature occurring on any 2 of the first 10 postpartum days, exclusive of the first 24 hours; foul, bloody discharge from vagina or incision; uterine tenderness; chills, malaise, lethargy, subinvolution of the uterus; lack of wound healing (REEDA).

- Implement standard precautions; aseptic technique during labor, birth, and postpartum period.
- Use good hand hygiene techniques to prevent transmission of infective material and provide clear instructions about wound care.
- Administer antibiotics.
- Address comfort needs related to hygiene, positioning, oral hygiene, and pain.
- A postpartum woman is at increased risk for developing urinary tract problems because of normal postpartum diuresis, increased bladder capacity, decreased bladder sensitivity from stretching or trauma, and possibly inhibited neural control of the bladder following the use of anesthetic agents. The nurse needs to assess for burning during urination, avoid urinary catheterization when possible, and encourage the woman to void frequently,
- Mastitis is an inflammation of the breast seen primarily in breastfeeding women. Symptoms such as cracking, plugged ducts, and redness and pain in the breast seldom occur before the fourth postpartum week. It is important to teach mother proper latching-on techniques and breast care. Continuation of breastfeeding is recommended as part of the treatment plan.
- Thromboembolic disease originating in the veins of the leg, thigh, or pelvis may occur antepartum or postpartum and carries with it the potential for creating a life-threatening pulmonary embolus. Nursing assessments of all body systems include: frequent vital signs and peripheral pulses assessments, check CMS, and assessment for Homans sign each shift. Thrombophlebitis signs and symptoms include: pain and swelling in the lower extremities and localized heat and redness. To prevent thromboembolic disease, the nurse will: assess lower extremities for signs of thrombophlebitis, encourage early ambulation, and assess for pulmonary embolus.
- Although many different types of psychiatric problems may be encountered in the postpartum period, postpartum blues is the most common. Postpartum blues episodes (feelings of overwhelming sadness and lack of desire to care for baby) occur

frequently in the week after birth, are associated with hormonal fluctuations, and are typically transient.

- Risk factors for postpartum depression should be screened for routinely during pregnancy and the postpartum period. Nurses should be alert to the risk of suicide and infanticide in cases of severe postpartum depression or psychosis.

- Telephone calls and home visits are effective measures for extending comprehensive care into the home setting of the postpartum family at risk. Support groups in which child care is available also can be an invaluable community service by professional nurses.

Clinical Reasoning in Action

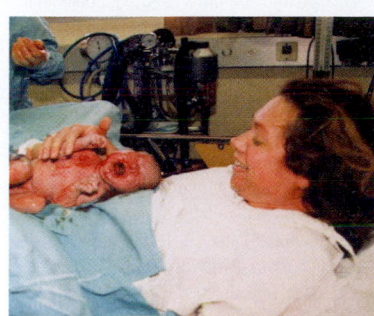

Betty Jones, a 32-year-old G4P2012, is admitted to the postpartum unit after a precipitous birth of a preterm (35 weeks' gestation) 4-lb baby girl followed by a postpartum tubal ligation. Betty's vital signs and postpartum assessment are within normal limits. She has an abdominal dressing that is dry and intact and she is able to void. Her IV with 10 units of oxytocin (Pitocin) is infusing well in her lower left arm. She admits to 3 on a pain scale of 10. Betty admits to active use of crack cocaine throughout her pregnancy, and smoked it most recently 5 hours before she gave birth. She is HIV positive with a CD4 count of 726 cells/mm³ and was treated with zidovudine during the pregnancy, labor, and birth. She also has a history of genital herpes and had been treated for chlamydial infection during the pregnancy. Her newborn has been admitted to the special care nursery because of her preterm status. Betty anticipates her baby will be taken into foster care when discharged from the nursery. Wishing to establish as much of a relationship with her baby as possible before that happens, she asks if she can breastfeed the baby while she is in the hospital.

1. What is your response to Betty's request to breastfeed her newborn?

2. Over the course of the first postpartum day, Betty appears lethargic and spends most of her time sleeping. After her evening visitors leave, you observe that she is highly energetic and excitable. Would urine testing be useful to help determine if Betty has used cocaine this evening?

3. Discuss supportive nursing care for newborns born of HIV positive mothers.

4. Betty wishes for an early discharge from the hospital. What physical criteria must be met before leaving the hospital?

5. Discuss when she should contact her healthcare provider after her discharge.

References

Acosta, C. D., Kurinczuk, J. J., Lucas, D. N., Tuffnell, D. J., Sellers, S., & Knight, M. (2014). *Severe maternal sepsis in the UK, 2011–2012: A national case-control study.* Retrieved from http://www.Plosmedicine.org/article/info%3Adoi%2F10.1371%2Fjournal.pmed.1001672

Albacar, G., Sans, T., Martín-Santos, R., García-Esteve, L., Guillamat, R., Sanjuan, J., . . . Vilella, E. (2011). An association between plasma ferritin concentrations measured 48h after delivery and postpartum depression. *Journal of Affective Disorders, 131*(1–3), 136–142. doi:10.1016/j.jad.2010.11.00

American College of Obstetrics & Gynecology (ACOG). (2011). *Thromboembolism in pregnancy.* Practice Bulletin No. 123. *Obstetrics & Gynecology, 118*, 718–29.

American College of Obstetrics & Gynecology (ACOG) Committee on Patient Safety and Quality Improvement (2014). Preparing for clinical emergencies in obstetrics and gynecology. Committee Opinion No. 590. *Obstetrics & Gynecology, 123*, 722–725.

American Psychiatric Association (APA). (2013). *Diagnostic and statistical manual of mental disorders: DSM-5* (5th ed.). Arlington, VA: Author.

Ayadi, A. M., Robinson, N., Geller, S., & Miller, S. (2013). Advances in the treatment of postpartum hemorrhage. *Expert Review of Obstetrics & Gynecology, 8*(6), 525–537.

Beck, C. T. (2002). Revision of the postpartum depression predictors inventory. *Journal of Obstetric, Gynecologic, and Neonatal Nursing (JOGNN), 31*(4), 394–402.

Beck, C. T. (2008). *Postpartum mood and anxiety disorders: Case studies, research, and nursing care* (Practice Bulletin) (2nd ed.). Washington, DC: AWHONN.

Beck, C., & Watson, S. (2010). Subsequent childbirth after a previous traumatic birth. *Nursing Research, 59*(4), 241–249. doi:10.1097/NNR.0b013e3181e501fd

Bianco, A., Roccia, S., A., Pileggi, C., & Pavia, M. (2013). Postdischarge surveillance following delivery: The incidence of infections and associated factors. *American Journal of Infection Control, 41*(6), 549–553. doi:10.1016/j.ajic.2012.06.011

Burt, V. K., & Stein, K. (2013). Treatment of women. In R.E. Hales, S.C. Yudofsky, & L.W. Roberts (Eds.), *The American psychiatric publishing textbook of psychiatry* (6th ed.). Arlington, VA: American Psychiatric Publishing.

Cunningham, F. G., Leveno, K. J., Bloom, S. L., Spong, C. Y., Dashe, J. S., Hoffman, B. L., . . . Sheffield, J. S. (2014). *Williams obstetrics* (24th ed.). New York, NY: McGraw-Hill.

Distefano, M., Casarella, L., Amoroso, S., Di Stasi, C., Scambia, G., & Tropeano, G. (2013). Selective arterial embolization as a first-line treatment for postpartum hematomas. *Obstetrics & Gynecology, 121*(2 Pt 2 Suppl 1), 443–447. doi:10.1097/AOG.0b013e31827d90e1

Duff, P. (2014). Maternal and fetal infectious disorders. In R. K. Creasy & R. Resnik (Eds.), *Maternal–fetal medicine: Principles and practice* (7th ed., pp. 802–851). Philadelphia, PA: Saunders.

Fletcher, S., Grotegut, C. A., & James, A. H. (2012). Lochia patterns among normal women: A systematic review. *Journal of Women's Health (15409996), 21*(12), 1290–1294. doi:10.1089/jwh.2012.3668

Francois, K. E., & Foley, M. R. (2012). Antepartum and postpartum hemorrhage. In S. G. Gabbe, J. R. Niebyl, J. L. Simpson, M. B. Landon, H. L. Galan, E. R. Jauniaux, & D. A. Driscoll (Eds.), *Obstetrics: Normal and problem pregnancies.* (6th ed.). Philadelphia, PA: Saunders.

Hale, T. W., & Rowe, H. E. (2014). *Medications & mothers' milk 2014.* (16th ed.). Plano, TX: Hale Publishing.

Harvey, C. J., & Dildy, G. A. (2013). Obstetric hemorrhage. In N. H. Troiano, C. J. Harvey, & B. F. Chez (Eds.), *AWHONN's high-risk & critical care obstetrics* (3rd ed., pp. 246–273). Philadelphia, PA: Lippincott.

Jahanfar, S., Ng, C. J., & Teng, C. L. (2013). Antibiotics for mastitis in breastfeeding women. *Cochrane Database of Systematic Reviews,* Issue 2. Art. No.: CD005458. doi: 10.1002/14651858.CD005458.pub3

James, D. C. (2014). Postpartum care. In K. R. Simpson & P. A. Creehan (Eds.), *AWHONN's perinatal nursing* (4th ed., pp. 530–580). Philadelphia, PA: Lippincott Williams & Wilkins.

Kellner, C., Greenberg, R., Murrough, J., Bryson, E., Briggs, M., & Pasculli, R. (2012). ECT in treatment-resistant depression. *American Journal of Psychiatry, 169*(12), 1238–1244. doi:10.1176/appi.ajp.2012.12050648

Kim, H. G., Geppert, J., Quan, T., Bracha, Y., Lupo, V., & Cutts, D. B. (2012). Screening for postpartum depression among low-income women using an interactive voice response system. *Maternal and Child Health Journal, 16*(4), 921–928. doi:10.1007/s10995-011-0817-6

Lawrence, R. M., & Lawrence, R. A. (2014). The breast and the physiology of lactation. In R. K. Creasy & R. Resnik (Eds.), *Maternal–fetal medicine: Principles and practice* (7th ed., pp. 112–130). Philadelphia, PA: Saunders.

Liberto, T. L. (2012). Screening for depression and help-seeking in postpartum women during well-baby pediatric visits: An integrated review. *Journal of Pediatric Healthcare, 26*(2), 109–117. doi:10.1016/j.pedhc.2010.06.012

Leung, A. N., & Lockwood, C. J. (2014). Thromboembolic disease in pregnancy. In R. K. Creasy & R. Resnik (Eds.), *Maternal–fetal medicine: Principles and practice* (7th ed., pp. 906–916). Philadelphia, PA: Saunders.

Logsdon, M., Tomasulo, R., Eckert, D., Beck, C., & Lee, C. (2012). Identification of mothers at risk for postpartum depression by hospital-based perinatal nurses. *MCN: The American Journal of Maternal Child Nursing, 37*(4), 218–225. doi:10.1097/NMC.0b013e318251078b

Mousa, H., Blum, J., Senoun, G., Shakur, H., & Alfirevic, Z. (2014). Treatment for primary postpartum haemorrhage. *Cochrane Database of Systematic Reviews,* Issue 2. Art. No.: CD003249.

Oberg, A., Hernandez-Diaz, S., Palmsten, K., Almqvist, C., & Bateman, B. (2014). Patterns of recurrence of postpartum hemorrhage in a large population-based cohort. *American Journal of Obstetrics and Gynecology, 210*(229), e1–e8.

Pessel, C., & Tsai, M. C. (2013). The normal puerperium. In A. H. DeCherney, L. Nathan, N. Laufer, & A. S. Roman (Eds.), *Current diagnosis & treatment: Obstetrics & gynecology* (11th ed., pp. 190–213). New York, NY: McGraw-Hill.

Poggi, S. B. (2013). Postpartum hemorrhage and abnormal puerperium. In A. H. DeCherney, L. Nathan, N. Laufer, & A. S. Roman (Eds.), *Current diagnosis & treatment: Obstetrics & gynecology* (11th ed., pp. 349–368). New York, NY: McGraw-Hill.

Robbins, K. S., Martin, S. R., & Wilson, W. C. (2014). Intensive care considerations for the critically ill parturient. In R. K. Creasy & R. Resnik (Eds.), *Maternal–fetal medicine: Principles and practice* (7th ed., pp. 1182–1214). Philadelphia, PA: Saunders.

Rouse, D. J. (2013). What is new in postpartum hemorrhage? *Obstetrics & Gynecology, 122*, 693–694. doi:10.1097/AOG.0b013e3182a2c357

Rowe, H., Baker, T. E. C., & Hale, T. W. (2016). Drug therapy and breastfeeding. In K. Wambach & J. Riordan (Eds.), *Breastfeeding and human lactation* (5th ed., pp. 171–206). Burlington, MA: Jones & Bartlett Learning.

Sosa, M. E. (2014). Bleeding in pregnancy. In K. R. Simpson & P. A. Creehan (Eds.), *AWHONN's perinatal nursing* (4th ed., pp. 143–162). Philadelphia, PA: Lippincott Williams & Wilkins.

Thorp, J. M., & Laughton, S. K. (2014). Clinical aspects of normal and abnormal labor. In R. K. Creasy & R. Resnik (Eds.), *Maternal–fetal medicine: Principles and practice* (7th ed., pp. 673–706). Philadelphia, PA: Saunders

Vossbeck-Elsebusch, A. N., Freisfeld, C., & Ehring, T. (2014). Predictors of posttraumatic stress symptoms following childbirth. *BMC Psychiatry, 14*, 200. doi:10.1186/1471-244X-14-200

Walker, M. (2014). Common breastfeeding problems. In R. G. Jordan, J. L. Engstrom, J. A. Marfell, & C. L. Farley (Eds.), *Prenatal and postnatal care: A woman-centered approach.* (pp.499–513). Ames, IA: John Wiley & Sons.

Wambach, K. (2016). Breast-related problems. In K. Wambach & J. Riordan (Eds.), *Breastfeeding and human lactation* (5th ed., pp. 319–357). Burlington, MA: Jones & Bartlett Learning.

Wetta, L. A., Szchowski, J. M., Seals, S., Mancuso, M. S., Biggo, J. R., & Tita, A. T. N. (2013). Risk factors for uterine atony/postpartum hemorrhage requiring treatment after vaginal delivery. *American Journal of Obstetrics and Gynecology, 209*(51), e1–6.

Whitmer, T. (2016). Physical and psychologic changes after childbirth. In S. Mattson & J. E. Smith (Eds.). *Core curriculum for maternal-newborn nursing* (6th ed. pp. 297-313). Philadelphia, PA: Association of Women's Health, Obstetric and Neonatal Nurses/Elsevier.

Witcher, P. M., & Hamner, L. (2013). Venous thromboembolism in pregnancy. In N. H. Troiano, C. J. Harvey, & B. F. Chez (Eds.), *AWHONN's high-risk & critical care obstetrics* (3rd ed., pp. 285–301). Philadelphia, PA: Lippincott.

Zaccardi, J. E. (2013). Managing urinary tract infections in women. *Clinical Advisor for Nurse Practitioners, 16*(2), 24–32.

Appendix A
Common Abbreviations in Maternal–Newborn and Women's Health Nursing

ABE	Acute bilirubin encephalopathy
AC	Abdominal circumference
accel	Acceleration of fetal heart rate
AFAFP	Amniotic fluid alpha-fetoprotein
AFI	Amniotic fluid index
AFP	Alpha-fetoprotein
AFV	Amniotic fluid volume
AGA	Average for gestational age
AHT	Abusive head trauma
AI	Amnioinfusion *or* adequate intake
AMOL	Active management of labor
AOP	Apnea of prematurity *or* Anemia of prematurity
ARBD	Alcohol-related birth defects
ARBOW	Artificial rupture of bag of waters
ARND	Alcohol-related neurodevelopmental disorder
AROM	Artificial rupture of membranes
ART	Assisted reproductive technology
AUB	Abnormal uterine bleeding
BAM	Becoming a mother
BAT	Brown adipose tissue (brown fat)
BBOW	Bulging bag of water
BBT	Basal body temperature
β-hCG	Beta-human chorionic gonadotropin
BL FHR	Baseline fetal heart rate
BL VAR	Baseline variability
BOW	Bag of waters
BPD	Biparietal diameter *or* Bronchopulmonary dysplasia
BPP	Biophysical profile
BRB	Bright red bleeding *or* Breakthrough bleeding
BR CA	Breast cancer
BSE	Breast self-examination
BSST	Breast self-stimulation test
BV	Bacterial vaginosis
cal	Calorie
CC	Chest circumference *or* Cord compression
CD	Cycle day

CEI	Continuous epidural infusion
cffDNA	Cell-free fetal DNA
CHL	Crown–heel length
CID	Cytomegalic inclusion disease
CLD	Chronic lung disease
CMV	Cytomegalovirus
CNM	Certified nurse-midwife
CNS	Clinical nurse specialist
COCs	Combined oral contraceptives
CPAP	Continuous positive airway pressure
CPD	Cephalopelvic disproportion *or* Citrate-phosphate-dextrose
CRL	Crown–rump length
CRNP	Certified registered nurse practitioner
C/S	Cesarean section (or C-section)
CST	Contraction stress test
CVS	Chorionic villus sampling
D&C	Dilatation and curettage
D&E	Dilatation and evacuation
DA	Ductus arteriosus
decels	Deceleration of fetal heart rate
DFMR	Daily fetal movement response
dil	Dilatation
DNP	Doctor of Nursing Practice
DPNB	Dorsal penile nerve block
DRI	Dietary reference intake
DTR	Deep tendon reflexes
DUB	Dysfunctional uterine bleeding
DVT	Deep vein thrombosis
EAB	Elective abortion
EASI	Extra-amniotic saline infusion
ECMO	Extracorporeal membrane oxygenator
ECV	External cephalic version
EDB	Estimated date of birth
EDC	Estimated date of confinement
EDD	Estimated date of delivery
EFM	Electronic fetal monitoring
EFW	Estimated fetal weight
EIA	Enzyme immunoassay

ELBW	Extremely low birth weight
ELF	Elective low forceps
ELISA	Enzyme-linked immunosorbent assay
EOS	Early onset sepsis
EP	Ectopic pregnancy
epis	Episiotomy
FAB	Fertility awareness–based methods
FAD	Fetal activity diary
FAS	Fetal alcohol syndrome
FASD	Fetal alcohol spectrum disorder
FBM	Fetal breathing movements
FBS	Fetal blood sample *or* Fasting blood sugar test
FCC	Family-centered care
FECG	Fetal electrocardiogram
fFN	Fetal fibronectin
FGM	Female genital mutilation
FHR	Fetal heart rate
FHT	Fetal heart tones
Fhx	Family history
FISH	Fluorescence *in situ* hybridization
FL	Femur length
FMC	Fetal movement count
FMH	Fetal–maternal hemorrhage
FMR	Fetal movement record
FO	Foramen ovale
FPG	Fasting plasma glucose test
FRC	Female reproductive cycle
FSE	Fetal scalp electrode
FSH	Follicle-stimulating hormone
FSHRH	Follicle-stimulating hormone–releasing hormone
FSPO$_2$	Fetal arterial oxygen saturation
G *or* grav	Gravida
GDM	Gestational diabetes mellitus
GIFT	Gamete intrafallopian transfer
GnRF	Gonadotropin-releasing factor
GnRH	Gonadotropin-releasing hormone
GTD	Gestational trophoblastic disease
GTPAL	Gravida, term, preterm, abortion, living children; a system of recording maternity history
HA	Head–abdominal ratio *or* headache
HAI	Hemagglutination-inhibition test
HC	Head compression
hCG	Human chorionic gonadotropin
hCS	Human chorionic somatomammotropin (same as hPL)
hMG	Human menopausal gonadotropin
hPL	Human placental lactogen
HPTs	Home pregnancy tests
HPV	Human papilloma virus
HSG	Hysterosalpingography
HSV	Herpes simplex virus
HT	Hormone therapy
IAP	Intrapartum antimicrobial prophylaxis
IBCLC	International board-certified lactation consultant
ICSI	Intracytoplasmic sperm injection
IDM	Infant of a diabetic mother
IEM	Inborn errors of metabolism
IPV	Intimate partner violence
ISAM	Infant of a substance-abusing mother
IUC	Intrauterine contraception
IUD	Intrauterine device
IUFD	Intrauterine fetal death
IUGR	Intrauterine growth restriction
IUI	Intrauterine insemination
IUPC	Intrauterine pressure catheter
IUS	Intrauterine system
IVF	In vitro fertilization
kcal	Kilocalorie
LADA	Left-acromion-dorsal-anterior
LADP	Left-acromion-dorsal-posterior
LBC	Lamellar body count
LBW	Low birth weight
LDRP	Labor, delivery, recovery, and postpartum
LGA	Large for gestational age
LH	Luteinizing hormone
LHRH	Luteinizing hormone–releasing hormone
LMA	Left-mentum-anterior
LLLI	La Leche League International
LML	Left mediolateral (episiotomy)
LMP	Last menstrual period *or* Left-mentum-posterior
LMT	Left-mentum-transverse
LOA	Left-occiput-anterior
LOF	Low outlet forceps
LOP	Left-occiput-posterior
LOS	Length of stay
LOT	Left-occiput-transverse
L/S	Lecithin/sphingomyelin ratio
LSA	Left-sacrum-anterior
LSP	Left-sacrum-posterior
LST	Left-sacrum-transverse
MAS	Meconium aspiration syndrome
mec	Meconium
MEN	Minimal enteral nutrition
MHT	Menopausal hormone therapy
MLE	Midline episiotomy
MRA	Maternal role attainment

MSAF	Meconium-stained amniotic fluid		**primip**	Primipara
MSAFP	Maternal serum alpha-fetoprotein		**PROM**	Premature rupture of membranes
multip	Multipara		**PSI**	Prostaglandin synthesis inhibitor
NAS	Neonatal abstinence syndrome		**PTB**	Preterm birth
NBS	New Ballard Score		**PTL**	Preterm labor
NEC	Necrotizing enterocolitis		**PTSD**	Posttraumatic stress disorder
NFP	Natural family planning		**PUBS**	Percutaneous umbilical blood sampling
NICU	Neonatal intensive care unit		**RADA**	Right-acromion-dorsal-anterior
NNS	Nonnutritive sucking		**RADP**	Right-acromion-dorsal-posterior
NP	Nurse practitioner		**RDA**	Recommended dietary allowance
NSCST	Nipple stimulation contraction stress test		**RDS**	Respiratory distress syndrome
NST	Non-stress test *or* Nonshivering thermo-genesis		**REM**	Rapid eye movements
			RIA	Radioimmunoassay
NSVD	Normal sterile vaginal delivery		**RLF**	Retrolental fibroplasia
NT	Nuchal translucency		**RMA**	Right-mentum-anterior
NTD	Neural tube defects		**RMP**	Right-mentum-posterior
NTE	Neutral thermal environment		**RMT**	Right-mentum-transverse
NVP	Nausea and vomiting of pregnancy		**RNC**	Certified registered nurse
NTT	Nuchal translucency testing		**ROA**	Right-occiput-anterior
OA	Occiput anterior		**ROM**	Rupture of membranes
OCPs	Oral contraceptive pills		**ROP**	Right-occiput-posterior *or* Retinopathy of prematurity
OCT	Oxytocin challenge test		**ROT**	Right-occiput-transverse
OF	Occipitofrontal diameter of fetal head		**RPL**	Recurrent pregnancy loss
OFC	Occipitofrontal circumference		**RRA**	Radioreceptor assay
OGTT	Oral glucose tolerance test		**RSA**	Right-sacrum-anterior
OM	Occipitomental (diameter)		**RSP**	Right-sacrum-posterior
OP	Occiput posterior		**RST**	Right-sacrum-transverse
p	Para		**SAB**	Spontaneous abortion
PABC	Pregnancy-associated breast cancer		**SBS**	Shaken baby syndrome
Pap smear	Papanicolaou smear		**SET**	Surrogate embryo transfer
PAPP-A	Pregnancy-associated plasma protein A		**SGA**	Small for gestational age
PCA	Patient-controlled analgesia		**SIDS**	Sudden infant death syndrome
PCEA	Patient-controlled epidural analgesia		**SMB**	Submentobregmatic diameter
PCOS	Polycystic ovarian syndrome		**SOB**	Suboccipitobregmatic diameter *or* Shortness of breath
PDA	Patent ductus arteriosus			
PG	Phosphatidylglycerol *or* Prostaglandin		**SPA**	Sperm penetration assay
PGS	Preimplantation genetic screening		**SRBOW**	Spontaneous rupture of bag of waters
PID	Pelvic inflammatory disease		**SROM**	Spontaneous rupture of membranes
Pit	Pitocin		**SSC**	Skin-to-skin contact
PKU	Phenylketonuria		**STI**	Sexually transmitted infection
PMDD	Premenstrual dysphoric disorder		**STS**	Serologic test for syphilis
PMR	Perinatal mortality rate		**SUID**	Sudden unexpected infant death
PMS	Premenstrual syndrome		**SVE**	Sterile vaginal exam
PNV	Prenatal vitamins		**TAB**	Therapeutic abortion
POP	Persistent occiput-posterior (position)		**TcB**	Transcutaneous bilirubin
PPHN	Persistent pulmonary hypertension of the newborn		**TCM**	Transcutaneous monitoring
			TDI *or* **THI**	Therapeutic donor insemination (*H* designates husband is donor)
PPD	Postpartum depression			
PPROM	Preterm premature rupture of membranes		**TET**	Tubal embryo transfer

TI	Therapeutic insemination
TOL	Trial of labor
TOLAC	Trial of labor after cesarean
TORCH	Toxoplasmosis, rubella, cytomegalovirus, herpesvirus hominis type 2
TSS	Toxic shock syndrome
TTN	Transient tachypnea of the newborn
ū	Umbilicus
UA	Uterine activity
UAC	Umbilical artery catheter
UAU	Uterine activity units
UC	Uterine contraction
UNHS	Universal newborn hearing screening

UPI	Uteroplacental insufficiency
US	Ultrasound
UTI	Urinary tract infection
VBAC	Vaginal birth after cesarean
VDRL	Venereal Disease Research Laboratories
VIP	Voluntary interruption of pregnancy
VLBW	Very low birth weight
VTE	Venous thromboembolism
VVC	Vulvovaginal *candidiasis*
WIC	Supplemental food program for women, infants, and children
ZIFT	Zygote intrafallopian transfer

Appendix B
Conversions and Equivalents

Temperature Conversion

(Fahrenheit temperature − 32) × 5/9 = Centigrade temperature

(Centigrade temperature × 9/5) + 32 = Fahrenheit temperature

Selected Conversion to Metric Measures

KNOWN VALUE	MULTIPLY BY	TO FIND
inches	2.54	centimeters
ounces	28	grams
pounds	454	grams
pounds	0.45	kilogram

Selected Conversion From Metric Measures

KNOWN VALUE	MULTIPLY BY	TO FIND
centimeters	0.4	inches
grams	0.035	ounces
grams	0.0022	pounds
kilograms	2.2	pounds

Conversion of Pounds and Ounces to Grams

POUNDS	OUNCES 0	1	2	3	4	5	6	7	8	9	10	11	12	13	14	15
0	—	28	57	85	113	142	170	198	227	255	283	312	340	369	397	425
1	454	482	510	539	567	595	624	652	680	709	737	765	794	822	850	879
2	907	936	964	992	1021	1049	1077	1106	1134	1162	1191	1219	1247	1276	1304	1332
3	1361	1389	1417	1446	1474	1503	1531	1559	1588	1616	1644	1673	1701	1729	1758	1786
4	1814	1843	1871	1899	1928	1956	1984	2013	2041	2070	2098	2126	2155	2183	2211	2240
5	2268	2296	2325	2353	2381	2410	2438	2466	2495	2523	2551	2580	2608	2637	2665	2693
6	2722	2750	2778	2807	2835	2863	2892	2920	2948	2977	3005	3033	3062	3090	3118	3147
7	3175	3203	3232	3260	3289	3317	3345	3374	3402	3430	3459	3487	3515	3544	3572	3600
8	3629	3657	3685	3714	3742	3770	3799	3827	3856	3884	3912	3941	3969	3997	4026	4054
9	4082	4111	4139	4167	4196	4224	4252	4281	4309	4337	4366	4394	4423	4451	4479	4508
10	4536	4564	4593	4621	4649	4678	4706	4734	4763	4791	4819	4848	4876	4904	4933	4961
11	4990	5018	5046	5075	5103	5131	5160	5188	5216	5245	5273	5301	5330	5358	5386	5415
12	5443	5471	5500	5528	5557	5585	5613	5642	5670	5698	5727	5755	5783	5812	5840	5868
13	5897	5925	5953	5982	6010	6038	6067	6095	6123	6152	6180	6209	6237	6265	6294	6322
14	6350	6379	6407	6435	6464	6492	6520	6549	6577	6605	6634	6662	6690	6719	6747	6776
15	6804	6832	6860	6889	6917	6945	6973	7002	7030	7059	7087	7115	7144	7172	7201	7228
16	7257	7286	7313	7342	7371	7399	7427	7456	7484	7512	7541	7569	7597	7626	7654	7682
17	7711	7739	7768	7796	7824	7853	7881	7909	7938	7966	7994	8023	8051	8079	8108	8136
18	8165	8192	8221	8249	8278	8306	8335	8363	8391	8420	8448	8476	8504	8533	8561	8590
19	8618	8646	8675	8703	8731	8760	8788	8816	8845	8873	8902	8930	8958	8987	9015	9043
20	9072	9100	9128	9157	9185	9213	9242	9270	9298	9327	9355	9383	9412	9440	9469	9497
21	9525	9554	9582	9610	9639	9667	9695	9724	9752	9780	9809	9837	9865	9894	9922	9950
22	9979	10007	10036	10064	10092	10120	10149	10177	10206	10234	10262	10291	10319	10347	10376	10404

Appendix C
Guidelines for Working With Deaf Patients and Interpreters

1. First, remember that it requires trust on the part of the patient to allow nonsigning caregivers and an interpreter into her life.

2. It is important to use a registered interpreter. Medical interpreters are registered with the Registry of Interpreters for the Deaf. Although family members and friends may offer to interpret, it is best to use registered medical interpreters because they are required to translate the patients' and nurses' words accurately without adding in any other opinion.

3. Greet the patient and the family with handshakes and a body posture that indicates welcome. You may point to your name tag and use the American Sign Language (ASL) alphabet cards to spell out your name. The patient may wish to select cards to indicate her name. It is especially important as you work together to make the effort to provide a greeting as you would with speaking patients; greetings help develop rapport.

4. Once the interpreter is present, continue to look at the patient and speak directly to her. There will be a temptation to look at the interpreter, and it will help to remember that you are speaking to the patient.

5. Avoid phrasing your words as if you are talking to the interpreter (e.g., "Can you tell her . . . ?"). Instead, phrase your questions as you do with speaking patients (e.g., "I'm going to ask you some questions now.").

6. Depend on the deaf patient to ask questions.

7. Look at the patient's face for signs of difficulty in understanding. Deaf patients have a behavior of "gesturing" that involves shaking their heads as if to indicate "yes" even when they do not understand. If the patient is nodding "yes," ask her to repeat the directions you have just given.

8. Be as direct as possible. Keep to what you want to know or what you want to convey. Speak in short sentences, using nontechnical words. Avoid colloquial or slang words. Be sure to explain what you want to do before you do it. For instance, tell her you want to start an IV and explain the equipment. Then, with her permission, start the IV.

9. Be aware that deaf patients may have difficulty understanding when to take medications. It will be helpful to associate taking medications or completing some treatment or activity with meals. (For instance, while showing her the two capsules she is to take when she goes home, tell her to take the two capsules at breakfast and another two capsules at bedtime.) Avoid saying, "Take two capsules at 8:00 a.m., 2:00 p.m., and 12:00 a.m."

10. The difference in interpreting time may also affect obtaining a history. It is best to begin with a specific event in the past and work forward.

What to Do Until the Interpreter Arrives

1. Role-play as much as possible.

2. Demonstrate what you want the patient to do or what you want to do.

3. Be resourceful.

4. Remember that some deaf patients can read lips. Some may read written language, but use care in assuming the patient understands.

What to Do to Prepare for Working With a Deaf Patient

1. Contact local agencies that work with deaf patients to see what resources are available. Ask about classes in ASL. Being able to use some basic signs will be very helpful while waiting for an interpreter to arrive.

2. Read to learn more about the deaf culture. Contact your local agency or the National Information Center on Deafness, Silver Springs, Maryland, to get suggestions on books you might read.

3. Investigate your health facility. What is available to assist you? Look for videos used for teaching in the maternal–child unit and note if they have captions. Remember that many deaf patients do not read written language, so it will be important to review the content of the video with an interpreter present.

Prepared with the kind assistance of Mr. Gerald Dement, Interpreter Coordinator, Pikes Peak Center on Deafness, Colorado Springs, Colorado.

Sign Language for Healthcare Professionals

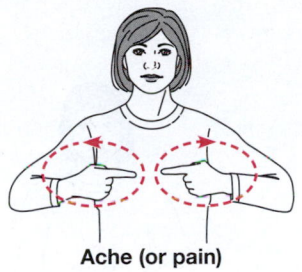

Ache (or pain)

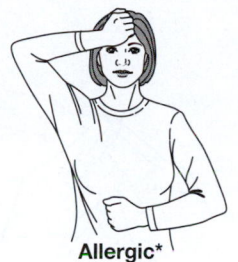

Allergic*

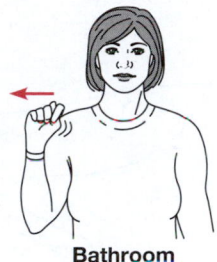

Bathroom

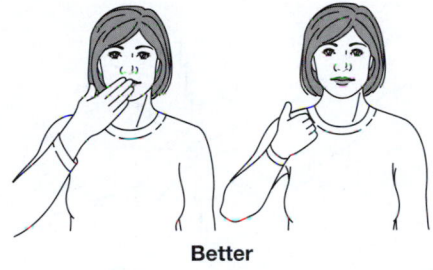

Better

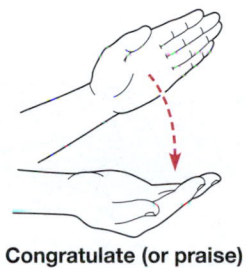

Congratulate (or praise)

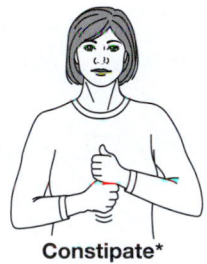

Constipate*

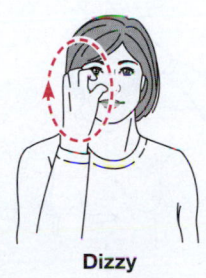

Dizzy

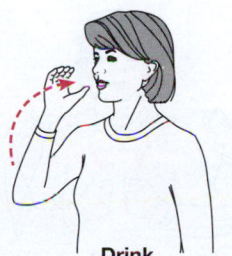

Drink

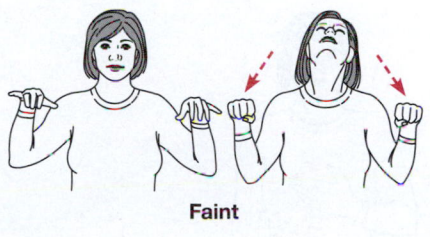

Faint

*Indicates signs that are in manually signed English. Those without an asterisk are in American Sign Language.

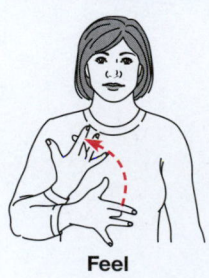

Feel

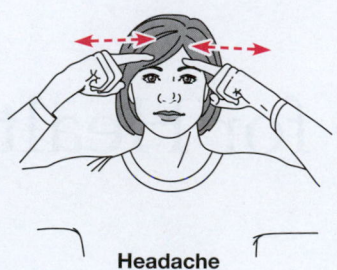

Headache

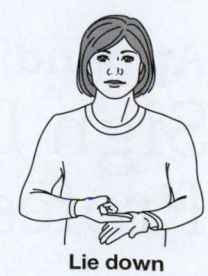

Lie down

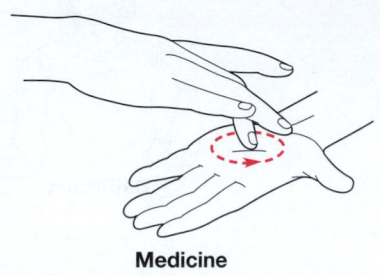

Medicine

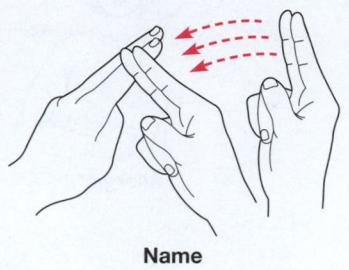

Name

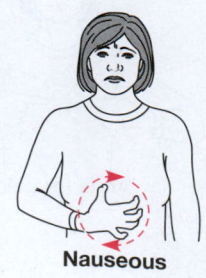

Nauseous

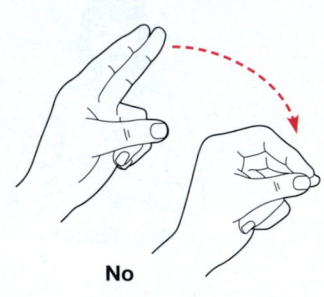

No

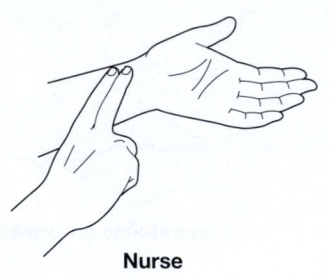

Nurse

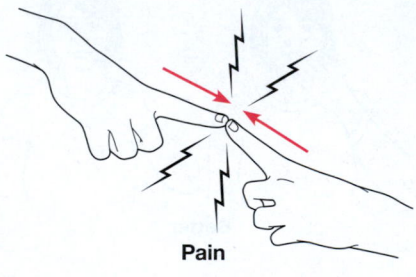

Pain

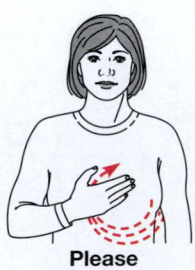

Please

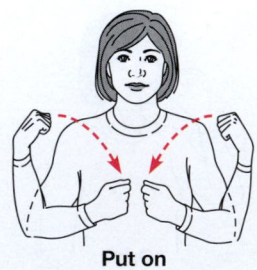

Put on

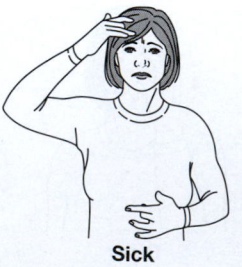

Sick

*Indicates signs that are in manually signed English. Those without an asterisk are in American Sign Language.

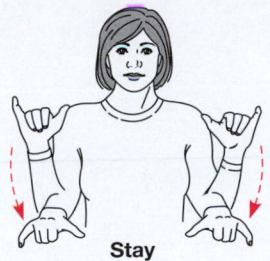

Stay

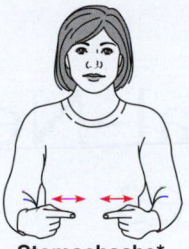

Stomachache*

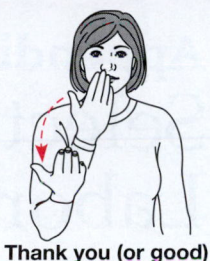

Thank you (or good)

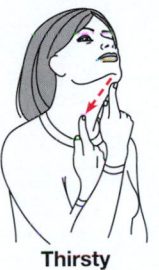

Thirsty

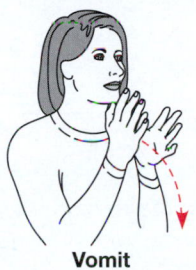

Vomit

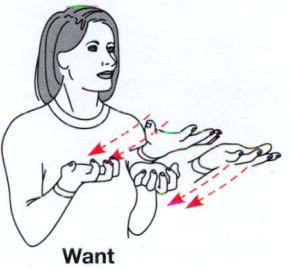

Want

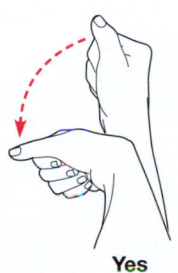

Yes

*Indicates signs that are in manually signed English. Those without an asterisk are in American Sign Language.

Appendix E
Selected Maternal–Newborn Laboratory Values

Normal Maternal Laboratory Values*

TEST	NONPREGNANT VALUES	PREGNANT VALUES
Hematocrit	37%–47%	32%–42%
Hemoglobin	12–16 g/dL**	10–14 g/dL**
Platelets	150,000–350,000/mm^3	Significant increase 3–5 days after birth (predisposes to thrombosis)
Partial thromboplastin time (PTT)	12–14 seconds	Slight decrease in pregnancy and again in labor (placental site clotting)
Fibrinogen	250 mg/dL	400 mg/dL
Serum glucose		
Fasting	70–80 mg/dL	65 mg/dL
2-hour postprandial	60–110 mg/dL	Less than 140 mg/dL
Total protein	6.7–8.3 g/dL	5.5–7.5 g/dL
White blood cell total	4500–10,000/mm^3	5000–15,000/mm^3
Polymorphonuclear cells	54%–62%	60%–85%
Lymphocytes	38%–46%	15%–40%

*All maternal and newborn laboratory values are approximate. Consult your local laboratory for guidelines as to normal values.
**At sea level.

Normal Term Neonatal Cord Blood Laboratory Values*

TEST	NORMAL VALUES
Hematocrit	35%–60%**
Hemoglobin	14–20 g/dL
Platelets	150,000–350,000/mm^3
Reticulocyte	3%–7%
White blood cell total	16,200–31,500/mm^3
White blood cell differential	
Polymorphonuclear (segs)	40%–80%
Lymphocytes	20%–40%
Monocytes	3%–10%
Serum glucose	55–96 mg/dL**
Serum electrolytes	
Sodium	129–144 mEq/L**
Potassium	3.4–10.0 mEq/L**
Chloride	100–121 mEq/L**
Carbon dioxide	13–29 mmol/L
Bicarbonate	18–23 mEq/L
Calcium	8.2–11.1 mg/dL
Total protein	4.8–7.3 g/dL

Note: Data from Fanaroff, A. A., & Martin, R. J. (Eds.). (2015). *Neonatal–perinatal medicine* (10th ed.). Philadelphia, PA: Elsevier Saunders.
*All maternal and newborn laboratory values are approximate. Consult your local laboratory for guidelines as to normal values.
**At sea level.

Glossary

A

Abortion   Loss of pregnancy before the fetus is viable outside the uterus; miscarriage.

Abruptio placentae (placental abruption)   Partial or total premature separation of a normally implanted placenta.

Accelerations   Periodic increases in the baseline fetal heart rate normally caused by fetal movement.

AIDS   Acquired immunodeficiency syndrome; immunologic disorder caused by infection with the human immunodeficiency virus (HIV) and characterized by increasing susceptibility to opportunistic infections and rare cancers.

Acrocyanosis   Cyanosis of the extremities.

Acrosomal reaction   Breakdown of the hyaluronic acid in the corona radiata by enzymes from the heads of sperm; allows one spermatozoon to penetrate the ovum zona pellucida.

Active acquired immunity   Formation of antibodies by the pregnant woman in response to illness or immunization.

Active management of labor (AMOL)   Medical protocol for augmentation of labor that includes (1) a strict criterion for labor admission, (2) early amniotomy, (3) high-dose oxytocin infusion for inefficient labor contractions, and (4) a commitment to provision of continuous nursing care.

Acute bilirubin encephalopathy (ABE)   Refers to the deposition of indirect or unconjugated bilirubin in the basal ganglia of the brain and to the permanent neurologic sequelae of untreated elevation of bilirubin level (hyperbilirubinemia). Also called *kernicterus*.

Adequate intake (AI)   A value cited for a nutrient when there are not sufficient data to calculate an estimated average requirement.

Adjustment reaction with depressed mood   A maternal adjustment reaction occurring in the first few postpartum days, characterized by mild depression, tearfulness, anxiety, headache, and irritability. Also called *postpartum blues*.

Afterpains   Cramplike pains due to contractions of the uterus that occur after childbirth. They are more common in multiparas, tend to be most severe during breastfeeding, and last 2 to 3 days.

Alternative therapy   Any procedure or approach that is used in place of conventional medicine.

Amenorrhea   Suppression or absence of menstruation.

Amniocentesis   Removal of amniotic fluid by insertion of a needle into the amniotic sac; amniotic fluid is used to assess fetal health or maturity.

Amnioinfusion (AI)   Procedure used to infuse a sterile fluid (such as normal saline) through an intrauterine catheter into the uterus in an attempt to increase the fluid around the umbilical cord to decrease or prevent cord compression during labor contractions; also used to dilute thick meconium-stained amniotic fluid.

Amnion   The inner of the two membranes that form the sac containing the fetus and the amniotic fluid.

Amniotic fluid   The liquid surrounding the fetus in utero. It absorbs shocks, permits fetal movement, and prevents heat loss.

Amniotic fluid embolism syndrome   An obstetric emergency that occurs when a bolus of amniotic fluid, fetal cells, hair, or other debris enters the maternal circulation and then the maternal lungs; the cause is unknown but has a 60% to 80% mortality rate. Also called *anaphylactoid syndrome of pregnancy*.

Amniotic fluid index (AFI)   A method of reporting fluid volume. The AFI is calculated by dividing the maternal abdomen into four quadrants with the umbilicus as the reference point. Then the deepest vertical pocket is measured. These measurements are summed to calculate the AFI.

Amniotomy   The artificial rupturing of the amniotic membrane.

Ampulla   The outer two thirds of the fallopian tube; fertilization of the ovum by a spermatozoon usually occurs here.

Anaphylactoid syndrome of pregnancy   An obstetric emergency that occurs when a bolus of amniotic fluid, fetal cells, hair, or other debris enters the maternal circulation and then the maternal lungs; the cause is unknown but has a 60% to 80% mortality rate. Also called *amniotic fluid embolism syndrome*.

Aneuploidy   An abnormal number of chromosomes that is often responsible for genetic defects.

Antepartum   Time between conception and the onset of labor; usually used to describe the period during which a woman is pregnant.

Apgar score   A scoring system used to evaluate newborns at 1 minute and 5 minutes after birth. The total score is achieved by assessing five signs: heart rate, respiratory effort, muscle tone, reflex irritability, and color. Each of the signs is assigned a score of 0, 1, or 2. The highest possible score is 10.

Areola   Pigmented ring surrounding the nipple of the breast.

Artificial rupture of membranes (AROM)   Use of a device such as an amnihook or Allis forceps to rupture the amniotic membranes.

Assisted reproductive technology (ART)   Term used to describe the highly technologic approaches used to produce pregnancy.

Autosomes   Chromosomes that are not sex chromosomes.

B

Bag of waters (BOW)   The membrane containing the amniotic fluid and the fetus.

Ballottement   A technique of palpation to detect or examine a floating object in the body. In obstetrics, the fetus, when pushed, floats away and then returns to touch the examiner's fingers.

Barlow maneuver   A test designed to detect subluxation or dislocation of the hip. A dysplastic joint will be felt to be dislocated as the femur leaves the acetabulum.

Baseline rate   The average baseline fetal heart rate (BL FHR) observed during a 10-minute period of monitoring.

Baseline variability (BL VAR)   Changes in the fetal heart rate that result from the interplay between the sympathetic and the parasympathetic nervous systems.

Becoming a mother (BAM)   Process by which a woman learns mothering behaviors and becomes comfortable with her identity as a mother. Also called *maternal role attainment*.

Bereavement   To have suffered the *event* of loss.

Biophysical profile (BPP)   Assessment of five variables in the fetus that help to evaluate fetal risk: breathing movement, body movement, tone, amniotic fluid volume, and fetal heart rate reactivity.

Birth rate Number of live births per 1000 population.

Birthing rooms Single rooms where the woman and her partner or other family members or support persons will stay for the labor, birth, recovery, and possibly the postpartum period.

Blastocyst The inner solid mass of cells within the morula.

Bloody show Pink-tinged mucus secretions resulting from rupture of small capillaries as the cervix effaces and dilates.

Boggy uterus A term used to describe the uterine fundus when it is not firmly contracted after the birth of the baby and in the early postpartum period; excessive bleeding occurs from the placental site, and maternal hemorrhage may occur.

Braxton Hicks contractions Intermittent painless contractions of the uterus that may occur every 10 to 20 minutes. They occur more frequently toward the end of pregnancy and are sometimes mistaken for true labor signs.

Brazelton Neonatal Behavioral Assessment Scale A brief examination used to identify a newborn's behavioral states and responses.

Breasts Mammary glands.

Broad ligament The ligament extending from the lateral margins of the uterus to the pelvic wall; keeps the uterus centrally placed and provides stability within the pelvic cavity.

Brown adipose tissue (BAT) Fat deposits in newborns that provide greater heat-generating activity than ordinary fat. Found around the kidneys, adrenals, and neck; between the scapulas; and behind the sternum. Also called *brown fat.*

C

Calorie Amount of heat required to raise the temperature of 1 kg of water 1°C.

Capacitation Removal of the plasma membrane overlying the spermatozoa's acrosomal area with the loss of seminal plasma proteins and the glycoprotein coat. If the glycoprotein coat is not removed, the sperm will not be able to penetrate the ovum.

Caput succedaneum Swelling or edema occurring in or under the fetal scalp during labor.

Cardinal ligaments The chief uterine supports, suspending the uterus from the side walls of the true pelvis.

Cardinal movements The positional changes of the fetus as it moves through the birth canal during labor and birth. The positional changes are descent, flexion, internal rotation, extension, restitution, and external rotation. Also called *mechanisms of labor.*

Cardiopulmonary adaptation Adaptation of the newborn's cardiovascular and respiratory systems to life outside the womb.

Cell-free fetal DNA Screening tool used to test for trisomy 13, 18, and 21. The test detects circulating fetal deoxyribonucleic acid (DNA) within the maternal serum.

Cephalohematoma Subcutaneous swelling containing blood found on the head of a newborn several days after birth; it usually disappears within a few weeks to 2 months.

Cephalopelvic disproportion (CPD) A condition in which the fetal head is of such a shape or size, or in such a position, that it cannot pass through the maternal pelvis.

Cerclage Surgical procedure in which a stitch is placed in the cervix to prevent a spontaneous abortion or premature birth.

Certified nurse–midwife (CNM) An RN who has received special training and education in the care of the family during childbearing and the prenatal, labor and birth, and postpartum periods. After a period of formal education, the nurse–midwife takes a certification test to become a CNM.

Certified registered nurse (RNC) A registered nurse who has shown expertise in a specific field by passing a national certification examination.

Cervical insufficiency Painless dilatation of the cervix without contractions because of a structural or functional defect of the cervix.

Cervical ripening Softening of the cervix; occurs normally as a physiologic process before labor or is stimulated to occur through the process of induction of labor.

Cervix The "neck" between the external os and the body of the uterus. The lower end of the cervix extends into the vagina.

Cesarean birth Birth of fetus accomplished by performing a surgical incision through the maternal abdomen and uterus.

Chemical conjunctivitis Irritation of the mucous membrane lining of the eyelid; may be due to instillation of silver nitrate ophthalmic drops.

Chlamydial infection Caused by *Chlamydia trachomatis*, this infection is the most common bacterial sexually transmitted infection in the United States.

Chloasma (melasma gravidarum) Brownish pigmentation over the bridge of the nose and the cheeks during pregnancy and in some women who are taking oral contraceptives. Also called *mask of pregnancy.*

Chorion The fetal membrane closest to the intrauterine wall that gives rise to the placenta and continues as the outer membrane surrounding the amnion.

Chorionic villus sampling (CVS) Procedure in which a specimen of the chorionic villi is obtained from the edge of the developing placenta at about 8 weeks' gestation. The sample can be used for chromosomal, enzyme, and DNA tests.

Chromosomes The threadlike structures within the nucleus of a cell that carry the genes.

Circumcision Surgical removal of the prepuce (foreskin) of the penis.

Cleavage Rapid mitotic division of the zygote; cells produced are called *blastomeres.*

Clinical nurse specialist (CNS) A nurse possessing a master's degree and specialized knowledge and competence in a specific clinical area.

Clinical practice guidelines Comprehensive interdisciplinary care plans for specific conditions that describe the sequence and timing of interventions that should result in expected patient outcomes.

Coitus interruptus Method of contraception in which the male withdraws his penis from the vagina before ejaculation.

Cold stress Excessive heat loss resulting in compensatory mechanisms (increased respirations and nonshivering thermogenesis) to maintain core body temperature.

Colostrum Secretion from the breast before the onset of true lactation; contains mainly serum and white blood corpuscles. It has a high protein content, provides some immune properties, and cleanses the newborn's intestinal tract of mucus and meconium.

Colposcopy The use of an instrument inserted into the vagina to examine the cervical and vaginal tissues by means of a magnifying lens.

Complementary therapy Any procedure or product that is used together with conventional medical treatment.

Condom Rubber sheath that covers a man's penis to prevent conception or disease.

Conduction Loss of heat to a cooler surface by direct skin contact.

Condylomata acuminata Known also as genital or venereal warts, they are a common sexually transmitted infection caused by the human papilloma virus (HPV).

Congenital dermal melanocytes   Macular areas of bluish black or gray-blue pigmentation found on the dorsal area and the buttocks of newborns. Also called *Mongolian blue spots*.

Conjugate vera   The true conjugate, which extends from the middle of the sacral promontory to the middle of the pubic crest.

Continuous epidural infusion (CEI)   A combination of opioid and local anesthesia medication that is continually administered via an electric pump.

Contraction stress test (CST)   A method of assessing the reaction of the fetus to the stress of uterine contractions. This test may be utilized when contractions are occurring spontaneously or when contractions are artificially induced by oxytocin challenge test (OCT) or breast self-stimulation test (BSST).

Convection   Loss of heat from the warm body surface to cooler air currents.

Cornua   The elongated portions of the uterus where the fallopian tubes open.

Corpus   The upper two thirds of the uterus.

Corpus luteum   A small yellow body that develops within a ruptured ovarian follicle; it secretes progesterone in the second half of the menstrual cycle and atrophies about 3 days before the beginning of menstrual flow. If pregnancy occurs, the corpus luteum continues to produce progesterone until the placenta takes over this function.

Cosleeping   A baby sleeping in close social and/or physical contact with a committed caregiver (usually the mother).

Cotyledons   Rounded portions into which the placenta's uterine surface is divided, consisting of a mass of villi, fetal vessels, and an intervillous space.

Couplet care   A family-centered approach for maternal–child nursing where both the mother and her baby are cared for by the same nurse, with the baby remaining at the mother's bedside. Also called *mother–baby care*.

Couvade   In some cultures, the male's observance of certain rituals and taboos to signify the transition to fatherhood.

Crowning   Appearance of the presenting fetal part at the vaginal orifice during labor.

Culture   The beliefs, values, attitudes, and practices that are accepted by a population, community, or an individual.

Cystitis   Inflammation of the bladder.

Cystocele   The downward displacement of the bladder, which appears as a bulge in the anterior vaginal wall.

D

Date rape   Rape in which the assailant is someone with whom the victim has had previous nonviolent interaction or which occurs between a dating couple.

Decelerations   Periodic decreases in the baseline fetal heart rate.

Decidua basalis   The part of the decidua that unites with the chorion to form the placenta. It is shed in lochial discharge after childbirth.

Decidua capsularis   The part of the decidua surrounding the chorionic sac.

Decidua vera (parietalis)   Nonplacental decidua lining the uterus.

Depo-Provera   A long-acting, injectable progestin contraceptive.

Diagonal conjugate   Distance from the lower posterior border of the symphysis pubis to the sacral promontory; may be obtained by manual measurement.

Diaphragm   A flexible disk that covers the cervix to prevent pregnancy.

Diastasis recti abdominis   Separation of the recti abdominis muscles along the median line. In women, it is seen with repeated childbirths or multiple gestations. In the newborn, it is usually caused by incomplete development.

Dietary reference intakes (DRIs)   Specific allowances for pregnant and lactating women, DRIs are subdivided into the recommended dietary allowance (RDA) and adequate intake (AI).

Dilatation of the cervix   Expansion of the external os from an opening a few millimeters in size to an opening large enough to allow the passage of the baby.

Dilation and curettage (D&C)   Stretching of the cervical canal to permit passage of a curette, which is used to scrape the endometrium to empty the uterine contents or to obtain tissue for examination.

Diploid number of chromosomes   Containing a set of maternal and a set of paternal chromosomes; in humans, the diploid number of chromosomes is 46.

Domestic violence   Defined as the collective methods used to exert power and control by one individual over another in an adult intimate relationship. Forms of abuse typically fall into three categories: psychologic abuse, physical abuse, and sexual abuse.

Doula   A supportive companion who accompanies a laboring woman to provide emotional, physical, and informational support and acts as an advocate for the woman and her family.

Ductus arteriosus (DA)   A communication channel between the main pulmonary artery and the aorta of the fetus. It is obliterated after birth by rising PO_2 and changes in intravascular pressure in the presence of normal pulmonary functioning. It normally becomes a ligament after birth but sometimes remains patent (patent ductus arteriosus, a treatable condition).

Ductus venosus   A fetal blood vessel that carries oxygenated blood between the umbilical vein and the inferior vena cava, bypassing the liver; it becomes a ligament after birth.

Dysmenorrhea   Painful menstruation.

Dyspareunia   Painful intercourse.

Dystocia   Difficult labor due to mechanical factors produced by the fetus or the maternal pelvis or due to inadequate uterine or other muscular activity.

E

Early adolescence   A term referring to adolescents who are age 14 and under.

Early deceleration   Periodic change in fetal heart rate pattern caused by head compression; deceleration has a uniform appearance and early onset in relation to maternal contraction.

Early (primary) postpartum hemorrhage   Profuse bleeding (loss of blood of greater than 500 mL) that occurs in the first 24 hours after childbirth, primarily caused by uterine atony.

Early term   Birth occurring between 37 weeks 0 days and 38 weeks 6 days.

Eclampsia   A major complication of pregnancy. Its cause is unknown; it occurs more often in the primigravida and is accompanied by elevated blood pressure, albuminuria, oliguria, tonic and clonic convulsions, and coma. It may occur during pregnancy (usually after the 20th week of gestation) or within 48 hours after childbirth.

Ectoderm   Outer layer of cells in the developing embryo that gives rise to the skin, nails, and hair.

Ectopic pregnancy (EP)   Implantation of the fertilized ovum outside the uterine cavity; common sites are the abdomen, fallopian tubes, and ovaries. Also called *oocyesis*.

Electronic fetal monitoring (EFM) A method of placing a fetal monitor on the fetus in order to obtain a continuous tracing of the fetal heart rate, which allows many characteristics of the FHR to be observed and evaluated.

Emancipated minors Minors who are legally considered to have assumed the rights of an adult. An adolescent may be considered emancipated if he or she is self-supporting and living away from home, married, pregnant, a parent, or in the military.

Embryo The early stage of development of the young of any organism. In humans the embryonic period is from about 2 to 8 weeks' gestation and is characterized by cellular differentiation and predominantly hyperplastic growth.

Embryonic membranes The amnion and chorion.

En face An assumed position in which one person looks at another and maintains his or her face in the same vertical plane as that of the other.

Endoderm The inner layer of cells in the developing embryo that give rise to internal organs such as the intestines.

Endometriosis Ectopic endometrium located outside the uterus in the pelvic cavity. Symptoms may include pelvic pain or pressure, dysmenorrhea, dyspareunia, abnormal bleeding from the uterus or rectum, and sterility.

Endometrium The mucous membrane that lines the inner surface of the uterus.

Engagement The entrance of the fetal presenting part into the superior pelvic strait and the beginning of the descent through the pelvic canal.

Engrossment Characteristic sense of absorption, preoccupation, and interest in the newborn demonstrated by fathers during early contact with their babies.

Epidural block Regional anesthesia effective through the first and second stages of labor.

Episiotomy Incision of the perineum to facilitate birth and to avoid laceration of the perineum.

Epstein's pearls Small, white blebs found along the gum margins and at the junction of the hard and soft palates; commonly seen in the newborn as a normal manifestation.

Erb-Duchenne paralysis (Erb palsy) Paralysis of the arm and chest wall as a result of a birth injury to the brachial plexus or a subsequent injury to the fifth and sixth cervical nerves.

Erythema toxicum Innocuous pink papular rash of unknown cause with superimposed vesicles; it appears within 24 to 48 hours after birth and resolves spontaneously within a few days.

Erythroblastosis fetalis Hemolytic disease of the newborn characterized by anemia, jaundice, enlargement of the liver and spleen, and generalized edema. Caused by isoimmunization due to Rh incompatibility or ABO incompatibility.

Estimated date of birth (EDB) During a pregnancy, the approximate date when childbirth will occur; the "due date."

Estrogens The hormones estradiol and estrone, produced by the ovary.

Ethnicity A social identity that is associated with shared beliefs, behaviors, and patterns.

Ethnocentrism An individual's belief that the values and practices of his or her own culture are the best ones.

Evaporation Loss of heat incurred when water on the skin surface is converted to a vapor.

Evidence-based practice An approach to problem solving and decision making based on the consideration of data from research, statistical analysis, quality measures, risk management measurements, and other sources of reliable information.

External cephalic version (ECV) Procedure involving external manipulation of the maternal abdomen to change the presentation of the fetus from breech to cephalic.

F

Fallopian tubes Tubes that extend from the lateral angle of the uterus and terminate near the ovary; they serve as a passageway for the ovum from the ovary to the uterus and for the spermatozoa from the uterus toward the ovary. Also called *oviducts* and *uterine tubes*.

False pelvis The portion of the pelvis above the linea terminalis; its primary function is to support the weight of the enlarged pregnant uterus.

Family Two or more persons who are joined together by bonds of sharing and emotional closeness and who identify themselves as being part of a family.

Family-centered care An approach to health care based on the concept that a hospital can provide professional services to mothers, fathers, and newborns in a homelike environment that will enhance the integrity of the family unit.

Female reproductive cycle (FRC) The monthly rhythmic changes in sexually mature women.

Fetal alcohol spectrum disorder (FASD) An umbrella term that includes all categories of prenatal alcohol exposure, including fetal alcohol syndrome (FAS); it is not meant to be used as a clinical diagnosis.

Fetal alcohol syndrome (FAS) Syndrome caused by maternal alcohol ingestion and characterized by microcephaly, intrauterine growth restriction, short palpebral fissures, and maxillary hypoplasia.

Fetal attitude Relationship of the fetal parts to one another. Normal fetal attitude is one of moderate flexion of the arms onto the chest and flexion of the legs onto the abdomen.

Fetal blood sampling (FBS) Blood sample drawn from the fetal scalp (or from the fetus in breech position) to evaluate the acid–base status of the fetus.

Fetal bradycardia A fetal heart rate less than 110 beats per minute during a 10-minute period of continuous monitoring.

Fetal breathing movements (FBM) Intrauterine practice respiratory movements that begin around the 17th to 20th week of gestation.

Fetal lie Relationship of the cephalocaudal axis (spinal column) of the fetus to the cephalocaudal axis (spinal column) of the woman. The fetus may be in a longitudinal or transverse lie.

Fetal movement count (FMC) A method for tracking fetal activity taught to pregnant women. Also called *fetal movement record (FMR)*.

Fetal position Relationship of the landmark on the presenting fetal part to the front, sides, or back of the maternal pelvis.

Fetal presentation The fetal body part that enters the maternal pelvis first. The three possible presentations are cephalic, shoulder, and breech.

Fetal tachycardia A fetal heart rate of 161 beats per minute or more during a 10-minute period of continuous monitoring.

Fetus The child in utero from about the seventh to ninth week of gestation until birth.

Fibrocystic breast changes Benign breast changes characterized by bilateral, cyclic breast pain and breast nodularities that may be unilateral or bilateral, and often in the upper outer quadrants of the breasts.

Fimbria Any structure resembling a fringe; the fringelike extremity of the fallopian tubes.

First-trimester combined screening Utilizes nuchal translucency testing (NTT) and serum testing to increase accuracy by testing for pregnancy-associated plasma protein-A (PAPP-A) and free beta human chorionic gonadotropin (βhCG) to determine if a fetus is at risk for trisomies 13, 18, and 21.

Folic acid   An important vitamin directly related to the outcome of pregnancy and to maternal and fetal health.

Follicle-stimulating hormone (FSH)   Hormone produced by the anterior pituitary during the first half of the menstrual cycle, stimulating development of the graafian follicle.

Fontanelles   In the fetus, the unossified spaces, or soft spots, consisting of a strong band of connective tissue lying between the cranial bones of the skull.

Foramen ovale   Special opening between the atria of the fetal heart. Normally, the opening closes shortly after birth; if it remains open, it can be repaired surgically.

Forceps-assisted birth   A birth in which a set of instruments, known as forceps, are applied to the presenting part of the fetus to provide traction or to enable the fetal head to be rotated to an occiput-anterior position. Forceps-assisted birth is also known as *instrumental delivery*, *operative delivery*, or *operative vaginal delivery*.

Forceps marks   Reddened areas over the cheeks and jaws caused by the application of forceps. The red areas usually disappear within 1 to 2 days.

Foremilk   Breast milk obtained at the beginning of the breastfeeding episode.

Full term   Birth occurring between 39 weeks 0 days and 40 weeks 6 days.

Fundus   The upper portion of the uterus between the fallopian tubes.

Funic presentation   A complication of labor in which the umbilical cord is interposed between the cervix and the presenting part.

G

Gametes   Female or male germ cells; contain a haploid number of chromosomes.

Gamete intrafallopian transfer (GIFT)   Retrieval of oocytes by laparoscopy; immediately combining oocytes with washed, motile sperm in a catheter; and placement of the gametes into the fimbriated end of the fallopian tube.

Gametogenesis   The process by which germ cells are produced.

General anesthesia   A state of induced unconsciousness that may be achieved through intravenous injection, inhalation of anesthetic agents, or a combination of both methods.

Genotype   The genetic composition of an individual.

Gestation   Period of intrauterine development from conception through birth; pregnancy.

Gestational age assessment tools   Systems used to evaluate the newborn's external physical characteristics and neurologic and/or neuromuscular development to accurately determine gestational age. These replace or supplement the traditional calculation from the woman's last menstrual period.

Gestational diabetes mellitus (GMD)   A form of diabetes of variable severity with onset or first recognition during pregnancy.

Gestational trophoblastic disease (GTD)   Disorder classified into two types: benign (hydatidiform mole) and malignant.

Gonadotropin-releasing hormone (GnRH)   A hormone secreted by the hypothalamus that stimulates the anterior pituitary to secrete FSH and LH.

Graafian follicle   The ovarian cyst containing the ripe ovum; it secretes estrogens.

Gravida   A pregnant woman.

Grief   An individual's *reaction* to loss, including physical symptoms, thoughts, feelings, functional limitations, and spiritual responses.

H

Habituation   Newborn's ability to diminish innate responses to specific repeated stimuli.

Haploid number of chromosomes   Half the diploid number of chromosomes. In humans there are 23 chromosomes, the haploid number, in each germ cell.

Harlequin sign   A rare color change that occurs between the longitudinal halves of the newborn's body, such that the dependent half is noticeably pinker than the superior half when the newborn is placed on one side; it is of no pathologic significance.

HELLP syndrome   A cluster of changes including *h*emolysis, *e*levated *l*iver enzymes, and *l*ow *p*latelet count; sometimes associated with severe preeclampsia.

Hemolytic disease of the newborn   Hyperbilirubinemia secondary to Rh incompatibility.

Herpes genitalis   A lifelong, recurrent sexually transmitted infection caused by the herpes simplex virus (HSV).

Hindmilk   Breast milk released after initial let-down reflex; high in fat content.

Human chorionic gonadotropin (hCG)   A hormone produced by the chorionic villi and found in the urine of pregnant women.

HIV   Human immunodeficiency virus; causes a progressive disease that ultimately results in the development of *acquired immunodeficiency syndrome (AIDS)*.

Hydatidiform mole   Degenerative process in chorionic villi, giving rise to multiple cysts and rapid growth of the uterus, with hemorrhage.

Hydramnios   An excess of amniotic fluid, leading to overdistention of the uterus. Frequently seen in pregnant women who have diabetes, even if there is no coexisting fetal anomaly. Also called *polyhydramnios*.

Hydrops fetalis   Fetal edema caused by anemia.

Hyperbilirubinemia   Excessive amount of bilirubin in the blood; indicative of hemolytic processes due to blood incompatibility, intrauterine infection, septicemia, neonatal renal infection, and other disorders.

Hyperemesis gravidarum   Excessive vomiting during pregnancy, leading to dehydration and starvation.

Hypoglycemia   Abnormally low level of sugar in the blood.

Hysterectomy   Surgical removal of the uterus.

Hysterosalpingography (HSG)   Testing by instillation of radiopaque substance into the uterine cavity to visualize the uterus and fallopian tubes.

I

In vitro fertilization (IVF)   Procedure during which oocytes are removed from the ovary, mixed with spermatozoa, fertilized, and incubated in a glass petri dish; then up to four viable embryos are placed in the woman's uterus.

Inborn errors of metabolism   Hereditary deficiency of specific enzymes needed for normal metabolism of specific chemicals.

Infant mortality rate   Number of deaths of infants under 1 year of age per 1000 live births in a given population per year.

Infant of diabetic mother (IDM) At-risk baby born to a woman previously diagnosed as having diabetes or who develops symptoms of diabetes during pregnancy.

Infant of substance-abusing mother (ISAM) A baby born to a mother who abuses or is addicted to drugs or alcohol; formerly called *infant of an addicted mother*.

Infertility Diminished ability to conceive.

Informed consent A legal concept that protects a person's rights to autonomy and self-determination by specifying that no action may be taken without that person's prior understanding and freely given consent.

Infundibulopelvic ligament Ligament that suspends and supports the ovaries.

Intimate partner violence (IPV) A pattern of coercive behaviors and methods used to exert power and control by one individual over another in an adult domestic or intimate relationship

Intrapartum The time from the onset of true labor until the birth of the neonate and expulsion of the placenta.

Intrauterine contraception (IUC) Small metal or plastic form that is placed in the uterus to prevent implantation of a fertilized ovum.

Intrauterine fetal surgery Surgery performed on a fetus to correct anatomic lesions that are not compatible with life if left untreated.

Intrauterine growth restriction (IUGR) Fetal undergrowth due to any etiology, such as intrauterine infection, deficient nutrient supply, or congenital malformation. A term used to describe fetuses falling below the 10th percentile in ultrasonic estimation of weight at a given gestational age.

Intrauterine pressure catheter (IUPC) A catheter that can be placed through the cervix into the uterus to measure uterine pressure during labor. Some types of catheters may be inserted for the purpose of infusing warmed saline to add additional intrauterine fluid when oligohydramnios is present.

Intrauterine resuscitation Corrective measures used to optimize the oxygen exchange within the maternal–fetal circulation that are implemented when signs of nonreassuring fetal status are detected during labor.

Involution Rolling or turning inward; the reduction in size of the uterus following childbirth.

Ischial spines Prominences that arise near the junction of the ilium and ischium and jut into the pelvic cavity; used as a reference point during labor to evaluate the descent of the fetal head into the birth canal.

Isthmus The straight, narrow part of the fallopian tube with a thick muscular wall and an opening (lumen) 2 to 3 mm in diameter; the site of tubal ligation. Also, a constriction in the uterus that is located above the cervix and below the corpus.

J

Jaundice Yellow pigmentation of body tissues caused by the presence of bile pigments.

K

Karyotype The set of chromosomes arranged in a standard order.

Kegel exercises Perineal muscle tightening that strengthens the pubococcygeus muscle and increases its tone.

Kernicterus An encephalopathy caused by deposition of unconjugated bilirubin in brain cells; may result in impaired brain function or death. Also called *acute bilirubin encephalopathy (ABE)*.

Kilocalorie (kcal) Equivalent to 1000 calories, it is the unit used to express the energy value of food.

L

La Leche League International (LLLI) Organization that provides information on and assistance with breastfeeding.

Labor induction The stimulation of uterine contractions before the spontaneous onset of labor, with or without ruptured fetal membranes, for the purpose of accomplishing birth.

Lactase deficiency A condition characterized by difficulty digesting milk and dairy products. Results from an inadequate amount of the enzyme lactase, which breaks down the milk sugar lactose into smaller digestible substances. Also called *lactose intolerance*.

Lacto-ovovegetarians Vegetarians who include milk, dairy products, and eggs in their diets and occasionally fish, poultry, and liver.

Lactovegetarians Vegetarians who include dairy products but no eggs in their diets.

Lanugo Fine, downy hair found on all body parts of the fetus, with the exception of the palms of the hands and the soles of the feet, after 20 weeks' gestation.

Laparoscopy Procedure that enables direct visualization of pelvic organs.

Large for gestational age (LGA) Excessive growth of a fetus in relation to the gestational time period.

Late adolescence A term referring to adolescents who are ages 18 to 19 years.

Late deceleration Symmetrical decrease in fetal heart rate beginning at or after the peak of the contraction and returning to baseline only after the contraction has ended, indicating possible uteroplacental insufficiency and potential that the fetus is not receiving adequate oxygenation.

Late preterm Births that occur between 34 0/7 through 36 6/7 weeks' gestation.

Late-preterm newborns Babies born between 34 0/7 and 36 6/7 weeks' gestation. These babies are at a greater risk for increases in mortality and morbidity because they are not physically mature and are more prone to have physiologic and metabolic complications

Late (secondary) postpartum hemorrhage Profuse bleeding (loss of blood of greater than 500 ml) that occurs from 24 hours to 6 weeks after childbirth.

Late term Births occurring between 41 weeks 0 days through 41 weeks 6 days.

Lecithin/sphingomyelin (L/S) ratio Lecithin and sphingomyelin are phospholipid components of surfactant; their ratio changes during gestation. When the L/S ratio reaches 2:1, the fetal lungs are thought to be mature and the fetus will have a low risk of respiratory distress syndrome (RDS) if born at that time.

Leopold maneuvers A series of four maneuvers designed to provide a systematic approach whereby the examiner may determine fetal presentation and position.

Let-down reflex Pattern of stimulation, hormone release, and resulting muscle contraction that forces milk into the lactiferous ducts, making it available to the newborn. Also called *milk ejection reflex*.

Leukorrhea Mucous discharge from the vagina or cervical canal that may be normal or pathologic, as in the presence of infection.

Lightening Moving of the fetus and uterus downward into the pelvic cavity.

Linea nigra The line of darker pigmentation extending from the umbilicus to the pubis noted in some women during the later months of pregnancy.

Local infiltration anesthesia Injection of an anesthetic agent into the intracutaneous, subcutaneous, and intramuscular areas of the perineum.

Lochia Maternal discharge of blood, mucus, and tissue from the uterus; may last for several weeks after birth.

Lochia alba   White vaginal discharge that follows lochia serosa and that lasts from about the 10th to the 21st day after birth.

Lochia rubra   Red, blood-tinged vaginal discharge that occurs following birth and lasts 2 to 4 days.

Lochia serosa   Pink, serous, and blood-tinged vaginal discharge that follows lochia rubra and lasts until the 7th to 10th day after birth.

Luteinizing hormone (LH)   Anterior pituitary hormone responsible for stimulating ovulation and for development of the corpus luteum.

M

Macrosomia   A condition seen in newborns of large body size and high birth weight (more than 4000 to 4500 g [8 lb, 13 oz to 9 lb, 14 oz]), such as those born of mothers who are diabetic or prediabetic.

Malposition   An abnormal position of the fetus in the birth canal.

Malpresentations   Various presentations of the fetus into the birth canal that is not "normal"—that is, brow, face, shoulder, or breech presentation.

Mammogram   A soft-tissue radiograph of the breast without the injection of a contrast medium.

Mastitis   Inflammation of the breast.

Maternal mortality rate   The number of maternal deaths from any cause during the pregnancy cycle per 100,000 live births.

Maternal role attainment (MRA)   Process by which a woman learns mothering behaviors and becomes comfortable with her identity as a mother. Also called *becoming a mother*.

Mature milk   Breast milk that contains 10% solids for energy and growth.

McDonald sign   A probable sign of pregnancy characterized by an ease in flexing the body of the uterus against the cervix.

Meconium   Dark green or black material present in the large intestine of a full-term newborn; the first stools passed by the newborn.

Meconium aspiration syndrome (MAS)   Respiratory disease of term, postterm, and small-for-gestational-age newborns caused by inhalation of meconium or meconium-stained amniotic fluid into the lungs; characterized by mild to severe respiratory distress, hyperexpansion of the chest, hyperinflated alveoli, and secondary atelectasis.

Meiosis   The process of cell division that occurs in the maturation of sperm and ova that decreases their number of chromosomes by one half.

Menarche   Beginning of menstrual and reproductive function in the female.

Mendelian (single-gene) inheritance   A major category of inheritance whereby a trait is determined by a pair of genes on homologous chromosomes.

Menopausal hormone therapy (MHT)   Administration of hormones, usually estrogen and a progestin, to alleviate the symptoms of menopause.

Menopause   The permanent cessation of menses.

Menstrual cycle   Cyclic buildup of the uterine lining, ovulation, and sloughing of the lining occurring approximately every 28 days in nonpregnant females.

Mesoderm   The intermediate layer of germ cells in the embryo that gives rise to connective tissue, bone marrow, muscles, blood, lymphoid tissue, and epithelial tissue.

Middle adolescence   A term referring to adolescents who are ages 15 to 17 years.

Milia   Tiny white papules appearing on the face of a newborn as a result of unopened sebaceous glands; they disappear spontaneously within a few weeks.

Miscarriage   Abortion that occurs naturally. Also called *spontaneous abortion*.

Mitosis   Process of cell division whereby both daughter cells have the same number and pattern of chromosomes as the original cell.

Molding   Shaping of the fetal head by overlapping of the cranial bones to facilitate movement through the birth canal during labor.

Monosomies   A genetic condition that occurs when a normal gamete unites with a gamete that is missing a chromosome.

Morning sickness   A term that refers to the nausea and vomiting that a woman may experience in early pregnancy. This lay term is sometimes used because these symptoms frequently occur in the early part of the day and disappear within a few hours.

Morula   Developmental stage of the fertilized ovum in which there is a solid mass of cells.

Mosaicism   Condition of an individual who has at least two cell lines with differing karyotypes.

Mother–baby care   Also called couplet care, a family-centered care approach in which the newborn remains at the mother's bedside and both are cared for by the same nurse.

Mottling   Discoloration of the skin in irregular areas; may be seen with chilling, poor perfusion, or hypoxia.

Mourning   The *process* by which individuals incorporate the loss experience into their lives, it is influenced by many factors including personality, gender, family dynamics, and social, religious, and cultural norms.

Mucous plug   A collection of thick mucus that blocks the cervical canal during pregnancy. Also called *operculum*.

Multigravida   Woman who has been pregnant more than once.

Multipara   Woman who has had more than one pregnancy in which the fetus was viable.

Multiple gestation   More than one fetus in the uterus at the same time.

Myometrium   Uterine muscular structure.

N

Nägele's rule   A method of determining the estimated date of birth (EDB): after obtaining the first day of the last menstrual period, subtract 3 months and add 7 days.

Neonatal morbidity   The number of potential cases per year of a disease, illness, or complication occurring in the neonatal period.

Neonatal mortality risk   The chance of death within the newborn period.

Neonatal transition   The first few hours of life, in which the newborn stabilizes his or her respiratory and circulatory functions.

Neutral thermal environment (NTE)   An environment that provides for minimal heat loss or expenditure.

Nevus flammeus   A capillary angioma directly below the epidermis; it is nonelevated, sharply demarcated, red-to-purple area of dense capillaries. Also called *port-wine stain*.

Nevus vasculosus   Raised, clearly delineated, dark-red, rough-surfaced birthmark commonly found in the head region. Also called *strawberry mark*.

New Ballard score (NBS)   A postnatal gestational age assessment tool, it is a refinement of a previous Ballard score tool with added criteria for more accurate assessment of the gestational age of newborns between 20 and 28 weeks' gestation and less than 1500 g.

Newborn screening tests   Tests that detect inborn errors of metabolism that, if left untreated, cause intellectual disability and physical handicaps.

Nidation Implantation of a fertilized ovum in the endometrium.

Nipple A protrusion about 0.5 to 1.3 cm in diameter in the center of each mature breast.

Non-Mendelian (multifactorial) inheritance The occurrence of congenital disorders that result from an interaction of multiple genetic and environmental factors.

Non-stress test (NST) An assessment method by which the reaction (or response) of the fetal heart rate to fetal movement is evaluated.

Nuchal translucency testing (NTT) A combination of an ultrasound and maternal serum test that is used to screen fetuses between 11 weeks and 1 day and 13 weeks and 6 days to determine if a fetus is at risk for a chromosomal disorder, such as Down syndrome (trisomy 21) or trisomy 18.

Nulligravida A woman who has never been pregnant.

Nullipara A woman who has not given birth to a viable fetus.

Nurse practitioner A professional nurse who has received specialized education in either a master's degree program or a continuing education program and thus can function in an expanded role.

Nurse researcher A professional nurse who has an advanced doctoral degree, typically a doctor of philosophy (PhD), and assumes a leadership role in generating new research.

O

Obstetric conjugate Distance from the middle of the sacral promontory to an area approximately 1 cm below the pubic crest.

Oligohydramnios Decreased amount of amniotic fluid, which may indicate a fetal urinary tract defect.

Orientation Newborn's ability to respond to auditory and visual stimuli in the environment.

Ortolani maneuver A manual procedure performed to rule out the possibility of developmental dysplastic hip.

Osteoporosis A condition most common in postmenopausal women that is characterized by decreased bone strength related to diminished bone density and bone quality. It is thought to be associated with lowered estrogen and androgen levels. Osteoporosis puts an individual at increased risk for fractures of the hip, forearm, and vertebrae.

Ovarian ligaments Ligaments that anchor the lower pole of the ovary to the cornua of the uterus.

Ovaries Female sex glands in which the ova are formed and in which estrogen and progesterone are produced. Normally there are two ovaries, located in the lower abdomen on each side of the uterus.

Ovulation Normal process of discharging a mature ovum from an ovary approximately 14 days before the onset of menses.

Oxytocin Hormone normally produced by the posterior pituitary, responsible for stimulation of uterine contractions and the release of milk into the lactiferous ducts.

P

Para A woman who has borne offspring who reached the age of viability.

Parent–newborn attachment Close affectional ties that develop between parent and newborn.

Passive acquired immunity Transfer of antibodies (IgG) from the mother to the fetus in utero.

Patient-controlled analgesia (PCA) A method of pain control where anesthesia, usually morphine or meperidine, is initially administered by the anesthesiologist and subsequent doses are self-administered by pushing a button controlled by a special IV pump system.

Pedigree Graphic representation of a family tree.

Pelvic cavity Bony portion of the birth passages; a curved canal with a longer posterior than anterior wall.

Pelvic cellulitis (parametritis) Infection involving the connective tissue of the broad ligament or, in severe cases, the connective tissue of all the pelvic structures.

Pelvic diaphragm Part of the pelvic floor composed of deep fascia and the levator ani and the coccygeal muscles.

Pelvic inflammatory disease (PID) An infection of the fallopian tubes that may or may not be accompanied by a pelvic abscess; may cause infertility secondary to tubal damage.

Pelvic inlet Upper border of the true pelvis.

Pelvic outlet Lower border of the true pelvis.

Pelvic tilt Exercise designed to reduce back strain and strengthen abdominal muscle tone. Also called *pelvic rocking*.

Perimenopause A term referring to the period of time before menopause during which the woman moves from normal ovulatory cycles to cessation of menses.

Perimetrium The outermost layer of the corpus of the uterus. Also known as the *serosal layer*.

Perinatal loss Death of a fetus or neonate from the time of conception through the end of the newborn period 28 days after birth.

Perineal body Wedge-shaped mass of fibromuscular tissue found between the lower part of the vagina and the anal canal.

Periodic breathing Sporadic episodes of apnea, not associated with cyanosis, that last for about 10 seconds and commonly occur in preterm newborns.

Periods of reactivity Predictable patterns of newborn behavior during the first several hours after birth.

Peripartum major mood episodes Clinical depression, as categorized by the *Diagnostic and Statistical Manual of Mental Disorders* (DSM-5) as Major Depressive Disorder with Peripartum Onset. Also called *postpartum depression*.

Peritonitis Infection involving the peritoneal cavity.

Persistent occiput-posterior (OP) position Malposition of the fetus in which the fetal occiput is posterior in the maternal pelvis.

Phenotype The whole physical, biochemical, and physiologic makeup of an individual as determined both genetically and environmentally.

Phenylketonuria A common metabolic disease caused by an inborn error in the metabolism of the amino acid phenylalanine.

Phosphatidylglycerol (PG) A phospholipid present in fetal surfactant after about 35 weeks' gestation.

Phototherapy The treatment of jaundice by exposure to light.

Physiologic anemia of infancy Result of the normal gradual drop in hemoglobin after birth due to higher oxygen levels resulting from initiation of breathing.

Physiologic anemia of the newborn A harmless condition in which the hemoglobin level drops in the first 6 to 12 weeks after birth, then reverts to normal levels.

Physiologic anemia of pregnancy Apparent anemia that results because during pregnancy the plasma volume increases more than does the number of erythrocytes.

Physiologic jaundice A harmless condition caused by the normal reduction of red blood cells, occurring 48 or more hours after birth, peaking at the 5th to 7th days, and disappearing between the 7th and 10th days.

Pica The eating of substances not ordinarily considered edible or to have nutritive value.

Placenta Specialized disk-shaped organ that connects the fetus to the uterine wall for gas and nutrient exchange. Also called *afterbirth.*

Placenta previa Abnormal implantation of the placenta in the lower uterine segment. Classification of type is based on proximity to the cervical os: *total*—completely covers the os; *partial*—covers a portion of the os; *marginal*—is in proximity to the os.

Polycystic ovarian syndrome (PCOS) The most common endocrine disorder affecting women of reproductive age, marked by menstrual dysfunction, androgen excess, obesity, hyperinsulinemia, and infertility.

Postconception age periods Period of time in embryonic/fetal development calculated from the time of fertilization of the ovum (about 266 days [38 weeks] or 9 1/2 calendar months). Also called *fertilization age.*

Postmature newborn A baby born after 42 completed weeks of gestation.

Postmaturity A term describing the newborn who is born after 42 completed weeks of gestation and also demonstrates characteristics of postmaturity syndrome.

Postpartum After childbirth.

Postpartum blues A maternal adjustment reaction occurring in the first few postpartum days, characterized by mild depression, tearfulness, anxiety, headache, and irritability. Also called *adjustment reaction with depressed mood.*

Postpartum depression Severe depression that occurs within the first year after giving birth with increased incidence at about the fourth week postpartum, just before resumption of menses, and upon weaning. Also called *peripartum major mood episodes.*

Postpartum endometritis (metritis) A reproductive tract infection limited to the uterus and associated with childbirth that occurs at any time up to 6 weeks postpartum.

Postpartum home care Visits for postpartum families that occur in the home setting. This provides opportunities for expanding information and reinforcing self-care and newborn/infant care techniques initially presented in the birth setting.

Postpartum mood episodes with psychotic features The most serious of postpartum psychiatric disorders and is considered an emergency, given the risk of infanticide or suicide. Also called *postpartum psychosis.*

Postpartum psychosis Psychosis occurring within the first 3 months after birth and is considered an emergency, given the risk of infanticide or suicide. Also called *postpartum mood episodes with psychotic features.*

Postterm Births occurring after 42 weeks' gestation.

Postterm labor Labor that occurs after 42 weeks' gestation.

Postterm newborn A baby born after 42 weeks' gestation.

Postterm pregnancy A pregnancy that extends more than 294 days or 42 weeks past the first day of the last menstrual period.

Posttraumatic stress disorder (PTSD) Intense psychologic distress resulting from a traumatic event and evidenced by recurrent, intrusive thoughts; flashbacks, persistent avoidance of stimuli associated with the trauma; a generalized feeling of "numbness"; and persistent signs of arousal. Also called *posttraumatic stress syndrome (PTSS).*

Precipitous birth (1) Unduly rapid progression of labor. (2) A birth in which no physician is in attendance.

Precipitous labor Labor lasting less than 3 hours.

Preeclampsia Toxemia of pregnancy, characterized by hypertension, albuminuria, and edema.

Pregnancy-related death The death of a woman while pregnant or within 1 year of the termination of pregnancy.

Premature rupture of membranes (PROM) Spontaneous rupture of the membranes before the onset of labor.

Premenstrual syndrome (PMS) Cluster of symptoms experienced by some women, typically occurring from a few days up to 2 weeks before the onset of menses.

Presenting part The fetal part present in or on the cervical os.

Preterm newborn Any baby born before 37 weeks' gestation.

Preterm labor Labor that occurs after 20 weeks' but before completion of 37 weeks' gestation

Primary infertility Refers to a woman with no prior pregnancies who is having difficulty conceiving.

Primigravida A woman who is pregnant for the first time.

Primipara A woman who has given birth to her first child (past the point of viability), whether or not that child is living or was alive at birth.

Professional nurse A person who has graduated from an accredited basic program in nursing, has successfully completed the nursing licensure examination (NCLEX), and is currently licensed as a registered nurse (RN).

Progesterone A hormone produced by the corpus luteum, adrenal cortex, and placenta whose function is to stimulate proliferation of the endometrium to facilitate growth of the embryo.

Prolactin A hormone secreted by the anterior pituitary that stimulates and sustains lactation in mammals.

Prolapsed umbilical cord Umbilical cord that becomes trapped in the vagina before the fetus is born.

Prostaglandins (PGs) Complex lipid compounds synthesized by many cells in the body.

Pseudomenstruation Blood-tinged mucus from the vagina in the female newborn; caused by withdrawal of maternal hormones that were present during pregnancy.

Psychologic disorders Abnormal mental or emotional conditions characterized by alterations in thinking, mood, or behavior.

Ptyalism Excessive salivation.

Pubis Pertaining to the pubes or pubic area.

Pudendal block Injection of an anesthetizing agent at the pudendal nerve to produce numbness of the external genitals and the lower one third of the vagina to facilitate childbirth and permit episiotomy if necessary.

Puerperal infection Infection of the reproductive tract associated with childbirth and occurring any time up to 6 weeks postpartum.

Puerperal morbidity A maternal temperature of 38°C (100.4°F) or higher on any 2 of the first 10 postpartum days, excluding the first 24 hours. The temperature is to be taken by mouth at least four times per day.

Puerperium The period after completion of the third stage of labor until involution of the uterus is complete, usually 6 weeks.

Pyelonephritis Inflammatory disease of the kidneys.

Q

Quadruple screen The most widely used test to screen for Down syndrome (trisomy 21), trisomies 13 and 18, and neural tube defects (NTDs). The serum test assesses for appropriate levels of alpha-fetoprotein (AFP), human chorionic gonadotropin (hCG), unconjugated estriol (UE3), and dimeric inhibin-A.

Quickening The first fetal movements felt by the pregnant woman, usually between 16 and 18 weeks' gestation.

R

Radiation Heat loss incurred when heat transfers to cooler surfaces and objects not in direct contact with the body.

Rape Sexual activity, often intercourse, against the will of the victim.

Reciprocity An interactional cycle that occurs simultaneously between mother and newborn. It involves mutual cueing behaviors, expectancy, rhythmicity, and synchrony.

Recommended dietary allowance (RDA) Government recommended allowances of various vitamins, minerals, and other nutrients.

Rectocele Condition that develops when the posterior vaginal wall is weakened; the anterior wall of the rectum can then sag forward, ballooning into the vagina, pushing the weakened posterior wall of the vagina in front of it.

Recurrent pregnancy loss (RPL) Three or more consecutive pregnancy losses before 24 weeks' gestation.

Regional analgesia The temporary and reversible loss of sensation produced by injecting an anesthetic agent (called a local anesthetic) into an area that will bring the agent into direct contact with nervous tissue.

Regional anesthesia Injection of local anesthetic agents so that they come into direct contact with nervous tissue.

Respiratory distress syndrome (RDS) Respiratory disease of the newborn characterized by interference with ventilation at the alveolar level, thought to be caused by the presence of fibrinoid deposits lining the alveolar ducts. Formerly called *hyaline membrane disease*.

Retained placenta Retention of the placenta beyond 30 minutes after birth.

Rh immune globulin (RhoGAM) An anti-Rh(D) gamma globulin given after birth to an Rh-negative mother of an Rh-positive fetus or child. Prevents the development of permanent active immunity to the Rh antigen.

Risk factors Any findings that suggest a pregnancy may have a negative outcome, for either the woman or her unborn child.

Round ligaments Ligaments that arise from the side of the uterus near the fallopian tube insertion to help the broad ligament keep the uterus in place.

Rupture of membranes (ROM) Rupture may be PROM (premature), SROM (spontaneous), or AROM (artificial). Some clinicians may use the abbreviation RBOW (rupture of bag of waters).

S

Sacral promontory A projection into the pelvic cavity on the anterior upper portion of the sacrum; serves as an obstetric guide in determining pelvic measurements.

Secondary infertility Condition in which couples are unable to conceive after one or more successful pregnancies.

Self-quieting ability Newborn's ability to use personal resources to quiet and console himself or herself.

Sepsis neonatorum Infections experienced by a newborn during the first month of life.

Sexual assault A broad term that refers to a variety of types of unwanted sexual touching or penetration without consent, from unwanted sexual contact or touching of an intimate part of another person to forced anal, oral, or genital penetration.

Sexually transmitted infection (STI) An infection ordinarily transmitted by direct sexual contact with an infected individual.

Shaken baby injuries Collection of symptoms and serious injuries caused by vigorously shaking a baby.

Skin turgor Elasticity of skin; provides information on hydration status.

Small for gestational age (SGA) Inadequate weight or growth for gestational age; birth weight below the 10th percentile.

Spermatogenesis The process by which mature spermatozoa are formed, during which the number of chromosomes is halved.

Spermicide A cream, foam, jelly, or suppository that, when inserted into the vagina before intercourse, destroys sperm or neutralizes any vaginal secretions and thereby immobilizes sperm.

Spinal block Injection of a local anesthetic agent directly into the spinal fluid in the spinal canal to provide anesthesia for vaginal and cesarean births.

Spontaneous rupture of membranes (SROM) The breaking of the "water" or membranes marked by the expulsion of amniotic fluid from the vagina.

Station Relationship of the presenting fetal part to an imaginary line drawn between the pelvic ischial spines.

Sterilization An inclusive term that refers to surgical procedures that permanently prevent pregnancy. In the male, sterilization is achieved through a procedure called a vasectomy. In the female, sterilization is done by tubal ligation.

Stillbirth The birth of a dead baby.

Striae Stretch marks; shiny purplish lines that appear on the abdomen, breasts, thighs, and buttocks of pregnant women as a result of stretching of the skin.

Subconjunctival hemorrhages Hemorrhages on the sclera of a newborn's eye, usually caused by changes in vascular tension during birth.

Subfertility A couple who has difficulty conceiving because both partners have reduced fertility.

Subinvolution Failure of a part to return to its normal size after functional enlargement, such as failure of the uterus to return to normal size after pregnancy.

Sudden unexpected infant death (SUID) The sudden death of an infant; the primary cause of infant death beyond the neonatal period in the United States.

Supine hypotensive syndrome (vena caval syndrome, aortocaval compression) A condition that can develop during pregnancy when the enlarging uterus puts pressure on the vena cava when the woman is supine. This pressure interferes with returning blood flow and produces a marked decrease in blood pressure with accompanying dizziness, pallor, and clamminess, which can be corrected by having the woman lie on her left side.

Surfactant A substance composed of phospholipid, which stabilizes and lowers the surface tension of the alveoli during extrauterine respiratory exhalation, allowing a certain amount of air to remain in the alveoli during expiration.

Sutures Fibrous connections of opposed joint surfaces, as in the skull.

Symphysis pubis Fibrocartilaginous joint between the pelvic bones in the midline.

Syphilis A chronic, sexually transmitted infection caused by the spirochete *Treponema pallidum*.

T

Taboo A behavior or object that is avoided by individuals or groups.

Telangiectatic nevi Small clusters of pink-red spots appearing on the nape of the neck and around the eyes of newborns; localized areas of capillary dilatation. Also called *stork bites*.

Term The normal duration of pregnancy.

Testosterone The male hormone; responsible for the development of secondary male characteristics.

Therapeutic insemination Procedure to produce a pregnancy in which sperm obtained from a woman's husband or from a donor is deposited in the woman's vagina.

Thermogenesis The newborn's physiologic mechanisms that increase heat production.

Thrombophlebitis Inflammation of a vein wall, resulting in thrombus.

Thrush A fungal infection of the oral mucous membranes caused by *Candida albicans*. Most often seen in newborns; characterized by white plaques in the mouth.

Tocolysis Use of medications to arrest preterm labor.

Total bilirubin Sum of conjugated (direct) and unconjugated (indirect) bilirubin.

Toxic shock syndrome (TSS) Infection caused by *Staphylococcus aureus*, found primarily in women of reproductive age.

Transitional milk Breast milk produced from the end of colostrum production until about 2 weeks postpartum.

Transverse diameter The largest diameter of the pelvic inlet; helps determine the shape of the inlet.

Trichomoniasis A sexually transmitted infection caused by *Trichomonas vaginalis*, a microscopic motile protozoan that thrives in an alkaline environment.

Trimester Three months, or one third of the gestational time for pregnancy.

Trisomies Abnormalities of chromosomal number, in this case, the presence of three homologous chromosomes rather than the normal two.

Trophoblast The outer layer of the blastoderm that will eventually establish the nutrient relationship with the uterine endometrium.

True pelvis The portion that lies below the linea terminalis, made up of the inlet, cavity, and outlet.

Tubal embryo transfer (TET) Procedure in which eggs are retrieved and incubated with the man's sperm then transferred back into the women's body at the embryo stage.

Tubal ligation Sterilization of a woman accomplished by transecting or occluding the fallopian tubes.

Tummy time Prone positioning of the newborn while awake.

U

Ultrasound High-frequency sound waves that may be directed, through the use of a transducer, into the maternal abdomen. The ultrasonic sound waves reflected by the underlying structures of varying densities allow identification of various maternal and fetal tissues, bones, and fluids.

Umbilical cord The structure connecting the placenta to the umbilicus of the fetus and through which nutrients from the woman are exchanged for wastes from the fetus.

Umbilical velocimetry Noninvasive ultrasound test that measures blood flow changes that occur in maternal and fetal circulation in order to assess placental function. Also known as *Doppler blood flow studies*.

Urinary tract infection (UTI) Significant *bacteriuria* in the presence of symptoms.

Uterine atony Relaxation of uterine muscle tone following birth.

Uterine rupture A nonsurgical disruption of the uterine cavity.

Uterosacral ligaments Ligaments that provide support for the uterus and cervix at the level of the ischial spines.

Uterus The hollow muscular organ in which the fertilized ovum is implanted and in which the developing fetus is nourished until birth.

V

Vacuum-assisted birth An obstetric procedure used to assist in the birth of a fetus by applying suction to the fetal head with a soft suction cup attached to a suction bottle (pump) by tubing and placing the device against the occiput of the fetal head.

Vagina The musculomembranous tube or passageway located between the external genitals and the uterus of a woman.

Vaginal birth after cesarean (VBAC) Practice of permitting a trial of labor and possible vaginal birth for women following a previous cesarean birth for nonrecurring causes such as fetal distress or placenta previa.

Variability Baseline fluctuations of two cycles per minute or greater in the FHR and classified by the visually quantified amplitude of peak-to-trough in beats per minute.

Variable decelerations Periodic changes in fetal heart rate caused by umbilical cord compression; decelerations vary in onset, occurrence, and waveform.

Vasectomy Surgical removal of a portion of the vas deferens (ductus deferens) to produce infertility.

Vegans Strict vegetarians; those who consume no food from animal sources.

Vulva The external structure of the female genitals, lying below the mons veneris.

W

Wandering baseline Fetal heart rate fluctuates between 120 and 160 beats/min in an unsteady wandering pattern and can be associated with neurologic impairment of the fetus or a preterminal event.

Wharton jelly Yellow-white gelatinous material surrounding the vessels of the umbilical cord.

Z

Zygote A fertilized egg.

Zygote intrafallopian transfer (ZIFT) Retrieval of oocytes under ultrasound guidance, followed by in vitro fertilization and laparoscopic replacement of fertilized eggs into the fimbriated end of the fallopian tube.

Index

Page numbers followed by f, t, and b indicate figures, tables, and boxes, respectively.

S

Guide to Special Features

EVIDENCE-BASED PRACTICE

HEALTH PROMOTION

KEY FACTS TO REMEMBER